Contact Dermatitis

Contact Dermatitis

Etain Cronin FRCP
Consultant Dermatologist
St John's Hospital for Diseases of the Skin
London

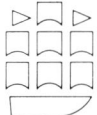

CHURCHILL LIVINGSTONE
EDINBURGH LONDON AND NEW YORK 1980

CHURCHILL LIVINGSTONE
Medical Division of Longman Group Limited

Distributed in the United States of America by
Churchill Livingstone Inc., 1560 Broadway, New York,
N.Y. 10036, and by associated companies, branches
and representatives throughout the world.

First published 1980
  Reprinted 1982
  Reprinted 1983

ISBN 0 443 02014 0

British Library Cataloguing in Publication Data
Cronin, Etain
    Contact dermatitis.
    1. Contact dermatitis
    I. Title
    616.5 RC593.C6 79-41434

Printed and bound in Great Britain by
William Clowes (Beccles) Limited, Beccles and London

Preface

The aim of this book has been twofold. One was to write an account of the clinical features of allergic contact dermatitis and the other was to try to make it a comprehensive reference to the literature on each particular aspect of the subject. Inevitably the attempt has fallen far short of the aims and, in particular, the collection of references has been hampered by my ignorance of different languages. The omission of references has therefore been a regrettable oversight rather than any deliberate exclusion.

The book has been written for practising dermatologists in an endeavour to make patch testing more comprehensible and encourage greater use of this investigation. I hope it will also be of use to those in industry who are concerned with the dermatological safety of products and environment.

As the knowledge and practice of patch testing becomes more widespread, reports of the geographical variation in incidences of sensitivity to various allergens are becoming more frequent. By including these results in the text I have tried to show that, although the allergens may differ, contact dermatitis occurs and is an important cause of eczema in every country. It is not a parochial affliction of communities who by chance happen to have a dermatologist interested in patch testing.

The Contact Clinic at St John's was started in 1953 by Dr C.D. Calnan and Dr R.H. Meara, since when this method of investigation has been a special interest of Dr Calnan and in the hospital generally. The results from this clinic have been included as it was thought they would be of value in showing the types and incidence of contact dermatitis seen in London over the years. By a quirk of timing, the Contact Clinic year has followed the financial year, running from March 31st to April 1st; thus the figures for 1976 ended in March 1977. At the time of finishing this book the 1977 figures, which ended in March 1978, were not complete and so could not be included in the text.

There are many compounds for which the patch test concentration is not established; when such a doubt exists I have queried the dilution and sometimes suggested more than one concentration for patch testing. For the errors and omissions which must exist, I apologise and I should be grateful if anyone takes the trouble to enlighten me.

I hope this book will be of some value to those already interested in contact dermatitis, but most of all I hope it will be a useful account of the subject for those for whom it is not easy to look up diverse and scattered references.

London, 1980 *E.C.*

Acknowledgements

To all those who have helped me in the preparation of this book I offer my most sincere thanks — firstly to Dr Arthur Rook, without whose constant encouragement I would never have written it, and who read much of the typescript. I am also greatly indebted to Dr John Mitchell who worked so hard to smooth out the errors of my writing and include punctuation, and was persuaded to write the chapters on plants and woods. The many references made me frequently resort to our librarian Mrs Hildegaard Freyhan, who patiently and willingly tracked down obscure papers, translated the German literature and never complained when yet another reference was needed, and always in a hurry. The typing was a considerable task and I sincerely thank Miss Linda Salmon and Mrs Helen Dilnot for labouring through it and also Mrs Doreen Summers who so generously helped. Sister Clifford in the Contact Clinic very kindly got out endless patch test forms and the many formulae were done by Mrs Mary Manley and Mr Steven Kyte in the Photographic Department.

For permission to publish the St John's data, I am most grateful to Dr Calnan, Dr Rycroft and the many registrars who worked in the Contact Clinic and have allowed me to use the results of all the patients they have investigated. I also thank the staff of St John's and the many dermatologists who have referred patients for investigation. For much technical information I am indebted to the members of the many firms who helped me when I consulted them, often in a state of great ignorance.

Finally I acknowledge with much gratitude the patience of my family, my friends and all those with whom I work, who thought that 'the book' would never be finished.

Contents

1. **Technique of Patch Testing**   1
   Introduction, Patch Test Unit, Allergens, Time of Reading, Recording of Results, Photopatch Tests, Standard Series, Allergic Reactions, Irritant Reactions, Interpretation of Patch Tests, Relevance, False Positive Reaction, False Negative Reaction, Effect of Prednisone on Patch Test Reactions, Complications of Patch Testing, Open Test, Usage Test.

2. **General**   20
   Age, Atopy, Seasonal Variations, Contact Urticaria, Systemic Absorption of Contact Allergens, Erythema Multiforme, Histology, Allergen Replacement.

3. **Clothing and Textiles**   36
   Dyes, Resins, Shoes and Rubber Boots, Hat Bands, Leather Accessories, Dry Cleaning, Fibreglass, Fire Retardants, Fluorescent Whitening Agents, Preservatives, Textile Fibres, Textile Purpura.

4. **Cosmetics**   93
   Creams, Deodorants and Antiperspirants, Eye Cosmetics, Hair Preparations, Lipsticks, Nail Preparations, Perfume.

5. **Foods**   171
   Proteins, Additives (antimicrobials, antioxidants, sequestrants, surface active agents), Colours, Flavouring Agents and Spices, Flour and Grains, Plants, Additives in Animal Feeds.

6. **Medicaments**   192
   Anaesthetics (local), Antibiotic and Antibacterial Compounds, Antifungal and Anticandidal Compounds, Antihistamines, Antimitotic Compounds, Dyes (tri-phenylmethane) Ethylenediamine, Corticosteroids, Vitamins, Other Medicaments.

7. **Metals**   279
   Antimony, Arsenic, Beryllium, Cadmium, Carbon, Chromium. Cobalt, Copper, Gold, Iron, Lead, Nickel, Nickel and Chromate and Cobalt, Palladium, Platinum, Selenium, Silica, Silver, Tellurium, Uranium, Zinc, Zirconium.

8. **Pesticides**   391
   Fungicides (phenols, nitrophenols, quinones, dithiocarbamates and thiurams, captan and similar chemicals, chloronitrobenzenes, mercury compounds, organotin compounds, mercaptobenzothiazole, phosphothioate), Herbicides (amides, bipyridyliums), Insecticides (pyrethroids, organothiocyanates, DDT, DD, Lindane, cyclodienes, organophosphorous compounds, carbamates, omite, dazomet), Rodenticides (Warfarin, Antu).

9. **Photosensitisers**   414
Phototoxic (topical, systemic), Photoallergic (topical, systemic), Phototoxic and Photoallergic, Sunscreens.

10. **Plants** *J.N.S. Mitchell*   461
General considerations, Plant families: Alliaceae, Alstroemeriaceae, Amaryllidaceae, Anacardiaceae, Araceae, Araliaceae, Aspidiaceae, Begoniaceae, Boraginaceae, Bromeliaceae, Cactaceae, Cannabidaceae, Capparidaceae, Compositae, Cruciferae, Euphorbiaceae, Geraniaceae, Gesneriaceae, Ginkgoaceae, Gramineae, Hydrophyllaceae, Iridaceae, Labiatae, Lauraceae, Leguminosae, Liliaceae, Moraceae, Myrtaceae, Orchidaceae, Polygonaceae, Primulaceae, Ranunculaceae, Rosaceae, Rubiaceae, Rutaceae, Saxifragaceae, Solanaceae, Umbelliferae, Urticaceae, Zingiberaceae, Miscellaneous.

11. **Woods** *J.N.S. Mitchell*   548
General Considerations, Plant Families: Apocynaceae, Betulaceae, Bignoniaceae, Burseraceae, Combretaceae, Cupressaceae, Ebenaceae, Fagaceae, Flindersiaceae, Hernandiaceae, Lauraceae, Leguminosae (Caesalpinioideae, Mimosoideae, Papilionoideae), Meliaceae, Moraceae, Naucleaceae, Pinaceae, Proteaceae, Rutaceae, Salicaceae, Sapotaceae, Sterculiaceae, Taxaceae, Thymelaeaceae, Ulmaceae, Verbenaceae, Lichens, Liverworts and Mosses.

12. **Plastics**   575
Monomers which Sensitise (acrylic, epoxy, formaldehyde), Resin Systems which cause Dermatitis (polyester—unsaturated, allyl), Resin Systems which rarely cause Dermatitis (polyester—saturated (alkyd), polyurethane), Monomers Non Allergic but Sensitising Additives (cellulose acetate, vinyl polymers, polyvinyl chloride, polyvinyl acetate, vinyl carbazole, vinyl pyridine, polyvinylidene chloride), Other Polymers (polystyrene, polyolefins, polyamides, fluoropolymers)

13. **Preservatives and Antibacterials**   664
Parabens, Phenolic Compounds, Mercury, Quaternary Ammonium Compounds, Bronopol, Chlorhexidine, Chloroacetamide, Chlorbutanol, Dimethoxane, Domiphen Bromide, Ethylenediaminetetraacetate, Ethylene Oxide, Imidazolidinyl Urea Compounds, Irgasans, Nordihydroguaiaretic Acid, Potassium Metabisulphite, Sorbic Acid, Tocopherols.

14. **Rubber**   714
Sources and Structure, Sensitisers, Incidence of Sensitivity, Sources of Sensitivity, Clinical Features, Patch Testing.

15. **Other Allergens**   771
Lanolin, Colophony, Formaldehyde and Glutaraldehyde, Oil of Turpentine, Alcohols and Glycols, Surfactants, Matches, Tattoos.

16. **Miscellaneous Occupational**   839
Oils, Papers, Copying, Printing and Duplicating, Inks, Photography, Fluxes, Chemical Depigmentation, Barrier Creams.

17. **Irritants and Sensitisers in Various Occupations**   879
Allergens for Selected Patients
Miscellaneous Compounds

Index   895

1.

Technique of patch testing

Introduction
Patch test unit
  Site of application
  Adhesive tape
  Marking the test site
Allergens
  Concentration
  Vehicle
  Amount
  Storage
  Deterioration
Time of reading
Recording of results
Photopatch tests
Standard series
Allergic reactions
Irritant reactions
Interpretation of patch
tests

Relevance
False positive reaction
False negative reaction
Effect of prednisone on
patch test reactions
Complications of patch
testing
  Severe reactions
  Plaster reactions
  Active sensitisation
  Focal flare
  Alteration in pigment
  Scars and keloids
  Systemic absorption
  Inoculation herpes simplex
Open test
Usage test

Introduction

Jadassohn (1896) was the first to establish the concept of allergic contact dermatitis when he reported to the German Dermatological Society in Graz (Austria) in 1895 that iodoform applied to the normal skin of five sensitised subjects reproduced their dermatitis.

Bloch, in Basel in 1911, described in detail the technique of patch testing. The allergen should be applied to a linen strip which is put on the back, covered with a slightly larger piece of gutta percha and fixed in place with zinc oxide adhesive plaster; the test should then be left for 24 hours. He graded the stages of the skin reaction from simple erythema to necrosis and ulceration, and stressed that a normal and a sensitised subject differ fundamentally in that only the latter reacts.

Bonnevie (1939) working at the Finsen Institute in Copenhagen established the value of the patch test in the investigation of patients suspected of having an allergic contact dermatitis. The patch test and its importance were accepted early in the Scandinavian countries.

Sulzberger in the U.S.A. gave a detailed description of the technique of patch testing (Sulzberger and Wise, 1931) and endeavoured to stress its importance in the investigation of patients with eczema.

It is important to standardise the technique of patch testing so that results may be validly compared from patient to patient, centre to centre and country to country. The results of patch testing are influenced by the test unit, the site of application and the adhesive tape.

Patch test unit

Several patch test units have been described including the pressure test by Fernstrom (1954) and the Al-test by Fregert. A comparison by Magnusson and Hersle (1965) of these and four other units did not indicate a best method but showed that the intensity of reactions varies with the different units. Recently a modification of the chamber method has been described by Pirilä (1975).

Al-test unit

Wide experience has been gained in the use of the Al-test by the International Contact Dermatitis Research Group (Fregert, 1969) and the North American Contact Dermatitis Group (1973). In general it is an effective and usually non-irritant test unit. It consists of aluminium foil covered with polythene with a 10 mm central disc of filter paper adhered by heat and not by glue. The units are supplied in rolls by Al-test Imeco Astra Agency AB, through the following agencies:

Austria:	Hermal Chemie, Kurt Herrmann & Co. GmbH, Gunterstrasse 11, A-1150 Wien, Austria.
Japan:	Kaigai Gijutsu Koeki Co. Ltd, 18 Sankyo Building 8F, 16-3, 2-chome, Nihonbashi, Chuo-ku, Tokyo, Japan.
Switzerland:	Imal Pharmaceutica AG, Postfach 163, CH-8030 Zurich, Switzerland.
United Kingdom:	Astra Chemicals Ltd, Watford, WD 17 QR, England.
USA, Canada, Italy:	Hollister-Stier Laboratories, Box 3145, Spokane, Washington 99220, USA.
Italy also:	Bayropharm Italiana S.p.A., Via Polidoro da Caravaggio 33, C.A.P. 201 56 Milano, Italy.
Sweden and elsewhere:	Imeco Astra Agency Co AB, S-151 85 Södertälje, Sweden.

Disadvantages of the Al-test unit

Reactions to the Al-test. Reactions to the polythene covering on the aluminium foil occasionally occur, causing erythema and slight oedema around the filter paper discs. Usually only some units, possibly a strip, are affected but occasionally all the tests are involved to a greater or lesser extent. The redness is most pronounced at two days; although it fades, it generally has not gone completely by four days. This reaction is a distinct disadvantage because by increasing the irritability of the test area it makes false positive reactions more likely, and adds to the difficulty of interpreting the test results.

The cause of the reaction is unknown. Fregert (1972) suggested that excess heat or ozone may have oxidised one patch of polythene during its fixation to the aluminium. Polythene aged by ultraviolet light and oxygen is changed in the same way. These oxidation products give a characteristic peak with infrared-spectrography which corresponds to carbonyl groups. Some, but not all, patients with an Al-test reaction are sensitive to colophony but only a few colophony sensitive patients react to the Al-test. It is possible that colophony and aged polythene have an allergen in common; it is also possible that in at least some patients the effect is an irritant one. In Japan, this reaction is not infrequent and has been attributed to the high humidity in summer (Hayakawa *et al.*, 1975).

Spread of the reaction. Strong reactions may not be localised to the test area of the filter paper disc and may even be accompanied by a considerable flare of erythema around the test site.

Occlusive tape. The Al-test requires an occlusive tape, which is more uncomfortable for the patient and causes more plaster reactions than does a non-occlusive tape.

Finn Chamber
A chamber, which is an effective test unit, has been devised by Pirilä (1975). The chambers are made of stiff aluminium and have a diameter of 8 mm and a depth of 0.5 mm; a filter paper is only required when testing with solutions.

The particular advantage of this chamber is its tight apposition to the skin which is apparent from the indented ring seen on the skin surface when the unit is removed. The presence of these rings indicates that the chambers have been correctly applied. Distinct advantages for the patient accrue from this tight occlusion; it allows the use of a porous tape and it localises the reactions to the test sites and diminishes their spread beyond. This containment of positive responses permits the allergens to be placed more closely together and a smaller area is required for patch testing.

The close proximity of the allergens makes accurate marking and re-marking of the test sites essential. The manufacturers distribute the chambers already attached to a porous tape and a special plastic plate marking the position of the chambers facilitates the readings. A dispenser for the chambers has also been devised (Pirilä, 1975).

In England the Finn Chamber test units are supplied as two rows of five chambers mounted on an oblong strip of Scanpor.
The distributors are:
  Chas. F. Thackray Ltd., P.O. Box 171, Park Street, Leeds LS1 1RQ, England
  Associated Hospital Supply, P.O. Box 4, Pershore, Worcestershire, England
Scanpor is made by:
  Norgesplaster A/S, Postboks, 158, Skøyen, Oslo 2. Norway.

Duhring Chamber

The Duhring chamber, designed by Frosch and Kligman (1979), is an enlarged aluminium unit measuring 18 mm across with an inner diameter of 12 mm and a capacity of 250 μl and six to eight can be fixed to the flexor surface of each forearm. For routine testing, its claimed advantage of greater reproducibility of results must be offset against its size, which limits the number that can be applied.

The choice of test unit depends on the preference of the clinician. The ICDRG used selected allergens to compare the Al-test and Finn Chamber and the incidence of positive reactions was the same with both (Cronin, 1978).

SITE OF APPLICATION

To establish the best site to apply patch tests Magnusson and Hersle (1965) compared reactions on the upper and lower back, on the flexor surfaces of the upper arm and forearm and on the extensor aspect of the thigh. The strongest responses both to irritants and to allergens occurred on the upper back, probably due to the pressure of clothes and the weight of the body when lying down.

The patch tests are applied in strips of five units and taped on to the back in vertical rows, beginning over the left scapula and continuing over the right but avoiding the skin over the vertebral column. Further tests can be applied to the back as downward extensions of these strips, and to the upper outer arms.

ADHESIVE TAPE

With a non-occlusive patch test unit, such as the Al-test, an occlusive adhesive tape facilitates absorption of the test material. Allergens in aqueous solution must be occluded if false negative responses are to be avoided, but when the base is petrolatum, which is an occlusive material, reactions occur whether or not the adhesive tape is occlusive. In contrast, an occlusive tape always potentiates an irritant whether in aqueous solution or petrolatum (Magnusson and Hersle, 1966). Prior to testing, each patient should be questioned as to previous plaster reactions; in the majority none has occurred and an occlusive tape can be used for routine testing. But for those who have reacted before, acrylic tapes, which are non-occlusive but almost non-allergenic, are used instead.

When the patch test unit is of itself occlusive, as is the Finn chamber, then a porous tape can be used routinely.

MARKING THE TEST SITES

It is essential not only to mark but to mark accurately the patch test sites, otherwise identification of positive reactions is impossible. When the patch tests are applied dots are made on the skin at the sides of the tape exactly opposite each filter paper disc or patch test unit. The dots are renewed, if the marks are faint, when the patches are removed at two days.

Various indelible markers have been used but none is entirely satisfactory because they all rub off to some extent.

Caucasian skin
  (i) Red felt tipped marking pen
 (ii) Gentian violet liquid or pen
(iii) Dihydroxyacetone (DHA)
           20 g of DHA dissolved in 50 ml of water
           Washable ink   5 ml
           Acetone   to 100 ml.

The ink is added to colour the solution, otherwise it is invisible when first applied; the acetone acts as preservative and facilitates rapid drying.

Dihydroxyacetone, an artificial sun-tan, gradually stains the skin brown and the colour remains for several days despite washing (Epstein, 1967). It can also be used to disguise vitiligo. One woman who applied DHA 1 per cent in glycerin, spirit and water to her neck for this purpose developed an acute erythema which was attributed to the DHA. This was not an allergic reaction because she subsequently painted the same preparation on other patches of vitiligo without an adverse effect (Harman, 1961).

Negro skin
The darker the skin the more difficult it is to mark. For Asian patients and those who are lightly pigmented Gentian violet or red ink is suitable.

For very dark skin a fluorescent marking ink is probably best, the dots being located by a Wood's light in a dark room (Jordan, 1971).

The allergen

The concentration of the allergen, the base in which it is diluted and the amount applied will each affect the results.

CONCENTRATION

The correct concentration of an allergen will give a moderate reaction in a sensitised person but none in controls. With bland chemicals this concentration is easy to determine but for the many allergens which also are irritants the concentration necessary to elicit an allergic reaction may differ very little from that producing an irritant response. Failure to appreciate this causes misinterpretation of results and is the major stumbling block in patch testing.

For all the standard allergens the correct patch test concentrations are known and lists have been published (Fregert and Hjorth, 1972). For a non-established allergen the correct concentration has to be determined. For most chemicals an initial test concentration of 0.1–1.0 per cent is suitable for clinical use, but for known irritants it should be weaker. If the results are negative the concentration can be increased. A positive reaction which looks allergic should be checked by using this same concentration to test about 50 controls. Many substances used in daily life, such as cosmetics and medicaments, can be applied without dilution but under the conditions of patch testing some are mild irritants.

It is convenient to give the concentration of allergens as percentages but such values are misleading as regards molecular concentrations which are clearly expressed in molality units. By using the molality system it becomes apparent that if the patch test concentration of dichromate is taken as unity then nickel is ten and formaldehyde is fifteen (Benezra *et al.*, 1978).

VEHICLE

Petrolatum is bland and occlusive and is the most suitable base for most allergens. Allergy to petrolatum is almost unknown but one patient who reacted to yellow soft parraffin was described by Malten (1969). The sensitivity was detected because the patient reacted to many allergens in the patch test series but not when they were repeated using a white soft paraffin base. A patch test with yellow soft paraffin was positive. Another patient (Grimalt and Romaguera, 1978) appeared to be sensitive to both white and yellow soft paraffin. Maibach (1978) has reported a case of chronic dermatitis and hyperpigmentation from petrolatum (white and yellow) but the mechanism, whether irritant or allergic, was not established.

Ethyl alcohol was compared with petrolatum as a patch test vehicle for some perfume ingredients and it improved the results slightly but not very greatly (Marzulli and Maibach, 1976). The influence of vehicles on the phototoxicity of methoxsalen and coal tar was studied by Suhonen (1976) and found to be considerable. The effect of emulsifiers was investigated by Rudzki *et al.* (1976) and though they increased the release of dichromate from petrolatum they varied in their enhancement of patch test reactions.

Water is the diluent for formaldehyde, whereas olive oil is the base for turpentine and for diluting perfumes. Methyl ethyl ketone is a non-irritant organic solvent and can be used for special test materials, as can alcohol and acetone. These solvents have the disadvantage of readily evaporating and thus concentrating the test material.

AMOUNT

A standard amount of test material should be used for each patch test; an excess should be avoided because it contaminates the surrounding unit and may spread beyond it.

For allergens in petrolatum stored in syringes, one strip of material is dispensed across the 10 mm diameter of the filter paper disc of the Al-test unit or across the 8 mm diameter of the Finn chamber.

For liquids one drop is dispensed on to the filter paper disc.

STORAGE OF ALLERGENS

Allergens in petrolatum are most conveniently stored in and dispensed from 5 ml polypropylene syringes. Solutions are kept in glass pipette bottles with well-fitting screw-top caps. Rubber in caps or syringes must be avoided because it contaminates the test material. Chemicals can be protected from light by covering syringes with aluminium foil and by using dark-coloured bottles.

DETERIORATION OF TEST SUBSTANCES

Deterioration, evaporation and contamination of test substances is prevented by storing them in polypropylene syringes (Trolle-Lassen and Hjorth, 1966). They can then be kept for about one year. Turpentine and *p*-phenylenediamine are particularly susceptible to oxidation, which changes their allergenic activity; *p*-phenylenediamine is also unstable in the light. Turpentine is protected by being kept in a brown, all-glass pipette bottle and *p*-phenylenediamine by being stored in a syringe covered with aluminium foil.

SUPPLY OF ALLERGENS

In order to make a valid comparison of results from different centres it is desirable that the allergens be obtained from a common source. The mid-Japan Contact Dermatitis Research Group (1976) compared the results of patch tests with selected Japanese allergens and those supplied by Trolab* and found that most of the Danish allergens were more reactive.

To obviate such discrepancies it is recommended that whenever possible patch test allergens be obtained from Trolab*.

Time of reading

Patch tests should be left on for at least one day, but as most work has been done with the allergens *in situ* for two days this is the standard procedure at St John's. Exposure times of one and two days were compared by Skog and Forsbeck (1978) but the initial results were inconclusive and the study is continued.

1st reading
Patients return two days after the tests are applied; the patches are removed by the nurse in the clinic and the identification marks are renewed. But the tests should not be read until ½–1 hour later. This allows sufficient time for the pressure effect of the patch to wear off and for positive reactions to become manifest.

At this first reading doubtfully positive tests are repeated and, if indicated by the initial results, further patch tests are applied.

2nd reading
The second reading is done at four days. Another reading at 6–7 days is an advantage (Mitchell, 1978) but is not routine practice at St John's.

Patch tests applied before a weekend are removed by the patient on the second day and read in the clinic on the third and fifth days.

If the patient can return to the clinic only once, then it must be for the four-day reading. This is essential because reactions to allergens such as neomycin often take longer than two days to become positive whereas any test reac-

*Trolab, Karen Trolle-Lassen, Cand. Pharm., 6B A.N. Hansens Alle — 2900 Hellerup, Denmark.

tions positive at two days will, if allergic, still be present at four days. Mathias and Maibach (1979) would not agree; they have reported significant reactions present only at the two day reading.

Recording results

It is most important for patch tests to be scored according to the reaction seen and not according to the interpretation placed on the reaction by the reader. Irritant reactions should be recorded as positive irritant and not as negative.

To facilitate understanding of patch test results from different centres, Wilkinson *et al.* (1970) recommended the following scheme:

–	Negative
?+	Doubtful reaction
+	Weak (non-vesicular) reaction
++	Strong (oedematous or vesicular) reaction
+++	Extreme (bullous or ulcerative) reaction
NT	Not tested
IR	Irritant.

A ?+ is a faint or macular erythema and is not interpreted as a proven allergic reaction;
+ is a palpable erythema.

Photopatch tests are graded similarly with the prefix Ph:
Ph–   *Ph?+*   *Ph+*   *Ph++*   *Ph+++*   *PhNT*

Photopatch tests

The technique for photopatch testing is the same as for ordinary patch tests except that photo-allergens are applied in duplicate, one series being irradiated. To be certain of differentiating between a contact dermatitis and a photocontact dermatitis the non-irradiated series should be kept constantly covered with black material from the time of application to the final reading. These patch tests should be removed in the dark at two days and after being read in artificial light the black cover should be re-applied until the final four-day reading.

The patch tests on the sites to be irradiated are also removed and read at two days and this series is then exposed to long-wave ultraviolet radiation (UVR), so-called 'black light'. A suitable spectrum of long-wave UVR is provided by Philips TL 20 W/08 fluorescent tubes, and four of these, secured in a wooden box and covered with 3 mm window glass, are a suitable source. The glass filter screens the very small amounts of short-wave UVR (290–320 nm) emitted by 'black light' lamps which may cause a reaction in very sensitive persons (Kobza, Ramsay and Magnus, 1973). The distance between the patient and the light sources is 20 cm.

If possible, the patient's tolerance to the long-wave ultraviolet source should have been previously established. Once a series of exposures to the UVR source alone has determined the patient's threshold, an exposure time just short of that giving a threshold reaction should be used for photopatch testing. Most patients can tolerate exposures of 20–30 minutes but this may have to be reduced to 2–5 minutes for very sensitive persons.

The irradiated tests are left uncovered, and all the tests are finally read at four days. The appearance of the reactions and the method of recording the results are the same as for contact allergens except that, as noted above, the prefix Ph is used to denote a photopatch test.

Standard series (battery)

There are distinct advantages in patch testing all patients to a standard series (battery) of about 20 allergens, to which can be added selected substances indicated by the history.

A standard series should include:
  all the common allergens (e.g. nickel, chromate, rubber)
  allergens likely to be unsuspected (e.g. lanolin, parabens)
  allergens relevant to the local community (e.g. plants, medicaments).

Such a series of substances was used by Agrup *et al.* (1970) to test 140 patients with hand eczema; one-third of them had positive reactions. The advantages in using a standard series are that sensitisation to common allergens is not missed and the incidence of sensitivity to the various allergens is monitored. An unexpected increase in numbers of cases sensitive to an allergen indicates a fresh exposure in the environment; this occurred with formaldehyde in clothing and ethylenediamine in a medicament.

A standard series should be under constant review, the infrequent allergens being discarded and others being added to assess their significance.

Selected batteries for particular occupations or dermatoses, e.g. hairdressers, dentists, nurses, shoes, clothing, ensure that patch testing is complete, and relevant allergens are not forgotten. Such batteries also need constant revision.

St John's
  Each patient is at present tested to the following 22 allergens in the order listed:

1.	Nickel	5 per cent in petrolatum
2.	Balsam of Peru	25 per cent in petrolatum
3.	Colophony	20 per cent in petrolatum
4.	Chlorocresol	2 per cent in petrolatum
5.	*p*-Phenylenediamine	1 per cent in petrolatum
6.	Mercaptobenzothiazole	1 per cent in petrolatum
7.	Formaldehyde	2 per cent in water
8.	Potassium dichromate	0.5 per cent in petrolatum
9.	Wool alcohols	30 per cent in petrolatum
10.	Epoxy resin	2 per cent in petrolatum
11.	Primula leaf	

12. Neomycin	20 per cent in petrolatum
13. Cobalt chloride	1 per cent in petrolatum
14. Turpentine peroxide	0.3 per cent in olive oil
15. Parabens	15 per cent in petrolatum
16. Thiuram-mix	
17. Mercapto-mix	
18. Perfume-mix	
19. PPD-mix	
20. Carba-mix	
21. Vioform	5 per cent in petrolatum
22. Ethylenediamine	1 per cent in petrolatum

Allergic reactions

Allergic reactions have the following clinical features:

red, raised, palpable
vesicular ⎫ depending upon intensity
bullous ⎭

persist for four days or longer
intensity may increase from 2–4 days.

Itching is a characteristic but very subjective feature. Some patients with moderate reactions complain bitterly while others tolerate even severe responses.

Spread along lymphatics
Very occasionally a thin line of erythema is seen leading away from a strongly positive patch test. This must reflect diffusion of the allergen from a draining lymphatic, causing an overlying eczema.

Irritant reactions

Irritant reactions tend to correspond exactly with the site of application of the test substance. They may have any of the following clinical features:

Look exactly the same as an allergic reaction
Soap reaction: the skin is slightly red, glazed and wrinkled; it may be brownish
Pustules
Necrosis: the epidermis slides off the underlying dermis
Pustular bulla: a bulla forms, often containing sterile pus
Ulceration: in severe reactions the skin ulcerates
Soreness rather than irritation
The intensity usually diminishes once the patch is removed and weak reactions fade or disappear by four days. However, with some irritants the intensity may remain unchanged or even increase between the first and the second reading (Björnberg, 1968).

Histology
When there is difficulty in differentiating clinically between an irritant and an allergic reaction, histology is no help as it is equally equivocal.

Treatment
Strong reactions, whether allergic or irritant, are best treated topically with a fluorinated steroid.

Interpretation of patch tests

Clinical experience is the best guide to the interpretation of patch tests. In doubtful reactions the patch test should be repeated: allergic reactions are reproducible whereas irritant responses are much more variable. The features of an obvious irritant response are quickly recognised. The difficulty arises when the morphology of the positive reaction fails to differentiate between an allergic and an irritant response. This is not uncommon and is the major reason for the misinterpretation of patch tests. All unknown allergens should be checked by:
  (i) Testing with dilutions: reactions to an allergen gradually diminish in severity, the weaker the solution; reactions to an irritant stop abruptly below a certain concentration.
  (ii) Test approximately 50 controls: this is by far the best method.

Relevance

At the conclusion of patch testing the relevance of the positive reactions should be assessed and recorded as:

present
past
unexplained.

Present relevance may mean that the allergen is the entire cause of the eczema, as in a primula dermatitis. More often the allergen is only an aggravating factor, as occurs with medicaments or with rubber glove sensitivity in a patient with hand eczema.

Past relevance implies a contact dermatitis in the past from an allergen to which the patient is no longer exposed.

Relevance unexplained usually implies an ignorant physician.

The two great errors in patch testing are false positive and false negative reactions.

False positive reaction

A false positive reaction is caused by an irritant.

1. *Test substance is wrong*
   - (i) Irritant used as a patch test   (unfamiliar or unknown compound)
   - (ii) Concentration is too high
   - (iii) Contamination   (by another allergen or by an irritant)
   - (iv) Pressure   (solids — wood, leather).

2. *Skin is hyper-irritable*
   - (i) Adjacent to a strong positive ⎫
   - (ii) Plaster reaction   ⎬ angry back syndrome (Mitchell, 1975).
   - (iii) Status eczematicus   ⎭

3. *'Rogue' positive* (Fisher)
   Very occasionally a test with a known substance is strongly positive but, when repeated, is completely negative. The usual causes of irritancy do not explain this response and why it occurs is obscure.

4. *Artefact*
   Very occasionally a patient, usually when seeking compensation, may try to simulate a positive reaction by scratching or otherwise irritating the skin (Meigel and Koops, 1976).

Patch testing large numbers with high concentrations of likely irritants will undoubtedly give many 'false' positive reactions, as reported by Kligman and Leyden (1979), but few would have difficulty in interpreting such results.

Status eczematicus
The presence of active eczema renders the whole skin more irritable and may thereby cause false positive reactions to allergens and increased reactivity to irritants, even when the tests are applied at a distant site. The more widespread the eczema, the greater is this influence. This hyper-reactivity of the skin of the patch test sites has been called 'the angry back syndrome' by Mitchell (1975) and he stressed that it is produced by even one strongly positive patch test reaction.

Ideally patch testing should be done only when the patient's eczema is quiescent but as this is rarely practicable the eczema should at least be limited and under good control. Patients with spreading or widespread eczema should never be patch tested because false positive reactions invalidate the results and because the application of the tests may irritate the back and make it eczematous.

Six patients with contact dermatitis and eight with atopic eczema were patch tested twice with the same series of allergens by Wilson (1955). Relevant reactions in the contact dermatitis patients were positive on both occasions; however, any non-relevant positive tests were, in both groups of patients, either negative on the second occasion or were shown to be irritant by serial testing.

The irritancy of a toilet soap, potassium palmitate and Neutrogena in 1 per cent and 5 per cent concentrations and of Teepol in 1 per cent concentration were compared in eczematous and normal subjects by patch testing (Bettley, 1964). A greater number of reactions occurred in the patients with eczema. Some patients with extensive and active eczema reacted strongly to the 1 per cent soap solution which is rare in normal subjects; a few were re-tested once their eczema was quiescent and their response was then weaker. The presence of active hand eczema was found by Björnberg (1968) to increase reactivity to some but not all irritants. The enhancement was most marked with benzalkonium chloride. Spread of eczema beyond the hands broadened the range of irritants to which the patients reacted.

False negative reaction

A false negative reaction is one in which the patch test is negative despite the patient being sensitive to the allergen. It is practically always the test substance which is at fault.

1. *Test substance*
   (i) Concentration is too low   (by dilution or in a product)
   (ii) Amount applied is too small   (fear of a strong reaction)
   (iii) Poor absorption of the allergen
   (iv) A corticosteroid combined with a medicament suppresses the reaction
   (v) Pieces of material   (insufficient allergen is released)
   (vi) Filter paper retains the allergen*
   (vii) Wrong ingredient of a product is applied.

2. *Patch test technique*
   (i) Non-occlusion   (insufficient absorption)
   (ii) Patch test falls off
   (iii) Reading too early.

3. *Patient*
   (i) Refractory state
   Immediately after a very severe allergic contact dermatitis the patient fails to respond to the dilute allergen but reacts when retested several weeks later. This must be extremely rare but has occurred with poison ivy dermatitis (Kligman, 1968).

Contact thermography has been found useful in the detection of weak reactions, in reducing the incidence of false negative reactions and in facilitating the interpretation of responses in dark skinned patients (Jarisch, Dièm and Kucera, 1976).

*Retention of the allergen by the filter paper disc has been reported with synthetic primin by Fregert, Hjorth and Schulz (1968) and with an alcoholic solution of hop tree leaves by Lynne-Davies and Mitchell (1974).

Effect of prednisone on patch test reactions

The effect of graded doses of oral prednisone on patch test reactions was studied by O'Quinn and Isbell (1969) and Feuerman and Levy (1972). Doses of 40 and 30 mg daily reduced or completely suppressed some reactions, while leaving others unaffected. With 20 mg daily negation of the test was much less likely but the intensity of the response was reduced. In another study with dilutions of *Rhus* antigen (Condie and Adams, 1973) the patch tests were repeated three weeks after stopping prednisone and the reactivity was found to have returned to the pre-steroid level.

These results suggest that prednisone 15 mg daily or less will not suppress patch test reactions and may have little effect on their intensity. A higher dose will affect the results.

Complications of patch testing

Even with the most careful technique patch testing may cause adverse reactions. These include:

Severe reactions to the test substances
Plaster reactions
Active sensitisation
Focal flare
Alteration in pigment
Scars and keloids
Systemic absorption
Inoculation herpes simplex.

Severe reactions to the test substances
Very occasionally many severe reactions turn a normal back into a veritable battleground and they may exacerbate or disseminate the patient's eczema. They are usually unexpected and therefore unavoidable, but if anticipated they should be prevented by reducing the amount and concentration of the allergen.

Plaster reactions
A mild plaster reaction due to irritation by an occlusive zinc oxide strapping is not uncommon. It is usually patchy and does not occur under every piece of plaster; sometimes it is pustular. Men with greasy, sweaty backs and small follicular lesions seem particularly prone to develop this reaction.

Severe eczematous plaster reactions are generally avoided by using a non-occlusive tape when enquiry reveals a previous adverse reaction. But a few patients, unaware of their allergy, have an occlusive strapping applied and develop an eczematous reaction. The appearance is characteristic: the outline of every piece of plaster is imprinted on the patient's back as eczema, and there is usually an associated reaction to colophony.

Active sensitisation

Active sensitisation is sensitisation to a chemical induced by the application of a patch test. It is a complication of patch testing but is not a hazard and it should not be used as an excuse by the indolent for eschewing this investigation. To reject patch testing is the greater disservice to the patient.

The frequency of active sensitisation is not known. It is detected either by

(i) The patch test becoming positive 10–14 days after application (flare-up) and on being repeated the test is positive in 2–4 days, or by

(ii) Systematically re-testing patients after an interval.

The most frequent cause of active sensitisation is the use of too high a concentration of the test substance; of lesser importance are the amount applied and how long the patch test remains on.

In 1968 Agrup reported the results of re-testing 379 hand eczema patients with 11 substances first applied 6–21 months previously. In 281 (74 per cent) the results were unchanged, in 73 (19 per cent) tests had become positive, in 19 (5 per cent) tests had become negative and in 6 (2 per cent) some tests had become positive while others became negative. The allergens for which there was a statistically significant change were potassium dichromate (0.29 per cent in water), cobalt chloride (2.4 per cent in water), p-phenylenediamine (2.2 per cent in ethanol), p-aminoazobenzene (0.9 per cent in MEK) and diaminodiphenylmethane (2 per cent in MEK).

Among the 79 patients thought to have been sensitised by the patch tests 20 per cent had healed, 52 per cent had improved, 20 per cent were the same, 8 per cent were worse.

The course of the hand dermatitis was the same whether or not the tests had sensitised. In these patients, therefore, the clinical course was unaffected by patch testing and they were not harmed by the investigation.

To study this risk, Meneghini, Rantuccio and Lomuto (1972) re-patch tested 181 patients with eczema and 100 patients with non-eczematous dermatoses. New positive tests were found in 31 patients with eczema and in four of the other group. It was considered more likely that sensitisation had been due to further environmental exposure than to patch test active sensitisation.

The crucial importance of the patch test concentration was shown by Skog (1965) when he reported that more subjects were sensitised by p-phenylenediamine 8 per cent in petrolatum than by 2 per cent in the same base. He diagnosed sensitisation when a flare (delayed positive response) occurred at the patch test site and not by re-testing.

An ether extract of *Primula obconica* is a potent allergen and it was found by re-testing to have sensitised 10 per cent of 234 patients with hand eczema (Agrup, Fregert and Rorsman, 1969). Vitamin E (*d,l*-alpha-tocopherol) 20 per cent in petrolatum sensitised 1 of 97 consecutive patients tested by Roed-Petersen and Hjorth (1975).

St John's

Active sensitisation is induced occasionally both by the standard allergens and by rare sensitisers of unsuspected potency. The diagnosis is made by the patient returning to report that a patch test has become positive. Such tests are practically always repeated, the sensitisation being confirmed by their being positive at 2–4 days. In recent years they are not known to have caused dermatitis.

In 1967, Calnan reported that the following allergens had sensitised patients:

Allergen	Number	Concentration %
Tetramethylthiuram disulphide	15	1
p-Phenylenediamine	10	2 and 0.5
Methyl methacrylate	5	100
Mercaptobenzothiazole	3	1
Neomycin	2	50
p-Hydroxybenzoates	2	9
Diglycidyl ether	2	10
Chlorpromazine	1	25
Potassium dichromate	1	0.5
Phosphorus sesquisulphide	1	1
Primula	1	
p-tert-Butylphenol formaldehyde	1	10
Cycloaliphatic diepoxide	1	5
Diethylaminopropylamine	1	10

Two women sensitised to tetramethylthiuram disulphide subsequently developed dermatitis from rubber suspender buttons.

Focal flare (flare-up)

The term focal flare or flare-up is imprecise; it has been used to describe two occurrences:

(i) A late reaction at the patch test site denoting active sensitisation
(ii) Reactivation of an eczema at its original site by a strong, relevant positive patch test.

Donor site flare in two patients with skin grafts has been described by Jordan and Finn (1974). The first man developed an infectious eczematoid dermatitis on the recipient site and the second an allergic medicament dermatitis in the grafted skin and in both men the donor sites flared simultaneously with the grafted areas.

Alteration in pigment

Particularly in more pigmented patients, strongly positive tests may cause post-inflammatory hyperpigmentation and possibly depigmentation. Patch testing with compounds such as monobenzyl ether of hydroquinone may depigment the skin.

Scars and keloids

Indiscriminate patch testing with too high concentrations of unknown substances, which turn out to be strong irritants, may cause scar or keloid formation. When patch testing is done by those trained in this technique such a complication must be extremely rare and has not been seen in St John's.

Systemic absorption

In general the amount of allergen absorbed from patch test sites is insufficient to produce any systemic effect, but it is not known how much the flare of an eczema induced by a strong allergic positive reaction is due to absorption from the patch test.

Toxic material can be absorbed and cause systemic effects. A spray containing nicotine was applied as a patch test and within fifteen minutes the man, who was a non-smoker, complained of nausea, vomiting, weakness, vertigo, pallor and sweating. The test was repeated in a man who was a smoker and despite being left on for two days it caused no symptoms (Epstein, 1942).

Inoculation herpes simplex

Active sensitisation was suspected when the site of a mascara patch test became red and swollen two weeks after application. The test was repeated but was negative at two days, by which time the original reddened patch test had become pustular. Herpes simplex was diagnosed and confirmed by cytology. The patient had had a recent herpes simplex lesion on her lip, which had not entirely healed (Calnan, 1971).

Open tests and usage tests are useful methods of investigation but the terminology and the techniques have not been standardized.

Open test

In an open test the test substance is applied to a delineated area of skin and the site is left uncovered. It simulates environmental exposure more closely than does a patch test; it reduces irritancy but it also reduces absorption.

The test substance may be applied once or several times. In this clinic a circle is drawn on the flexor surface of the patient's forearm and the patient is asked to apply the test substance twice a day for two days, stopping if there is any reaction. Occasionally, when the material is applied only once, this is done in the clinic, usually on the back. The test is read at two days. Some objective sign such as erythema, papules or a stronger reaction is required for the test to be positive.

This is a useful procedure for checking patch test reactions of doubtful significance particularly to a cosmetic, medicament or household substance, when it is uncertain if the response obtained by the patch test is irritant or allergic.

Open tests may also be used to assess the effect of unknown substances before, or instead of, applying them as patch tests.

Usage test

If an open test or patch test to a strongly suspected test substance is negative, the patient should be asked to use the preparation again as they would normally. This is particularly valuable in deciding whether a specific cosmetic or garment has been the cause of a contact dermatitis.

References

Agrup, G. (1968) Sensitisation induced by patch testing. *British Journal of Dermatology*, 80, 631.

Agrup, A., Dahlquist, I., Fregert, S. and Rorsman, H. (1970) Value of history and testing in suspected contact dermatitis. *Archives of Dermatology*, 101, 212.

Agrup, G., Fregert, S. & Rorsman, H. (1969) Sensitisation by routine patch testing with ether extract of *Primula obconica, British Journal of Dermatology*, 81, 897.

Benezra, C., Andamson, J., Chabeau, C., Ducombs, G., Foussereau, J., Lachapelle, J.M., Lacroix, M. and Martin, P. (1978) Concentrations of patch test allergens; Are we comparing the same things? *Contact Dermatitis*, 4, 103.

Bettley, F.R. (1964) Non-specific irritant reactions in eczematous subjects. *British Journal of Dermatology*, 76, 116.

Björnberg, A. (1968) *Skin Reactions to Primary Irritants in Patients with Hand Eczema*, Thesis, pp. 124, 132, Göteborg, Sweden. Oscar Isacsons Tryckeri AB.

Bloch, B. (1911) Experimentelle Studien über das Wesen der Jodoformidiosynkrasie, *Zeitschrift für Experimentelle Pathologie und Therapie*, 9, 509.

Bonnevie, P. (1939) *Aetiologie und Pathogenese der Ekzemkrankheiten*. Copenhagen: Arnold Busck.

Calnan, C.D. (1967) Studies in contact dermatitis: XX Active sensitisation. *Transactions of the St John's Hospital Dermatological Society*, 53, 128.

Calnan, C.D. (1971) Inoculation herpes simplex as a complication of patch tests. *Contact Dermatitis Newsletter*, 10, 232.

Condie, M.W. & Adams, R.M. (1973) Influence of oral prednisone on patch test reaction to *Rhus* antigen. *Archives of Dermatology*, 107, 540.

Cronin, E. (1978) Comparison of Al-test and Finn Chamber. *Contact Dermatitis*, 4, 301.

Epstein, E. (1942) Untoward reactions to patch tests. *Journal of Investigative Dermatology*, 5, 55.

Epstein, E. (1967) Marking paint for patch tests. *Contact Dermatitis Newsletter*, 2, 8.

Fernstrom, Å.I.B. (1954) Patch test studies: 1. A new patch test technique. *Acta Dermatovenereologica*, 34, 203.

Feuerman, E. & Levy, A. (1972) A study of the effect of prednisone and an antihistamine on patch test reactions. *British Journal of Dermatology*, 86, 68.

Fregert, S. (1972) Side-reactions to Al-test. *Contact Dermatitis Newsletter*, 11, 256.

Fregert, S. & Hjorth, N. (1972) The principal irritants and sensitisers. *Textbook of Dermatology*, 2nd ed, ed. Rook, A., Wilkinson, D.S. and Ebling, F.J.G. p. 415 Oxford: Blackwell.

Fregert, S., Hjorth, N., Magnusson, B., Bandmann, H-J., Calnan, C.D., Cronin, E., Malten, K., Meneghini, C.L., Pirilä, V. & Wilkinson, D.S. (1969). Epidemiology of contact dermatitis. *Transactions of the St John's Hospital Dermatological Society*, 55, 17.

Fregert, S., Hjorth, N. & Schulz, K-H. (1968) Patch testing with synthetic primin in persons sensitive to *Primula obconica*. *Archives of Dermatology*, 98, 144.

Frosch, P.J. & Kligman, A.M. (1979) The Duhring chamber. An improved technique for epicutaneous testing of irritant and allergic reactions. *Contact Dermatitis*, 5, 73.

Grimalt, F. & Romaguera, C. (1978) Sensitivity to petrolatum. *Contact Dermatitis*, 4, 377.

Harman, R.R.M. (1961) Severe contact reaction to dihydroxyacetone. *Transactions of the St John's Hospital Dermatological Society*, 47, 157.

Hayakawa, R., Kobayashi, M., Ueda, H. & Morikawa, F. (1975) Clinical evaluation of Al-test patch test. *Journal of Dermatology*, 2, 111.

Jadassohn, (1896) Zur Kenntniss der Arzneiexantheme. *Archiv für Dermatologie und Syphylis*, 34, 103.

Jarisch, R., Diem, E. & Kucera, H. (1976) Verbesserte Diagnostik des Epikutantests mittels Kontaktthermographie. *Hautarzt*, 27, 595.

Jordan, W.P. (1971) Fluorescent marking ink for patch test site identification. *Contact Dermatitis Newsletter*, 10, 229.

Jordan, W.P. & Finn, J.W. (1974) Flare dermatitis. Occurrence in skin transplant donor site following sensitisation in recipient site. *Archives of Dermatology*, 109, 884.

Kligman, A.M. (1958) Poison ivy (*Rhus*) dermatitis: An experimental study. *Archives of Dermatology*, 77, 149.

Kligman, A.M. & Leyden, J.J. (1979) 'Reactions' to standard patch test materials. *Acta Dermatovenereologica*, 59, Suppl. 85, p. 101.

Kobza, A., Ramsay, C.A., & Magnus, I.A. (1973) Photosensitivity due to the 'sunburn' ultraviolet content of white fluorescent lamps. *British Journal of Dermatology*, **89**, 351.

Lynne-Davies, G. & Mitchell, J.C. (1974) Photopatch testing with Al-test and Duke 71 (plastic) patch. *Contact Dermatitis Newsletter*, **16**, 484.

Magnusson, B. & Hersle, K. (1965) Patch test methods: I. A comparative study of six different types of patch tests. *Acta Dermato-venereologica*, **45**, 123.

Magnusson, B. & Hersle, K. (1965) Patch test methods: II. Regional variations of patch· test responses. *Acta Dermato-venereologica*, **45**, 257.

Magnusson, B. & Hersle, K. (1966) Patch test methods: III. Influence of adhesive tape on test response. *Acta Dermato-venereologica*, **46**, 275.

Maibach, H. (1978) Chronic dermatitis and hyperpigmentation from petrolatum. *Contact Dermatitis*, **4**, 62.

Marzulli, F.N. & Maibach, H.I. (1976) Effects of vehicles and elicitation concentration in contact dermatitis testing. *Contact Dermatitis*, **2**, 325.

Malten, K.E. (1969) A case of contact eczema to yellow soft paraffin. *Contact Dermatitis Newsletter*, **5**, 106.

Mathias, C.G.T. & Maibach, H.I. (1979) When to read the patch test? *International Journal of Dermatology*, **18**, 127.

Meigel, W.N. & Koops, D.H. (1976) Skarifikationsartefakte der Testreaktion bei einer berufsdermatologischen Begutachtung. *Der Hautarzt*, **27**, 349.

Meneghini, C.L., Rantuccio, F. & Lomuto, M. (1972) A propos de réactions de sensibilisation active aprés l'éxecution des tests diagnostiques épicutanés: Observations sur 281 Cas. *Annales de Dermatologie et de Syphilographie*, **99**, 161.

Mitchell, J.C. (1975) The angry back syndrome: eczema creates eczema. *Contact Dermatitis*, **1**, 193.

Mitchell, J.C. (1978) Day 7 (D7) patch test reading — valuable or not? *Contact Dermatitis*, **4**, 139.

North American Contact Dermatitis Group (1973) Epidemiology of contact dermatitis in North America: 1972. *Archives of Dermatology*, **108**, 537.

Mid-Japan Contact Dermatitis Research Group (1976) Standardization of patch tests in Japan. *Contact Dermatitis*, **2**, 205.

O'Quinn, S.E. & Isbell, K.H. (1969) Influence of oral prednisone on eczematous patch test reactions. *Archives of Dermatology*, **99**, 380.

Pirilä, V. (1975) Chamber test versus patch test for epicutaneous testing. *Contact Dermatitis*, **1**, 48.

Roed-Petersen, J. & Hjorth, N. (1975) Patch test sensitisation from *d*, *l*-alpha-tocopherol (Vitamin E). *Contact Dermatitis*, **1**, 391.

Rudzki, E., Zakrzewski, Z., Prokopczyk, G. & Kozlowska, A. (1976) Application of emulsifiers for the patch test. *Dermatologica*, **153**, 333.

Skog, E. (1965) Sensitisation to *p*-phenylenediamine. *Archives of Dermatology*, **92**, 276.

Skog, E. & Forsbeck, M. (1978) Comparison between 24-hour and 48-hour exposure time in patch testing. *Contact Dermatitis*, **4**, 362.

Suhonen, R. (1976) Photoepicutaneous testing. Influence of the vehicle, occlusion time and concentration of the test substances on the results. *Contact Dermatitis*, **2**, 218.

Sulzberger, M.B. & Wise, F. (1931) The contact or patch test in dermatology. *Archives of Dermatology*, **23**, 519.

Trolle-Lassen, C. & Hjorth, N. (1966) Deterioration of substances used for patch testing. *Berufsdermatosen*, **14**, 176.

Wilkinson, D.S., Fregert, S., Magnusson, B., Bandmann, H-J., Calnan, C.D., Cronin, E., Hjorth, N., Maibach, H.I., Malten, K.E., Meneghini, C.L. & Pirilä, V. (1970) Terminology of contact dermatitis. *Acta Dermato-venereologica*, **50**, 287.

Wilson, H.T.H. (1955) Standard patch tests in eczema and dermatitis. *British Journal of Dermatology*, **67**, 219.

2.

General

AGE
ATOPY
SEASONAL VARIATIONS
CONTACT URTICARIA

SYSTEMIC ABSORPTION OF CONTACT
ALLERGENS
ERYTHEMA MULTIFORME
HISTOLOGY
ALLERGEN REPLACEMENT

Age

ALLERGIC CONTACT DERMATITIS IN CHILDREN

With the possible exception of poison ivy dermatitis, allergic contact dermatitis is uncommon in children. Whether this is due to their lack of exposure or to their failure to become sensitised is uncertain. They readily respond to some irritants because Marcussen (1963) patch tested children with nickel sulphate 5 per cent and formaldehyde 4 per cent and many had irritant reactions, especially those aged 0–1 year.

Poison ivy
In 1931, Straus showed that it is possible to sensitise newborn infants to poison ivy and thirty years later Epstein (1961) sensitised children aged 1–12 months but found them less susceptible than children over the age of 3 years, who resembled adults in their reactivity, while children aged 1–3 years were intermediate between the two groups. In Northern California, *Rhus* plants (including poison ivy) are the commonest cause of contact dermatitis in children (Epstein, 1971). It was the opinion of Fries and Lightstone (1962) that although poison ivy dermatitis occurs in children sensitisation by other contact allergens was infrequent and Mobley and Mansmann (1974) stated that in their clinical experience even sensitivity to poison ivy is seldom seen in children under 5 years of age.

Balsam of Peru
During their routine patch testing of eczematous patients Fregert and Möller (1963) patch tested 101 children under the age of 15 years and 24 per cent reacted to balsam of Peru (25 per cent in petrolatum) a significantly higher incidence than the 6 per cent found in the 2824 adults tested. The sensitisation was

thought to have followed the ubiquitous exposure to compounds related to balsam of Peru in medicaments, perfumes and flavourings.

Nickel

Sensitisation to nickel has been described in young children. Four such children, reported by Reiffers *et al.* (1974), were a baby 7 months old sensitised by fasteners on rubber pants, a girl aged 18 months by metal on her bed, a boy aged 4 years ?from toys and another boy aged 7 years by an intravenous drip needle. Each had a positive patch test to nickel 3 per cent. It is not uncommon for teenage girls to be sensitised by nickel in cheap jewellery (p. 347).

Shoes

Children occasionally become sensitised to rubber and the adhesive, *para-tertiary* butyl phenol formaldehyde, in their shoes. Some are sensitised by leather as was the child described by Reiffers *et al.* (1973) who reacted on patch testing to potassium dichromate 0.5 per cent.

Medicaments

Phenyl mercuric borate (Merfen) sensitivity has been described in a baby and 2 young children by Reiffers *et al.* (1973). Merthiolate allergy in a boy aged 3 years was thought initially to be impetigo. Ethylene diamine in aminophylline suppositories and Mycolog cream sensitised an asthmatic boy aged 5 years causing pruritus ani, and benzocaine dermatitis simulated a photodermatitis in a girl aged 7 years (Fisher, 1975). In California, Epstein (1971) thought neomycin, ethylenediamine and thiomersal were the most frequent medicament sensitisers in children (thiomersal because it is a popular topical remedy). Difficulty in the removal of a tracheostomy tube from a baby aged 3 months was attributed to a contact allergy of the tracheal mucosa due to the benzalkonium chloride used for disinfecting the tube. A patch test with a 0.1 per cent solution of benzalkonium chloride was positive (Padnos, Horwitz and Wunder, 1965).

CONTACT DERMATITIS IN ELDERLY PATIENTS

Allergens

It is not known whether elderly patients have a diminished tendency to be sensitised to contact allergens. That they are sensitised is common clinical experience as exemplified by medicament sensitisation in those with stasis eczema. Rather unexpectedly, Coenraads, Bleumink and Nater (1975) found the incidence of positive patch test reactions to common allergens increased with age.

Irritants

In industry advancing age seems to increase susceptibility to minor irritants, and failure to recover after exposure leads to recurrent and chronic dermatitis. Reactions to irritants in various age groups were studied by Coenraads, Bleumink and Nater (1975). They found the number of responses to croton oil (20 per cent in mineral oil) was less among the elderly but reactions to thymoquinone (1 per cent in ethanol) and crotonaldehyde (7.5 per cent with sodium lauryl sulphate 4 per cent in water) were similar in all age groups.

Atopic eczema

Irritant dermatitis
Patients with atopic eczema are undoubtedly susceptible to irritants and atopics are prone to develop irritant dermatitis. Agrup (1969) in her study of hand eczema found that a history of atopic dermatitis was significantly more frequent in patients with irritant hand dermatitis than in those with an allergic contact eczema. To help young atopics to avoid training for unsuitable types of employment, Wilkinson (1975) has suggested that the school and the employment medical services guide these children in their choice of jobs. The family doctor and parents should also be given guidance notes on this problem.

The irritability of atopic skin is reflected in their discomfort from woollen clothes; this wool intolerance was found in over 40 per cent of atopics by Hambly, Levia and Wilkinson (1978).

Allergic dermatitis
Opinions differ as to whether or not patients with atopic eczema are susceptible to sensitisation by contact allergens. The evidence, now accumulating, suggests that atopics do not have a constitutional predisposition to develop an allergic contact dermatitis. The discrepancies in the patch test results reported may be due to differing criteria, both for the diagnosis of atopy and for the selection of patients for investigation.

In 1964, Epstein and Mohajerin patch tested various groups of patients and found that of 100 atopics 28 had significant positive reactions, whereas of 100 psoriatics only 9 reacted, and of 20 patients with acne none had positive patch tests. They concluded that contact dermatitis was frequent in patients with atopic dermatitis. These results were supported by the finding that of 120 patients sensitive to neomycin 55–75 per cent were atopics (Epstein, 1965). Malten (1968) patch tested 80 atopic patients and reported that 34 per cent were sensitive to one or more of the allergens. Human dander has been reported to give positive patch tests in atopics (Uehara and Ofuji, 1976). Six patients with immediate-type hypersensitivity to algae and lichens were investigated by Champion (1971): five had atopic eczema, which was aggravated by inhaling or contacting the algae, and three had positive patch tests to lichens. The contact allergen was thought to be in the fungus component of the lichen.

Other investigations provide no evidence that atopics are particularly likely to develop allergic contact dermatitis (Sulzberger et al., 1932). In a European study, 4000 eczematous patients, of whom 233 had atopic eczema, were patch tested. Among the atopics 26 per cent had positive patch tests and this number did not differ significantly from the incidence in patients with discoid or seborrhoeic eczema (Cronin et al., 1970). In Warsaw, Rudzki and Grzywa (1975) patch tested 93 atopic dermatitis patients and found a diminished number of reactions to several allergens including potassium dichromate 0.5 per cent (aqueous), formaldehyde 2 per cent (aqueous), turpentine 10 per cent (arachis oil) and p-phenylenediamine 2 per cent (petrolatum), but an increased frequency of responses to neomycin 40 per cent (petrolatum) and oxytetracycline 50 per cent (petrolatum). This increased frequency of neomycin sensitivity among atopics was also reported by Epstein (1965) and Bandmann, Breit and Leutgeb (1972) who found some increase for neomycin but not for other allergens. It was not confirmed by Magnusson et al. (1969) or Wereide (1970). Evidence of an atopic background was sought but not found by Caron (1964) in 37 patients who were sensitive to nickel. There is evidence that atopics have a diminished incidence of sensitisation to common contact allergens. In the U.S.A. patch tests with *Rhus* oleoresins were positive in 6 out of 40 (15 per cent) atopic subjects compared with 27 out of 44 (61 per cent) normal controls, and the patch test actively sensitised one-third of 24 controls but only one of 16 atopics (Jones, Lewis and McMartin, 1973).

Suppression of cell mediated immunity was demonstrated in two adults with severe active atopic eczema and during a clinical remission the response to phytohaemagglutinin returned to normal in one of the patients (Lobitz, Honeyman and Winkler, 1972). Similar hyporeactivity of cell mediated immunity in patients with atopic eczema was reported by Hovmark (1975) and the impairment has been correlated with the severity of the dermatitis (Forsbeck, Hovmark and Skog, 1976). The presence of a factor in atopic serum which depresses the function of the patient's own, but not normal, lymphocytes has been reported by Andersen and Hjorth (1975). It is possible that the excessive production of IgE antibodies in atopics is associated with the demonstrable depression of their thymus dependent delayed type hypersensitivity (McGeady and Buckley, 1975; Rachelefsky et al., 1976).

The incidence of positive patch test reactions in 101 children with eczema was investigated by Fregert and Möller (1963). They found no significant differences in the number of positive reactions in the 37 children with atopic eczema and the rest of the group. Similarly in other young children with atopic eczema positive patch tests to common contact allergens were rare and children were found to be less readily sensitised than adults to DNCB (Meneghini and Rantuccio, 1967; Meneghini, 1969).

The relatives of patients with contact dermatitis have been intensively studied by Forsbeck, Skog and Ytterborn. In 1966 they reported a 43 per cent incidence of atopy among the children of patients with contact dermatitis. They continued this study (1971) but found only a slight increase in atopy among all the relatives of patients with contact dermatitis as compared with the patients themselves and a control group. However, there was a high incidence (41 per cent) of atopy among the daughters of men with contact dermatitis. In a further investigation (1968) of 101 pairs of twins they reported no correlation between atopy and the incidence of positive patch tests.

Pustular patch test reactions
Pustular patch test reactions to 5 per cent nickel sulphate were studied in atopic patients by Uehara, Takahashi and Ofuji (1975). They found that pustular responses occurred when the tests were applied to skin containing follicular papules or to sites which were eczematous, lichenified or traumatised. They were rare on normal skin.

Seasonal variations

The cold weather and low humidity of winter causes chapping, dryness and itching of the skin and predisposes to irritant dermatitis. Similarly, the low humidity in centrally-heated hospital wards may be a significant factor in the development of the xerosis which so many patients acquire while in hospital (Mitchell, 1972). A seasonal effect is much less obvious in allergic contact dermatitis.

In Copenhagen, Hjorth (1967, 1975) studied the incidence of reactions to common allergens for each month of the period 1935–1961. If primula sensitivity was excluded, the overall incidence of positive reactions was similar throughout the year but individual allergens had a seasonal variation which, with some, paralleled exposure. Reactions to primula were frequent in summer when sales of the plant are high; rubber reactions peaked in late summer and were explained by shoe dermatitis. Nickel sensitivity was most frequent in mid-autumn and late spring and Hjorth related this to a higher incidence of hand dermatitis at these times. Reactions to dichromate were frequent in late summer. Responses to formaldehyde and mercuric chloride were most frequent in winter, but some may have been false positives due to a heightened irritability of the skin in winter.

A definite seasonal variation in cement dermatitis in Kuwait was reported by Kanan (1972). He studied a series of 191 men, of whom all except two were immigrants from neighbouring Middle Eastern countries. Of these, 104 had worked with cement in their own countries and only 16 had a history of mild cement dermatitis; 87 had no previous contact with cement. The majority (105) were plasterers. The dermatitis began within one year in 87, within five years in 71 and the period was longer in the rest. All had positive patch tests to potassium dichromate 0.5 per cent and 13 reacted to cobalt chloride 5 per cent. The cement dermatitis had been present for over two years in 112 men and of these 84 (75 per cent) had exacerbations only during the hot months from May to mid-November and were virtually free during the rest of the year. The greatest attendance at the clinic was in September when the temperature was high and the humidity was rising.

Contact urticaria

Contact urticaria is a weal and flare response elicited by the application of certain compounds to intact skin. There are 3 major types:
 (i) Non-immunologic
 (ii) Immunologic
(iii) Uncertain mechanism.
   The features of each have been described by Maibach and Johnson (1975) and in a further review the following substances were listed as producing contact urticaria.

Medicaments
Horse serum
Streptomycin
Chlorpromazine
Cod liver oil
Penicillin
Cetyl and stearyl alcohol
Aspirin
Monoamylamine
DMSO
Diethyltoluamide (insect repellent)
Benzophenone
Tetanus antitoxin
Phenylmercuric propionate
Oestrogenic cream
Mechlorethamine hydrochloride
Cobalt chloride
Bacitracin

Industrial Contactants
Castor bean pomace
Platinum salts
Aliphatic polyamines
Ammonia
Sulphur dioxide
Formaldehyde
Sodium sulphide
Aminothiazole
Lindane
Acrylic monomer
Exotic woods

Cosmetics
Nail polish
Hair sprays
Hair bleach
Perfumes

Textiles
Wool
Silk

Physical Agents
Cold (acquired contact)
Heat
Water
Light (UV and visible)

Animals
Dog and cat saliva
Animal danders
Arthropods
Marine animals

Plants
Uren urticaria (nettles)
Cactus
Marine plants
Rhus

Foods
Wheat
Carrots
Potato
Flour
Spices

(Odom and Maibach, 1976)

These reactions are usually investigated by applying the suspected compounds to normal skin but scratch and prick tests have been used in some patients.

Non-immunologic
This non-immunological type of reaction may be produced by contact with a variety of compounds. These include plants such as stinging nettles and the sap of *Agave americana* mistakenly applied by a patient as a hair restorer (Kerner, Mitchell and Maibach, 1973), arthropods as exemplified by certain caterpillars and chemicals including tetrahydrofurfuryl ester of nicotinic acid (Trafuril) and dimethyl sulfoxide. Cobalt chloride 10 per cent in 95 per cent isopropyl alcohol was used as a colour indicator in a sweat provocation test and elicited urticaria in the subject to whom it was applied (Smith, Odom and Maibach, 1975).

Immunologic

A few subjects develop an immediate type of hypersensitivity after cutaneous contact with a particular compound and further skin contact elicits urticaria which may be localised or widespread and is sometimes associated with features of anaphylaxis. Compounds which have induced this reaction include:

Medicaments: Nitrogen mustard (Daughters and Maibach, 1973; Grunnet, 1976; Sanchez Yus and Suarez Martin, 1977)

cephalosporins (Tuft, 1975); bacitracin (Comaish and Cunliffe, 1967);

aminopyrine (Castellas Rodellas, 1974);

monoamylamine (Tharp, 1973).

Foods: Potato (Pearson, 1966)

fruits and vegetables (Hannuksela and Lahti, 1977)

eggs (Rudzki and Grzywa, 1977).

Hair dye: (Calnan, 1967).

Insect repellant: Diethyltoluamide (Maibach and Johnson, 1975).

Silk: (Rudzki, 1977).

Balsam of Peru: (Temesvári, *et al.*, 1978).

Teak: (Schmidt, 1978).

Animal fur: (Rudzki and Grzywa, 1978).

Dermatitis associated with immediate type hypersensitivity

Dermatitis of the hands in chefs and sandwich makers, associated with immediate type hypersensitivity to proteins in foods, has been described by Hjorth and Roed-Petersen (1976). A similar case in a woman, sensitised to fresh shrimps (*Pandalus*), was reported by Mitchell (1974). Another woman who reacted repeatedly to turkey skin was investigated by Maibach (1976), and a patient of Fisher and Stengel's (1977) had an occupational dermatitis of the hands from calf's liver. The same effect has been caused by balsam of Peru and cinnamic aldehyde (Rudzki and Grzywa, 1978).

Polyethylene glycol in an antifungal preparation induced contact urticaria and caused dermatitis of the feet in another patient described by Fisher (1977a).

Uncertain mechanism

The mechanism by which ammonium persulphate elicits urticaria in certain subjects (Calnan and Shuster, 1963) is not understood. The reaction is not due to the liberation of histamine (Mahzoon, Yamamoto and Greaves, 1977).

Reactions to the systemic absorption of contact allergens

Contact allergens given orally or systemically to sensitised persons can cause dermatitis. This effect, which is provoked in some but not all subjects, may be an important factor in the chronicity of eczema. Many of the reactions have been described in other sections of this book and the subject has been reviewed by Cronin (1972 and 1975).

Medicaments

Antibiotics
Sulphonamides: During the Second World War many of the troops were sensitised by topical suphonamides, usually suphanilamide (Grant Peterkin, 1945) and subsequently if given oral sulphonamides some developed generalised eruptions, the severity of which depended upon the sensitivity of the subject and the dose of sulphonamide given (Park, 1944). An unusual feature was the negative patch test reactions in many of these patients. Sulzberger *et al.* (1947) found that only 31 per cent of their patients with dermatitis from sulphonamides had positive patch test responses but of those with severe eruptions all reacted.

Streptomycin: When streptomycin was introduced for the treatment of tuberculosis the hazard of contact dermatitis among the nursing staff was not at first appreciated and some were sensitised. Desensitisation by courses of injections was successful but caused eczema and urticaria during the treatment. Patch tests which had previously evoked responses with low dilutions then failed to react with concentrations of 50 per cent and 20 per cent (Crofton, 1953; Wilson, 1958).

Penicillin: (p. 216).

Quinolines: (p. 220).

Neomycin and bacitracin: A patient of Pirilä and Rantanen (1960) who was sensitised to neomycin and bacitracin by a topical application suffered stomatitis from their use in throat tablets, a systemic reaction when they were inserted into a root canal, and 1.3 g of oral neomycin provoked diarrhoea and dermatitis. Ekelund and Möller (1969) also induced reactions with oral neomycin in sensitised subjects. In contrast, subjects sensitised to neomycin by the Draize test were challenged by Maibach (1971) with neomycin 1 g daily for five days, and none reacted.

Phenothiazines
Nurses, pharmacists and those manufacturing chlorpromazine are at risk of being sensitised. A nurse who was desensitised by an oral course of the drug developed oedema and irritation of the eyelids during the procedure (Morris-Owen, 1963). Promethazine (p. 237).

Ethylenediamine (p. 244)
This compound is used as a stabiliser in Mycolog cream (U.S.A.) and Tri-Adcortyl cream (Great Britain). It is an allergen and sensitised patients have developed dermatitis after receiving aminophylline which contains ethylenediamine and theophylline (Provost and Jillson, 1967). The antihistamines antazoline, promethazine and pyribenzamine are derivatives of ethylenediamine and carry the same risk (Fisher, 1973).

Antimitotic compounds
Chlorambucil (p. 238). Nitrogen mustard (p. 238).

Vitamins
Thiamine (p. 249). Vitamin B_{12} (p. 320).

Organic arsenical
Vuletić (1934) and his assistant developed a contact dermatitis from arsphenamine which was confirmed by patch testing. Inhalation of neosalvarsan then caused asthma in both doctors and one also had fever, urticaria and gastrointestinal symptoms.

Turpentine
Turpentine-sensitive subjects were challenged with a proprietary medicament containing turpentine (Ozothin). Three used it in suppository form and two developed peri-anal dermatitis; six were given it orally or intravenously and none reacted (Klaschka, 1975).

Foods
Azo dyes: Subjects found to be sensitive to azo dyes on patch testing were fed large amounts of the appropriate dye and though some reacted so did a few controls and the effects were not reproducible (Baer and Leider, 1949).

Flavours: Patients sensitive to balsam of Peru have had their eczema provoked by eating fruits, ices and orange marmalade (Hjorth, 1961, 1971) and vanilla sugar (Pirilä, 1970). Cinnamon has had similar effect on a sensitised patient (Leifer, 1951).

p-Aminobenzoic acid (PABA): A brewer, who was found on patch testing to be sensitive to PABA, healed his palmar eczema by avoiding contact with beer at work and by stopping drinking it (Malten, 1970).

Thiuram chemicals
Antabuse (tetraethylthiuram disulphide) caused a violent reaction and a widespread eczema in a patient sensitised by dipentamethylenethiuram disulphide in a rubber contraceptive (Wilson, 1962). In a similar patient (Pirilä, 1957) the reaction occurred within four hours and a thiuram patch test was reactivated.

Metals

Nickel
Urticaria and anaphylactoid reactions have been described in nickel-sensitive patients who received intravenous infusions through nickel-plated cannulae (p. 349) and in a patient after the insertion of Smith-Petersen vitallium nail (p. 351).

Widespread eczema has been attributed to orthopaedic screws (p. 349) and a localised dermatitis and suppuration to an underlying osteotomy plate (p. 350).

Chromium (p. 311).

Cobalt (p. 320).

Copper (p. 327).

Erythema multiforme

An erythema multiforme-like eruption is very occasionally a manifestation of an allergic contact sensitivity; it generally arises *de novo* and not as a sequel of a primary eczematous focus. The eruption, which may be bullous, usually affects the face and arms, sometimes the hands and spread occurs to the trunk and thighs. Ulceration of the mouth has been described (Chanial, Wertheimer and Tolot, 1961). The histology of the lesions has been that of erythema multiforme but the changes of toxic epidermal necrolysis were seen in one patient (Holst, Kirby and Magnusson, 1976). Patch testing shows the patient to be extremely sensitive to the responsible chemical.

The following allergens have caused erythema multiforme: primula (Hjorth, 1966), the tropical woods Rio rosewood, Pao Ferro and *Eucalyptus saligna* (Holst, Kirby and Magnusson, 1976), terpenes (Kirby and Darley, 1978), *p*-chlorbenzenesulfonylglycolic acid nitrile (Richter and Scholz, 1970), a phenyl sulphone derivative (Roed-Petersen, 1975), an epoxy resin compound ? the accelerator (Chanial, Wertheimer and Tolot, 1961), and 9-bromofluorine which caused a bullous eruption with some erythema multiforme-like lesions (Powell, 1968). It has also occurred as a secondary spread in patients with nickel dermatitis (Calnan, 1956).

The histology of patch test reactions

Early work on the histology of patch test reactions suggested that a clear distinction could be made between an irritant and an allergic reaction on the basis of the cell type in the inflammatory infiltrate, mononuclear cells predominating in sensitisation and polymorphonuclear leucocytes in irritant responses (Nexmand, 1949, 1950; Baer and Yanowitz, 1952). Further studies have shown other histological differences between definite allergic and definite irritant reactions. Bandmann (1965) studied the histology of allergic patch test reactions and found within 6–9 hours of the allergen being applied there was a perivascular infiltrate in the dermis and cells had already penetrated through the basal layer. By 20–40 hours there was marked oedema of the supra-basal layer, sometimes with vesiculation, and at sites of marked inflammation the basement membrane had disappeared. The dermal infiltrate was thought to consist predominantly of immature lymphocytes and reticulum cells. In an irritant reaction from machine oil the basement membrane was still intact at 6 hours. It was found helpful by Grosshans *et al.* (1968) to combine histological and cytological examination in the identification of allergic reactions. They noted three features which were characteristic of allergic reactions: an abundance of acid mucopolysaccharides in the oedema fluid, preservation of the epidermal filaments, and an infiltrate composed of monocytes and lymphocytes. The value of cytology has been confirmed by Song, Achten and Oleffe (1972): after 72 hours they observed blast cells in the infiltrate of allergic but not of irritant reactions. The ^{3}H-thymidine labelling index differs in the two reactions: it is significantly higher in an allergic reaction compared with an irritant response (Lachapelle, 1973).

Biopsies from positive patch tests elicited by different allergens were studied by Martin Pascual (1976); a feature common to all the reactions was participation of the sweat ducts and pilosebaceous follicles.

The light and electron microscopic changes in allergic and irritant reactions to DNCB in the guinea-pig were reported by Flax and Caulfield (1963). In an allergic response the changes in the dermis were oedema, vasodilatation and an increase in mononuclear cells; in the epidermis there was an invasion of mononuclear cells accompanied by extracellular oedema and damage to the epidermal tonofilaments and desmosomes. In a toxic reaction there was a slight increase in mononuclear cells but the principal changes were intracellular oedema of the epidermal cells with neither extracellular oedema nor changes in the tonofilament-desmosome complexes. A parallel study by Medenica and Rostenberg (1971) showed that in sensitisation there was a dermal infiltrate of mononuclear cells and basophils, the epidermis was invaded by cells and was oedematous, and in the keratinocytes there were secondary lysosomes, swollen mitochondria and aggregated tonofilaments. In irritant reactions they found an accumulation of polymorphonuclear cells in the dermis, damaged vessels and focal splitting of the epidermis from the dermis. In the epidermis the nuclei were particularly affected with loss of chromatin and cytoplasmic organelles. However Groth (1978) described, in allergic reactions in the guinea-pig, a significant increase in polymorphonuclear cells in the dermis. A study in man by Metz (1972) confirmed that in allergic reactions the epidermal cells show minimal change but there is intercellular oedema with disintegration of the desmosomes and disappearance of the basement membrane, where inflammatory cells invade the epidermis. In contrast, in irritant reactions there is major damage to the epidermal cells with intracellular vesicle formation and cytolysis of cells. The electron microscopic changes seen after patch tests with vehicles and with chromates have been studied by Forslind and Wahlberg (1978).

Histology would be a most valuable asset if it could resolve clinical doubt as to whether a patch test reaction is irritant or allergic. This it can not do; when the morphological features of the response are indeterminate the histology is not diagnostic (Wilhelm, Sarkany and Calnan, 1958) and with reactions to DNCB (?relatively mild) Hartman, Hoedemaeker and Nater (1976) did not find the histology distinctive of either irritation or sensitisation.

Allergic reactions to DNCB have been studied in man by Dvorak et al. (1974) and Dvorak, Mihm and Dvorak (1976). They found in addition to mononuclear cells in the dermis, infiltration and degranulation of basophil leucocytes, degranulation and replication of mast cells, increased vascular permeability and deposition of fibrin. The microvascular changes consisted of the development of gaps between the endothelial cells of the superficial capillary venules in the dermal papillae, caused possibly by degranulation of basophils and mast cells. The vessels of the superficial plexus of veins were cuffed by inflammatory cells, there was marked hypertrophy of endothelial cells and pericytes and some endothelial cells were necrotic and some were in mitosis. New basal lamina was laid down but in an abnormal way. Mast cells in mitosis were seen and immature mast cells were present in the dermis. In contrast low basophil counts in the infiltrate were found by Rantuccio et al. (1978).

Evidence is accumulating that Langerhans cells play an important role in allergic contact dermatitis. In man (Silberberg, 1973) and in guinea-pigs (Silberberg, Baer and Rosenthal, 1974b; Hunziker and Winkelmann, 1978) Langerhans cells have been found in apposition to mononuclear cells in allergic but not in toxic reactions. In guinea-pigs passively sensitised to DNCB, Langerhans cells have been identified in lymphatic vessels at the sites of allergic reactions (Silberberg, Baer and Rosenthal, 1974a; Silberberg et al., 1975). These experimental findings have been reviewed by Silberberg, Baer and Rosenthal (1976). More recently they have demonstrated in guinea-pigs, sensitised to ferritin, and to a lesser extent in control animals, that Langerhans cells carry the ferritin to the marginal sinus and cortex of draining lymph nodes (Silberberg-Sinakin et al., 1976). In a symposium on the Langerhans cell, the origin, nature and function of these cells was discussed by Shelley and Juhlin (1978) and their visualisation with a histofluorescence method after the uptake of L-dopa and catechloamines was described by Sjöborg et al. (1978).

Allergen replacement

Once sensitisation is established the ideal is to remove the allergen completely from the patient's environment. The practice is not so simple. Many allergens are ubiquitous and it is difficult for patients to recognise their presence and to accept that materials they have handled previously with impunity are now causing their dermatitis.

Gloves give some protection but they are more effective against irritants than sensitisers. Moursiden and Faber (1973) have shown that allergens penetrate through both rubber and plastic gloves.

Allergen replacement, a term first used by Calnan (1970), is the replacement of a dermatitic compound by a less sensitising but effective alternative. Among possible substitutions he discussed acetylated lanolin, perfumes without specific sensitisers, hardwoods unrelated to teak, esterification of colophony, turpentine free of Δ^3-carene, purified eosin, the hair dye ortho-nitro-para-phenylenediamine, plastic instead of rubber, polyamide hardeners in epoxy resin systems, aminoacid based fluxes instead of hydrazine, and molybdate instead of chromate in primer paints. He criticised the use of dinitrochlorbenzene in re-circulating water systems and advised scrupulous care not to introduce dermatitic plants into new areas.

Alternatives to allergens, particularily for patients in the U.S.A., are given by Fisher (1977b) and replacements and substitutions for sensitisers in industry are discussed by Adams (1977).

References

Adams, R.M. (1977) Allergen replacement in industry. *Cutis*, **20**, 511.
Agrup, G. (1969) Hand eczema. *Acta Dermato-venereologica*, **49**, Suppl. 61, p. 59.
Andersen, E. & Hjorth, N. (1975) B-lymphocytes, T-lymphocytes and phytohaemagglutinin responsiveness in atopic dermatitis. *Acta Dermato-venereologica*, **55**, 345.

Baer, R.L. & Leider, M. (1949) The effects of feeding certified food azo dyes in para-phenylenediamine hypersensitive subjects. *Journal of Investigative Dermatology*, 13, 223.

Baer, R.L. & Yanowitz, M. (1952) Differential cell counts in the blister fluid of allergic eczematous and irritant bullous lesions. *Journal of Allergy*, 23, 95.

Bandmann, H-J. (1965) Histopathology of allergic cutaneous test reactions. Sixth European Congress of Allergology. *Acta Dermato-venereologica (Stockholm)*, p. 3.

Bandmann, H-J., Breit, R. & Leutgeb, Chr. (1972) Kontakt-allergie und dermatitis atopica. *Archiv für Dermatologische Forschung*, 244, 332.

Calnan, C.D. (1956) Nickel dermatitis. *British Journal of Dermatology*, 68, 229.

Calnan, C.D. (1967) Hair dye reaction. *Contact Dermatitis Newsletter*, 1, 16.

Calnan, C.D. (1970) Studies in contact dermatitis. XXIII. Allergen replacement. *Transactions of the St John's Hospital Dermatological Society*, 56, 131.

Calnan, C.D. & Shuster, S. (1963) Reactions to ammonium persulphate. *Archives of Dermatology*, 88, 812.

Caron, G.A. (1964) Nickel sensitivity and atopy. *British Journal of Dermatology*, 76, 384.

Castellas Rodellas, A., Grimalt Sancho, F., Castel Rodó, T. & Piñol aguadé, J. (1974) Urticaria por contacto. *Medicina Cutanea*, 11, 417.

Champion, R.H. (1971) Atopic sensitivity to algae and lichens. *British Journal of Dermatology*, 85, 551.

Chanial, G., Wertheimer, J. & Tolot, F. (1961) Dermite professionelle par inducteur épicote, á type d'érythémepolymorphe. *Archives des Maladies Professionelles de Médicine der Travail et de Sécurité Sociale*, 22, 171.

Coenraads, P.J., Bleumink, E. & Nater, J.P. (1975) Susceptibility to primary irritants. Age dependence and relation to contact allergic reactions. *Contact Dermatitis*, 1, 377.

Comaish, J.S. & Cunliffe, W.J. (1967) Absorption of drugs from varicose ulcers: A cause of anaphylaxis. *British Journal of Clinic Practice*; 21, 97.

Crofton, J. (1953) Desensitisation to streptomycin and P.A.S. *British Medical Journal*, ii, 1014.

Cronin, E. (1972) Contact dermatitis XVII. Reactions to contact allergens given orally or systemically. *British Journal of Dermatology*, 86, 104.

Cronin, E. (1975) Ekzematöse reaktionen bei innerlicher Aufnahme von Kontakt-allergenen. *Hautarzt*, 26, 68.

Cronin, E., Bandmann, H-J., Calnan, C.D., Fregert, S., Hjorth, N., Magnusson, N., Maibach, H., Malten, K., Meneghini, C., Pirila, V. & Wilkinson, D.S. (1970) Contact dermatitis in the atopic. *Acta Dermato-venereologica*, 50, 183.

Daughters, D. & Maibach, H.I. (1973) Urticarial and anaphylactoid reactions to the topical applications of nitrogen mustard. *Contact Dermatitis Newsletter*, 13, 359.

Dvorak, A.M., Mihm, M.C. & Dvorak, H.F. (1976) Morphology of delayed-type hypersensitivity reactions in man. II. Ultrastructural alterations affecting the microvasculature and the tissue mast cells. *Laboratory Investigation*, 34, 179.

Dvorak, H.F., Mihm, M.C., Dvorak, A.M., Johnson, R.A., Manseau, E.J., Morgan, E. & Colvin, R.B. (1974) Morphology of delayed-type hypersensitivity reactions in man. I. Quantative description of the inflammatory response. *Laboratory Investigation*, 31, 111.

Epstein, E. (1971) Contact dermatitis in children. *Pediatric Clinics of North America*, 18, 839.

Epstein, S. (1965) Neomycin sensitivity and atopy. *Dermatologica*, 130, 280.

Epstein, S. & Mohajerin, A.H. (1964) Incidence of contact sensitivity in atopic dermatitis. *Archives of Dermatology*, 90, 284.

Epstein, W.L. (1961) Contact-type delayed hypersensitivity in infants and children: Induction of *rhus* sensitivity. *Pediatrics*, 27, 51.

Fisher, A.A. (1973) The broad implications of allergic sensitisation to ethylenediamine hydrochloride. *Contact Dermatitis Newsletter*, 14, 418.

Fisher, A.A. (1975) Childhood allergic contact dermatitis, *Cutis*, 15, 635.

Fisher, A.A. (1977a) Contact urticaria due to polyethylene glycol. *Cutis*, 19, 409.

Fisher, A.A. (1977b) Allergen replacements in allergic dermatitis. *International Journal of Dermatology*, 16, 319.

Fisher, A.A. & Stengel, F. (1977) Allergic occupational hand dermatitis due to calf's liver. An urticarial 'immediate' type hypersensitivity. *Cutis*, 19, 561.

Flax, M.H. & Caulfield, J.B. (1963) Cellular and vascular components of allergic contact dermatitis. *American Journal of Pathology*, 43, 1031.

Forsbeck, M., Hovmark, A. & Skog, E. (1976) Patch testing, tuberculin testing and sensitisation with dinitrochlorobenzene and nitrosodimethylaniline of patients with. atopic dermatitis. *Acta Dermato-venereologica*, 56, 135.

Forsbeck, M. Skog, E. & Ytterborn, K.H. (1966) The frequency of allergic diseases among relatives of patients with allergic eczematous contact dermatitis. *Acta Dermato-venereologica*, 46, 149.

Forsbeck, M., Skog, E. & Ytterborn, K.H. (1968) Delayed-type of allergy and atopic disease among twins. *Acta Dermato-venereologica*, **48**, 192.

Forsbeck M., Skob, E. & Ytterborn, K.H. (1971) Allergic disease among relatives of patients with allergic contact dermatitis. *Acta Dermato-venereologica*, **51**, 123.

Forslind, B. & Wahlberg, J.E. (1978) The morphology of chromium allergic skin reactions at electron microscopic resolution. Studies in man and guinea-pig. *Acta Dermato-venereologica*, **58**, Suppl. 79, p. 43.

Fregert, S. & Möller, H. (1963) Contact allergy to balsam of Peru in children. *British Journal of Dermatology*, **75**, 218.

Fries, J.H. & Lightstone, A.C. (1962) Pediatric allergy: A critical review of the literature. *Annals of Allergy*, **20**, 282.

Grant Peterkin, G.A. (1945) Sulphonamide rashes: An analysis of 500 cases seen in North Africa and Italy. *British Medical Journal*, ii, 1.

Grosshans, E., Mayer, S., Foussereau, J. & Basset, A. (1968) Contribution á l'étude histologique et cytologique des test épicutanés. *Bulletin de la Société Francaise de Dermatologie et de Siphiligraphie*, **75**, 371.

Groth, O. (1978) The cellular infiltrate and its measurement in contact dermatitis. *Acta Dermato-venereologica*, **58**, Suppl. 79, p. 57.

Grunnet, E. (1976) Contact urticaria and anaphylactoid reaction induced by topical application of nitrogen mustard. *British Journal of Dermatology*, **94**, 101.

Hambly, E.M., Levia, L. & Wilkinson, D.S. (1978) Wool intolerance in atopic subjects. *Contact Dermatitis*, **4**, 240.

Hannuksela, M. & Lahti, A. (1977) Immediate reactions to fruits and vegetables. *Contact Dermatitis*, **3**, 79.

Hartman, A., Hoedemaeker, Ph.J. & Nater, J.P. (1976) Histological aspects of DNCB sensitisation and challenge tests. *British Journal of Dermatology*, **94**, 407.

Hjorth, N. (1961) *Eczematous Allergy to Balsams*, p. 171. Copenhagen: Munksgaard.

Hjorth, N. (1966) Primula dermatitis. *Transactions of the St. John's Hospital Dermatological Society*, **52**, 207.

Hjorth, N. (1976) Seasonal variations in contact dermatitis. *Acta Dermato-venereologica*, **47**, 409.

Hjorth, N. (1971) Allergy to balsams. *Spectrum*, **8**, 97.

Hjorth, N. (1975) Jahreszeitliche Schwankungen der Kontaktekzeme. *Hautarzt*, **26**, 75.

Hjorth, N. & Roed-Petersen, J. (1976) Occupational protein contact dermatitis in food handlers. *Contact Dermatitis*, **2**, 28.

Holst, R., Kirby, J. & Magnusson, B. (1976) Sensitisation to tropical woods giving erythema multiforme-like eruptions. *Contact Dermatitis*, **2**, 295.

Hovmark, A. (1975) An *in vivo* and *in vitro* study of cell-mediated immunity in atopic dermatitis. *Acta Dermato-venereologica*, **55**, 181.

Hunziker, N. & Winkelman, R.K. (1978) Langerhans cells in contact dermatitis in the guinea-pig. *Archives of Dermatology*, **114**, 1309.

Jones, H.E., Lewis, C.W. & Mcmartin, S.L. (1973) Allergic contact sensitivity in atopic dermatitis. *Archives of Dermatology*, **107**, 217.

Kanan, M.W. (1972) Cement dermatitis and atmospheric parameters in Kuwait. *British Journal of Dermatology*, **86**, 155.

Kerner, J., Mitchell, J. & Maibach, H.I. (1973) Irritant contact dermatitis from *Agave americana* L. *Archives of Dermatology*, **108**, 102.

Kirby, D.J. & Darley, C.R. (1978) Erythema multiforme associated with a contact dermatitis to terpenes. *Contact Dermatitis*, **4**, 238.

Klaschka, F. (1975) Allergy to turpentine: Examination of systemic trigger action. *Contact Dermatitis*, **1**, 319.

Lachapelle, J.M. (1973) Comparative histopathology of allergic and irritant patch test reactions in man. *Archives Belge de Dermatologie*, **28**, 83.

Leifer, W. (1951) Contact dermatitis due to cinnamon. Recurrence of dermatitis following oral administration of cinnamon oil. *Archives of Dermatology*, **64**, 52.

Lobitz, W.C., Honeyman, J.F. and Winkler, N.W. (1972) Suppressed cell-mediated immunity in two adults with atopic dermatitis. *British Journal of Dermatology*, **86**, 317.

Mahzoon, S., Yamamoto, S. & Greaves, M.W. (1977) Response of skin to ammonium persulphate. *Acta Dermato-venereologica*, **57**, 125.

Malten, K.E. (1968) The occurrence of hybrids between contact allergic eczema and atopic dermatitis (and vice versa) and their significance. *Dermatologica*, **136**, 404.

Malten, K.E. (1970) Source of PABA exposure. *Contact Dermatitis Newsletter*, **7**, 160.

Magnusson, B., Fregert, S., Hjorth, N., Høvding, G., Pirilä, V. & Skog, E. (1969) Routine patch testing: V. Correlation of reactions to the sites of dermatitis and the history of the patient. *Acta Dermato-venereologica*, **49**, 556.

Maibach, H.I. (1971) Personal communication.

Maibach, H.I. (1976) Immediate hypersensitivity in hand dermatitis. *Archives of Dermatology*, **112**, 1289.

Maibach, H.I. & Johnson, H.L. (1975) Contact urticaria syndrome. *Archives of Dermatology*, **111**, 726.

Marcussen, P.V. (1963) Specificity of epicutaneous tests in children. *Acta Dermato-venereologica*, **43**, 219.

Martin Pascual, A. (1976) Histopatologia del eczema de contacto. *Actas dermo-sifiliograficas*, **67**, 403.

Mcgready, S.J. & Buckley, R.H. (1975) Depression of cell-mediated immunity in atopic eczema, *Journal of Allergy and Clinical Immunology*, **56**, 393.

Medenica, M. & Rostenberg, A. (1971) A comparative light and electron microscopic study of primary irritant contact dermatitis and allergic contact dermatitis. *Journal of Investigative Dermatology*, **56**, 259.

Meneghini, C.L. (1969) Patch tests in atopic dermatitis children. *Contact Dermatitis Newsletter*, **6**, 132.

Meneghini, C.L. & Rantuccio, F. (1967) Eczematous contact hypersensitivity in children. *Contact Dermatitis Newsletter*, **2**, 23.

Metz, J. (1972) Elektronenmikroskopische Untersuchungen an allergischen und toxischen Epicutan-testreaktionen des Menschen. *Archiv fur Dermatologische Forschung*, **245**, 125.

Mitchell, J.C. (1972) Per cent humidity of the air in a dermatological ward, xerosis of the skin and irritant contact dermatitis. *Contact Dermatitis Newsletter*, **11**, 287.

Mitchell, J.C. (1974) Contact urticaria from a shrimp, *Pandalus*. *Contact Dermatitis Newsletter*, **16**, 486.

Mobley, S.L. & Mansmann, H.C. (1974) Current status of skin testing in children with contact dermatitis. *Cutis*, **13**, 995.

Morris-Owen, R.M. (1963) 'Cover-dose' management of contact sensitivity to chlorpromazine. *British Journal of Dermatology*, **75**, 167.

Moursiden, H.T. & Faber, O. (1973) Penetration of protective gloves by allergens and irritants. *Transactions of the St. John's Hospital Dermatological Society*, **59**, 230.

Nexmand, P.H. (1949) The cellular content of exudates from eczematous and toxic patch test reactions. *Journal of Investigative Dermatology*, **13**, 85.

Nexmand, P.H. (1950) Skin sensitisation to nitrogen mustard with reference to the cytologic differences between primary-irritant and eczematous reactions. *Dermatologica*, **100**, 73.

Odom, R.B. & Maibach, H.I. (1976) Contact urticaria: A different contact dermatitis. *Cutis*, **18**, 672.

Padnos, E., Horwitz, I.D. & Wunder, G. (1965) Contact dermatitis complicating tracheostomy. *American Journal of Diseases of Children*, **109**, 90.

Park, R.G. (1944) Sulphonamide Allergy. *British Medical Journal*, i, 781.

Pearson. R.S.B. (1966) Potato sensitivity, an occupational allergy in housewives. *Acta Allergologica*, **21**, 507.

Pirilä, V. (1957) Dermatitis due to rubber. *Acta Dermato-venereologica. Proceedings of the 11th national Congress of Dermatology*, Vol. 11, 252.

Pirilä, V. (1970) Endogenic contact eczema *Allergie und Asthma*, **16**, 15.

Pirilä, V. & Rantanen, A.V. (1960) Root canal treatment with bacitracin-neomycin as cause of flare-up of allergic eczema. *Oral Surgery*, **13**, 589.

Powell, E.W. (1968) Skin reactions of 9-bromofluorene. *British Journal of Dermatology*, **80**, 491.

Provost, T.T. & Jillson, O.F. (1967) Ethylenediamine contact dermatitis. *Archives of Dermatology*, **96**, 231.

Rachelefsky, G.S., Opelz, G., Mickey, M.R., Kiuchi, M., Terasaki, P.I., Siegel, S.C., & Stiehm, E.R. (1976) Defective T cell function in atopic dermatitis. *Journal of Allergy and Clinical Immunology*, **57**, 569.

Rantuccio, F., Sinisi, D., Scardigno, A. & Conte, A. (1978) Histologic aspects of patch test reactions in allergic contact dermatitis. *Contact Dermatitis*, **4**, 338.

Reiffers, J., Hunziker, N., Brun, R. & Vidmar, B. (1973) Sensibilisations cutanées allergique peu communes. *Dermatologica*, **148**, 285.

Richter, G. & Schloz, H. (1970) Kontaktekzem und makuloses Exanthem bei *p*-Chlor-benzosulfonylglykolsäurenitril-allergie. *Berufsdermatosen*, **18**, 70.

Roed-Petersen, J. (1975) Erythema multiforme as an expression of contact dermatitis. *Contact Dermatitis*, **1**, 270.

Rudzki, E. (1977) Contact urticaria from silk. *Contact Dermatitis*, **3**, 53.

Rudzki, E. & Grzywa, Z. (1975) Contact sensitivity in atopic dermatitis. *Contact Dermatitis*, **1**, 285.

Rudzki, E. & Grzywa, Z. (1977) Contact urticaria from egg. *Contact Dermatitis*, **3**, 103.

Rudzki, E. & Grzywa, Z. (1978) Two types of contact urticaria and immediate reactions to patch-test allergens. *Dermatologica*, **157**, 110.

Sanchez Yus, E. & Suarex Martin, E. (1977) Urticaria de contacto y reacción anafilactoide inducidas por applicacion topica de mostaza nitrogenada. *Actas Dermo-Sifiliograficas*, **68**, 39.

Schmidt, H. (1978) Contact urticaria to teak with systemic effects. *Contact Dermatitis*, **4**, 176.

Shelley, W.B. & Juhlin, L. (1978) The Langerhans cell: its origin, nature and function. *Acta Dermato-venereologica*, **58**, Suppl. 79, 7.

Silberberg, I. (1973) Apposition of mononuclear cells of Langerhans cells in contact allergic reactions: an ultrastructural study. *Acta Dermato-venereologica*, **53**, 1.

Silberberg, I., Baer, R.L. & Rosenthal, S.A. (1974a) Circulating Langerhans cells in a dermal vessel. *Acta Dermato-venereologica*, **54**, 81.

Silberberg, I., Baer, R.L. & Rosenthal, S.A. (1974b) The role of Langerhans cells in contact allergy: 1. An ultrastructural study of actively-induced contact dermatitis in guinea pigs. *Acta Dermato-venereologica*, **54**, 321.

Silberberg, I., Baer, R.L. & Rosenthal, S.A. (1976) The role of Langerhans cells in allergic contact hypersensitivity. A review of findings in man and guinea pigs. *Journal of Investigative Dermatology*, **66**, 210.

Silberberg, I., Baer, R.L., Rosenthal, S.A., Thorbecke, G.J. & Berezowsky, V. (1975) Dermal and intravascular Langerhans cells at sites of passively-induced allergic contact sensitivity. *Cellular Immunology*, **18**, 435.

Silberberg-Sinakin, I., Thorbecke, G.J., Baer, R.L., Rosenthal, S.A. & Berezowsky, V. (1976) Antigen-bearing Langerhans cells in skin, dermal lymphatics and in lymph nodes. *Cellular Immunology*, **25**, 137.

Sjöborg, S., Axelsson, S., Falck, B. Jacobsson, S. & Ringberg, A. (1978) A new method for the visualisation of the epidermal Langerhans cell and its application on normal and allergic skin. *Acta Dermato-venereologica*, **58**, Suppl. 79, 23.

Smith, J.D., Odom, R.B. & Maibach, H.I. (1975) Contact urticaria from cobalt chloride. *Archives of Dermatology*, **111**, 1610.

Song, M., Achten, G. & Oleffe, J. (1972) Utilite du dermogramme dans le diagnostic des dermatoses professionelles. *Archives Belges de Dermatologie*, **28**, 223.

Straus, H.W. (1931) Artificial sensitisation of infants to poison ivy. *Journal of Allergy*; **1**, 137.

Sulzberger, M.B., Kanoff, A., Baer, R.L. & Lowenberg, C. (1947) Sensitisation by topical application of sulfonamide. *Journal of Allergy*, **18**, 92.

Sulzberger, M.B., Spain, W.C., Sammis, F. & Shahon, H.I. (1932) Studies in hypersensitiveness in certain dermatoses: 1. Neurodermatitis (disseminated type). *Journal of Allergy*, **3**, 423.

Temesvári, E., Soós Gy., Podányi, E., Kovács, I. & Németh, I. (1978) Contact urticaria provoked by balsam of Peru. *Contact Dermatitis*, **4**, 65.

Temesvári, E., Soós, Gy., Podányi, E. Kovács, I. & Németh, I. (1978) Kontakturtikaria durch Perubalsam. *Dermatosen in Beruf und Umwelt*, **26**, 81.

Tharp, C.K. (1973) Contact urticaria to monoamylamine. *Contact Dermatitis Newsletter*, **14**, 391.

Tuft, L. (1975) Contact urticaria from cephalosporins. *Archives of Dermatology*, **111**, 1609.

Uehara, M. & Ofuji, S. (1976) Patch test reactions to human dander in atopic dermatitis. *Archives of Dermatology*, **112**, 951.

Uehara, M., Takahashi, C. & Ofuji, S. (1975) Pustular patch test reactions in atopic dermatitis. *Archives of Dermatology*, **111**, 1154.

Vuletić, A. (1934) Uber Salvarsanüberempfindlichkeit und akute salvarsan Intoxikation infolge beruflicher Benetzungen der Finger mit Salvarsanlösungen. *Archiv für Dermatologie und Syphilis*, **169**, 436.

Wereide, K. (1970) Neomycin sensitivity in atopic dermatitis and other eczematous conditions. *Acta Dermato-venereologica*, **50**, 114.

Wilhelm, E., Sarkany, I. & Calnan, C.D. (1958) Studies in contact dermatitis: VI. Histology in the diagnosis of patch tests, *Transactions of the St. John's Hospital Dermatological Society*, **41**, 31.

Wilkinson, D.S. (1975) Careers advice to youths with atopic dermatitis. *Contact Dermatitis*, **1**, 11.

Wilson, H.T.H. (1958) Streptomycin dermatitis in nurses. *British Medical Journal*, i, 1378.

Wilson, H.T.H. (1962) Side-effects of disulfiram. *British Medical Journal*, ii, 1610.

3.

Clothing and textiles

DYES
  Clothing
  Stockings, tights (panty hose), socks
  Hair nets
RESINS
  Clothing
  Sheets
SHOES and RUBBER BOOTS
HAT BANDS
LEATHER ACCESSORIES

DRY CLEANING
  Retexing, stain repellants, fabric softeners
FIBREGLASS
FIRE RETARDANTS
FLUORESCENT WHITENING AGENTS
PRESERVATIVES
  Mothproofing
TEXTILE FIBRES
TEXTILE PURPURA

Pigments and dyes

A *pigment* is a compound containing molecules with a colour bearing group, the chromophore. Most pigments are inorganic oxides, insoluble salts or lakes, and are made by precipitating soluble vegetable or synthetic dyes with aluminium hydroxide or a suitable metal salt. Well known pigments are white lead which has been used for centuries, and Prussian Blue which is ferric ferrocyanide; the natural pigments haem in blood and chlorophyll in plants are both porphyrins.

A *dye*, which also is coloured, is characterised by its ability to attach to fibres, usually by an acidic or basic group. It withstands removal by washing, retains its colour and resists the action of light.

The difference between a dye and a pigment is in their ability to attach to fibres; a pigment with this property can be used as a dye.

Mordants
A mordant is a chemical which can combine both with a dye and with a fabric and can thus fasten a dye to a fabric for which it has little intrinsic affinity. Material is soaked in a soluble salt of aluminium, chromium or iron, which is then hydrolysed to the metallic hydroxide. In this form it will link to an acid dye to give an insoluble colour.

Textile dyes

Prior to the 1850s, dyes were natural extracts of vegetables, animals, and minerals. Vegetable dyes were imported into Britain for the textile industry from many parts of the world. The woad of Western Europe was superseded by the blue indigo of tropical Asia, madder for browns and reds came from France, logwood dyes for blacks and navy from South America, orchil for deep red from Italy and the coasts of Africa, safflower for orange-red from the Middle East and yellow fustic from the West Indies. Many of the natural dyes were red, other colours being limited or non-existent; green had to be compounded by mixing blue and yellow. Scarcity could mean status. The costly purple dye obtained from whelks in the Eastern Mediterranean became known as Imperial Purple and was the origin of the phrase 'born in the purple'; it can now be synthesised and is no longer desirable. Dependence on imports of these natural products threatened the expansion of the textile industry.

In 1856, William Henry Perkins, a young scientist, then aged 18 years, attempted to synthesise quinine in a home-made laboratory. He failed, but instead produced Mauve or Aniline Purple (C.I. 846) and revolutionised the dye industry. Dyes were synthesised in rapid succession from the coal tar derivatives benzene, naphthalene and anthracene. In 1859 Magenta (C.I. 677) was made, in 1868 Alizarine (C.I. 1027), the colour in madder, and in 1858 Greiss made his momentous discovery of the diazo reaction which led to the synthesis of its first important members, Bismark Brown in 1863 and the yellow-brown dye Chrysoidine in 1876. Within 50 years, new dyeing processes were introduced and the limited number of natural colours were replaced by synthetic dyes of every hue.

Early dyes, being water-soluble, were unsuitable for the synthetic water-repellent fibres nylon and terylene; for these, insoluble disperse-type azo dyes were developed. These dyes are applied as dispersions in combination with an emulsifier.

The vast number of dyes has made their nomenclature and classification difficult. The same dyes are frequently made by many companies and carry a variety of trade names. Only by referring to the Standard Colour Index and finding the standard colour index name and number of these dyes can they be recognised as being identical chemically.

Dye chemists classify dyes according to the conditions and reactions of the dyeing process and not by chemical structure. They are divided into basic, acidic, mordant, direct cotton, sulphur, azo and vat dyes.

For dermatologists there are two important chemical groups, azo and anthraquinone dyes.

1. *Azo dyes*
These are derivatives of azobenzene, the azo bridge being $-N=N-$

When coupled with amines they form basic dyes, and with phenols they become acidic dyes. Azo compounds can be linked to give a double azo (diazo) compound such as Bismark Brown, for which there are now three different structures. The simplest is:

Bismark Brown (Basic Brown 1 C.I. 21000)

2. Anthraquinone dyes

These dyes are synthesised from the anthracene derivative anthraquinone:

Complexing of these molecules produces a range of dyes: Alizarin, the red-brown dye of madder is an anthraquinone:

Alizarin (Ç.I. 1027)

Vat dyes

Vat dyes are so called because the solutions were originally stored in wooden vats. They are reduced by alkali to a soluble colourless leuco form and as such are applied to the fibre; the insoluble coloured dye is regenerated by acid oxidation. Most are azo or anthraquinone derivatives; a few are polycyclic compounds (Whittaker and Wilcox, 1950; Gibbs, 1961).

CLOTHING

Incidence of sensitivity

Although many hundreds of dyes are used in the textile industry, they rarely sensitise; and since 1930, only small series and individual cases have been described. The reports for various types of clothing have been summarised by Cronin (1968) and for trousers by Sim-Davies (1972).

St John's

From 1970–1976, 21 women and 26 men have been seen with dermatitis from dyes in clothing, an incidence of three women and approximately four men each year (Table 3.1). In both the women seen in 1971 the dermatitis had occurred in the past.

Table 3.1 Numbers of patients seen each year with dermatitis from dyes in clothing. St John's 1970–1976.

	1970	1971	1972	1973	1974	1975	1976	Total
Women	4	2	2	5	2	4	2	21
Men	6	3	2	4	3	5	3	26

Garments causing sensitivity

St John's

Women

Dresses, blouses and summer suits, made entirely or partially of synthetic fibres, have been the most frequent source of dye sensitivity among women's clothes. Lining materials are sometimes responsible, underclothes rarely. However, in 1970, a woman was seen with dermatitis from a blue brassière and a blue crimplene suit, and, in the 1968 series (Cronin, 1968), two patients reacted to their black petticoats and one to underwear she had dyed herself. Scarves rarely cause dermatitis.

Men

Trousers with a synthetic fibre component are by far the commonest source of dye sensitivity among men's clothes, and it may be a separate pair of trousers rather than those of a suit which is responsible. In the 1972 series of 15 patients (Sim-Davies, 1972) a suit was the source in only two men but of the 13 men seen from 1972–1976, the trousers of a suit were to blame in six.

Dyes in shirts and pyjamas rarely cause dermatitis, although green striped pyjamas sensitised one man reported by Sim-Davies (1972) and brightly coloured shirts another (Cronin, 1968). Among the 26 men seen from 1970–1976 two had dermatitis from shirts, one from a blue singlet and another from mauve underpants.

Trouser pocket dermatitis. In Barcelona, 16 men have been seen with dermatitis on their thighs under the nylon fabric of their trouser pockets. The allergen was not identified but the skin healed when the material of the pockets was changed (Grimalt, Romaguera, Pinol Aguadé, 1976).

Clinical features

St John's

Women

Age. Teenage girls and women of any age may be affected; of 19 patients seen at St John's from 1970 to 1976, six were aged 17–20 years (Table 3.2). In two patients the sensitivity had occurred in the past and their ages at the time of that dermatitis were not recorded.

Table 3.2. Ages of 19 women with clothing dermatitis due to dyes. St John's 1970–1976.

Age, years	17–20	21–30	31–40	41–50	51–60	61–70	71–80
No. Patients	6	2	0	6	2	2	1

Length of history. This dermatitis usually demands attention and consequently the histories are relatively short; half of the patients (11 of 19) had had symptoms for less than three months (Table 3.3).

Table 3.3. Lengths of history in 19 women with clothing dermatitis due to dyes. St John's 1970–1976.

Duration of History	0–1 mth	> 1–3 mths	> 3–12 mths	> 1–3 yrs	> 8 yrs +
No. Patients	3	8	5	2	1

Distribution. The distribution of the eruption mirrors the responsible garment(s), and a feature to be sought is sparing of skin protected by underclothes. The dermatitis may be so acute that the red sheeted eczema replicates the pattern of the garment on the patient's skin, making the diagnosis obvious. In the majority, however, the eczema is less dramatic. Dresses, blouses and sweaters usually cause dermatitis of the axillae (in 13 of the 19 patients seen at St John's) particularly their borders rather than their vaults, the trunk above the brassière or petticoat is affected and also the neck; the dermatitis on the arms corresponds with the lengths of the sleeves of the garment. A petticoat affects the gap between pants and brassière, and a brassière involves the breasts and the back. Careful delineation of the extent of the eczema may suggest a likely garment.

Hand eczema — knitting wool. In 1969, one week after starting to knit a wine-coloured pure wool sweater, a woman aged 55 years developed a patchy eczema first on her right hand then on her left hand and face. The distribution corresponded to her way of holding the wool and her knitting. On patch testing she reacted to the wine coloured wool and Wool Red B, one of its constituent dyes.

Men

Age. Most patients were middle-aged (Table 3.4).

Table 3.4. Ages of 26 men with clothing dermatitis due to dyes. St John's 1970–1976.

Age, years	21–30	31–40	41–50	51–60	61–70	71–80
No. Patients	2	3	11	3	4	3

Length of history. The duration of symptoms tends to be longer in men than women, probably because the symptoms are usually less acute and the diagnosis is slow in coming to mind. In the present series 24 of the 26 patients had histories of up to one year (Table 3.5).

Table 3.5. Lengths of history in 26 men with clothing dermatitis due to dyes. St John's 1970–1976.

Duration of History	0–1 mth	> 1–3 mths	> 3–12 mths	> 1–3 yrs	> 8+ yrs
No. Patients	2	5	17	1	1

Distribution. Trousers cause dermatitis at sites of sweating, pressure and friction: these are the inner or posterior thighs, the popliteal fossae and the lower legs. Skin under socks and underpants is spared, and sometimes the line of demarcation is striking. The eczema is often sheeted, and the diagnosis is easily missed if trouser dye dermatitis is not considered in men with leg eczema.

The backs of the hands were affected by contact with material at the pocket edge in 7 of 15 patients (Sim-Davies, 1972). It is rare for the eczema to spread to the arms and face, or to become widespread.

When a suit is the cause of the dermatitis there may be bands of eczema on the wrists from contact with the cuffs of the jacket; other areas, being protected by the shirt, are spared.

Dermatitis from pyjamas can be mistaken for an erythroderma of other origin. Such a patient (Sim-Davies, 1972) was admitted to hospital where his dermatitis cleared; it relapsed after he was discharged, and by the time he returned to the clinic he had made the diagnosis himself.

Shirts cause eczema initially of the neck and borders of the axillae and it may then spread more widely.

Sensitising dyes

The sensitising dyes, present in both men's and women's clothes, practically all belong to the Disperse group which was developed for use on synthetic fibres. Chemically, disperse dyes are of three main classes: aminoazobenzene, aminoanthraquinones and nitrodiarylamines. The majority of the sensitisers are azo dyes, but many are anthraquinones; nitro dyes sensitise occasionally, and Disperse Yellow 39, a Methine dye, was responsible for a small spate of trouser dermatitis (Sim-Davies, 1972). Disperse dyes are unlikely to be used for cotton, rayon or wool. The propensity of disperse dyes to sensitise is probably related to the difficulty of making them fast on a synthetic fibre, whereas natural fibres hold dyes more readily.

Vat dyes are used for cotton, rayon and linen but not for synthetic fibres.

It is possible but time-consuming, and dependent upon the good-will of the manufacturer, to trace the dyes present in a particular garment. The sensitising dyes have been identified in only a few reports.

Four of 20 nursing sisters in one hospital and another from a different hospital were sensitised to Vat Green 1, an anthraquinoid dye used as a shading component in their navy-blue uniforms. It accounted for 5–10 per cent of the colour in the cloth. This dye is sometimes used for making green operating theatre material and then accounts for 50 per cent of the colour (Wilson and Cronin, 1971).

Mordants (Chromate)

In 1967, in Vienna, textile dermatitis was attributed to chromate sensitivity in five patients. The one man and two of the women had been pre-sensitised, but the other two women were thought to have acquired the allergy from the textiles (Ebner, 1967). It was not stated specifically that the chromate was present as a mordant. Two men, sensitised to chromate by cement, developed dermatitis from chromium dyes in green military uniform. Chemical analysis confirmed the presence of chromium in the fabric and it continued to be released in six successive launderings (Fregert et al., 1978).

Patch testing

Clothing

Patch testing with pieces cut from clothing may be unreliable either because the concentration of allergen in the sample is too low to elicit a reaction, or sometimes because the wrong garments are tested.

Allergens can be extracted by solvents such as 4-methoxy-4-methyl-2-pentanol. The use of such extracts for patch testing gave reactions in 51 patients in whom the sensitising material gave no response. Four of these patients were women sensitive to dress material (Fregert, 1964).

St John's

Pieces of clothing

Positive patch tests to pieces cut from clothing have been relied upon to make the diagnosis, and every patient has reacted to one or more of their garments. As patients often do not suspect their clothing, it is not always easy to persuade them that they need to be tested with material from all their clothing, new and old. Patch testing with a few chosen garments, selected by the patient, is often inconclusive. Coloured underclothes are tested only if there is an appropriate pattern of eczema.

Occasionally the patch tests are equivocal; when this occurs the patient is asked to wear the suspected garment again and to return to the clinic.

Para-phenylenediamine

The sensitising dyes so often belong to groups of chemicals other than azo dyes that PPD is completely unreliable as a detector of this dermatitis. It does not always elicit a positive reaction even in those sensitised to azo dyes: only five of eight patients sensitised by azo or nitro dyes in the 1968 series gave definite reactions and of 15 patients with trouser dermatitis only two had positive patch tests to PPD (Cronin, 1968; Sim-Davies, 1972).

In the present series 45 of the 47 patients were patch tested with PPD in petrolatum (0.5 per cent in 1970 and 1 per cent in 1971–1976). Eight (20 per cent) of the patients reacted (Table 3.6).

Table 3.6. Reactions to *para*-phenylenediamine (0.5–1.0 per cent) in 45 patients with clothing dye dermatitis. St John's 1970–1976.

	Tested	**+**
Women	21	4
Men	24	4
Total	45	8 (20%)

[The male patients seen in 1970 and 1971 have already been reported by Sim-Davies (1972)]

A selected series of dyes

The dyes known to sensitise most frequently (Cronin, 1968; Sim-Davies, 1972) have been grouped as a patch test series and used since 1973 to test patients suspected of having a clothing dye dermatitis (Table 3.7).

Seventeen patients, 6 women (Nos. 8–13) and 11 men (Nos. 5–15) have been tested with this series and 16 of the patients reacted to one or more of these dyes. In one woman (No. 11) the series was negative and the sensitising dye in her green blouse was later identified through the help of the manufacturers as Disperse Yellow 64, a quinoline dye (Calnan, 1977). Among the women the most frequent sensitiser in the series was Disperse Blue 124 (azo) whereas among the men it was Dispersed Red 11 (anthraquinone) and Disperse Orange 76 (azo) (Table 3.7).

It seems to be a valid assumption for our patients that if they fail to react to this series and to their garments, a clothing dye dermatitis has probably been excluded.

Other dyes
In a few patients in this series the actual dyes used in the manufacture of the garment were identified and the patients were patch tested with them. The dyes to which the patients reacted are listed below:

		Colour Index No.
Women Patient No. 1	Disperse Red 17 (azo)	11210
No. 6	Disperse Yellow 54 (quinoline)	—
	Disperse Orange 1 (azo)	11080
No. 11	Disperse Yellow 64 (quinoline)	47023
Men. Patient No. 2	Disperse Blue 26 (anthraquinone)	63305
	Disperse Red 11 (anthraquinone)	62015
	Acid Black 48 (anthraquinone)	65005
No. 3	Foron Blue	

Each dye was tested at a concentration of 1 per cent in petrolatum.

St John's
The following dyes have been identified as sensitisers; the majority have already been reported (Cronin, 1968; Sim-Davies, 1972):

Disperse Yellow 3: (C.I. 11855, Azo)

Disperse Yellow 4: (C.I. 12770, Azo)

Disperse Yellow 9: (C.I. 10375, Nitro)

Disperse Yellow 39: (Indole indigo)

Disperse Yellow 54: (Quinoline)

Disperse Yellow 64: (C.I. 47023, Quinoline)

Disperse dyes

Table 3.7. Results of patch testing patients with clothing dye dermatitis with a selected series of dyes. St John's 1973–1976. Concentration of each dye was 1 per cent in petrolatum

Patients	PPD	Yellow				Orange		Red		Blue				Black		Clothing
		3	4	9	39	3	76	1	11	3	7	35	124	1	2	+
	az	az	az	nitro	meth	az	az	az	aq	aq	aq	aq	az	az	az	
Women																
1	—	—	NT	NT	NT	NT	NT	+	NT	—	NT	NT	NT	NT	NT	Navy blouse
2	—	—	—	—	—	—	+	—	—	—	—	—	+	—	—	Black blouse
3	—	—	NT	NT	NT	NT	NT	NT	NT	NT	NT	NT	NT	NT	NT	Grey dress
4	+	—	—	+	+	+	NT	—	—	+	+	+	NT	+	+	Brown lining / Black dress
5	—	—	NT	NT	NT	—	NT	NT	NT	+	+	NT	NT	NT	NT	Blue materials
6	—	—	—	—	+	+	NT	—	—	—	—	—	NT	—	—	Black trousers
7	—	—	—	—	—	—	—	—	—	—	+	—	+	—	—	Dress: scarf
8	—	—	—	—	+	—	—	—	—	—	—	—	—	—	—	Blue wool sweater
9	+	—	—	—	—	+	—	—	—	—	—	—	+	—	—	Brown trousers / Navy jersey
10	—	—	—	—	—	—	+	—	—	—	—	—	+	—	—	Navy lining blazer
11	—	—	—	—	—	—	—	—	—	—	—	—	—	—	—	Green blouse
12	—	—	—	—	—	—	—	+	—	—	—	—	+	—	—	Brown lining
13	+	—	—	—	—	—	—	—	—	—	—	+	+	—	—	Blue lining
Total	$\frac{3}{13}$	$\frac{0}{13}$	$\frac{0}{10}$	$\frac{1}{10}$	$\frac{3}{10}$	$\frac{3}{11}$	$\frac{2}{8}$	$\frac{2}{11}$	$\frac{0}{10}$	$\frac{2}{12}$	$\frac{3}{11}$	$\frac{2}{10}$	$\frac{5}{8}$	$\frac{1}{10}$	$\frac{1}{10}$	

Patients	PPD	Yellow				Orange		Red				Blue		Black		Clothing
		3	4	9	39	3	76	1	11	3	7	35	124	1	2	+
Men																
1	−	−	NT	NT	NT	NT	NT	−	NT	−	NT	NT	NT	NT	NT	Blue suit / Green trousers
2	NT	−	NT	NT	+	NT	NT	+	+	+	NT	NT	NT	NT	NT	Trousers
3	−	NT	NT	NT	NT	NT	NT	NT	NT	NT	+	NT	NT	NT	NT	Trousers
4	+	−	NT	NT	NT	NT	NT	−	NT	−	NT	NT	NT	NT	NT	Trousers
5	−	−	−	−	−	−	NT	−	+	+	−	−	NT	−	−	Trousers
6	−	−	−	−	−	−	NT	−	+	+	−	−	NT	−	−	Underpants
7	−	−	−	−	+	−	+	−	−	−	−	−	−	−	−	Black trousers
8	−	−	−	−	−	−	+	−	+	+	−	+	−	−	−	Trousers
9	−	−	−	+	−	−	−	−	+	+	+	+	−	−	−	Trousers
10	−	+	+	+	+	+	+	+	+	+	+	+	+	+	+	Trousers
11	−	−	−	−	−	−	NT	−	−	−	+	+	−	−	−	Uniform
12	−	−	−	−	−	−	+	−	−	−	−	−	−	−	−	Trousers / *Other clothes*
13	−	−	−	−	−	−	−	−	−	−	−	−	−	−	−	3 shirts —
14	+	+	−	−	−	+	+	+	+	−	−	−	+	+	+	Blue singlet +
15	−	−	−	−	−	−	−	+	−	−	−	−	−	−	−	NT
Total	$\frac{2}{14}$	$\frac{2}{14}$	$\frac{0}{11}$	$\frac{2}{11}$	$\frac{3}{11}$	$\frac{2}{11}$	$\frac{5}{8}$	$\frac{4}{14}$	$\frac{7}{12}$	$\frac{6}{14}$	$\frac{3}{12}$	$\frac{3}{11}$	$\frac{2}{9}$	$\frac{2}{11}$	$\frac{2}{11}$	

NT = Not Tested

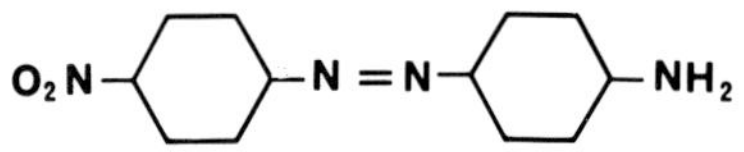

O_2N—⬡—$N=N$—⬡—NH_2

Disperse Orange 3: (C.I. 11005, Azo)

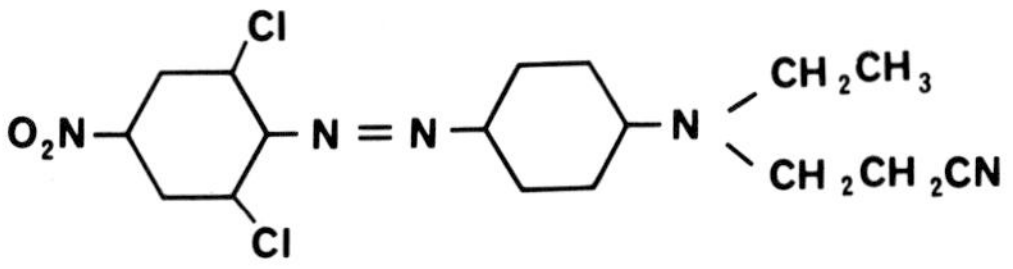

Disperse Orange 76: (Monoazo)

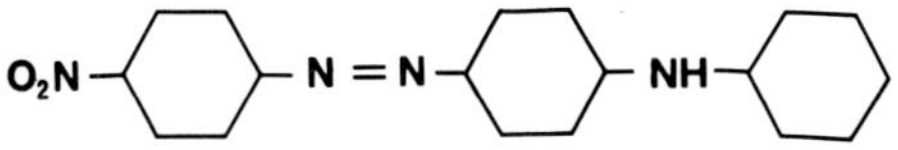

O_2N—⬡—$N=N$—⬡—NH—⬡

Disperse Orange I: (C.I. 11080, Azo)

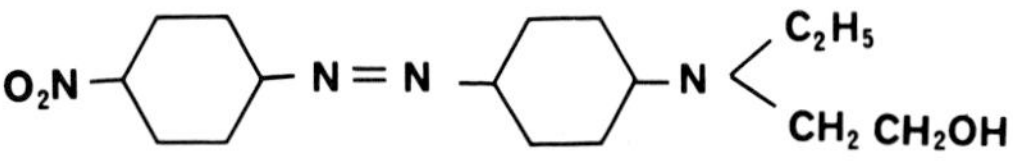

Disperse Red 1: (C.I. 11110, Monoazo)

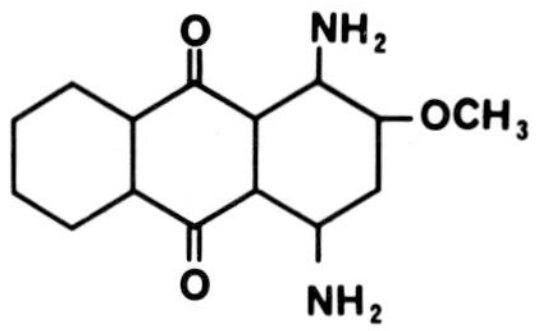

Disperse Red 11: (C.I. 62015, Anthraquinone)

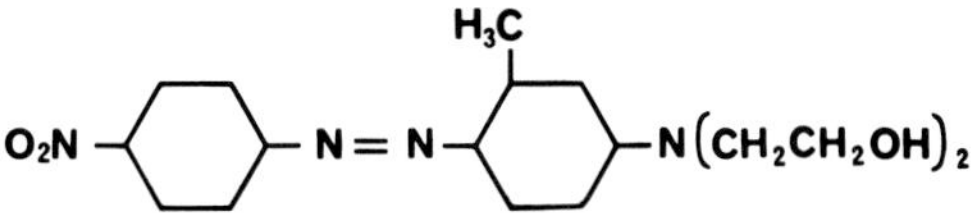

Disperse Red 17: (C.I. 11210, Monoazo)

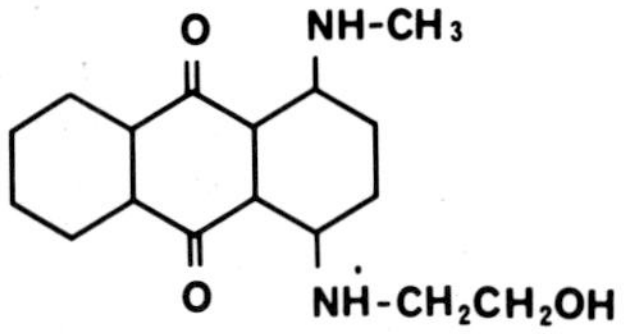

Disperse Blue 3: (C.I. 61505, Anthraquinone)

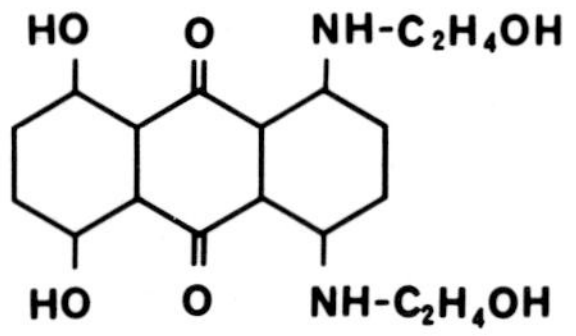

Disperse Blue 7: (C.I. 62500, Anthraquinone)

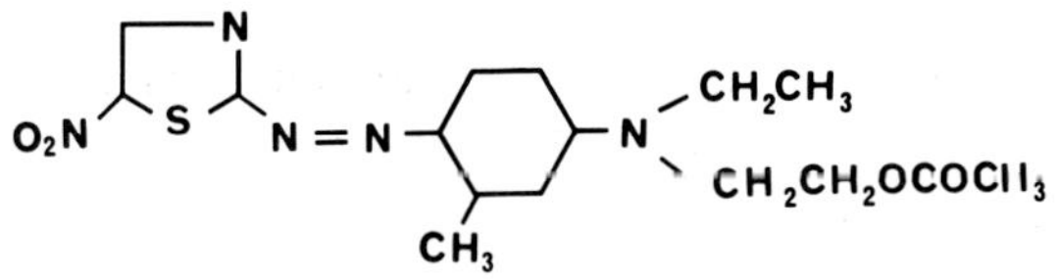

Disperse Blue 124: (Monoazo)

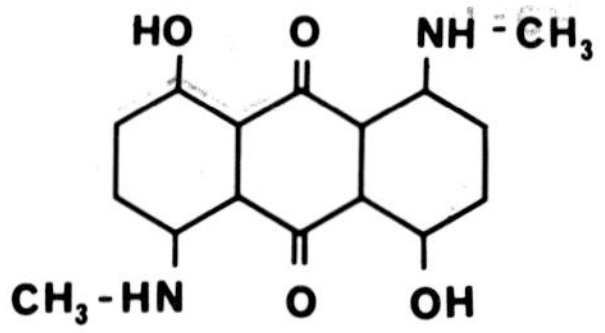

Disperse Blue 26: (C.I. 63305, Anthraquinone)

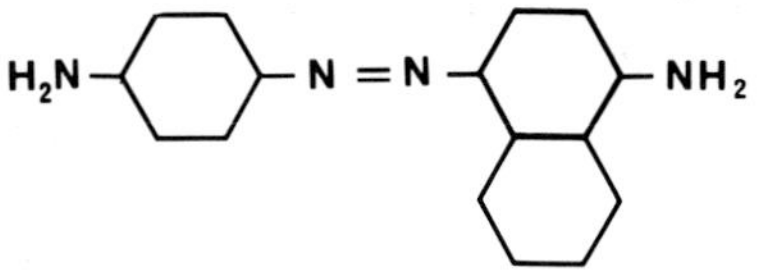

Disperse Black 1: (C.I. 11365, Azo)

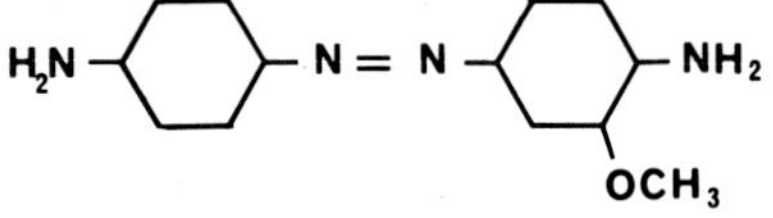

Disperse Black 2: (C.I. 11255, Azo)

Acid Black 48: (C.I. 65005, Anthraquinone)

For routine patch testing
1. Pieces, about 7 mm × 7 mm, from all the patient's coloured clothes
2. The 14 dyes tabulated or a similar series each diluted to 1 per cent in petrolatum
3. PPD 1 per cent in petrolatum.

The most essential of these are the clothing patch tests. Coarse fabrics may irritate the skin and cause a mild erythema at the two day reading but the redness has generally faded by four days.

Alternatives
Patients sensitised to Disperse dyes should be advised to wear clothes made of the natural fibres cotton, rayon or wool, and to avoid textiles made partially or wholly of synthetic yarns.

Most patients react to dyes of several colours and inspection of a fabric gives little indication of its colour composition. Nevertheless one woman seen at St John's (Patient No. 5, Selected Dye Series), who preferred blue materials, reacted to two blue dyes. She was advised to choose other colours.

In most cases, the dermatitis resolves once the sensitising garment has been discarded. A few patients, however, return with repeated relapses after buying new clothes and in Ebner's (1975) experience exclusion of the allergen can be difficult in textile dermatitis.

Phototoxic textile dermatitis. A phototoxic hypopigmentation from bikini bathing suits occurred in two women and was attributed to Disperse Blue 35 in the fabric (Hjorth and Moller, 1976) (pp. 49 and 423).

Occupational dermatitis

Fur trade
Among fur workers, asthma is the greatest hazard, but some develop dermatitis. In 1959, 80 fur workers were studied in New York: contact dermatitis occurred as the only symptom in ten, and in association with other allergies in eight. The ten, with contact dermatitis only, had been at work for at least a year, but most for 10–15 years. Six of this group were patch tested with *para*-phenylenediamine: each reacted to 3 per cent in water, and five to 2 per cent in petrolatum (Silberman and Sorrell, 1959).

St John's

Case 1. A man, aged 25 years, who had been a furrier for ten years, tacked wet fur on to boards in the process of making fur garments and the dye from them blackened his fingers. In 1969 he developed a fissured eczema which began on the palmar aspect of his fingers and spread over both palms. He attended the clinic a year later and was patch tested; he reacted to a black Persian fur, to a black mink fur, to PPD 0.5 per cent and weakly to Disperse Red 1. Tests with natural coloured furs were negative. He was advised to work with undyed skins only, and his hands improved provided he took this advice but they relapsed immediately he handled dyed fur. Seven months later, he changed his job on account of his dermatitis. In 1976 he returned to the clinic because for six months he had had a recurrent dermatitis of the eyes and face. For the previous four years he had worked in a drawing office and for one year had made photocopies using the diazo process. Patch tests: he had a positive response to the diazo chemical in the paper and still reacted to PPD and Disperse Red 1.

Case 2. A man, aged 66 years, had been a fur cutter for four years, when he developed a patchy eczema on the backs of his hands; this spread to his face, scalp, arms and legs. He said he had left this job because the dermatitis cleared at home and relapsed at work. The eruption, when seen four months after it had first appeared, looked like discoid eczema. On patch testing he reacted to PPD (0.5 per cent) and to Disperse Yellow 3 (1 per cent); he brought only one fur and did not react to it.

By the time he was seen again, five weeks after he had stopped work, his skin had improved but it had not healed. It was thought that his eczema was partly occupational and partly constitutional.

Textile industry

Dermatitis in the textile industry has been reviewed in an excellent monograph by Cywie *et al.* (1977). They emphasise that the vast numbers of dyes, their many trade names and their impurity make for great difficulty in accurate diagnosis. The report describes many dyes and gives their structural formulae.

In the 1950s, the greatest hazard for wool textile workers was not from dyes but from potassium chromate, used as a mordant. It caused chrome holes and dermatitis (Hellier, 1958).

In 1956, an outbreak of contact dermatitis occurred in a Dutch cotton-printing mill where the printing was done by hand. Many men developed an incapacitating eczema after being sensitised by the dye diazotised ice red TR (Malten, 1957).

Employees in the dyeing and finishing shops of textile factories have been found frequently to develop dermatitis where potassium dichromate, triethanolamine and carbamol are used in the technological processes (Venediktova and Gudina, 1976).

Formaldehyde resins acting as pigment binders were found to be the cause of dermatitis of the hands and arms in a man working in a textile printing shop. Patch tests: he reacted to dichromate, formaldehyde, urea formaldehyde and some pigments. The allergen was identified as the resin and not the colours, because the pigments, to which the patient reacted, were shown by chemical analysis to be those which contained the formaldehyde resin binders (Herve-Bazin, Foussereau and Cavelier, 1977).

Pigmented contact dermatitis. Naphthol AS, an azo dye coupling compound, caused an outbreak of pigmented contact dermatitis in a textile mill in Mexico. The hyperpigmentation was spotty and affected principally the exposed sites. Fifty-three workers in contact with the compound were patch tested with Naphthol AS 5 per cent in water and 24 reacted (Ancona-Alayón *et al.*, 1976).

Clothing factory
In a small factory making blue denim boiler suits five of the women machinists were sensitised by an unidentified blue azo dye in the fabric. During sewing the material was held by the right hand, steadied by the left arm and then fell over the left thigh and foot. The affected women complained of severe irritation of these sites although clinically their dermatitis was slight. The five women were patch tested: four reacted to the blue denim, four to its blue azoic dye, but only one to the fabric after double washing. It was agreed by the manufacturers to double rinse the material and no further cases of dermatitis occurred (Newhouse, 1974).

Dye manufacture —phototoxic —Disperse Blue 35
Over a period of ten years, about 130 workers, employed in a chemical factory making the anthraquinone dye Disperse Blue 35, developed a photocontact dermatitis from the complete dye. The eruption appeared only in summer, affected only the light-exposed skin and was not severe. On photopatch testing the reactions could be elicited both in workers exposed to the dye and in unexposed controls (Gardiner *et al.*, 1971). These results suggest that the reaction was phototoxic and not photoallergic.

NYLON STOCKINGS, TIGHTS (PANTY HOSE) AND SOCKS

Incidence of sensitivity
Dermatitis from stockings, tights (panty hose) and socks is probably unusual in most countries. The early cases were reviewed by Cronin (1968), since when 11 patients have been reported from Zürich (Suter, 1965) and 10 were seen in Strasbourg from 1966–1970 (Foussereau *et al.*, 1971; Foussereau *et al.*, 1972).

St John's
Each year, between three and six women are seen with dermatitis from the dyes in nylon stockings or tights (panty hose). Sock dermatitis in men is rare, either one or no patients being seen each year (Table 3.8).

Table 3.8. Numbers of patients seen each year with dermatitis from the dyes in nylon stockings, tights (panty hose) or socks. St John's 1970–1976.

	1970	1971	1972	1973	1974	1975	1976	Total
Stockings and tights	3	5	3	5	5	4	6	31
Socks	1	0	1	1	1	0	0	4

Sensitisers

Dyes
Disperse dyes are the sensitisers in nylon hosiery.

Rubber
The elastic in the waistband of tights is securely sleeved with nylon thread and tights are laddered and discarded long before this covering breaks down. Occasionally the rubber in elastic stockings causes dermatitis (p. 750)

Finishes
Formaldehyde resins are not used in stocking manufacture, and other finishes have not been incriminated as a cause of dermatitis.

Clinical features

Stockings and tights (panty hose)

Age and length of history. From 1970–1976 at St John's, a diagnosis of hosiery dermatitis was made in 31 women. Their ages ranged from 17 to 66 years. The length of history was 3–12 months in 22 patients, shorter in 3 and longer in 6.

Distribution: characteristic pattern. The characteristic pattern affects the dorsa of the feet under the shoes, the heels and sometimes the soles; the popliteal fossae; the thighs, particularly the medial and posterior aspects; and, when due to tights, there may be a band of eczema round the waist. Very occasionally the whole leg is eczematous. This distribution, with all or at least several sites affected, is typical and, when present, the diagnosis is straightforward.

Feet only. The dermatitis may be confined to the feet. With this localisation the diagnosis is difficult and uncertain and is readily mistaken for shoe dermatitis. The eczema was predominant on the dorsa of the toes in one of the six cases investigated in Strasbourg (Foussereau *et al.*, 1972). An interesting sequence of events was reported by Maibach (1975). A woman while being treated for an acute fungus infection of the toe webs developed a vesicular eczema of the dorsa of her toes which was shown to be due to sensitisation to the azo and anthraquinone dyes in her panty hose. Such patients are detected at St John's because many patients with recalcitrant foot eczema are referred for patch testing and they are tested with a series of allergens which includes the yellow stocking dye specifically to identify this dermatitis. The frequency with which this pattern occurred in the 1968 series (Cronin, 1968) and during the period 1970–1976 is shown in Table 3.9. Among the 31 women seen from 1970 to 1976 the dermatitis was confined to the feet in seven.

Lichenoid dermatitis. A most unusual lichenoid dermatitis caused by the dyes in black stockings has been described from Southern Italy (Meneghini, 1971). A woman, aged 40 years, whilst in mourning developed a pruriginous eruption,

Table 3.9. Numbers of patients with stocking or tights dermatitis in whom the feet only were affected. St John's 1954–1966 and 1970–1976.

	1954–66	1970	1971	1972	1973	1974	1975	1976	Total 1970–76
No. patients with stocking dermatitis	34	3	5	3	5	5	4	6	31
Feet only	2	2	1	0	0	1	1	2	7

first on her legs and then on her thighs. The condition persisted for two years but flared up when her father died and she again wore black stockings. She then had a verrucous papular eczema on the fronts of her shins and on the dorsa of her feet. On patch testing she reacted to PPD, benzocaine and triethanolamine.

Socks

St John's
From 1970–1976, a diagnosis of sock dermatitis was made in only four men; two incriminated new socks. Three of the men had had eczema for three to four months and the fourth for three years. The eczema was confined to the feet in two, and in the other two it also affected their lower legs under their socks.

Sensitising dyes

Brown stockings and tights
The colour of brown nylon stockings is compounded by mixing a red, a yellow and a blue dye. The proportions are varied to achieve different shades, and other dyes may be added to produce particular colours.

In England the principal dyes are:

Disperse Yellow 3 (C.I. 11855) Azo
Disperse Red   1 (C.I. 11110) Azo
Disperse Blue 3 (C.I. 61505) Aq.

Imported hosiery will contain other dyes.

Disperse Yellow 3 is the principal and most frequent sensitiser. It was first reported, as Colour F, from New York in 1947 (Dobkevitch and Baer) and was the yellow azo dye which sensitised five women investigated in London in 1956 (Calnan and Wilson).

France. Six women investigated in Strasbourg were sensitive to Disperse Yellow 3, and it was confirmed that the dye, not an impurity, was the allergen (Foussereau *et al.*, 1972).

Denmark. Danish stockings may also contain Disperse Orange 3 (C.I. 11005) to which cases of sensitivity have been reported (Hjorth and Rothenburg, 1967).

Switzerland and Austria. Disperse Red 17 is used in Swiss and Austrian stockings and sensitivity to it has been reported from Zürich (Suter, 1965).

U.S.A. In California, panty hose containing *para*-amino-acetanilide-*para*-cresol (an azo dye) and methylamino-4-(2-hydroxymethylamino) anthraquinone sensitised a young woman reported by Maibach (1975).

St John's

Disperse Yellow 3 was the most frequent sensitiser in the period 1954– 1966; 30 of 33 patients with stocking dermatitis reacted to it at that time and since then the allergen has not changed. From 1970– 1976, of 31 women with hosiery dermatitis 27 were allergic to this dye. PPD is a poor detector of this sensitisation. In the recent series only 7 of 31 reacted to it, 17 of 27 reacted to Disperse Red 1, and two of 27 reacted to Disperse Blue 3 (Table 3.10).

Table 3.10. Frequency of reactions to D. Yellow 3, D. Red 1, D. Blue 3 and *para*-phenylenediamine in patients with dermatitis from brown nylon stockings or tights. St John's 1954– 1966 and 1970– 1976.

Year	No. Patients	D. Yellow 3 Tested	+	D. Red 1 Tested	+	D. Blue 3 Tested	+	PPD Tested	+
1954– 66	34	33	30	30	21	30	5	30	19
1970– 76	31	31	27	27	17	27	2	31	7

Disperse Red 17 was the sensitiser in one woman, who reacted also to PPD but was negative to the other stockings dyes. Another woman reacted to Disperse Orange 3 and also to PPD, D. Yellow 3 and D. Red 1.

Black stockings

A woman with dermatitis from black nylon stockings and positive patch tests to a black and a yellow azo dye was described by Calnan and Wilson (1956). In Zürich, Suter (1965) reported six women with stocking dermatitis, who reacted to an unidentified Disperse Black stocking dye. Three of these women and another similar patient reacted also to Disperse Red 17.

In Italy, particularly in the South, it is the custom for women to wear mourning for many months. An allergic contact dermatitis of the legs and body from PPD and related compounds is consequently not unusual (Meneghini, 1971).

Socks

Dyes

In Strasbourg two men with sock dermatitis were sensitive to Disperse Yellow 3; one also reacted to a PPD chemical in his rubber boots (Foussereau *et al.*, 1972). In Vancouver a man with acute dermatitis caused by black socks was mistakenly patch tested with food dyes and reacted to an azo dye, Citrus Red No. 2; subsequent tests with other azo dyes were negative. The dyes in his socks were not identified (Mitchell, 1972).

Mordant (Chromate)

A coal miner with mild constitutional eczema developed dermatitis of his feet and legs while working in a wet seam. Patch testing showed that he was sensitive to chromate. His socks were reduced to ash which, on analysis, showed a high chromate content. A chrome mordant was thought to be the most likely source of this chromate and the cause of the dermatitis (Mitchell, 1967).

St John's

> Of the four men with sock dermatitis, three reacted to Disperse Yellow 3, two to Disperse Red 1 and two to PPD: the fourth man reacted repeatedly to his navy socks but was negative to all the dyes tested.

Patch testing

Stockings and tights
Dyes, extracted with a solvent from the stocking, elicited reactions in 16 women who had failed to react to the stocking itself (Fregert, 1964). The incidence of direct reactions has also been increased by steaming a fragment of stocking before applying it as a patch test (Sidi and Arouete, 1959).

St John's

> The dyes in brown nylon stockings and tights are known, and patch testing with them is relied upon to make the diagnosis. Patients have to be tested with the fabric when the stockings or tights in question are black, coloured or not made of nylon. The dyes are then unknown and the material has to be relied upon for patch testing.

PPD is not a good diagnostic indicator of this dermatitis (Table 3.10).

For routine testing
1. Disperse Yellow 3 (1 per cent in petrolatum)
2. Disperse Orange 3 (1 per cent in petrolatum)
3. Disperse Red 1 (1 per cent in petrolatum)
4. Disperse Red 17 (1 per cent in petrolatum)
5. Disperse Blue 3 (1 per cent in petrolatum)
6. PPD (1 per cent in petrolatum)
7. Pieces of the stocking, particularly if a colour other than brown or if the thread is not nylon.

In the U.K., 1 and 7 are the most important of this series, but testing with 2 and 4 helps to detect dermatitis from imported hosiery.

Socks. The dyes in socks are unknown.

For routine testing
1. Pieces approximately 7 mm × 7 mm from every sock
2. The 5 nylon stocking dyes
3. PPD 1 per cent in petrolatum.

Alternatives

Stockings and tights. Non-allergic stockings and tights are specially made for these patients by Aristoc. They currently contain the following dyes:

    Disperse Yellow 1 (C.I. 10345) nitro
    Disperse Red   11 (C.I. 62015) anthraquinone
    Disperse Blue   3 (C.I. 61505) anthraquinone
  The stockings = NCSI
  The tights   = NCNI

Socks. Men can wear white socks of any fabric, or coloured socks made of wool or cotton.

Occupational dermatitis

Five men working in a stocking factory developed a hyperkeratotic, fissured eczema mainly of the palms, with lesser involvement of the sides and backs of the fingers. Each man worked on a rotating stand removing dyed stockings from hot metal frames. They were tested with all the ingredients of the dye tank. Four men reacted to Disperse Yellow 3, and four to a red azo dye. All the other constituents evoked no response (Cronin, 1968).

HAIR NETS

Brown nylon hair nets have become unfashionable but they are still worn by some older women and hair net dermatitis, although infrequent, does still occur.

In 1958, 27 cases were reported from London (Calnan, Marten and Wilson, 1958). Twenty-three of the women were over 40 years old; they presented with a red, scaly, sometimes exudative eczema behind the ears, on the nape of the neck and along the frontal hairline. In some patients the rash spread beyond these sites, a vesicular eczema of the upper half of the ears being particularly characteristic. Sometimes, the condition simulated seborrhoeic eczema or lichen simplex of the neck so closely that the diagnosis was clarified only by patch testing.

Similar dyes caused stocking dermatitis in six of these patients and hair dye dermatitis in another two of the women.

The dyes in the hair nets were not identified but it was established that they were of the azo and anthraquinone groups because these patients gave positive patch test reactions to PPD and to three Disperse nylon stocking dyes. The positive patch tests in these 27 patients were as follows:

Hair net	PPD	D. Yellow 3 (azo)	D. Red 1 (azo)	D. Blue 3 (aq.)
26	18	15	10	5

The patient who failed to react to the brown nylon mesh of her hair net was sensitive to its elastic band.

St John's

Between 1970 and 1976, six women have been seen with hair net dermatitis; two in 1970, two in 1975 and two in 1976. The dermatitis affected the hairline, particularly the nape of the neck and the ears. Three of the women also had nylon stocking dermatitis, and one of them had, in addition, dermatitis from her clothes and her brown nylon gloves.

The positive patch test results in these six patients were as follows:

Hair net	PPD	D. Yellow 3 (azo)	D. Red 1 (azo)	D. Blue 3 (aq.)
3	0	6	5	0

The concentration of each Disperse dye was 1 per cent in petrolatum, and the concentration of PPD was increased in 1970 from 0.5 per cent to 1 per cent.

Resins in textiles

TECHNOLOGY

The first patent for strengthening cellulose fabrics with formaldehyde was taken out in Germany in 1908 and, by the 1920s, urea and melamine formaldehyde were being used to achieve crease-resistance. As cotton and rayon are weakened by a high resin content, production of treated fabrics was limited until the 1950s when synthetic fibres were introduced and acclaimed for their rapid drying and inherent resistance to creasing. This threat to the cotton fabric market galvanised the expansion in textile resin technology. These resins were developed to endow cellulose with the assets of man-made fibres while retaining the advantages of cotton, namely the absorption of sweat and good wearing properties. Synthetic fibres do not absorb moisture and they attract dirt.

Easy-care clothing resins are all formaldehyde polymers, these being the only resins which react safely with cellulose. All resins weaken the fibres to some extent, but this defect is counter-balanced by the properties they confer. Treated fabrics resist creasing, shrinking and stretching, and their feel and drape may be improved, as may be their absorption of dyes and resistance to light. Cloth can be made waterproof and also be permanently pleated.

Types of resin

There are two different types of resin treatment.

The earlier process involved polycondensation, in which urea and melamine formaldehyde are polymerised within the interstices of the fibres, any reaction between the fibre and the resin being minimal. These resins have disadvantages. They absorb chlorine from bleaches to form chloramides. The melamine formaldehyde chloramide, being yellow, causes discolouration, whereas the urea formaldehyde chloramide breaks down with heat, particularly ironing, to release hydrochloric acid, which damages the fabric. Another defect is their limited wash-fastness: during laundering water lost during polymerisation is reabsorbed into the resin molecule breaking it down and the resin is gradually washed out of the cloth.

The second method was introduced in the 1960s. In this process, reactive resins, the cyclic ureas, are made to combine directly with the fibre. The formaldehyde (methylol) groups of the resin cross-link with the hydroxyl groups of the cellulose to form stable atomic bonds. These resins have a greatly improved wash- and chlorine-fastness. In chemical structure they consist of either

5-membered rings	or	6-membered rings
ethylene urea		propylene urea
dihydroxyethylene urea		dihydroxypropylene urea
		triazones

To confer reactivity these molecules must be combined with methylol (formaldehyde) groups.

Dimethylol alkyl carbamate resins are effective and have been used particularly for white shirts. They have the advantage of giving a soft feel to fabrics, but, as they require high temperatures and liberate large amounts of formaldehyde during post-cure processing, working conditions are difficult.

In Britain, urea formaldehyde and dimethyloldihydroxyethylene urea are most commonly used. In the U.S.A., too, dimethyloldihydroxyethylene urea is used, as are dimethylol alkyl carbamates (Jordan, 1972).

Processing
A fabric is treated with resin in three stages. Initially, the cloth is soaked in an aqueous solution of resin and a catalyst, such as ammonium dihydrogen phosphate; secondly, excess fluid is squeezed out and the resin is cured or polymerised by heating the fabric to about 120° C for approximately three minutes; finally, in the after-wash free formalin, excess resin and other residues are removed. This process of washing and re-drying an already dried cloth is expensive and, regrettably, it is being omitted with increasing frequency.

Application
The reactive resins are preferred for their stability and chlorine fastness, but expense limits their use. However, the cost of a fabric or a garment to the consumer is no criterion whatsoever of the type of resin used in its manufacture.

Polyester cotton. Cotton is added to a polyester for the comfort of the wearer but it requires a resin finish; in about 90 per cent of fabrics this will be either dihydroxydimethylolethylene urea (2–5 per cent resin 'add-on'), or another resin of the reactive type. When this type of cloth is used for shirts the polyester to cotton ratio is 2:1, and when it is used for blouses, dresses, trousers, overalls and sheets this ratio is 1:1. Sheets, because of frequent and heavy laundering, particularly require the reactive resins.

Pure cotton. About half the pure cotton fabrics contain the reactive resins and most of the rest contain urea or perhaps melamine formaldehyde. Mercerised cotton is made by swelling the cotton yarn or fabric in a concentrated (25 per cent) solution of caustic soda, subjecting it to high tension and then washing out the caustic soda. This imparts lustre, and allows greater penetration of resins and of dyes, the latter enhancing the depth of colour which can be produced.

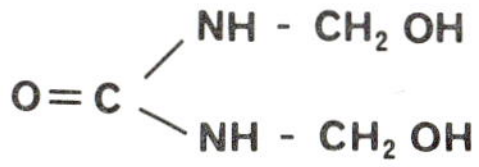

Dimethylol urea (urea formaldehyde)

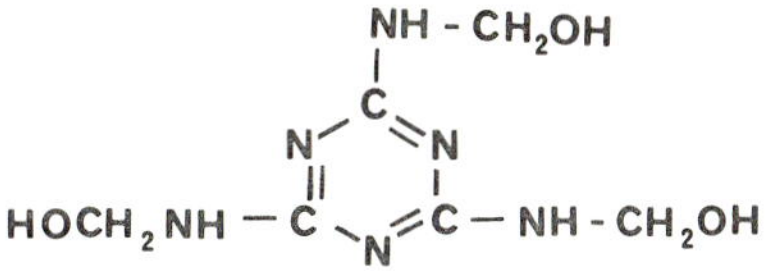

Trimethylolmelamine (melamine formaldehyde)

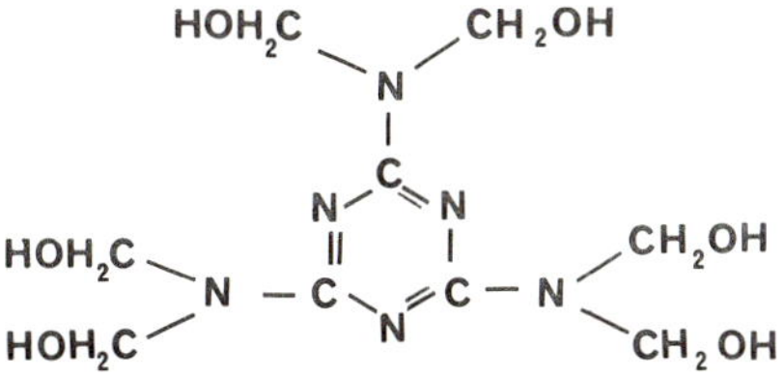

Hexamethylolmelamine (melamine formaldehyde)

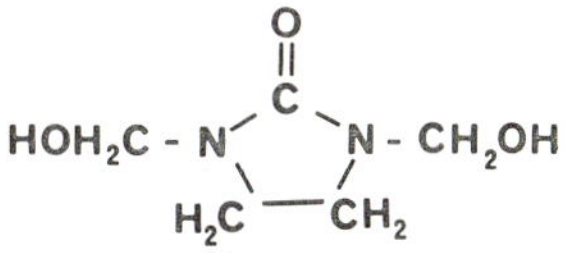

Dimethylolethylene urea

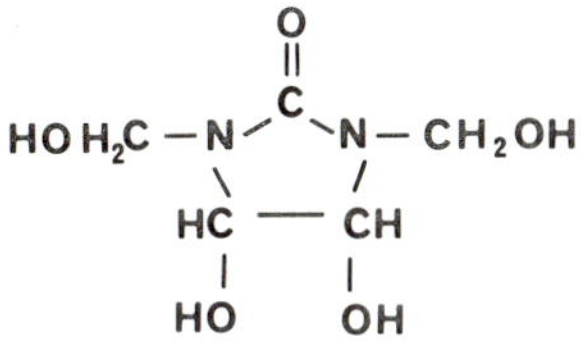

Dimethyloldihydroxyethylene urea

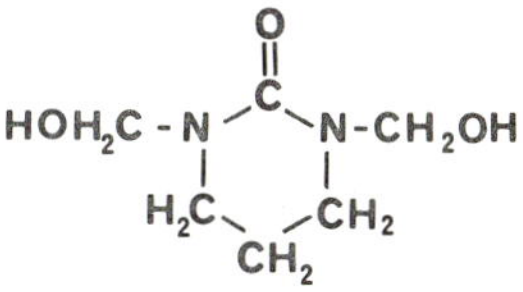

Dimethylolpropylene urea

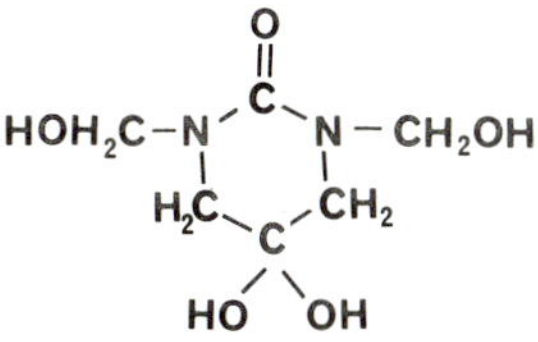

Dimethyloldihydroxypropylene urea

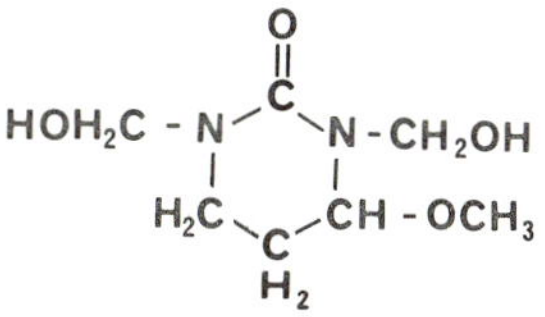

Dimethylolmethoxypropylene urea

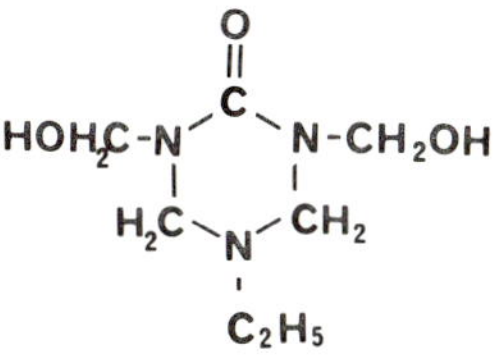

Dimethylolethyltriazone

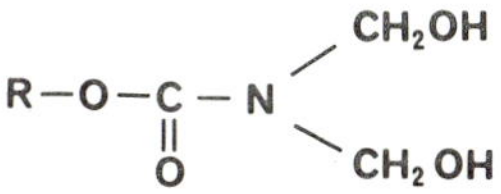

R = alkyl, hydroxyalkyl or alkoxyalkyl

Dimethylol carbamates

Viscose rayon. Rayon is a generic term for fibres derived from natural polymers. Viscose rayon is made from cellulose, and acetate rayon is produced from cellulose acetate. Urea formaldehyde, in quite high concentrations (10–12 per cent resin 'add-on'), is used for about 80 per cent of these materials; they rarely contain the reactive resins. If oil (the ultimate source of synthetic fibres) becomes scarce, it is possible that increasing amounts of rayon, which is cheap, will be produced both alone and blended with other fibres.

Rain wear. Polyester with cotton or rayon is often made waterproof by a finish of melamine formaldehyde (3–5 per cent resin 'add-on').

Glazed material. This effect is achieved with melamine formaldehyde.

Children's clothes. These are likely to contain urea or melamine formaldehyde.

Cotton interlining fabrics. These stiffeners, such as are used in shirt collars, are treated with a specialised melamine-ethylene urea formaldehyde resin.

Nylon taffeta. This fabric is used for stiff underskirts and petticoats. The effect is achieved by a high content (up to 20 per cent resin 'add-on') of melamine formaldehyde.

Wool. It is rare for wool to contain these resins, but they are added very occasionally for waterproofing. If a trend develops for Permanent Press woollen garments this situation may change.

Fabrics not resin-treated

Pure synthetic fibres. The inherent properties of man-made fibres make resin treatment unnecessary. Garments made of the following fabrics do not contain resins:

polyamide (nylon, with the exception of 'paper' petticoats)
polyester   (Terylene, Crimplene, Dacron)
acrylics   (Acrilan, Courtelle, Orlan, Dralon).

Although these fabrics do not themselves contain resins, lace trimmings on slips and nightdresses may be stiffened with melamine formaldehyde and the resin also acts as a flame retardant.

Silk. Silk fibres have a low abrasion resistance and break easily. Resins are avoided because they accentuate this defect.

The level of free formaldehyde in textiles
All fabrics treated with resin contain some free formaldehyde, the amount depending mainly on the after-wash. Other factors influencing the concentration are the level of free formaldehyde in the resins used, the degree of cure and the air extraction during drying. If the afterwash is omitted during manufacture,

new garments may have very high levels and 1000 p.p.m. may not be unusual (Jordan, 1972). Polyester-cotton sheeting, correctly treated with a resin containing 1 per cent free formaldehyde but with no afterwash, can show 800–1000 p.p.m.; a wash in the factory would reduce this to less than 100 p.p.m. Cutters, machinists and pressers handling such material can find the formaldehyde very unpleasant. The level can be effectively reduced by standing garments in a well ventilated warehouse for a few weeks before distribution for sale. Laundering does wash out free formaldehyde, but it is replenished by the prolonged slow release from resin broken down during wear, washing and ironing. Man can smell free formaldehyde in a concentration as low as 200 p.p.m. An acceptable level of formaldehyde for textiles has not been generally established; in Japan legislation has been introduced which strictly regulates the formaldehyde content of clothing; in particular no free formaldehyde is allowed in any fabric for use by children.

In 1959, in Norway, the free and combined formaldehyde was estimated in aqueous extracts of 256 samples of new textiles. Rayon fabrics were found to be heavily contaminated with free formaldehyde, the majority containing 5000–12 000 p.p.m.; the amount in cotton materials varied from 100–8000 p.p.m. (Høvding, 1959). In Utrecht, in 1964, patients' clothes were examined for free formaldehyde: the rayon specimens contained approximately 5000 p.p.m., while in cotton and linen the level was about 500 p.p.m. (Berrens, Young and Jansen, 1964). The free formaldehyde content of 112 American fabrics was estimated by Schorr, Keran and Plotka (1974), and they confirmed high levels in rayon, in cotton and in blends of these with synthetic fibres. Rayon contained up to 3500 p.p.m., polyester-cotton mixtures up to 2900 p.p.m. and cotton 1500 p.p.m. Pure nylon and acrylic contained less than 30 p.p.m. and the level in wool was below 200 p.p.m.

Other resins and additives

Acrylates in an aqueous dispersion improve crease recovery and allow a reduction in the amount of formaldehyde resin used in the fabric.

Polyterpene resins may be used as a textile finish.

Anionic silicates are used on cotton and rayon to enhance the smoothness and feel of the fabric.

Softeners are usually cationic products.

Resin catalysts, such as citric or formic acid, may remain in the textile but are removed by the first wash.

CLOTHING

Incidence of sensitivity

Dermatologists in Scandinavia were the first to recognise and to draw attention to clothing dermatitis caused by the formaldehyde treatment of fabrics, and most of the case reports have emanated from these countries.

Denmark and Norway

At the Finsen Institute in Copenhagen, the first of these patients was seen in 1934, and sensitisation was ascribed to the formaldehyde fixation of a dye. Four cases, seen between 1939 and 1945, had been sensitised by casein fibres hardened with formaldehyde. In 1950, 0.04 per cent of all cases patch tested at the Finsen Institute had formaldehyde clothing dermatitis, and by 1958 the number had risen to 0.4 per cent. At this time, pre-sensitisation by formaldehyde deodorants was important and had occurred in seven of 26 women (Marcussen, 1959). Despite the disappearance of these deodorants by 1960, the number of cases of clothing dermatitis continued to increase (Marcussen, 1962). In Oslo, in 1954, the incidence of formaldehyde clothing dermatitis among inpatients was 1.8 per cent (8/439) and by 1961 it was 8.4 per cent (49/585) (Weireide, 1964).

In different clinics a similar proportion of all patients with formaldehyde sensitivity had acquired the allergy from clothing. At the Finsen Institute, in 1960, this proportion was 36 per cent (35/96) (Marcussen, 1959); in 1958, in Bergen, it was 33 per cent (45/137) (Høvding, 1961); and in Oslo, the proportion rose from 10 per cent in 1954 to 42 per cent in 1961 (Wereide, 1964).

Australia

In 1973, a report from Adelaide described 1000 cases of allergic contact dermatitis; of the 41 patients allergic to formaldehyde, 34 (83 per cent) had been sensitised by clothing (Burry *et al.*, 1973).

United States

Few cases have been seen in the U.S.A.; three were reported from New Orleans in 1965 (O'Quinn and Kennedy, 1965), three from San Francisco in 1966 (Epstein and Maibach, 1966) and another case was shown at a clinical meeting in Chicago in 1966 (Shellow and Altman, 1966). This strange dearth is unexplained. One suggestion is that American fabrics are washed more thoroughly during manufacture (Fisher, Kanof and Biondi, 1962). Despite this paucity of clothing dermatitis the incidence of formaldehyde sensitivity is comparable to that in Europe. Formaldehyde sensitivity among eczematous patients in North America was 4 per cent in 1972 (North American Contact Dermatitis Group, 1973) and in Europe it was 3.5 per cent in 1969 (Fregert *et al.*, 1969); both series had been tested with 2 per cent formaldehyde in water.

St John's

Fifteen years ago only patients suspected of having a contact dermatitis were patch tested and during the six years from 1956 to 1961, 30 patients were seen with formaldehyde textile dermatitis. Since then there has been a greater tendency to patch test patients with persistent eczema and each is tested with a standard series which includes formaldehyde 2 per cent in water. It is therefore likely that our recognition of this dermatitis is greater and mild cases which previously would have remained unrecognised are now diagnosed. In the seven years from 1970–1976, 33 cases have been seen (Table 3.11). This apparent similarity in incidence over the past 20 years is erroneous because the selection of patients and the method of patch testing have changed. This type of clothing dermatitis is now infrequent.

Table 3.11. Yearly incidence of formaldehyde resin textile dermatitis. St John's 1956–1976.

1956–58	59–61	Total	70	71	72	73	74	75	76	Total
7	23	30	7	8	2	5	5	4	2	33

Clinical features

Sex incidence

In all the published series this dermatitis is more common in women, probably because they have a greater variety of resin-treated clothes, most of which are worn close to the skin giving sweat an opportunity to leach out formaldehyde. In Bergen, all 45 patients reported were women (Høvding, 1961); in Oslo, the ratio of women to men was 3:1 (Wereide, 1964), in Copenhagen 6:1 (Marcussen, 1962) and in Holland 2:1 (Malten, 1964).

St John's

> In the series of 30 patients seen from 1956 to 1961 there were 25 women and 5 men, a ratio of 5:1. Among the 33 patients seen from 1970 to 1976 there were 27 women and 6 men, again a ratio of approximately 5:1.

Age

This allergy seems not to occur in children but has been described in a 17-year-old boy (Shellow and Altman, 1966).

St John's

> In this clinic the dermatitis is not uncommon in young women. In the 1963 series (Cronin, 1963) there were two girls aged 15 and 17 years and of the 33 patients seen from 1970 to 1976, eight (24 per cent) were aged 17–20 years (Table 3.12).

Table 3.12. The ages of women and men with textile dermatitis from formaldehyde resins. St John's 1970–1976.

Ages Years	17–20	21–30	31–40	41–50	51–60	61–70
F	8	5	5	5	3	1
M			1	2	3	

Clinical patterns

The dermatitis occurs at sites of sweat and friction (Fig. 3.1). Dresses, blouses and shirts usually initiate the dermatitis and it remains a predominantly axillary eczema affecting especially the borders of the axillae with sparing or a lesser degree of involvement of the vaults. The eczema may spread to the sides of the neck, elbow flexures, arms and parts of the upper trunk not covered by underclothes. In the Copenhagen series the sides and back of the neck were most frequently affected (Marcussen, 1962). Occasionally the eruption becomes generalised (Høvding, 1961) and even the face has been involved (Malten, 1964). In two patients described by Uehara (1978), the lesions, which were intensely itchy, were discrete, red, follicular papules.

Skirts cause eczema of the knees and calves (Malten, 1964) and under the waist band if a slip is not worn.

Trousers produce an eczema in the gluteal folds, the popliteal fossae and the inner thighs.

The jacket of a suit may cause dermatitis of the wrists (Malten, 1964).

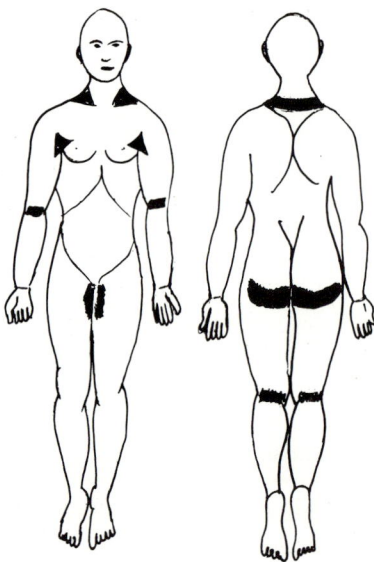

Fig. 3.1 Sites affected in textile dermatitis from formaldehyde resins

St John's

In the 1963 series (Cronin, 1963) 27 of the 30 patients had axillary dermatitis. Of the 33 patients seen from 1970 to 1976, 25 (75 per cent) had eczema of the axillae, which in 19 were the initial sites and in the other 6 were involved later.

In contradistinction to dye dermatitis, formaldehyde eczema usually is a sub-acute, grumbling dermatitis which is easily overlooked and dismissed as a constitutional eczema. It does not produce on the skin a striking imprint of the responsible garment as may occur with allergy to a dye in clothing.

Patients' histories have varied from 2 weeks to 10 years (Høvding, 1961), 3 years (Malten, 1964) and 10 years (O'Quinn, 1965).

St John's

The lengths of history were recorded in 29 of the 33 patients; they tended to be long for a dermatitis due entirely to a contact allergen. In 18 (62 per cent) the eczema had been present for more than a year and in only 5 (17 per cent) of the patients was the history less than three months (Table 3.13). The duration of symptoms was not recorded in three patients, and another woman with hand eczema had had a clothing dermatitis in the past which she had recognised herself, and had cured by avoiding drip dry clothes.

Table 3.13. Lengths of history in 29 patients with formaldehyde resin textile dermatitis. St John's 1970–1976.

	Weeks		Months	Years		
	0–6	7–12	4–12	>1–3	>3–10	>10
Duration symptoms						
No. patients	1	4	6	8	6	4

The follow-up of these patients has been poor and in many of those with long histories, the allergy had probably been superimposed upon an existing eczema.

Presensitisation

St John's

In the 1963 series of 30 patients (Cronin, 1963) three were presensitised to formaldehyde, two by a glue and one by an unknown source. In the recent group of 33 patients one young woman reacted to a formaldehyde plantar wart remedy, with an exudative eczema of her foot. One month later she developed axillary dermatitis. Patch tests: she reacted to formaldehyde (2 per cent aq.), dimethylolmethoxypropylene urea (10 per cent pet.), dimethoxypropylene urea (10 per cent pet.) and a mixture of ethylene urea and melamine formaldehyde (10 per cent pet.).

Patch testing

Formaldehyde
Reactions to formaldehyde occur in some but not all patients with formaldehyde resin textile dermatitis. Patients sensitised by the cyclic urea resins are unlikely to be sensitive to formaldehyde.

The irritancy of formaldehyde must also be taken into account when patch testing; too high a concentration gives misleading false positive reactions (Epstein and Maibach, 1966).

Formaldehyde textile resins
In 1964, in Nijmegen, 27 patients with clothing dermatitis were patch tested with textile resins with the following results:

Dimethylol urea (urea formaldehyde)	50% aq.	13 positive
Melamine formaldehyde	50%–70% aq. or in acetone	9 positive
Dimethylolethylene urea	50%–70% aq. or in acetone	8 positive
Dimethyloldihydroxyethylene urea	50% aq.	7 positive
Formaldehyde	5% aq.	7 positive

The reaction to formaldehyde was considered to be of secondary importance and due to a group reaction (Malten, 1964).

Pieces of fabric
Patch testing with pieces of fabric cannot be relied upon to make this diagnosis

and a negative reaction does not invalidate the diagnosis. It has been estimated that the concentration of free formaldehyde in such patch test samples is insufficient to elicit a reaction in the majority of patients (Berrens *et al.*, 1964). Materials producing negative patch tests in sensitised subjects have been found to contain formaldehyde on chemical testing (Cronin, 1963).

St John's

Since 1956, patients suspected of having clothing dermatitis have been patch tested with
  (i) Formaldehyde 2 per cent aqueous
  (ii) Formaldehyde textile resins 10 per cent in soft paraffin
(iii) Pieces of clothing.
   The fabric is included to avoid missing a dye dermatitis.
1956–1961: During this time 30 patients were diagnosed and they gave the following positive reactions (Cronin, 1963):

Formaldehyde 2% aq.	Urea and/or Melamine formaldehyde 10%	Pieces of clothing
29/30	19/26	4/20

1970–1976: From 1970 onwards this patch test series was widened to include the reactive resins, the cyclic ureas, and since 1974 the patients have been tested with each of the following resins:

1. Dimethylolmethoxypropylene urea
2. Dimethyloldihydroxyethylene urea
3. Dimethylolpropylene urea
4. Ethylene urea and melamine formaldehyde
5. Urea formaldehyde
6. Melamine formaldehyde.

   The 33 patients seen during this period gave the following results:

	Formaldehyde (2% aqueous)	Resins 10% in petrolatum					
		1	2	3	4	5	6
Tested	33	11	33	11	11	33	11
+	29	3	4	8	8	29	6

   These patch tests results show that in this clinic:

  (i) Formaldehyde 2 per cent (aq.) detects the majority but not all cases
 (ii) Urea formaldehyde is still the most frequent resin sensitiser in textiles
(iii) Reactive resins, the cyclic ureas, should be used for testing.

Criteria for diagnosis

The criteria for diagnosis are:
1. A pattern of eczema consistent with a clothing dermatitis
2. A positive patch test reaction to formaldehyde or to a formaldehyde clothing resin, or both.

Patch test series

The following is an adequate patch test series; samples of the patients' coloured clothing are included to avoid missing a dye dermatitis:

1. Formaldehyde	2 per cent in water
2. Urea formaldehyde	10 per cent in petrolatum
3. Melamine formaldehyde	10 per cent in petrolatum
4. Dimethylolpropylene urea	10 per cent in petrolatum
5. Dimethylolmethoxypropylene urea	10 per cent in petrolatum
6. Dimethyloldihydroxyethylene urea	10 per cent in petrolatum
7. Pieces from each coloured garment	

Tests for formaldehyde in textiles

Chromotropic acid in sulphuric acid reacts with formaldehyde to give a violet colour. This reaction is specific and sensitive.

Schiff's reagent becomes pink-purple in colour in the presence of free aldehydes. This test is less specific, but as formaldehyde is the only aldehyde likely to be present in textiles it probably is adequate.

Free formaldehyde can be detected in fabrics either by aqueous extraction (Høvding, 1959; Berrens *et al.*, 1964) or by its gaseous diffusion in a confined space (Blohm, 1959; Fisher *et al.*, 1962). Chromotropic acid is used as the indicator.

Free and combined formaldehyde are detected by acidic extraction; the following two methods are simple procedures:

Chromotropic acid (Marcussen, 1962)
(4,5-Dihydroxy-2,7-naphthalenedisulphonic acid. It should be pure for this test)
   (i) Bring the samples of fabric to boiling in 5 ml of 1 per cent sulphuric acid
   (ii) Stand for 5 minutes
   (iii) Add 1 drop to 2 ml of 72 per cent sulphuric acid containing a few small crystals of chromotropic acid
   (iv) Heat the mixture over a flame.
An intense red-purple colour indicates a positive test.

Schiff's reagent
   (i) Cut small strips of material approximately 1 cm × 6 cm
   (ii) Rinse all test tubes in 0.1 N hydrochloric acid
   (iii) Immerse the strips in about 5 ml of 0.1 N hydrochloric acid
   (iv) Heat the test tubes in a water bath for 5–10 minutes
   (v) Cool, then remove and discard the material
   (vi) Add 5 drops of Schiff's reagent to the acid in the test tube.
A pink-purple colour indicates a positive test. If the dye runs, a comparison must be made between two extracts, one with and one without Schiff's reagent; this colour comparison is not always easy.

Management of patients

To cure the dermatitis all the patient's clothes which contain formaldehyde must be identified. Rayons, cottons and mixtures of natural and synthetic fibres are the textiles to be sought, rather than pure synthetic fabrics, woollen sweaters or tweed jackets and dresses. Once the offending garments have been eliminated from routine wear, the symptoms are relieved (Marcussen, 1962); this applies particularly to garments with a high level (over 0.05 per cent; 500 p.p.m.) of free formaldehyde (Berrens *et al.*, 1964). In the acute stage, it is helpful to persuade women to wear an old formalin-free blouse as an undergarment to protect the skin from inadvertent contact with formalin-containing outer clothes. To screen clothes, it probably is preferable to use the acid extraction methods, which identify free and combined formaldehyde. Although free formaldehyde is the greater danger, any textiles which contain resin should be avoided while the patient has eczema.

It is not possible to remove the resin from a garment by frequent laundering.

Once the skin has healed patients seem to tolerate garments identified as containing only small amounts of formaldehyde. They are asked to wear these for only short periods, at least initially, and to avoid hot atmospheres which may cause sweating.

Prophylaxis. It is impracticable for most patients and most clinicians to test new clothes for the presence of these resins. The patients are advised to avoid drip-dry, crease-resistant cottons and rayons as much as possible. They should be strongly urged to wash, when practicable, all new clothes before wearing them. This greatly reduces the level of free formaldehyde and compensates for an after-wash omitted in manufacture.

Despite the present impossibility of avoiding these resins, this dermatitis does not appear to become chronic. Once the eczema has healed, patients seem not to suffer recurrent relapses; at least they do not return to the clinic with any. This is probably because, in most cases, formaldehyde and textile resins act as weak allergens. Patients sensitised by formaldehyde from other sources rarely develop textile dermatitis, even when wearing garments known to contain free formaldehyde (Fisher *et al.*, 1962).

Industrial dermatitis

In a Czechoslovakian textile plant using urea and melamine formaldehyde, dermatitis occurred in 63 workers (5.25 per cent of all employees). Most of the patients were seamstresses. Their faces, eyelids, hands and arms were affected. Some had conjunctivitis, oral ulceration and upper respiratory tract inflammation.

These changes were attributed to free formaldehyde in the cloth; it was suggested that working conditions could be improved by reducing dust, by air extraction and by controlling the level of formaldehyde in fabrics (Kachlik, 1968).

After 47 years, a seamstress, who steamed clothes containing formaldehyde, developed burning of her eyes and a hyperkeratotic eczema on her palms and soles. A patch test with formaldehyde was positive at 1 but negative at 2 days. Formaldehyde was, however, considered to be relevant in the aetiology (Roth, 1969).

Dermatitis from a textile finish

In the 1940s, a finish on underwear shorts caused a sharp outbreak of dermatitis in the U.S.A. Adolescents, who had worn the unwashed shorts for 2–3 days, developed a well-demarcated dermatitis under the pants, with pain, swelling and irritation of the genitalia and several required catheterisation. Patch tests with the unwashed fabric were positive in the patients and in 7 of 95 controls. Constituents of the finish were applied as patch tests: abietic acid produced no reaction in either patients or controls; 0.3 per cent oleoresin elicited reactions in 8 of 95 controls and all 4 patients tested. The clinical history and the results of these tests suggest that this was an irritant rather than an allergic dermatitis (Neilson and Reiches, 1941).

The manufacturers recalled the shorts and shipped them to South America. As further cases of dermatitis occurred there, the pants were returned to the U.S.A., only to produce a second wave of dermatitis there. The last case was seen in about 1961 (Birmingham and Weber, 1966).

SHEETS

In Canada, in 1971 and 1972, there was an explosive outbreak of contact dermatitis caused by the resin in permanently-pressed coloured sheets and pillowcases. The sheets, made of 50 per cent cotton and 50 per cent polyester, were manufactured by one particular company and the dermatitis erupted after they changed their technique of applying the resin to the fabric from a slow cold method to a hot flash process (Wilkinson, 1976). Once the implicated process was stopped, the incidence of cases dropped abruptly.

Hundreds were affected but usually only one person in each family. The time interval between buying the sheets and the onset of the dermatitis varied between 10 and 60 days. All the patients developed widespread, extremely itchy, follicular papules which were most marked on the arms and legs, with sparing of the palms, soles and scalp. Some patients also had scattered patches of erythema which characteristically affected the pinnae including the lobes of the ears. Oedema of the eyes and face occurred sometimes, as did crusted eczematous lesions. Even when the sheets were discarded, the eruption took eight weeks to clear in some patients.

Patch testing with (i) the sheets was positive in six patients and negative in three, (ii) 2 per cent formaldehyde was always negative, (iii) a permanent press monomer was positive in four of eleven patients tested. The manufacturers would not disclose the identity of this monomer (Panaccio, Montgomery and Adam, 1973).

In Montreal (Wilkinson, 1973), 5 of 11 patients reacted to the perma-press resin *N,N*-dimethylol-4-methoxy-5,5-dimethylpropylene urea, and none reacted either to formaldehyde or to other additives. A new substitute resin also gave negative responses in those patients tested. Many launderings failed to remove the allergen, and prolonged baking of the sheets increased it. Gel column chromatography identified the main allergen as a compound with a molecular weight over 1500 but also showed that other compounds, with molecular weights over 5000, were reactive too. It was concluded that the permanent press resin used on these sheets was unstable to heat and moisture and that a fragment of the polymer was the allergen, which, because of its large size, penetrated the skin through the pilosebaceous follicles.

A case of dermatitis from non-iron sheets and pillowcases has been reported also from Lund in Sweden (Fregert and Tegner, 1971). This patient did not react to formaldehyde but did to dimethyloldihydroxyethylene urea.

St John's

This dermatitis was first seen in 1973 in an isolated patient who had bought coloured Canadian sheets in a shop and slept in them for a week before the eruption developed. The store denied any other complaints. No further cases occurred until April 1975, when nine patients were seen in the following 18 months (Rycroft, Cronin and Calnan, 1976). They had all bought brightly coloured Canadian Wabasso bed sheets at cheap prices in street markets or from dealers. After sleeping in the sheets for 3–14 days one or several members of the family including children, developed on the body and sometimes the face an itching, burning eruption which, in some patients, was severe and in others mild. The follicular lesions were striking. The dermatitis was easily mistaken for scabies and one or two patients only escaped this diagnosis by querying the safety of their new sheets.

Patch tests: of all these patients four reacted to their sheets and five did not; none reacted to formaldehyde 2 per cent in water. With different sheets the rash took 3–4 weeks to clear. The patients were advised to discard the sheets but one patient found them comfortable after three launderings.

It seemed likely that in these patients the dermatitis was of two types. The resin probably acted as an irritant in those who had developed the eruption after sleeping in the sheets for only three days, whereas it sensitised those who required longer exposure times and had positive patch tests to the sheets.

As stated by Rycroft *et al.* (1976) it would be interesting to know how sheets which were made unsaleable in Canada because of their hazard were able to be offloaded on to the markets of England and probably other countries.

Shoes and boots

Sensitisation from a component of a shoe or fashion boot is not uncommon but it is one of the most difficult types of contact dermatitis to diagnose accurately. Shoes are always in high fashion, they are made by numerous manufacturers in many countries and their design and the materials used in their manufacture are constantly changing. Consequently it is difficult to establish, even with the help of the manufacturers, the composition of any particular part of a shoe.

Sensitisers in shoes

Rubber

Outer soles. The outer sole may be made of rubber, or a rubber resin or rubber leather composition. However, in the U.K. polyurethane and polyvinyl chloride are being used with increasing frequency for soling. Bedroom slippers may have rubber soles.

Heel stiffeners. Bedroom slippers are particularly likely to have rubberised heel stiffeners.

Plimsolls (track shoes). Plimsolls and track shoes are made largely of rubber and fabric.

Elastic. Elastic gussets and pieces of elastic are easily overlooked in shoes; they may be inset in the sides of men's slip-on shoes, under flaps on the fronts of women's shoes or inside the heel bands of sling-back shoes.

At the present time mercaptobenzothiazole (MBT) is the commonest sensitiser in patients with shoe dermatitis investigated in the U.S.A. The following incidences have been reported: 15 of 35 patients (Adams, 1972), 9 of 25 patients (Jordan, 1972) and 13 of 42 patients (Dahl, 1975). Similarly at St John's, MBT is the most frequent sensitiser in shoes (Cronin, 1966).

However, this is not so in Greece, where only 6 of 25 patients with shoe dermatitis were sensitised by MBT (Varelzides *et al.*, 1974).

Tetramethylthiuram disulphide sensitivity is less frequent; the number of patch test reactions reported was 3 of 35 patients by Adams (1972), 5 of 25 patients by Jordan (1972), 9 of 42 patients by Dahl (1975) and 5 of 25 patients by Varelzides *et al.* (1974). Diphenylguanidine and monobenzyl ether of hydroquinone each sensitised two patients in Adams' (1972) series.

The release of rubber chemicals from insoles was investigated by Hegyi and Šaršúnová (1974) and although they were able to extract them with ether and hexane they were not able to do so with water or synthetic sweat.

In Iran, the soles of the traditional cloth Maleki shoes are now being made with used car tyres. A man wearing such shoes developed dermatitis of the soles and on patch testing he reacted to the PPD rubber-mix. The individual components of the mix were not available for testing but isopropylphenyl-*para*-phenylenediamine (IPPD) was thought to be the most likely sensitiser (Leppard and Parhizgar, 1977).

Adhesives

Para-tertiary-butylphenol formaldehyde (PTBP resin). PTBP resin is used in neoprene (synthetic rubber) adhesives to bond the outer sole to the upper of the shoe (p. 616). Although other compounds are being introduced PTBP resin is still used in the making of shoes.

Dodecyl mercaptan. Dodecyl mercaptan is also used in neoprene adhesives.

Thiurams and mercaptobenzothiazole. The linings and inner socks of shoes are secured by latex adhesives and some are formulated with thiurams and mercaptobenzothiazole.

Colophony (rosin) may be present as a tackifier in shoe cements (Jordan, 1972).

Ethyl butyl thiourea has been used in a neoprene-based adhesive.

PTBP resin sensitises about 10–20 per cent of patients with shoe dermatitis in the U.S.A. [4 of 35 patients (Adams, 1972) 4 of 25 patients (Jordan, 1972) and 8 of 42 patients (Dahl, 1975)]. Similarly at St John's a few patients, including children, are seen, each year, with shoe dermatitis caused by this resin glue.

Dodecyl mercaptane has been found to be a frequent cause of shoe dermatitis in Spain, one source of contact being its addition to some Neoprene adhesives (Romaguera Sagrera, Grimalt Sancho and Pinol Aguadé, 1974; Grimalt and Romaguera, 1975). In 1976, at St John's, 20 patients thought to have shoe dermatitis were patch tested with dodecyl mercaptane but none reacted.

Latex adhesives may be the source of sensitisation to thiurams and mercaptobenzothiazole (Jordan, 1972; Dahl, 1975).

Colophony (rosin) sensitised one of 25 patients in Jordan's (1972) series.

Ethyl butyl thiourea was the allergen in a rubber adhesive used to secure the nylon cover to the rubber insoles of athletic shoes. The patients had positive patch tests to the insole, the adhesive and ethyl butyl thiourea (1 per cent pet.) (Roberts and Hanifin, 1979).

Leather

The chemicals used to tan leather sensitise and in many countries leather still remains the most frequent cause of shoe dermatitis. Chromium compounds and vegetable tans are the most likely allergens but formaldehyde and glutaraldehyde are also possible sensitisers.

The trivalent chromium compounds, used to tan leather, can be leached from the leather by sweat but although Samitz and Gross (1960) and Samitz, Katz and Gross (1960) identified hexavalent chromate in sweat extracts of shoe leather, the finding of chromate in similar aqueous extracts was not confirmed by Fregert and Gruvberger (1970). Whichever of the chromium compounds is the actual sensitiser, potassium dichromate (Cr_6) is the most reliable chemical to use for diagnostic patch testing.

In Greece, the majority of the people wear chrome tanned leather shoes and chrome compounds are the most frequent cause of shoe dermatitis. In Athens, 16 of 25 patients with shoe dermatitis were sensitised to dichromate (Varelzides *et al.*, 1974). In three reports from the U.S.A. approximately 20 per cent of the patients in each series was sensitive to dichromate [7 of 35 patients (Adams, 1972), 5 of 25 (Jordan, 1972), 9 of 42 (Dahl, 1975)]. In the tropics chrome tanned leather sandals have caused dermatitis in British Naval seamen and in servicemen's wives (Scutt, 1966; Hindson, 1969). In contrast to these reports, at St John's chromate is not a frequent allergen in patients with shoe dermatitis and patients sensitised to chromate from other sources do not have shoe dermatitis.

Vegetable tanned leather imported from East India into Britain caused positive patch test reactions in patients with shoe dermatitis seen at St John's, but the sensitiser was not identified (Cronin, 1966). Later a particular type of sandal made of Indian buffalo hide caused dermatitis in several countries. In the U.S.A. six cases were reported by Lynch and Rudolph (1969) and similar patients were seen by Adams (1972) and Spoor (1973). Another girl (Minkin, Cohen and Frank, 1971) initially developed dermatitis from these sandals and subsequently from the leather lining of an American shoe. It was ascertained that this lining leather, supplied by a British firm, had been imported from India. Similar patients with Indian sandal dermatitis were seen in Australia, in Denmark (Rothenborg and Hjorth, 1971) and also in England.

Formaldehyde patch test reactions, in patients with shoe dermatitis, have been reported by Adams (1972), Jordan (1972), Dahl (1975) and Varelzides *et al.* (1974). However, formaldehyde allergy in a patient with shoe dermatitis was considered to have little significance by Epstein (1969).

Glutaraldehyde is an effective tanning agent and some of the leather so prepared is used for the uppers of shoes. Glutaraldehyde-tanned leather elicited positive patch test reactions in five patients sensitised through occupational or therapeutic exposure. Although these patients did not have shoe dermatitis this finding confirms that glutaraldehyde in leather is released and is a potential source of dermatitis (Jordan, Dahl and Albert, 1972).

Dyes

In Jordan's (1972) series of 25 patients he lists 5 as being sensitive to 'dyes' and 4 to *para*-phenylenediamine (PPD). Likewise among the 42 patients investigated by Dahl (1975) 5 reacted to dyes and 5 to PPD. Without naming the specific dyes to which his patients reacted, Dahl listed the dyes he used for testing:

Wood Orange A 1 per cent
Calcozine Black 1 per cent
Solvent Red 2G 0.5 per cent
Euchrysine GGA 0.5 per cent
New Blue RS concentrate 1 per cent
PPD 1 per cent
Nigrosine B 1 per cent

Disperse Orange 0.5 per cent
Bismark Brown 1 per cent
Calcocid Orange 2G 1 per cent
Oil Yellow 1 0.5 per cent
Leather Brown 5RTA 0.5 per cent
Bismark Brown R 1 per cent

Each diluted in white petrolatum.

One of Adam's patients (1974) reacted to a Bismark Brown.

In Fisher's (1973a) experience dermatitis from dyes in leather shoes is extremely rare, which he attributes to the firm fixation of the dyes to the leather, but he has found that re-dyed shoes, in which the colour is not so fast, do cause dermatitis. Dyes in fabric shoes bleed and have likewise caused dermatitis in his patients, most of whom also reacted to *para*-phenylenediamine. At St John's there have been no cases in which a shoe dermatitis was proved to be due to a dye.

Plastics

In some countries polyvinyl chloride (PVC) and polyurethane are displacing leather and rubber in shoe manufacture. PVC is made into uppers, linings, socks (innermost sole lining) and outer soles, and polyurethane is used principally for soles, foam socks and foam linings and occasionally for uppers.

Polyurethane resins and dodecyl mercaptane, added to plastics to stop polymerisation, have caused shoe dermatitis in Spain (Romaguera Sagrera *et al.*, 1975; Grimalt and Romaguera, 1975). At St John's several patients have been seen who were sensitised, some acutely, by PVC linings in their shoes but the allergen in the plastic is proving very difficult to identify.

Toe-puffs (stiffeners)
Toe-puffs, formerly made of nitrocellulose in the U.K. and sometimes of rubberised material in the U.S.A., are now being made of plastics such as nylon or polyester. Film toe-puffs are simply adhesives sprayed directly on to the shoe fabric and moulded and stiffened by heat.

Heel stiffeners
Heel stiffeners vary in composition; they may contain leather, cellulose fibres, binders, waxes and colours. Some of the stiffeners for women's shoes are made in a similar way to toe-puffs and those of bedroom slippers may be rubberised.

Nickel
Nickel in metal fasteners and in trimmings, such as buckles, may cause patches of dermatitis on the feet.

Clinical features
Shoe dermatitis occurs in both children and adults and should be considered in every patient with eczema of the feet. However, when the eczema consists of tiny closely set vesicles confined entirely to the insteps a contact dermatitis is then very unlikely.

Typically the upper of a shoe causes dermatitis of the dorsa of the feet and toes with sparing of the web spaces and delimitation by the upper margin of the shoe. The sole of a shoe causes dermatitis of the weight bearing areas of the sole with sparing of the instep; very occasionally only the anterior part of the sole is involved. A toe-puff produces eczema of the dorsa of the toes and dermatitis from a heel stiffener wraps around the heel. The straps of a sandal may be imprinted as eczema on the feet.

Many patients do not have these typical patterns; the eczema may be patchy, and asymmetrical, it may affect particularly the dorsa and medial sides of the great toes, the web spaces may be involved and it may be superimposed upon an existent constitutional foot eczema. It is only by careful patch testing and follow-up of these patients that the diagnosis can be clarified.

Leucoderma of the dorsa of the feet, from the depigmenting action of monobenzyl ether of hydroquinone in rubber, occured in one of Adams' (1972) patients and a patch test with the chemical reproduced this effect.

In the patients with Indian sandal dermatitis seen at St John's the clinical presentation was striking in that the dermatitis which was under the leather around the great toe and on the dorsum of the foot was severe and in some patients vesicular and bullous. The pruritus was always intense and the pruriginous eczema often spread over the ankles and up the legs. These features were also described by Adams (1972).

Patients with shoe dermatitis may have eczema of other sites, particularly the hands (Calnan and Sarkany, 1959; Epstein, 1969).

Eczema of the feet is not uncommon in children and they should be patch tested although the results are frequently negative. Silvers and Glickman (1968) suggest that an atopic diathesis in these children makes them unduly susceptible to irritation from wearing shoes and may explain their eczema. Juvenile plantar dermatosis is now a recognised clinical picture and is well described by Shrank (1979) and Neering and van Dijk (1978).

Patch testing
Patch testing with shoes is time consuming and it can not be done in a hurry. As the chemical allergens in shoes are often unknown, careful patch testing with each shoe is the most important part of the investigation.

1. *Pieces of each shoe*
The patient should be asked, and if necessary persuaded, to bring one of every pair of shoes, including new shoes, old shoes, gardening shoes, sports shoes and bedroom slippers. It is then necessary carefully and diligently to remove with a scalpel various pieces from each shoe corresponding with the pattern of dermatitis on the patient's feet. It is important not to damage the shoes (they may not be the cause of the patient's eczema); the pieces removed should be thin slithers about 7 mm × 7 mm in surface area. If the samples excised are thick their pressure causes false positive patch test reactions. All layers of the shoes should be tested and when the dermatitis is on the soles, shavings should be taken from the outer as well as the inner soles of the shoes. It is usually difficult to reach the toe-puff area. Epstein (1969) has found that scraping this site with a mastoid curette is an effective method of obtaining samples. In an unlined shoe scraping the upper leather with a scalpel blade produces a fine powder, which is a suitable test material.

2. *Tanning compounds*
Potassium dichromate	0.5 per cent
Glutaraldehyde	0.25 per cent and 1 per cent in water
? Formaldehyde	2.0 per cent in water

Vegetable tans or a piece of vegetable tanned leather, if available.

3. *Adhesives*
PTBP resin	10 per cent
Dodecyl mercaptan	0.1 per cent in toluene, this concentration is a mild irritant (Romaguera, 1974)
Mercaptobenzothiazole	1.0 per cent
Thiuram-mix	
Colophony	20 per cent

4. *Rubber*
    Thiuram-mix
    Mercapto-mix
    PPD-mix
    Carba-mix

5. *Dyes*
    *Para*phenylenediamine   1 per cent
    Shoe dyes if available
    D. Yellow 3   1 per cent ⎤
    D. Red   1   1 per cent ⎬ to exclude a contact dermatitis
    D. Blue   3   1 per cent ⎦ from nylon stocking dyes

The diluent is petrolatum unless stated.

Alternative shoes
In the U.S.A. allergen-free shoes are made by several companies, the details of which are given by Fisher (1973a).

In the U.K. special shoes are not made for these patients but shoe companies are helpful in advising which of their shoes are free of particular allergens.

In general the following advice is given to patients:

Discard the shoes to which they reacted on patch testing and wear those which elicited no response:
    if rubber sensitive — a shoe preferably with a leather or alternatively a plastic sole; track shoes made of plastic are available
    if leather sensitive — an all plastic or fabric shoe
    if PVC sensitive   — an all leather or fabric shoe
    if sensitive to
    PTBP resin   — shoe companies will supply lists of their shoes free of this resin glue. Moccasins, if the patient will wear them, are a way of avoiding all shoe glues.

Control of hyperhidrosis. Fisher (1973b) has found that controlling hyperhidrosis of the feet with tannic acid foot baths and powder enables some patients to wear shoes containing chemicals to which they are sensitive, without developing dermatitis.

Occupational disease
Dermatitis is frequent in the tanning industry. The preparation of skins is a wet, messy job and in addition workers are exposed to trivalent chromium compounds in the tanning liquors and to hexavalent chromate salts in the preparatory procedures. Bulikowski and Tyras (1976) investigated the exposure to chromium compounds in a tannery and found their concentration in the air to be below the permitted level. They concluded from the levels of chromium in the urine of the tanners that absorption occurred through both the skin and the respiratory tract. Epidermal tests on 70 workers showed that 6 were sensitive to

chromium compounds. All the types of occupational hazard in the tanning industry have been reviewed by Sommer, Hincker and Mehl (1971). Apart from dermatoses the workers are at risk of developing various kinds of infections, poisoning, eye lesions and diseases of the upper respiratory tract.

A survey in Northamptonshire, a centre of the boot and shoe industry, has given evidence of an association between nasal cancer and work in this industry (Acheson, Cowdell and Jolles, 1970).

In Italy polyneuropathy occurs in shoe and leather workers, and it has been attributed by Buiatti *et al.* (1978) to exposure to solvents in glues. Three cases in shoe factory workers in the U.S.A. were thought to be caused by methyl ethyl ketone (Dyro, 1979).

RUBBER BOOTS

Contact dermatitis from rubber boots usually occurs in men and is acquired at work by wearing boots for prolonged periods. Cases have been reported in the gold mining industry of South Africa (Lowenthal, Levy and Hins, 1968) and among fishermen and other occupations in Newfoundland (Ross, 1969).

The dermatitis from rubber boots usually involves the dorsa of the feet and the soles and may extend up the legs to the top of the boot. The dermatitis on the dorsa of the feet is sometimes severe, with exudation, vesiculation and even blister formation. Occasionally the dorsa of the feet are spared and only the soles are affected. In some of the patients seen by Lowenthal *et al.* (1968) the eczema disseminated to other parts of the body.

Sensitisers

Mercaptobenzothiazole (MBT) and thiurams
In England mercaptobenzothiazole (MBT) is a commoner sensitiser than tetramethythiuram disulphide (TMTD) in rubber boots. Among 15 men with rubber boot dermatitis patch tested at St John's, 7 reacted to MBT 2 per cent (pet.), 4 to TMTD 2 per cent (pet.) and 4 reacted to both chemicals. In the South African series of Lowenthal *et al.* (1968) of 26 men patch tested, 8 reacted to MBT and 2 to TMTD. However, in Czechoslovakia only one of 109 patients with boot dermatitis was sensitised by MBT (Jirásek, Kalenský and Sevcová, 1975).

Isopropylaminodiphenylamine (IPPD)
In Prague (Jirásek, Kalenský and Sevcová, 1975) 109 patients employed as miners, concrete mixers, farmers and washerwomen, developed an allergic contact dermatitis from rubber boots. The sensitiser was *N*-phenyl-*N*-isopropyl-PPD (IPPD) in all except two; of these exceptions one was sensitised by MBT and the other by phenyl-β-naphthylamine. Among the patients sensitised by IPPD 38 per cent had a purpuric eczema due to a toxic capillaritis, several had purpura without eczema and one patient had generalised purpura. This staining of the skin persisted for months or even for years. Two Englishmen, who worked in the same dyers and cleaners, developed a striking purpuric eczema of the feet and widespread purpura on the body from sensitisation to IPPD in rubber boots

(Calnan and Peachey, 1971). Another adult male and a girl aged five years were also sensitised to this chemical by rubber boots (Vollum and Marten, 1968) and a further two patients were reported by Crow (1967).

Patch testing
1. A thin shaving about 7 mm × 7 mm from the boot
2. The four rubber mixes (p. 74).

Alternative boots
Plastic boots are suitable for these patients. In the U.K. such boots are made by Futura Footwear Ltd. Stalybridge, Cheshire.

Hat bands

Hat bands used to be made of leather but nowadays they are as likely to be made of fabric or plastic. Occasionally men develop an allergic contact dermatitis of the forehead from a hat band.

In those made of leather dichromate is sometimes but not always the sensitiser (Bett, 1958). Hat bands made from Indian (Madras) sheep skins have caused dermatitis in Prague; 17 of 24 patients reacted to the leather but only two of 16 were sensitive to chromium (Novák and Schwank, 1976).

Laurel oil is used to give lustre to felt hats and the reports of its causing dermatitis have been summarised by Foussereau, Benezra and Ourisson (1967). Some hat bands are finished with a varnish containing colophony which may cause dermatitis.

Leather accessories

Contact dermatitis from various leather articles occurs occasionally. A man sensitised by his watch strap was tested with a series of vegetable tans and reacted to myrabolam and quebracho extract powder. Myrabolam contains chebulinic acid 12 per cent and chebulagic acid 2 per cent (Calnan and Cronin, 1978). Orthodichlorobenzene was identified as the sensitiser in the dye of a black leather gun belt which caused dermatitis in an American policeman (Wright, 1979).

Dry cleaning

Textiles are dry cleaned with fat solvents and small amounts of detergent. In Great Britain, and probably in most countries, perchloroethylene is the principal chemical employed.

Perchloroethylene (tetrachloroethylene)
$$Cl_2C = C\,Cl_2$$
This solvent is used in closed machines for about 80 per cent of this work.

Trifluorotrichloroethane (Arklone, ICI; Valclene, Dupont)

$$F_2Cl \; CC \; Cl_2 \; F$$

This compound and similar newer chemicals are said to be less toxic, to be better solvents, and to dry at a lower temperature; they constitute about 15 per cent of these solvents.

Trichloroethylene (Trilene)

$$ClHC = C \; Cl_2$$

Trilene has been replaced because of its toxicity (p. 890) and now constitutes only about 5 per cent of these chemicals. It is still used in closed systems for special purposes such as the cleaning of dirty factory overalls.

White spirit is rarely used.

Dry cleaning is done in stages in a closed system. The textile load is immersed in solvent for the removal of solid dirt and short-chain fatty acids. The solvent is then cleansed by filtration and a long-chain anionic detergent and water are added to remove soluble stains. The textile is then rinsed in solvent and, if required, retexing is carried out at this stage. Finally, the garment is dried by heat.

If the dry cleaning solvent is not adequately cleansed during re-cycling, short-chain fatty acids may actually be deposited on the fabrics. This is more likely to occur with coin-operated machines than with professional cleaners.

Dermatitis from cleaned clothes

These chemicals are irritants but probably not allergens. If drying of a garment is incomplete, solvent will remain in the fabric particularly where there are several thicknesses of material. The polythene wrapping, so often used, aggravates the situation by preventing evaporation. When first worn after cleaning, such a garment may cause an irritant dermatitis, but, as the solvent evaporates, this effect disappears.

Occupational dermatitis

Dermatitis of the hands in a metal worker was attributed by Vail (1974) to allergy to perchloroethylene. Patch testing with perchloroethylene 1 per cent in olive oil was positive at two days but an open test was negative. He had no dermatitis provided he avoided this chemical.

St John's

A self-employed man, aged 38 years, had worked as a dry cleaner for four years, applying perchloroethylene and other detergents and solvents manually to noticeable stains on fabrics. He did not wear gloves. He developed thickening and discomfort of the pulps of several fingers and the skin under their nails. When seen four months after the onset of the symptoms, there was gross thickening of the distal part of the right index finger nail and bed, with lesser involvement of the right thumb and middle finger, and of the same fingers of the left hand. On patch testing he did not react to perchloroethylene 1 per cent but did to a piece of rubber; this was attributed to his recently wearing gloves. Open tests with undiluted perchloroethylene and another cleaner were negative. The condition was thought to be an irritant dermatitis. He remained at work but wore plastic gloves and used spatulas for applying the solvents. After three months, his fingers had healed but the thickening of his right index finger nail remained.

Toxicity
A male aged 19 years, employed in a dry cleaning business, developed a connective tissue disorder, similar to vinyl chloride disease. It was attributed to his exposure to perchloroethylene (Sparrow, 1977).

Re-texing
Textile finishes and sizes, which give body to fabrics, together with fibres broken during wear, are lost in dry cleaning. The fabric consequently loses substance and feels limp; re-texing coats the fibres and restores body to the fabric. About 50–60 per cent of garments are re-texed after cleaning.

Waxes. Approximately 80 per cent of re-texing compounds are waxes; paraffin wax is the commonest but carnuba wax or silicones may be used, and lanolin is sometimes included as a softening agent. Esters of titanium and aluminium are added as improvers in that they help to fix the wax coating to the fibre. A waxy material is always used for a water-repellent finish.

Resins. Resin constitutes about 20 per cent of these agents. They usually are polyterpenes, although coumarone-indene resins have been used; the polyvinyl acetate emulsions, tried at one time, have been almost completely discontinued.

Skin reactions
Dermatitis, if it ever occurs, must be extremely rare.

Stain repellants
These preparations are not intended to make fabrics withstand soiling but to make stains easier to remove.
   'Scotchgard', a stain and water repellant, was used in the manufacture of a pair of slacks which caused contact dermatitis in a wearer. Patch tests with treated fabrics were positive and those with untreated cloth were negative. The stain repellant contained a fluorocarbon, acrylates and rubber materials, but the exact sensitiser was not identified (Eskelson and Goodman, 1963).

Fabric softeners
These are often quaternary ammonium compounds, particularly distearyl-dimethylammonium chloride. Other cationic chemicals such as the acetates and hydrochlorides of amidoamines also achieve this effect.

Fibre glass

Fibre glass is an irritant, not a sensitiser. It has been shown by Heisel and Hunt (1968) that the irritation caused by fibre glass is dependent upon the diameter of the filaments; if very fine, they cause no discomfort. Susceptibility to this itch also differs amongst individuals but the reasons for this variation was not found by Björnberg et al. (1979). The histology of patch test reactions to fibre glass shows changes due to minor trauma and also features of eczema (Cuypers et al., 1975).

Curtain materials are sometimes made with fibre glass and, if inadvertently laundered with clothing, can produce outbreaks of fibre glass dermatitis in a family. The first account (Madoff, 1962) described episodes of acute irritation in three small siblings in New England, and the next came from New York reporting a mother and her three children (Abel, 1966). The diagnoses were made retrospectively. In 1967, two families were seen in London; the diagnosis was suspected and confirmed clinically (Peachey, 1967). In each report fibre glass curtains had been washed in an automatic washing machine with, or in one instance before, the family's clothes. The glass particles lodge in the textiles and cause severe itching within minutes of the garments being worn: a pricking sensation is characteristic. Scratch marks are the principal physical sign, and a mild erythema may also be present. In one 6 year-old girl the particles induced foreign body granulomas on the buttocks, legs and feet (Lechner and Hartmann, 1977).

The glass particles can be seen microscopically in Sellotape skin strippings taken from irritable areas. They can be similarly demonstrated in the laundered clothes (Peachey, 1967). These particles have been seen, with some difficulty, in biopsies from skin exposed experimentally to fibre glass (Fisher and Warkentin, 1969). They were demonstrated in the foreign body granulomas of the child described above.

Symptoms are quickly relieved by bathing and a change of clothes. It is, however, difficult, even with several washes, to remove the glass fibre from contaminated clothing.

Fibre glass, used to reinforce the plastic of a school chair, was the cause of chronic eczematous patches on the backs of a schoolgirl's thighs. Glass particles were seen in a potassium hydroxide preparation of scrapings from the eczematous areas (Eby and Jetton, 1972).

Occupational dermatitis

Workers handling fibre glass often experience considerable discomfort and irritation from the glass spicules. Of 1847 employees making plastic reinforced with glass fibre, 14.6 per cent had an occupational dermatitis. The changes were both irritant and allergic, being attributed to the glass fibre and to synthetic resins respectively (Antoniev and Vilchinsky, 1972). Workers in the fibre glass industry were also investigated by Cuypers, Bleumink and Nater (1975) and their conclusions were similar. Fifty-six of the spinners were carefully examined and only four were free of symptoms; the skin changes varied from burns, traumatic lesions and a few vesicles to a widespread erythemato-papular eruption on the limbs, face and neck. Epoxy resin was the commonest allergen, 36 of 66 (54 per cent) patch tested being sensitive. They found that showering did not remove the glass fibres from the skin.

St John's

Patients with fibre glass dermatitis are rarely seen. A coach builder complained that, for three months, fibre glass at work had caused irritation of his neck, arms and legs. A papule on his arm was biopsied but glass was not seen in the sections.

Rockwool

Rockwool is a similar fibrous glass wool made from a mineral, coke and lime-stone, compounded with a mineral oil, a silicone compound and a phenolformal-dehyde resin. Patch test reactions with this material, although caused by mechanical irritation, simulate in appearance allergic responses (Björnberg and Löwhagen, 1975).

Fire retardants

The ease and rate with which objects burn is very variable. Flame retardants increase fire resistance in one of two ways. In one the solid is altered to make it less flammable, so that the article chars rather than burns; phosphates and phosphonium compounds act in this way. In the second the gases which are emitted and burn are extinguished; antimony chloride acts by forming a dense vapour which will not burn.

Domestic textiles

Phosphorus and phosphonium compounds

The flammability of cotton fabrics is reduced by phosphorus based compounds (Pyrovatex, Ciba-Geigy; Proban, Albright and Wilson). The treatment is limited because it is expensive. Proban is a polymer produced by cross-linking the condensate of tetrakis (hydroxymethyl) phosphonium chloride (THPC) and urea with ammonia followed by oxidation to convert the trivalent phosphorus to the pentavalent form. This finish has been used in the U.K. for children's night-dresses for about fifteen years. It is effective on cotton materials but is limited with blends of cotton and synthetic fibres. It gives a soft feel to the fabric, gives more body to the material and the colour is maintained but it makes the material more friable. However, the domestic market for fire retardant treated fabric is small compared to its use in industrial and instituitional areas.

In 1964, legislation was introduced requiring that children's nightdresses pass tests for low flammability; pyjamas and fabrics which might be used to make nightdresses were not controlled. Proban is used to treat cotton winceyette, a very common nightdress material. Brushed nylon does not require a flame retardant and has replaced winceyette in the U.K. market.

Dermatitis — case reports: Two children have been described, one of whom developed eczema and the other urticaria, while wearing Proban-treated night-dresses. Both reacted to patch tests with the treated fabric but neither was tested with the phosphonium salt. A hundred control children with eczema gave negative reactions when patch tested with this material (Martin-Scott, 1966).

Tris(2,3-dibromopropyl)phosphate (Firemaster LVT 23P)
Tris(2,3-dibromopropyl)phosphate (TDB P), a phosphate ester, is used in clothing and furnishing fabrics for its flame retardant properties. In 1976 the International Contact Dermatitis Research Group added TDB P 5 per cent in petrolatum to their standard series and two of 1103 (0.2 per cent) routine patients reacted. One was a chemical worker with dermatitis from a fire protective suit and the second was a woman with spectacle frame dermatitis. These frames did not contain TDB P but another phosphate ester and it was assumed to be the primary sensitiser (Andersen, 1977).

In the United States Tris has been used to treat children's nightwear made of polyester and acetate but since being shown to cause neoplasms of the kidney in rats its use in wearing apparel is likely to be universally banned.

Industrial textiles
Industrial overalls, tarpaulins and similar fabrics may be treated with antimony oxide and a chlorinated compound. Timonox (Associated Lead Manufacturers Limited) is such an emulsion. Antimony chloride cannot be applied directly to the fabric as it releases hydrochloric acid which damages the material.

The cotton lining of uniforms for military firemen may be treated in this way, as were uniforms for use in the Vietnam war. The cotton linings are treated, not the outer woollen fabric, as wool has an innate fire resistance. Proban is also extensively used for treatment of cotton uniforms and linings.

Fluorescent whitening agents

The whitening of fabrics has been thought desirable since pre-historic times. Bleaches are effective but they damage the fibres, and blueing with dyes, though it masks the natural yellow colour, gives a dull finish. In the 1930s, the industrial development of fluorescent whitening agents began, and they now total 10 per cent of the dyes manufactured (Furvick, 1973). Fluorescent whitening agents (FWAs) absorb ultraviolet light and emit instead visible light in the blue region of the spectrum. Materials appear whiter than white and, as more visible light is emitted than received, the fabric has a brilliant quality. These whiteners cause fabrics to glow in ultraviolet light.

At a symposium on fluorescent whitening agents held in Stockholm in 1973, Gold listed their six basic structures as (i) stilbene, (ii) coumarin and carbostyril, (iii) diphenylpyrazoline, (iv) naphthalic acid imide, (v) combinations of benzoxazole with ethylene structures and aromatics and (vi) compounds built from hetero-aromatics, and ethylene or aromatics, or both. Because different brighteners bind to natural and to synthetic fibres, several are present in most detergents. The majority are stilbene derivatives.

The world production, about 30 million kilograms each year, is used in the following ways: in detergents 58 per cent, by the paper industry 25 per cent, in textile finishing 12 per cent, and in plastics and other materials 5 per cent (Furvick, 1973).

Fluorescent whiteners disguise the yellowing of a fabric; they do not hide

dirt. In common with dyes, they have an affinity for textile fibres and are relatively fast to washing. They are applied as a textile finish but some loss occurs
during laundering and wear; the whiteners in detergents replace this loss and
maintain the whiteness and brilliance of a fabric (Carter, 1973).

DERMATITIS

Fluorescent whitening agents in detergents have caused a limited amount of
dermatitis among consumers. They have not been reported as causing trouble in
industry.

Photosensitivity

In 1957, Burckhardt reported two isolated cases of allergic photosensitivity
caused by blankophores or whitening agents in detergents. In both, their skin
was treated with the detergents then irradiated with light; each gave an
eczematous response. Re-exposure to the detergent caused a relapse and, though
one patient recovered, one remained light sensitive. The responsible whitener
was not identified. The absence of other cases was probably due to this whitener
having had a localised and limited sale in Switzerland.

There is no evidence that other fluorescent whiteners have caused photodermatitis in man (Calnan, 1973) nor have they been found to be phototoxic in
hairless mice (Forbes and Urbach, 1975).

Textile dermatitis

The fluorescent whiteners in detergents have caused localised 'epidemics' of textile dermatitis in Copenhagen and Barcelona. They have not caused dermatitis
of the hands in housewives.

Osmundsen recognised the condition in 1969 (Osmundsen, 1969) and in that
year, the whitener was the commonest contact allergen in Denmark. In 16
months, 167 patients of both sexes were seen at the Finsen Institute (Osmundsen, 1973) and 103 patients were diagnosed in Barcelona (Piñol Aguadé et al.,
1971).

The diagnosis was easily missed until the characteristics of the eruption were
defined. Itching, particularly at night, was a marked feature. The distribution
was that of a textile dermatitis, the sites of predilection being the inner part of
the upper arms, axillary borders, flexor forearms, neck, trunk and thighs. In
some of the Spanish patients seborrhoeic eczema was simulated. The skin
changes were sometimes so slight as to be overlooked, and the patients were
classified as having 'pruritus'. Typical lesions were faint red macules with a
finely wrinkled surface which joined to form a reticulate pattern. Petechiae and
infiltration occurred in some patients, and those severely affected had a widespread eczema (Osmundsen, 1969).

Pigmented contact dermatitis

An extraordinary pigmentation occurred in nearly half of the Spanish patients
and in nine of the 167 Danish patients. It affected not only the sites of dermatitis but also the cheeks and earlobes. In some of the Danish patients, the

pigmentation was preceded by eczema, but in others pigmentation was their only symptom; they were described as dark complexioned Caucasians who tanned easily. Biopsies showed pigmentary incontinence (Osmundsen, 1970).

This observation means that a contact dermatitis can present as pigmentation only.

Patch testing

Denmark
All 167 patients, including those who had pigmentation, reacted to the whitener Tinopal CH 3566, 0.1 per cent or 1 per cent in soft paraffin. Benzyl salicylate 5 per cent, an ingredient of soap perfumes (Rothenborg and Hjorth, 1968), elicited a reaction in 16 of 88 patients tested. Thirteen patients were tested with nylon washed with the detergent: seven reacted and six did not (Osmundsen, 1973).

The brightener was added to the routine series of patch tests and seven more cases were diagnosed (Osmundsen, 1969).

Spain
A pyrazoline whitener was the most frequent sensitiser; of 103 patients tested, 83 (80 per cent) reacted to 10 per cent, and 69 (67 per cent) to 1 per cent. Five stilbene whiteners, in a concentration of 1 per cent, were used for patch testing more than half of these patients; a few reacted (Piñol Aguadé *et al.*, 1971).

The sensitiser
Tinopal is a trade name for several fluorescent whiteners of differing chemical structures. Tinopal CH 3566 is a mixture of two pyrazolines:

1 CPY = the monochlorodiphenylpyrazoline

1 CPY = the monochlorodiphenylpyrazoline 1-(3-chlorphenyl)-3-phenyl-pyrazoline

2 CPY = the dichlorodiphenylpyrazoline 1-(3-chlorphenyl)-3-(4-chlorphenyl)-pyrazoline

It was added to the detergent for whitening nylon.

The Danish patients were tested with a series of pyrazoline derivatives 1 per cent in soft paraffin; of 64 tested, 60 reacted to the monochloropyrazoline and 63 to the dichloropyrazoline.

Cross-reactions were blocked by an ethyl group in the 4 position in the pyrazoline ring and by substitutions in the *para* position in the 1-benzyl ring (Osmundsen and Alani, 1971).

Sensitising potential

The manufacturers, using the Shelanski-Shelanski repeated insult human patch test, had failed to detect the brightener as a sensitiser, whereas Osmundsen and Alani (1971) sensitised 16 of 20 guinea-pigs to the commercial brightener by using the maximisation test and thereby graded it as a strong sensitiser. In defence of industry, Philp (1971) reported that the brightener had been identified as an allergen by the Draize test.

Prognosis

It took 2–3 weeks for the dermatitis to improve once obvious contact with Tinopal CH 3566 ceased; this probably was the time required for the whitener to be washed out of clothes. The pigmentation may persist for years.

The whitener was withdrawn from the Danish market and the 'epidemic' ceased.

Other countries

Exposure to Tinopal CH 3566 must have been limited because outbreaks of dermatitis were not reported elsewhere. It is not marketed in Great Britain, or in the U.S.A. (Osmundsen, 1972).

Rigorous predictive patch testing by industry ensures that, in general, allergenic fluorescers are discarded (Griffith, 1973).

St John's

Many patients with light sensitive eruptions and with textile dermatitis have been investigated in the Contact Clinic, but in none has a fluorescer been identified as an allergen.

A series of 200 consecutive patients were tested with three stilbene and two pyrazoline derivatives, each 2 per cent in petrolatum; all the tests were negative. Tinopal CH 3566 was not included in this study (Calnan, 1973).

Carcinogenicity and toxicity

A coumarin and two stilbene whiteners were shown by Bingham and Falk (1970) to increase the action of ultraviolet radiation in producing cutaneous carcinomas in mice. However, in similar studies on hairless mice Forbes and Urbach (1975) found no evidence that the brighteners which they used were either phototoxic or capable of enhancing photocarcinogenesis. The data on the toxicity of FWA's used in soaps, detergents and textiles has been reviewed by Gloxhuber and Bloching (1978) and they concluded that, with some exceptions, they are a safe group of compounds.

Preservatives in textiles

Germicidal chemicals are added to textiles to prevent odour, rotting and mildew.

Cotton, silk and synthetic fibres: Quaternary ammonium compounds, dichlorophen (particularly for acrylics) and phenyl mercuric compounds, which have been used in nylon shirts.

Wool: Dichlorophen, pentachlorophenol and pentachlorophenyl laurate prevent mildew during storage. Most of the chemical is removed during wet processing but residues may remain in the finished material.

Shoe linings: Pentachlorophenyl laurate is replacing phenyl mercuric acetate.

Protective clothing: Tributyltin oxide, dichlorophen and pentachlorophenyl derivatives.

Industrial fabrics, including tents and tarpaulins: Sodium salicylanilide has been used as an anti-mildew agent; copper and zinc naphthenate, hydroxyquinolates, pentachlorophenol and derivatives.

Dermatitis

Tributyltin oxide
A solution containing 0.5 per cent tributyltin oxide (TBTO) and 2.5 per cent of a quarternary ammonium compound was used during laundering to disinfect soldiers' socks. One summer it was mistakenly added in too high a concentration so that prior to drying, the water in the socks contained 0.01 per cent TBTO instead of the usual 0.001 per cent. This batch of socks caused an acute dermatitis of the feet in 70 young soldiers, who had worn them for long marches during hot weather. Patch tests with TBTO 0.01 per cent and 0.001 per cent (aqueous) and the quaternary ammonium compound were negative in the 14 men tested confirming that the TBTO had acted as an irritant (Molin and Wahlberg, 1975).

MOTH PROOFING

Clothes moths and carpet beetles cause much damage to clothing, carpets and upholstery. To protect against them the following chemicals are used:

Sodium fluosilicate and DDT (dichlorodiphenyltrichloroethane)
Dieldrin is less frequently used for textiles but is still applied to carpet and upholstery yarns
Eulan: chloro-bis-(dichloro-hydroxyphenyl)-*o*-toluene sulphonic acid.
Mitin FF: dichlorophenyl-(chlorophenoxy-sulphonic acid)-chlorophenyl urea.

Fumigants for use in confined spaces are *para*-dichlorobenzene and naphthalene.

Textile fibres

Textile fibres themselves are extremely rare sensitisers. One report incriminated virgin nylon as the cause of a dermatitis provoked by nylon stockings and a nylon blouse. Patch tests with virgin nylon were positive (Morris, 1960). Another woman reported by Rudzki (1977) developed urticaria every time she wore silk; she had first noticed it when she was seven years old and at the age of 56 years a piece of silk wrapped round her arm elicited contact urticaria.

Occupational dermatitis
Factory workers may develop an irritant dermatitis from fibres of various kinds.

Nylon factories
Caprolactam, from which nylon is made, is a hygroscopic, fat soluble and irritant compound. Elizarov (1959) found that many men working with it in Russia developed dermatitis of the finger tips, hands and arms, which had a tendency to become secondarily infected and sometimes spread to the body. Workers in a Rumanian nylon factory were similarly found to develop not only dry palms and hand eczema but also oil folliculitis (Nastase and Munteanu, 1964). Caprolactam, being hygroscopic, was thought to have caused the dryness, peeling and fissuring of the palms; the polyamide polymer had the same effect. Rubber gloves and an emollient cream were effective prophylactically. In a special section of the factory, where fibre extension and reeling were carried out, oil was used for greasing the fibres and caused dermatitis in 19 of the workers. The emulsifier was thought to be responsible. In the same section, 30 women developed oil folliculitis.

Methylol chloroacetamide in a nylon spin finish has caused dermatitis (p. 699).

Cotton mill
A fibre called Bokomake caused dermatitis in 136 of 853 women working in a Japanese cotton mill. The cotton fibres, which pervaded the atmosphere, settled on exposed skin and by pricking caused itchy, red papules on the hands, arms and neck. Patch tests were negative. Rubber gloves prevented the lesions and the skin healed while the women remained at work (Matsuo and Imamura, 1964).

Fishing nets
In Polish fishing net factories, women developed callosities on their fourth and fifth fingers due to friction from the coarse hemp, sisal and nylon fibres. Jellyfish sticking to the nets also caused dermatitis (Schwann, 1963).

Cancer of the mouth and pharynx in textile workers
There is an increased incidence of oral and pharyngeal cancers in male textile workers, except for those who are weavers or knitters. The amount of dust exposure is significant and fibre preparing, which is a dusty job, carries the greatest risk (Moss and Lee, 1974).

Textile purpura

Toxic

During the 1939–1945 World War hundreds of British soldiers developed a purpuric eruption from wearing woollen khaki shirts. The dermatitis consisted of papules, areas of erythema, scaly patches and a striking purpura, accentuated at sites of pressure and friction. At its onset, the rash was often symptomless and was confined to the shirt area. In some cases it cleared rapidly, in others the purpuric papules spread, particularly to the feet and ankles and in yet other cases, the soldiers required weeks of hospital treatment (Hodgson and Hellier, 1946; Grant Peterkin, 1946).

The cause was not determined. Patch tests were unhelpful, DDT was exonerated (Hodgson and Hellier, 1946; Grant Peterkin, 1946), and it was postulated that an unknown toxic chemical impregnating the woollen fabric was responsible.

Pressure

Petechiae are sometimes produced on men's skin by vests made of a lattice pattern of small perforations. The fine purpuric dots are often linear; they occur particularly over the scapulae, below the axillae and at sites of pressure. Patients are unaware of these marks. In one man, scrutinised in the Contact Clinic at St John's, the purpura appeared to be under the threads but not under the holes of his string vest.

In Rhodesia, this type of cellular vest has caused petechiae in children. Pressure from the sharp edges of the perforations was thought to be the cause (Kibel, 1965).

Stockings

One summer in the London area a curious, transient, purpuric eruption occurred on the legs of female traffic wardens. Allergy to black nylon stockings was excluded, and the cause remained obscure; prolonged standing in hot weather was thought to be significant (Marks and Savin, 1968). Although it was not suggested by these authors, the pressure of a slightly coarse regulation stocking on mildly oedematous legs may have been a factor.

RUBBER PURPURA

Sensitisation

Sensitivity to the rubber antioxidant isopropylaminodiphenylamine has caused purpura. In Bulgaria this chemical was used in elastic for underclothes and caused allergic contact dermatitis. In some patients the eczema was purpuric, and in nine women a secondary purpuric eruption appeared on the shoulders, chest, back, buttocks and thighs. Purpuric streaks occurred from pressure. In three patients positive patch tests intensified the purpura. The capillary fragility was thought to be due to the absorption of the rubber chemical (Batschvarov and Minkov, 1968).

St John's

Two men were sensitised by isopropylaminodiphenylamine in their rubber boots. Their eczema was purpuric, and both developed a widespread purpura (Calnan and Peachey, 1971).

References

Abel, R.R. (1966) Washing machine and fibreglass. *Archives of Dermatology*, **93**, 78.

Acheson, E.D., Cowdell, R.H. & Jolles, B. (1970) Nasal cancer in the Northamptonshire boot and shoe industry. *British Medical Journal*, **i**, 385.

Adams, R.M. (1972) Shoe dermatitis. *California Medicine*. **117**, 12.

Ancona-Alayón, A., Escobar-Márques, R., González-Mendoza, A., Bernal-Tapia, J.A., Macotela-Ruíz, E. & Jurado-Mendoza, J. (1976) Occupational pigmented contact dermatitis from Naphthol AS. *Contact Dermatitis*, **2**, 129.

Andersen, K.E. (1977) Sensitivity to a flame retardant, Tris(2,3-dibromopropyl)phosphate (Firemaster LVT 23 P). *Contact Dermatitis*, **3**, 297.

Antoniev, A.A. & Vilchinsky, M.P. (1972) Occupational skin disease in workers engaged in the production of glass-fibre reinforced plastics. *Klinicheskaya Meditsina (Moscow)*, **50**, 111.

Batschvarov, B. & Minkov, D.M. (1968) Dermatitis and purpura from rubber in clothing. *Transactions of the St John's Hospital Dermatological Society*, **54**, 178.

Berrens, L., Young, E. & Jansen, L.H. (1964) Free formaldehyde in textiles in relation to formalin contact sensitivity. *British Journal of Dermatology*, **76**, 110.

Bett, D.C.G. (1958) The potassium dichromate patch test. *Transactions of the St John's Hospital Dermatological Society*, **40**, 41.

Bingham, E. & Falk, H.L. (1970) Combined action of optical brightners and ultraviolet light in the production of tumours. *Food and Cosmetic Toxicology*, **8**, 173.

Birmingham, D.J. & Weber, L.F. (1966) Dermatitis from formaldehyde resins — discussion. *Archives of Dermatology*, **94**, 800.

Björnberg, A. & Löwhagen, G-B. (1975) Patch test reactions to rockwool. *Contact Dermatitis*, **1**, 242.

Björnberg, A., Lowhagen, G-B & Tengberg, J.E. (1979) Skin reactivity in workers with and without itching from occupational exposure to glass fibres. *Acta Dermato-venereologica*, **59**, 49.

Blohm, S.G. (1959) Formaldehyde contact dermatitis. 1. A simple method for determination of small amounts of formaldehyde. *Acta Dermato-venereologica*, **39**, 450.

Buiatti, E., Cecchini, S., Ronchi, O., Dolara, P. & Bulgarelli, G. (1978) Relationship between clinical and electromyographic findings and exposure to solvents, in shoe and leather workers. *British Journal of Industrial Medicine*, **35**, 168.

Bulikowski, W. & Tyras, H. (1976) Dermatological evaluation of occupational exposure of tanners to chromium compounds. *Berufsdermatosen*, **24**, 132.

Burckhardt, W. (1957) Photoallergische Ekzeme durch Blankophore (optische Aufheller). *Hautarzt*, **8**, 486.

Burry, J.N., Kirk, J., Reid, J.G. & Turner, T. (1973) Environmental dermatitis: patch tests in 1000 cases of allergic contact dermatitis. *Medical Journal of Australia*, **2**, 681.

Calnan, C.D. (1973) Dermatitis from optic bleachers in detergents MVC-Report 2. *Fluorescent Whitening Agents*, p. 99. NFR Swedish Natural Science Research Council.

Calnan, C.D. (1973) Hazards of optic bleaches. *Transactions of the St John's Hospital Dermatological Society*, **59**, 275.

Calnan, C.D. (1977) Textile dye Disperse Yellow 64. *Contact Dermatitis*, **3**, 209.

Calnan, C.D. & Cronin, E. (1978) Vegetable tans in leather. *Contact Dermatitis*, **5**, 295.

Calnan, C.D., Marten, R.H. & Wilson, H.T.H. (1958) Nylon hair-net dermatitis. *British Medical Journal*, **ii**, 544.

Calnan, C.D. & Peachey, R.D.G. (1971) Allergic contact purpura. *Clinical Allergy*, **1**, 287.

Calnan, C.D. & Wilson, H.T.H. (1956) Nylon stocking dermatitis. *British Medical Journal*, **i**, 147.

Calnan, C.D. & Sarkany, I. (1959) Studies in contact dermatitis. IX. Shoe dermatitis. *Transactions of the St John's Hospital Dermatological Society*, **43**, 8.

Carter, P. (1973) Fluorescent whitening agents for the soap and detergent industry. MVC-Report 2. *Fluorescent Whitening Agents*, p. 51. NFR Swedish Natural Science Research Council.

Cronin, E. (1963) Formalin textile dermatitis. *British Journal of Dermatology*, **75**, 267.

Cronin, E. (1966) Shoe dermatitis. *British Journal of Dermatology*, **78**, 617.

Cronin, E. (1968) Studies in contact dermatitis: XVIII. Dyes in clothing. *Transactions of the St John's Hospital Dermatological Society*, 54, 156.

Cronin, E. (1968) Studies in contact dermatitis: XIX. Nylon stocking dyes. *Transactions of the St John's Hospital Dermatological Society*, 54, 165.

Crow, K.D. (1967) Contact dermatitis from Nonox ZA. *Contact Dermatitis Newsletter*, 2, 12.

Cuypers, J.M.C., Bleumink, E. & Nater, J.P. (1975) Dermatologische Aspekte der Glasfaserfabrikation (1). *Berufsdermatosen*, 23, 143.

Cuypers, J.M.C., Hoedemaeker, Ph. J., Nater, J.P. & Jong, de M.C.J.M. (1975) The histopathology of fibreglass dermatitis in relation to von Hebra's concept of eczema. *Contact Dermatitis*, 1, 88.

Cywie, P.L., Herve-Bazin, B., Foussereau, J., Cavelier, C. & Coirier, A. (1977) Les eczemas allergiques professionnels dans L'industrie textile. Rapport No 244/RI, No ISSN 0397-4529, *Institut National De Recherche et De Securite*. Vandoeuvre; France: Centre de Recherche.

Dahl, M.V. (1975) Allergic contact dermatitis from footwear. *Minnesota Medicine*, 58, 871.

Dobkevitch, S. & Baer, R. (1947) Eczematous cross-hypersensitivity to azodyes in nylon stockings and to paraphenylenediamine. *Journal of Investigative Dermatology*, 9, 203.

Dyro, F.M. (1978) Methyl ethyl ketone polyneuropathy in shoe factory workers. *Clinical Toxicology*, 13, 371.

Ebner, H. (1967) Chromatkontaktallergie als ursache von Bekleidungsekzemen. *Dermatologica*, 135, 355.

Ebner, H. (1975) Kontaktekzeme durch Kleidung. *Hautarzt*, 26, 72.

Eby, C.S. & Jetton, R.L. (1972) School desk dermatitis. *Archives of Dermatology*, 105, 890.

Elizarov, G.P. (1959) Klinik, Prophylaxe und Therapie der Kaprolaktam Dermatitis. Gigiena truda i professional nýe zabôlevaniya. *Moskva*, 3, 20 (Summary Berufsdermatosen (1960) 8, 233).

Epstein, E. (1969) Shoe contact dermatitis. *Journal of the American Medical Association*, 209, 1487.

Epstein, E. & Maibach, H.I. (1966) Formaldehyde allergy. *Archives of Dermatology*, 94, 186.

Eskelson, Y.D. & Goodman, L.S. (1963) Contact dermatitis from 'Scotchgard', a stain repellant for fabrics. *Journal of the American Medical Association*, 183, 136.

Fisher, A.A. (1973a) *Contact Dermatitis*. 2nd ed. pp. 157, 159, 160 Philadelphia: Lea and Febiger.

Fisher, A.A. (1973b) Prevention of shoe dermatitis by controlling hyperhidrosis with tannic acid. *Cutis*, 12, 493.

Fisher, A.A., Kanof, N.B. & Biondi, E.M. (1962) Free formaldehyde in textiles and paper. *Archives of Dermatology*, 86, 753.

Fisher, B.K. & Warkentin, J.D. (1969) Fibre Glass Dermatitis. *Archives of Dermatology*, 99, 717.

Forbes, P.D. & Urbach, F. (1975) Experimental modification of photocarcinogenesis. 1. Fluorescent whitening agents and short UVR. 2. Fluorescent whitening agents and simulated solar UVR. 3. Simulation of exposure to sunlight and fluorescent whitening agents. *Food and Cosmetic Toxicology*, 13, 335, 339, 343.

Foussereau, J., Benezra, Cl. & Ourisson, G. (1967) Contact dermatitis from laurel. I. Clinical aspects. *Transactions of the St John's Hospital Dermatological Society*, 53, 141.

Foussereau, J., Sengel, D., Tanahashi, Y., Limam-Mestiri, S. & Malleville, J. (1971) L'allergie au disperse yellow 3 de colorants vestimentaires (bas et chaussettes). *Bulletin de la Société Francaise de Dermatologie et de Syphiligraphy*, 78, 70.

Foussereau, J., Tanahaski, Y., Grosshans, E., Liman-Mestiri, S. & Khochnevis, A. (1972). Allergic eczema from disperse yellow 3 in nylon stockings and socks. *Transactions of the St John's Hospital Dermatological Society*, 58, 75.

Fregert, S. (1964) Extraction of allergens for patch testing. *Acta Dermato-venereologica*, 44, 107.

Fregert, S. & Gruvberger, B. (1970) Chromium in leather. *Contact Dermatitis Newsletter*, 8, 174.

Fregert, S., Gruvberger, B., Göransson, K. & Normark, S. (1978) Allergic contact dermatitis from chromate in military textiles. *Contact Dermatitis*, 4, 223.

Fregert, S., Hjorth, N., Magnusson, B., Bandmann, H-J., Calnan, C.D., Cronin, E., Malten, K., Meneghini, C.L., Pirilä, V., & Wilkinson, D.S. (1969) Epidemiology of contact dermatitis. *Transactions of the St John's Hospital Dermatological Society*, 55, 17.

Fregert, S. & Tegner, E. (1971) Non-iron agents. *Contact Dermatitis Newsletter*, 9, 200.

Furvik, N.B. (1973) Fluorescent whitening agents in textile industry. MCV-Report 2. *Fluorescent Whitening Agents*, p. 43. NFR Swedish Natural Science Research Council.

Gardiner, J.S., Dickson, A., MacLeod, T.M. & Frain-Bell, W. (1971). The investigation of photocontact dermatitis in a dye manufacturing process. *British Journal of Dermatology*, 86, 264.

Gibbs, F.W. (1961) *Organic Chemistry Today*. Harmondsworth. Penguin Books Limited.

Gloxhuber, Ch. & Bloching, H. (1978) Toxicologic properties of fluorescent whitening agents. *Clinical Toxicology*, 13, 171.

Gold, H. (1973) The chemistry of the major structures of fluorescent whitening agents. MVC-Report 2. *Fluorescent Whitening Agents*, p. 23. NFR Swedish Natural Science Research Council.

Grant Peterkin, G.A. (1946) Purpuric type of contact dermatitis. *British Medical Journal*, i, 106.

Griffith, J.F. (1973) Fluorescent whitening agents: Tests for skin sensitising potential. *Archives of Dermatology*, 107, 728.

Grimalt, F. & Romaguera, C. (1975) New resin allergens in shoe contact dermatitis. *Contact Dermatitis*, 1, 169.

Grimalt, F., Romaguera, C. & Piñol Aguadé, J. (1976) Dermatitis de contacto por bolsillos de plástico de pantalones. *Medicina Cutanea I.L.A.*, 4, 7.

Hegyi, E. & Šaršunová, M. (1974) Experimental investigation of the dermatotropic effect of insole materials containing chemicals used in the rubber industry. *Československá dermatologie*, 49, 103.

Heisel, E.B. & Hunt, F.E. (1968) Further studies in cutaneous reactions to glass fibres. *Archives of Environmental Health*, 17, 705.

Hellier, F.F. (1958) Skin hazards in the wool textile industry. *Occupational Allergy*, p. 81. H.E. Stenfert Kroese N.V.-Leiden, Holland.

Herve-Bazin, B., Foussereau, J. & Cavelier, C. (1977) L'eczéma allergique au support de pigments textiles. *Berufsdermatosen*, 25, 113.

Hindson, T.C. (1969) Chrome leather dermatitis in Singapore. *Contact Dermatitis Newsletter*, 6, 120.

Hjorth, N. & Möller, H. (1976) Phototoxic textile dermatitis ('bikini dermatitis'). *Archives of Dermatology*, 112, 1445.

Hjorth, N. & Rothenborg, H.W. (1967) Zur Häufigkeit der Nylonstrumpfekzeme. *Zeitschrift für Haut und Geschlechtskrankheiten*, 42, 717.

Hodgson, G.A. & Hellier, F.F. (1946) Dermatitis caused by shirts in B.L.A. *Journal of the Royal Army Medical Corps*, 87, 110.

Høvding, G. (1959) Free formaldehyde in textiles. *Acta Dermato-venereológica*, 39, 357.

Høvding, G. (1961) Contact eczema due to formaldehyde in resin finished textiles. *Acta Dermato-venereologica*, 41, 194.

Jirásek, L., Kalenský, J. & Sevcová, M. (1975) Gumové holinky-přičina profesionálního eczému. Alergogenni a kapilarotoxické působeni Antioxidantu 4010NA. *Československá Dermatologie*, 50, 303.

Jordan, W.P. (1972) Clothing and shoe dermatitis. *Postgraduate Medicine*, 52, 143.

Jordan, W.P., Dahl, M.V. & Albert, H.L. (1972) Contact dermatitis from glutaraldehyde. *Archives of Dermatology*, 105, 94.

Kachlik, Z. (1968) Hromadný výskyt profesionálnich kóznich onemocněni v konfekčnim závodě přizpracováni látek nemačkavé úpravy. *Pracovni Lékařstvi*, 20, 154.

Kibel, M.A. (1965) Petichiae from vests. *British Medical Journal*, ii, 521.

Leblanc, R.B. (1968) Flammability and fire resistance of textiles. *American Dyestuff Reporter*, 57, 35.

Lechner, W. & Hartmann, A.A. (1979) Glass fibre-induced foreign body granulomas. *Hautarzt*, 30, 100.

Leppard, B.J. & Parhizgar, B. (1977) Contact dermatitis to PPD rubber in Maleki shoes. *Contact Dermatitis*, 3, 91.

Loewenthal, L.J.A., Levy, S.J. & Hins, S. (1968) Rubber dermatitis in the gold-mining industry. *South African Medical Journal*, 42, 1327.

Lynch, P.J. & Rudolph, A.J. (1969) Indian sandal strap dermatitis. *Journal of the American Medical Association*, 209, 1906.

Madoff, M.A. (1962) Dermatitis associated with fibrous glass material. *Tufts Folia Medical*, 8, 100.

Maibach, H. (1975) Panty hose dermatitis resembling and complicating tinea pedis. *Contact Dermatitis*, 1, 329.

Malten, K.E. (1957) Eczema in a cotton-printing mill. *Acta Dermato-venereologica*. Proceedings of the XI International Congress of Dermatology, Vol. 2, 353.

Malten, K.E. (1964) Textile finish contact hypersensitivity. *Archives of Dermatology*, 89, 215.

Marcussen, P.V. (1959) Contact dermatitis due to formaldehyde in textiles, 1934–1958. *Acta Dermato-venereologica*, 39, 348.

Marcussen, P.V. (1962) Dermatitis caused by formaldehyde resins in textiles. *Dermatologica*, 125, 101.

Marks, R. & Savin, J.A. (1968) Purpuric dermatosis of female traffic wardens. *Transactions of the St John's Hospital Dermatological Society*, 54, 183.

Martin-Scott, I. (1966) Contact textile dermatitis (with special reference to fire proof fabrics). *British Journal of Dermatology*, 78, 632.

Matsuo, T. & Imamura, S. (1964) An observation on cotton fibre dermatitis called 'Bokomake'. *Acta Dermatologica (Kyoto)*. 59, 114.

Meneghini, C. (1971) Lichenoid contact dermatitis. *Contact Dermatitis Newsletter*, 9, 194.

Minkin, W., Cohen, H.J. & Frank, S.B. (1971) Contact dermatitis to East Indian leather. *Archives of Dermatology*, 103, 522.

Mitchell, J.C. (1972) Allergic contact dermatitis from a certified food dye presenting as 'sock dermatitis'. *Contact Dermatitis Newsletter*, 11, 247.

Mitchell, J.C. (1967) Personal communication.

Molin, L. & Wahlberg, J.E. (1975) Toxic skin reactions caused by tributyltin oxide (TBTO) in socks. *Berufsdermatosen*, 23, 138.

Morris, G.E. (1960) Nylon dermatitis. *New England Journal of Medicine*, 263, 30.

Moss, E. & Lee, W.R. (1974) Occurrence of oral and pharyngeal cancers in textile workers. *British Journal of Industrial Medicine*, 31, 224.

Nastase, G. & Munteanu, M. (1963–1964) Occupational diseases of the skin. *Australian Journal of Dermatology*, 7, 153.

Neering, H. & van Dijk, E. (1978) Juvenile plantar dermatosis. *Acta Dermato-venereologica*, 58, 531.

Neilson, A.W. & Reiches, A.J. (1941) Contact dermatitis due to underwear. *Archives of Dermatology*, 44, 218.

Newhouse, M.L. (1974) Dermatitis in a clothing factory. *Contact Dermatitis Newsletter*, 16, 478.

North American Contact Dermatitis Group (1973) Epidemiology of contact dermatitis in North America: 1972. *Archives of Dermatology*, 108, 537.

Novák, M. & Schwank, R. (1976) Contact dermatitis caused by sweat bands. *Ceskoslovenská Dermatologie*, 51, 31.

O'Quinn, S.E. & Kennedy, C.B. (1965) Contact dermatitis due to formaldehyde in clothing textiles. *Journal of the American Medical Association*, 194, 593.

Osmundsen, P.E. (1969) Contact dermatitis due to an optical whitener in washing powders. *British Journal of Dermatology*, 81, 799.

Osmundsen, P.E. (1970) Pigmented contact dermatitis. *British Journal of Dermatology*, 83, 296.

Osmundsen, P.E. (1972) Contact dermatitis from an optical whitener in washing powders. *Cutis*, 10, 59.

Osmundsen, P.E. (1973) Contact dermatitis due to an optical whitener in washing powders. MCV-Report 2. *Fluorescent Whitening Agents*, p. 69. NFR Swedish Natural Science Research Council.

Osmundsen, P.E. & Alani, M.D. (1971) Contact allergy to an optical whitener, 'CPY', in washing powders. *British Journal of Dermatology*, 85, 61.

Panaccio, F., Montgomery, D.C. & Adam, J.E. (1973) Follicular contact dermatitis due to coloured permanent-pressed sheets. *Canadian Medical Association Journal*, 109, 23.

Peachey, R.D.G. (1967) Glass fibre itch: A modern washday hazard. *British Medical Journal*, ii, 211.

Philp, J. McL. (1971) Contact allergy to an optical whitener. *British Journal of Dermatology*, 85, 495.

Pinol Aguadé, J., Grimalt, F., Romaguera, C., Mascaro, J.M. & Cisneros, J.L. (1971) Dermitis por blanqueadores ópticos. *Medicina Cutánea*, 5, 249.

Roberts, J.L. & Hanifin, J.M. (1979) Athletic shoe dermatitis. *Journal of the American Medical Association*, 241, 275.

Romaguera Sagrera, C., Grimalt Sancho, F. & Piñol Aguadé, J. (1974) Nuevos alergenos, pertenecientes al grupo de las resinas, en la dermatitis de contacto al calzado. Medicina Cutanea. *Ibero-Latino-Americana*, 11, 201.

Ross, J.B. (1969) Rubber boot dermatitis in Newfoundland: A survey of 30 patients. *Canadian Medical Association Journal*, 100, 13.

Roth, W.G. (1969) Tylotisches Ekzem der Palmae und Plantae durch Dunsten Formalinhaltiger Kleidung. *Berufsdermatosen*, 17, 263.

Rothenborg, H.W. & Hjorth, N. (1968) Allergy to perfumes from toilet soaps and detergents in patients with dermatitis. *Archives of Dermatology*, 97, 417.

Rothenborg, H.W. & Hjorth, N. (1971) Indian sandal dermatitis. *Ugeskrift fer Laeger*, 133, 802.

Rudzki, E. (1977) Contact urticaria from silk. *Contact Dermatitis*, 3, 53.

Rycroft, R.J.G., Cronin, E. and Calnan, C.D. (1976) Canadian sheet dermatitis. *British Medical Journal*, ii, 1175.

Samitz, M.H. & Gross, S. (1960) Extraction by sweat of chromium from chrome tanned leathers. *Journal of Occupational Medicine*, 2, 12.

Samitz, M.H., Katz, S. & Gross, S. (1960) Nature of the chromium extracted from leather by sweat. *Journal of Occupational Medicine*, 2, 435.

Schorr, W.F., Keran, E. & Plotka, E. (1974) Formaldehyde allergy: The quantitative analysis of American clothing for free formaldehyde and its relevance in clinical practice. *Archives of Dermatology*, 110, 73.

Schwann, J. (1963) Berufsstigmata und Dermatitiden bei der Herstellung von Fischnetzen. *Berufsdermatosen*, 11, 8.

Scutt, R.W.B. (1966) Chrome sensitivity associated with tropical footwear in the Royal Navy. *British Journal of Dermatology*, 78, 337.

Shellow, H. & Altman, A.T. (1966) Dermatitis from formaldehyde resin textiles. *Archives of Dermatology*, **94**, 799.

Shrank, A.B. (1979) The aetiology of juvenile plantar dermatosis. *British Journal of Dermatology*, **100**, 641.

Sidi, E. & Arouete, J. (1959) Sensibilisation aux colorant azoïques et au groupe de la para. *La Presse Medicale*, **67**, 2067.

Silberman, D.E. & Sorrell, A.H. (1959) Allergy in fur workers with special reference to paraphenylenediamine. *Journal of Allergy*, **30**, 11.

Silvers, S.H. & Glickman, F.S. (1968) Atopy and eczema of the feet in children. *American Journal of Diseases of Children*, **116**, 400.

Sim-Davies, D. (1972) Studies in contact dermatitis: XXIV, Dyes in trousers. *Transactions of the St John's Hospital Dermatological Society*, **58**, 251.

Sommer, D., Hincker, E. & Mehl, J. (1971) Pathologie professionnelle dans les tanneries. *Archives des Maladies Professionnelles de Medicine du Travail et de Sécurité Sociale (Paris)*, **32**, 723.

Sparrow, G.P. (1977) A connective tissue disorder similar to vinyl chloride disease in a patient exposed to perchlorethylene. *Clinical and Experimental Dermatology*, **2**, 17.

Spoor, H.J. (1973) Indian leather dermatitis. *Cutis*, **11**, 805.

Suter, H. (1965) Untersuchungen über das Polyamidstrumpfekzem. *Dermatologica*, **130**, 411.

Uehara, M. (1978) Follicular contact dermatitis due to formaldehyde. *Dermatologica*, **156**, 48.

Vail, J.T. (1974) False negative reactions to patch testing with volatile compounds. *Archives of Dermatology*, **110**, 130.

Varelzides, A., Katsambas, A., Georgala, S. & Capetanakis, J. (1974) Shoe dermatitis in Greece. *Dermatologica*, **149**, 236.

Venediktova, K.P. & Gudina, R.V. (1976) Clinico-immunological characteristics of allergic dermatitis and eczema in textile workers. *Vestnik Dermatologii i Venerologii*, No. 10, 32.

Vollum, D.I. & Marten, R.H. (1968) Dermatitis from 4-isopropylaminodiphenylamine. *Transactions of the St John's Hospital Dermatological Society*, **54**, 73.

Wereide, K. (1964) Formaldehyde as a contact allergen in textiles. *Acta Allergologica*, **19**, 351.

Whittaker, C.M. & Wilcock, C.C. (1950) *Dyeing with Coal-Tar Dyestuffs*. London: Bailliére, Tindall and Cox.

Wilkinson, R.D. (1973) Sheet dermatitis. *Canadian Medical Association Journal*, **109**, 14.

Wilkinson, R.D. (1976) Personal communication.

Wilson, H.T.H. & Cronin, E. (1971) Dermatitis from dyed uniforms. *British Journal of Dermatology*, **85**, 67.

Wright, R.C. (1979) Dermatitis from orthodichlorobenzene in a leather dye. *Contact Dermatitis*, **5**, 124.

4.

Cosmetics

CREAMS
  Astringents
DEODORANTS AND ANTIPERSPIRANTS
  Feminine hygiene sprays
EYE COSMETICS
  Mascara
  Eye shadow
  Eye liners
  Eye creams
HAIR PREPARATIONS
  Dyes
  Bleaches
  Permanent waving
  Setting lotions

Hair sprays
Tonics, stimulants and restorers
Shampoos
Hairdressers
Men's hair creams
Shaving preparations
LIPSTICKS
  Rouge, blush-on
NAIL PREPARATIONS
  Nail varnish
  Nail base coats
  Synthetic nail covers
  Artificial nails (p. 583)
  Nail hardeners
PERFUME

The accurate diagnosis of cosmetic dermatitis is often a problem. Women use many different types of cosmetics and some are mild irritants when used for patch testing, which can make the results of these investigations difficult to interpret. In addition many cosmetics have complicated formulations; the irritancy of some of the constituents may be unknown and yet it is essential to avoid irritant concentrations when using the separate ingredients for patch testing. In the U.K. dermatologists are greatly helped in these investigations in having the cooperation of cosmetic manufacturers who readily disclose the composition of their preparations and supply samples for patch testing. The labelling of cosmetic ingredients, according to the nomenclature of the Cosmetic Ingredient Dictionary (now enforced in the U.S.A.) will greatly facilitate the investigation of patients with cosmetic dermatitis (Larsen, 1977; Menkart, 1977). The programme for the investigation and regulation of cosmetics in the United States has been detailed by Eiermann (1978).

In the United States, the cosmetics which caused dermatitis in 57 women and 13 men were listed by Schorr (1974) as:

creams and lotions (31)
hair dye and colour rinses (6)
eye makeup (5)
multiple cosmetics (4)
shampoos (2)
skin fresheners (1)

perfumes and colognes (9)
deodorants (6)
facial makeups (5)
after shave lotions (3)
nail preparations (1)

The sensitiser in the cosmetic was not always identified but the allergens to which this group of patients reacted were:

parabens (8)

mercurials (5)

ethylenediamine — EDTA (2)

eugenol (1)

oil of clove (1)

balsam of Peru (3)

sorbic acid (4)

dichlorophene (6)

lanolin (5)

isoeugenol (2)

cinnamic aldehyde (3)

oil of eucalyptus (1)

formalin (3)

hexachlorophene (1)

Brij 30 and 72 (2)

oil of bergamot (1)

lavender oil (2)

Among these 70 patients 40 per cent had a previous history either of a contact dermatitis, unrelated to cosmetics, or of stasis dermatitis.

Pigmented cosmetic dermatitis

In Japan pigmented cosmetic dermatitis has been related to perfumes (p. 613) and to coal tar dyes, particularly brilliant lake red R in various coloured cosmetics (Sugai, Takahashi and Takagi, 1977). In a further study 64 patients with pigmented and 98 with non-pigmented cosmetic dermatitis were patch and photopatch tested with 11 coal tar dyes. The incidence of allergic reactions was: brilliant lake red R (D and C Red 31) 8.6 per cent, toluidine red (D and C Red 35) 1.9 per cent, lithol red calcium salt (D and C Red 11) 1.9 per cent, permanent orange (D and C orange 17) 1.9 per cent, carbanthrene blue (D and C Blue 9) 1.4 per cent, and erythrosine (FD and C Red 3) 0.7 per cent (Mid Japan Contact Dermatitis Research Group, 1978).

Creams

Cosmetic creams are of many types and their consistency varies from a firm texture to quite a thin liquid. The majority belong to one of the following categories: foundation, moisturising, cleansing, night, body, bath, hand and baby creams. Despite this variety basically they all consist of oily compounds, water, emulsifiers, preservatives and perfume. Other additives may be present depending upon the claims and purpose of the preparation.

1. *Oily compounds*

   Oils: Liquid paraffin, almond oil, glyceryl monostearate, isopropyl myristate, isopropyl palmitate, propylene glycol and polyethylene glycol.

   Fats: Petrolatum and stearic acid.

   Waxes: Lanolin, beeswax, paraffin wax, lanette wax, candelilla wax, carnauba wax and ceresin (ozokerite).

2. *Emulsifiers*

The emulsifiers are divided into groups of chemicals, each containing many compounds; a few examples are:

A. Ionic surface active agents:
   Anionic: soap, sodium lauryl sulphate.
   Cationic: quaternary ammonium compounds.
B. Non-ionic surface active agents:
   Glyceryl monostearate and sorbitan compounds (sorbitan being a mixture of anhydrides of sorbitol).

Spans are partial esters of long chain fatty acids (such as lauric, palmitic, stearic or oleic acid) and hexitol anhydrides such as sorbitan. They are usually oil- but not water-soluble, although they can be dispersed in water.

Tweens are condensation products of a Span with ethylene oxide, a polyoxyethylene derivative. They are soluble in water. Tween 80 is polyoxyethylene sorbitan monooleate; Crillet 3 is polyoxyethylene sorbitan monostearate; Arlacel 83 is sorbitan sesquioleate; and Arlacel A is mannide monooleate.

C. Amphoteric surface active agents:
   Miranols.

3. *Preservatives*
These include the paraben esters, phenolic compounds, formaldehyde, bronopol, sorbic acid, quaternary ammonium compounds, organic mercurials, edetates, betaines (Ambiteric and Tego) and miranols (see p. 97).

4. *Anti-oxidants*
Butylated hydroxyanisole, butylated hydroxytoluene, di-*tert*-butyl hydroquinone and metabisulphites.

5. *UVR absorbers*
Some creams contain an ultraviolet light absorber such as hydroxymethylphenylbenzotriazole (Tinuvin P) to prevent spoilage by UV radiation.

6. *Perfume*

7. *Water*

8. *Additives*
These vary depending upon the purpose of the cream.

Emollients are one of the commonest additives in creams, being included to slow the evaporation of water from the emulsion and to promote hydration of the skin. They include:

Wax esters:	lanolin, spermaceti and beeswax
Steroid alcohols:	cholesterol and lanolin alcohols
Fatty alcohols:	lauryl, cetyl, olelyl and stearyl alcohols
Triglyceride esters:	animal and vegetable fats and oils
Phospholipids:	lecithin and cephalin
Polyhydric alcohol esters:	glycols and sorbital
Fatty alcohol ethers:	cetyl, stearyl and oleyl ethers
Alkyl fatty esters:	hydrocarbon oils and waxes
Lanolin derivatives:	beeswax derivatives; silicone oils.

Vitamins

Hormones

Colours

Detergents and soaps (in cleansing creams and lotions)

Antiseptics (dichlorophen, chloroxylenol, quaternary ammonium compounds)

Foaming agents (miranols)

Astringents (zinc phenol sulphonate)

Constituents of cosmetics may have several actions, and the list given is not intended to be comprehensive but is meant to give an idea of characteristic components of cream preparations (Sagarin, 1957).

DERMATITIS

Eczema of the face and irritation of the eyelids are not uncommon in women, and, when they occur, the question of allergy to cosmetics is immediately raised by the patient and frequently by the dermatologist. Since 1965 at St John's, numerous women have been tested to many and varied cosmetics, but the incidence of allergy to creams and similar preparations is low; and there are few cases reported in the literature.

A. Preservatives

Paraben esters (p. 665)
The most widely used preservatives in creams and lotions are the methyl, ethyl, propyl, butyl and benzyl esters of *p*-hydroxybenzoic acid. They are added to the formulations in concentrations of 0.1–0.3 per cent, or less. Although allergens, the incidence of sensitivity induced primarily by paraben esters in a cosmetic must be extremely small, and Schorr (1970a) has never seen this happen from a cosmetic applied to normal skin. Similarly, Hjorth and Trolle-Lassen (1962) thought that, in cosmetics, these esters have a low sensitising potential.

St John's
From 1965–1976 seven women have been investigated in whom paraben esters in cosmetic creams were thought to have been the source of their parabens sensitivity and the cause of their dermatitis. One man was sensitised by a sun-protective cream (p. 670).

Phenols (p. 673)
These include dichlorophen, hexachlorophane, bithionol, *o*-phenylphenol, chlorocresol and chloroxylenol *p*-chloro-*m*-xylenol (PCMX).

Dichlorophen has been reported as the cause of an allergic cosmetic contact dermatitis (Epstein, 1966; Schorr, 1970b) (p. 677).

Formaldehyde-Releasing Agents Dowicil 200 (p. 695) and Bronopol (p. 695) are of themselves preservatives and in addition they release formaldehyde. These and other formaldehyde releasers are discussed by Fisher (1978).

Chloroxylenol (PCMX) (p. 675).

St John's

> *Chloroxylenol (PCMX)* in an emollient lotion was thought to be the cause of one woman's hand eczema and an aggravating factor in another (p. 676)

> *o-Phenylphenol* in one particular foundation cream sensitised two women (p. 681)

Imidazolidinyl urea compounds (Germall 115)
Allergic contact dermatitis from this preservative in moisturising lotions and liquid eyeliners has been reported in one patient by Mandy (1974) and in two patients by Fisher (1975a). Patch tests with 1 per cent imidazolidinyl urea in petrolatum or solution were positive in each patient.

Miranols

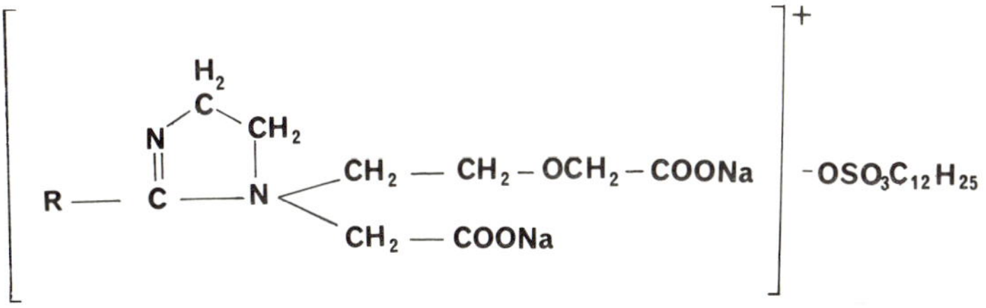

Miranol C2M (lauroylcycloimidinium-1-ethoxyethionic acid-2-ethionic acid) + lauryl sulphate group

Miranols are imidazole derivatives and it is claimed that they reduce the irritant effect of some synthetic detergents. The basic compound is Miranol C2M conc. but its foaming properties are limited. Miranol C2M is combined with sodium lauryl sulphate to form Miranol MSA, a non-irritant complex.

These compounds are used mainly in shampoos on account of their excellent foaming properties, but they may be included in creams as emulsifiers and as mild preservatives. A woman was sensitised to Miranol MSA [2-nonyl-2-imidazolinium lauryl sulphate-1-(2-hydroxyethyl)-1-carboxymethyl disodium salt] contained in a facial cleansing cream which caused facial swelling; subsequently, she developed a more severe dermatitis from this chemical in a cleansing mousse. She was patch tested with Miranol MSA 3 per cent in water and was positive. She was then patch tested with other Miranols, each at a concentration of 3 per cent, and it seemed likely that these patch tests caused active sensitisation (Verbov, 1969).

Patch testing
Miranols 1 per cent in water.

Other preservatives
Sorbic acid, organic mercurials, quaternary ammonium compounds and edetates have not been reported as the identified cause of a cosmetic dermatitis in a particular patient. However, in Schorr's (1974) study patients with cosmetic dermatitis reacted to patch tests with all of them, except quaternary ammonium compounds which were not included in that particular series.

St John's

Chloroacetamide in one particular foundation cream sensitised three women (p. 699).

Di-tert-butyl hydroquinone. This anti-oxidant is sometimes used in cosmetics as a preservative; or it may have already been added to the oils used in the cosmetic formulation to prevent the oils going rancid.
   A woman aged 56 years complained of a recurrent dermatitis of her eyelids for one year; on the last occasion her neck was also affected. Patch testing, which included an array of her cosmetics, evoked a weak reaction to one night cream. This she applied to one of her antecubital fossae without producing a reaction, but when she used it on her face the original dermatitis relapsed. When tested with the constituents of this cream, she reacted only to di-*tert*-butyl hydroquinone 1 per cent.

B. Lanolin
Despite the vast amount of lanolin and its various derivatives which are used in the manufacture of cosmetics, sensitisation from these preparations is most infrequent but has been reported (Cronin, 1966). Lanolin in such creams is probably innocuous because they are applied to normal skin, whereas lanolin in medicaments sensitises because they are applied to eczematous or otherwise damaged skin.

St John's
During the 14 years 1953–1966, 40 lanolin sensitive patients were seen in the clinic. Thirteen were women with facial eczema; of these, seven had noticed that one particular proprietary cream or Ung. Aquosum B.P., which contains 3 per cent wool alcohols (Cronin, 1966), had precipitated or aggravated their symptoms. Once they discarded all lanolin-containing preparations, all these patients recovered. Patients sensitised by a medicament, however, did not complain of cosmetic dermatitis.
   The diagnosis of lanolin cosmetic dermatitis in the patients seen subsequently from 1966–1976 was based on the sudden onset of eczema involving mainly or exclusively the face of a woman who uses cosmetics and who, by patch testing, is shown to be sensitive to wool alcohols.

Incidence
From 1966–1976, 0–4 women have been seen each year with this dermatitis (Table 4.1); the diagnosis has been made only once in a man. In the 11 years, 1966–1976, 9283 women were investigated in the Contact Clinic, and in only 26 was this diagnosis made — an incidence of 0.3 per cent.

Table 4.1. Numbers of women and men seen each year with cosmetic dermatitis due to 'lanolin' (1966–1976).

Year	1966	1967	1968	1969	1970	1971	1972	1973	1974	1975	1976	Total
No. of women	3	0	2	4	2	2	1	4	2	4	2	26
No. men	0	0	0	0	0	0	0	0	1	0	0	1

Clinical features

Age. The allergy affects the young and old alike: the ages of these patients ranged from 13 to 78 years (Table 4.2).

Table 4.2. Ages of 27 patients with cosmetic dermatitis due to 'lanolin' (1966–1976).

Age Years	11–20	21–30	31–40	41–50	51–60	61–70	71–80
No. Pts.	2	6	4	5	6	3	1

Length of history. The length of history was very variable, being as short as one week or as long as 25 years, but in nearly half (13 of the 27 cases) the duration was between one and six months. In one woman the sensitisation was of past relevance, her facial rash having occurred 20 years previously from a popular cosmetic cream (Table 4.3).

Table 4.3. Length of history in 27 patients with cosmetic dermatitis due to 'lanolin' (1966–1976).

Length of History	1 month	>1–6 months	>6 mths–5 yrs	>5 yrs	No Inf.	Past Relevance
No. Patients	2	11	9	3	1	1

Pattern of eczema. The eczema was confined to the face in 18 of these 26 women, and involved the face, neck or ears in seven. In the other case, the eruption had initially affected the face and neck but had cleared, only to be followed later by an acute transient eczema of the left eye, the hands and the feet for which no definite cause was found.

The one man complained of irritation of the face particularly after playing squash; he was in the habit of using his wife's cosmetic creams and his sensitisation and dermatitis were attributed to them.

The history is characteristically episodic, the patient complaining of recurrent attacks of redness and swelling of her face. Occasionally the oedema is so pronounced and the epidermal change so slight that a mistaken diagnosis of angio-oedema is made. The eyelids particularly are affected by swelling, redness, scaling and irritation, and in 12 of the 26 women involvement of the eyes was the dominant feature.

Three of the women had a past history of stasis eczema, of a stasis ulcer or of both.

Patch testing
The results of patch tests in these 26 women and one man were as follows:

	Tested	*Positive*
Wool alcohols 30 per cent in petrolatum	27	25
Hydrogenated lanolin	16	11
Cosmetics	17	11

to one containing
'lanolin' or a derivative

Two women did not react to wool alcohols 30 per cent, although one of them reacted to Ung. Aquosum B.P. containing 3 per cent wool alcohols and the other to hydrogenated lanolin. Negative patch tests to lanolin-containing cosmetics are probably explained by their relatively low concentration of lanolin or of a lanolin derivative. It is also likely that some of the patients were tested with the wrong cosmetics. Because such false negative reactions occur, it is insufficient to rely on patch testing with cosmetics alone to make this diagnosis.

Follow-up. Only 16 of the 27 patients kept follow-up appointments and of these 15 had remained clear for intervals of one week to one year. The exception was a woman who described an episode of reddening of her face in the absence of any obvious lanolin contact.

The failure of these patients to attend the clinic, especially as they had facial eczema, does suggest that their skin remained clear.

C. Perfumes

Practically all cosmetics, other than those which are claimed to be non-allergic, contain small amounts of perfume. The low concentration probably accounts for the infrequent occurrence of primary perfume sensitivity from this source.

D. Triethanolamine

Triethanolamine in hand lotions produced a contact dermatitis of the hands in 27 patients described by Thyresson, Lodin and Nilzen (1956). As this hand lotion, containing the triethanolamine, had been on the market for several years, the authors thought the outbreak of dermatitis might have been due to household detergents acting synergistically to facilitate penetration of the skin by the allergen. On patch testing, the patients reacted to the hand lotion and to 10–80 per cent triethanolamine.

Tea Coco hydrolysed protein is the standard name for the triethanolamine salt of the condensation product of coconut fatty acids with polypeptides and amino acids derived from collagen. It is a mild surfactant and may be used in shampoos and cleansers. A woman, who developed a severe facial dermatitis from this fatty acid polypeptide condensate in a skin cleanser, was described by Emmett and Wright (1976). Patch tests confirmed her sensitisation: she reacted strongly to the cleanser and to the Tea Coco hydrolysed protein 50 per cent and 5 per cent aqueous.

St John's

Between 1965–1976 this allergy was seen in only two women. One, sensitised by a face cream, gave only weak reactions to a patch test and to an open test with the cream, but had definite discomfort when she used it on her face. A new cream caused an acute relapse; patch testing with this cream was positive, and when she was patch tested with its ingredients she reacted to triethanolamine 5 per cent. She subsequently used a cream without triethanolamine and her face healed.

The second woman, who had acute hand eczema, was patch tested with her new hand cream and she reacted on two of three occasions. She was then tested with its ingredients and reacted strongly to triethanolamine 10 per cent. She also had positive patch tests to nickel, cobalt, balsam of Peru, wool and coal tars.

Patch testing
Triethanolamine 5 per cent in petrolatum.

E. Beeswax (Propolis)

Propolis (bee glue) is a dark yellow-brown adhesive resin which bees mix with wax to form a cementing substance in their hives and may also use it for embalming slain intruders (Bunney, 1968). Propolis is a known sensitiser in bee-keepers but neither propolis nor beeswax has been reported as a cause of cosmetic dermatitis. Beeswax present in an adhesive plaster sensitised two men reported by Schwartz and Peck (1935) and two women developed stomatitis and perioral eczema from chewing propolis; both had positive patch tests to propolis and one, tested with balsam of Peru, was negative (Wanscher, 1976). A woman, employed in moulding art objects from beeswax, developed chronic palmar eczema; a strongly positive patch test to natural beeswax established the cause, which had previously been unsuspected (Camarasa, 1975).

In bee-keepers the incidence of propolis dermatitis was found to be significant by Bunney (1968) and the allergens were thought to be derived mainly from poplar resins. In her series of 13 bee-keepers with positive patch tests to their own propolis, seven cross-reacted to balsam of Peru. A bee-keeper described by Rothenborg (1967) reacted to raw, unpurified beeswax but not to purified beeswax. The raw wax was thought to have been contaminated by poplar tree resins to which he was sensitive. Similarly, Borlin (1947) reported a bee-keeper who reacted repeatedly to crude but not to purified beeswax.

St John's
A man aged 30 years developed swelling, itching and scaling of his face after he had started to use a proprietary cold cream. When he stopped using it, his face healed, but on re-applying it, the symptoms recurred. Several patch tests with the cold cream were positive, and of its ingredients he reacted to beeswax.

Patch testing
Beeswax — as is.

F. Emulsifiers

In Helsinki, Hannuksela, Kousa and Pirilä (1976) patch tested approximately 1206 eczematous patients with eight emulsifiers, and reported that 121 (10 per cent) had irritant reactions and 25 (2.1 per cent) allergic reactions. Their results were as follows:

	Conc. %(pet.)	Reactions Allergic	Toxic
Lanette N	20	8	4
Arlacel 83 (sorbitan sesquioleate)	20	6	5
Span 60 (sorbitan monostearate)			
Span 80 (sorbitan monooleate)+	5+5	5	4
Atlas G 2162 (polyoxyethylene oxypropylene stearate)	20	4	0
Atlas G 1441 (polyoxyethylene sorbital lanolin derivative)	20	5	1
Tween 40 (polyoxyethylene sorbitan monopalmitate)+	5+5	2	2
Tween 80 (polyoxyethylene sorbitan monooleate)+			
Aldo 33 (glycerol monostearate)	20	0	2
Triethanolamine stearate	5	5	108

(Triethanolamine stearate and Atlas G 1441 were tested in 1132 cases)

Patch tests with preparations containing the sensitising emulsifiers were positive in the 14 subjects tested and they were applied topically by two patients and both reacted. Cross reactions occurred between sorbitan sesquioleate (Arlacel 83) and sorbitan monostearate and monooleate (Spans).

A patient who reacted to glyceryl monostearate in a cream deodorant was reported by Schwartzberg (1961). Patch tests with the deodorant and glyceryl monostearate were positive. Two controls had negative patch tests to glyceryl monostearate.

G. UVR absorbers
2-(2'-Hydroxy-5'-methylphenyl) benzotriazole (Tinuvin P) is a standard ultraviolet light absorber used particularly in plastics to prevent their discolouration by light.

St John's
During the period 1974–1976 four women were seen with an allergic contact dermatitis from Tinuvin P in a face cream. Each had eczema of the face, although in one woman it was confined to the eyelids, and two women had used it on other areas and these too were affected. Patch tests: Each reacted to Tinuvin P 1 per cent (petrolatum); three were tested with their face cream and two reacted.

Three of the patients had used one particular brand of cosmetics and the manufacturers have since withdrawn Tinuvin P from their products.

Patch testing
Tinuvin P 1 per cent in petrolatum.

G. White mineral oil

St John's
Since 1970, three women have been found to react to the mineral oil component of a face cream, a foundation cream and a baby lotion.

The first patient, who had constitutional eczema, was investigated because she had recently developed eczema of her face. A patch test and open test with her complexion cream were positive, and of its constituents she reacted only to the mineral oil, but did so on two occasions. It was ascertained from the manufacturers that the oil contained no additives.

The second patient had recently developed eczema of her eyelids. A patch test with her foundation cream was quite strongly positive, and of its constituents only the mineral oil elicited a definitely positive response; but, she attended for only the two-day reading.

The third patient had an acute exudative eczema of her face. On patch testing she had several positive reactions one of which was to a baby lotion; she was tested to the ingredients and had irritant reactions to propylene glycol and sodium dioctyl sulphosuccinate, both undiluted, but she was also positive to the mineral oil which had been applied well away from the irritant patch tests.

It seems improbable that white mineral oil could act as a sensitiser, and the more reasonable interpretation of these results is that they were mild irritant reactions. Control series with the mineral oils were not done.

Cosmetic patch testing positive — ingredients negative

Occasionally patch tests with cosmetic creams are positive and yet the patient fails to react to the ingredients when tested separately. The investigation of 11 such patients is tabulated below.

Cosmetic patch test +	Open test	Ingredients patch tests 2d	4d	Repeat P.T. Cosmetic	Usage test
F1 Night Cream	—	—	—	—	+
F2 Cleansing Milk	—	—	ND	—	+
F3 Foundation Cream) same	—	—	ND	ND	+
F4 Foundation Cream)	+	—	—	ND	ND
F5 Foundation Cream	—	—	—	+	+
F6 Foundation Cream	ND	—	—	ND	ND
F7 Baby Lotion	+	—	ND	—	ND
F8 Pancake Powder	ND	—	ND	ND	ND
F9 Moisture Cream	—	—	—	+	+
F10 Cleansing Milk	—	—	—	—	+
M1 Lanolin Cream	—	—	—	—	ND

+ = Reaction   – = No reaction   ND = Not done

An open test, in which the cosmetic is applied 2–3 times a day to the same place on a forearm, was usually done immediately after the initial patch tests; it was positive in two and negative in seven patients.

Usage test. Six patients, all with negative open tests and negative tests with the ingredients, used the cosmetic on their faces. Four said that, as a result, the rash had recurred and two that their faces had become red or itchy. None of these patients was seen with the relapse.

The interpretation of these results is speculative. Calnan (1975) has called this anomaly compound allergy and suggested that the allergen is a combination of more than one constituent. Among the 11 patients detailed above it is likely that the man's initial patch test response was irritant because all subsequent tests were negative. In the 10 women the positive usage and open tests make the explanation less certain. Weak allergens may have been missed by testing the individual constituents in too low a concentration. Equally the cosmetics may have been acting as a mild irritant and it is possible that two or more of the ingredients acting together may have an irritant effect, whereas acting individually, as in ingredient testing, they are innocuous.

Intolerance of cosmetics

Very occasionally a rather fussy type of woman is seen who describes discomfort from any and every type of cosmetic and yet on patch testing reacts to none.

One such patient, a woman aged 37 years, complained of having had swelling of her eyes and a patchy rash on her face for two years. She was tested with all her cosmetics and with the ingredients of a cleansing cream and was negative to all of them. Subsequently she continued to use a variety of different cosmetics but after a time complained that all produced discomfort. Another woman, aged 34 years, said that for 18 years cosmetics had made her face tingle and irritate and had caused headaches. Ordinary lipsticks made her lips sore and cracked, whereas non-allergic ones were comfortable. Every time she was seen, her face was normal. She was negative to all patch tests, including her cosmetics and 50 per cent eosin.

These patients are advised to use cosmetics with moderation and to wear them for short periods only but it is very unlikely that they take the slightest notice of this recommendation.

Stinging compounds.

Some cosmetics, toiletries and medicaments cause an unpleasant stinging sensation in a few susceptible individuals. Especially prone are women with fair complexions, who tan poorly. The discomfort, which is subjective, occurs particularly around the nasolabial folds and on the cheeks. It begins within a couple of minutes, intensifies and then abates in about 15 minutes. Compounds which cause this stinging response were identified by Frosch and Kligman (1977) and they classified them as:

Slight: benzene 1 per cent, phenol 1 per cent, salicylic acid 5 per cent, resorcinol 5 per cent, phosphoric acid 1 per cent.

Moderate: sodium carbonate 15 per cent, trisodium phosphate 5 per cent, propylene glycol, propylene carbonate, propylene glycol diacetate, dimethylacetamide, dimethylformamide, dimethylsulphoxide (each undiluted), diethyltoluamide, dimethyl phthalate, 2-ethyl-1, 3-hexanediol (each 50 per cent), benzoyl peroxide lotion 5 per cent and gel 10 per cent.

Severe: crude coal tar 5 per cent, phosphoric acid 3.3 per cent, hydrochloric acid 1.2 per cent, sodium hydroxide 1.3 per cent, 2-ethoxyethyl-*p*-methoxy-cinnamate 2 per cent.

Patch testing

1. Creams are applied and undiluted
2. Paraben-mix 15 per cent in petrolatum

3. Wool alcohols 30 per cent in petrolatum
4. Hydrogenated lanolin or another lanolin preparation.

Weak positive patch test reactions to creams may be due to mild irritation, and differentiation from weak allergic responses may be impossible on a clinical basis. They should be checked by:

(i) Repeating the original patch test. An irritant reaction is much less likely to be reproducible than an allergic one.

(ii) An open test. The cosmetic is applied 2–3 times daily to the same site on the flexor surface of one forearm. This test is of most help when it is positive because it confirms the significance of the positive patch test.

   A negative open test does not exclude sensitisation to the cosmetic and it should always be confirmed by the usage test.

(iii) A usage test. The patient is asked to apply the cosmetic to her face or to use it as she would normally. This test is important because the usage test may be positive when an open test has been misleadingly negative and subsequent testing with the constituents demonstrates sensitisation to one of them.

Patch testing with the constituents
In the U.K., cosmetic manufacturers are of the greatest help in their willingness to supply for patch testing each ingredient of any of their cosmetic preparations. The patient can then be patch tested with:

   Suitable dilutions of each constituent
   The whole cosmetic can be repeated.

Re-testing with the whole cosmetic is most important because it establishes whether or not the patient is still reacting to it.

Alternatives

Parabens. Cosmetics without parabens preservatives have been practically non-existent and patients were almost completely restricted to a pharmaceutical emollient cream, the few proprietary creams known not to contain parabens and to a loose face powder. Fortunately manufacturers are now beginning to produce ranges of cosmetics with alternative preservatives.

Lanolin. In the U.K., cosmetic manufacturers are most cooperative in supplying lists of their products which do not contain lanolin or one of its derivatives. Many such preparations are available, and each patient should be given a comprehensive list so that she can buy a satisfactory armamentarium of suitable cosmetics.

Perfume. So-called 'non-allergic' cosmetics do not contain perfume.

Other allergens. Discarding the particular cosmetic seems to be sufficient.

ASTRINGENTS

Astringents are used in the pious hope of removing wrinkles, closing enlarged pores and reducing excessive grease.

They usually are lotions but may be formulated as creams. The lotions are aqueous or dilute alcoholic solutions of mildly acidic salts such as potassium aluminium sulphate, zinc phenolsulphonate, zinc sulphate and aluminium chlorohydrate, or lactic acid. Alcohol in a concentration of 20–50 per cent is itself astringent. Witch hazel (an aqueous extract of twigs of *Hamamelis virginiana*) is credited, perhaps falsely, with being astringent.

Skin fresheners are mildly alkaline astringents containing 10–20 per cent alcohol, witch hazel and borax.

Astringent solutions with a high alcohol content may be self-preserving but others may require the addition of parabens as preservatives.

Patch testing

Astringents applied to the skin undiluted probably are mildly irritant. They should be diluted possibly to 50 per cent or even to 20 per cent for patch testing.

DEODORANTS AND ANTIPERSPIRANTS

Deodorants

The distinctive axillary odour is due to the breakdown of apocrine sweat by Gram-positive bacteria to produce acrid-smelling compounds.

Shelley, Hurley and Nichols (1953) have shown that apocrine sweat is sterile when secreted, but that, on reaching the skin surface, it is contaminated by bacteria whereupon its breakdown commences. If the sterility of the apocrine sweat is maintained, the production of these malodorous compounds is prevented. They found that washing, shaving and the application of antibacterial compounds rendered the axillae socially acceptable. Ten years later, Shehadeh and Kligman (1963) demonstrated that it was the Gram-positive but not the Gram-negative bacteria which changed the apocrine sweat to produce its characteristic smell.

Deodorants contain antibacterial compounds, and their effect depends upon reduction of the axillary bacterial flora. Until recently, hexachlorophane was the most popular (Harry's Cosmeticology), but with increased recognition of its toxicity its use has become greatly restricted. Other effective chemicals include quaternary ammonium compounds, quinolines, trichlorocarbanilide and aluminium salts; in the U.S.A., neomycin has been allowed in these preparations. Deodorants do not influence the amount of axillary sweating, and if this is considerable the effect of the deodorant will be diminished by dilution.

ANTIPERSPIRANTS

Antiperspirants are used to try to reduce the quantity of eccrine axillary sweating; aluminium salts have been found to be particularly efficacious in this respect; they have the added advantage of being active against Gram-positive bacteria. Salts of aluminium, including the sulphate, chloride and phenol sulphonates, act as antiperspirants but, on account of their low pH (2.5–3.0), they cause skin irritation and rotting of fabrics. They have now been replaced by aluminium chlorohydrate or chlorhydrol $(Al_2(OH)_5Cl)_x$, which is less acidic (pH 4 approximately) and is less damaging to clothes; it is added to formulations usually in a 20 per cent concentration (Harry's Cosmeticology, p. 264). A statistically accurate method for evaluating antiperspirants is described by Wooding and Finklestein (1975).

A fascinating account of the efficacy of anhydrous aluminium chloride as an antiperspirant is given by Shelley and Hurley (1975). They found that the axillae could be made dry provided that the details of the method they had devised were followed meticulously. The three essential facets were:

(i) to apply aluminium chloride hexahydrate 25 per cent in absolute ethyl alcohol to the axillae
(ii) the axillae must then remain dry and non-sweating for 6–8 hours
(iii) the skin must be closely occluded with vinyl chloride for 2–8 hours.

As axillary sweating virtually stops during sleep, these conditions were best achieved at night. The site of action was shown to be superficial in the terminal sweat duct yet below the stratum corneum. They suggested that the aluminium combines with the keratin fibrils of the sweat duct effecting a functional closure which blocks the delivery of sweat to the surface. The bactericidal action of the aluminium prevents the formation of miliaria, the duct remains intact and as the intraductal pressure rises secretion from the sweat gland ceases. They found little to support the hypothesis of Papa and Kligman (1967) that aluminium salts cause permeability of the sweat ducts so that they leak sweat despite the ductal pore remaining patent. The efficacy of aluminium chloride was found to vary from one individual to another by Majors and Wild (1974) and in his evaluation of the effectiveness of antiperspirant preparations Steed (1975) confirmed this observation.

Incidence of sensitivity

Discomfort from one deodorant, alleviated by changing to another, is not uncommon. Aluminium salts, acting as irritants but not as sensitisers, probably account for these transitory symptoms.

Reports of sensitisations are not infrequent.

St John's

From 1971–1974, 2–4 cases of proven sensitisation to deodorants were seen each year; for no obvious reason the numbers rose to 9 in both 1975 and 1976. During this period a further 15 patients were thought to have significant patch test reactions to a deodorant but sensitisation was not confirmed by testing with the ingredients (Table 4.4).

Table 4.4. Incidence of contact dermatitis due to deodorants. St John's 1971–1976.

	1971	1972	1973	1974	1975	1976	Total
Cases, proven	2	4	3	2	9	9	29
Cases, ingredients not tested	1	3	1	2	3	5	15

Sex incidence
Of the 29 proven cases, 24 were women and 5 were men.
Of the 15 suspected cases, 12 were women and 3 were men.

Clinical features

The presenting feature is a bilateral axillary dermatitis, particularly of the vaults, and, if severe, it may spread down the arms and to other areas of the body. When antiperspirants are applied to a constitutional eczema of the axilla, they may cause considerable skin irritation or even sensitise and give a false impression that the whole condition is a deodorant dermatitis.

Case reports — sensitisation

Sensitisation has been reported from cetalkonium chloride, Irgasan DP300, perfume, vitamin E and zirconium; *n*-butyl phthalate, and propellants in deodorant sprays, have also been found to be sensitisers.

Contact dermatitis from cetalkonium chloride in a deodorant was reported by Shmunes and Levy (1972); on patch testing, the patient reacted to the deodorant and to 0.1 per cent benzalkonium chloride. He was not tested to cetalkonium chloride, which is a very similar compound.

Irgasan DP300 has been reported as a sensitiser in deodorants by Roed-Petersen, Auken and Hjorth (1975) and by Wahlberg (1976).

After using an aerosol antiperspirant for one week, a man developed an acute axillary eczema which, within weeks, became a generalised exfoliative dermatitis. On subsequent patch testing, he reacted to the aerosol and, of the ingredients, to the perfume; patch tests on ten control subjects were negative (Wishart, 1974).

In the U.S.A. an aerosol deodorant containing *dl*-alpha-tocopherol has caused severe contact dermatitis. Minkin, Cohen and Frank (1973) described the generalised spread of the eruption which occurred in their three patients, each of whom required systemic steroids. Another three men seen by Aeling, Panagotacos and Andreozzi (1973) were patch tested and each reacted to vitamin E oil 4 per cent.

Zirconium in deodorant sticks has caused granulomas.

N-Dibutyl phthalate, included as an emollient in an aerosol antiperspirant deodorant, caused acute axillary dermatitis in a woman on the three occasions she used this new product. A patch test with the aerosol was positive and, of the ingredient, she reacted to *N*-dibutyl phthalate. She was tested with dimethyl phthalate and diethyl phthalate, and these were negative. The rapid onset of symptoms indicated that she was presensitised, but the source of the sensitivity was not traced (Sneddon, 1972). Unusual sensitisers in three patients were the deodorant spray propellants, Freon 11 (trichloromonofluoromethane) and Freon

12 (dichlorodifluoromethane). Patch tests: Each patient reacted to Froen 11 and one to Froen 12; two were tested to ethyl chloride and both had positive responses. These latter reactions were thought more likely to be an independent sensitisation rather than cross-reactions. Fifteen controls were tested with the three compounds and none reacted (Ketel, 1976).

St John's

From 1971–1976, sensitisation to a constituent of a deodorant has been confirmed in 29 patients. Each patient had a positive patch test to their deodorant and subsequently 10 were tested with each ingredient of the deodorant and 19 only with the suspected allergens in the formulation. The results in these 29 patients were as follows:

Allergen	P.T. conc.%	No. positive
Perfume	2–10	26
Formaldehyde	2	1
Fentichlor	0.5	1
Irgasan DP300	2	2

One patient reacted to both the perfume and Irgasan DP300. The patient sensitised by Fentichlor has been reported by Calnan (1975). The perfume in one particular deodorant caused many of these cases of sensitisation.

Patch testing

Deodorant and antiperspirant — 'As Is'.

When used as a closed patch test, these preparations may be mild irritants; the significance of a positive result should be confirmed by a positive open test and by subsequent testing with the ingredients appropriately diluted.

FEMININE HYGIENE SPRAYS

This rather precious title has been given to so-called vulval deodorants, which were introduced about 1969 and have had a considerable vogue particularly in the U.S.A. They are usually formulated as aerosols and contain only a perfume, an emollient and a propellant. Antibacterials, which initially were included, are now often omitted (Fisher, 1973).

Irritancy

After these sprays had been on the market for about a year, gynaecologists reported seeing patients with irritation of the vulva from their use (Kaye, 1970). By 1972, reports of 26 severe local reactions had been received by the F.D.A. (Gowdy, 1972). Fisher (1973) clarified the problem by patch testing such patients; his conclusion was that the commonest reaction is irritation from the propellants, which reached the skin as a result of too close an application of the spray.

Sensitisation

Thirty women and two men with a history of reactions were patch tested

(Fisher, 1973). Four of the women and one man had positive patch tests to the sprays. They were tested with the constituents and the sensitisers were found to be:

Benzethonium chloride: One woman and one man reacted to a 1/1000 aqueous solution and both reacted also to benzalkonium chloride.

Chlorhexidine: had sensitised one woman, she reacted to a 1 per cent aqueous solution.

Isopropyl myristate: One woman was sensitive to this emollient, concentration not specified.

Perfume: A woman, known to be sensitive to perfumes, reacted immediately she applied the deodorant. She reacted when patch tested to its perfume, whereas three controls did not.

Two of the four women had a previous history of skin disease; seborrhoeic eczema in one, and 'prickly heat' in the other.

Patch testing

Spray 'As Is'.

Sanitary napkins. Perfumed sanitary napkins are now being made and a patient who reacted to cinnamaldehyde and cinnamic alcohol in the perfume of the pad is described by Larsen (1979).

Eye cosmetics

MASCARA

Mascara is prepared in cake, cream or liquid form and has the following formulation:

1. A base, which is waxy and may be soapy
2. Preservatives
3. Perfume
4. Pigments
5. Colophony, or derivative sometimes
6. Solvents, as softening agents, in the cream and liquid forms.

Incidence of sensitivity

St John's
    Although mascara is frequently blamed by patients as being the cause of dermatitis of the eyelids, sensitisation seems to be extremely uncommon. In some women mascara probably acts as an irritant.
    From 1964–1976, only four women have been traced who were possibly sensitised to an ingredient of their mascara.

Clinical features

The patients complain of irritation, redness, soreness and swelling of the eyelids.

Case reports —

Sensitisation

Allergic contact dermatitis due to a precise constituent of a mascara has not been described recently, if ever. Calnan (1976) listed the sources of sensitisation to perfumes in 102 patients seen at St John's and in two it was mascara; one of these patients is described below (Case 3).

St John's

> *Case 1.* A young woman, aged 18 years, had had erythema of her eyelids for five months. On patch testing she reacted repeatedly to a black mascara and subsequently, on two occasions, to the wax base which contained a mixture of undecylenic acid 1 per cent and beeswax 3 per cent. Unfortunately she did not return for further tests to determine which, if either, was the allergen (Cronin, 1967).

> *Case 2.* A woman, aged 37 years, complained of recurrent eyelid dermatitis for two years. Patch tests: She reacted to her mascara and of its ingredients the test with beeswax was positive. A usage test with the mascara caused slight irritation; she changed to another make and had no further trouble. However, of 69 controls tested with the beeswax 3 of 69 were positive, putting the diagnosis in the original patient in some doubt.

> *Case 3.* A 20-year-old woman had had, for two weeks, soreness and scaling of her eyelids which had become progressively more swollen and uncomfortable. She changed to a different brand of mascara, and the condition cleared. She reacted to a patch test with the original mascara; when subsequently tested with its constituents, she was found to be sensitive to the perfume 1 per cent. She reacted neither to balsam of Peru nor to wood or coal tars.

> *Case 4.* A woman aged 30 years described having had, for eighteen months, an unexplained recurrent swelling of her eyelids. Patch tests: she reacted to colophony in the standard series, and of her many cosmetics to one particular mascara. When tested with the ingredients the allergen was identified as hydroabietyl alcohol (abitol) (patch test concentration 20 per cent in petrolatum). Subsequently 3 similar cases were seen, sensitised by the same mascara and the same allergen; of these one reacted to colophony but two did not.
>   Abitol is added to the mascara as a film former so that water or moisture runs off the lashes.

Irritant

St John's

> Eight patients who reacted to a patch test with their mascara were subsequently tested with each constituent and none reacted. Six of these patients were re-patch tested with the mascara, and five had positive responses.

Patch tests
Mascara 'As Is'.

Solvents are used particularly in the manufacture of cream and liquid mascara, and Epstein (1965) reported that occlusive patch tests with these preparations give misleading false positive responses. The liquid mascaras were the most likely to cause these irritant reactions, and although many of the positive tests were sharply demarcated and looked irritant, others were identical in appearance to a mild allergic response. The cream mascaras were less irritant.

Drying the patch test before application, to volatilise the solvents, removed the irritancy from the creams and from some, but not all, of the liquids, whereas the use of a covered but non-occlusive patch test eliminated it from both the cream and the liquid mascaras. Epstein attributed these toxic effects to the volatile solvents in these cosmetics.

St John's
Many mascaras applied as patch tests have similarly been found to be irritant, and a one-plus reaction to a mascara is interpreted with caution.

Open tests and usage tests
These may help to differentiate between an irritant and an allergic response, but they are not as reliable with mascara as they are with other cosmetics. They may be positive even when subsequent testing with the constituents excludes sensitisation.

If the mascara is fractionated, testing with the solvents should be done with some care, as some of them, if applied undiluted, are quite strong irritants. Reactions to 1 per cent coded samples can also be misleading as, even at this concentration, mascara ingredients can be irritants.

EYE SHADOWS

Eye shadow is essentially a cream, a creamy liquid or a powdery cake which spreads easily and contains pigments. It consists of ingredients such as:

1. A base: composed of waxes, oils and sometimes lanolin
2. Antioxidants: butylated hydroxyanisole, di-*tert*-butyl hydroquinone
3. Preservatives: commonly paraben esters
4. Pigments
5. Lightening powders may be added: titanium dioxide, zinc oxide
6. Binding compounds: including colophony
7. Pearlisers: aluminium powder, bismuth oxychloride, titanium-coated mica
8. Solvents and emulsifiers may be added
9. Perfume.

Incidence of sensitivity

St John's
Eye shadows are rare sensitisers: from 1960–1975, only five patients have been seen who were allergic to an ingredient of their eye shadow.

Clinical features

Irritation and swelling starts on the eyelids and may spread to involve the whole face; in one of the patients seen at St John's the eruption became generalised. The eye shadow is often suspected by the patient, who may establish it as the cause by changing from one make to another. However, eye cosmetics are frequently incriminated wrongly as a source of irritation and dermatitis of the eyelids; only patch testing can decide whether they are, in fact, responsible.

Case reports

Sensitisation

Lanolin. The glossy type of eye cosmetics, which contains lanolin, caused dermatitis in three patients reported from the U.S.A. (Schorr, 1973). Two of the patients also had lanolin lipstick cheilitis, and the third reacted to isoeugenol, an ingredient of her cosmetic perfumes.

Colophony

St John's

Three patients have been seen, each of whom had used one particular make of eye shadow in which colophony was present as a binding agent. It has been reformulated without colophony.

Case 1. Three weeks after starting to use a new eye shadow, an 18-year-old girl suddenly developed irritation of her eyelids which became swollen overnight; the condition subsequently spread to her whole face. It subsided within a week; she changed her eye shadow and remained well. On patch testing, she repeatedly reacted to one of her eye shadows, and when tested with the diluted ingredients, a constituent mixture containing 0.07 per cent colophony was positive at 2 days but negative at 4 days; she reacted to colophony 20 per cent. She was seen over the next two years and had no recurrence.

Case 2. A woman, aged 21 years, had had itchy scaly patches on her hands and face, especially round her eyes, for five years, and similar patches on her abdomen and thighs for one month. She had been sensitive to adhesive plaster since the age of 7 years. On patch testing she reacted to colophony 20 per cent in petrolatum, to her eye shadow and to red azo dye 1 per cent aqueous. It was ascertained from the manufacturers that the eye shadow did contain colophony (Calnan, 1971).

Case 3. A girl, aged 16 years, developed swelling, itching and scaling of both eyelids. Within a week, her face became swollen and she developed a generalised eruption which cleared in ten days. After a few weeks, she again used an eye shadow and once more her eyelids swelled. On patch testing, she reacted to two eye shadows and to colophony 20 per cent. She discarded these eye shadows and remained well (Cronin, 1972).

Di-tert-butyl hydroquinone

A woman, aged 41 years, who had had swollen eyelids for one week, reacted on patch testing to three eye shadows, all of the same make. Of the ingredients, she was positive to di-*tert*-butyl hydroquinone 1 per cent in petrolatum (Calnan, 1973).

St John's

A 55-year-old woman had had scaling of her eyelids for four weeks and hand eczema for three weeks. On patch testing, she reacted repeatedly to her green eye shadow cream, and when tested with its components reacted to the antioxidant, 2, 5-di-*tert*-butyl hydroquinone 1 per cent in MEK. The concentration in the cream was 0.52 per cent (Calnan, 1973). Controls were tested and were negative. The patient's eyes healed but her hand eczema persisted.

A third case of sensitivity to this anti-oxidant has been seen, the source being a cream cosmetic (p. 98).

Diisopropanolamine DIPA: $(CH_3CHOHCH_2)_2NH$

Diisopropanolamine may also be used in cosmetic gloss formulations to 'set up' the gel.

St John's

A girl, aged 15 years, complained of irritation of her eyelids and face for six months and attributed this to her cosmetics. When patch tested, she reacted only to her eye gloss; she was then tested to its ingredients, and reacted to diiso-propanolamine, undiluted. This substance also gave a positive open test; as it is an irritant, it should have been diluted for patch testing. It was, in fact, tested undi-luted on 24 control subjects of whom six gave irritant responses. Nevertheless, the patient's reaction did not look irritant, it was eczematous and spread beyond the patch test site; for this reason it was considered to be an allergic response (Cronin, 1973).

It was also the sensitiser in a blushing gel (p. 149).

Irritant patch test reactions

St John's

Eye shadows do not usually give irritant patch tests, but six women with positive patch tests to their eye shadows failed to react to the ingredients. Four were retested with the whole eye shadows; two reacted once more, but two were nega-tive.

Patch testing

Eye shadow 'As Is'.

Lead in an Asian eye cosmetic

Raised serum lead levels, in two Asian infants, were traced to the presence in their eyes of a black Asian eye cosmetic called surma a fine powder which is applied to the conjunctivae. It contained 90 per cent lead sulphide and had been obtained, as is most surma, on a visit to India or Pakistan (Pearl, 1977). The use of surma is common in Asian families and the raised blood lead concentra-tions have been studied by Ali, Smales and Aslam (1978).

EYELINERS

These cosmetics are used to emphasise the eyes by outlining the lid margins; although usually a dark colour, they are also made in paler shades. They may be formulated as a cake or a fluid, and they consist of a base, preservatives and pigment. They seem to have the same tendency as mascara to produce irritant patch tests.

St John's
From 1966 to 1976 six patients have been seen with positive patch tests to these cosmetics. Three young women were investigated. In two, patch tests with the eyeliner were positive, those with the constituents were negative. The third patient reacted to her eyeliner when patch tested, but she had a negative open test, and when she subsequently used it daily on her eyelids she had no further trouble.

Patch testing
Eyeliner 'As Is'.
   A weak positive response may be irritant; it should be checked by an open test and then by a usage test.

EYE CREAMS

Creams are sometimes marketed as 'eye creams'. They probably have a formulation similar to that of other creams, but they may contain an astringent.

Case reports
Contact dermatitis from an eye cream was reported by Calnan (1971). The patient complained of irritation, redness and swelling of her eyelids, and, on patch testing, she reacted to her eye cream and subsequently to a mixture of chloroacetamide and sodium benzoate 1 per cent; she failed to react to sodium benzoate 1 per cent on its own. The chloroacetamide was probably added to the formulation as a preservative.

Patch testing
Eye cream 'As Is'.

Hair preparations

HAIR DYES

The practice of colouring hair with natural vegetable dyes dates back to antiquity and is still a popular method of dyeing hair in some parts of the world. In Western countries, however, vegetable extracts have been almost entirely superseded by synthetic dyes, and, since the 1960s, the tinting of hair has been done not only by experts at the hairdressers but also as a popular home cosmetic procedure. It has been estimated that about 40 per cent of women in the U.S.A. use hair colours (Corbett and Menkart, 1973).

To be acceptable, a hair dye has to be harmless to the skin and it must dye rapidly and effectively. To be permanent it needs to penetrate the hair, not just coat it, and in doing so it should alter neither the structure nor the appearance of the hair.

Hair dyes belong to one of three groups: vegetable dyes, metallic dyes and synthetic organic dyes (Harry's Cosmeticology).

Vegetable dyes

Henna

Henna is derived from the dried leaves and stems of *Lawsonia inermis* plants which grow in Egypt, Tunis, Iran and India. The active principle, lawsone, is 2-hydroxy-1, 4-naphthoquinone.

2-Hydroxy-1, 4-naphthoquinone (lawsone)

Henna dyes the hair red, but the shade produced is not admired in all societies; and it also stains the finger nails. It can be combined with indigo to give a black colour.

Henna causes immediate type hypersensitivity. At *St John's* a hairdresser was seen who developed wheezing and coryza when she handled henna; a prick test with henna 1 per cent in water was positive (Cronin, 1979). Reports of dermatitis have not been traced.

Chamomile

Chamomile is a yellow dye extracted from the dried flower heads of *Anthemis nobilis* (Roman chamomile) and *Matricaria chamomilla* (German chamomile). The dye, apigenin, which is 4', 5, 7-trihydroxyflavone, is also present in parsley and celery.

4',5,7-Trihydroxyflavone (chamomile)

It is sometimes used in shampoos and hair rinses, but its efficacy is doubtful. It is a potential sensitiser, as allergic contact dermatitis has occurred in people handling the plant, *Anthemis nobilis*, or who have used compresses of chamomile or chamomile ointment (Mitchell and Rook, 1979).

Metallic dyes

Metallic dyes coat the hair, giving it a metallic sheen. They make the hair brittle and impair subsequent permanent waving.

Lead dyes, which are called colour restorers, usually contain lead acetate. They change grey hair to a yellow, brown or black colour, depending upon the technique and the frequency of application.

Salts of bismuth, silver, copper, nickel and cobalt may be used to give a range of colours.

One series of dyes contains an ion of a metal, such as nickel or chromium securely chelated within a complex molecule. Irgalan dyes have this structure; they have been used as semi-permanent colours to dye grey hair.

The demand for any of these dyes is extremely small, and, because of anxiety about lead toxicity, the concentration of lead salts permitted in them may be restricted, as may be their sale.

Synthetic organic dyes

Temporary Dyes

These preparations, often called colour rinses, contain a mixture of dyes which simply coat the hair and are removed by shampooing. Such dyes may be anthraquinone colours (Acid Violet 43) of the type used to dye wool, azo dyes (Tartrazine Yellow) and Eosin YS Red (Corbett and Menkart, 1973). Dyes from the range permitted in foods, drugs and cosmetics are also suitable.

They are usually prepared as aqueous solutions to be combed through the hair, but they may be formulated as shampoos or aerosol sprays.

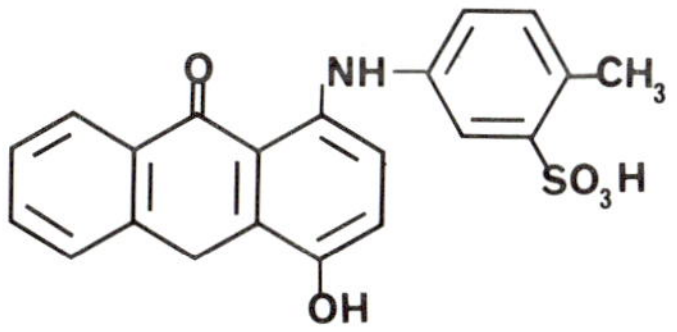

Acid Violet 43

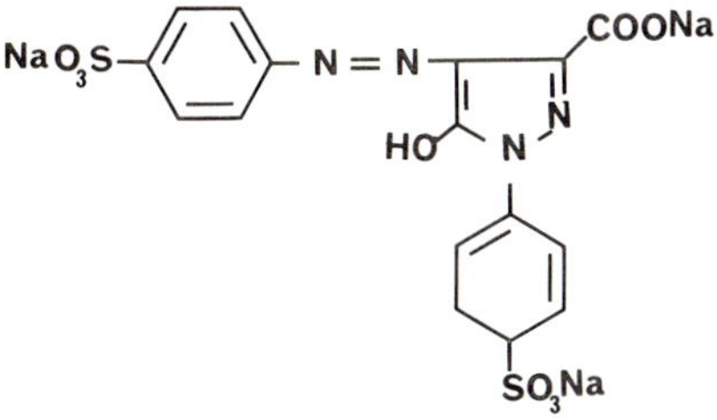

Tartrazine (C.I. Acid Yellow 23)

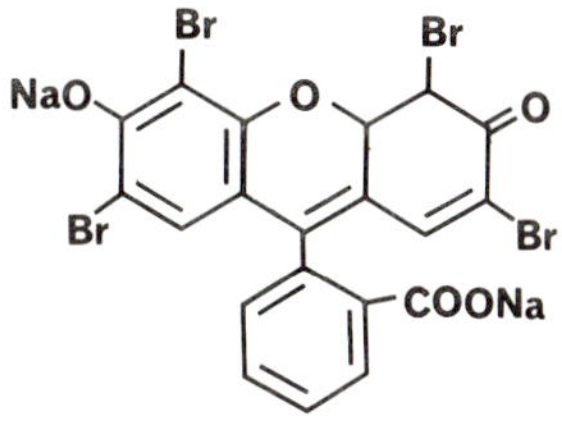

Eosin YS (Red)

Semi-permanent dyes

Semi-permanent dyes are low molecular weight chemicals which penetrate the hair shaft but are retained for about five to ten shampoos only. They are coloured compounds and do not require the use of hydrogen peroxide. Shades are achieved by blending red and yellow nitro dyes for red and blonde tints, and adding blue anthraquinone dyes for brown colours. The penetration of these blue dyes into normal hair is restricted by their large molecular size, but if the hair is made porous by permanent waving or bleaching an excess may be absorbed into the hair shaft and produce a calamitous green colour (Harry's Cosmeticology, p. 447). The final commercial preparation contains approximately 9–10 dyes dispersed in a shampoo base. It is applied to freshly washed hair, left on for 20–40 minutes and then rinsed off.

Chemically, these dyes are nitrophenylenediamines, nitroaminophenols and anthraquinones (Corbett and Menkart, 1973).

This group of hair colourants is the most popular of those used in Great Britain.

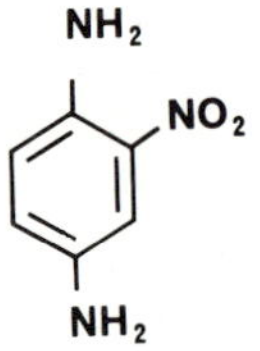

o-Nitro-p-phenylenediamine (ONPPD)

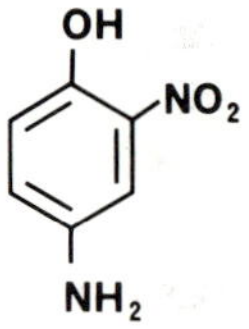

Nitroaminophenol

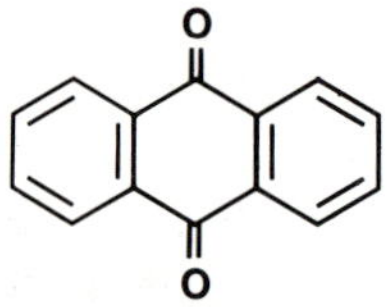

Anthraquinone

Sensitisation by nitro dyes

St John's

Sensitisation by nitro dyes is extremely uncommon; however, positive patch tests to nitro dyes are not uncommon in patients sensitised by para dyes.

From 1965 to 1976, only 5 patients have been seen who were sensitised by nitro-PPD dyes only; 3 were women who had used hair colours and 2 were hairdressers.

Case 1. A 41-year-old woman, who was in the habit of using a permanent hair dye containing PPD and nitro dyes, developed dermatitis. She changed to a semipermanent dye containing nitro dyes, and had a worse attack of dermatitis than before, with swelling of the face and tightness of the scalp.

Patch tests: Initially, she reacted to PPD 0.5 per cent, but, when seen again ten weeks later for further tests, the results were as follows:

PPD 1%	negative
p-toluylenediamine 1%	negative
o-nitro-PPD 1%	positive

and ingredients of the semipermanent dye, nitro-PPD 1 per cent positive.

Case 2. A 62-year-old woman, with hand eczema for five years, complained of swelling of the left eye for one month and irritation of the hair line for one week.

Patch tests: PPD 1 per cent and *p*-toluylenediamine 1 per cent both very weakly positive; *o*-nitro-PPD 1 per cent positive.

Case 3. A 16-year-old girl was referred with hand eczema which had begun, 18 months previously, after using a colour shampoo.

Patch tests: PPD 0.5 per cent, negative; *p*-toluylenediamine 1 per cent, negative; *o*-nitro-PPD 2 per cent, positive; 1 per cent, positive.

Case 4. A 16-year-old hairdresser had had hand eczema for six months.

Patch tests: PPD 0.5 per cent, negative; *p*-toluylenediamine 1 per cent, negative; *o*-nitro-PPD 1 per cent, positive.

Case 5. A 19-year-old hairdresser had an 18 month history of hand eczema.

Patch tests: PPD 1 per cent, negative; *p*-toluylenediamine 1 per cent, negative; *o*-nitro-PPD 1 per cent, positive (p. 000).

Permanent dyes

These are the 'para' or oxidation dyes and form the most important group of hair colourants. They disguise grey hair, add red tints to brown hair and can change the original colour through a range of browns to black. In the development of these dyes, hydrogen peroxide is used; as it bleaches melanin, it makes it possible, if so desired, for a lighter shade than the original colour to be obtained.

The dyes, which are known as primary intermediates, have little colour; they are oxidised, possibly within the hair shaft, by hydrogen peroxide or a similar oxidant, to form colourless quinone-diimines. These are rapidly polymerised in the presence of a coupler, also called a modifier, to produce indo dyes, which are large, coloured molecules held within the hair shaft and are difficult to remove. As a result the hair remains permanently coloured.

'Para' dyes (primary intermediates)

p-Phenylenediamine (PPD)

p-Benzoquinone diimine

p-Aminophenol

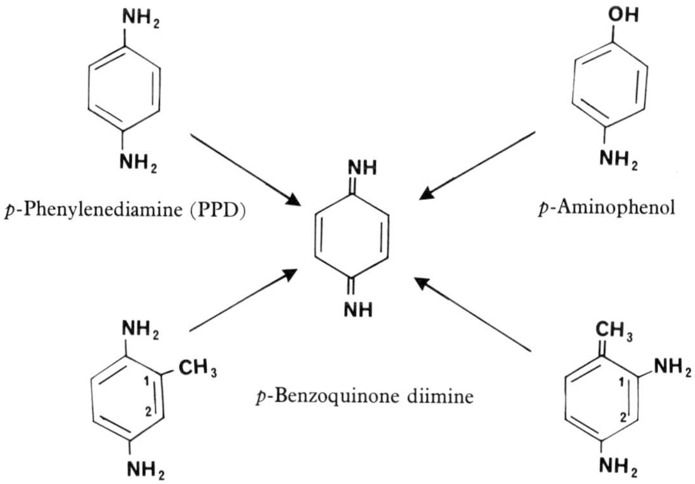

p-Toluylenediamine PTD; 2-methyl-*p*-phenylenediamine)   *m*-Toluylenediamine (MTD; 2,4-diaminotoluene)

Para-phenylenediamine and the toluylenediamines have a similar affinity for hair; they are used in various combinations in hair dyes because PPD gives a black shade and the toluylenediamines a redder colour. A few black dyes may contain only PPD. A multiplicity of dyes is used in the final products so as to satisfy the demand for a wide range of colours and shades. Ammonia is added to the formulation not only because an alkaline medium facilitates the release of oxygen from hydrogen peroxide but also because it causes the hair to swell and increases penetration of the dye.

Oxidant. Hydrogen peroxide (H_2O_2) is stable in an acid medium at pH 3. It is packed separately and is only added to the dye immediately before use.

Couplers (Modifiers)	Hair colour
Resorcinol	green-brown
m-Aminophenol	light brown
Pyrogallol	gold
2, 4-Diaminoanisole	purple-blue
Hydroquinone	light grey-brown
Catechol	grey-brown
(Corbett and Menkart, 1973)	

Dye base. This is usually an ammonium oleate soap with a small amount of detergent and free ammonia; the final pH is about 9.5 (Corbett and Menkart, 1973).

The dyes are marketed in two packs, one containing the dye and its couplers, the other the hydrogen peroxide.

Sensitising potential

Sensitisation by PPD has, in the past, been considered so great a hazard that its use in hair dyes was banned in Germany in the early 1900s; it was subsequently prohibited in France, and in 1964 in Sweden (Fregert, 1972). It is no longer held that these dyes constitute a great hazard, and in the light of the proposed regulations for the European Economic Community, which allows up to 6 per cent PPD in hair dyes (Corbett and Menkart, 1973), these restrictions are likely to be rescinded.

Para-phenylenediamine 10 per cent sensitised all 24 subjects exposed to the maximisation test by Kligman (1966). Each reacted to a challenge concentration of 0.5 per cent; PPD was graded as 5, which includes the most potent allergens.

Para-toluylenediamine (PTD) has never been banned because it has always been considered a weaker allergen than *para*-phenylenediamine (PPD). This is now being questioned. Magnusson (1974) sensitised guinea-pigs to PPD and PTD by

(i) intradermal injections of 0.1 ml PPD or PTD in propylene glycol, and
(ii) a topical application of 0.1 ml PPD or PTD in ethanol.

The animals were challenged by open tests with 0.5 per cent, 1.0 per cent and 5.0 per cent PPD or PTD in 95 per cent ethanol. The results were as follows:

Allergen	Route of Administration	
	Intradermal	Topical
PPD	11/20 sensitised	10/20 sensitised
PTD	20/20 sensitised	18/20 sensitised

St John's

These experimental findings are not reflected clinically in our patch test results. As many of the modern permanent dyes contain both PPD and toluylenediamines, users are often exposed to both allergens simultaneously. From 1965 to 1976, 45 patients presenting with hair dye dermatitis were tested, both with PPD and with *p*-toluylenediamine (PTD); 43 reacted to PPD, whereas 21 were sensitive to PTD. Similarly, in hairdressers there is a greater incidence of reactions to PPD than to PTD (p. 137).

In contrast to the findings in guinea-pigs Epstein and Taylor (1979), using the maximisation test in man, sensitised nearly half (15/34) with 2 per cent aqueous PPD but none (0/31) with PTD 2 per cent aqueous. Those sensitised reacted to open and closed tests with commercial dyes developed with hydrogen peroxide.

Incidence of sensitivity

Most cases of sensitisation occurred in the 1930s, at which time patients with severe dermatitis were reported in the literature (Schwartz and Barban, 1952). Despite the steadily increasing popularity of hair dyes, the incidence of dermatitis has fallen considerably and remains low.

The safety of these modern oxidation dyes has been attributed by Corbett and Menkart (1973) to five factors:

1. The high purity of the *p*-phenylenediamine.
2. The use of stable hydrogen peroxide which ensures efficiency of the reaction during application.
3. Precision in formulation allows rapid consumption of imines.
4. The shampoo base facilitates washing away excess dye.
5. The marketing of packs ensures that the chemicals are used in the correct proportions.

The provision of cautionary notices on the bottle, awareness of the risks, patch testing, and improvements in the technique of application of these dyes have probably all contributed to the reduction in the number of cases of dermatitis.

St John's

Each year from 1965–1976, two to six patients with existing hair dye dermatitis have been investigated in the Contact Clinic, and a further nought to six patients gave a history of having had this dermatitis in the past (Table 4.5).

During this time, four patients had positive patch tests to PPD and, despite using hair dyes, two of them had no history of hair dye dermatitis and in the other two the relevance of the reaction to their eczema was very doubtful. Two other patients who reacted to PPD were a man and a woman each with a four-year history of hand eczema. The man had acquired the sensitivity by occasionally dyeing his wife's hair, and the woman had developed her eczema after dyeing her mother's hair (Table 4.5.).

Hairdressers are not included in this series of patients.

Table 4.5. Yearly incidence of patients with present and past hair dye dermatitis (St John's, 1965–1976). (Included are four patients sensitive to hair dyes but without a relevant history and two with hand eczema.)

	1965	1966	1967	1968	1969	1970	1971	1972	1973	1974	1975	1976	Total
Present Dermatitis	2	6	6	6	5	6	4	6	3	4	6	5	59
Past Dermatitis	4	4	1	2	0	2	0	3	1	1	0	6	24
No Relevance	0	1	1	0	2	0	0	0	0	0	0	0	4
Hand Eczema	0	0	0	0	0	1	0	0	1	0	0	0	2

Sex incidence

Among Caucasians hair dye dermatitis is probably more common in women than men but in Asian countries it is more frequently seen in men. From 1965–1976, 64 women sensitised to hair dyes were seen as compared with 25 men (Table 4.6). Of the 25 men 9 were Asian patients.

Table 4.6. Sex incidence of patients sensitised to hair dyes (St John's, 1965–1976).

	1965	1966	1967	1968	1969	1970	1971	1972	1973	1974	1975	1976
Women	5	9	7	6	5	8	1	6	5	4	1	7
Men	1	2	1	2	2	1	3	3	0	1	5	4

Clinical features

Age

It is strikingly a dermatitis of the middle-aged and elderly; 70 of the 89 patients (80 per cent) were over the age of 40 years (Table 4.7).

Table 4.7 Ages of 89 women and men sensitised to hair dyes (St John's, 1965–1976).

	11–20	21–30	31–40	41–50	51–60	61–70	71–80
Women	2	3	6	23	15	15	0
Men	0	2	6	6	9	2	0

Patterns of dermatitis

Modern hair dyes give colours which look so natural that their use is rarely obvious; patients must, therefore, be asked directly whether a tint or dye has been applied.

The dermatitis may begin within a few hours of the dye being used or may appear on the following day. The severity of the eczema varies considerably. There may be intense oedema of the face, particularly of the eyes, with exudation of the scalp; erythema and swelling may extend down the neck on to the upper chest and upper arms, and can even become generalised. The swelling of the face may be so striking that a mistaken diagnosis of angioneurotic oedema is made.

Usually the features are less dramatic, the patient complaining of intermittent swelling and irritation of the eyes, face, scalp and neck. Occasionally the irritation is generalised, which is possibly explained by systemic absorption of the dye.

When periodic swelling of the eyes is the only symptom, the patient may fail to connect it with having her hair 'tinted'.

Occasionally there is nothing more than irritation at the scalp margins, as can happen when the tinting is done by experts at a hairdresser's. They limit skin contamination to the periphery of the scalp where it is unavoidable if all visible hair is to be coloured.

Patients applying the dye themselves wear gloves, but, even so, their hands and arms may be affected.

Two patients had hand eczema as a result of dyeing a relative's hair.

Two men had eczema of the arms due to contact with their wife's or girlfriend's dyed hair. One of the Asian patients had eczema from dyeing his beard and not his scalp.

Beard dermatitis

Men use hair dyes to colour their beards and sensitisation causes the same types of dermatitis as when the dyes are applied to scalp hair. In a similar way the intensity of the reaction varies from exudation to slight erythema and itching around the beard margins. It is suprising how reluctant men may be, even after patch testing, to accept the diagnosis.

Patch testing

Patients suspected of having hair dye dermatitis are patch tested to:

p-phenylenediamine	(PPD)	1 per cent in petrolatum
p-toluylenediamine	(PTD)	1 per cent in petrolatum
o-nitro-p-phenylenediamine	(ONPPD)	1 per cent in petrolatum.

Hair dyes

The hair dyes themselves are sometimes applied, but as they are formulated in a shampoo base they are irritant and the results may be difficult to interpret.

Patch test results. The patch test results in the 89 patients seen from 1965–1976 were as follows:

Dye	No. Tested	Positive	%
PPD	89	84	(94%)
PTD	53	24	(45%)
ONPPD	49	15	(31%)

The five patients negative to PPD had the following reactions:

PPD – ve	PTD + ve	1
PPD – ve	PTD – ve ONPPD + ve	3
PPD – ve	Scratch test to PPD + ve	1

(In 1971 the concentration of PPD used for patch testing was increased from 0.5 per cent to 1 per cent.)

Patch testing

The following series of chemicals is suggested for patch testing a patient suspected of having hair dye dermatitis:

1. p-Phenylenediamine 1 per cent in petrolatum
2. p-Toluylenediamine 1 per cent petrolatum

3. *m*-Toluylenediamine 1 per cent in petrolatum
4. *o*-Nitro-*para*-phenylenediamine 1 per cent in petrolatum
5. Resorcinol 2 per cent in petrolatum
6. *m*-Aminophenol 1 per cent in petrolatum
7. Hydroquinone 1 per cent in petrolatum
8. The dye, diluted possibly to 10 per cent in water (this dye may also be applied as an open test to the forearm).

Cross-reactions. Cross sensitivity between para-dyes and some antihistamines has been reported as protracting dermatitis caused by hair dye (Mackie and Mackie, 1964). Cross-reactions have been reported to be frequent between the hair dye *p*-aminodiphenylamine and the rubber anti-oxidant 4-isopropylaminodiphenylamine (Schønning and Hjorth, 1969) (See hairdresser's patch tests, p. 137).

Immediate-type hypersensitivity to p-phenylenediamine

St John's
An Asian man, aged 28 years, had been using a permanent dye regularly and without trouble for four years, but on the last occasion he developed severe oedema and irritation of his eyes and face, and he noticed difficulty in breathing. The symptoms subsided rapidly. A patch test with PPD 0.5 per cent was negative, but a scratch test gave an immediate weal (Calnan, 1967).

Systemic absorption
Hair dye is absorbed systemically as was confirmed in a woman who noticed darkening of her urine for five hours after her hair was dyed. The absorption spectrum of her dark urine was the same as that of normal urine with added hair dye (Marshall and Palmer, 1973). Dye was detected in the urine of four of eight volunteers after dyeing their hair (Maibach, Leaffer and Skinner, 1975) and these results although queried as being artefacts (Yare and Garcia, 1977) were held to be valid (Maibach, Leaffer and Skinner, 1977). A puzzling case of dark urine was traced to the use of a hair dye (Peter, 1975).

Allergenicity of dyed hair
The dye, once fully polymerised inside the hair, is inert and harmless, thus dyed hair is non-allergenic and does not cause dermatitis in those sensitised. This was confirmed by Reiss and Fisher (1974) when they patch tested 20 subjects, including three hairdressers all known to be strongly positive to PPD, with hair that had been dyed the previous day with PPD dyes. None reacted to the hair. This observation is of particular importance to hairdressers, who so frequently handle dyed hair.

However, hair dyed at home may not be so harmless and unreacted dye may remain on the hair, probably due to faulty technique. Four unusual cases of such sensitisation have been reported; three were men. One man presented with patches of discoid eczema on his trunk and upper arms. Patch tests: he reacted to *p*-phenylenediamine 1 per cent and to *p*-toluylenediamine 1 per cent, both in petrolatum, and to his wife's black dyed hair. She regularly dyed her own hair, and the pattern of her husband's dermatitis was attributed to her habit of reading in bed with her head resting near his axilla (Mitchell, 1972). A dental hygienist developed dermatitis of her left arm from contact with patients' hair. On patch resting she reacted to *o*-nitro-*p*-phenylenediamine 2 per cent but was negative to *p*-phenylenediamine (Hindson, 1975).

St John's

A man with exudative discoid eczema on his arms queried whether his wife's dyed black hair might be implicated. Patch tests: he reacted to PPD 1 per cent and his wife's hair dye (Cronin, 1973). Since then a similar patient has been seen, with eczema of the left forearm. Patch tests: he was positive to PPD 1 per cent and his girl friend's hair dye but he was negative to her dyed hair (Warin, 1976).

Dyeing hair in those sensitised

Some patients weakly sensitised to *p*-phenylenediamine (PPD) are known to be able to continue dyeing their hair with PPD with impunity (Reiss and Fisher, 1974). However, this cannot be taken as a general rule for all PPD-sensitive patients, because, despite every care in technique and application, dermatitis may certainly result.

Alternatives

There is no satisfactory alternative to the permanent dyes, and sensitised patients should be advised to stop using them and to try to become reconciled to their natural colour. Henna can be used, but its characteristic red colour is rarely acceptable; brown dyes, some of which are premetallised chemicals, are available, but they are not so effective as the para-group; blue and pink rinses for grey hair are safe.

Legislation

In Great Britain it is required by law that, if a dye contains *p*-phenylenediamine, toluylenediamine or similar para-dyes, its container must be labelled with the word 'Caution'. Moreover, it must be stated that the dye can cause inflammation, and instructions on skin testing must be included.

Hairdressers are supposed to do skin tests prior to dyeing or tinting hair, but this is frequently overlooked, particularly in women having their hair dyed regularly.

Other dyes, including the semipermanent nitro-dyes, are outside the poisons regulations: their containers are not required to carry a poison label, nor is a skin test required.

Carcinogenicity of hair dyes

At the present time there is no definite evidence that hair dyes are carcinogenic in man; however laboratory work has proved that they are mutagens and has established that their carcinogenic potential requires further study.

In 1969, it was reported from Japan that carcinomas of the liver could be induced in rats by feeding them with *m*-toluylenediamine (Ito, Hiasa, Konishi and Marugami, 1969). Nitro-phenylenediamines and the oxidative phenylenediamines were then shown, in the United States and England, to produce mutants in certain sensitive bacteria and to cause breakage of chromosomes in cultures of human lymphocytes (Ames, Kammen and Yamasaki, 1975; Searle, Harnden, Venitt and Gyde, 1975). These findings have been confirmed (Benedict, 1976). In the study of Burnett *et al*. (1975) the topical application of three oxidation hair dyes mixed with hydrogen peroxide produced no ill-effects in mice. However Searle and Jones (1977) reported that in one particular strain of mice the appearance of tumours was accelerated and their incidence was increased following repeated painting with one of two coloured shampoos, one of which contained nitrophenylenediamines and the other an azo-dye-metal complex and aminonitrophenol.

A study in Oxford (Kinlen *et al*., 1977) detected no difference in the use of hair dyes between 191 women with breast cancer and 561 matched controls and in an American series (Hennekens *et al*., 1979) the 20 year period following the first use of permanent hair dyes was cleared of a cancer risk.

Green hair
Hair made excessively porous by thioglycollates or bleaches may turn green with dyes (p. 118) or from the deposition of copper. Such a colour change in two children was due to copper in chlorinated swimming water (Lampe, Henderson and Hansen, 1977). The source of the copper is either algicides or corrosion of copper pipes as in the dormitory water which caused green hair (Nordlund, Hartley and Fister, 1977). Quaternary ammonium compounds inhibit the absorption of copper by hair and prevent the discolouration. Shampooing will not remove the green colour (Bhat *et al*., 1979).

Repigmentation of hair
The spontaneous repigmentation of grey hair on the scalp, beard and arms following a photosensitive dermatitis was reported by Bhutani *et al*. (1978).

HAIR BLEACHES

Hair colour can be lightened by applying hydrogen peroxide. Although not sensitising, the procedure always damages the hair to some extent and if carried out to excess, the hair becomes dull and brittle. Bleaches are sold in twin packs; in one there is a stable acidic solution of hydrogen peroxide and in the other an alkaline preparation, usually containing ammonia. Prior to use, the two are mixed, releasing oxygen from the peroxide in the alkaline medium. Persulphates are effective bleaches and are also frequently used to decolourise hair.

The changes in hair damaged by bleaching and cold waving have been studied with the scanning electron microscope by Selze and Wolff (1976).

Ammonium persulphate
Ammonium persulphate is a strong oxidiser and can be added to hydrogen peroxide to enhance the bleaching effect. As well as being used in hairdressing salons it is included in some packs for application at home. It is a powder, and it is added as such to the peroxide.

Ammonium persulphate is an irritant and a sensitiser and it causes immediate urticarial-type reactions and dermatitis both in persons having their hair bleached and in the hairdressers applying it.

$$NH_4 - O - \overset{\overset{O}{\|}}{S} \begin{smallmatrix} \diagup O \\ \mid \\ \diagdown O \end{smallmatrix}$$

$$NH_4 - O - \underset{\underset{O}{\|}}{S} \begin{smallmatrix} \diagup O \\ \mid \\ \diagdown O \end{smallmatrix}$$

Ammonium peroxydisulphate (ammonium persulphate)

Immediate type reactions

Subjects having their hair bleached. In 1963, Calnan and Shuster reported that ammonium persulphate can produce an effect like histamine release. Two of their patients were women who had had their hair bleached. During the procedure, one had developed redness and swelling of her face and had temporarily lost consciousness. The second said that every time she had applied the bleach she felt hot, her face became red and swollen, her scalp and vulva were intensely itchy and she developed a headache and felt drowsy. After a short sleep, the symptoms had disappeared on each occasion. Five hairdressers with hand eczema were investigated; in each case a saturated solution of ammonium persulphate applied to the intact skin caused a weal and flare which took 15 minutes to appear. The weal was larger if the skin had been scratched, but its appearance was still delayed. The effect was reduced or suppressed by antihistamines, and it did not occur in skin depleted of histamine by 48/80. Ammonium persulphate was scratched into the skin of 57 controls, and three developed large weals. It was concluded that ammonium persulphate is a weak histamine liberator but it was not established that the effect was due to sensitisation. *In vitro* studies by Mahzoon, Yamamoto and Greaves (1977) confirmed that ammonium persulphate is a poor histamine liberator but that the reason for the abnormal reactivity of skin mast cells in susceptible individuals, whether immunological or an inherent property of the cells, remains to be clarified.

Hairdressers. Occasionally hairdressers develop an immediate type hypersensitivity to ammonium persulphate. Three hairdressers with asthma each of whom reacted strongly to scratch tests with persulphate powder were reported by Gaultier, Gervais and Mellerio (1966). Another with rhinitis and asthma was described by Fisher and Dooms-Goosens (1976); this patient developed a weal and mild asthma when scratch tested with 1 per cent aqueous solution of ammonium persulphate.

Some hairdressers complain that bleaches make their hands irritable; this is probably due to the non-specific histamine release effect of the persulphate.

Dermatitis

Subjects having their hair bleached – irritant. If the persulfate is applied for too long a time (Gaultier, Gervais and Mellerio, 1966) or in too high a concentration it can cause an erythema of the scalp and forehead which may weep and crust and be associated with breaking of the hair. This reaction can occur the first time a bleach is applied; the onset is rapid and the patient may feel burning of the scalp while still in the hairdressers and by then erythema of the scalp may already be apparent. Such a case was described by Fisher and Dooms-Goosens (1976). Patch tests with ammonium persulphate are negative in these patients.

St John's

A woman whose hair was dyed too dark a shade returned to the hairdressers to have the colour removed. It took six hours to have her hair bleached and washed twice and finally tinted, by which time there was erythema of her scalp, forehead and temples. Six hours later exudation had begun on the scalp and weeping and crusting continued for three days; by ten days the skin had healed. The hair did not break but the patient had exceptionally coarse hair. Patch tests with the standard series, hair dyes and ammonium persulphate 2.5 per cent in petrolatum were all negative. A scratch test with ammonium persulphate crystals was also negative.

Allergic

St John's

Persulphates can cause an allergic contact dermatitis, but this is rare. A woman, when bleaching her hair, used potassium persulphate to boost the effect of hydrogen peroxide, and five hours later she developed itching, burning and swelling of her scalp, ears and forehead and to a lesser extent of her face. The next day, the skin around her hairline was red and weeping. On recovery, scratch tests with potassium and ammonium persulphate were positive, and she had positive patch tests to 1 per cent and 5 per cent potassium persulphate.

Hairdressers — Irritant. Hairdressers are said to develop irritant hand eczema from persulphates (Gaultier, Gervais and Mellerio, 1966; Fisher and Dooms-Goosens, 1976). Certainly some hairdressers with hand eczema notice that contact with bleaching powder aggravates the condition.

Allergic. A few hairdressers with hand eczema develop a delayed-type hypersensitivity to persulphates. It was the entire cause of the hand eczema in a hairdresser reported by Fisher and Dooms-Goosens (1976), and it has caused pronounced worsening of the hands, accompanied by sneezing and rhinitis, in an atopic hairdresser (Widstrom, 1977).

St John's

Very occasionally a hairdresser is seen who is thought to have a delayed type hypersensitivity to ammonium persulphate (p. 137).

Scratch testing

Ammonium persulphate crystals, moistened with water, are applied to a small superficial scratch on the forearm and are left there for 15 minutes. A positive reaction is a large weal and flare extending well beyond the line of the scratch.

If a high degree of allergy is suspected the test should be done with a 1 per cent aqueous solution of ammonium persulphate.

Patch testing
Ammonium persulphate 2.5 per cent and 1 per cent in petrolatum (A concentration of 5 per cent is irritant).

Carbamide perhydrate
The ready decomposition of carbamide perhydrate to urea and hydrogen peroxide bleached and damaged the hair of three workers making or packaging this compound in a pharmaceutical factory (Bolck, Ziegler and Sieler, 1977).

PERMANENT WAVING

Cold waving chemicals have almost entirely replaced the previously used hot waving processes. Practically all modern permanent cold wave reducing solutions contain ammonium thioglycollate, but thioglycerol has been used and other effective chemicals include beta-mercaptopropionic acid, thiomalic acid and thiourea (Harry's Cosmeticology).

The usual reducing solution contains 5–6 per cent ammonium thioglycollate ($SH-CH_2COONH_4$), to which ammonia is added because a pH of 9–9.5 is critical; at a lower pH the chemical is less effective, and at a higher pH it is depilatory. The thioglycollate is applied to the hair to break the cystine cross linkages within the keratin; it does so by reducing the disulphide (-S-S-) bonds to form cysteine sulphydril (-SH) groups. In this softened state, the hair is wound on to small curlers to assume a new and kinked configuration. The reducing solution is left on for about 10–40 minutes, and then the hair is rinsed and the cystine bonds are restored by applying a neutraliser, which is a mild oxidising agent. The choice of oxidiser for use by hairdressers is usually a weak solution of hydrogen peroxide, whereas for home packs it is sodium perborate or sodium borate. After neutralisation the hair is unwound and then washed and set.

Traumatic breakage of the hair does occur occasionally. This chemical rearrangement of the hair structure always weakens the shaft to some extent and if the curlers are wound too tightly, or if the solution is left on too long, the hair will break. Bleached hair is particularly vulnerable and the scanning electron microscopic appearance of such damaged hair has been described by Selzle and Wolff (1976). The breakage may occur as the hair is unwound from the curler or it may be a more gradual process, the shafts breaking as a result of combing during the succeeding days.

Dermatitis
At the time that both thioglycerol and ammonium thioglycollate were being used in cold wave solutions, Downing (1951) assessed them and found each compound to be irritant and sensitising, but the thioglycerol was the more sensitising of the two.

In persons having their hair permed sensitisation to thioglycollates must be exceedingly rare, if it ever occurs. Whereas an irritant dermatitis does happen occasionally due to a careless technique in which there is excessive contamination of the scalp by the thioglycollate solution.

Among hairdressers, too, sensitisation to thioglycollate is unusual. In the 1950s allergic contact dermatitis in hairdressers from thioglycerol in cold wave solutions was reported (Burckhardt, 1953).

Necrosis of the scalp has followed hairdressing procedures. Ippen and Seubert (1975) suggest the following explanation: if, instead of a bleach or dye, a thioglycollate solution is mistakenly applied, and the hairdresser, on realising the error, uses a borate neutraliser instead of the usual hydrogen peroxide, heat is generated and borium released, which causes the necrosis.

Hair straighteners
Hair may be straightened by the same chemicals as are used for permanent waving. The hair is kept straight by the viscosity of the formulation which contains the reducing agent, which is usually ammonium thioglycollate.

Depilatories
Many depilatories contain thioglycollates. By raising the pH of the formulation to 10–12.5, the thioglycollate activity is enhanced sufficiently to break the hair. Sensitisation to thioglycerol in an epilating cream has been recorded by Foussereau and Benezra (1970).

Patch testing
Ammonium thioglycollate 1 per cent and 2.5 per cent in petrolatum. The reducing solution itself should not be used because it is irritant.

HAIR SETTING LOTIONS

Setting lotions are used to maintain the style in which the hair is set. The earlier ones contained gum or mucilage, but these have now been replaced by aqueous or alcoholic solutions of a resin, usually polyvinylpyrrolidone. Colour and perfume are added.

Reports of sensitivity to this type of preparation have not been traced.

However, hair dyes are occasionally added to the formulation and may then sensitise, as in the four women who developed severe dermatitis from a coloured setting lotion reported by Osmundsen (1975). Patch tests with the setting lotion were positive and each reacted strongly to a coded dye (2424c) 0.1 per cent in petrolatum.

Patch tests
Setting lotion undiluted.

HAIR SPRAYS

Hair sprays are designed to form a plastic film around the hairs to hold them in place without making the hair look too set or feel too hard and tacky. Hair sprays consist of:

1. Resin:

Shellac (resinous excretion of insects living on resin trees in India) was used initially but it was found to be too hard and brittle.

Polyvinylpyrrolidone was an improvement but, being hygroscopic, it becomes sticky; this drawback is only partially counteracted by the addition of isopropyl myristate or dimethylphthalate.

Polyvinyl acetate/crotonic acid polymer overcomes many of these faults and is now popular. The acid monomer is neutralised by 2-amino-2-methyl-1-propanol (AMP) or 2-amino-2-methyl-1,3-propanediol (AMPD), both of which have a pH 10–11 at 0.1 molar.

$$H_3C - \underset{\underset{CH_3}{|}}{\overset{\overset{NH_2}{|}}{C}} - CH_2OH \qquad\qquad HOCH_2 - \underset{\underset{CH_3}{|}}{\overset{\overset{NH_2}{|}}{C}} - CH_2OH$$

2-Amino-2-methyl-1-propanol   2-Amino-2-methyl-1,3-propanediol

The degree of neutralisation of the resin controls its water solubility, so that, by adjusting the proportion of resin to amine, the normal and the hard-to-hold sprays are formulated.

Dimethylhydantoin formaldehyde is sometimes used.

2. Industrial Methylated Spirit:
This is often denatured by the addition of diethyl phthalate or Bitrex solution (denatonium benzoate) in order to give the alcohol an unpleasant bitter taste.

$$\left[\underset{CH_3}{\overset{CH_3}{\bigcirc}} - NHCOCH_2 \underset{\underset{C_2H_5}{|}}{\overset{\overset{C_2H_5}{|}}{N^+}} - CH_2 - \bigcirc \right] \quad (C_6H_5COO)^-$$

Benzyldiethyl[(2,6-xylylcarbamoyl)methyl] ammonium benzoate (Denatonium benzoate; Bitrex)

3. Propellants: Arctons 11 and 12

4. Perfume

5. Additives: lanolin

St John's

Women readily incriminate hair sprays as the cause of a dermatitis of their face and neck. Despite patch testing many such patients with hair sprays, none has reacted, and no case of sensitivity has been diagnosed. One woman had a positive patch test to her hair spray, but patch testing with the constituents supplied as coded samples was completely unsatisfactory; irritant reactions were produced and no allergen was identified. In the case of another woman, in which there was strong circumstantial evidence, patch testing with the hairspray and with each constituent separately was negative, as was an open test to the whole spray.

Patch testing
Hair Spray 'As Is'.

HAIR TONICS, STIMULANTS AND RESTORERS

Hair tonics, stimulants and restorers are used to try to improve existing hair; men also use them in the pious hope that baldness may, as a result, be prevented or even cured.

These preparations may contain sulphur derivatives, resorcinol, vitamins, β-naphthol, quinine, oil of Cade (Juniper Tar oil), capsicum, pilocarpine and cantharides (Harry's Cosmeticology).

Irritant dermatitis
A man, having used a Cactus Juice Shampoo for male pattern baldness, subsequently applied to his scalp the juice from what he thought was a cactus. Within minutes, he felt a severe burning, and in two days he had an exudative dermatitis. The plant was in fact *Agave americana* L. (Century plant) and its sap is incorrectly called cactus juice. The sap is a strong irritant and produces both urticaria and eczema; open tests were positive and were identical in the patient and two controls (Kerner, Mitchell and Maibach, 1973).

Pigmentation
Pigmentation of a man's palms, temples and hair margins by a hair tonic was attributed to photoactivation of phenols and diphenyls in the formulation to form coloured quinonoid compounds (Forman, 1975).

Patch testing
These preparations may be irritants if applied as formulated.

SHAMPOOS

Shampoos are meant to remove oil and dirt from the hair, but their degreasing effect must be limited to avoid excessive drying. Soap is generally unsuitable because, being alkaline, it reacts with mineral salts in hard water to produce insoluble soaps which are deposited on the hair. The alkyl sulphates, such as the mixture sodium lauryl ether sulphate, are the most commonly used substances. They are anionic detergents which clean the hair while retaining its lustre and leaving it manageable. The alkyl benzene sulphonates, used in washing-up liquids, are effective, but they do not leave the hair in such good condition.

The additives in shampoos, which have been detailed by Spoor (1973) and others, are included in the following list:

Preservatives: formalin, bronopol, parabens, cresols, fentichlor, tetrasodium salt of EDTA

Anti-dandruff and medicinal compounds: selenium sulphide, zinc pyrithione, iodoquinolines, quaternary ammonium compounds, coal tar solution

Conditioners (to coat and lubricate the hair): lanolin, silicones, glycols, egg derivatives, amino acids, polypeptides

Foam builders (stabilise the lather): coconut monoethanolamide

Stabilisers: stearyl alcohol, spermaceti, glycerine

Cosmetics: perfumes, dyes.

Shampoos are in contact with the skin for so short a time that they have little opportunity to cause dermatitis, and in fact they rarely do so. Medicated shampoos may bleach colour from dyed hair (Spoor, 1977).

Bird's nest hair
Very occasionally matting of the scalp hair occurs after a shampoo; the hair becomes irreversibly tangled and has to be cut off (Howell, 1956). Three women in whom this happened after a cetrimide shampoo were reported by Dawber and Calnan (1976) who investigated the factors responsible for this disaster.

St John's
At least three patients have been tested with every constituent of a shampoo, and all the tests were negative in each patient. A cetrimide shampoo caused an irritant dermatitis of the fingers, face and neck in one woman (p. 693).

Occupational dermatitis

Allergic
A woman in charge of packing shampoos in polyvinyl chloride tubes developed dermatitis of the hands, arms, face and neck. Patch tests: she reacted to formaldehyde (present as a preservative in the shampoo) and epoxy resin (used as a plasticiser in the PVC containers) (Ancona-Alayon, Jiminez-Castilla and Gomez-Alvarez, 1976).

Irritant
From a company making shampoos, Sheffrin (1974) reported in a letter that, each year, 2.7 per cent of the women employed on the automated lines filling containers received treatment at the medical centre for mild and transient dermatitis of their hands. Most cases occurred when a mechanical fault caused the shampoos to leak onto the filling lines, thereby contaminating the containers. Once their hands were clear the girls were able to resume this work. Pre-

employment exclusion of girls with previous eczema or xeroderma was thought to reduce the incidence.

Patch tests
Undiluted shampoos cause mild irritant soap reactions; the appearances, particularly at the second reading, are easily differentiated from those of a true allergic reaction.

HAIRDRESSERS

During the three or four years of their apprenticeship, hairdressers are taught the techniques of shampooing, cutting, styling, permanent waving, dyeing, tinting and bleaching hair. In the first year, their main occupation is washing hair, and they may be required to do more than 20 shampoos a day. In general, they cannot wear rubber gloves when shampooing because the rubber pulls the hair, and is uncomfortable for the customer.

The greatest insult to hairdressers' hands takes place, therefore, during their early apprenticeship, when their hands are immersed in shampoos for many hours each day.

In Munich, Borelli et al. (1965) studied young hairdressers over a four-year period. They found that the greatest number of reactions to the alkali resistance test and to patch testing occurred in second year apprentices; reactions during the third and fourth years were met less frequently and were not so pronounced. Reichenberger (1972) reported from Essen, that one apprentice hairdresser in three had skin involvement during their first year and that more than two in three were affected by the end of their training. On the basis of a survey, by questionnaire, of dermatologists in the United Kingdom, Black and Russell (1973) concluded that irritant hand dermatitis from shampoos was a considerable hazard among young apprentice hairdressers. Many do 20–30 shampoos a day, but at a busy time, some may have to cope with up to 40.

Allergy to thioglycollates among hairdressers was studied by Schulz (1961); the hydrazide ester was found to be a particularly strong sensitiser and its sale was therefore banned. Of those sensitised by the hydrazide compound, 60 per cent reacted to the amide of thioglycollic acid, 57 per cent to the glycollic ester and 35 per cent to ammonium thioglycollate. Topical application of the hydrazide, and of other esters, was successful in sensitising guinea-pigs.

Sensitisation to nickel is common among young female hairdressers. Wahlberg (1975) studied 35 hairdressers and found that 14 (40 per cent) were sensitive to nickel and he thought that their continual handling of metal objects at work was a significant source of nickel contact. The prognosis in these 14 patients was bad as all had had to leave hairdressing. A personal history of atopy was less frequent in those with nickel sensitivity than in the rest of the group. Ammonium thioglycolate facilitates the release of nickel from hair clips and plated metal (Dahlquist, Fregert and Gruvberger, 1979).

Formaldehyde, used as a preservative in shampoos, has caused allergic contact dermatitis in hairdressers (Schorr, 1971) and hair dander has also been described. A scratch test with an acetone extract of the dander was positive Mikkelsen and Thomsen (1978).

Ineral

In 1970, a new preparation, called Ineral, was introduced to strengthen hair weakened and damaged by either perming or bleaching. It is available only in hairdressing salons. The product consists of two parts; the original powder contained formaldehyde cyanoguanidine compounds, and the liquid was an acidic solution of polyvinylpyrrolidone. When these were mixed, an activated liquid was obtained which, if applied to hair within half an hour, combined with the keratin to strengthen it.

Hairdressers massaged the solution into wet hair without wearing gloves, and some developed hand eczema and nail dystrophy with onycholysis. The dermatitis characteristically affected the second and third fingers of the left hand. In some patients all the nails were affected, but in most it was just the left second and third fingernails; occasionally, the thumbnails or the right second and third fingernails were involved (Lépine and Fachot, 1971). The nails became discoloured and thickened, with separation of the distal half from the nail bed. Investigations in France showed that hairdressers had positive patch tests to Ineral (Lépine and Fachot, 1971) and established that the formaldehyde cyanoguanidine (monomethylol dicyandiamide) compound was both a sensitiser and an irritant (Bourgeois-Spinasse and Grupper, 1971). In Copenhagen, five hairdressers had positive patch tests to a 10 per cent aqueous solution of the mixture, and follow-up confirmed that the onycholysis was reversible (Hjorth and Niordson, 1972).

Following the appearance of these cases, the formulation of the Ineral powder was changed. In 1973, Hjorth reported that a hairdresser with a vesicular dermatitis of her hands had positive patch tests to both the new and the old Ineral powders diluted to 10 per cent in petrolatum.

St John's

Hairdressing as an industry was described in detail by James and Calnan (1959), who examined and patch tested 100 hairdressers with hand eczema. There were 68 women and 32 men; 63 were aged between 15 and 25 years; 61 had an irritant dermatitis of the hands, 16 had a combination of constitutional and irritant dermatitis and 23 were allergic to hairdressing allergens. These sensitisers were ammonium thioglycollate in eight patients, PPD in eight, rubber gloves in three, and the reaction was both to PPD and to thioglycollate in two patients; a further two reacted both to PPD and to rubber gloves. Despite the low dilution of ammonium thioglycollate (1 per cent was used for patch testing), it was considered difficult to be certain that the reactions to this chemical were allergic and not irritant.

During the three years 1971 to 1973, a total of 106 hairdressers were investigated in the Contact Clinic. They have been divided into the following three groups:

A. Hairdressers with hand eczema   84
B. Patients with hand eczema who had once been hairdressers   10
C. Hairdressers with skin disease other than hand eczema   12

A. Hairdressers with hand eczema (84 cases)

Sex

There were 72 females and 12 males; a ratio of 6 females to 1 male.

Age
The very young age, particularly of the girls, was striking; 46 (64 per cent) of them were aged 17 years or less (Table 4.8).

Table 4.8. Ages of 72 female and 12 male hairdressers with hand eczema.

Age, Years	15	16	17	18–20	21–30	31–40	41–70	Total
Females	8	17	21	11	11	2	2	72
Males	1	2	1	0	5	0	3	12

Site
The hands were the principal site of the eczema; in 71 (85 per cent) of the patients the eczema was confined to the hands and arms, and in only 13 (15 per cent) had it spread to other areas.

Time of onset
The hand eczema began within one year of starting work in 52 (62 per cent) of the patients, and it had, in fact, begun within 1–3 months in 24 (29 per cent). During the second and third years, the onset of eczema was less frequent, beginning then in only 9 (11 per cent) patients, but the incidence rose again to 20 (24 per cent) in those who had been at work for more than three years (Table 4.9).

Table 4.9. The time interval between starting work and the onset of hand eczema in 84 hairdressers.

	1–3 mths	>3–6 mths	>6–12 mths	>2–3 yrs	>3+ yrs	No Info.
No. of Patients	24	16	12	9	20	3

Prior to leaving school, some of these girls had already started doing shampoos in their free time, and even at this stage a few had noticed dryness and chapping of their hands. The intervals cited above have been measured from the commencement of full-time work. The breakdown of the skin in the first year reflects the heavy load of shampooing done in this period.

Results of patch testing
The results of patch testing these 84 patients with sensitising hairdressing chemicals are tabulated below:

48 (57 per cent) had positive reactions
36 (43 per cent) had negative reactions

	Concentration %	Tested	+	%
Hair dyes	1 (pet.)	84	27	32
Ammonium persulphate	5–1 (pet.)	78	12	15
Ammonium thioglycollate	5–1 (pet.)	77	2	3
Thiuram	1 (pet.)	84	2	2
Mercaptobenzothiazole	2 (pet.)	84	0	
Formaldehyde	2 (aqueous)	84	1	1
Nickel (total positive)	2.5 (pet.)	84	16	19
(Nickel = only positive)			(9)	(11)

Dyes

Three dyes were tested: *p*-phenylenediamine (PPD), *p*-toluylenediamine (PTD) and *o*-nitro-*p*-phenylenediamine (ONPPD) each 1 per cent in petrolatum.

There was a surprisingly high incidence of reactions to PPD and PTD among the junior apprentices. Of those aged 15–17 years, 21 of 50 tested were sensitive to PPD, 10 of 45 to PTD and 6 of 45 to ONPPD (Table 4.10). One girl, aged 19 years, reacted only to ONPPD.

Presumably the irritant hand dermatitis caused by shampoos predisposed these young girls to sensitisation. It is very likely that they were often careless about wearing gloves in all stages of dyeing and tinting and that their eczematous hands were often contaminated by the dyes.

It is usually impossible to predict clinically those who are sensitised.

Table 4.10 Positive patch tests to dyes in hairdressers of various ages.

Ages yrs	15–16		17		18–20		21–30		31–40		41–70		Total		
	Tested	+	Tested	+	Tested	+	Tested	+	Tested	+	Tested	+	Tested	+	%
PPD	28	11	22	10	11	1	16	1	2	1	5	2	84	26	31
PTD	24	6	21	4	8	0	15	1	2	1	3	0	73	12	16
ONPPD	24	2	21	4	9	1	15	0	2	0	4	2	75	9	12

PPD = *p*-phenylenediamine 1 per cent in petrolatum
PTD = *p*-toluylenediamine 1 per cent in petrolatum
ONPPD = *o*-nitro-*p*-phenylenediamine 1 per cent in petrolatum

PPD mix of rubber chemicals. None of these patients cross-reacted to the mix of PPD rubber additives.

Ammonium thioglycollate and ammonium persulphate
Seventy-five patients were patch tested with ammonium thioglycollate 5 per cent in water, one with 2.5 per cent and one with 1 per cent; two reacted to 5 per cent but, as mild irritant reactions occur with this concentration, they probably were not sensitised.

Seventy-five patients were patch tested with ammonium persulphate 5 per cent in petrolatum; 11 were recorded as positive, but these responses are difficult to interpret and some may have been irritant reactions. Another patient was negative to 2.5 per cent and of two patients tested with 1 per cent, one reacted quite strongly and was probably sensitised.

Nickel
All 84 patients were tested with nickel sulphate 5 per cent or 2.5 per cent in petrolatum, and 16 (19 per cent) reacted. Most were young, 12 being only 15–17 years old (Table 4.11).

Table 4.11 Ages of 16 hairdressers sensitive to nickel.

Age yrs	15–17	18–20	21–30	31–70	Total
No Tested	50	11	16	7	84
+ve	12	2	2	0	16

Dermatitis from jewellery had occurred in 12 of these 16 patients; in three no information concerning the source of sensitisation had been recorded, and one girl, aged 15 years, had no history of nickel dermatitis from jewellery or from clothing.

It is difficult to assess the importance of this nickel sensitisation in the aetiology of these young patients' hand eczema but contact with scissors and other metal objects used in hairdressing is probably significant once they have developed an irritant shampoo dermatitis.

Rubber

All the patients were screened for sensitivity to rubber gloves by routine testing with a series of thiurams, mercaptobenzothiazole and carbamates. Only two of the 84 patients had positive tests, and they both reacted to thiurams. One was a girl aged 17 years who reacted to tetraethylthiuram disulphide (TETD) and to dipentamethylthiuram disulphide (PTD). The other was a woman, aged 22 years, who reacted to TETD, PTD and tetramethylthiuram monosulphide (TMTM). The concentration of these chemicals was 1 per cent in petrolatum.

Formaldehyde

Each of the 84 patients was tested with formaldehyde 2 per cent in water. One girl aged 17 years reacted. She had no history of contact with formalin, and although the sensitivity may have been acquired from shampoos, the evidence was circumstantial. She was also positive to nickel and to cobalt, having been sensitised by the buckle of a watch strap, two years previously.

B. Patients with hand eczema who had been hairdressers in the past (10 cases)

In this group of 10 patients, there were 9 females all of whom had acquired hand eczema while hairdressing, and in whom it had continued despite changing jobs (4) or becoming full-time housewives (5). Their ages ranged between 15 and 20 years in 4, and between 21 and 30 years in 5.

There was one man; he was 66 years old and had retired, but had had, for 17 years, a generalised fluctuating dermatitis.

Patch testing with hairdressing allergens

PPD: Four women reacted (one reacted also to ONPPD; none to PTD). The one man also was sensitive.

PPD-mix of ruber chemicals: Two of the women and the man, all of whom were sensitive to PPD, reacted also to a mixture containing the three rubber additives: isopropylaminodiphenyleneamine, phenylcyclohexyl-PPD and diphenyl-PPD.

Rubber: One woman aged 20 years reacted to TMTD.

Nickel: Two women reacted; their respective ages were 19 and 26 years.

C. Hairdressers with skin disease other than hand eczema (12 cases)

In this group there were 9 women whose ages ranged between 23 and 29 years and who had the following diagnoses: contact dermatitis to red-headed matches (1), eczema of the eyelids (3), eczema of the face and neck (1), otitis externa and hypostatic eczema (1), widespread eczema (1), urticaria (1) and traumatic hair loss (1).

There were three men: one was 22 years old and had contact dermatitis from nickel jewellery (his hands were unaffected); the second was 30 years old and had hypostatic dermatitis; the other was 40 years old and had contact dermatitis of his face from epoxy resin.

Patch testing with hairdressing allergens
None of these patients had hand eczema and none had been sensitised by hairdressing chemicals.

Each one was tested with PPD, nickel and formaldehyde: the man with epoxy resin dermatitis reacted to PPD as a cross-reaction to sulphonamides which had been used 20 years previously to treat a leg ulcer; another man had been sensitised to nickel by jewellery.

About half the group were tested with PTD, ONPPD, thioglycollate and persulphate; in none was any test positive.

Patch testing

Hairdressers should be patch tested with:

1. *p*-Phenylenediamine 1 per cent in petrolatum
2. *p*-Toluylenediamine 1 per cent in petrolatum
3. *o*-Nitro-*p*-phenylenediamine 1 per cent in petrolatum
4. Ammonium thioglycollate 2.5 per cent in water
5. Ammonium persulphate 2.5 per cent in petrolatum
6. Formaldehyde 2 per cent in water
7. Nickel sulphate 5 per cent in petrolatum
8. Cobalt chloride 1 per cent in petrolatum
9. Rubber chemicals — thiurams, MBT, carbamates
10. Resorcinol 1 per cent in petrolatum
11. *p*-Aminophenol 1 per cent in petrolatum
12. Hydroquinone 1 per cent in petrolatum
13. Pyrogallol 1 per cent in petrolatum
14. Balsam of Peru 25 per cent

Recommendations
It seems reasonable to advise young apprentices with hand eczema to give up hairdressing in order to try to avoid the eczema becoming chronic and self-perpetuating. Trained hairdressers can usually continue at work with the aid of topical therapy, providing they dry their hands frequently and avoid allergens to which they are sensitive.

Atopic subjects do particularily badly and should be advised against hairdressing as a choice of career (Wilkinson and Hambly, 1978).

Interdigital hair sinuses
Men's barbers, but not ladies' hairdressers, develop pits, inflammatory nodules and even sinuses in the interdigital spaces of their fingers due to penetration of short, sharp hairs into the skin. A case in a dog groomer has been reported by Price and Popkin (1976), and they reviewed the literature.

MEN'S HAIR CREAMS

Men use hair creams to keep their hair tidy and to make it look glossy. These preparations are usually emulsions, but they may be brilliantines based on an oil, grease or, occasionally, polyethylene or polypropylene glycol. Mucilages and gels are also made.

Most formulations include a perfume and a colour; other constituents include lanolin, beeswax and other waxes, triethanolamine and an alcohol. The emulsions contain an emulsifier and may require a preservative such as chlorocresol or parabens, whereas the liquid brilliantines may contain a deodorised kerosene or isopropyl myristate (Harry's Cosmeticology).

A few hair creams contain a germicide.

Contact dermatitis
Sensitisation must be extremely rare.

St John's
　Fentichlor in hair creams has caused allergic photosensitisation (p. 436). Several
　men have been tested with the separate constituents of hair creams, but all the
　tests have been negative.

Patch testing
Hair Cream 'As Is'.

A hair cream, like any other cosmetic cream, may occasionally cause a mild irritant reaction. This can be checked by an open test and then by a usage test in which the patient is asked to use the preparation again as he would normally.

SHAVING PREPARATIONS

Preparations are available for use before, during and after shaving; the choice varies according to whether a safety razor or an electric razor is used. The following account is based on Harry's Cosmeticology.

Pre-shave preparations

(a) *Safety razor*. These are applied to soften the beard and are intended mainly for use with brushless shaving creams. They also reduce the irritant effect of shaving. They are based on a soap and a detergent but may contain surface active agents, urea or a sequestering agent. Most contain a perfume.

(b) *Electric razor*. As the face must be dry for an electric shave, these preparations are rapidly-drying lotions which stiffen the beard and lubricate the skin. They usually contain 70–80 per cent alcohol and a perfume; the oily effect is achieved by adding either isopropyl myristate or, sometimes, hexadecyl alcohol.

Shaving creams
These are used only for wet shaving with a safety razor or other blade.

(a) *With a brush*. Shaving creams used with a brush must not only form a good lather, but also be non-irritant and easily washed off. They are based on a soap and contain stearic acid, coconut oil, potassium and sodium hydroxides and a perfume; glycerine or sorbitol syrup is added to prevent too rapid drying. Other oils and emollients such as lanolin or cetyl alcohol may be added to the formulation.

(b) *Brushless*. These creams do not form a lather: they moisten and lubricate the beard, and, after shaving, they are not washed off but are rubbed into the skin. They have a formulation similar to that of vanishing creams. Most contain stearic acid and a perfume; in addition, oils, lanolin, triethanolamine and sometimes a surface active agent may be included.

After-shave lotions

These perfumed lotions are very similar to those for use before electric shaving, but their alcohol content is below 50 per cent. They may also contain a germicide, aluminium chlorohydroxide, menthol, camphor or, as an emollient, glycerine. A barber sensitised by an after-shave lotion has been described (p. 163).

Contact dermatitis

St John's

The only shaving preparations which have definitely been proved to be the cause of allergic contact dermatitis are after-shave lotions; the perfume is the allergen (p. 162).

Patch testing

Undiluted, many of these shaving preparations cause irritant soap reactions. Testing with various dilutions, open test and usage tests will distinguish between an allergic and an irritant response, and by testing with the constituents individually, an allergen can be identified.

Lipsticks

Ordinary lipsticks are composed of:

1. Mineral oils
2. Waxes
3. Castor oil
4. Lanolin
5. Preservatives
6. Perfume
7. Colours.

The oils and waxes form the basis of the stick; the waxes give solidity, the castor oil is present as a solvent for the dyes, and the lanolin is added as an emollient and to improve the texture. Two sorts of colour are used: the staining dyes to give a permanent effect, and the pigments, including lakes, to achieve a wide range of colours. In the past, the halogenated fluoresceins were the most commonly used staining dyes, but nowadays those azo dyes which conform to the American Food, Drugs and Cosmetic Regulations are also used, in free sulphonic acid forms (Wilsmann, 1965).

Sensitisers in lipsticks

The sensitiser in lipstick usually is a colour but occasionally is lanolin or perfume; cases have been reported in which it was oleyl alcohol or azulene.

Colours

Eosin (D & C Red 21; 2,4,5,7-tetrabromofluorescein)

Eosin is made by first condensing resorcinol with phthalic anhydride to produce fluorescein, which is then brominated to form eosin.

Bromofluorescein derivatives were established as a principal cause of lipstick cheilitis by Sulzberger *et al.* in 1938. That the allergen is not eosin itself but an impurity in it was first shown by Hecht, Schwarzschild and Sulzberger (1939) and Sulzberger and Hecht (1941); this was confirmed by Calnan (1959). They all found that sensitised patients gave weaker patch test reactions to eosin purified by crystallisation than to the original impure dye. Variations in the purity of eosin in different lipsticks accounted for patients being able to use one lipstick and not another. The exact chemical identity of the allergen is unknown.

Incidence of sensitivity

St John's

In 1957, when Calnan and Sarkany described lipstick cheilitis, it was the commonest type of cosmetic dermatitis, and sensitisation must have occurred quite frequently because they saw 110 cases in four and a half years. The condition was a contact dermatitis due to the eosin in lipstick and not a photosensitivity (Calnan and Sarkany, 1957).

The incidence of eosin sensitivity fell rapidly after 1960 (Table 4.12). Thirteen patients have been seen since 1966 but in nine the allergy was a legacy of a lipstick cheilitis 10–20 years previously. Three patients with cheilitis due to eosin were seen from 1970–1972 but their histories were long, being 10, 8 and 4 years respectively. However, the woman seen in 1975 had had irritation, soreness and exudation of her lips for only one year. Patch tests showed her to be sensitive to eosin, and it was ascertained that her lipstick contained eosin; she avoided such lipsticks and two months later she was greatly better.

Table 4.12. Yearly incidence of patients sensitive to eosin (St John's, 1960–1976).

Year	1960	61	62	63	64	65	66	67	68	69	70	71	72	73	74	75	76
No. patients	20	2	7	2	3	6	0	2	0	0	2	1	4	1	0	1	2

The fall in incidence is due in part to a change in the fashion of lipstick colours;

in the mid-1940s, dark red, long-lasting shades containing eosin in high concentrations (2 per cent or more) were worn. It was during this period that lipstick cheilitis due to eosin was so common. In the past fifteen years, paler shades of lipstick have become much more popular, and many of these lighter colours do not require the addition of eosin. Consequently, it may be omitted from the formulation, or, if present, it is in too low a concentration (0.05 per cent — 0.5 per cent) to sensitise. A few, dark, traditional shades may contain as much as 1 per cent or even more eosin. Another important factor is the use, nowadays, of a much purer eosin compared with that available in the past. As impurities in eosin are the sensitisers, the refined eosin, currently in use, is much less allergenic.

Clinical features
The clinical features of eosin lipstick cheilitis were reported by Calnan and Sarkany (1957). They described discomfort and soreness of the lips with scaling, cracking and dryness of the vermillion part, and occasionally there were more severe changes with exudation. The corners of the mouth were spared, and the skin beyond the lip margins was rarely involved because lipstick is not applied to these areas.

Other pigments
Other pigments, particularly lakes, are used in lipsticks to give a wide range of colours. Lakes are insoluble pigments formed by the interaction of a soluble dye and a metallic oxide such as aluminium oxide or calcium oxide (Calnan and Sarkany, 1957). The sensitising potential of these pigments must be very low because lipstick cheilitis has become a clinical rarity, and reports of sensitisation to individual colours are rare.

Case reports
In 1938, Sulzberger *et al.* studied 14 patients with lipstick cheilitis; of these, seven reacted to azo dyes present in their lipsticks. The following dyes were identified as sensitisers.

(i) *1-Sulpho-β-naphthalene-azo-β-naphthol*

Seven of the 14 women reacted to this dye.

(ii) *p-Nitrobenzene-azo-β-naphthol* (para red dark)

Three of the 14 patients reacted to this dye; an almost identical dye caused reactions in these three women and in another patient.

(iii) *Sodium salt of m-xylene-azo-β-naphthol-3, 6-disulphonic acid*

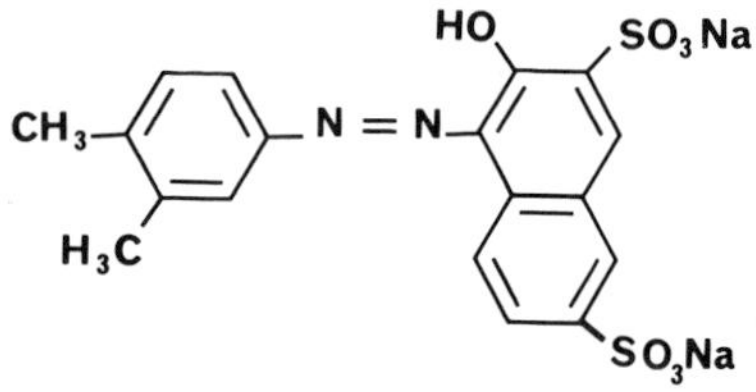

Three women reacted to this azo dye.

Carmine

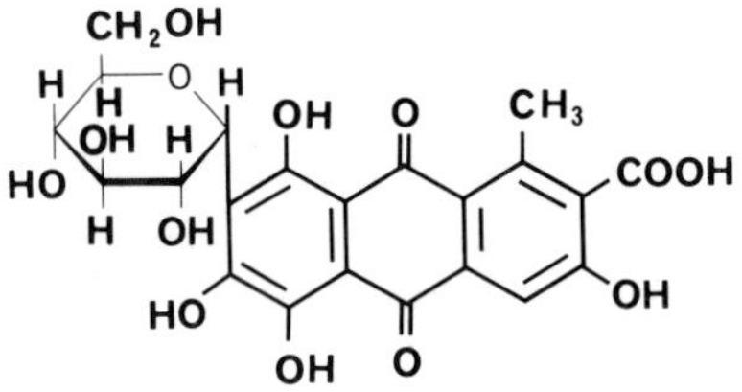

Carminic acid (the essential constituent of carmine). Carmine is the aluminium lake of the pigment cochineal which is derived from the dried bodies of female insects reared on cacti in Mexico. It was the allergen in three patients sensitised by lip salves (Sarkany, Meara and Everall, 1961).

St John's

From 1955–1976, only 12 patients have been seen with lipstick cheilitis caused by sensitivity to lakes and other colours; of these, five were sensitised by D and C Yellow 11 (Quinazoline Yellow SS) during the years 1973–1975.

D and C Red no. 36 (Permaton Red; Fire Red 2513)

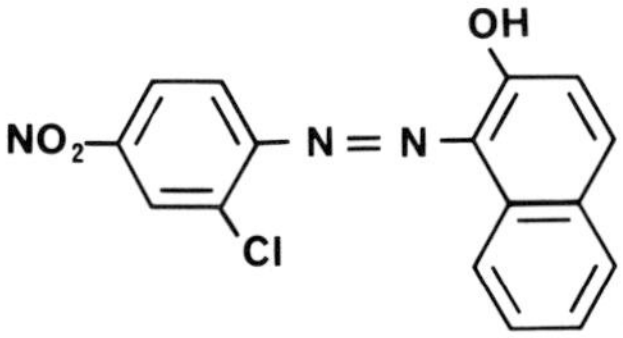

1-(*o*-chloro-*p*-nitrophenylazo)-2-naphthol

This pigment sensitised two patients, one of whom not only had lipstick cheilitis but also had a facial rash due to the same dye in a face powder (Calnan, 1967). A third patient aged 55 years was seen in 1969; she complained of having had dry, sore lips for one year. On patch testing she reacted to her own lipstick but not to eosin 50 per cent; on fractionating the lipstick and testing with the ingredients, she reacted to 1 per cent D and C Red no. 36.

The only difference between this dye and the 'para red dark', reported by Sulzberger *et al.* in 1938, is the presence in the former of a chlorine atom.

D and C Red no. 31 (Brilliant Lake Red R.) Calcium salt of 3-hydroxy-4-phenylazo-2-naphthoic acid.

This lake was the allergen in two patients reported previously (Cronin, 1967). In 1972 a third woman, aged 64 years, was diagnosed. She complained that, 18 months previously, after getting new dentures, she had immediately developed discomfort of her tongue, gums and lips. Patch tests with her lipstick were positive but were negative with eosin 50 per cent and when tested with the constituents, she reacted to D and C Red no. 31, 1 per cent in petrolatum.

D and C Red no. 19 (Rhodamine B; Tetraethylrhodamine; C.I. Basic Violet 10; C.I. 45170)

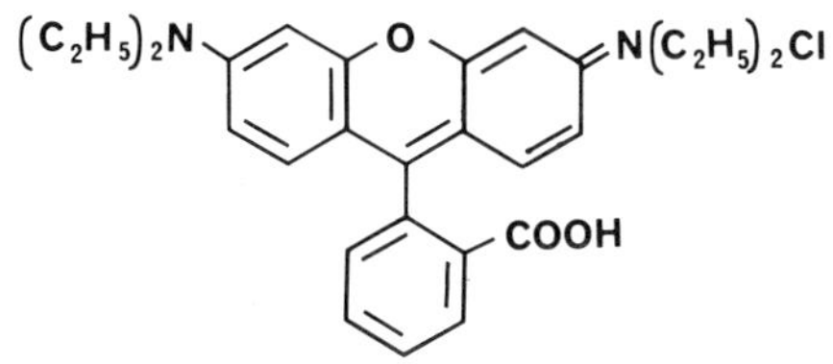

3-Ethochloride of 9-*o*-carboxyphenyl-6-diethylamino-3-ethylimino-3-isoxanthine.

This lake was a second sensitiser in the lipstick of one of the above patients who reacted to D and C Red no. 31 (Cronin, 1967).

D and C Red no. 17 (Toney Red; Sudan III; C.I. Solvent Red; C.I. 26100)

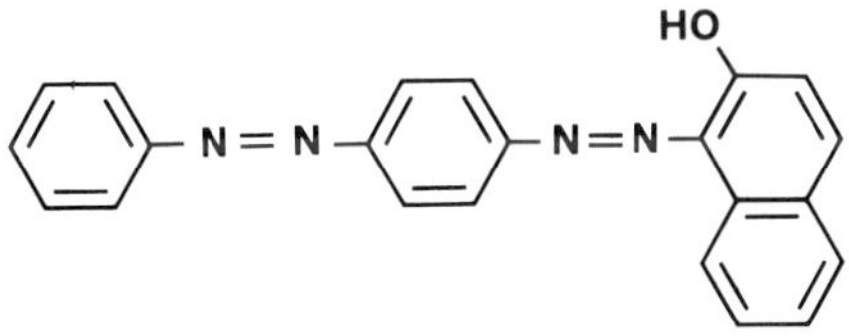

1-(*p*-phenylazophenylazo-2-naphthol)

Two of the five patients sensitised by Quinazoline Yellow, described below, were also sensitised by this colour in the lipstick.

D and C Yellow no. 11 (Quinazaline Yellow SS; C.I. 47000) is a mixture of components 1 and 2

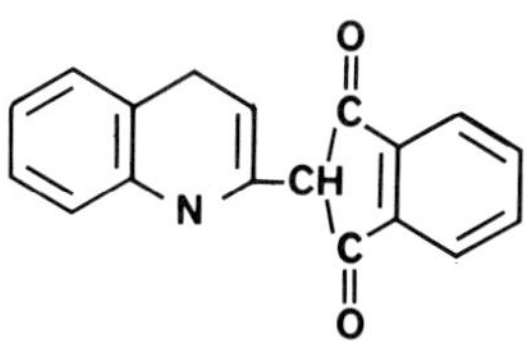

Component 1

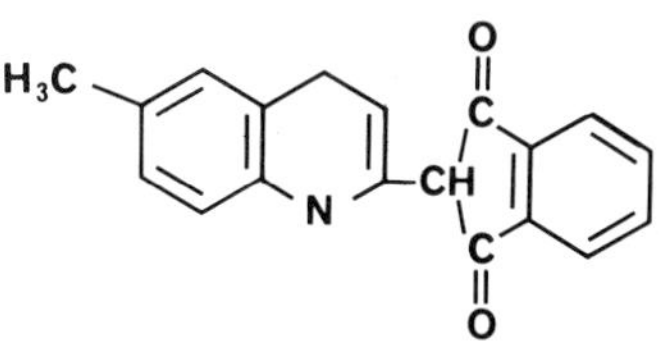

Component 2

Quinazoline Yellow (D and C Yellow 11) is a mixture of two compounds; it is only slightly soluble in alcohol or in oils. Although rarely used in lipsticks, it has the advantage of giving a more even colour than other dispersed pigments. It is sometimes added to nail lacquers, colognes and other lotions and it may be used in the coating of tablets. In the U.S.A. it is not allowed in foods but may be permitted for drugs.

Sulphonation of Quinazoline Yellow produces D and C Yellow 10 (E 104), a colour approved by the EEC regulations for use in foods, drugs and cosmetics. In the U.S.A. it is not permitted in foods.

Quinazoline Yellow is a severe sensitiser and has caused dermatitis when used in a lipstick (Calnan, 1976) and in rouges (Larsen, 1975; Calnan, 1976).

St John's

In the three years 1973–1975, five women were seen who had been sensitised to Quinazoline Yellow by one particular lipstick containing 4 per cent of this colour. Three of these patients have been described in detail by Calnan (1976). In the initial patients the diagnosis was difficult because the severity of the dermatitis made it quite unlike a usual lipstick cheilitis. After applying the lipstick a few times each woman developed severe oedema of the lips, face and eyes. In two patients the reaction spread to the neck. A third woman had a widespread eruption accompanied by malaise, and in a fourth patient each attack of cheilitis was followed by erythema multiforme. Three of the patients required systemic steroids. The first woman seen also used the lipstick as a rouge and on one occasion developed a severe reaction on her face without involvement of her lips. The second patient at the time of sensitisation developed a focal flare on her left wrist where the lipstick had been applied, to show its colour, at the time of purchase a week before. Patch tests: all five women were positive to the lipstick, and to Quinazoline Yellow; two reacted to another dye in the lipstick D and C Red 17, and three were negative. Initially the colours were applied undiluted but in the last two patients at a concentration of 1 per cent in petrolatum. One patient reacted less strongly to another make of lipstick which was found not to contain the sensitisers. This apparently anomalous reaction was due to contamination by the sensitising lipstick which had been caused by her habit of wearing two lipsticks simultaneously.

Active sensitisation

At least two patients have been actively sensitised by patch tests with Quinazoline Yellow, the first with 1 per cent in petrolatum and the second with 0.1 per cent in petrolatum.

D and C Orange no. 17 (Permanent Orange)

1-(2,4-Dinitrophenylazo)-2-naphthol

This lake was the sensitiser in another patient reported by Calnan (1967).

Lanolin

Lipsticks with a glossy appearance are now popular in the U.S.A. They may contain 46 per cent lanolin oil and other lanolins. Two patients with dermatitis from these lipsticks reacted to the routine wool wax alcohol 30 per cent (Schorr, 1973).

St John's

One patient has been seen, in whom lanolin was thought to be the cause of her cheilitis. This was a 29-year-old woman with atopic dermatitis whose face was severely affected; she said that she was allergic to lipstick. On being patch tested, 50 per cent eosin produced no response, but she reacted weakly both to wool alcohols 30 per cent and to one of her lipsticks; she did not react to five other lipsticks, all of the same brand. It was ascertained that the lipstick to which she was sensitive contained lanolin or a derivative, and that the other lipsticks contained neither lanolin nor wool alcohols.

Perfume

A patient with cheilitis, who was investigated by Baer (1938), produced vesicular reactions to patch tests with her lipsticks. Subsequently, she was tested further and she reacted to the base and perfume together but not to the base itself, or to other constituents. Of the perfume ingredients, she reacted strongly to methyl heptine carbonate (? undiluted). This is a synthetic chemical which smells of violets. It was shown in controls that this chemical is an irritant, but the intensity of the patient's patch test reaction to it, even when it was diluted in the lipstick, suggested that she was allergic to it.

St John's

The perfume was the sensitiser in one woman who has already been reported (Cronin, 1967). This patient had negative patch tests to eosin, but she reacted to two lipsticks of the same make; on subsequent testing she reacted strongly to the lipstick perfume 5 per cent.

Oleyl alcohol

St John's

Oleyl alcohol in the lipstick base was the sensitiser in three patients with lipstick dermatitis reported by Calnan and Sarkany (1960).

Azulene

St John's

Azulene (cyclopentacycloheptene) has been used as an anti-irritant in lipsticks and has sensitised one patient; she reacted quite strongly to azulene 1 per cent (Cronin, 1967).

Propyl Gallate

St John's

Propyl gallate was the unexpected allergen in another patient with mild but persistent lipstick cheilitis (Cronin, 1980).

False positive patch tests to lipsticks

St John's

In 1968, a 39-year-old atopic patient attended the clinic complaining that her lips had been sore and cracked for five days. When patch tested, she gave a strong reaction to her lipstick, but did not react either to eosin 50 per cent or to the standard series of allergens. She was subsequently re-tested with the same lipstick and with each of its constituents; all these tests, including that with the lipstick, were negative. She was asked to wear the lipstick again and did so without trouble.

Intolerance of lipstick

St John's

Occasionally, patients are seen who complain of discomfort caused by lipsticks but they fail to react to patch tests with their lipsticks. One such case, a 25-year-old patient, was patch tested with the individual constituents of her lipstick to ensure that she was not allergic to any of them and these tests were also negative. Another patient complained that lipsticks made only her top lip uncomfortable; she also had negative patch tests. It was thought that the discomfort of the lipstick caused her to suck and bite her upper lip, and that this made it sore, scaly and cracked.

These patients seem to have a physical intolerance of lipsticks but are not allergic to them. They can usually wear a lipstick for short but not for prolonged periods.

Patch tests

1. All lipsticks
2. Eosin 50 per cent in a bland base or soft paraffin
3. Wool alcohols 30 per cent in petrolatum.

When eosin cheilitis was prevalent, it was found that the patch test technique was important. For patch testing purposes, no reliance could be placed on the small concentration (1–2 per cent, or less) of eosin present in lipsticks, because the dye combines strongly with keratin and insufficient penetrates through to the dermis to elicit a positive result. To ensure sufficient absorption of eosin, 50 per cent in a colourless lipstick base, applied directly and firmly to the skin, was used routinely for patch testing (Calnan and Sarkany, 1957).

This same method is still used, and the patient is tested, at the same time, with all her lipsticks to avoid missing an allergen other than eosin.

Alternatives

Non-allergic lipsticks are available, which contain neither eosin nor perfume. If other allergens, such as a pigment or lanolin, have to be avoided, cosmetic firms are most helpful in giving information about lipsticks which do not contain them.

ROUGE — BLUSH-ON

The older name rouge has been largely superseded by the euphemism blush-on. These cosmetics are made as creams, compressed powders, colour sticks and sometimes as transparent gels. It also has to be remembered that women may use their lipsticks as a rouge.

Rouges rarely cause dermatitis but the colours, colophony and a preservative have been known to sensitise.

D and C Yellow 11 and D and C Red 17

The colour D and C Yellow 11 is a strong sensitiser and the severity of the reactions it evokes is a reflection of the allergen rather than a feature of rouge dermatitis. It has also caused lipstick dermatitis (p. 145). Its concentration was 0.075 per cent and 0.05 per cent in the rouge sticks used by the two patients reported by Calnan (1976).

A girl used a new rouge and two days later developed an acute contact dermatitis of her face, particularly around her eyes.

Patch tests: she reacted to the rouge and, of its constituents, to D and C Yellow 11 (Larsen, 1975a).

St John's

Two similar patients were reported by Calnan (1976). The oedema of the face was a striking feature in both women, and the first patient who also had swelling of her eye-lids developed an urticarial rash on her neck. The diagnosis of a contact dermatitis was not immediately obvious in either case.

Patch tests: both patients reacted to their rouge and D and C Yellow 11 1 per cent in petrolatum. The first patient also reacted to D and C Red 17 (1 per cent in petrolatum) another of the colours in her rouge stick.

Colophony

A woman developed an acute contact dermatitis of the face 10 days after applying a rouge to her whole face. Patch tests were positive to the rouge and to colophony, one of its ingredients (Foussereau, 1975).

Dowicil 200 and Di-isopropanolamine

Dowicil 200 is an isomer of 1-(3-chloroallyl)-3,5,7-triaza-1-azonia-adamantane chloride; it releases formaldehyde (p. 695).

Di-isopropanolamine in an eye gloss sensitised another patient (p. 114).

St John's

Dermatitis of the cheeks in a girl aged 17 years was traced to her use of a blushing gel.

Patch tests: she was tested with the standard series, the gel and its ingredients and reacted to the blushing gel, Dowicil 200 10 per cent (aq.), di-isopropanolamine 1 per cent (aq.) and formaldehyde 2 per cent (aq.) She did not react to Dowicil 200 1 per cent or di-isopropanolamine 0.5 per cent. She also had hand eczema, which was unrelated to this allergy.

A series of 168 controls were patch tested with Dowicil 200 10 per cent (aq.). Only one man with clothing dermatitis reacted; he was also sensitive to formaldehyde and formaldehyde clothing resins. None of the 61 controls reacted to di-isopropanolamine 1 per cent (aq.).

Patch testing

Dowicil 200 1 per cent in petrolatum.

Nail preparations

Nail polish is an abrasive powder used for polishing nails with a chamois leather buffer. It consists of finely divided particles of stannic oxide, talc, silica, kaolin or precipitated chalk (Calnan and Sarkany, 1958) and is harmless to the skin. Nowadays it is seldom used, having been almost completely replaced by nail varnish.

Nail varnish is now a commonly used cosmetic. Included with varnishes are base coats, top coats and coloured and colourless lacquers, all of which have a similar composition:

(i) Film former: cellulose nitrate, as pyroxylin, which consists chiefly of nitrocellulose, is used almost exclusively because it is hard, tough, stable and waterproof; however, it has drawbacks in that it gives a poor gloss, tends to shrink and it does not adhere well to the nail. These defects are remedied by the addition of a resin which improves adhesion and gloss, and of a plasticiser which reduces shrinkage and gives flexibility.

(ii) Resin: the most commonly used compound is aryl-sulphonamide formaldehyde resin (Santolite, Monsanto), made by reacting *p*-toluenesulphonamide with formaldehyde. It improves the gloss, adhesion, hardness and flow of the varnish.

(iii) Plasticisers: prevent wrinkling and distortion of the film of varnish; they include dibutyl phthalate, dioctyl phthalate, tricresyl phosphate, triphenyl phosphate, camphor and castor oil.

(iv) Solvents: constitute about three-quarters of the finished product. Many solvents are used and include ethyl, butyl and amyl acetates, acetone, methyl ethyl ketone, various alcohols, hexane, toluene and xylene.

(v) Colours: soluble colours are not used because they stain the nailplates and the hands; insoluble pigments are used instead, as they can be suspended in the lacquer without dissolving in it.

(vi) Pearlised or frosted effects are produced by the addition of crystals of guanine (2-amino-6-hydroxypurine); this chemical is obtained from fish scales, usually of herrings or sardines. A synthetic pearliser sometimes used is bismuth oxychloride. Colours and pearlising compounds are added to only some nail varnishes.

Base coat. This is applied before the varnish to help to prevent it chipping. The resins it contains are of the methylmethacrylate, phenol formaldehyde, sulphonamide formaldehyde or alkyd variety; these all form a better base for the nitrocellulose varnish to adhere to than does the nailplate. Compared with the lacquer, it contains more resin, dries more rapidly and forms a harder film.

Top coat. This is applied after the lacquer to improve its wearing properties and to increase the gloss. It contains more nitrocellulose and plasticiser and less resin than does the nail varnish.

Nail varnish remover consists of a solvent such as methyl ethyl ketone or ethyl acetate; to counteract its drying effect, an oily substance such as olive oil, castor oil or butyl stearate may be added.

Cuticle remover: Many of these are dilute solutions of sodium or potassium hydroxide; more elaborate formulations are also sold which include perfumes, preservatives and dyes.

Nail hardeners: These may contain a specific chemical such as formaldehyde or have a formulation very similar to a nail varnish.

   Most of the information on the formulation of these products has been taken from Alexander (1966), Klarmann (1962) and Sagarin (1957).

NAIL VARNISH

Incidence of sensitivity

St John's
   At St John's, sensitivity to nail varnish has been seen only in women. In 1958 Calnan and Sarkany reported 56 cases investigated during the previous five years, an average of about 11 patients a year. From 1965–1970 approximately six patients were seen each year and from 1971–1976, nine patients a year (Table 4.13).

Table 4.13. Incidence of nail varnish dermatitis. St John's 1965–1976.

Year	1965	66	67	68	69	70	71	72	73	74	75	76
No. patients	4	5	5	10	6	7	9	10	9	7	9	7

p-Toluenesulphonamide formaldehyde.
(X = the number of repeating limits)

Sensitiser—the resin

   Sensitivity to nail varnish was first described in 1925 (Miller and Taussig), and by the early 1940s it had already been established that the resin (Palmer, 1941), an aryl-sulphonamide formaldehyde polymer, was the antigen (Simon, 1943). At this time, Keil (1943) investigated 19 patients with this dermatitis and found that 18 of them had positive patch tests to *p*-toluene sulphonamide formaldehyde resin. In further investigations, Keil and Van Dyck (1944) found that, of four patients tested with sulphanilamide, one reacted, and that, of 21 patients tested with 2 per cent formaldehyde, 9 had positive responses.

In 1958, Calnan and Sarkany described the clinical features of 56 patients seen at St John's and recorded the results of their patch test investigations. Of 30 patients patch tested, all had positive reactions to their nail varnish, 20 reacted to the aryl sulphonamide resin, 2 to a glyceryl phthalate resin and 8 reacted to both. Twelve patients were tested with formaldehyde and all were negative; similarly, four patients tested with sulphanilamide did not respond.

Colophony is mentioned by Foussereau (1975) as a cause of nail varnish dermatitis.

Clinical features
The condition occurs principally in women, but two men sensitised by their colourless nail lacquer have been reported by Fisher (1974). The diagnosis can be missed even by clinicians aware of its features; this is a pity as it is easily cured. The patient rarely suspects her nail varnish and sometimes, wishing to reject what seems to her a very unlikely possibility, may deny using it. It is important to ask the direct question 'Do you ever wear coloured or colourless nail varnish?', and it is worth examining the nails for traces of nail varnish, as remnants have been seen despite a categorical denial that it has been worn.

Age

St John's
The ages of the 88 patients seen since 1965 have been scattered through the decades; about half were between 16 and 30 years, the youngest person was 16 years old, and the oldest 71 years (Table 4.14).

Table 4.14. Ages of patients with nail varnish dermatitis. St John's 1965–1976.

Age (years)	16–20	21–30	31–40	41–50	51–60	61–70	71–80
No. patients	17	25	9	18	12	6	1

Length of history

St John's
The length of history was recorded in 86 patients and ranged from three weeks to nine years. In the majority (62) the diagnosis was made within a year of the first symptom, but in 5 patients it was delayed for 4–5 years and in one woman for 9 years (Table 4.15).

Table 4.15. Length of history in 86 patients with nail varnish dermatitis (St John's 1965–1976).

	Weeks		Months		Years		
	0–6	7–11	3–6	7–12	> 1–3	4–5	6–10
No. patients	13	9	25	15	18	5	1

Distribution
In the majority of patients the condition is a dermatitis of the face and neck.

Nail folds
The skin around the nails is rarely affected because the lacquer is applied only to the impermeable nailplate. If the surrounding skin is inadvertently painted, the varnish is immediately wiped off because this smudging is cosmetically unattractive. However, dermatitis of the fingers can occur: Burgess (1940) described a case, and Palmer (1941) described another woman who experienced itching around her nails whenever she applied lacquer.

St John's
Since 1965, four women not only had involvement of the usual sites of nail varnish dermatitis, but also had dry cracked nail folds. One said that she tended to smudge the nail varnish on to her fingers when she was removing it.

Skin
The three principal sites of dermatitis were described by Calnan and Sarkany (1958):

1. *The eyelids*. The upper eyelids are the most commonly affected site. They become itchy, red and scaly but can occasionally be moist and exudative. Usually both eyes are affected but sometimes the eczema is unilateral.

2. *The lower half of the face*. Especially affected are the corners of the mouth and the chin. The eczema is blotchy, consisting of ill-defined, slightly red, scaly patches.

3. *The sides of the neck and upper chest*. These sites may have similar red scaly patches.

In a few patients the imprints of the fingernails can be seen as four or five oval, red areas on the sides of the face or neck, on the upper chest or, as in one patient, on the inner upper arms. This pattern of dermatitis is probably produced by resting the face or chin on the fingers for prolonged periods, or by sleeping with the hands in one position so that the nails always touch the same part of the skin. Such discrete eczematous patches on the neck are not always due to nail varnish as they can be closely simulated by a constitutional eczema; but in these latter patients the face is usually spared whereas in those with nail varnish dermatitis the face is usually affected.

Rare patterns of dermatitis

Otitis externa. The dermatitis may start in the external auditory meatus then spread behind the ears and subsequently involve the neck, face and upper chest. It is extremely easy to overlook the diagnosis in these patients and to misdiagnose the condition as seborrhoeic dermatitis.

Among the patients seen since 1965, in addition to the usual sites, the pinnae were involved in four, the skin behind the ears in six, and five had otitis externa.

Cheilitis and 'cracks'. Cheilitis, perlèche and cracking of the corners of the eyes occur occasionally as part of the dermatitis. Eight patients were recorded as having had involvement of the lips or angles of the mouth and in one of them the cheilitis was pronounced owing to her habit of pressing her nails against her lips.

Another patient complained of fissuring in the corners of her eyes, mouth and around her ears for four years and of red patches on her face for one year. She had been referred initially to an ophthalmic hospital. Once she stopped wearing nail varnish the condition cleared.

Widespread involvement. The dermatitis was confined to the head and neck in 68 (80 per cent approx.) of the patients seen since 1965, but in the remaining 20 (20 per cent approx.) it had spread to involve other areas. There was eczema of the upper chest in nine women and it had spread to the shoulders and arms in six of them and, in four the antecubital fossae were also affected. The thighs were involved in two women, the groins in one and the inner knees or popliteal fossae in four. In a further four patients, patches of eczema were present on the trunk. One patient had eczema of her nape, shoulders and axillae in addition to pruritus vulvae. She stopped using nail varnish and within a month her skin was clear.

Generalised dermatitis. In a few patients the eruption is almost generalized, covering large areas of the body including the face, trunk, buttocks, arms and legs. A case of this type was described by Shellow (1941). In another case, reported by Burgess (1940), there was typical eczema of the face and neck associated with generalised itching and pruritus ani; all these symptoms cleared when she stopped using nail varnish.

The elderly patient, who was 71 years old when she was first seen, had such an extensive eczema of her face, neck, ears and trunk that she was admitted to hospital; there the condition cleared, only to relapse immediately on her discharge. The diagnosis was subsequently made by a clinician who previously had had a similar case with widespread involvement; in both instances the patient's bright red nails had suggested the diagnosis (Calnan, 1971).

Patch testing
1. Several nail varnishes
2. Aryl-sulphonamide formaldehyde (Santolite) resin 10 per cent in petrolatum.

The nail varnish should be painted all over the disc of filter paper or lint and allowed to dry. This drying is important because not only does it evaporate solvents, which are irritants, but it also prevents the patch sticking to the skin and avoids the misleading erythema caused by pulling off an adherent patch. Drying can be hastened by putting the patches on a warm surface such as the top of a steriliser or on a radiator.

Results

When a patch test with nail varnish or the resin is positive it produces a disc of erythema which is usually slightly thickened. The reaction is rarely vesicular or exudative. Although the patient may not react to all her lacquers, in order to make this diagnosis patch tests with at least one nail varnish or the resin must be positive.

Formaldehyde allergy has been attributed to nail polish. This was the case in a woman who had eczema of her hands and arms and who reacted to patch tests with formaldehyde, nail varnish, neomycin and tripelennamine hydrochloride (Epstein and Maibach, 1966).

St John's

The patch test results in the 88 patients seen since 1965 are shown below; four patients were not tested with nail varnish, and in nine the resin was omitted. The equivocal and negative responses to the resin were probably false negative reactions.

	Tested	+	?+	—
Nail Varnish	84	82	2	0
Resin 10 per cent in petrolatum	79	73	3	3
Formaldehyde 2 per cent in water	87	4	0	83

Four women reacted to formaldehyde. In three patients it was probably due to an associated clothing resin dermatitis, and in the fourth patient the most likely source was her use of solutions for a duplicating machine.

Patient 1. A woman, aged 40 years, had a three-year history of irritation and soreness which had started on her lips and had subsequently spread to her eyelids and chin and to the sides of her neck; by the time she was patch tested, she had lichenified eczema on the sides of her neck. She also complained of her limbs and body being itchy. On being patch tested, she reacted not only to her nail varnish, nail varnish resin 10 per cent, and formaldehyde 1 per cent, but also to the clothing resin urea-formaldehyde 10 per cent. Her clothes were tested for formalin; she was then advised not to wear those which contained formaldehyde and was told that she should stop wearing nail varnish. Her eczema cleared and, over the course of a year, the irritation of her body gradually subsided.

Patient 2. A woman, aged 24 years, had had itchy patches on her neck, around her ears, and in her axillae and elbow flexures for two years. She was aware that perfumes and cheap jewellery irritated her skin. On patch testing she was sensitive to nail varnish, nail varnish resin 10 per cent, perfumes, nickel sulphate 2.5 per cent and formaldehyde 2 per cent. She was given a special nail varnish and all the eczema cleared except for the patches in her axillae; these were thought to be due to formaldehyde resins leached from her clothes.

Patient 3. A woman, aged 68 years, had had eczema on the neck, hands and arms for nine months. On patch testing, she reacted to her nail varnish, to nail varnish resin 10 per cent and to formaldehyde 2 per cent. She then wore only non-allergic nail varnish and her eczema appeared to clear, but six months later it recurred particularly on the extensor surfaces of her elbows and on her thighs. She was re-tested and was found to be sensitive to dimethylol urea formaldehyde 10 per cent, plastic and plasticisers. Her skin greatly improved when she avoided contact with plastic, but the possibility of an associated textile dermatitis was not investigated further.

Patient 4. A woman aged 34 years related that three years previously she had had attacks of eczema of her hands, eyes and face, and because patch testing showed her to be sensitive to nail varnish she wore a non-allergic lacquer and her eczema cleared for two years. It then recurred as before.

Patch tests: she reacted to aryl-sulphonamide formaldehyde nail varnish resin, her non-allergic lacquer, formaldehyde, nickel and cobalt. The non-allergic enamel did not contain formaldehyde or a formaldehyde resin. She used a duplicating machine, and as one of the solutions used in the process is known to contain formaldehyde, this was thought to be the source of her formaldehyde sensitisation. She was not investigated further.

Prognosis
This is uniformly good; once the patient stops wearing nail varnish the condition heals.

Alternatives
As the resin is the sensitiser the patient cannot wear any ordinary type of nail varnish and this includes coloured and colourless lacquers, base coats and top coats. In our experience advising the patient simply to allow the lacquer to dry completely on the nails as suggested by Fisher (1974) is quite ineffective.

Various cosmetic companies make non-allergic varnishes which are formulated without the sensitising resin, and these are suitable for such patients.

Dermatitis from guanine in pearlised lacquer
As described, guanine from fish scales is added to nail lacquer to produce a pearly or frosted appearance. Four women who were sensitive only to pearlised lacquers were reported by Stritzler (1958). They were tested with the ingredients of the lacquer and reacted only to the pearly material; in addition, they were found to react to pure guanine and to powdered defatted scales from sardines.

Non-allergic discolouration of nails
Staining of the nail plate by pigments in the varnish sometimes occurs. An orange discolouration of the nails caused by browner shades of nail varnish was described by Calnan (1967). One of the colours responsible was Transparent Yellow Lake 16901, a lake of Naphthol Lake Yellow FYS (Colour Index No. 10316). Calnan was unable to reproduce this effect in volunteers by using either the lacquer or the pigment. A pronounced brown staining of the nail plate, which was produced by resorcinol on lacquered but not on unlacquered nails, was reported by Loveman and Fliegman (1955). The development of the colour seemed to require the presence of nitrocellulose in the lacquer base, but the mechanism by which the resin facilitated the discolouration remained uncertain.

Pigmentation of the nails has also been reported to result from contact with 5 per cent ammoniated mercury ointment used therapeutically (Butterworth and Strean, 1963).

Nail preparations rarely damage the nails, but when they do the cosmetic disfigurement is so obvious and unsightly that the dermatologist soon learns of the condition. A spate of reports suddenly appears in the literature; but it as suddenly ceases once the product has been withdrawn from the market.

NAIL BASE COATS

A base coat is applied before the coloured nail varnish to help to prevent chipping of the lacquer. A base coat containing phenol formaldehyde resin and synthetic rubber was formulated over 25 years ago in the U.S.A.; this caused subungual haemorrhages, red-brown discolouration of the nail plate, onycholysis and hyperkeratosis under the nail. The associated symptoms were sometimes slight, and some patients failed to notice the changes occurring under their coloured lacquer. The condition usually began after using the base coat weekly for about three months, and the nails grew out normally within 3–4 months of stopping it. Patch testing with the base coat was positive; in one series of 12 patients, some reacted to the resin, some to the rubber solution and others reacted to neither (Sulzberger et al., 1948). In another group of 32 women, Rein and Rogin (1950) found that most (27) were sensitive to the phenol formaldehyde resin. Other reports have confirmed the occurrence of sensitivity to base coat (Laymon et al., 1948; Fanberg et al., 1948). To determine the mechanism, Mitchell (1949) applied the base coat to toe nails removed from cadavers and found that phenol penetrated through the nail plate. It was his opinion that all these base coats were similar and that each contained about 1 per cent phenol.

In 1959, a newly introduced undercoat caused similar changes in the nails of a patient reported by Reisch, but in this case the patch tests were negative. The effect was thought to have been due to occlusion by the non-permeable film of base coat.

SYNTHETIC NAIL COVERS

In about 1958, coloured adhesive films which could be stuck onto nails were introduced as a substitute for nail varnish. In the U.S.A. they were withdrawn from the market because they damaged nails, and in the U.K. similar nail plate disruption was reported (Calnan, 1958). The film was made of polyvinyl chloride and contained plasticisers, stabilisers and colours, and the adhesive was similar to that used in ordinary strapping. The effect on the nail was traumatic and not allergic. Samman (1961) attempted to determine how the damage was produced and concluded that the most likely explanation was a combination of the impermeability of the adhering film and the cumulative trauma to the nail plate when the film was repeatedly pulled off.

ARTIFICIAL NAILS

(See p. 583)

NAIL HARDENERS

A minor but annoying nail abnormality is lamellar splitting of the distal edge of the nail plate. It is probably quite common in women, and, because the nail breaks easily, it is impossible to grow fashionably long nails. Any cosmetic marketed as a cure is bound to sell.

In the latter half of the 1960s, nail hardeners, which were basically solutions of formaldehyde, appeared on the market. They caused paronychia, subungual hyperkeratosis, leuconychia and onycholysis. Once the hardener was no longer applied, the nails grew out normally. These changes were reported from the U.S.A. (March, 1966; Jawny and Spada, 1967; Rice, 1968), and one patient had such severe pain in her fingers that she was given systemic corticosteroids (Lazar, 1966). The condition was also seen in Canada (Danto, 1968). In addition to the nail dystrophy, three women developed small haemorrhages on their lips as a result of biting their nails (Huldin, 1968). In the U.S.A. several hardeners have been withdrawn because of these reactions.

St John's

At St John's, about six cases have been seen (Samman, 1971). They showed a rather dramatic whitening of the distal half of the nail plate with onycholysis and a little subungual hyperkeratosis but this was not a marked feature. These patients had usually, but not always, used the hardener more frequently than was recommended by the manufacturers.

Patch testing

The American patients and the one in Canada had positive patch tests to the hardener, but these reactions may have been due to the formaldehyde acting as an irritant rather than an allergen. The patient reported by Rice (1968) also had a vesicular reaction to formaldehyde 2 per cent.

Some of the patients seen at St John's were patch tested with the hardener and gave irritant responses; none was thought to be allergic.

Occupational

A persistent eczema of the right hand in a manicurist was traced to her sensitisation to the orange wood stick traditionally used for applying cuticle remover. She changed to an ivory stick and her hand healed (Brun, 1978).

Perfumes

Perfumes are complex mixtures of fragrances, and their composition, and the art of compounding them, are closely guarded trade secrets. They are widely used in cosmetics, soaps and domestic cleaners including polishes, detergents, scouring powders, disinfectants and household sprays. In cosmetics and soaps they are added to enhance the attraction of the product, whereas in household cleaners they may be used either for this purpose or to disguise an unpleasant odour.

A perfume is an alcoholic solution, usually of denatured ethanol, containing

15–25 per cent perfume oils. A toilet water contains 3–5 per cent of these oils, a cologne about 1–2 per cent and cosmetics less than 0.5 per cent.

A perfume oil consists of:

(i) Fragrances which may be natural or synthetic. Natural fragrances are either essential oils obtained from plants by pressing or by steam distillation (orange, clove, bergamot, pine needles, cinnamon and vetiver), or flower oils extracted from plants by solvents, usually alcohol. Known as 'absolutes' (purified concretes), these include jasmin absolute and rose absolute. Synthetic fragrances are organic substances and may be alcohols, aldehydes or ketones.

(ii) Fixatives to hold the fragrances. Three are secretions from the sexual scent glands of animals — castor from beavers, civet from skunks and musk from deer — and a fourth, ambergris, is a waxy material derived from the intestinal tract of the sperm whale (Klarmann, 1962).

Sensitising chemicals

The complexity of perfumes and the difficulty of obtaining information about their composition has meant that until recently comparatively little was known of the chemical sensitisers they contain. As each perfume is usually composed of a large number, even hundreds, of ingredients, patch testing patients with such series, even with the cooperation of the manufacturers, is only rarely practicable.

The Research Institute of Fragrance Materials (RIFM) has reported (Opdyke, 1975) on the toxic, irritant, allergic and phototoxic properties of hundreds of perfume ingredients. However, in Calnan's (1976) opinion, rather than advise against the use of single ingredients it is preferable to establish safe upper limits for their concentrations.

On the basis of his personal experience Fisher (1975b) has listed over a hundred potential sensitisers in perfumes, and their concentrations and diluents for patch testing. He included as photosensitisers the essential oils of bergamot, lavender, cedarwood, neroli and petitgrain. An eye cream perfume consisting of 94 constituents, and the 12 which elicited patch test reactions in a sensitised patient, have been reported by Larsen (1975b). He later patch tested 20 perfume-sensitive patients with several series of perfume ingredients and found that most reactions were elicited by jasmin synthate 10 per cent (18 patients), cinnamic alcohol 5 per cent (15 patients) and hydroxycitronellal 4 per cent (9 patients). Only nine patients reacted to balsam of Peru 25 per cent. Petrolatum was the diluent for each test material (Larsen, 1977).

Tropical grasses of the genus *Cymbopogon* are grown in India, Ceylon and Java and are the sources of fragrant volatile oils including oil of citronella, lemongrass oil, and palmarosa and ginger grass.

Oil of citronella

Contact dermatitis from oil of citronella was investigated in detail by Keil (1947). He concluded that the principal allergen is the aldehyde citronellal.

Oil of lemon

Oil of lemon is obtained from the peel of *Citrus medica* var. *limonum* (Rutaceae), which is grown in Mediterranean countries and in California.

Another patient described by Keil (1947) reacted to oil of lemon.

Lemongrass oil

The main constituent of lemongrass oil is the diolefinic aldehyde, citral. From it are derived ketones called ionones, which are used in perfumes and cosmetics. Sensitivity to lemongrass oil had been reported and investigated by Mendelsohn (1944, 1946). He described an outbreak of dermatitis in eight of 30 men who were working on a boat from India. Part of the cargo was lemongrass oil, some of which had been spilled. The eight men developed a contact dermatitis mainly of the face and arms; one man's wife was also affected and the wife and daughter of another were sensitised. As samples of the lemongrass oil could not be obtained, four of the men were tested with pine wood which has been contaminated by the fragrant oil and each reacted. Mendelsohn (1964) later obtained samples of lemongrass oil and used them for patch testing 20 patients. He found the undiluted oil to be a strong irritant and that at a concentration of 10 per cent it actively sensitised one in ten; he concluded that a 1 per cent dilution was suitable for patch testing. He did not obtain positive reactions with the ionones derived from citral.

Cinnamic aldehyde

Cinnamic aldehyde is a common ingredient of the perfumes used for household products, and alpha-amyl cinnamic aldehyde is often added to jasmin absolute. It is also used as a flavour and is present in many toothpastes, sweets, chewing gums, soft drinks and cakes. The chemistry and uses of cinnamic aldehyde have been reviewed by Collins and Mitchell (1975).

As a perfume ingredient, cinnamic aldehyde is a frequent allergen and cases of sensitisation have been reported by Schorr (1975) and Ogier and Duverneuil (1977). Tolerance of perfumes containing this aldehyde by a patient known to be sensitive to it was reported by Fisher and Dooms-Goosens (1976), and they suggested that this quenching phenomenon may relate to the low concentration of the aldehyde, or its reaction with an amine or an alcohol, or to its oxidation to cinnamic acid.

Cinnamic aldehyde used as a flavour in toothpastes has caused dermatitis (p. 180).

Benzyl Salicylate

In order to assess the incidence of sensitivity to perfumes in toilet soaps and detergents, Rothenborg and Hjorth (1968) routinely patch tested 1943 eczematous patients to two detergent and two soap perfumes. (A toilet soap contains 0.2–2 per cent perfume.) The soap perfumes were applied separately as 5 per cent in petrolatum, and the detergent perfumes were combined as 2.5 per cent of each in petrolatum. In this series 78 patients (4 per cent) reacted to one or more of the perfumes; men equalled women in the number who were positive, and in both sexes the older patients reacted more frequently.

Only one of the detergent perfume manufacturers would disclose the ingredients and gave samples for patch testing; the makers of one of the toilet soap perfumes gave limited information. It was found that benzyl salicylate was the most frequent sensitiser in these two perfumes. Benzyl salicylate is a pleasant-smelling organic solvent which is widely used for blending the perfume into the greasy soap.

In this group of perfume-sensitive patients, 46 per cent were also positive to wood tars, whereas only 23 per cent reacted to balsam of Peru. This contrasts with those who were negative to perfume among whom only 3.6 per cent were sensitive to wood tars. The authors concluded that, in the majority, this perfume sensitivity was likely to be an aggravating factor superimposed upon an existing eczema rather than a primary cause. In three sensitised patients there was a direct correlation between using the perfumed soap or detergent and a relapse of their eczema.

At the Finsen Institute, benzyl salicylate was used in the standard series for routine patch testing of patients with eczema. In their investigation of 167 patients sensitised to the optical whitener 'CPY', Osmundsen and Alani (1971) found that 18 per cent also reacted to benzyl salicylate. The importance of this allergy was uncertain, but it was thought probable that it relates to perfumes in household products.

Phenylacetaldehyde (α-toluic aldehyde, hyacinthin)
This chemical is used in perfumes and as a flavouring agent for foods in a concentration of less than 2 ppm. Fregert (1970) patch tested 275 routine eczematous patients to 0.5 per cent in alcohol: four were positive, and a further two patients were sensitised by the patch test. There was no cross-reaction between the balsams and phenylacetaldehyde. Fregert concluded that because of its sensitising potential this chemical should not be added to perfumes.

Methyl heptine carbonate
Methyl heptine carbonate has caused dermatitis in a lipstick perfume (p. 147), and in an after-shave lotion (p. 163).

Methylanisate
Sensitisation to methylanisate and parabens in a patient with a stasis ulcer was considered by Malten (1977) to be a group reaction.

Costus absolute
Costus root oil derived from *Saussurea lappa*, a Compositae plant, is used in perfumes. It is a potent sensitiser in the guinea-pig (Maibach and Mitchell, 1975). It has caused dermatitis of the face in Japan and it elicits reactions in those sensitised to Compositae plants (Mitchell, 1974). Its principal allergens are sesquiterpene lactones (Mitchell and Epstein, 1974) (p. 510).

Jasmin, cananga and ylang-ylang oils
In Japan, Nakayama has shown that jasmin, cananga and ylang-ylang oils are the common perfume sensitisers, whereas reactions to balsam of Peru are rare (reported by Mitchell, 1975).

Balsam of Peru
Balsam of Peru is obtained from trees growing in El Salvador. It is a thick, transparent liquid of variable composition containing many compounds, and smells of vanilla and cinnamon. This balsam is used by the pharmaceutical, cosmetic and flavouring industries. It is included in the standard patch test series principally to detect patients sensitised to perfumes and essential oils. However, only about half such patients will react to it, and its use does not obviate the necessity of testing with suspected perfumes or flavours. Hjorth's (1961) study is the standard work on this and other balsams. Ebner (1974) has recorded his patch test results with various balsams.

Balsam of Tolu
The chemicals present in balsam of Tolu have been listed by Mitchell (1975).

Incidence of sensitivity
Sensitisation to perfume ingredients is probably not uncommon but it is difficult to state a frequency because of the lack of a reliable test substance to screen for this allergy.

Causes of sensitisation
In women, perfumes and deodorants are the most frequent sources of sensitisation and in men after-shave lotions and deodorants are usually responsible.

St John's
The sources of sensitisation in 102 patients with a proven allergy to perfumes were listed by Calnan (1976) as:

Perfume	76	Moisture cream	2
Deodorants	14	Mascara	2
Eau de Cologne	11	Foundation	1
Talcum powder	7	Sun tan oil	1
After-shave	7	Cleansing creams	1
Hand cream	2	Freshener pads	1
Lipsticks	2	Tonic lotion	1

Medicaments
Perfumes are an unnecessary addition to medicaments and should be omitted because they add to the risk of sensitisation. Although Mycolog® cream contains only 0.1 per cent perfume there are three reports of it causing a contact dermatitis (Goldberg, 1972; Coskey and Bryan, 1975; Larsen, 1977). Ten patients sensitised by the perfume in one particular ointment were reported by Novák (1974).

Other sources
The perfume Violet 3567, in a black shoe polish, caused a contact dermatitis (Broughton, 1969). Allergy to the perfume in toilet paper was suggested as a cause of perianal irritation, but the diagnosis was not proved by patch testing (Keith, Reich and Bush, 1969).

Clinical features

Women develop red itchy eczematous patches at sites where perfume has been applied. This is usually behind the ears, on the neck, the upper chest and sometimes the elbow flexures and wrists. Occasionally it is used more widely and the eruption is then more diffuse. If the sensitivity is acute the eczema may be vesicular. Women frequently realise that they have become sensitive to perfume and a history of this allergy is given when they are seen for treatment of another pattern of eczema.

Men usually develop this sensitivity from after-shave lotions and present with a red eczematous eruption of the beard area and the adjacent part of the neck; the forehead is sometimes involved. They frequently do not relate their after-shave to their dermatitis. Eczema of the fingers in a barber was traced to an after-shave lotion; he had positive patch tests to methyl heptine carbonate (0.5 per cent pet.), hydroxycitronellal (10 per cent pet.) and cinnamic alcohol (5 per cent pet.). Chromatography confirmed their presence in the after-shave lotion (van Ketel, 1978). Facial eczema in a man may also result from the rare occurrence of his becoming sensitive to his wife's cosmetics.

Deodorant perfumes cause an axillary dermatitis (p. 109).

Pigmented cosmetic dermatitis

In Japan, Nakayama, Harada and Toda (1976) have proved that a common disfiguring pigmentation of the face may be due to an allergic contact dermatitis from cosmetics. The causative allergens were benzyl salicylate, ylang-ylang oil, cananga oil, jasmin absolute, hydroxycitronellal, methoxycitronellal, sandalwood oil, Red 219, benzyl alcohol, cinnamic alcohol, lavender oil, geraniol/geranium oil, trichlorocarbanilide and Irgasan CF_3. The patients were cured or greatly improved by adhering to an Allergen Controlled System (ACS) in which they used the harmless cosmetics recommended and a bland cleanser.

Patch testing

Perfume oil	10 per cent in olive oil
Perfume	undiluted
Toilet water	undiluted
Eau de Cologne	undiluted
After-shave lotion	undiluted
Balsam of Peru	25 per cent in petrolatum

Perfume series

Cinnamic aldehyde	1 per cent in petrolatum
Cinnamic alcohol	5 per cent in petrolatum
Benzyl salicylate	2 per cent in petrolatum
Methyl salicylate	2 per cent in petrolatum
Benzyl benzoate	2 per cent in petrolatum
Benzyl alcohol	5 per cent in petrolatum
Musk ambrette	5 per cent in ethanol
Eugenol	2 per cent in petrolatum
Isoeugenol	2 per cent in petrolatum

Coumarin	5 per cent in petrolatum
Hydroxycitronellal	4 per cent in petrolatum
Jasmin absolute	10 per cent in petrolatum
Jasmic synthetic	10 per cent in petrolatum
Costus root oil	0.1 per cent in petrolatum
Oil of Sandalwood	2 per cent in petrolatum

(Larsen, 1977)

Balsam series and components of Balsam of Peru

Pine resin	25 per cent in petrolatum
Spruce resin	25 per cent in petrolatum
Vanillin	10 per cent in petrolatum
Benzyl benzoate	5 per cent in petrolatum
Benzyl cinnamate	5 per cent in petrolatum
Methyl cinnamate	5 per cent in petrolatum
Cinnamyl alcohol	5 per cent in petrolatum
Cinnamic acid	5 per cent in petrolatum
Cinnamic aldehyde	1 per cent in petrolatum
Benzyl salicylate	2 per cent in petrolatum
Eugenol	2 per cent in petrolatum

References

Aeling, J.L., Panagotacos, P.J. & Andreozzi, R.J. (1973) Allergic contact dermatitis to vitamin E aerosol deodorant. *Archives of Dermatology*, **108**, 579.

Alexander, P. (1966) Hand preparations. Part One: Formulation of nail varnishes. *Manufacturing Chemist and Aerosol News*, June, p. 37.

Ali, A.R., Smales, O.R.C. & Aslam, M. (1978) Surma and lead poisoning. *British Medical Journal*, **ii**, 915.

Ames, B.N., Kammen, H.O. & Yamasaki, E. (1975) Hair dyes are mutagenic: identification of a variety of mutagenic ingredients. *Proceedings of the National Academy of Sciences of the United States of America*, **72**, 2423.

Ancona-Alayon, A., Jimenez-Castilla, J.L. & Gomez-Alvarez, E.M. (1976) Dermatitis from epoxy resin and formaldehyde in shampoo packers. *Contact Dermatitis*, **2**, 356.

Baer, H.L. (1935) Lipstick dermatitis. *Archives of Dermatology*, **32**, 726.

Benedict, W.F. (1976) Morphological transformation and chromosome abberations produced by two hair dye components. *Nature*, **260**, 368.

Bhat, G.R., Lukenbach, E.R., Kennedy, R.R. & Parreira, R.M. (1979) The green hair problem: a preliminary investigation. *Journal of the Society of Cosmetic Chemists*, **30**, 1.

Bhutani, L.K., Minocha, Y.K., Dhir, G.G. & Rao, D.S. (1978) Repigmentation of hair following photosensitive dermatitis. *Dermatologica*, **156**, 101.

Black, M.M. & Russell, B.F. (1973) Shampoo dermatitis in apprentice hairdressers. *Journal of the Society of Occupational Medicine*, **23**, 120.

Bolck, F., Ziegler, V. & Sieler, H. (1977) Bleaching of hair by carbamide perhydrate. *Contact Dermatitis*, **3**, 214.

Borelli, S., Moormann, J., Dungemann, H. & Manok, M. (1965) Ergebnisse einer vierjährigen Untersuchungsreihe bei Berufsanfangern des Friseurgewerbes. *Berufsdermatosen*, **13**, 216.

Borlin, von E. (1947) Berufsekzeme bei bienenzuchtern. *Dermatologica*, **94**, 109.

Bourgeois-Spinasse, J. & Grupper, M.Ch. (1971) Insuffisance des tests prophétiques. nouvelles méthodes d'investigation allergique. *Bulletin de Dermatologie et de Syphiligraphie*, **78**, 571.

Broughton, R.H. (1969) Perfume in shoe polish. *Contact Dermatitis Newsletter*, **6**, 115.

Brun, R. (1978) Contact dermatitis to orangewood in a manicurist. *Contact Dermatitis*, **4**, *315*.

Bunney, M.H. (1968) Contact dermatitis in beekeepers due to propolis (Bee glue). *British Journal of Dermatology*, **80**, 17.

Burckhardt. W. (1953) Coiffeurekzem verursacht durch ein neues Kaltdauerwellenwasser. *Dermatologica*, **107**, 253.

Burgess, J.F. (1940) Nail polish dermatitis. *Canadian Medical Association Journal*, **43**, 544.

Burnett, C., Lanman, B., Giovacchini, R., Wolcott, G., Scala, R. & Keplinger, M. (1975) Long-term toxicity studies on oxidation hair dyes. *Food and cosmetics toxicology*, **13**, 353.

Butterworth, T. & Stream, L.P. (1963) Mercurial pigmentation of nails. *Archives of Dermatology*, **88**, 55.

Calnan, C.D. (1957) Dermatitis cosmetica. *Praxis*, **36**, 782.

Calnan, C.D. (1958) Onychia from synthetic nail coverings. *Transactions of the St John's Hospital Dermatological Society*, **41**, 66.

Calnan, C.D. (1959) Allergic sensitivity to eosin. *Acta Allergologica*, **13**, 493.

Calnan, C.D. (1967) Hair dye reaction. *Contact Dermatitis Newsletter*, **1**, 16.

Calnan, C.D. (1967) Reactions to artificial colouring materials. *Journal of the Society of Cosmetic Chemists*, **18**, 215.

Calnan, C.D. (1971) Chloracetamide dermatitis from a cosmetic. *Contact Dermatitis Newsletter*, **9**, 215.

Calnan, C.D. (1971) Colophony in eyeshadow. *Contact Dermatitis Newsletter*, **10**, 235.

Calnan, C.D. (1971) Personal Communication.

Calnan, C.D. (1973) Ditertiarybutylhydroquinone in eyeshadow. *Contact Dermatitis Newsletter*, **13**, 368.

Calnan, C.D. (1973) Ditertiarybutyl hydroquinone. *Contact Dermatitis Newsletter*, **14**, 402.

Calnan, C.D. (1975) Compound allergy to a cosmetic. *Contact Dermatitis*, **1**, 123.

Calnan, C.D. (1975) Dihydroxydichlorodiphenylmonosulphide in a deodorant. *Contact Dermatitis*, **1**, 127.

Calnan, C.D. (1976) Quinazoline yellow SS in cosmetics. *Contact Dermatitis*, **2**, 160.

Calnan, C.D. (1976) Dermatocosmetic relations. *Journal of the Society of Cosmetic Chemists*, **27**, 491.

Calnan, C.D. & Sarkany, I. (1957) Studies in contact dermatitis; ii. Lipstick cheilitis. *Transactions of the St John's Hospital Dermatological Society*, **39**, 28.

Calnan, C.D. & Sarkany, I. (1958) Studies in contact dermatitis; iii. Nail varnish. *Transactions of the St John's Hospital Dermatological Society*, **40**, 1.

Calnan, C.D. & Sarkany, I. (1960) Studies in contact dermatitis; xii. Sensitivity to oleyl alcohol. *Transactions of the St John's Hospital Dermatological Society*, **44**, 47.

Calnan, C.D. & Shuster, S. (1963) Reactions to ammonium persulphate. *Archives of Dermatology*, **88**, 812.

Camarasa, G. (1975) Occupational dermatitis from beeswax. *Contact Dermatitis*, **1**, 124.

Collins, F.W. & Mitchell, J.C. (1975) Aroma chemicals. Reference sources for perfume and flavour ingredients with special reference to cinnamic aldehyde. *Contact Dermatitis*, **1**, 43.

Corbett, J.F. & Menkart, J. (1973) Hair Colouring. *Cutis*, **12**, 190.

Coskey, R.J. & Bryan, H.G. (1975) Contact dermatitis due to perfume in mycolog cream. *Archives of Dermatology*, **111**, 131.

Cronin, E. (1966) Lanolin dermatitis. *British Journal of Dermatology*, **78**, 167.

Cronin, E. (1967) Contact dermatitis from cosmetics. *Journal of the Society of Cosmetic Chemists*, **18**, 681.

Cronin, E. (1972) Clinical prediction of patch test results. *Transactions of the St John's Hospital Dermatological Society*, **58**, 153.

Cronin, E. (1973a) Dermatitis from wife's dyed hair. *Contact Dermatitis Newsletter*, **13**, 363.

Cronin, E. (1973b) Di-isopropanolamine in an eyeshadow. *Contact Dermatitis Newsletter*, **13**, 364.

Cronin, E. (1979) Immediate-type hypersensitivity to hema. *Contact Dermatitis*, **5**, 198.

Cronin, E. (1980) Lipstick dermatitis due to propyl gallate. *Contact Dermatitis* (to be published).

Dahlquist, I., Fregert, S. & Gruvberger, B. (1979) Release of nickel from plated utensils in permanent wave liquids. *Contact Dermatitis*, **5**, 52.

Danto, J.L. (1968) Allergic contact dermatitis due to a formaldehyde fingernail hardener. *Canadian Medical Association Journal*, **98** (ii), 652.

Dawber, R.P.R. & Calnan, C.D. (1976) Bird's nest hair. Matting of scalp hair due to shampooing. *Journal of Clinical and Experimental Dermatology*, **1**, 155.

Downing, J.G. (1951) Dangers involved in dyes, cosmetics and permanent wave lotions applied to hair and scalp. *Archives of Dermatology*, **63**, 561.

Ebner, H. (1974) Perubalsam und Parfums. Untersuchungen uber allergologische Beziehungen zwischen diesen Substanzen. *Hautarzt*, **25**, 123.

Eiermann, H.J. (1978) Cosmetic regulatory activities in the United States: past present and future. *Contact Dermatitis*, **4**, 157.

Emmett, E.A. & Wright, R.C. (1976) Allergic contact dermatitis from tea-coco hydrolysed protein. *Archives of Dermatology*, **112**, 1008.

Epstein, E. (1965) Misleading mascara patch tests. *Archives of Dermatology*, **91**, 615.

Epstein, E. (1966) Dichlorophene allergy. *Annals of Allergy*, **24**, 437.

Epstein, E & Maibach, H. (1966) Formaldehyde allergy. *Archives of Dermatology*, **94**, 186.

Epstein, W.L. & Taylor, M.K. (1979) Experimental sensitisation to paraphenylenediamine and paratoluenediamine in man. *Acta Dermato-venereologica*, **59**, Suppl. 85, p. 55.

Fanberg, S.J. & Sharlit, H. (1948) Hyperkeratosis and onycholysis after use of new nail cosmetic. *Journal American Medical Association*, **137**, 785.

Fisher, A.A. (1973) Allergic reaction to feminine hygiene sprays. *Archives of Dermatology*, **108**, 801.

Fisher, A.A. (1974) Unique features of nail polish sensitisation. *Cutis*, **14**, 327.

Fisher, A.A. (1975a) Allergic contact dermatitis from Germall 115, a new cosmetic preservative. *Contact Dermatitis*, **1**, 126.

Fisher, A.A. (1975b) Patch testing with perfume ingredients. *Contact Dermatitis*, **1**, 166.

Fisher, A.A. (1978) Dermatitis due to formaldehyde-releasing agents in cosmetics and medicaments. *Cutis*, **22**, 655

Fisher, A.A. & Dooms-Goosens, A. (1976a) The effect of perfume 'ageing' on the allergenicity of individual perfume ingredients. *Contact Dermatitis*, **2**, 155.

Fisher, A.A. & Dooms-Goosens, A. (1976b) Persulfate hair bleach reactions. *Archives of Dermatology*, **112**, 1407.

Forman, L. (1975) Pigmentation of the palms and scalp probably due to proprietary hair tonics containing various phenols and phenolic derivatives. *British Journal of Dermatology*, **93**, 718.

Foussereau, J & Benezra, Cl. (1970) *Les Eczémas Allergiques Professionals*, p. 385. Paris, Masson et Cie.

Foussereau, J. (1975) A case of allergy to colophony in a facial cosmetic. *Contact Dermatitis*, **1**, 259.

Fregert, S. (1970) Sensitisation to phenylacetaldehyde. *Dermatologica*, **141**, 11.

Fregert, S. (1972) Chemischer Nachweis von Paraphenylendiamin in Haarfärbemitteln. *Hautarzt*, **23**, 393.

Frosch, P.J. & Kligman, A.M. (1977) A method for appraising the stinging capacity of topically applied substances. *Journal of the Society of Cosmetic Chemists*, **28**, 197.

Gaultier, M., Gervais, P. & Mellerio, F. (1966) Deux causes d'asthme professionnel chez les coiffeurs: persulfate et soie. *Archives des Maladies Professionnelles de Médecine du Travail et de Sécurité Sociale*, **27**, 809.

Goldberg, H.S. (1972) Allergic contact dermatitis from the perfume in Mycolog cream. *Archives of Dermatology*, **105**, 896.

Gowdy, J.M. (1972) Feminine deodorant sprays. *New England Journal of Medicine*, **287**, 203.

Hannuksela, M., Kousa, M. & Pirilä, V. (1976) Contact sensitivity to emulsifiers. *Contact Dermatitis*, **2**, 201.

Harry, R.G. (1973) *Harry's Cosmeticology*, Revised by J.B. Wilkinson *et al.*, 6th edn. Leonard Hill Books, London.

Hecht, R., Schwarzschild, L., & Sulzberger, M.B. (1939) Sensitisation to simple chemicals. V. Comparison between reactions to commercial and to purified dyes. *New York State Journal of Medicine*, **39**, (ii), 2170.

Hennekens, C.H., Speizer, F.E., Rosner, B., Bain, C.J., Belanger, C. & Peto, R. (1979) Use of permanent hair dyes and cancer among registered nurses. *Lancet*, **i**, 1390.

Hindson, C. (1975) *o*-Nitro-paraphenylenediamine in hair dye — an unusual dental hazard. *Contact Dermatitis*, **1**, 333.

Hjorth, N. (1961) *Eczematous Allergy to Balsams*. Copenhagen, Munksgaard.

Hjorth, N. (1973) Occupational dermatitis from Ineral (new formula). *Contact Dermatitis Newsletter*, **13**, 385.

Hjorth, N & Niordson, A-M, (1972) Occupational dermatitis with onycholysis in hairdressers. *Contact Dermatitis Newsletter*, **11**, 254.

Hjorth, N. & Trolle-Lassen, C. (1962) Skin reactions to preservatives in creams. *American Perfumer and Cosmetics*, **77**, 146.

Howell, R.G. (1956) Matting of the hair by shampoo. *British Journal of Dermatology*, **68**, 99.

Huldin, D.H. (1968) Haemorrhages of the lips secondary to nail hardeners. *Cutis*, **4**, 709.

Ippen, H. & Seubert, A. (1975) Kopfhautnekrosen durch Haarbehandlung — eine Erklarungsmöglichkeit. *Hautarzt*, **26**, 598.

Ito, N., Hiasa, Y., Konishi, Y. & Marugami, M. (1969) The development of carcinoma in liver of rats treated with m-toluylenediamine and the synergistic and antagonistic effects with other chemicals. *Cancer Research*, **29**, 1137.

James, J. & Calnan, C.D. (1959) VII. Dermatitis in ladies' hairdressers. *Transactions of the St John's Hospital Dermatological Society*, **42**, 19.

Jawny, L. & Spada, F. (1967) Contact dermatitis to a new nail hardener. *Archives of Dermatology*, **95**, 199.

Kaye, B.M. (1970) Hazards of hygienic deodorant sprays for women. *Journal of the American Medical Association*, **212**, 2121.

Keil, H. (1943) Dermatitis due to hair lacquer and nail polish. *Journal of the American Medical Association*, **123**, 857.

Keil, H. (1947) Contact dermatitis due to oil of citronella. Report of 3 cases with experimental studies on ingredients and related substances. *Journal of Investigative Dermatology*, **8**, 327.

Keil, H. Van Dyck, L.S. (1944) Dermatitis due to nail polish. A study of twenty-six cases with the chief allergenic component toluene sulphonamide formaldehyde resin and related substances. *Archives of Dermatology*, **50**, 39.

Keith, L., Reich, W. & Bush, I.M. (1969) Toilet paper dermatitis. *Journal of the American Medical Association*, **209**, 269.

Kerner, J., Mitchell, J. & Maibach, H.I. (1973) Irritant contact dermatitis from *Agave Americana* L. *Archives of Dermatology*, **108**, 102.

Ketel, W.G. van (1976) Allergic contact dermatitis from propellants in deodorant sprays in combination with allergy to ethyl chloride. *Contact Dermatitis*, **2**, 115.

Ketel, W.G. van (1978) Dermatitis from an aftershave. *Contact Dermatitis*, **4**, 117.

Kinlen, L.J., Harris, R., Garrod, A. & Rodriguez, R. (1977) Use of hair dyes by patients with breast cancer: a case-control study. *British Medical Journal*, **ii**, 366.

Klarmann, E.G. (1962) Cosmetic Chemistry for Dermatologists, p. 55, 92 American Lecture Series. Springfield, Illinois', Thomas.

Kligman, A. (1966) The identification of contact allergens by human assay. *Journal of Investigative Dermatology*, **47**, 393.

Lampe, R.M., Henderson, A.L. & Hansen, G.H. (1977) Green hair. *Journal of the American Medical Association*, **237**, 2092.

Larsen, W.G. (1975a) Cosmetic dermatitis due to a dye (D and C yellow No. 11). *Contact Dermatitis*, **1**, 61.

Larsen, W.G. (1975b) Cosmetic dermatitis due to a perfume, *Contact Dermatitis*, **1**, 142.

Larsen, W.G. (1977) Perfume dermatitis. A study of 20 patients. *Archives of Dermatology*, **113**, 623.

Larsen, W.G. (1977) Cosmetic ingredient labeling. *International Journal of Dermatology*, **16**, 580.

Larsen, W.G. (1979) Sanitary napkin dermatitis due to the perfume. *Archives of Dermatology*, **115**, 363.

Laymon, C.W. & Rusten, E.M. (1948) Disturbance of the nails produced by base coats. *Minnesota Medicine*, **31**, 1218.

Lazar, P. (1966) Reactions to nail hardeners. *Archives of Dermatology*, **94**, 446.

Lépine, M.J. & Fachot, M-L. (1971) Dermatite allergique des mains des coiffeurs par un nouveau produit capillaire: l'Ineral. *Bulletin de Dermatologie et de Syphiligraphie*, **78**, 250.

Loveman, A.B. & Fliegelman, M.T. (1955) Discolouration of the nails. *Archives of Dermatology*, **72**, 153.

MacKie, B.S. & MacKie, L.E. (1964) Cross-sensitisation in dermatitis due to hair dyes. *Australian Journal of Dermatology*, **7**, 189.

Magnusson, B. (1974) The allergenicity of paraphenylenediamine versus that of paratoluenediamine. *Contact Dermatitis Newsletter*, **15**, 432.

Mahzoon, S., Yamamoto, S. & Greaves, M.W. (1977) Response of skin to ammonium persulphate. *Acta Dermato-venereologica*, **57**, 125.

Maibach, H.I., Leaffer, M.A. and Skinner, W.A. (1975) Percutaneous penetration following use of hair dyes. *Archives of Dermatology*, **111**, 1444.

Maibach, H.I., Leaffer, M.A. & Skinner, W.A. (1977) Reply. *Archives of Dermatology*, **113**, 1610.

Maibach H.I. & Mitchell, J.C. (1975) Costus absolute (Saussurea): Predictive assay for allergic contact sensitisation in guinea pigs. *Contact Dermatitis*, **1**, 184.

Majors, P.A. & Wild, J.E. (1974) The Evaluation of antiperspirant efficacy—Influence of certain variables. *Journal of the Society of Cosmetic Chemists*, **25**, 139.

Malten, K.E. (1977) Sensitisation to solcoseryl and methylanisate (fragrance ingredient). *Contact Dermatitis*, **3**, 219.

Mandy, S.H. (1974) Contact dermatitis to substituted imidazolidinyl urea—A common preservative in cosmetics. *Archives of Dermatology*, **110**, 463.

March, C.H. (1966) Allergic contact dermatitis to a new formula to strengthen nails. *Archives of Dermatology*, **93**, 720.

Marshall, S. & Palmer, W.S. (1973) Dark urine after hair colouring. *Journal of the American Medical Association*, **226**, 1010.

Mendelsohn, H.V. (1944) Dermatitis from lemon grass oil (*Cymbopogon citratus* or *Andropogon citratus.*) *Archives of Dermatology*, **50**, 34.

Mendelsohn, H.V. (1946) Lemon grass oil. *Archives of Dermatology*, **53**, 94.

Menkart, J. (1977) Cosmetic ingredient labeling. *Cutis*, **20**, 585.

Mid-Japan Contact Dermatitis Research Group (1978) Incidence of allergic reactions to coal tar dyes in patients with cosmetic dermatitis. *Journal of Dermatology*, 5, 291.

Mikkelsen, F. & Thomsen, K. (1978) Occupational contact dermatitis to human hair. *Contact Dermatitis*, 4, 165.

Miller, H.E. & Taussig, L.R. (1925) Cosmetics. *Journal of the Americal Medical Association*, 84, 1999.

Minkin, W., Cohen, H.J. & Frank, S.B. (1973) Contact dermatitis from deodorants. *Archives of Dermatology*, 107, 775.

Mitchell, J.C. (1972) Allergic contact dermatitis from paraphenylenediamine presenting as 'nummular eczema'. *Contact Dermatitis Newsletter*, 11, 270.

Mitchell, J.C. (1974) Contact sensitivity to costusroot oil, an ingredient of some perfumes. *Archives of Dermatology*, 109, 572.

Mitchell, J.C. (1975) Contact hypersensitivity to some perfume materials. *Contact Dermatitis*, 1, 196.

Mitchell, J.C. & Epstein, W.L. (1974) Contact hypersensitivity to a perfume material, costus absolute. *Archives of Dermatology*, 110, 871.

Mitchell, J. & Rook, A. (1979) *Botanical Dermatology*. Lea & Febiger and Henry Kimpton, London. p. 187.

Mitchell, J.H. (1949) Nail changes following the use of 'base coats'. *Medical Clinics of North America*, 33, 95.

Nakayama, H., Harada, R. & Toda, M. (1976) Pigmented cosmetic dermatitis. *International Journal of Dermatology*, 15, 673.

Nordlund, J.J. Hartley, C. & Fister, J. (1977) On the cause of green hair. *Archives of Dermatology*, 113, 1700.

Novák, M. (1974) Contact sensitisation to constituents of perfume composition in antiphlogistic ointment. *Československá Dermatologie*, 49, 375.

Ogier, M & Duverneuil, G. (1977) Dermites allergiques a l'aldéhyde cinnamique. *Archives des Maladies Professionelles de Médecine du Travail et de Sécurité Sociale*, 38, 835.

Opdyke, D.L. (1975) The safety of fragrance ingredients. *British Journal of Dermatology*, 93, 351.

Osmundsen, P.E. (1975) Contact dermatitis from a hair dye. *Contact Dermatitis*, 1, 186.

Osmundsen, P.E. & Alani, M.D. (1971) Contact allergy to an optical whitener, 'CPY', in washing powders. *British Journal of Dermatology*, 85, 61.

Palmer, R.B. (1941) Dermatitis from nail lacquer. *Archives of Dermatology*, 44, 13.

Papa, C.M. & Kligman, A.M. (1967) Mechanisms of eccrine anidrosis II. The antiperspirant effect of aluminium salts. *Journal of Investigative Dermatology*, 49, 139.

Pearl, K.N. (1977) Lead hazard in Asian eye cosmetic. *Lancet*, 1, 315.

Peter, J.B. (1975) Pigmentation from 'Loving Care' hair dye. *New England Journal of Medicine*, 293, 458.

Price, S.M. & Popkin, G.L. (1976) Barbers' interdigital hair sinus. *Archives of Dermatology*, 112, 523.

Reichenberger, M. (1972) Befunde bei Erstuntersuchungen von Hautkranken im Friseurgewerbe unter besonderer Berucksichtigung der Dyshidrosis. *Berufsdermatosen*, 20, 124.

Rein, C.R. & Rogin, J.R. (1950) Allergic eczematous reactions of the nail bed due to 'Under Coats'. *Archives of Dermatology*, 61, 971.

Reisch, M. (1959) Nail changes due to new base coat. *Archives of Dermatology*, 80, 230.

Reiss, F. & Fisher, A.A. (1974) Is hair dyed with paraphenylenediamine allergenic? *Archives of Dermatology*, 109, 221.

Rice, E.G. (1968) Allergic reactions to nail hardeners. *Cutis*, 4, 971.

Roed-Petersen, J., Auken, G. & Hjorth, N. (1975) Contact sensitivity to Irgasan DP300. *Contact Dermatitis*, 1, 293.

Rothenborg, H.W. (1967) Occupational dermatitis in beekeeper due to poplar resins in Beeswax, *Archives of Dermatology*, 95, 381.

Rothenborg, H.W. & Hjorth, N. (1968) Allergy to perfumes from toilet soaps and detergents in patients with dermatitis. *Archives of Dermatology*, 97, 417.

Sagarin, E. (1957) *Cosmetics, Science and Technology*. New York: Interscience Publishers Inc.

Samman, P.D. (1961) Onychia due to synthetic nail coverings; Experimental studies. *Transactions of the St John's Hospital Dermatological Society*, 46, 68.

Samman, P.D. (1971) Personal communication.

Sarkany, I., Meara, R.H. & Everall, J. (1961) Cheilitis due to carmine in lip salve. *Transactions of the St John's Hospital Dermatological Society*, 46, 39.

Schønning, L. & Hjorth, N. (1969) Cross sensitisation between hair dyes and rubber chemicals. *Berufsdermatosen*, 17, 100.

Schorr, W.F. (1970a) Allergic skin reactions from cosmetic preservatives. *American Perfumer and Cosmetics*, 85, 39.

Schorr, W.F. (1970b) Dichlorophen (G-4) allergy. *Archives of Dermatology*, **102**, 515.

Schorr, W.F. (1971) Formaldehyde in shampoos and toiletries. *Contact Dermatitis Newsletter*, **9**, 220.

Schorr, W.F. (1973) Lip gloss and gloss-type cosmetics. *Contact Dermatitis Newsletter*, **14**, 408.

Schorr, W.F. (1974) Cosmetic allergy: Diagnosis, incidence and management. *Cutis*, **14**, 844.

Schorr, W.F. (1975) Cinnamic aldehyde allergy. *Contact Dermatitis*, **1**, 108.

Schulz, K.H. (1961) Durch Thioglykoesaurederivate ausgeloste Kontaktekzeme im Friseurberuf. *Berufsdermatosen*, **9**, 244.

Schwartz, L. & Barban, C. (1952) Paraphenylenediamine hair dyes. *Archives of Dermatology*, **66**, 233.

Schwartz, L & Peck, S.M. (1935) The irritants in adhesive plaster. *Public Health Reports*, **50**, 811.

Schwartzberg, S. (1961) Allergic eczematous contact dermatitis caused by sensitisation to glyceryl monostearate. *Annals of Allergy*, **19**, 402.

Searle, C.E., Harnden, D.G., Venitt, S. & Gyde, O.H.B. (1975) Carcinogenicity & mutagenicity tests of some hair colourants and constituents. *Nature*, **255**, 506.

Searle, C.E., & Jones, E.L. (1977) Effects of repeated application of two semi-permanent hair dyes to the skin of a and DBAF mice. *British Journal of Cancer*, **36**, 467.

Selzle, D. & Wolff, H.H. (1976) Exogener Haarschaden durch Bleichen & Kaltwelle. *Hautarzt*, **27**, 453.

Sheffrin, S. (1974) Shampoo dermatitis. *Journal of the Soceity of Occupational Medicine*, **24**, 31.

Shehadeh, NH. & Kligman, A.M. (1963) The effect of topical antibacterial agents on the bacterial flora of the axilla. *Journal of Investigative Dermatology*, **40**, 61.

Shelley, W.B. & Hurley, H.J. (1975) Studies on topical antiperspirant control of axillary hyperhidrosis. *Acta Dermato-Venereologica*, **55**, 241.

Shelley, W.B., Hurley, H.J. & Nichols, A.C. (1953) Axillary odour. Experimental study of the role of bacteria, apocrine sweat and deodorants. *Archives of Dermatology*, **68**, 430.

Shellow, H. (1941) Generalised dermatitis from nail polish. *Archives of Dermatology*, **44**, 463.

Shmunes, E. & Levy, E.J. (1972) Quaternary ammonium compound contact dermatitis from a deodorant. *Archives of Dermatology*, **105**, 91.

Simon, F.A. (1943) Nail polish eczema. *Southern Medical Journal*, **36**, 157.

Sneddon, I.B. (1972) Dermatitis from dibutylphthalate in an aerosol antiperspirant & deodorant. *Contact Dermatitis Newsletter*, **12**, 308.

Spoor, H.J. (1973) Shampoos. *Cutis*, **12**, 671.

Spoor, H.J. (1977) Shampoos and hair dyes. *Cutis*, **20**, 189.

Steed, M.W. (1975) Evaluation of antiperspirant preparations under normal conditions of use. *Journal of the Society of Cosmetic Chemists*, **26**, 17.

Stritzler, C. (1958) Dermatitis of the face caused by guanine in pearly nail lacquer. *Archives of Dermatology*, **78**, 252.

Sugai, T., Takashashi, Y. & Takagi, T. (1977) Pigmented cosmetic dermatitis and coal tar dyes. *Contact Dermatitis*, **3**, 249.

Sulzberger, M.B., Goodman, J., Byrne, L.A. & Mallozzi, E.D. (1938) Acquired specific hypersensitivity to simple chemicals. II. Cheilitis, with special reference to sensitivity to lipsticks. *Archives of Dermatology*, **37**, 597.

Sulzberger, M.B. & Hecht, R. (1941) Acquired specific hypersensitivity to simple chemicals. VI. Further studies on the purification of dyes in relation to allergic reactions. *Journal of Allergy*, **12**, 129.

Sulzberger, M.B., Rein, C., Fanburg, S.J., Wolf, M., Shair, M.H. & Popkin, G.L. (1948) Allergic eczematous reactions of the nail bed. Persistent subungual and ungual changes based on contact with 'undercoats' containing artificial resins and rubbers. *Journal of Investigative Dermatology*, **11**, 67.

Thyresson, N., Lodin, A., & Nilzen, A. (1956) Eczema of the hands due to triethanolamine in cosmetic hand lotions for housewives. *Acta Dermato-venererologica*, **36**, 355.

Verbov, J.L. (1969) Contact dermatitis from Miranols. *Transactions St John's Hospital Dermatological Society*, **55**, 192.

Wahlberg, J.E. (1975) Nickel allergy and atopy in hairdressers. *Contact Dermatitis*, **1**, 161.

Wahlberg, J.E. (1976) Routine patch testing with Irgasan DP300. *Contact Dermatitis*, **2**, 292.

Wanscher, B. (1976) Contact dermatitis from propolis. *British Journal of Dermatology*, **94**, 451.

Warin, A.P. (1976) Contact dermatitis to partner's hair dye. *Clinical and Experimental Dermatology*, **1**, 283.

Widstrom, L. (1977) Allergic reactions to ammonium persulphate in hair bleach. *Contact Dermatitis*, **3**, 343.

Wilkinson, D.S. & Hambly, E.M. (1978) Prognosis of hand eczema in hairdressing apprentices. *Contact Dermatitis*, **4**, 63.

Wilsmann, H. (1965) Replacement of bromo acids in lipsticks by water soluble FDC and DC colours. *Journal of the Society of Cosmetic Chemists*, **16**, 105.

Wishart, J.M. (1974) Generalised exfoliative dermatitis due to contact with an antiperspirant. *British Journal of Clinical Practice*, **28**, 264.

Wooding, W.M. & Finklestein, P. (1975) A critical comparison of two procedures for antiperspirant evaluation. *Journal of the Society of Cosmetic Chemists*, **26**, 255.

Yare, R.S. & Garcia, M. (1977) Percutaneous penetration following use of hair dyes. *Archives of Dermatology*, **113**, 1610.

5.

Foods

PROTEINS
ADDITIVES
  Antimicrobials
    Sodium benzoate
    Paraben esters
    Sorbic acid and salts
    Propionic acid and salts
    Sulphur dioxide and sulphites
    Acetic acid and salts
    Nitrites and nitrates
    Ethylene and propylene oxides
    Diethyl pyrocarbonate
    Propylene glycol
    Antibiotics
  Antioxidants
    Butylated hydroxyanisole
    Butylated hydroxytoluene
    Gallate esters
    Tocopherols
  Sequestrants
  Surface active agents
COLOURS
FLAVOURING AGENTS AND SPICES
  Foods
  Toothpastes

FLOUR AND GRAINS
PLANTS
  Chicory
  Endive
  Garlic (p. 471)
  Lettuce
  Onion (p. 471)
  Potato
  Green Coffee
ADDITIVES IN ANIMAL FEEDS
  Cobalt
  Dinitolmide
  Ethoxyquin
  Ethylenediamine dihydroiodide
  Furazolidone
  Nitrofurazone
  Halquinol
  Hydroquinone
  Quindoxin (p. 440)
  Spiramycin
  Tylosin
  Virginiamycin

Protein

The term 'eczema hybrids' was coined by Malten (1967, 1968) to describe atopic patients with an associated contact sensitivity, and patients with contact dermatitis who had positive intracutaneous tests to inhalant and other reaginic allergens. He suggested that in such patients healing of a contact eczema may be retarded by reaginic proteins penetrating the damaged epidermis.

This conception of protein as a cause of allergic contact dermatitis was verified by Hjorth and Weismann (1972) when they found that a combination of Type I and Type IV sensitivities caused occupational hand eczema in people preparing food. In 1976, Hjorth and Roed-Petersen reported their detailed investigation of 24 female sandwich-makers or kitchen workers and nine male chefs with hand eczema. The patients presented with eczema of the finger tips of the left hand, corresponding to the sites of contact with the food during its preparation. They had noticed that handling fish or certain vegetables caused, within 10–30 minutes, irritation which was sometimes followed by redness and vesicles. On investigation, 10 of the patients had positive scratch tests only and were designated as having protein contact dermatitis. In another 15, both scratch and patch tests were positive and, of the remaining eight, six had plain Type IV contact dermatitis and two an irritant dermatitis. Applying the incriminated food for 20 minutes to skin healed of eczema caused, within half an hour, erythema and itching and sometimes vesicles. In the Type I group, fish and shellfish were the most frequent allergens; in the Type IV group, metals, onion and garlic predominated, while a few were sensitive to cucumber, horseradish, leek, parsley and tomato. It was stressed that patch tests will not diagnose this Type I variety of contact dermatitis. Suspected foods must be used for scratch tests and also as 20-minute applications to normal skin and sites of previous eczema. The authors concluded that protein can not only cause a primary allergic dermatitis (protein contact dermatitis), but also aggravate an existing dermatitis and may exacerbate an atopic eczema.

In 1948 Bonnevie described 'mussel itch', an occupational hand dermatosis occurring in Danish factories making mussel preserves. In some factories up to half the workers were affected. They developed red, itchy, scabies-like papules on the hands, particularly in the finger webs, which subsided after 1–2 days away from work. The lesions probably occurred at sites of shell scratches. A few employees developed urticaria or asthma, possibly from inhaling mussel fumes from the autoclaves. Sensitivity to raw and autoclaved mussel was confirmed by positive intradermal and passive transfer tests.

An interesting case (Mitchell, 1974a) was that of a young Indonesian housewife with hand eczema, which had begun when she was a hairdresser. At home she prepared shrimps frequently and had noticed that the raw, but not the cooked, flesh made her fingers itchy. A scratch test with raw shrimp flesh (*Pandalus*) (family Pandalidae) was positive, while that with the cooked flesh was negative. Once the hand eczema had healed, she could handle raw shrimps without discomfort, although scratch tests with raw shrimp remained positive. This contact urticaria was thought to have aggravated rather than caused the patient's eczema. A patient of Klehr and Milbradt (1978) had a positive reaction to the muscle of pig but not to its kidney. The antigens were thought to be the muscle amino-acids 3-methyl-histidine, monomethyl lysin and tri-methyl lysin.

Mitchell (1974b) made a strong plea that in reports of sensitivity to animal protein the correct zoological names be used so that records from centres in different places can be validly compared.

Patch and scratch tests

The following foods were recommended by Hjorth (1975) for investigating chefs and other kitchen workers; additional foods reported as contact allergens have been included in the list:

Artichoke	Fish
Asparagus	Flour
Carrot	Meats
Chives	Poultry skin and flesh

Cucumber
Endive
Garlic
Horseradish
Cheese

Shellfish
Leek
Lemon peel
Lettuce
Onion (various).

Food additives

A food additive is a compound, other than a food, which is deliberately added to improve storage, processing, production or packaging of the food. An interesting and comprehensive account of these substances, which range from enzymes and vitamins to colours, is given in the Handbook of Food Additives (1972) and much of the information given below is taken from this source. In the United States, compounds categorised as GRAS ('generally recognised as safe') are included in a GRAS list which exempts them from the Federal law requiring safety clearance before marketing. Regulations concerning these food additives differ from country to country. Food additives have been reviewed by Jukes (1977).

Antimicrobials
Despite the widespread consumption of antimicrobials in food, their presence seems not to be an appreciable hazard. They are added to protect the carbohydrate and protein content of foods from attack by micro-organisms, rather than the fats which are not so vulnerable.

Sodium benzoate
Sodium benzoate is more active against bacteria and yeasts than against moulds. In concentrations of 0.05–0.1 per cent it is added to acidic foods such as drinks, syrups, fruits, jams, jellies, salted margarine, pickles and pie fillings.

Paraben esters (p. 665)
The paraben esters inhibit the growth of moulds and yeasts; this activity increases with their chain length, but their water solubility proportionally decreases. In concentrations up to 0.1 per cent they are added to cakes, particularly fruit cakes, pies and fillings, soft drinks, beer, creams and pastes, and fruit products.

The paraben esters are well known topical sensitisers (p. 666) but their presence in food seems not to cause trouble, even in those sensitised (Schorr, 1972).

Sorbic acid and its salts
Sorbic acid and its salts are more active against yeasts and moulds than against bacteria. Concentration limits are set for only certain foods: in cheese it may not exceed 0.3 per cent by weight. Sorbic acid and sorbates may be added directly to the food or used as a spray, dip or coating on wrapping material. They are used for cheese and cheese products, fruit products including dried fruit, and pickles. Added to wines, sorbates reduce the requirement of sulphur dioxide,

and in combination with sodium benzoate they are added to beverages and fruit juices. Potassium sorbate is permitted in margarine.

Dermatitis from sorbates is rare (p. 707).

Propionic acid and its salts
Propionates are active against moulds. They are allowed in some cheese products.

Sulphur dioxide and sulphites
Sulphur dioxide and sulphites are effective against many organisms, but their use is limited by their taste. As fumes and vapour, sulphur and sulphur dioxide are used to preserve dried fruit and vegetables, and vegetables may be dipped into solutions of sulphites and bisulphites. These compounds are also important in wine making.

Potassium metabisulphite has caused dermatitis (p. 706).

Acetic acid and its salts
Vinegar is impure acetic acid. Both the acid and its acetates have antimicrobial activity: they are used in sauces and pickles where their taste is desirable.

Nitrites and nitrates
Nitrites and nitrates are curing salts. Saltpetre is potassium nitrate. Nitrites are added to cured meats as preservatives, colour fixatives and for flavouring. They are potentially toxic and the possibility of their being carcinogenic, through the production of nitrosamines, is being questioned.

Ethylene and propylene oxides
Ethylene oxide and propylene oxide are used for the gaseous sterilisation of some foods. It is important to remove residual gases as they are irritants, ethylene oxide more so than propylene oxide.

Diethyl pyrocarbonate (Pyrocarbonic acid diethyl ester)
Diethyl pyrocarbonate is especially effective against yeasts. Its use in soft drinks, wines and beers is limited by the regulations of different countries.

Propylene glycol (p. 809)
Propylene glycol inhibits the growth of moulds and fungi.

Antibiotics
Several antibiotics have been investigated but little used as food preservatives.

Antioxidants
Antioxidants are added to foods principally to prevent the lipid component from being broken down into low molecular-weight compounds by atmospheric oxygen. The unpleasant taste and smell of rancid foods is due to degraded fats. Antioxidants must not affect the taste or colour of the food and they are required to withstand heat and long storage.

Many of the natural and synthetic antioxidants added to foods are phenols, including propyl gallate, octyl gallate, dodecyl gallate (lauryl gallate), butylated hydroxyanisole (BHA) and butylated hydroxytoluene (BHT). Antioxidants have a synergistic effect and usually several are used together. As combinations of the synthetic antioxidants — BHA, BHT and propyl gallate — are most effective, they are often used, particularly for animal fats. They are added in concentrations of 100 ppm for the gallates and 200 ppm for BHA or BHT or their mixtures. Nordihydroguaiaretic acid and propyl gallate are more effective antioxidants for unsaturated vegetable oils. The naturally occurring tocopherols and gum guaiac are less potent antioxidants; they are added in concentrations of 1000 ppm.

Chelators
Metal salts (e.g., of iron and copper) catalyse auto-oxidation, and to prevent this, metal chelators are frequently included with the antioxidants. Citric acid is often used but to make it fat-soluble it has to be added in propylene glycol. Phosphoric acid or isopropyl citrate are sometimes preferred, but the latter is a less effective chelator. Ethylenediaminetetraacetic acid, though a good chelator for other foods, is insoluble and ineffective in lipids.

Packaging
Antioxidants are often added to the waxy layer on the inner side of packaging material.

Butylated hydroxyanisole (BHA) and *Butylated hydroxytoluene* (BHT)

Butylated hydroxyanisole is an antioxidant used especially for fats and oils in foods and sometimes on packaging. Butylated hydroxytoluene has a much wider application and is added to foods, food packaging and animal feeds and also to petroleum products, jet fuels, rubber and plastics.

To investigate a possible depigmenting effect of BHT (Vollum, 1971), subjects were examined after single (Bentley-Phillips and Bayles, 1974) and repeated (Maibach, Gellin and Ring, 1975) patch tests with concentrations of BHT up to 3 per cent in cream bases. No depigmentation occurred, but there was irritation at the patch test sites (p. 871).

Butylated hydroxyanisole (BHA) and BHT have been included in two standard series and the results were as follows:

	%	Diluent	Tested	+	
BHA	5	Petrolatum	360	1	(Meneghini *et al.*, 1971)
BHT	5	Petrolatum	360	0	(Meneghini *et al.*, 1971)
BHA	2	Petrolatum	112	3	(Roed-Petersen & Hjorth, 1976)
BHT	2	Petrolatum	112	3	

Case reports
Case reports of sensitivity to BHA or BHT are rare. Two sensitised women with relevant histories were described by Roed-Petersen and Hjorth (1976). Both had

hand eczema. Patch tests: one reacted to several allergens including BHT 2 per cent in petrolatum but not to BHA 2 per cent in petrolatum; the other reacted to BHA, to BHT and to nordihydroguaiaretic acid (NDGA). In each patient the eczema cleared with topical medicaments and an antioxidant-free diet. Oral provocation tests caused a recurrence of the hand eczema in both. The first patient reacted to 10 mg of BHA with 10 mg of BHT, then to 20 mg of BHA over four days; the second reacted to 20 mg of BHA over four days. Alcoholic solutions of BHA (5 per cent) and BHT (5 per cent) were painted on the first patient's fingers, and after 15 minutes the areas itched and then became urticarial. A third patient with a leg ulcer and many positive patch tests reacted to BHT, BHA and NDGA (each 2 per cent in petrolatum), but she had no dermatitis.

A cook with chronic hand eczema who developed cheilitis and circum-oral eczema after eating mayonnaise was investigated by Fisher (1975b). Patch tests with the mayonnaise (known to contain BHA) and with 2 per cent BHA were positive. The cook avoided mayonnaise and his hands and mouth healed.

A woman sensitised by a miconazole cream containing 0.005 per cent BHA was reported by Degreef and Verhoeve (1975). Patch tests: she reacted to miconazole nitrate 2 per cent and to BHA 5 per cent, each in petrolatum.

BHA and BHT have been reported as a cause of vasomotor rhinitis and asthma (Fisherman and Cohen, 1973): oral challenge reproduced the clinical symptoms and altered the bleeding time.

Patch testing
BHA 2 per cent in petrolatum
BHT 2 per cent in petrolatum.

Gallate esters

Propyl gallate   Lauryl gallate

The esters of gallic acid are used as antioxidants in edible oils and fats and may also be added to cosmetic and pharmaceutical preparations. They are sometimes present in paints, varnishes, boot polishes and plastics (Brun, 1970). Concentrations of 100 ppm are permitted in food and up to 200 ppm in topical products.

Sensitising potential. It has been shown experimentally that guinea-pigs and man are readily sensitised by propyl gallate (Kahn, Phanuphak and Claman, 1974). Prior feeding of the guinea-pigs with propyl gallate suppressed the induction of sensitisation. It was suggested that man's oral intake similarly induces tolerance to a compound which is potentially a strong sensitiser.

Case reports

Eczematous patients were investigated for sensitisation to antioxidants by Roed-Petersen and Hjorth (1976) and they found one who reacted to lauryl (dodecyl) gallate 2 per cent in olive oil, but none reacted to propyl gallate.

Sensitivity to lauryl gallate in margarine was detected as the cause of occupational hand eczema in five bakers and pastry cooks by Brun (1964, 1970). The hand eczema was characteristically chronic and hyperkeratotic. The first patient (Brun, 1964) reacted on patch testing to the margarine and subsequently to lauryl gallate 0.2 per cent in alcohol, this being its concentration in the margarine. The other four patients (Brun, 1970) also reacted to this concentration. Another five patients who had been sensitised by gallic acid esters in margarine were reported by Buckhardt and Fierz (1964). A food shop assistant attributed her dermatitis to margarine and on patch testing she reacted to lauryl gallate and octyl gallate 0.25 per cent but not to the margarine (Rudzki and Baranowska, 1975).

Octyl gallate is used as an antioxidant in margarine and peanut butter. A man employed in mixing octyl gallate into peanut butter developed dermatitis of the hands and face, which was related to his doing this job. Patch tests: he reacted to octyl gallate 1 per cent and 0.1 per cent in olive oil, but had no reaction to the same concentrations of lauryl (dodecyl) gallate; he was not tested with the peanut butter. Thirty control patients were tested with octyl gallate 1 per cent and none reacted (van Ketel, 1978).

Patch testing

Gallate ester 0.1 per cent and 1 per cent in petrolatum or olive oil.

Gallate esters are irritant and Rudzki and Baranowska (1975) reported toxic reactions with propyl gallate 1 per cent, lauryl gallate 0.25 per cent and octyl gallate 0.25 per cent.

Tocopherols

Antioxidants occur in both plant and animal tissues, and of the group the most important are the tocopherols. The higher concentration in plants accounts for vegetable oils being more stable than animal fats. Tocopherols are yellow oils, and, having long side chains, are fat-soluble. They are degraded by heat, light and oxygen and during the storage and preparation of food they are easily oxidised to tocoquinones which are not antioxidants. The acetate esters of the tocopherols are more stable and d- and dl-alpha-tocopheryl acetates are sold commercially.

Sensitisation by tocopherols in topical applications has been reported (p. 000), but not as yet in food. Roed-Petersen and Hjorth (1976) reported one patient who reacted on routine patch testing to 20 per cent dl-alpha-tocopherol, but the relevance and source of sensitisation was unknown. They also described a man who was actively sensitised by a patch test with dl-alpha-tocopherol 20 per cent in petrolatum; he did not cross-react to d-alpha-tocopherol or d-alpha-tocopherol-succinate, both tested at 5 per cent and 20 per cent in petrolatum.

Patch testing

dl-alpha-tocopherol 10 per cent in petrolatum.

Sequestrants

The presence of metals in foods increases oxidation and hastens deterioration. Thus, traces of copper and iron (0.1–5 ppm) speed the rancidity of fats; metals catalyse the oxidation of vitamins; and the presence of copper, iron and chromium accelerates the discolouration of fruit and vegetables.

Sequestrants act synergistically with antioxidants; they are chosen with regard to their toxicity, colour, effect on flavour and their compatibility with the substrate. The most useful technically are citrates, pyrophosphates and ethylenediaminetetraacetate (EDTA).

Surface active agents

The use of surface active agents in culinary preparations has enabled much longer storage and transport of foods. The principal action of these surfactants is to emulsify, but they also act as wetting compounds and as suspending and solubilising agents. Naturally-occurring surface active agents are lecithin in eggs and soybeans, and saponin in liquorice. Synthetic surfactants include sucrose esters, sorbitan esters, polyoxyethylene sorbitan esters, polyoxyethylene esters, polyglycerol esters, glycerol mono-esters and propylene glycol mono-esters.

An emulgator, ME18, was incriminated as the likely cause of the outbreak of Margarine Disease which occurred first in West Germany in the late 1950s and then in the Netherlands in 1960 (Mali and Malten, 1966). In Holland there was good evidence that those affected had eaten the margarine, but in Germany the association was more nebulous. The emulgator was added, not to emulsify but to maintain the dispersion of water in the margarine at high temperatures and to prevent the fat spattering in a frying pan. In each epidemic the patients developed an acute, toxic erythema and some were systemically ill. Serological investigations demonstrated the presence of circulating antibodies which were present only at the height of the patient's illness. An adduct in the emulgator was thought to be the sensitiser.

COLOURS IN FOODS

Colours are added to foods to replace those destroyed by preservatives, processing, heat or light, to disguise unattractive colours produced during processing (e.g. canned peas would naturally be yellow or brown), to enhance the appearance of a pale or colourless product and to ensure uniformity of colour between different batches of food.

Natural colouring agents may be plant pigments (e.g. carotenoids, chlorophylls, flavonoids and anthocyanins), animal pigments (e.g. cochineal) or metals and metallic oxides. Synthetic dyes belong to the following groups: azo, triarylmethane, indigoid, xanthene, anthraquinone, quinoline and artificial caramels. Occasionally spices (e.g. turmeric) are used for their colour rather than for their flavour (Fairweather and Swann, 1978).

Urticaria, angio-oedema and purpura have been described following the ingestion of food dyes and preservatives. The azo dyes reported as causing such reactions are tartrazine (C.I. 19140), sunset yellow (C.I. 15985), new coccine (C.I. 16255) and amaranth (C.I. 16185). The preservatives provoking these effects are sodium benzoate and 4-hydroxybenzoic acid; aspirin has a similar action (Michaëlsson and Juhlin, 1973; Michaëlsson, Pettersson and Juhlin, 1974).

In contrast, contact dermatitis from food dyes seems to be extremely rare.

Oranges

In the United States the skin of oranges is dyed in Florida but not in California. In 1937 Traub, Gordon and Dyke reported two cases of sensitisation to the dye Yellow O B (*ortho*-toluene-azo-*beta*-naphthylamine), a colour then permitted on Florida oranges. Their evidence was that the first patient had a strongly positive patch test reaction to a 25 per cent solution of the dye, but a doubtful response to 1 per cent; the second patient was not tested with the dye but reacted to a patch test with the dyed orange rind. About the same time, Schwartz (1938) investigated the causes of dermatitis in the citrus fruit industry but found no cases of dermatitis from the dyes used on oranges. In the discussion of a paper, Rothman (1949) cited a doctor whose eyelid eczema had been attributed to the dye on Florida oranges and a relapse to contact with a similar azo dye in Nembutal capsules. Citrus red 2 is now used to colour oranges in Florida. A chef with an allergic contact dermatitis from his black socks was found on patch testing to react to citrus red 2 (2 per cent in petrolatum). There was no history relevant to this food dye and the response was probably a cross-reaction to the clothing dye (Mitchell, 1972).

Bakers

Eczema in a baker was found to be due to sensitivity to the food dye Ponceau Red 6 R (Bandmann and Nasemann, 1961).

Patch testing

Dye 2 per cent in petrolatum (orange peel is irritant).

FLAVOURING AGENTS AND SPICES

Flavouring agents, spices, volatile oils and perfumes all belong to a group of substances called balsams, which are sweet-scented extracts of various trees, shrubs, fruits and plants. Each balsam contains many compounds, some of which are common to several balsams. Direct botanical exposure to balsams occurs but usually contact is through perfumes and flavouring materials.

Foods

A detailed study of allergy to balsams, allied perfumes and flavouring agents was made by Hjorth (1961); otherwise sensitivity to flavours in foods is rarely reported.

In a confectionery factory, eight cases of occupational contact eczema were investigated by Heygi (1971). Patch tests with the flavourings undiluted were carried out and reactions occurred to ethyl acetate, lemon, diacetyl and strawberry; of 102 controls tested, six reacted to these or other flavours. Another confectioner sensitised to cardamom, reacted to cardamom powder, oil of cardamom (2 per cent) turpentine peroxides and terpenoids, including dipentene (limonene 2 per cent) and borneol (2 per cent) in the dried seeds (Mobacken and Fregert 1975).

Lovage is used as a flavour for tobaccos, liqueurs, cordials, confectionery, foods and medicaments. Sensitisation of a perfume laboratory technician was reported by Calnan (1969); the man had a positive patch test to the lovage concentrate, whereas eight controls were negative.

Synthetic oil of mustard in a liniment caused contact dermatitis in a patient described by Gaul (1964). A patch test with oil of mustard 0.1 per cent in petrolatum was positive. Synthetic oil of mustard (allyl isothiocyanate) is irritant and should be diluted to 0.1 per cent for patch testing.

Oil of juniper is used as a spice in sausages; it caused both occupational dermatitis and asthma in a case reported by Rothe, Heine and Rebohle (1973).

Monosodium glutamate (MSG)
Monosodium glutamate is derived from beet sugar, the gluten of wheat and corn, or it can be synthesised. Its property of enhancing the flavour of protein foods was first recognised in Japan in the early 1900s and the use of MSG has been especially associated with food in Chinese restaurants. It is now widely used in frozen foods containing meat or fish, canned foods and dry soup mixes. In small quantities it is tasteless.

About 15–25 minutes after eating MSG a few susceptible people develop a burning sensation in the back of the neck, which spreads over the arms and thorax and is associated with infra-orbital discomfort. The symptoms last about 45 minutes (Shaumburg and Byck, 1968).

Toothpaste
Flavours in toothpastes very occasionally sensitise, causing stomatitis, cheilitis and eczema of the hand which holds the brush. Cinnamon is a well-known sensitiser and this flavour in a toothpaste has caused oral symptoms and dermatitis in patients in Britain, Sweden and the United States. Cinnamic aldehyde was the allergen, the patients reacting to patch tests with 1 per cent in petrolatum; the majority of those tested did not react to balsam of Peru (25 per cent in petrolatum) (Magnusson and Wilkinson, 1975; Kirton and Wilkinson, 1975; Drake and Maibach, 1976).

In another case of toothpaste stomatitis and dermatitis reported from Copenhagen, the sensitisers were oil of spearmint (which contains 50 per cent carvone), carvone and anethole (anise camphor) (Hjorth and Jervøe, 1967).

Immediate-type hypersensitivity to caraway seed oil in toothpastes has been described by Heygi and Doležalóva (1976).

Patch testing
Balsam of Peru, which is a composite mixture, is used to screen for sensitivity to flavours, but although a positive reaction is helpful, failure to react does not exclude sensitivity to a flavouring agent.

Flavour 1–5 per cent in petrolatum
Balsam of Peru 25 per cent in petrolatum.

FLOUR AND GRAINS

Bakers

Bakers run the risk of developing rhinitis, asthma and eczema; these occupational diseases have been reviewed by Bonnevie (1958) and Young (1974).

Immediate-type hypersensitivity
In Berlin, Herxheimer (1967) found that 8 per cent of apprentice bakers reacted to prick tests with rye and wheat flours within a month of starting work. In half of them the reaction subsequently disappeared, while other apprentices, initially negative, became positive. At the end of three years, 23 per cent of the 177 apprentices followed had a positive skin test to flour, and this compares with an 18 per cent incidence among adult bakers. There was no direct correlation between the results of these tests and the presence of the disease.

An analysis of wheat flour demonstrated 40 antigens, some of which are related to antigens in rye flour and grass pollen. Bakers with respiratory symptoms were shown to react (*in vitro* or *in vivo*) to an extract of wheat flour (Blands *et al.*, 1976). Sera from two bakers with asthma was examined by Baldo and Wrigley (1978) using the radioallergosorbent test (RAST). IgE antibodies to wheat flour components were present, the strongest reactions being to wheat albumins and globulins.

In Helsinki, 25 per cent of 234 bakery employees were found to have atopic disease, 54 (23 per cent) had allergic rhinitis, 21 (9 per cent) had asthma and 11 (5 per cent) had atopic eczema. Flour dusts were the specific allergens in the asthmatic patients being wheat (9), rye (7), barley (5) and oats (2). Bakery work is therefore definitely unsuitable for anyone with a personal and probably for those with a family history of atopy (Järvinen *et al.*, 1979).

Dermatitis

Irritant: The sticky dough, sugars, peels and other ingredients of bread and cakes, as well as the detergents and soap used for cleansing, may cause an irritant hand eczema in bakers.

Allergic: In the 1920s ammonium and potassium persulphates and benzoyl peroxide were added to flour to inhibit proteolytic enzymes from attacking the gluten films which surround the carbon dioxide bubbles. These form during fermentation and determine the lightness of bread. Both chemicals are sensitisers and their introduction increased the incidence of bakers' eczema. Persulphates, thought to be the greater hazard, were banned, initially in Switzerland, Belgium and Denmark (Bonnevie, 1958). In Germany persulphate sensitivity became a considerable problem and after their use was prohibited in 1957, the incidence of bakers' eczema fell (Wagner, 1959; Preyss, 1960).

Ammonium persulphate and benzoyl peroxide are still permitted in flour in the Netherlands (Young, 1974) and in the U.K., but although benzoyl peroxide is still widely used many millers have replaced persulphates with potassium bromate, which is equally efficient and easier to handle.

Flavours were significant allergens in 4 bakers with hand eczema patch tested by Malten (1979). Each reacted to several of the following compounds eugenol (8 per cent), dihydrocoumarin (5 per cent), citral = neral (0.5 per cent), phenyl acetaldehyde (2 per cent), methyl heptine carbonate (0.5 per cent), cinnamic alcohol (5 per cent), cinnamic aldehyde (0.5 per cent), o-methoxy cinnamic aldehyde (4 per cent), benzylidene acetone (0.5 per cent), amyl cinnamate (32 per cent), benzyl cinnamate (8 per cent), cinnamyl benzoate (10 per cent) and cinnamyl-cinnamate (8 per cent), each in petrolatum.

'Contact urticaria'

In bakers with immediate-type hypersensitivity to flour and hand eczema Bonnevie (1958) suggested that contact with the flour could provoke urticarial reactions which prolonged the duration of their dermatitis. Similarly, inhalation of flour has elicited eczema (Heyl and Reinert-Dilthey, 1968; Heyl, Wolff and Osten, 1970).

Patch tests

Ammonium persulphate 2.5 per cent in petrolatum
Benzoyl peroxide 1 and 5 per cent in petrolatum
Flavours
Essences.

Scratch tests

Grains

A girl in a test bakery developed eczema of the fingers and when patch tested she reacted twice to malt flour; she did not react to bread flour, malt, barley or gibberelic acid 2 per cent in petrolatum. Malt flour is derived from barley (*Hordeum vulgare*); gibberelic acid is one of its natural constituents and is present in a final concentration of 0.3 ppm (Calnan, 1973).

A docker who unloaded cattle fodder developed eczema of the hands and eyelids. On the basis of positive patch tests it was attributed to contact with brans, vitamins, beetpulp, maize and barley. He transferred to other work and his skin healed (Malten, 1970). Similarly, a farm stockman with eczema of the arms was patch tested and found to react to rolled barley and rolled oats. He avoided all contact with them and his skin healed (Solomons, 1971). A farm labourer, with a dry fissured eczema of the dorsa of his hands, wrists and forearms was found on patch testing to react to barley dust (a scratch test was negative). He left the farm to work in a garage and his skin recovered (Cronin, 1979).

PLANTS

Chicory: *Cichorium intybus* [Compositae]
Hand eczema in a Danish grocer was found to be caused entirely by sensitivity

to *Cichorium intybus* var. *foliosum*. Patch tests: he reacted to a leaf and an ether extract of the leaves (Friis *et al.*, 1975). These authors also described an American supermarket manager who had eczema of his hands and arms which was caused by sensitivity to *Cichorium intybus*, *C. endiva* (endive) and *Lactuca sativa* (lettuce). Patch tests: he reacted to the leaves of each plant and to the sesquiterpene lactone alantolactone 0.1 per cent in petrolatum, an allergen of the Compositae family. Chicory is used as a coffee substitute and has caused occupational dermatitis in workers gathering the plant and in others cleaning and drying it in the factories (Bonnevie, 1948).

Endive: *Cichorium endiva* [Compositae]
The patient reported by Friis *et al.* (1975) was sensitive to *Cichorium endiva* (escarole, broad leaved endive).

Lettuce: *Lactuca sativa* [Compositae]
Lettuces cultivated for food include:

> *Lactuca sativa* var. *longifolia* (Romaine)
> *Lactuca sativa* var. *foliosa* (Cabbage lettuce)
> *Lactuca sativa* var. *capitata* (Iceberg)

The patient reported by Friis *et al.* (1975) reacted on patch testing to a leaf of *Lactuca sativa* var. *longifolia*; and a gardener who was sensitised by *Lactuca sativa* (?variety) was reported by Krook (1973).

In 1932, Rinkel and Balyeat described a salad maker with severe eczema of her hands, arms and face, which cleared completely when she stopped handling and eating lettuce. A patch test with the lettuce was positive, but subsequently became negative when an intradermal test was positive.

Patch tests
Leaf 'As Is'

Miscellaneous foods

Potato: *Solanum tuberosum* [Solanaceae]
Atopic housewives may develop immediate-type hypersensitivity to potatoes. Cleaning potatoes precipitates rhinorrhoea, sneezing, wheezing or urticaria. Inhalation of the allergen causes irritation of eczematous patches, and handling the raw potato aggravates hand eczema. The majority, but not all the patients, can eat cooked potatoes. The allergen is unknown (Bruce Pearson, 1966; Nater and Zwartz, 1967; Cronin, 1973).

Three cases of occupational dermatitis in a potato crisp factory were described by Inman (1965). The allergens were flavouring powders dusted on to the crisps. The patients were patch tested with the wheat filler, and the onion and cheese powders, and reacted to one or more of them. None of the five controls reacted.

Green coffee: *Coffea* [Rubiaceae]
Coffee workers who inhale the dust of green (raw) coffee beans may develop an allergic asthma and rhinitis. The allergen in these unroasted beans was thought

by Freedman *et al.* (1964) to be chlorogenic acid, a phenolic compound present in green coffee beans, oranges (*Citrus sinensis*), castor beans (*Ricinus communis*) and many other plants and they sensitised laboratory animals to it. These findings were refuted by Layton *et al.* (1965) and Layton, Panzani and Cortese (1968), who suggested that a protein in the green coffee bean is the likely sensitiser. Lehrer, Karr and Salvaggio (1978) tried to identify this allergen but were not successful. The existence of a sensitiser in green coffee beans is not disputed, it is the identity of the allergen which is in doubt. Roasting the beans destroys the allergen.

ADDITIVES IN ANIMAL FEEDS

The allergens in animal feeds are compounds added for nutritional, medicinal or other purposes, rather than the feed itself. Sensitisation is more likely to occur in those manufacturing the feed, who are exposed to high concentrations of the additives, than in those handling the final mixtures in which the sensitisers are greatly diluted.

Compounds added to feeds have been listed by Burrows (1975) and Neldner (1972). They include:

Antibiotics and drugs of all types, both as growth promoters and therapeutically: Tylosin; nitrofurazone; sulphacetamide and sulphamethazine; chlortetracycline and oxytetracycline; neomycin and bacitracin, especially for swine; organic arsenicals; ethylenediamine dihydroiodide; phenothiazine, piperazine and thiabendazole as anthelminthics; stilboestrol and progesterone compounds.

Antioxidants: gallate esters — octyl, dodecyl and propyl
  butylated hydroxyanisole (BHA)
  butylated hydroxytoluene (BHT)
  ethoxyquin.

Colours.

Vitamins.

Trace elements: cobalt, iodine, iron, manganese, molybdenum, selenium, zinc.

Emulsifiers, stabilisers and binders: lecithins, alginates, flours, gum.
  Sorbitan esters and EDTA (disodium ethylenediaminetetraacetate).

A few of these compounds have been reported as causing allergic contact dermatitis in those manufacturing the foodstuffs, in those feeding the animals and in veterinary surgeons.

Cobalt

A man developed an occupational dermatitis from cobalt while working in a factory making mineral mixtures for addition to animal feeds. Patch tests: he reacted to cobalt nitrate 2 per cent, nickel sulphate 5 per cent and potassium dichromate 0.5 per cent (Breucker and Höfs, 1966).

Dinitolmide

3,5 Dinitro-*o*-toluamide; 2 methyl-3,5-dinitrobenzamide; Dot; Zoalene.
  Dinitolmide is added to chicken feed to prevent coccidioidomycosis.

A man in a poultry food factory developed eczema of the hands, and when patch tested he reacted to dinitolmide 1 per cent in petrolatum; tests on five controls were negative. He did not react to other dinitrobenzene compounds (Bleumink and Nater, 1973 a,b).

Patch testing
Dinitolmide 1 per cent in petrolatum.

Ethoxyquin 6-Ethoxy-1, 2-dihydro-2,2,4-trimethylquinoline; Santoquin; Kurasan. Ethoxyquin is an antioxidant used principally in animal feeds and for a few special purposes. In supplements of vitamins A and D_3 its concentration is 5 per cent, but in the final animal feed its level is reduced to 0.0001 per cent. Fish and bone meals and tallow are likely to contain ethoxyquin (Burrows, 1975). A dip or spray containing 0.3 per cent ethoxyquin is used to prevent scald (browning) of the skin of apples during storage (Wood and Fulton, 1972).

Occupational dermatitis

Manufacture of animal feed. Sensitivity to ethoxyquin has been reported in workers mixing and adding ingredients in the manufacture of animal feeds. This work is dusty, and powder settling on the skin and clothes predisposes to sensitisation.

In Germany sensitisation of a fodder-doser was described by Melhorn and Beetz (1971), and cases among other feedstuff workers were reported by Schubert, Göring and Gans (1973). In Sweden, Wahlberg (1974) found ethoxyquin to be the cause of dermatitis in three men mixing the ingredients of animal foodstuffs. Two were patch tested and reacted to ethoxyquin 0.125–0.5 per cent in water; tests in ten controls were negative. Wahlberg stressed that the dusty atmosphere determined the widespread pattern of the dermatitis which could be severe. Similarly, in Northern Ireland (Burrows, 1975), two men working in an animal feed mill were sensitised. One had a generalised eczema, worse on the face and arms, and the other had dermatitis of the hands and feet. Patch tests: both reacted to ethoxyquin 0.5 per cent in petrolatum. In Belgium, van Hecke (1977) saw the same type of dermatitis in a man working in a factory making animal feed, and in Czechoslovakia, Jirásek and Kalensky (1975) described sensitivity in 14 subjects doing the same sort of work.

Pig feed sensitised two Danish workers (Zachariae, 1978).

Farmer. A farmer was sensitised to ethoxyquin by a dusty calf food, which contained < 100 ppm of ethoxyquin. The eczema affected the exposed areas and resembled a photodermatitis. Patch tests: he reacted to the animal feed and ethoxyquin 0.2 per cent. The feed was supplied without the ethoxyquin and he used it and remained well (van Hecke, 1977). Neither this man, nor the one mentioned above (van Hecke, 1977), reacted to vioform.

Apple packers. In British Columbia, 25 apple packers developed dermatitis of their hands while handling apples still wet with ethoxyquin spray. Patch tests:

all 25 reacted to ethoxyquin 0.5 per cent in water. Tests on controls were negative (Wood and Fulton, 1972).

Patch testing
Ethoxyquin 0.5 per cent in petrolatum or water.

Ethylenediamine dihydroiodide
Ethylenediamine dihydroiodide is given to animals as a nutritional source of iodine, as an expectorant or as a treatment for 'foot rot' or 'lumpy jaw'.

A farmer who presented with a dermatitis resembling a photodermatitis was investigated by Fisher (1975a). Patch tests: the standard series revealed that he had been sensitised to ethylenediamine dihydrochloride in Mycolog cream. It was then ascertained that he fed ethylenediamine dihydroiodide to his cows. When patch tested with ethylediamine dihydroiodide 1 per cent in petrolatum he reacted. This allergy was considered to be a cross-reaction to the primary sensitiser, ethylenediamine dihydrochloride.

Patch testing
Ethylenediamine dihydroiodide 1 per cent in petrolatum.

Furazolidone 3-(5-Nitrofurfurylideneamino)-2-oxazolidinone; Furoxone; Nifuran
Furazolidone is a synthetic derivative of the nitrofurazone group. It is added to animal feeds as a growth-promoting factor.

In a factory making animal feeds it was added to the chicken fodder, and after two years a woman mixing the fodder developed hand eczema which she attributed to the furazolidone. Patch tests: she reacted to the undiluted furazolidone (Scharfenberg, 1967). In the Prague series of 32 patients with occupational dermatitis from animal food additives reported by Jirásek and Kalensky (1975), three were sensitive to furazolidone. One was later given the related drug Furantoin for a urinary infection and she developed a generalised eruption.

Patch testing
Furazolidone? 1 per cent in petrolatum.

Nitrofurazone Furacin (See p. 215)
Nitrofurazone (Furacin) is used in human (p. 215) and veterinary medicine, and it may also be added to animal feeds. It is a well known sensitiser.

A man who worked in a feed shop scooped feed from storage bins into sacks, raising clouds of dust in the process. He developed acute attacks of dermatitis of the hands, arms, face and neck. On patch testing he reacted to nitrofurazone 1 per cent; he then remarked that nitrofurazone was present in a chicken feed he sold (Caplan, 1969).

Sensitisation in a hog rancher with acute episodes of dermatitis (Neldner, 1972) was established by a positive patch test to a feed supplement containing nitrofurazone. He was also sensitive to Tylosin. Subsequently he accidentally used nitrofurazone to treat a pig with a salmonella infection and developed an acute relapse of his dermatitis.

Patch testing
Nitrofurazone 0.2 per cent in petrolatum.

Halquinol (p. 220)
Halquinol is added to pig feed to treat or prevent scour caused or complicated by *E. coli* and *Salmonella*.

A foreman in an animal feed mill added Quixalaud (a mixture containing halquinol 60 per cent and chalk 40 per cent) to animal feeds, and two weeks later developed dermatitis of the hands and wrists. Patch tests: he reacted to 1 per cent Quixalaud (Burrows, 1975).

Patch testing
Halquinol 5 per cent in petrolatum.

Hydroquinone
Sensitivity to the antioxidant hydroquinone was found in 12 workers engaged in feeding cattle and pigs (Jirásek and Kalensky, 1975).

Patch testing
Hydroquinone 1 per cent in petrolatum.

Quindoxin (p. 440)

Spiramycin
Spiramycin may be added to animals' drinking water or be given by injection.

Of the nine veterinary surgeons with eczema investigated by Hjorth and Weismann (1973), six reacted on patch testing to spiramycin 1–10 per cent in petrolatum or water.

Patch testing
Spiramycin 1–5 per cent in petrolatum.

Tylosin: *Tylan*
Tylosin is classified as a macrolide antibiotic; it may be added to the animal feed, to the drinking water or be given by injection.

A farm-hand with eczema of the hands and arms who had been sensitised by poultry food was reported by Preyss (1969). A more widespread dermatitis was described by Neldner (1972), in a girl who fed a pig each day, and in a hog rancher. Both patients reacted to patch tests with the crude feed supplement. Only the girl was tested with tylosin 1 per cent in water and she reacted. Nine veterinary surgeons with hand eczema which, in some, had spread to other sites, were investigated by Hjorth and Weismann (1973): six had positive patch tests to tylosin 1–10 per cent in petrolatum or water.

Patch testing
Tylosin 5–10 per cent in petrolatum.

Virginiamycin (p. 226)

A warehouseman, in a pharmaceutical factory, frequently entered a room where a virginiamycin food additive (Stafac®) for pigs and poultry was made and stored in barrels. The room was dusty and he developed dermatitis of the eyelids. Patch tests: he reacted to Stafac dust 20 per cent (pet.), virginiamycin 5 per cent (pet.), Factor M of virginiamycin 5 per cent (pet.) and pristinamycin 5 per cent (pet.) but not to Factor S of virginiamycin 5 per cent (pet.) (Tennstedt, Dumont-Fruytier and Lachapelle, 1978).

Patch testing (p. 226)

Patch testing

Antibiotics and medicaments including:

Ethylenediamine dihydroiodide	1 per cent in petrolatum
Dinitolmide	1 per cent in petrolatum
Furazolidone	? 1 per cent in petrolatum
Nitrofurazone (Furacin)	0.2 per cent in petrolatum
Spiramycin	1–5 per cent in petrolatum
Tylosin	5 and 10 per cent in petrolatum

Antioxidants including

Ethoxyquin	0.5 per cent in petrolatum or water
Hydroquinone	1 per cent in petrolatum

Trace elements

Cobalt chloride	1 per cent in petrolatum
Iodine	0.5 per cent in alcohol

Emulsifiers, stablisers and binders including

EDTA	1 per cent in petrolatum
Sorbic acid	2.5 per cent in petrolatum or water

Colours

Vitamins.

References

Baldo, B.A. & Wrigley, C.W. (1978) IgE antibodies to wheat flour components *Clinical Allergy*, **8**, 109.

Bandmann, H-J. & Nasemann, Th. (1961) Bäckerekzem durch eine Lebensmittelfarbe der Azofarb-stoffreihe. *Berufsdermatosen*, **9**, 79.

Bentley-Phillips, B. & Bayles, M.A.H. (1974) Butylated hydroxytoluene as a skin lightener. *Archives of Dermatology*, **109**, 216.

Blands, J., Diamant, B., Kallós, P., Kallós-Deffner, L. & Løwenstein, H. (1976) Flour allergy in bakers. *International Archives of Allergy and Applied Immunology*, **52**, 392.

Bleumink, E. & Nater, J.P. (1973a) Dermatitis from zoalene in poultry food. *Contact Dermatitis Newsletter*, **13**, 375.

Bleumink, E, & Nater, J.P. (1973b) Allergic contact dermatitis to dinitolmide. *Archives of Dermatology*, **108**, 423.

Bonnevie, P. (1948) Some experiences of war-time industrial dermatoses. *Acta Dermato-venereologica*, **28**, 231.

Bonnevie, P. (1958) Occupational allergy in bakery, p. 161. *Occupational Allergy*, Leiden, Holland. Stenfert Kroese N.V.

Breucker, G. & Höfs, W. (1966) Kobalthaltiges futtermittel für Wiederkäuer als berufliches Ekzematogen. *Dermatologische Wochenschrift*, **152** (1), 528.

Bruce Pearson, R.S. (1966) Potato sensitivity, an occupational allergy in housewives. *Acta Allergologica*, **21**, 507.

Brun, R. (1964) Kontaktekzem auf Laurylgallat und p-Hydroxy-benzoe-säureester. *Berufsdermatosen*, **12**, 281.

Brun, R. (1970) Eczéma de contact á un antioxidant de la margarine (gallate) et changement de metier. *Dermatologica*, **140**, 390.

Burckhardt, W. & Fierz, U. (1964) Antioxydantien in der Margarine als Ursache von Gewerbeekzemen. *Dermatologica*, **129**, 431.

Burrows, D. (1975) Contact dermatitis in animal feed mill workers. *British Journal of Dermatology*, **92**, 167.

Calnan, C.D. (1969) Lovage sensitivity. *Contact Dermatitis Newsletter*, **5**, 99.

Calnan, C.D. (1973) Malt flour dermatitis. *Contact Dermatitis Newsletter*, **14**, 390.

Caplan, R.M. (1969) Cutaneous hazards posed by agricultural chemicals. *Journal of the Iowa Medical Society*, **59**, 295.

Cronin, E, (1973) Immediate-type hypersensitivity to potato. *Contact Dermatitis Newsletter*, **13**, 358.

Cronin, E. (1979) Contact dermatitis from barley dust. *Contact Dermatitis*, **5**, 196.

Degreef, H. & Verhoeve, L. (1975) Contact dermatitis to miconazole nitrate. *Contact Dermatitis*, **1**, 269.

Drake, T.E. & Maibach, H.I. (1976) Allergic contact dermatitis and stomatitis caused by a cinnamic aldehyde flavored toothpaste. *Archives of Dermatology*, **112**, 202.

Fairweather, F.A. & Swann, C.A. (1978) Colouring agents added to food. *Health Trends*, **10**, 12.

Fisher, A.A. (1975a) Allergic contact dermatitis in animal feed handlers. *Cutis*, **16**, 201.

Fisher, A.A. (1975 b) Contact dermatitis due to food additives. *Cutis*, **16**, 961.

Fisherman, E.W. & Cohen, G. (1973) Chemical intolerance to butylated hydroxyanisole (BHA) and butylated hydroxytoluene (BHT) and vascular response as an indicator and monitor of drug intolerance. *Annals of Allergy*, **31**, 126.

Freedman, S.O., Shulman, R., Krupey, J. & Schon, A.H. (1964) Antigenic properties of chlorogenic acid. *Journal of Allergy*, **35**, 97.

Friis, B., Hjorth, N., Vail, J.T. & Mitchell, J.C. (1975) Occupational contact dermatitis from *Cichorium* (chicory, endive) and *Lactuca* (lettuce). *Contact Dermatitis*, **1**, 311.

Gaul, L.E. (1964) Contact dermatitis from synthetic oil of mustard. *Archives of Dermatology*, **90**, 158.

Handbook of food additives (1972) 2nd ed. Ed. Furia, T.E. Cleveland, Ohio: CRC Press.

Hecke, E. van. (1977) Contact dermatitis to ethoxyquin in animal feeds. *Contact Dermatitis*, **3**, 341.

Heygi, E. (1971) Contact sensitivity to flavourings. *Contact Dermatitis Newsletter*, **9**, 206.

Heygi, E. & Doležalová, A. (1976) Urticarial reaction after patch tests of toothpaste with a subshock condition: Hypersensitivity to caraway seed. *Československá dermatologie*, **51**, 19.

Herxheimer, H. (1967) Skin sensitivity to flour in bakers' apprentices. *Lancet*, **1**, 83.

Heyl, U. & Reinert-Dilthey, I. (1968) Neue Gesichtspunkte bei der Beurteilung des Bäckerekzems. *Berufsdermatosen*, **16**, 204.

Heyl, U., Wolff, U. & Osten, H. (1970) Inhalative Provokation und Lungenfunktion-sprüfung ekzemkranker Backer and Müller mit nachgewiesener Mehlallergie vom Cutan-vascularen typ. *Berufsdermatosen*, **18**, 77.

Hjorth, N. (1961) *Eczematous Allergy to Balsams, Allied Perfumes and Flavouring Agents*. Copenhagen, Denmark: Munksgaard.

Hjorth, N. (1975) Battery for testing of chefs and other kitchen workers. *Contact Dermatitis*, **1**, 63.

Hjorth, N. & Jervøe, P. (1967) Allergisk kontaktstomatitis og kontaktdermatitis fremkaldt af smagsstoffer I tandpasta. *Tandlægebladet*, **71**, 937.

Hjorth, N. & Roed-Petersen, J. (1976) Occupational protein contact dermatitis in food handlers. *Contact Dermatitis*, **2**, 28.

Hjorth, N. & Weismann, K. (1972) Occupational dermatitis in chefs and sandwich-makers. *Contact Dermatitis Newsletter*, **11**, 301.

Hjorth, N. & Weismann, K. (1973) Occupational dermatitis among veterinary surgeons caused by spiramycin, tylosin and penethamate. *Acta Dermato-venereologica*, **53**, 229.

Inman, P.M. (1965) Dermatitis in a crisp factory. *Acta Dermato-venereologica*, **45**, 295.

Järvinen, K.A.J., Pirilä, V., Björksten, F., Keskinen, H., Lehtinen, M. & Stubb, S. (1979) Unsuitability of bakery work for a person with atopy: a study of 234 bakery workers. *Annals of Allergy*, **42**, 192.

Jirásek, L. & Kalensky, J. (1975) Kontakni alergický ekzém z krmných směsi v živočisné výrobě. *Československá Dermatologie*, 50, 217.

Jukes, H. (1977) Current concepts in nutrition: Food additives. *New England Journal of Medicine*, 297, 427.

Kahn, G., Phanuphak, P. & Claman, H.N. (1974) Propyl gallate — Contact sensitisation and orally-induced tolerance. *Archives of Dermatology*, 109, 506.

Ketel, W.G. van (1978) Dermatitis from octyl gallate in peanut butter. *Contact Dermatitis*, 4, 60.

Kirton, V. & Wilkinson, D.S. (1975) Sensitivity to cinnamic aldehyde in a toothpaste, 2. Further studies. *Contact Dermatitis*, 1, 77.

Klehr, N. & Milbradt, R. (1978) Zur allergen-spezifität bei der proteindermatitis (Hjorth). *Dermatosen In Beruf Und Umwelt*, 26, 187.

Krook, G. (1973) Contact dermatitis due to lettuce. *Contact Dermatitis Newsletter*, 13, 346.

Layton, L.L., Greene, F.C., Panzani, R. & Corse, J.W. (1965) Allergy to green coffee. Failure of patients allergic to green coffee to react to chlorogenic acid, roasted coffee or orange. *Journal of Allergy*, 36, 84.

Layton, L.L., Panzani, R. & Cortese, T.A. (1968) Coffee — reaginic human sera tested in human volunteers & macaque monkeys. Absence of reactions to chlorogenic acid. *International Archives of Allergy*, 33, 417.

Lehrer, S.B., Karr, R.M. & Salvaggio, J.E. (1978) Extraction and analysis of coffee bean allergens. *Clinical Allergy*, 8, 217.

Magnusson, B. & Wilkinson, D.S. (1975) Cinnamic aldehyde in toothpastes. 1. Clinical aspects and patch tests. *Contact Dermatitis*, 1, 70.

Maibach, H.I., Gellin, G. & Ring, M. (1975) Is the antioxidant butylated hydroxytoluene a depigmenting agent in man? *Contact Dermatitis*, 1, 295.

Mali, J.W.H. & Malten, K.E. (1966) The epidemic of polymorph toxic erythema in the Netherlands in 1960. The so-called margarine disease. *Acta Dermato-venereologica*, 46, 123.

Malten, K.E. (1967) Eczema hybrids. *Contact Dermatitis Newsletter*, 1, 6.

Malten, K.E. (1968) The occurrence of hybrids between contact allergic eczema and atopic dermatitis (and vice versa) and their significance. *Dermatologica*, 136, 404.

Malten, K.E. (1970) Allergic contact dermatitis due to cattle fodder products. *Contact Dermatitis Newsletter*, 7, 158.

Malten, K.E. (1979) Four bakers showing positive patch-tests to a number of fragrance materials, which can also be used as flavors. *Acta Dermato-venereologica*, 59, Suppl. 85, 117.

Mehlhorn, H.Ch. & Beetz, D. (1971) Das Antioxydans Aethoxyquin als berufliches Ekzematogen bei einem Futtermitteldosierer. *Berufsdermatosen*, 19, 84.

Meneghini, C.L., Rantuccio, F. & Lomuto, M. (1971) Additives, vehicles and active drugs of topical medicaments as causes of delayed-type allergic dermatitis. *Dermatologica*, 143, 137.

Michaëlsson, G. & Juhlin, L. (1973) Urticaria induced by preservatives and dye additives in food and drugs. *British Journal of Dermatology*, 88, 525.

Michaëlsson, G., Pettersson, L. & Juhlin, L. (1974) Purpura caused by food and drug additives. *Archives of Dermatology*, 109, 49.

Mitchell, J.C. (1972) Allergic contact dermatitis from a certified food dye presenting as 'sock dermatitis'. *Contact Dermatitis Newsletter*, 11, 247.

Mitchell, J.C. (1974a) Contact urticaria from a shrimp, *Pandalus. Contact Dermatitis Newsletter*, 16, 486.

Mitchell, J.C. & Lynne-Davies, G. (1974 b) Zoological names for animal materials and products. *Contact Dermatitis Newsletter*, 16, 493.

Mobacken, H. & Fregert, S. (1975) Allergic contact dermatitis from cardamon. *Contact Dermatitis*, 1, 175.

Nater, J.P. & Zwartz, J.A. (1967) Atopic allergic reactions due to raw potato. *Journal of Allergy*, 40, 202.

Neldner, K.H. (1972) Contact dermatitis from animal feed additives. *Archives of Dermatology*, 106, 722.

Preyss, J.A. (1960) Zur Beurteilung des Bäckerekzems. *Berfusdermatosen*, 8, 68.

Preyss, J.A. (1969) Allergie gegen Tylosintartrat. *Berufsdermatosen*, 17, 166.

Rinkel, H.J. & Balyeat, R.M. (1932) Occupational dermatitis due to lettuce. *Journal of the American Medical Association*, 98, 137.

Roed-Petersen, J. & Hjorth, N. (1975) Patch test sensitisation from d,l-alpha-tocopherol (vitamin E). *Contact Dermatitis*, 1, 391.

Roed-Petersen, J. & Hjorth, N. (1976) Contact dermatitis from antioxidants. Hidden sensitisers in topical medications and foods. *British Journal of Cermatology*, 94, 233.

Rothe, A., Heine, A. & Rebohle, E. (1973) Wacholderbeeröl als Berufsallergen für Haut und Atemtrakt. *Berufsdermatosen*, 21, 11.

Rothman, S. (1949) The effects of feeding certified food azo dyes in paraphenylene-diamine-hypersensitive subjects. *Journal of Investigative Dermatology*, **13**, 223. Discussion p. 231.

Rudzki, E. & Baranowska, A. (1975) Reactions to gallic esters. *Contact Dermatitis*, **1**, 393.

Scharfenberg, B. (1967) Nitrofuranhaltiges Hühnerkukenfutter als berufliches Ekzematogen. *Dermatologische Wochenschrift*, **153**, 60.

Schaumberg, H.H. & Byck, R. (1968) Sin Cib-Syn: Accent on glutamate. *New England Journal of Medicine*, **279**, 105.

Schorr, W.F. (1972) The skin and chemical additives to foods. *Archives of Dermatology*, **105**, 131.

Schubert, von H., Göring, H-D., & Gans, U. (1973) Untersuchungen zur Sensibilisierungs-fähigkeit von Aethoxyquin und *p*-Pheneditin. *Dermatologische Monatsschrift*, **159**, 791.

Schwartz, L. (1938) Cutaneous hazards in the citrus fruit industry. *Archives of Dermatology*, **37**, 631.

Solomons, B. (1971) Sensitisation to oats and barley. *Contact Dermatitis Newsletter*, **10**, 231.

Tennstedt, D., Dumont-Fruytier, M. & Lachapelle, J.M. (1978) Occupational allergic contact dermatitis to virginiamycin, an antibiotic used as a food additive for pigs and poultry. *Contact Dermatitis*, **4**, 133.

Traub, E.F., Gordon, R.E. & Van Dyke, L.S. (1937) Dermatitis from dyed and otherwise treated citrus fruits. *Journal of the American Medical Association*, **108** (1), 872.

Vollum, D.I. (1971) Hypomelanosis from an antioxidant in polyethylene film. *Archives of Dermatology*, **104**, 70.

Wahlberg, J.E. (1974) Contact sensitivity to ethoxyquin — an antioxidant in animal foodstuffs. *Contact Dermatitis Newsletter*, **16**, 476.

Wagner, G. (1959) Eine Analyse von 500 allergischen Kontaktekzemen. *Berufsdermatosen*, **7**, 307.

Wood, W.S. & Fulton, R. (1972) Allergic contact dermatitis from ethoxyquin in appled packers. *Contact Dermatitis Newsletter*, **11**, 295.

Young, E. (1974) Allergic reactions among bakers. *Dermatologica*, **148**, 39.

Zachariae, H. (1978) Ethoxyquin dermatitis. *Contact Dermatitis*, **4**, 117.

6.

Medicaments

ANAESTHETICS (LOCAL)
- Amethocaine
- Benzocaine
- Procaine
- Proxymetacaine
- Amylocaine
- Cyclomethycaine
- Cinchocaine
- Lignocaine
- Prilocaine
- Falicain
- Propanidid
- Pentazocine

ANTIBIOTIC AND ANTIBACTERIAL COMPOUNDS
- Acriflavine: Proflavine: Aminoacridine
- Bacitracin
- Chloramphenicol
  - Azidoamphenicol
  - Chlorfenicone
- Clindamycin
- Erythromycin
- Framycetin
- Fucidin   (Sodium fusidate)
- Gentamicin
- Idoxuridine
- Isonicotinic
  - acid hydrazide   (INAH)
- Neomycin
- Nitrofurazone
- Penicillin
- Polymyxin B
- Quinolines   (Vioform)
- Streptomycin
- Sulphonamides
- Tetracyclines
  - Chlortetracycline   (Aureomycin)
  - Oxytetracycline   (Terramycin)
- Tromantadine hydrochloride
- Virginiamycin

ANTIFUNGAL AND ANTICANDIDAL COMPOUNDS
- Chlorphenesin   (Mycil)
- Clotrimazole   (Canesten)
- Dibenzthione   (Fungiplex)
- Haloprogin   (Halotax)
- Mesulphen   (Tineafax)
- Miconazole   (Daktarin)

- Pecilocin   (Variotin)
- Pyrrolnitrin   (Micturin)
- Tolnaftate   (Tinaderm)
  - Monoamylamine
- Chlordantoin
- Nystatin

ANTIHISTAMINES
- Antazoline   (Antistin)
- Diphenhydramine   (Benadryl)
- Mepyramine   (Anthisan)
- Pheniramine   (Trimeton)
- Promethazine   (Phenergan)

ANTIMITOTIC COMPOUNDS
- Chlorambucil   (Leukeran)
- 5-Fluorouracil
- Nitrogen Mustard
- Triaziquone   (Trenimon)

- Pigmentation
- Busulphan   (Myleran)

DYES — TRIPHENYLMETHANE
- Brilliant Green
- Gentian Violet
- Patent Blue Violet

ETHYLENEDIAMINE

CORTICOSTEROIDS
- Corticotrophin   (ACTH)
- Hydrocortisone
- Prednisone
- Triamcinolone

VITAMINS
- Vitamin A acid   (Retinoic Acid)
- Vitamin B₁   (Thiamine)
- Vitamin E   (Tocopherol)
- Vitamin K

OTHER MEDICAMENTS
- Apomorphine
- Benzoin, tincture
- Benzophenones
- Bufexamac
- p-Chlorobenzenesulphonylglycolic acid
  - nitrile
- Chromonar   (Carbocromen)
- Coumarin
- Crotamiton   (Eurax)
- Dimercaprol   (BAL)
- Ephedrine
  - Phenylephrine   (Metaoxedrine)

Epinephrine	Propantheline bromide	
Ichthammol	Quinidine	
Iodine	Quinine	
Diiodohydroxypropane (Iothion)	Resorcinol	
Meclofenoxate	Salicylates	
Nitroglycerin	Sesame Oil	
Phenylbutazone (Butazolidin)	Stilboestrol	(Diethyl)
p-Hydroxyphenylbutazone (Oxyphenbutazone; Tanderil)	Storax	(Mastic)
	Thioxolone	
Piperazine	Triafur	
Hydroxyzine	Triton X45	
Practolol	Xerumenex	
Propranolol		
Phenoxybenzamine		

Local anaesthetics

The nomenclature of local anaesthetics gives no guide to their sensitising potential; the suffix 'caine' signifies the anaesthetic property of the compound, not its structural formula or its sensitising potential. 'Caines' differ in their chemical type and their ability to sensitise. Thus the esters of *para*-aminobenzoic acid are notorious allergens, whereas the aminoacyl amides, such as lignocaine (Xylocaine), are allergically almost inert; the quinoline cinchocaine (dibucaine) is also a sensitiser.

BENZOIC ACID DERIVATIVES

Esters of p-aminobenzoic acid

Amethocaine	(tetracaine, Pantocaine)
Benzocaine	(Anaesthesin)
Procaine	(novocaine)

Ester of m-aminobenzoic acid

Proxymetacaine	(proparacaine)

Esters of benzoic acid

Amylocaine	(Stovaine)
Cyclomethycaine	(Surfacaine, Topocaine)

QUINOLINE DERIVATIVE

Cinchocaine	(dibucaine, Nupercaine, Percaine)

ANILIDES OR AMIDE DERIVATIVES

Lignocaine	(lidocaine, Xylocaine)
Prilocaine	(Citanest)

OTHER COMPOUNDS

Local anaesthetic — Falicain (propipocaine)
Intravenous anaesthetic — Propanidid (Epontol)
Analgesic — Pentazocine (Fortral)

Different 'caines' are used in different countries so that the incidence of reactions to a particular local anaesthetic varies geographically. In Great Britain topical anaesthetics are prescribed principally for the treatment of pruritus ani, haemorrhoids and occasionally pruritus vulvae; the sensitisers in these medicaments are amethocaine and cinchocaine. A few preparations, including some ear-drops, contain benzocaine.

St John's

Patch-testing with local anaesthetics is selective. From 1971–1976 inclusive, 52 patients in all were found to be sensitive to a local anaesthetic: the source in 48 was a medicament, and in four dentists it was occupational.

| | Medicament | | Dentists | |
	Men	Women	Men	Women
1971	4	3		
1972	5	4		
1973	3	2	1	
1974	6	1	2	
1975	5	7		
1976	2	6	1	
TOTAL	25	23	4	

The 48 patients in the medicament group were sensitised by:

amethocaine (18)
amethocaine and cinchocaine (4): cinchocaine (14)
amethocaine and benzocaine (1): benzocaine (8).

Three were not fully investigated.
The 4 dentists were sensitive to amethocaine.

AMETHOCAINE HYDROCHLORIDE (tetracaine hydrochloride; Pantocaine. Hydrochloride of 2-(dimethylamino)ethyl ester of *p*-butylaminobenzoic acid)

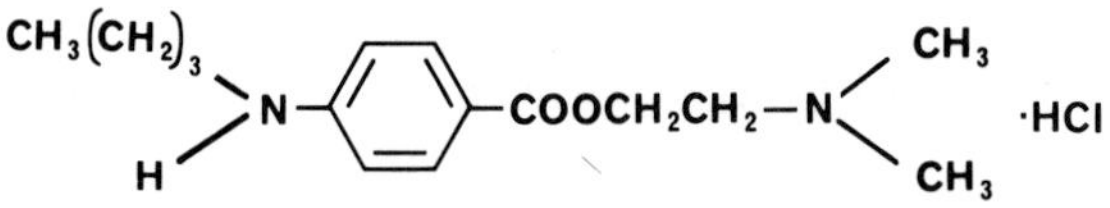

In Great Britain, amethocaine is the surface anaesthetic in many of the topical medicaments formulated for pruritus ani, and it not uncommonly sensitises.

Case report

Twenty patients with dermatitis due to local anaesthetic ointments were patch tested by Wilson (1966); 13 of the 16 with anogenital pruritus and three of the four with other patterns of eczema reacted to amethocaine 1 per cent in petrolatum.

Sensitised guinea-pigs show little cross-sensitivity to other para-compounds (Kalveram *et al.*, 1978).

Medicaments

St John's

Between 1971 and 1976, 23 patients (13 women and 10 men) were found to be sensitive to amethocaine, 19 had used Locan (Duncan and Flockhart), a cream containing amethocaine 0.8 per cent, cinchocaine 0.4 per cent and amylocaine 1 per cent.

The diagnoses in the 13 women were:

pruritus vulvae (6) eczema of the face (2) leg (1) hands (1) widespread (1) herpes zoster (1) and urticaria (1).

In the 10 men they were:

pruritus ani (9) and otitis externa (1).

Patch tests: the results were as follows:

Amethocaine		Cinchocaine		Amylocaine		PPD		Locan	
Tested	+	Tested	+	Tested	+	Tested	+	Tested	+
23	23	18	7	8	1	23	4	18	18

The anaesthetics and PPD were each 1 per cent in petrolatum.

Occupational — dentists

Amethocaine is added to a few dental surface anaesthetics to enhance and prolong the anaesthetic effect of lignocaine on mucosae. Dentists while applying these preparations to their patients' gums are at risk of being sensitised to amethocaine.

St John's

Between 1971 and 1976 four dentists were seen who had been sensitised by amethocaine used in this way. The clinical picture is characteristic: each had cracking and scaling of the finger pulps especially of the thumb, index and middle fingers.

Patch tests: each of the 4 reacted to amethocaine but not to procaine or to PPD (each allergen was 1 per cent in petrolatum).

An alternative is unnecessary; the dentist has to avoid formulations containing amethocaine.

Patch testing

Amethocaine hydrochloride 1 per cent in petrolatum.

BENZOCAINE (ethyl aminobenzoate; Anaesthesin; Orthesin)

$$H_2N-\langle\langle\ \rangle\rangle-COOC_2H_5$$

Sensitising potential

The sensitising potential of benzocaine was studied in humans by Kligman (1966) and in guinea-pigs by Magnusson and Kligman (1969). In both series it was a fairly weak sensitiser, being graded as 2 on a 1–5 scale.

Incidence of sensitivity

In many countries topical benzocaine is a popular remedy and the frequency of sensitisation varies with prescribing customs. In Europe and North America the incidence of sensitivity was 4–5 per cent of eczematous patients tested, whereas in Auckland, New Zealand, it was only 1.4 per cent. In Adelaide 25 of 327 (7.6 per cent) patients with dermatitis from medicaments were sensitive to benzocaine.

	P.T. conc.	No tested	+%	Reference
Europe	5%	4825	4	(Fregert *et al.*, 1969)
N. America	5%	1200	5	(North Am. Cont. Derm. Group, 1973)
Warsaw	5%	877	5.9	(Rudzki and Klieniewska, 1970)
Auckland	?	214	1.4	(Black, 1972)
		Medic. derm.		
Adelaide	?	327	7.6	(Burry *et al.*, 1973)

In the European study there were marked differences between centres: in Munich 77 of 800 (10 per cent) tested were sensitive compared with eight of 800 (1 per cent) in Copenhagen. In countries such as Italy and Germany benzocaine preparations are popular, particularly in the treatment of stasis ulcers and dermatitis, and sensitisation is quite frequent. In Warsaw, 15.2 per cent of patients with stasis dermatitis and 4.1 per cent of those with other forms of eczema had positive patch tests to benzocaine 5 per cent in petrolatum (Rudzki and Baranowska, 1974). Ointments for wounds, preparations for haemorrhoids and anogenital pruritus and salves for nipples may contain benzocaine.

St John's

In Great Britain, relatively few preparations contain benzocaine and consequently it is not a common allergen.

Between 1971 and 1976, nine patients (6 women and 3 men) were seen who had been sensitised by benzocaine. They had used it for the following conditions: pruritus ani (4) otitis externa (1) analgesic cream for back pain (1) and a salve for nipples (1). One patient had applied a benzocaine cream to her face and in another woman with hand eczema the source of contact was not traced.

Patch tests: each of the nine patients reacted to benzocaine 1–5 per cent in petrolatum, three of the nine reacted to PPD 1 per cent in petrolatum.

Patch testing

Benzocaine 5 per cent in petrolatum.

PROCAINE HYDROCHLORIDE (*p*-aminobenzoyldiethylaminoethanol hydrochloride; 2-diethylaminoethyl *p*-aminobenzoate hydrochloride; Novocaine; Syncaine; Anesthesol; Topokain)

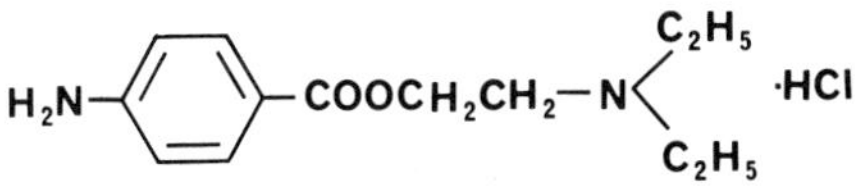

$$H_2N-\text{[benzene ring]}-COOCH_2CH_2-N\begin{array}{c}C_2H_5\\C_2H_5\end{array}\cdot HCl$$

Sensitising potential

The sensitising potential of procaine hydrochloride was studied by Kligman (1966); with an induction concentration of 25 per cent he sensitised six of 24 subjects, grading it as 2, a fairly weak sensitiser, on a 1–5 scale.

Case reports

Allergy to procaine was first reported in 1921 in three dentists (Lane, 1921), and the chemical groups responsible for sensitisation were studied by Goodman (1939) and Fish and Freedman (1964). Sensitivity to procaine in patients reacting to procaine penicillin was investigated by Fernstrom (1959, 1960a, b, c, 1962).

In Czechoslovakia there was a striking fall in the incidence of procaine sensitivity from 10.6 per cent in 1953–1957 to 0.5 per cent in 1963–1967 (Hegyi, 1969). In Helsinki, cases of procaine sensitivity reappeared following the purchase in Rumania and subsequent use of Gerovital applications, which contain procaine chloride (Förström *et al.*, 1977).

St John's

From 1971–1976 inclusive there were no cases of primary sensitisation.

Patch testing

Procaine hydrochloride 1–5 per cent in petrolatum.

PROXYMETACAINE   (3-amino-4-propoxybenzoic acid 2-(diethylamino)ethyl ester; proparacaine; Ophthaine; Ophthetic)

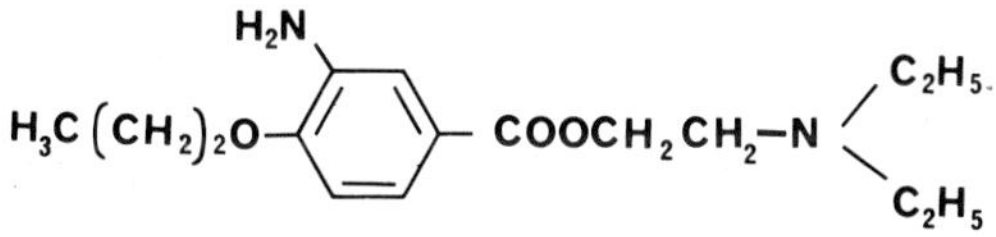

$$H_3C(CH_2)_2O-\text{[benzene ring, H_2N]}-COOCH_2CH_2-N\begin{array}{c}C_2H_5\\C_2H_5\end{array}$$

Proxymetacaine hydrochloride has approximately the same potency, as a local anaesthetic, as amethocaine (tetracaine); it is almost non-irritant, and in concentrations of 0.5 per cent is suitable for use in the eye.

Case reports

(1) An ophthalmologist developed dry, fissured finger tips first on the left hand and then on the right; the condition healed on holiday. Patch tests: of the medicaments he handled he reacted only to Ophthetic eye drops; and of the constituents he was sensitive to proparacaine. He changed to tetracaine (amethocaine) and remained well (March and Greenwood, 1968). (2) A doctor, who wore contact lenses, developed blepharitis and was treated with many ophthalmic solutions and ointments. Patch tests: he reacted to Chibro-Kerakain eye-

drops and of the constituents to proxymetacaine 2 per cent in water but not to benzalkonium chloride 0.05 per cent in water (Bandmann, Breit and Mutzek, 1974).

Patch testing
Proxymetacaine 2 per cent in water.

AMYLOCAINE HYDROCHLORIDE (1-(dimethylamino)-2-methyl-2-butanol benzoate hydrochloride; Stovaine).

Case report
In Wilson's (1966) report, two of twenty patients sensitised by ointments containing local anaesthetics reacted to amylocaine 1 per cent in petrolatum.

St John's
Between 1971 and 1976 inclusive, no case of primary sensitisation was seen. But of 8 patients allergic to amethocaine one also reacted to amylocaine (p. 195) which was present in the sensitising medicament.

Patch testing
Amylocaine hydrochloride 1 per cent in petrolatum.

CYCLOMETHYCAINE HYDROCHLORIDE (The *p*-cyclohexyloxybenzoic acid ester of *N*-(3-hydroxypropyl) pipecoline hydrochloride; Topocaine; Surfathesin)

Cyclomethycaine although little used in Great Britain is used in other countries. Reports of sensitisation have not been found.

Patch testing
Cyclomethycaine 1 per cent in petrolatum

CINCHOCAINE HYDROCHLORIDE (dibucaine hydrochloride; 2-butoxy-*N*-(2-diethylaminoethyl) cinchoninamide hydrochloride; Nupercaine; Percaine; Cincaine; Sovacaine)

Case reports
In Wilson's series (1966), nine of sixteen patients with anogenital pruritus, and two of four with eczema elsewhere, reacted to cinchocaine 1 per cent in petrolatum.

St John's
Between 1971 and 1976 inclusive, 18 patients (11 men and 7 women) were found to have been sensitised by cinchocaine, 8 through using a rectal ointment, Proctosedyl (Roussel), containing cinchocaine hydrochloride 0.5 per cent.
The diagnoses in the 11 men were:
pruritus ani (9), haemorrhoids (1) herpes zoster (1)
and in the 7 women:
pruritus vulvae (3) pruritus ani (2) sunburn (1) eczema of the face (1).

Patch tests

	Cinchocaine	1%	Vioform	5%
	Tested	+	Tested	+
	18	18	18	3

(both allergens were in petrolatum)

Cinchocaine is a quinoline derivative and cross-reactions to the *para*-amino compounds, PPD and amethocaine would not be expected; 3 of the 18 patients reacted to vioform, another quinoline derivative, but it is impossible to say whether these were cross-reactions or independent sensitisations.

Patch testing
Cinchocaine hydrochloride 1 per cent in petrolatum.

LIGNOCAINE (2-diethylamino-2', 6'-acetoxylidide; lidocaine; Xylocaine; Xylotox; Xylocitin; Duncaine)

Lignocaine is widely used as an intradermal local anaesthetic but sensitisation is extremely rare.

Case reports

Injections of Xylotox for dental anaesthesia produced severe swelling of the mouth in a man described by Noble and Pierce (1961); intradermal tests with xylocaine and other local anaesthetics were positive.

Generalised exfoliative dermatitis, presumed to be due to lidocaine hypersensitivity, was reported by Hofmann, Maibach and Prout (1975). Patch testing with lidocaine hydrochloride 20 per cent in petrolatum was negative and, although an intradermal test with 2 per cent lidocaine was negative at 45 minutes, the patient developed an eruption on the arms and shoulders 8 hours later.

Patch testing

Lignocaine ?5 per cent in petrolatum.

PRILOCAINE HYDROCHLORIDE (2-(propylamino)-*o*-propionotoluidide hydrochloride; Citanest; Xylonest)

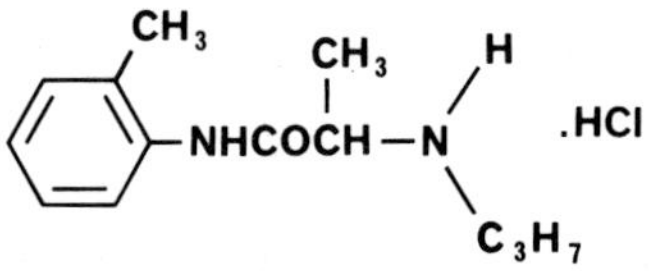

This local anaesthetic and lignocaine have similar properties, but prilocaine is less toxic and is used in dentistry and for spinal anaesthesia.

Contact sensitivity to prilocaine has not been reported but a case of an anaphylactoid reaction has been described by Göransson (1976). The patient, who had previously received prilocaine for dental anaesthesia without trouble, was given a further injection and 45 minutes later became itchy and nauseated and within 4 hours he was shocked and had generalised urticaria. He recovered and was later tested intracutaneously with prilocaine: he did not react to 0.02 mg/ml, gave a slight weal to 0.2 and 2 mg/ml at 1 hour and a definite reaction to 20 mg/ml, which began after 25 minutes and reached a maximum in 60 minutes. Because of the prolonged interval between the dental injection of prilocaine and the development of shock it was suggested that the antigen was not prilocaine but one of its metabolites.

Patch testing

Prilocaine 5 per cent in petrolatum.

FALICAIN (3-piperidino-4′-propoxypropiophenone hydrochloride; propipocaine)

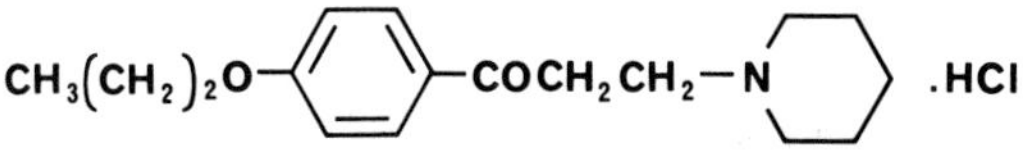

Falicain is a local anaesthetic used in Germany in rectal preparations, nose drops, oral solutions and antimicrobial lotions.

Case reports
In Berlin, Behrbohm and Lenzner (1975) saw 35 cases of sensitisation and during two years in Dresden, Scholz and Richter (1977) saw a further 28 cases. Most of the patients had perianal dermatitis which in some had generalised.
Sensitisation by nose drops simulated erysipelas of the face.
Patch tests: the patients reacted to falicain 1 per cent in petrolatum.

Patch testing
Falicain 1 per cent in petrolatum.

PROPANIDID ({4-[(diethylcarbamoyl) methoxy]-3-methoxyphenyl} acetic acid propyl ester; Epontol)

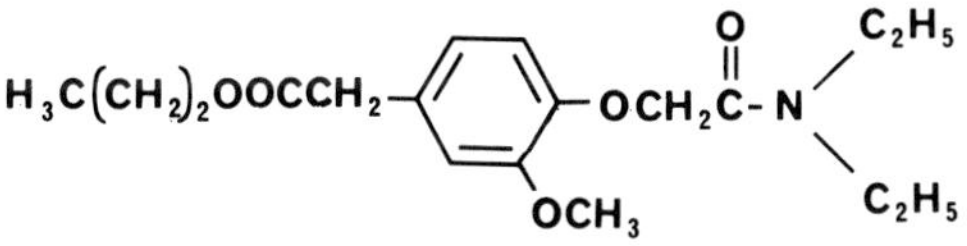

$$H_3C(CH_2)_2OOCCH_2 - \bigcirc - OCH_2\overset{\overset{O}{\parallel}}{C} - N \overset{C_2H_5}{\underset{C_2H_5}{<}}$$

OCH$_3$

Propanidid is a derivative of eugenol, which is obtained from oil of cloves. Being an intravenous anaesthetic, it can be used instead of barbiturates. It is formulated as a 5 per cent solution of propanidid suspended in camphor polyoxyethylated castor oil.

Case reports
Allergic contact dermatitis has been described in two anaesthetists. One (Case 1) had hand dermatitis (Bandmann and Doenicke, 1970) and the other (Case 2) had a severe recurrent dermatitis of the hands, eyes and face (Sneddon and Glew, 1973).

Patch tests

		Case 1	Case 2
Epontol	As Is	++	++
Propanidid	5% aqueous	++	
Propanidid	?		+++
Base		—	—
Eugenol	2% in petrolatum	NT	+
Cinnamon oil	5% in olive oil	NT	+ } 'mild positives'
Balsam of Peru	25% in petrolatum	—	+

Patch testing
Propanidid 5 per cent aqueous.

PENTAZOCINE (1,2,3,4,5,6-hexahydro-6,11-dimethyl-3-(3-methyl-2-butenyl)-2,6-methano-3-benzazocin-8-ol; Fortral; Sosigon; Talwin)

This analgesic has an effect comparable to that of morphine and pethidine but is less addictive.

Repeated injections into one site causes skin sclerosis with ulcer and sometimes nodule formation (Schlicher, Zuehlke and Lynch, 1971; Parks, Perry and Muller, 1971; Agache and Bidard de la Noë, 1972). Similar changes were produced experimentally in guinea-pigs by Parks et al. (1971); the histology of these lesions confirmed their suggestion that ischaemia due to the direct vaso-constrictive and vaso-occlusive effects of pentazocine was the cause. Such ischaemia may have caused the extensive skin ulceration of both lower legs described by Seymour and Raynor (1974) in an addict who injected the drug into his leg veins.

Antibiotic and antibacterial compounds

ACRIFLAVINE
Acriflavine is a mixture of 2,8-diamino-10-methyl acridinium chloride and 2,8-diaminoacridine

Once popular as a topical antiseptic, acriflavine is rarely used nowadays. Contact sensitivity was reported in the past (Beare, 1947).

Patch testing
Acriflavine ? 0.1 per cent in petrolatum.

PROFLAVINE DIHYDROCHLORIDE (3,6-Diaminoacridinium chloride hydrochloride)

Proflavine dihydrochloride, an acridine dye, was used in the past as a pre-operative surgical application and caused many cases of pigmented allergic contact dermatitis (Mitchell, 1972).

Patch testing
Proflavine hydrochloride ?0.1 per cent in petrolatum.

9-AMINOACRIDINE HYDROCLORIDE (aminacrine hydrochloride; Monacrin; Acramine Yellow)

Case report
A man, an habitual user of Acriflex cream (Allen and Hanbury Ltd.; containing 0.1 per cent aminoacridine hydrochloride), applied it to his scrotum and developed an acute contact dermatitis. Patch tests: he reacted to Acriflex and to aminacrine 0.1 per cent in petrolatum, but not to acriflavine or proflavine, both 0.1 per cent in petrolatum (Wilson, 1971).

St John's
Two patients were seen, one in 1973 and the other in 1976; both had used Acriflex (Allen and Hanbury Ltd), the first for haemorrhoids and the second to treat his grazed elbow. In this latter patient the reaction was severe with blistering. Patch tests: both men reacted to Acriflex and aminacrine hydrochloride 1 per cent in petrolatum.

Patch testing
Aminoacridine hydrochloride 1 per cent and 0.1 per cent in petrolatum.

BACITRACIN (ZINC SALT)

Bacitracin is a polypeptide produced by strains of *Bacillus subtilis* and *B. licheniformis*. It is active against a range of Gram-positive organisms and against spirochaetes.

Case reports
Direct sensitisation by bacitracin seems to be rare; the positive patch tests to bacitracin seen in many patients in Finland are considered by Pirilä and Rouhunoski (1960) to signify cross-reactions to neomycin (p. 214). Two patients, one with a stasis ulcer and the other with cheilitis, who were definitely sensitised by bacitracin and not by neomycin, were reported by Binnick and Clendenning (1978).

St John's
No case of sensitisation has been traced among the patients seen between 1971 and 1976.

Cross-reactions

Polymyxin B sulphate. A woman with contact dermatitis of her feet had positive patch test reactions to polymyxin B sulphate 1 per cent, 5 per cent and 30 per cent and to bacitracin 1 per cent, 5 per cent and 30 per cent, each in petrolatum. It was thought these might be cross-reactions rather than independent sensitisations (van Ketel, 1974).

Anaphylaxis
Fifteen minutes after applying an ointment containing bacitracin to her stasis ulcer a woman collapsed; she had a pricking sensation and swelling of her face, generalised itching, sweating, dyspnoea and hypotension. Later, she remembered that twice in the past she had had urticaria after her ulcer had been treated with other preparations containing bacitracin (Comaish and Cunliffe, 1967). Three months later, because a prick test with bacitracin 1/1000 was negative, 0.03 ml of bacitracin 1/1000 (2.3 units) was injected intradermally, and within 4 minutes she had a severe anaphylactic shock and lost consciousness. It was stressed that the concentration for intradermal testing should be 1000-fold less than that for prick tests.

In a similar case described by Roupe and Strannegård (1969), a 14-year-old atopic girl collapsed with anaphylactic shock after an ointment containing bacitracin was applied to her infected eczema. Two months previously a similar application had caused irritation and swelling of her lip. Prausnitz-Küstner tests done on monkeys and one human were positive.

Patch testing
Bacitracin 20 per cent in petrolatum.

CHLORAMPHENICOL (D(-)-threo-2,2-dichloro-N-[β-hydroxy-α-(hydroxymethyl)-p-nitrophenethyl] acetamide; Chloromycetin)

$$O_2N-\langle\bigcirc\rangle-\underset{\underset{CH}{|}}{CH}\underset{\underset{CH_2OH}{|}}{CH}-NH-\underset{\overset{O}{||}}{C}-CHCl_2$$

Chloramphenicol is produced by *Streptomyces venezuelae* and has a wide range of antimicrobial activity. It is mainly bacteriostatic, though under some conditions it is bactericidal.

Sensitising potential
With the human maximisation test Kligman (1966) sensitised none of the 22 subjects. In clinical practice, chloramphenicol is not a frequent sensitiser (Bandmann, 1972) but this may be a reflection of its limited use for eczema rather than its being a weak allergen.

Case reports
In 1963, Schwank and Jirásek reported 29 cases of contact sensitivity to

chloramphenicol, which had been used on the lower legs by 22 of the patients. Patch tests with chloramphenicol 1 per cent in petrolatum or in alcohol elicited reactions in all the patients but in nine of 149 controls. Six further patients, who worked in a plant making chloramphenicol, developed a contact dermatitis of the face and hands.

Cross-reactions to DNCB

Group reactions were studied in 30 patients and cross sensitivity to 2,4-dinitrochlorbenzene occurred in 40 per cent, to *p*-dinitrobenzene in 37 per cent and to *p*-nitrobenzoic acid in 17 per cent (Schwank and Jirásek, 1963). In Eriksen's (1978) study of 15 chloramphenicol sensitive patients, although three reacted to *p*-nitrobenzoic acid and two to *p*-dinitrobenzene none reacted to DNCB. In a further 27 patients primarily sensitised to DNCB neither chloramphenicol nor the *p*-nitro compounds elicited reactions.

Systemic reactions

A woman, who had used chloramphenicol topically in the past, was given 1 g by mouth and developed anaphylactic shock with oedema of the face and generalised urticaria. A week later a patch test with 1 per cent chloramphenicol produced the same reaction but to a lesser degree (Kozáková, 1976).

A positive patch test reaction to 50 per cent chloramphenicol was attributed to a previous drug eruption from intramuscular chloramphenicol (Rudzki, Grzywa and Maciejowska, 1976).

St John's

In 1973, 441 patients were routinely tested with chloramphenicol 5 per cent in petrolatum; only three reacted. Apart from this series, patch testing with chloramphenicol is selective. From 1971 to 1976 inclusive, 14 patients were found to be sensitive (seven men and seven women); in five the allergy was known to have resulted from eye medicaments. The allergy was of present relevance in 10 patients and of past relevance in four patients. One (Patient 11 below) denied having used chloramphenicol topically, but remembered being given it orally for an adhesive plaster dermatitis and subsequently developing a generalised eruption.

Patch tests

Patient	Age	Site or Diagnosis	Relevance	Chloramphenicol 5–10% pet.	1% cream	Other +
1. M	40	Eyes, face, hands	Present	+	+	Nil
2. M	50	Eye injury. Seb. derm.	present	NT	+	Neo. Lanolin
3. F	51	Conjunctivitis	Past	NT	+	Nil
4. M	67	Eyes, feet	Past	+	NT	Leathers
5. F	63	Eyes, face	Past	NT	+	Neomycin
6. F	77	Eyes, hand	?Present	+	NT	Thiurams Et. diamine
7. F	35	Otitis externa	Present	NT	+	Neo. Lanolin PPD Ethylene-diamine
8. M	52	Otitis externa	?Present	NT	+	Lanolin Colophony

Patient	Age	Site or Diagnosis	Relevance	Chloramphenicol 5–10% pet.	1%	Other + cream
9. M	48	Face, hands, feet	?Present	+	NT	Neo. Gentam. Et. diamine Turps. Colophony
10. F	26	Hands	?Present	NT	+	Nil
11. M	31	Hands	Past	+	NT	Nil
12. M	69	Hands	?Present	+	NT	Thiurams
13. F	60	Stasis	Present	NT	+	Neo. Framycetin PPD
14. F	21	Discoid	Present	+	+	Nil

Patch testing
Chloramphenicol 5 and 10 per cent in petrolatum.

In vitro tests
The reliability of *in vitro* tests and of different types of epicutaneous tests in the diagnosis of chloramphenicol sensitivity have been investigated by Wätzig and Ruffert (1977).

AZIDOAMPHENICOL   (D-(-)-threo-2-azido-N-[β-hydroxy-α-(hydroxymethyl)-p-nitrophenethyl]acetamide; azidamfenicol)

Azidoamphenicol is an antibiotic closely related to chloramphenicol. Eucortyl (Bayer) contains dexamethasone 0.01 per cent and azidoamphenicol 1.5 per cent.

Case report
Since 1968, Eucortyl has been a popular medicament in Norway where four cases of sensitivity to azidoamphenicol, confirmed by patch testing, have been reported by Wereide (1975). Three patients had lower leg eczema with spread to other sites, and the other had hand and arm eczema. Patch tests: all four patients reacted to Eucortyl and to azidoamphenicol 1–2 per cent.

Cross-sensitivity
Three of the four patients cross-reacted to chloramphenicol 2 per cent.

Patch testing
Azidoamphenicol ?5 per cent in petrolatum.

Wereide (1975) thought that cases of sensitivity are missed through Eucortyl giving false negative patch tests, and by testing with too low concentrations of azidoamphenicol. However, he did not suggest a reliable yet non-irritant patch test concentration.

Chlorfenicone
Chlorfenicone is a dichloracetylation derivative of chloramphenicol.

St John's

Case reports

Two women were sensitised by using Genetris pessaries (Carlo Erba) for a vaginal discharge. Both developed generalised eruptions and one required systemic corticosteroids. Patch tests: Both patients reacted to a Genetris suppository and to chlorfenicone 1 per cent in petrolatum (Cronin, 1969).

Patch testing
Chlorfenicone 1 per cent in petrolatum.

CLINDAMYCIN

Clindamycin has been formulated as a lotion and a case of contact dermatitis has been reported (Coskey, 1978). Patch test concentration: clindamycin hydrochloride 1 per cent aqueous.

ERYTHROMYCIN (Erythrocin; Erycin; Ilotycin).

This antibiotic has a spectrum of activity similar to that of benzyl penicillin.

Case report

Erythromycin has a low sensitising potential. Erythromycin base has been advocated as a substitute for neomycin by Fisher (1976, 1977) on the basis of his experience that none of 60 patients with stasis ulcers was sensitised by the topical application of erythromycin base 5 per cent in petrolatum. However, erythromycin stearate is not equally safe as a patient of van Ketel's (1976) with a leg ulcer was sensitised by pure erythromycin stearate 5 per cent in petrolatum. Patch tests: she reacted to erythromycin stearate 0.1 per cent, 1 per cent and 5 per cent in petrolatum. He also described immediate type hypersensitivity in a girl aged 7 years who developed urticaria after receiving erythromycin suspension for one week. A scratch test with the suspension elicited a reaction whereas a patch test gave no response.

Patch testing
Erythromycin stearate 1 per cent and 5 per cent in petrolatum.

FRAMYCETIN (Soframycin — framycetin sulphate)

Framycetin consists of neomycin B (99 per cent) neomycin C (1 per cent and neamine (0.2 per cent). Despite its close similarity to neomycin (p. 210) sensitivity to framycetin is infrequent. This apparent discrepancy is probably due to the much more frequent prescribing of neomycin. Patch test reactions have been reported but nearly always in patients sensitive to neomycin; reactions to framycetin alone are uncommon.

Case reports

In the series recorded by Kirton and Munro-Ashman (1965) 45 patients had positive patch test reactions both to neomycin and to framycetin (each 1 per cent in petrolatum); five reacted to framycetin only and four to neomycin only.

St John's

In the series reported by Carruthers and Cronin (1976), 450 consecutive patients were patch tested with neomycin and framycetin (each 20 per cent in petrolatum). Thirteen (2.9 per cent) reacted to both, 10 (2.2 per cent) reacted to neomycin alone and four (0.9 per cent) to framycetin alone. It was suggested that the combined reactions were due to sensitisation by neomycin B which is common to both neomycin and framycetin, the isolated reactions to neomycin by sensitivity to neomycin C or neamine, and those to framycetin alone by an allergy to an unidentified impurity.

Patch testing

Framycetin 20 per cent in petrolatum.

SODIUM FUSIDATE (Fusidic acid sodium salt; Fucidin)

Fusidic acid, isolated from the fungus *Fusidium coccineum*, is highly effective against staphylococci, and as 2 per cent sodium fusidate (Fucidin) it is used as a topical antibiotic.

Case reports

Two cases of sensitisation have been reported (Verbov, 1970; Dave and Main, 1973), both in women with stasis ulcers. One had used Fucidin ointment (Leo Labs. Ltd.) and the other Intertulle Fucidin (Leo Labs. Ltd.). The latter patient presented with an acute dermatitis of her eyelids and face, and the former recalled having had in the past a similar type of eczema and it recurred with patch testing. Patch tests: both reacted to sodium fusidate 2 per cent in water and neither responded to the base of the Fucidin ointment.

St John's

Only selected patients, usually those with stasis eczema, are tested with fucidin. From 1971–1976 inclusive, 12 women and 2 men were found to have been sensitised: 10 had stasis eczema, 2 otitis externa and 2 dermatitis medicamentosa of whom one had used Fucidin ointment for herpes simplex and the other for a graze on his leg. Patch tests: all these patients reacted to fucidin 2 per cent in petrolatum.

Patch testing

Sodium fusidate 2 per cent in petrolatum.

GENTAMICIN (Gentamycin)

GENTAMICIN SULPHATE (Cidomycin; Garamycin; Gentalyn; Genticin; Refobacin).

Gentamicin sulphate is produced by *Micromonospora purpura*, an Actinomycete. It is effective against Gram-positive and Gram-negative bacteria, including *Staphylococcus aureus*, *Streptococcus pyogenes*, species of *Pseudomonas*, *Proteus*, and *Escherichia coli*.

Gentamicin applied topically can sensitise, although most reports are of cross-sensitivity to neomycin rather than of direct sensitisation by gentamicin.

Case reports
In Munich, a series of 37 patients was patch tested with neomycin sulphate and with gentamicin sulphate, both 20 per cent in petrolatum. Thirty reacted to neomycin only, five to neomycin and to gentamicin, and two to gentamicin only. Of these latter two patients, one was a bacteriology technician who had been in contact with gentamicin sulphate, and the other was a patient whose leg ulcer had been treated with many ointments (Bandmann and Mutzek, 1973).

St John's
Only selected patients, usually those with stasis eczema, are tested with gentamicin. From 1971–1976 inclusive, 8 patients were found to be sensitive, of whom 7 had stasis eczema and one eczema of the eyelids. Three reacted to gentamicin but not to neomycin or framycetin. The patch test results were as follows:

Patients	gentamicin 20%	neomycin 20%	framycetin 10–20%
3	+	—	—
5	+	+	+

(diluent was petrolatum)

Toxicity
Deafness and vestibular and renal damage occur with parenteral therapy. Drake (1974) described a woman who developed tinnitus each time she treated her paronychia with gentamicin sulphate cream 0.1 per cent.

Patch testing
Gentamicin sulphate 20 per cent in petrolatum.

IDOXURIDINE (2'-deoxy-5-iodouridine; IDU; Herplex; Kerecid; Iduridin)

Idoxuridine is an antiviral agent used to treat herpes simplex.

Case reports

Sensitisation was first reported by Osmundsen (1975). He described two women who had used Iduridin ophthalmic ointment containing 0.2 per cent idoxuridine, one for recurrent herpes simplex of her abdominal wall and the other for troublesome perianal viral warts. Patch tests: both patients reacted to Iduridin and idoxuridine 1 per cent in petrolatum; 12 controls gave no reaction. Four cases were also reported by Amon, Lis and Hanifin (1975). Three were men with recurrent herpes progenitalis, one of whom was sensitised by an ointment containing 0.5 per cent idoxuridine and the other two by 5 per cent idoxuridine in dimethylacetamide. The fourth man had used an 0.5 per cent preparation for herpes keratitis. On patch testing, these patients reacted to idoxuridine and to brominated and chlorinated, but not fluorinated, pyrimidine analogues.

St John's

    In 1975, a woman was seen who had been sensitised by an ointment containing 0.5 per cent IDU, which she had used to treat a herpes simplex infection of her thigh. Patch tests: she reacted to the 0.5 per cent IDU preparation.

Patch testing

Idoxuridine 0.5 per cent in petrolatum.

ISONICOTINIC ACID HYDRAZIDE (INAH)

Case report

A nurse developed a contact eczema to isonicotinic acid hydrazide cones, which she was using to treat an ulcerated BCG reaction (Ippen, 1978).

NEOMYCIN SULPHATE

Neomycin was isolated in 1949 from certain strains of *Streptomyces fradiae* in culture. It consists of two active components, neomycin B (78–88 per cent) and neomycin C (16–10 per cent). A third component, present only in small amounts (5–2 per cent), is the degradation product neamine (neomycin A). Both neomycin B and C have two components, a deaminohexose (neosamine B or C) linked to *d*-ribose and a deaminohexose linked to 2-deoxystreptamine. Framycetin consists almost entirely (99 per cent) of neomycin B with small amounts of neomycin C (1 per cent) and traces of neamine.

    Neomycin is a broad-spectrum antibiotic used widely in topical preparations. It is a well-known contact sensitiser. The first cases were reported from the U.S.A. by Kile, Rockwell and Schwarz (1952) and Baer and Ludwig (1952), and from Great Britain by Calnan and Sarkany (1958).

Sensitising potential

In the human maximisation test using sodium lauryl sulphate as an adjuvant, Kligman (1966) sensitised seven of 25 subjects with neomycin, making it a fairly weak sensitiser, grade 2 on a 1–5 scale. This relatively low sensitising potential was confirmed by Marzulli and Maibach (1973) using the Draize procedure.

These results differed from those of the guinea-pig maximisation test in which 18 of 25 animals were sensitised, making it a grade 4 sensitiser on a 1–5 scale (Magnusson and Kligman, 1969).

Clinically, Hjorth and Thomsen (1968) found that neomycin, formulated as an ointment, sensitises more often than when in a cream, lotion or powder base.

Incidence of sensitivity
The frequency of sensitisation varies with prescribing habits, and the incidence reported is influenced by the pattern of eczema of the patients in particular series. Despite this, as can be seen in the following Table, the low incidence of 1.7 per cent in Warsaw contrasts strikingly with the 10.3 per cent reported from Auckland, New Zealand.

Country or City	Number Tested	Patch Test Conc. %	+%	Report
Scandinavia	5558	40	4.5	Magnusson et al. (1968)
Europe	4825	20	3.7	Fregert et al. (1969)
N. America	1200	20	6.0	N. American Cont. Derm. Grp. (1973)
Warsaw	1205	40	1.7	Rudzki and Kleniewska (1970)
Auckland	214	20	10.3	Black (1972)
Adelaide	50/327 pts + a medicament			Burry et al. (1973)

In Finland, neomycin preparations are sold without prescriptions and consequently neomycin is their commonest contact allergen. The incidence of sensitivity rose in 1968 to 19 per cent of all the patients tested (Forström and Pirilä, 1978).

St John's
Every patient attending the Contact Clinic is routinely patch tested with neomycin sulphate 20 per cent in petrolatum. The yearly incidence of sensitisation remained between 4–5 per cent during the period 1971 to 1976, the total numbers were similar in men (4.2 per cent) and in women (3.7 per cent) (Table 6.1).

Table 6.1. Yearly incidence of neomycin sensitivity. St John's 1971–1976.

	Total			Males			Females		
	+ Neo.	Tested	%	+ Neo.	Tested	%	+ Neo.	Tested	%
1971	76	1558	4.9	36	707	5.1	40	851	4.7
1972	63	1606	3.9	37	738	5.0	26	868	3.0
1973	60	1546	3.9	33	710	4.6	27	836	3.2
1974	57	1433	4.0	29	655	4.4	28	778	3.6
1975	61	1858	3.3	19	887	2.1	42	971	4.3
1976	80	1982	4.0	41	937	4.4	39	1045	3.7

Clinical features
The sensitivity is usually superimposed upon an existing eczema, and clinically the condition usually worsens gradually rather than deteriorating suddenly. Many neomycin formulations contain a corticosteroid which helps to suppress the irritation caused by the allergen, and so the unsuspecting patient continues to apply the preparation.

Patients with hypostatic eczema and ulcers (Stolze, 1966) or with chronic otitis externa (Jensen, Allen and Nordecai, 1966) are particularly prone to neomycin sensitisation (Kirton and Munro-Ashman, 1965). This is partly due to the large number of medicaments used by these particular patients.

St John's

To determine whether neomycin sensitises more often on its own or in association with the development of sensitivity to other topical medicaments, the 397 patients seen between 1971 and 1976 inclusive have been divided into:

(i) Those sensitive to neomycin only
(ii) Those sensitive to neomycin and also to vioform, lanolin, parabens, ethylenediamine or another medicament or base.

The numbers in the two groups were equal, half of the patients (52 per cent) were sensitive to neomycin only, and half (48 per cent) were additionally sensitised to another medicament or base (Table 6.2).

Table 6.2. Sensitisation to neomycin alone or in association with another medicament allergen (St John's 1971–1976).

	Sensitised neomycin only				Sensitised neo. + other med. allergen			
	Males	%	Females	%	Males	%	Females	%
1971	16/36	44	21/40	53	20/36	55	19/40	47
1972	24/37	64	12/26	46	13/37	35	14/26	54
1973	17/33	52	17/27	63	16/33	48	10/27	37
1974	18/29	62	20/28	71	11/29	38	8/28	29
1975	6/19	32	19/42	45	13/19	68	23/42	55
1976	22/41	54	15/39	39	19/41	46	24/39	62
Total	103/195	53%	104/202	52%	92/195	47%	98/202	49%
			207/397 52%				190/397 48%	

Patterns of eczema

The patterns of eczema in the neomycin sensitive patients are listed in Table 6.3. The predominance of hand eczema reflects the many patients who attend the clinic with this condition and does not incidate that hand eczema predisposes to neomycin sensitivity. It is interesting, and contrary to what might have been anticipated, that in

Table 6.3. Patterns of eczema in 397 patients sensitised to neomycin (St John's 1971–1976).

	Males	Females
Hands only	43	39
Hands + elsewhere	21	27
Face	18	41
Hypostatic	21	26
Otitis externa	10	7
Pruritus ani	12	4
Atopic	6	9
Discoid	5	0
Widespread	3	6
Other sites	56	43
Total	195	202

this group there were more patients with eczema confined to the hands than with hand eczema which had spread to other sites.

Patients with hypostatic eczema and otitis externa do develop neomycin sensitivity but the number of patients with this diagnosis seen in this clinic is relatively small. Pruritus ani, which occurs predominantly in men, is prone to be complicated by allergy to medicaments.

Ages of patients
The majority (82 per cent) of these patients were over 30 years of age but the allergy can occur in persons less than 20 years old, and in this series 3 boys, two aged 10 years and the other 8 years, were sensitive: two had foot eczema and one had atopic eczema (Table 6.4).

Table 6.4. Ages of 397 patients sensitive to neomycin (St John's 1971–1976).

Age (years)	0–10	11–20	21–30	31–40	41–50	51–60	61–70	71–90	Total
Males	3	9	16	28	54	43	38	4	195
Females	0	16	26	30	42	61	23	4	202

Length of history
The length of history was the same for both sexes: in about one-third (38 per cent) the duration of eczema was up to one year; in approximately one-third (29 per cent) it was 1–5 years; and in the other third (32 per cent) it was more than 5 years (Table 6.5). In eight patients the duration of the eczema was not recorded.

Table 6.5. Duration of eczema in 389 patients sensitive to neomycin (St John's 1971–1976).

	0–3 mths	>3–12 mths	>1–3 yrs	>3–5 yrs	>5 yrs	Total
Males	30	44	34	21	61	190
Females	29	46	34	24	66	199

Cross-reactions
The patterns of cross-sensitivity between various neomycins, kanamycin and streptomycin have been studied in guinea-pigs by Chung and Carson (1975).

1. *Framycetin (Soframycin).* The close similarity between framycetin and part of the neomycin complex explains their frequent cross-sensitisation. In the Hague, 12 patients sensitive to neomycin 5 per cent reacted also to framycetin 5 per cent; it was known that 11 had not used the latter antibiotic (Boonan and Waveren Hogervorst, 1964).

St John's
Framycetin is not included in the routine test series and it is likely to be used only when a medicament allergy is strongly suspected. During the 1971–1976 period, 76 of the neomycin sensitive patients were tested with framycetin 10–20 per cent in petrolatum and 66 (87 per cent) reacted. This high incidence is influenced by the selection of patients and may be partly due to independent sensitisation by the two antibiotics, because in 1976 450 consecutive patients were tested with both neomycin and with framycetin, each 20 per cent in petrolatum, and of the 23 (5 per cent) who were sensitive to neomycin, only 13 (57 per cent) also responded to framycetin (Carruthers and Cronin, 1976).

2. *Gentamicin*. In the various series reported, a quarter to a half of the patients sensitive to neomycin cross-reacted to gentamicin.

In Helsinki, of 100 patients sensitive to neomycin, 40 had positive patch tests to gentamicin sulphate 30 per cent in petrolatum, and it was known that none had been exposed to this antibiotic (Pirilä, Hirvonen and Rouhunkoski, 1968). In Heidelberg, 33 patients were found to be sensitive to neomycin, and eight reacted also to gentamicin (Braun and Schütz, 1969). In the U.S.A. 11 of 20 neomycin-sensitive patients had positive patch tests to gentamicin 10–30 per cent in petrolatum (Schorr, Wenzel and Hegedus, 1973).

St John's
> Only 41 of the neomycin sensitive patients were patch tested with gentamicin sulphate (20 per cent) and 17 (40 per cent) reacted.

3. *Kanamycin*. Neomycin and kanamycin have similar chemical structures and cross-react (Pirilä and Rouhunkoski, 1960; Epstein and Wenzel, 1963; Boonen and Waveren Hogervorst, 1964).

4. *Tobramycin*. In the United States, tobramycin is used in ophthalmic preparations; 20 neomycin sensitive patients were tested with tobramycin 20 per cent in petrolatum and 13 reacted (Schorr and Ridgway, 1977). In Helsinki, tobramycin was positive in 24.7 per cent of their neomycin sensitive patients (Forström and Pirilä, 1978).

5. *Streptomycin*. Cross-sensitivity between neomycin and streptomycin has been reported but the evidence, summarised by Epstein and Wenzel (1962), is conflicting.

6. *Bacitracin*. There is disagreement as to whether neomycin and bacitracin cross-react or whether sensitisation to each antibiotic occurs independently. In Finland, where patch test reactions to both antibiotics are frequent, Pirilä and Rouhunkoski (1960) thought that they do cross-react. In contrast, Epstein and Wenzel (1962, 1963) concluded, on the basis of animal experiments and clinical observation, that the sensitivities occur independently, a view supported by Boonen and Waveren Hogervorst (1964), and Binnick and Clendenning (1978).

7. *Cycloheximide (Actidione)*. A possible cross-reaction between neomycin and cycloheximide was reported in a man who used Neobacrin Ophthalmic Ointment and also came into contact with cycloheximide as a constituent of culture media. Patch tests: he reacted to neomycin 20 per cent and to cycloheximide 0.1 per cent and 0.01 per cent each in petrolatum (Black, 1971).

Cycloheximide (Actidione) is used in culture media and as an horticultural spray, particularly for roses and cherry trees.

Patch testing
Neomycin sulphate 20 per cent in petrolatum (the reaction may take 7 days to become positive).

NITROFURAZONE (5-nitro-2-furaldehyde semicarbazone; nitrofural; Furacin)

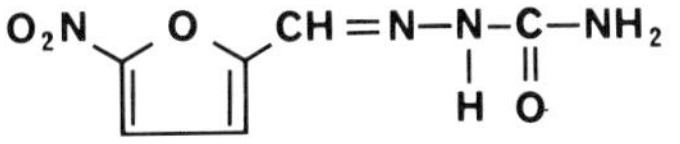

$$O_2N \quad O \quad CH=N-N-C-NH_2$$
$$\overset{|}{H} \quad \overset{\|}{O}$$

Nitrofurazone (Furacin) is an antibiotic used only topically; the concentration in most preparations is 0.2 per cent. (Nitrofurantoin, Furadantin, is a urinary antiseptic.)

Sensitising potential
In the human maximisation test Kligman (1966) used an induction concentration of 25 per cent in conjunction with sodium lauryl sulphate as adjuvant and sensitised 14 of 24 subjects, grading Furacin as a strong sensitiser (grade 4 on a 1–5 scale). In contrast, with the Draize procedure, using an induction and challenge concentration of 0.2 per cent (which is the concentration in topical preparations), Marzulli and Maibach (1973) sensitised only one of 93 subjects, suggesting that the reputation of Furacin as a potent sensitiser may be unwarranted. Although experimentally nitrofurazone may not be a potent allergen, clinical experience has shown it to produce intense sensitivity causing severe reactions.

Case reports
In Great Britain, Furacin is little used and cases of sensitisation have not been reported. In South Africa it is a popular remedy and many cases of sensitisation occur often with acute widespread eruptions requiring systemic steroids and admission to hospital. Patients with stasis eczema and ulcers or injury to the skin of the leg are particularly prone to sensitisation (Hull and Beer, 1977). In Heidelberg, 58 patients, many of whom had stasis eczema or ulcers, were sensitised by medicaments containing 0.2 per cent Furacin, and re-exposure to it had in some caused a generalised eczema (Braun and Schütz, 1968). Sensitisation has also been reported from Holland in 14 patients with leg ulcers (Bleumink, Lintum and Nater, 1974); each had a positive patch test to Furacin ointment containing 0.2 per cent nitrofurazone.

Nitrofurazone as an additive in animal feed sensitised a hog rancher in Denver, U.S.A. He reacted to a patch test with the feed but was not tested with nitrofurazone. By accident he was re-exposed to Furacin, when treating an infected pig, and he had an acute relapse (Neldner, 1972).

St John's
During the period 1971–1976 inclusive, 3 sensitised patients were seen:

Patient 1. A man aged 40 years applied only Furacin Soluble Ointment (Eaton Labs.) to his hypostatic ulcer and three weeks later he was admitted to hospital with a very severe widespread eczema, which was purpuric on his legs.

Patient 2. A man aged 65 years was prescribed Furacin ointment by a surgeon for a long standing ulcer on his sole. He developed swelling of the eyelids and a widespread eruption on the limbs and trunk which was still fluctuating six months later.

Patient 3. A 24-year-old man used Furacin ointment to treat his seborrhoeic eczema and a contact dermatitis from a nickel neck chain. He noticed no deterioration.

Patch tests

	Furacin ointment 0.2%	Other +
Patient 1	+++	Colophony, formalin, turps.
Patient 2	+++	Neomycin, TCP ointment
Patient 3	++	Nickel

Patch testing
Nitrofurazone 0.2 per cent in petrolatum.

PENICILLIN

Penicillin is a generic term for the whole group of natural and semi-synthetic penicillins; the largest source of penicillin is the mould — *notatum-chrysogenum* species of *Penicillium*. Penicillin G is a potent anti-microbial which in adequate concentrations is bactericidal: it is effective against many species of Gram-positive and Gram-negative cocci.

Sensitising potential
The potent allergenicity of topical penicillin was confirmed by Kligman (1966) with the human maximisation test in which 10 of 24 subjects were sensitised by penicillin G, giving it a grade 4 rating (on a 1–5 scale). In the guinea-pig maximisation test, penicillin G was graded as 5 because it sensitised all the test animals (Magnusson and Kligman, 1969).

Case reports
The first case of contact dermatitis reported was that of an Army medical officer in Chicago who, shortly after beginning to prepare and give injections of penicillin, developed an acute dermatitis first on his face and then on his hands. Patch tests with various penicillins were strongly positive (Pyle and Rattner, 1944).

The facility of topical penicillin to sensitise was realised during the 1939–1945 war when it was used in the treatment of war wounds; cases of contact dermatitis with positive patch tests to the relevant penicillin were reported by Michie and Bailie (1945) and Vickers (1946). In 1948, Brown wrote a comprehensive review of the then current literature on reactions to penicillin including many reports of contact dermatitis.

Penicillin in milk from cows treated for mastitis was thought to have caused dermatitis of the face, neck, hands and arms of a woman living on a farm; it was also blamed for a generalised eczema in a farmer. The woman had a previous history of dermatitis from penicillin; the man had not, but he had for two years used penicillin to treat his cows' mastitis. Both patients had positive patch tests, the woman reacting to penicillin 200 000 units per ml and the farmer to procaine penicillin 100 000 units per ml (Vickers, Bagratuni and Alexander, 1958).

Because of its strong sensitising potential the prescribing of topical penicillin has been largely abandoned but in Malaysia penicillin medicaments are available over the counter and penicillin is their most frequent cause of contact dermatitis from antibiotics (Nagreh, 1976).

AMPICILLIN

Ampicillin, a semisynthetic compound derived from 6-aminopenicillanic acid, is a broad-spectrum antibiotic.

Case report
In Hamburg, from 1967 to 1969 inclusive, 92 cases of occupational eczema occurred among members of the medical profession; sixty-one had an allergic contact dermatitis, principally from drugs. Ampicillin was the most frequent allergen, being the sensitiser in 24 of the cases, most of whom were nurses exposed occupationally. Patch tests: each reacted to ampicillin 5 per cent in water, and some to other penicillins. The lymphocyte transformation test was done in 16 of these cases and was positive in eight (Schülz, Schöpf and Wex, 1970).

POLYMYXIN B

Polymyxin B is used in the treatment of Gram-negative infections.

Case report
Sensitisation to polymyxin B sulphate has been reported (Möller, 1976) in patients with stasis ulcers and eczema treated with a Terramycin-Polymyxin B ointment. Patch tests: the patients reacted to polymyxin B 3 per cent in petrolatum. Polymyxin B may cross react with bacitracin (van Ketel, 1974).

Patch testing
Polymyxin B 3 per cent in petrolatum (Möller, 1976).

QUINOLINES

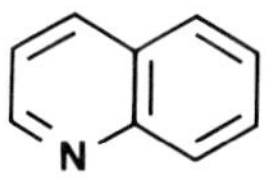

Quinoline (1-Benzazine)

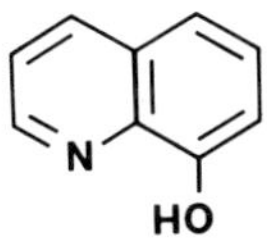

8-Hydroxyquinoline
(8-quinolinol; oxyquinoline)

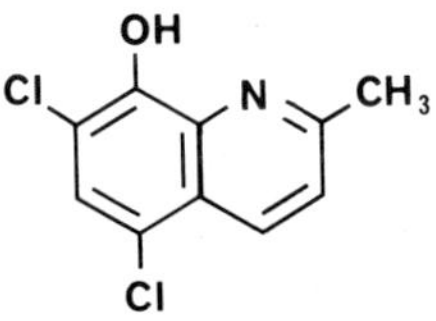

Chlorquinaldol (5,7-dichloro-
2-methyl-8-quinolinol;
Sterosan; Steroxin)

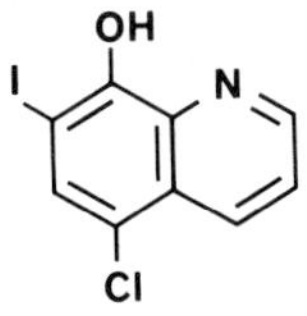

Iodochlorhydroxyquin (5-chloro-7-iodo-
8-quinolinol; Chinoform; clioquinol;
Entero-Vioform; Vioform)

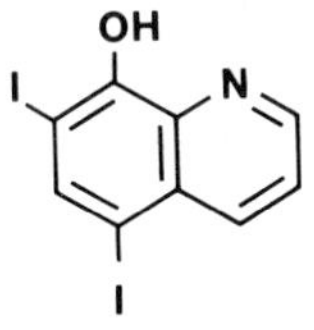

Diiodohydroxyquin (5,7-diiodo-
8-quinolinol; Diodoquin)

Halquinol (Quinolor; Quixalin; Quixalad) is a mixture of these three.

5,7-Dichloro-8-quinolinol
57-74 wt per cent (Chloroxine)

5-Chloro-8-quinolinol
23-40 wt per cent (Dermofongin A)

7-Chloro-8-quinolinol
3 wt per cent

Hydroxyquinolines are widely used topical antibacterial compounds; they are usually formulated in a concentration of 3 per cent, often in combination with a steroid. It has been estimated that 3–4 per cent of Vioform applied topically is absorbed and most is excreted as conjugated metabolites in the urine (Fischer and Hartvig, 1977).

Entero-Vioform and Diodoquin are also given systemically.

Sensitising potential

Experimentally, Vioform has been shown to be a weak allergen. In the human maximisation test Vioform 25 per cent with sodium lauryl sulphate as adjuvant failed to sensitise any of 23 subjects (Kligman, 1966). The maximisation test in guinea-pigs sensitised five of 25 animals (Magnusson and Kligman, 1969).

Incidence of sensitivity

Hydroxyquinolines sensitise, but infrequently. Vioform has been included in several large patch test series and low incidences of sensitisation were recorded; similar results were obtained with Sterosan.

Series	Allergen	Conc. %	Tested	+ %	Report
Scandinavia	Vioform + Sterosan	3	5251	2.4	Magnusson et al., 1968
Europe	Vioform	5	4825	1.7	Fregert et al., 1969
Spain	Sterosan	3	987	1.3	Garcia-Perez and Moran, 1975
Warsaw	Vioform	3	877	1.3	Rudzki and Kleniewska, 1970
Auckland	Vioform	?	214	3.7	Black, 1972

In Germany, patients with stasis ulcers and eczema become sensitised to Vioform, and a 3.1 per cent incidence has been reported in their patients. Sterosan is used in Germany as an antifungal medicament and 1 per cent of 4000 patients reacted to it (Breit and Bandmann, 1973).

St John's

Iodochlorhydroxyquin (Vioform) 5 per cent in petrolatum is included in the routine patch test series applied to every patient. From 1971 to 1976 inclusive, the sensitisation rate has been 1.2–2 per cent; approximately 2 per cent of the men and 1 per cent of the women are sensitised each year (Table 6.6).

Clinical features

Sensitivity to hydroxyquinolines is likely to be missed unless they are included

Table 6.6. Yearly incidence of vioform sensitivity (St John's 1971–1976).

	Total			Males			Females		
	+ Vioform	Tested	%	+ Vioform	Tested	%	+ Vioform	Tested	%
1971	31	1558	?	19	707	2.7	12	851	1.4
1972	30	1606	1.9	16	738	2.2	14	868	1.6
1973	24	1546	1.6	19	710	2.7	5	836	0.6
1974	23	1433	1.6	15	655	2.3	8	778	1.0
1975	24	1858	1.3	12	887	1.4	12	971	1.2
1976	24	1982	1.2	13	937	1.4	11	1045	1.1

in a standard patch test series. This is because they are relatively weak allergens, and sensitivity usually does not cause a dramatic exacerbation of an eczema. In addition the presence in the formulation of a steroid, which is often fluorinated, partially suppresses the irritation and inflammation.

St John's

From 1971 to 1976 inclusive a total of 156 patients sensitive to Vioform were seen; the majority (101) reacted to Vioform only, but 55 reacted also to another medicament, or to wool alcohols, parabens, chlorocresol or ethylenediamine (Table 6.7).

Table 6.7. Sensitisation to Vioform alone or associated with another medicament allergen (St John's 1971–1976).

	Vioform only		Vioform + another Medicament or Base	
	Males	Females	Males	Females
	66/94	35/62	28/94	27/62
Total	101/156 (65%)		55/156 (35%)	

Patterns of eczema

In these 156 patients there seemed to be no particular pattern of eczema that predisposed to Vioform sensitivity (Table 6.8). That the majority had hand eczema is due to the large number of such patients attending this clinic. Like neomycin sensitivity the allergy was no more frequent if the eczema had spread beyond the hands.

Table 6.8. Patterns of eczema in 156 patients sensitive to Vioform (St John's, 1971–1976).

	Males	Females
Hands only	15	10
Hands + elsewhere	19	7
Face	4	9
Stasis	6	10
Otitis externa	1	5
Pruritus ani	9	1
Atopic	0	2
Discoid	5	0
Widespread	5	3
Other sites	30	15
Total	94	62

Oral provocation

A deliberate oral provocation with clioquinol (Vioform) or chlorquinaldol (Sterosan) produced a generalised eruption in six of nine quinoline-sensitive patients (Ekelund and Möller, 1969). Entero-Vioform caused a similar eruption in a patient allergic to Vioform (Skog, 1975). One tablet of Diodoquin containing 210 mg of 5, 7-diiodo-8-hydroxyquinoline given to a Vioform-sensitive man elicited, within 12 hours, a severe relapse of his eczema (Leifer and Steiner, 1951).

St John's

In 1974 and 1975, two women experienced a generalised eruption after taking Entero-Vioform. One had hand eczema and although she had treated it with a fluorinated steroid preparation containing Vioform without discomfort, she took one tablet of Entero-Vioform, and developed an acute rash which lasted for 5 days. The other patient had rosacea and developed a severe reaction from a Vioform-hydrocortisone ointment. She recalled having had a generalised eruption while taking Entero-Vioform 8 years previously, but the sensitising application was not known. Patch tests: both patients reacted to Vioform 5 per cent in petrolatum.

Cross-sensitivity

Cross-reactions were studied by Leifer and Steiner (1951) in three patients — two sensitised by Vioform, the other by Diodoquin. Patch tests: each patient reacted to Vioform, Diodoquin, Quinolor and Sterosan. The conclusion was that for reactivity both the substituted quinoline and the hydroxyl group are essential but that the halogen substitutions are not important. It was postulated that halogenated hydroxyquinolines are degraded to carboxylated pyridines forming the antigenic complex.

A wide spectrum of cross-reactions was also reported by Allenby (1965) in three patients with stasis ulcers or eczema who reacted adversely to Remiderm containing halquinol. Each was thought to have been pre-sensitised by Vioform, which all had used previously. Patch tests: each reacted to halquinol and to other halogenated hydroxyquinolines. Cross-sensitivity between Vioform and Sterosan is said to be uncommon (Hjorth and Fregert, 1972).

A woman, known to react to ingested quinine, applied Nystaform HC cream (nystatin, iodochlorhydroxyquinoline (Vioform) 3 per cent and hydrocortisone 0.5 per cent) to her submammary intertrigo. Twelve hours after the first application she developed a generalised erythema and within hours had bronchospasm which required intravenous and oral steroids (Simpson, 1974). A quinoline ring is common to both quinine and Vioform.

Irritancy

Creams containing 3 per cent clioquinol may cause irritation and in Helsinki the ratio of allergic to irritant dermatitis was one to five. Irritancy depended upon the concentration of clioquinol and not its crystal size (Kero, Hannuksela and Sothman, 1979).

Patch testing

Iodochlorhydroxyquin (Vioform) 5 per cent in petrolatum
Chlorquinaldol (Sterosan)   5 per cent in petrolatum
Other quinolines   5 per cent in petrolatum.

QUINODERM

Quinoderm (Quinoderm Co.) is an acne preparation containing potassium hydroxyquinoline sulphate 0.5 per cent and benzoyl peroxide 10 per cent. Adverse reactions to it are usually an irritant effect but very occasionally it sensitises. Patch tests with Quinoderm are difficult to interpret because of its irritancy.

The sensitising potential of benzoyl peroxide was investigated by Poole, Griffiths and MacMillan (1970) using repeated insult patch tests on 69 human subjects. The induction was with 10 per cent benzoyl peroxide and 1 per cent sulphur in polyethylene glycol and the challenge was with 10 per cent benzoyl peroxide in the same base. Clinically it was thought that 40 per cent of the 69 subjects were sensitised but in only 10 was this verified by a challenge patch test; benzoyl peroxide 10 per cent in polyethylene glycol did not appear to be an irritant.

St John's

Three young women have been investigated in whom the patch test results suggested that the benzoyl peroxide in Quinoderm had sensitised them. Each reacted to Quinoderm and benzoyl peroxide (two to 5 per cent and one to 1 per cent in petrolatum) but not to potassium hydroxyquinoline sulphate 1 per cent in petrolatum, or to other ingredients of the base.

As benzoyl peroxide is an irritant, it is impossible to be absolutely certain of the validity of these reactions, but the response to 1 per cent was thought definitely to be significant.

Patch testing

Benzoyl peroxide 1 per cent and 5 per cent in petrolatum
Potassium hydroxyquinoline 1 per cent in petrolatum
Quinoderm (gives irritant reactions).

STREPTOMYCIN

Streptomycin is produced by the Actinomycete *Streptomyces griseus*. In high concentrations it is bactericidal and in low concentrations bacteriostatic. Its greatest application is in the treatment of tuberculosis.

Sensitising potential

So great is the sensitising capacity of streptomycin when applied to the skin that it has no place in topical medication. In the human maximisation test with an induction concentration of 25 per cent and a challenge concentration of 10 per cent Kligman (1966) sensitised 20 of 25 subjects grading it as a strong sensitiser (grade 4 on a 1–5 scale). In the guinea-pig maximisation test, too, it was a strong (grade 4) allergen.

In 1949, Marcussen showed the incidence of sensitisation among nurses to be correlated with their degree of exposure. One sensitised nurse gave herself a hormone injection with a streptomycin syringe and provoked a severe relapse at sites of a past dermatitis and a previously positive patch test.

Case reports (nurses)

Contact dermatitis among nurses giving streptomycin to patients with tuber-culosis was first reported by Strauss and Warring (1947a). Four of twelve nurses in a sanatorium developed dermatitis of their hands and eyelids and each had a positive patch test to 2 per cent streptomycin (Strauss and Warring, 1947b). In a study of 18 sensitised nurses, Wilson (1958) confirmed that the hands, arms and eyelids were most frequently affected; 17 had positive patch tests to strep-tomycin 5 per cent in water and one reacted only to an intradermal injection. He found that on wards where gloves and masks were worn for giving injections nurses escaped sensitisation, whereas on other wards where nurses were not so protected dermatitis occurred.

St John's

From 1971 to 1976 inclusive, two women seen had been sensitised by streptomycin in the past. One, aged 25 years, had, when 5 years old, played with bottles contain-ing streptomycin and developed a rash. The other, aged 36 years, had worked for a pharmaceutical firm when 17 years of age and had been sensitised to streptomycin. Patch tests: both patients reacted to streptomycin 1 per cent in petrolatum.

Patch testing

Streptomycin 1 per cent in petrolatum.

SULPHONAMIDES

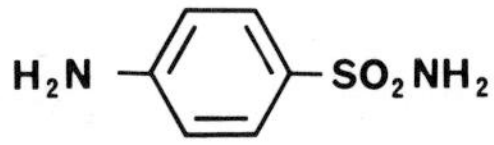

Sulphanilamide (sulfanilamide; *p*-amino-benzenesulfonamide)

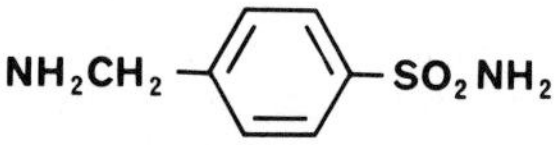

4-Homosulfanilamide (α-amino-*p*-toluenesulfonamide; mafenide; maphenide; Marfanil; Sulfamylon)

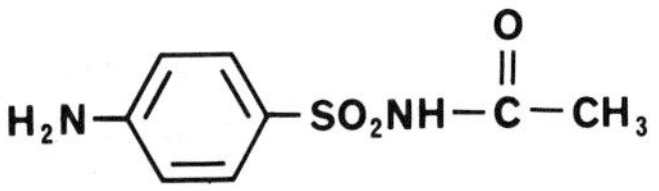

N'-Acetylsulphanilamide (Sulfacetamide; sulphacetamide; Albucid)

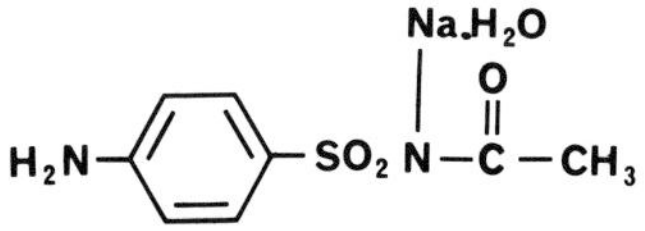

N'-Acetylsulphanilamide sodium (Albucid Soluble)

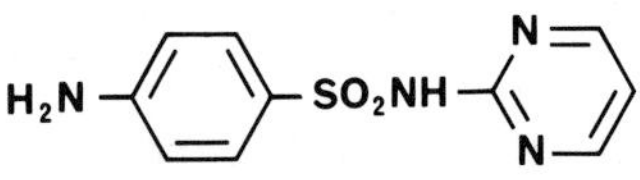

Sulphadiazine (sulfadiazine; 2-sulfanil-amidopyrimidine)

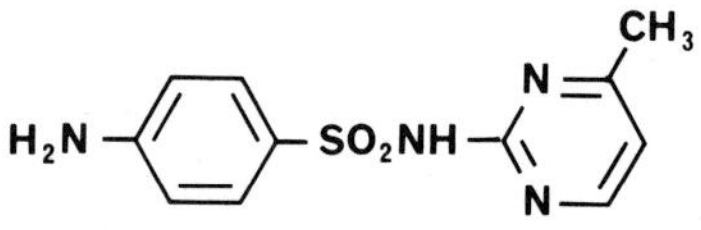

Sulphamerazine (sulfamerazine; *N'*-(4-methyl-2-pyrimidyl) sulfanilamide)

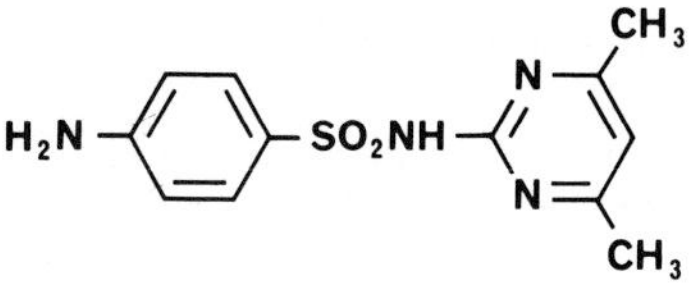

Sulphamethazine (sulfadimidine; sulfamethazine; *N'*-(4,6-dimethyl-2-pyrimidinyl)sulfanilamide)

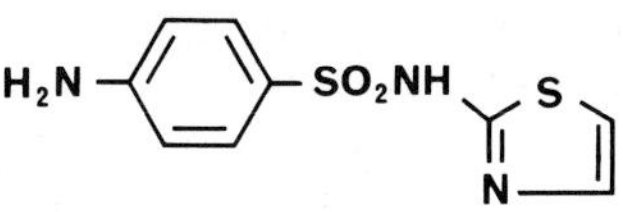

Sulphathiazole (sulfathiazole; *N'*-2-thiazolylsulfanilamide)

Sulphonamides are antibacterial compounds; applied topically they are notorious sensitisers.

Sensitising potential
In the human maximisation test, Kligman (1966) used sulphathiazole 25 per cent and sensitised only one of 15 subjects, and with sulphanilamide 25 per cent he sensitised five of 25 subjects. This low incidence of sensitisation (grade 1 and 2 respectively on a 1–5 scale) does not accord with clinical experience, but in the guinea-pig maximisation test sulphathiazole sensitised nine of 25 animals (grade 3). Marfanil was also used on the guinea-pigs and all 20 tested were sentised (grade 5) (Magnusson and Kligman, 1969). Marfanil (mafenide) was assessed by the Draize procedure on human subjects and an induction concentration of 5 per cent sensitised two of 93 (2 per cent) and an induction concentration of 20 per cent sensitised eighteen of 108 (16 per cent) (Marzulli and Maibach, 1973).

Incidence of sensitivity
The incidence of sensitisation will be a direct reflection of the use of topical sulphonamides in a community. In Germany and Italy they are frequently used and often sensitise; in Great Britain, apart from eye preparations, their topical use is minimal and cases of dermatitis are rarely seen.

In a series reported from Munich (Bandmann and Breit, 1974), 6.4 per cent of the men and 5.4 per cent of the women had positive patch tests to 10 per cent mafenide (4-homosulfanilamide), a popular antibiotic in Germany. In contrast, when sulphanilamide 5 per cent was included in a patch test series in Warsaw only 0.8 per cent of 621 patients were found to be sensitive (Rudzki and Kleniewska, 1970).

Case reports
Mafenide acetate 11.2 per cent in a cream base was found to be effective in controlling sepsis in patients with burns (Yaffee and Dressler, 1969). Four hundred patients treated with mafenide were studied and, though the incidence of skin complications was 9.5 per cent, none of the 11 patients patch tested with mafenide acetate 11.2 per cent in a cream base had reacted by the final two-day reading. The efficacy of mafenide in the treatment of burns was confirmed by Velasco and Africk (1971), but they described three patients who developed an eruption at the site of application, or more widely, during the treatment. Patch tests: all these reacted to mafenide acetate 8.5 per cent and to mafenide hydrochloride 5 per cent, but none reacted to sulphanilamide 8.5 per cent or to a mixture containing sulphadiazine, sulphamerazine and sulphamethazine.

St John's
Patients are tested with sulphonamides only if there is a relevant history. From 1971 to 1976, two women and one man were found to be sensitised; both women by eye drops containing 10 per cent sulphacetamide and the man from past use of a sulphanilamide preparation. Patch tests: each reacted to the relevant sulphonamide, but only one of the three to para-phenylenediamine.

A photosensitive patient reacted to sulphapyridine but no relevance was found for the response (p. 443).

Cross-reactions

Sulphonamides sometimes, but not always, cross-react one with another or with other amino compounds such as *p*-phenylenediamine.

Patch testing

No one sulphonamide will detect sensitivity to the whole group: the suspected sulphonamide must be used for patch testing.

Appropriate sulphonamide 5 per cent in petrolatum.

TETRACYCLINES

Contact dermatitis from the tetracyclines is rare; the relevant literature was reviewed by Dohn (1960).

CHLORTETRACYCLINE (Aureomycin; Biomycin)

St John's

Two cases of sensitisation have been seen. The first (Calnan, 1967) was a woman who had used Aureomycin ointment on a dermabraded tattoo and developed dermatitis. In the second patient an Aureomycin ointment had been used to treat her varicose ulcers. Patch tests: the first patient reacted to the Aureomycin ointment, chlortetracycline and demethylchlortetracycline, but there was no response to oxytetracycline, tetracycline and cymecycline (Calnan 1967). The second patient reacted to Aureomycin 0.5 per cent (in petrolatum).

Patch testing

Chlortetracycline 3 per cent in petrolatum.

OXYTETRACYCLINE (Terramycin)

4-(Dimethylamino)-1,4,4a,5,5a,6,11,12a-octa-hydro-3,5,6,10,12,12a-hexahydroxy-6-methyl-1,11-dioxo-2-naphthacenecarboxamide

Case reports

Nine patients sensitised by oxytetracycline, applied as a Terramycin-Polymyxin B ointment in the treatment of chronic stasis ulcers and eczema, have been reported by Bojs and Möller (1974), and Möller (1976). Patch tests: the first three patients reported were tested with a series of tetracyclines, 3.5 per cent in petrolatum; each one reacted to oxytetracycline, and two reacted also to tetracycline and methacycline. In addition they all had reactions to undiluted Polymyxin B sulphate, but it was then uncertain whether these were an irritant or an allergic effect (Bojs and Möller, 1974). The next six patients reacted to oxytetracycline, and to polymyxin B, both 3 per cent in petrolatum; these results confirmed polymyxin as an allergen (Möller, 1976).

St John's

In 1971, two women with leg ulcers were found to be sensitive to oxytetracycline. One, aged 43 years, had had hypostatic ulcers for 5 years and among other medicaments had used a spray containing oxytetracycline. The other was 59 years old and had had hypostatic ulcers for 24 years; an oxytetracycline ointment was one of many applications she had used. Both patients had had generalised eruptions but in neither was it associated with the use of the oxytetracycline preparation. Patch tests: Patient 1 reacted to the Terramycin-hydrocortisone spray she used, to oxytetracycline 5 per cent, neomycin 20 per cent and Soframycin 10 per cent, but not to chlortetracycline 3 per cent (Aureomycin ointment).

Patient 2 reacted to oxytetracycline 1 per cent, neomycin 20 per cent, soframycin 10 per cent, lanolin and parabens. Tests with the Terramycin-hydrocortisone ointment she had used, chlortetracycline 1 per cent (Aureomycin) and tetracycline 1 per cent (Achromycin) were negative.

Patch testing

Oxytetracycline 3 per cent in petrolatum.

TROMANTADINE HYDROCHLORIDE (*N*-2-Dimethylaminoethoxy-acetyl-aminoadamanto hydrochloride; Viru-Merz ointment)

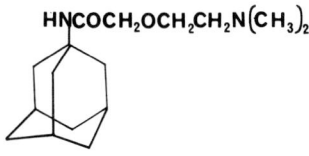

Tromantadine hydrochloride is a synthetic antiviral compound used topically in the treatment of herpes simplex.

Case report

A series of 240 patients with herpes simplex was treated with tromantadine hydrochloride 1 per cent in a gel base, and 20 developed local irritation. Patch tests with the preparation elicited a response in 12 of the 20 patients confirming their sensitisation. In the other eight patients the local reaction was considered irritant (Fanta and Mischer, 1976).

Patch testing
Tromantadine hydrochloride 1 per cent ? base.

VIRGINIAMYCIN (Staphylomycin; Stapolidex)

Virginiamycin and Pristinamycin are produced by strains of *Streptomyces* and belong to the streptogramin group of antibiotics. Chemically they have a macrocyclic peptide structure and each consists of a major fraction (a macrocyclic lactone) and a minor component (a depsipeptide).

The sensitiser
Virginiamycin consists of 2 factors, M and S, and so far all the patients sensitised by medicaments have reacted to the M fraction, and not to the S component.

One subject sensitised experimentally by virginiamycin reacted on subsequent patch testing to both the M and S fractions, each 5 per cent in petrolatum. An oral dose of virginiamycin caused quite a severe eruption (Lachapelle and Lamy, 1973).

Case reports
In some countries virginiamycin is available as a topical antibiotic. It has been used for burns, flexural dermatitis and impetigo, and cases of sensitivity have been reported from the Netherlands (Bleumink and Nater, 1972 a, b) and Belgium (Lachapelle and Lamy, 1973; Baes, 1974).

As an animal food additive it has caused dermatitis in Belgium (p. 188).

Patch testing
Various concentrations have been used for patch testing: Baes (1974) used virginiamycin and the M and S fractions each 1 per cent in petrolatum and obtained positive reactions in eight patients. However, Bleumink and Nater (1972 b) found the 0.5 per cent and 2 per cent concentrations present in Staphylomycin ointment and powder, respectively, to be too low for patch testing, giving false negative reactions. They recommended that a concentration of 5–10 per cent be used for the whole antibiotic, and for the M and S fractions.

PRISTINAMYCIN (Pyostacin)

Pristinamycin, like virginiamycin, contains two fractions (Ia and IIa). Chemically both antibiotics are very closely related, and all patients sensitised by virginiamycin have reacted to pristinamycin. This is not a cross-reaction but due to the fact that factor M of virginiamycin and factor IIa of pristinamycin are identical (Baes, 1974).

Case report
A man sensitised by virginiamycin in a topical preparation took one tablet of pristinamycin (250 mg) and 4 hours later had an anaphylactic reaction with stupor, urticaria and vomiting. Patch tests with virginiamycin, pristinamycin,

factors M and IIa, each 1 per cent in petrolatum, were all positive. He developed transient oedema of his eyes and lips, and weals adjacent to a positive patch test (Baes, 1974).

Patch testing

Virginiamycin	5 per cent in petrolatum
Factor M	5 per cent in petrolatum
Factor S	5 per cent in petrolatum
Pristinamycin	5 per cent in petrolatum
Factor 11a	5 per cent in petrolatum
Factor 1a	5 per cent in petrolatum.

Antifungal and anticandidal compounds

CHLORPHENESIN (3-(*p*-Chlorophenoxy)-1,2-propanediol; Mycil)

$$Cl \!-\!\!\langle \bigcirc \rangle\!\!-\! OCH_2 \overset{\overset{\displaystyle OH}{\displaystyle |}}{C}HCH_2OH$$

St John's
Two patients have been seen who were sensitised to chlorphenesin. The first, a woman aged 22 years, treated the macerated toe webs of her right foot with several antifungal applications, including Mycil ointment (Duncan Flockhart) containing chlorphenesin 0.5 per cent. After 8 weeks, the foot became swollen and bullous and later the other foot was affected. Her hands were itchy but no rash appeared. The second patient, a man aged 21 years, also used several antifungal preparations on his feet including a Mycil powder containing 1 per cent chlorphenesin: he developed eczema of the feet which spread to his hands. Patch tests: both patients reacted to their Mycil preparations and chlorphenesin 1 per cent in petrolatum; neither reacted to other anti-fungal medicaments.

Patch testing
Chlorphenesin 1 per cent and 0.5 per cent in petrolatum.

CLOTRIMAZOLE (diphenyl-2-chlorophenyl-1-imidazolyl-methane; canesten).

Case report
A man with pruritus ani, who was sensitised to clotrimazole in Canesten creame had positive patch tests to the cream and to clotrimazole one per cent in methyl ethyl ketone (Roller, 1978).

Patch testing
Clotrimazole 1 per cent in methyl ethyl ketone.

DIBENZTHIONE (3,5-Dibenzyltetrahydro-2H-1,3,5-thiadiazine-2-thione; sulbentine; Fungiplex)

Dibenzthione is a topical antifungal compound used also in deodorants.

Case reports
Sensitivity to dibenzthione and cross-reactivity with thiadiazine and triazine compounds were first reported by Behrhohm and Zschunke (1965) from Germany. Ten years later it was reported that two patients in Sweden had been sensitised by Fungiplex (Liden and Göransson, 1975). Patch Tests: both patients reacted to dibenzthione 3 per cent in petrolatum, whereas 17 controls did not.

Patch testing
Dibenzthione ?1-3 per cent in petrolatum.

HALOPROGIN (3-Iodoprop-2-ynyl 2,4,5-trichlorophenyl ether; Halotax).

Haloprogin, a topical antimicrobial agent, is effective against dermatophytes, yeasts and bacteria; it is a rare sensitiser.

Case report
One case of allergic contact dermatitis has been described by Rudolph (1975). The patient applied a 1 per cent haloprogin cream to a fungus infection and after one week she developed a local reaction. Patch tests: she reacted to 1 per cent, but not to 0.1 per cent, haloprogin in petrolatum.

Ethyl sebacate, a solubiliser in both the cream and lotion formulations of haloprogin, has caused contact dermatitis (Moss, 1974; Berlin and Miller, 1976).

Patch testing
Haloprogin 1 per cent in petrolatum.

MESULPHEN (2,7-Dimethylthianthrene; mesulfene; tineafax)

Mesulphen, a fungicide and scabicide, is a component of the antifungal oint-ment Tineafax (Burroughs Wellcome & Co.). It sensitises very occasionally.

Case reports
In Amsterdam, six patients with dermatitis of the feet were sensitised by mesul-phen in Tineafax ointment (van Ketel, 1967). Patch tests: all reacted to Tineafax ointment and to mesulphen 8 per cent in petrolatum, this being the concentration in Tineafax. The case of a man similarly sensitised by Tineafax ointment was reported by Connor (1973) from London. Patch tests: Tineafax ointment and mesulphen 8 per cent and 1 per cent in petrolatum gave positive tests, whereas those with each constituent of the base were negative.

St John's
Two patients were seen between 1971 and 1976 inclusive. One was a woman who in 1971 had applied Tineafax among other medicaments to a burn on her leg and developed eczema of the area which spread to other sites. The other, reported by Calnan (1972), used Tineafax for a supposed fungal infection of his feet and noticed that the condition was aggravated. Patch tests: both patients reacted to Tineafax and mesulphen 5 per cent in petrolatum.

Patch testing
Mesulphen 5 per cent in petrolatum.
(Tineafax is sometimes a mild irritant.)

MICONAZOLE NITRATE (1-[2,4-Dichloro-β-(2,4-dichlorobenzyloxy)-phenethyl] imidazole nitrate; Daktarin)

Miconazole nitrate is an antimycotic and is formulated as a 2 per cent cream and powder (Daktarin).

Case reports
Three cases of sensitivity have been reported. The first patient, a woman in Holland, used Daktarin cream for her tinea pedis and after 6 weeks developed dermatitis (van Ketel, 1974). Patch tests: she reacted to Daktarin cream and powder (both contain 2 per cent miconazole nitrate) and to miconazole nitrate 2

per cent in petrolatum and in water. Patch tests with the following imidazole compounds were negative: mebendazole, tinidazole and metronidazole, each 2 per cent and 10 per cent in petrolatum and in water; tests with histamine and pilocarpine 2 per cent in water also were negative.

In the second case, a woman in Belgium developed an extensive vesicular eczema after repeated application of Daktarin cream. Patch tests: she reacted to miconazole cream and to miconazole 2 per cent in petrolatum (Degreef and Verhoeve, 1975).

The third patient applied Daktarin gel to her hand; she was sensitised and developed a disseminated dermatitis (Samsoen and Jelen, 1977).

Patch testing
Miconazole nitrate 2 per cent in petrolatum
(Daktarin cream can be mildly irritant.)

PECILOCIN (N-(8'-hydroxy-6'-methyl-*trans-trans-cis*-dodeca-2',4',6'-trienoyl)-2-pyrrolidone; Variotin)

Pecilocin is an antifungal antibiotic derived from *Paecilomyces varioti Bainier* var. *antibioticus*.

Case reports
A series of 44 patients who had been treated with pecilocin (Variotin) were patch tested with it by Nørgaard (1977). Seven reacted but in only three was there a history of aggravation by the medicament. Contact dermatitis has also been described by Sundararajan (1970); his patient reacted strongly to a patch test with pecilocin 3000 units/g and none of 12 controls reacted. Another man who developed an acute eczema after applying Variotin ointment to an axillary fungus infection was reported by Groen, Bleumink and Nater (1974). Patch tests: he reacted to Variotin ointment and pecilocin 50 per cent and 10 per cent in petrolatum, but he gave no reaction to the 2 per cent concentration.

St John's
For four months a man used Variotin ointment to treat a fungal infection of his feet. After an initial improvement the condition deteriorated and he developed eczema over both feet which spread to his hands. Patch tests: he reacted to Variotin, and to pecilocin 1 per cent and 0.5 per cent but not to 0.1 per cent.
Fifty controls were patch tested with pecilocin 1 per cent in petrolatum and none reacted.

Patch testing
Pecilocin 1 per cent in petrolatum.
(Variotin ointment is mildly irritant.)

PYRROLNITRIN (Micturin)

Pyrrolnitrin inhibits the growth of fungi, is less active against yeasts and Gram-positive bacteria, and has no effect on Gram-negative organisms.

Case reports
Sensitisation caused an acute dermatitis in two patients who used Micturin cream for an inguinal dermatitis. Patch tests: both patients reacted strongly to the cream and to pyrrolnitrin 1 per cent in petrolatum, and had no response to the other components of the cream. One had a cross-reaction to chlorodinitrobenze (Meneghini and Angelini, 1975).

Patch testing
Pyrrolnitrin 1 per cent in petrolatum (Meneghini and Angelini, 1975).

TOLNAFTATE (*m,N*-dimethylthiocarbanilic acid *0*-2-naphthyl ester; Tinactin; Tinaderm; Tonoftal)

Tolnaftate 1 per cent as a lotion or in a cream base is widely used as an antimycotic, but sensitisation is very rare.

Case reports
Two cases of sensitisation have been reported from the U.S.A. (Gellin, Maibach and Wachs, 1972; Emmett and Mars, 1973). The first patient used a 1 per cent solution of tolnaftate for intertrigo of his groins, and the second used a 1 per cent tolnaftate cream for dermatitis of his foot. Patch tests: both patients reacted to their Tinactin preparation and to tolnaftate 1 per cent and 0.1 per cent in petrolatum; the first patient also reacted to tolnaftate diluted to 0.05 per cent and 0.01 per cent.

Another patient, described by Bowyer (1972), used Tinaderm for a fungal infection and a few days later developed an acute dermatitis while using it as a face cream. She had a positive patch test to the cream but was not tested separately with tolnaftate.

Patch testing
Tolnaftate 1 per cent and 0.1 per cent in petrolatum.

Monoamylamine
A woman who had used tolnaftate cream on her leg eczema was patch tested with the cream and its constituents. She reacted strongly to the tolnaftate (?concentration) and developed a weal under undiluted monoamylamine applied to her back. The weal subsided within 2 days. Similar tests in three controls were negative (Tharp, 1973).

CHLORDANTOIN ((5-(1-ethylpentyl)-3-(trichloromethylthio)hydantoin; clodantoin; Sporostacin)

$$CH_3(CH_2)_3CH—N—C=O$$

Chlordantoin as a 1 per cent cream is used to treat candidiasis of the vagina.

Case report
Two women were sensitised while using chlordantoin cream to treat their vaginitis. The first had used a variety of medicaments for many months but the second had used the cream for only 2 weeks. Patch tests: both patients reacted to the 1 per cent chlordantoin cream but not to the cream base; neither was tested with chlordantoin alone (Epstein, 1966).

Patch testing
Chlordantoin 1 per cent in ?petrolatum.

NYSTATIN

Nystatin is an antibiotic derived from cultures of *Streptomyces noursei*. It is active against fungi and yeasts and is used principally for the treatment of candidiasis of the skin and mucous membranes. Formulations generally contain 100 000 i.u. per g or ml.

Case reports
The first reported case of sensitisation (Wasilewski, 1970) was in a woman who developed pruritus vulvae after her husband had used Mycolog cream★; she

*Mycolog cream contains nystatin, neomycin, gramicidin, triamcinolone acetonide and ethylenediamine.

applied Nystaform-HC ointment** which exacerbated her symptoms. Patch tests: she reacted to Nystatin 100 000 i.u./ml in 70 per cent ethanol, to ethylenediamine 1 per cent in petrolatum, to Mycolog cream and to Nystaform-HC ointment.

Coskey (1971, a,b) described three further patients (2 men and one girl). One man had pruritus ani and the other intertrigo of his groins; both had used Mycolog cream. The girl had used nystatin vaginal pessaries. Patch tests: each reacted to nystatin 100 000 units in 1 g of Velvachol.

A further case was in a boy aged 3 years, sensitised by Mycolog ointment (Foussereau et al., 1971). Patch tests: he reacted to nystatin ointment (100 000 units per g) and to Mycolog ointment.

St John's

Patients are patch tested with nystatin or nystatin-containing medicaments only if indicated by the history. From 1971 to 1976 inclusive, three men and two women were found to be sensitive, the three men had used the medicament for eczema of the genitalia, pruritus ani and intertrigo of the groins, one woman had applied it to her hand eczema and the other to her stasis ulcer. Patch tests: each patient reacted to nystatin 100 000–350 000 i.u./g in plastibase or petrolatum.

The woman with hand eczema had noticed that it was exacerbated by a nystatin ointment. Subsequently she was given nystatin orally and after 4 days developed a generalised eruption; her mouth was unaffected.

Patch testing
Nystatin 100 000 i.u./g in petrolatum.

Antihistamines

The structural core of many antihistamines is a substituted ethylamine: $-CH_2CH_2N =$; most have the following skeletal structural formula:

There are 5 principal groups of antihistamines (Douglas, 1970).

HISTAMINE

**Nystaform-HC ointment contains nystatin, iodochlorhydroxyquin and hydrocortisone.

ETHANOLAMINES

e.g. Diphenhydramine, its hydrochloride (Benadryl) and its 8-chloro-theophyllinate (dimenhydrinate; Dramamine)

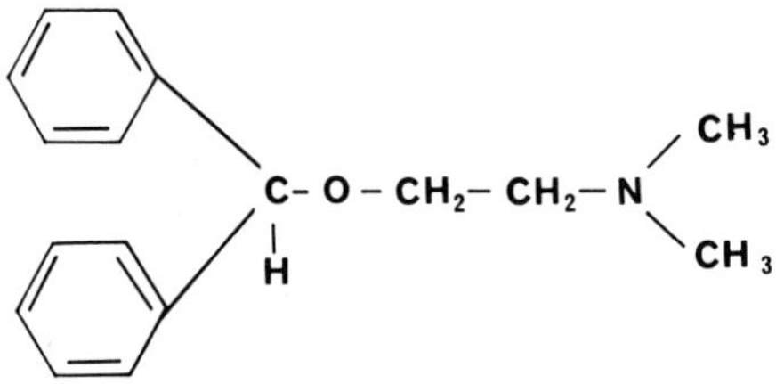

Diphenhydramine

ETHYLENEDIAMINES

e.g. Pyrilamine (mepyramine) and its maleate (Anthisan), antazoline and its hydrochloride (Antistin; Histostab)

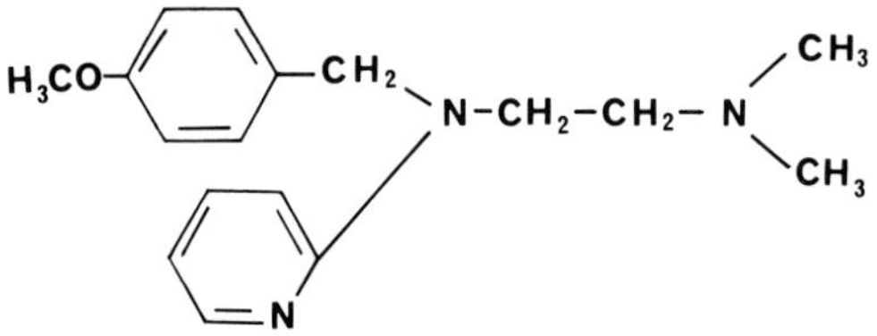

Pyrilamine

ALKYLAMINES

e.g. Chlorpheniramine and its maleate (Piriton); pheniramine; its aminosalicylate (Daneral) and its maleate (Trimeton)
Brompheniramine and its maleate (Dimotane)

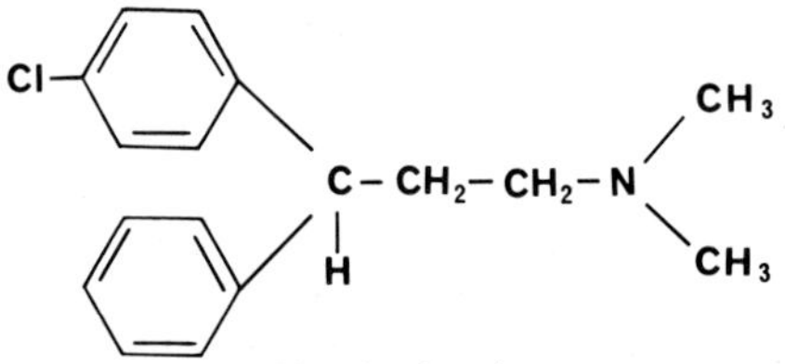

Chlorpheniramine

PIPERAZINES

e.g. Chlorcyclizine and its hydrochloride (Histantin). Cyclizine and its hydrochloride (Marezine)

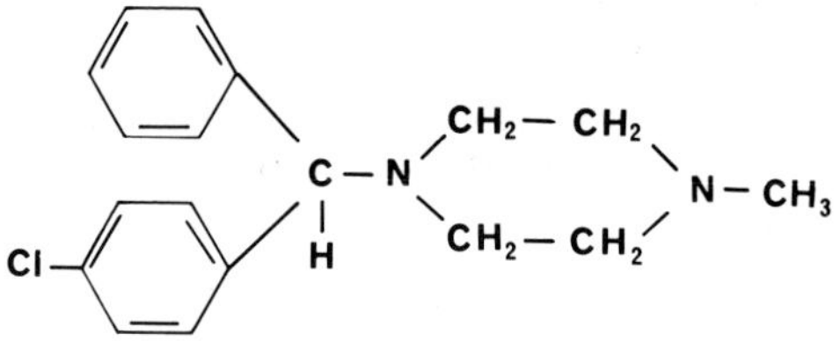

Chlorcyclizine

PHENOTHIAZINES

e.g. Promethazine and its hydrochloride (Phenergan); trimeprazine and its tartrate (Vallergan)

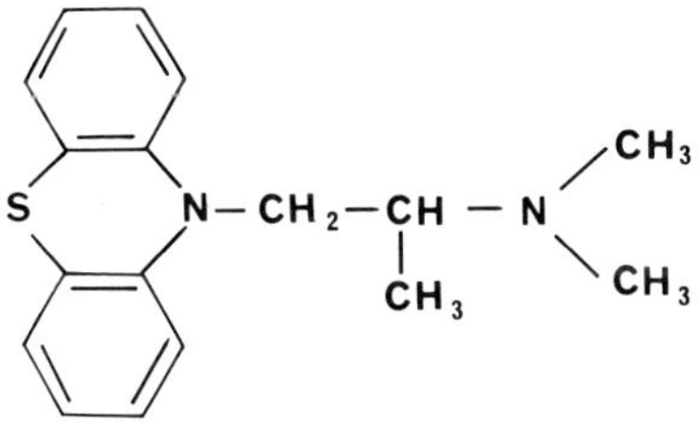

Promethazine

ANTAZOLINE (2-(*N*-Benzylanilinomethyl)-2-imidazoline; Antistin; Histostab; Antasten)

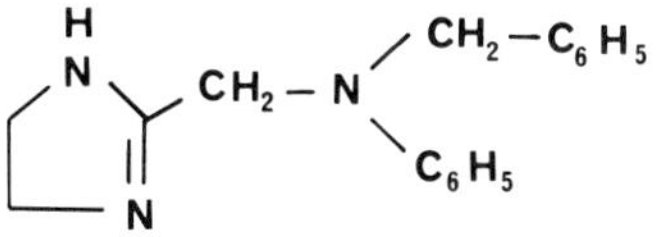

Antazoline

Case report

A man previously sensitised by Antasten ointment had a severe exacerbation when he used Antistin-Privine eye drops. Patch tests with a 2 per cent Antasten cream and with several other antihistamines were positive (Rajka and Pallin, 1964).

St John's

From 1971 to 1976 inclusive, about 21 patients, all women, have been seen with reactions, some severe, to one particular cream containing 2 per cent antazoline methanesulphonate. Patch tests with the cream usually elicited strong reactions and 3 blistered; but only 4 of 17 patients tested with antazoline methanesulphonate 1 per cent in petrolatum responded. One of the base ingredients was a surfactant; it was applied in concentrations of 1 per cent and 5 per cent to 16 patients and 9 reacted but many of the responses appeared to be irritant. Other ingredients of the base elicited no reactions in those tested.

This discrepancy between the clinical picture, the strongly positive patch tests to the cream and the weak responses to the ingredients were not explained. It may have been due to poor absorption of antazoline from the petrolatum base used for patch testing or to two compounds in the formulation acting synergistically; these possibilities were not investigated.

Patch testing

Antazoline 1 per cent ?? in petrolatum.

DIPHENHYDRAMINE (2-Diphenylmethoxy-*N*, *N*-dimethylethylamine; Benadryl) (Formula p. 234)

Case report

Topical application of Benadryl can cause allergic contact dermatitis. Schreiber and Naylor (1962) described the induction of photosensitivity by its oral administration. In another case, a man with atopic dermatitis, while taking Benadryl, developed a papular eruption and abnormal neurological signs which could be reproduced by exposure to the drug (Davenport and Wilhelm, 1965).

St John's

From 1971–1976, sensitivity to diphenhydramine was verified in 7 patients and seemed very probable in a further 6 patients.

The medicament had been used for a variety of pruritic conditions: stasis eczema (3) eczema (2) lichen simplex (1) insect bites (1) pruritus ani (2) itchy scalp (1), and 3 patients had applied it to prevent or treat sunburn. Patch tests: all 13 patients reacted to their proprietary medicament containing diphenydramine 1–2 per cent; 7 patients were tested with diphenhydramine 10 per cent in water or 5 per cent in petrolatum and each reacted.

Patch testing

Diphenhydramine 2 per cent in petrolatum.

MEPYRAMINE (2-[(2-Dimethylaminoethyl)(*p*-methoxybenzyl)amino]pyridine; pyrilamine; Anthisan). (Formula p. 234)

St John's

From 1971 to 1976 inclusive, two men and three women were seen who had been sensitised by one proprietary cream containing 2 per cent mepyramine maleate. The conditions for which it had been used were pruritus ani, a contact dermatitis of the face due to nail varnish and itchy eyes; two patients had used it on patches of eczema in the past and had found it made them worse. Patch tests: each of the 5 patients reacted to the proprietary cream containing 2 per cent mepyramine maleate; two were tested with mepyramine maleate 1 per cent in petrolatum and both reacted.

Patch testing

Mepyramine maleate 2 per cent in petrolatum.

PHENIRAMINE (2-[α-(2-Dimethylaminoethyl)benzyl]pyridine; Trimeton)

Case report

A woman who had previously taken Benadryl orally for pruritus vulvae was prescribed Trimeton and developed an eruption on her neck. She was then given an intravenous injection of Benadryl and the eruption became generalised and severe. Patch and scratch tests with a series of antihistamines including Benadryl were all negative except for a positive patch test with a Trimeton tablet (Epstein, 1949).

Patch testing
Pheniramine ?2 per cent in petrolatum.

PROMETHAZINE HYDROCHLORIDE (10-(2-Dimethylaminopropyl)-
phenothiazine hydrochloride; Phenergan)
(Formula p. 235)

Case report
Among the antihistamines used in France, Phenergan cream was reported to be
the principal sensitiser, having, in 1953, caused half the cases of dermatitis
medicamentosa in the series of Sidi, Hincky and Gervais (1955). It was
emphasised that patients sensitised by topical application may develop serious
photosensitivity if given the drug orally as an anti-pruritic. Patch tests: among
their patients, nine of 83 reacted to phenergan in water, 39 of 128 to
p-phenylenediamine, and three 3 of 11 to Largactil. The base was irritant in
many patients.

In Holland, Suurmond (1966) confirmed the irritancy of the Phenergan cream
base but thought that some patients had been sensitised by the triethanolamine
it contained. Patch tests: eight out of 22 reacted to promethazine 2 per cent in
lanette wax-cream; four of these eight also reacted to 5 per cent triethanolamine
and three to 1 per cent triethanolamine. Because only patients sensitised to
phenergan reacted to triethanolamine, it was thought this might be cross-
sensitisation as both are tertiary amines.

Photosensitivity from the topical use of Phenergan cream is a considerable
problem in Venezuela. Sensitivity to the sun may persist for six or more years
after the drug is stopped (Soto, 1968; Prisco, Soto and Herrera, 1968).

St John's
No cases of contact sensitivity to promethazine have been traced for the period
1971–1976 but photosensitive patients sometimes react to it (p. 443).

Patch testing
Promethazine hydrochloride 2 per cent in petrolatum.

Antimitotic compounds

CHLORAMBUCIL (Leukeran) (4-{*p*-[Bis(2-chloroethyl) amino]phenyl}butyric
acid)

$$\text{HOOC}-\text{CH}_2-\text{CH}_2-\text{CH}_2 - \underset{}{\bigcirc} - \text{N} \underset{\text{CH}_2-\text{CH}_2-\text{Cl}}{\overset{\text{CH}_2-\text{CH}_2-\text{Cl}}{<}}$$

Chlorambucil is an aromatic derivative of mechlorethamine (nitrogen mustard).

Case report

A woman with chronic lymphatic leukaemia was given chlorambucil 6 mg daily, and three weeks after starting it she developed a generalised maculopapular and urticarial eruption. An oral challenge with the drug caused generalised urticaria; a scratch test with chlorambucil was positive at 18–20 hours; and a patch test was positive at 3 days (Knisley, Settipane and Albala, 1971). In a similar patient (Millard and Rajah, 1977), although oral challenge elicited the urticarial eruption, patch, scratch and intradermal tests were negative.

5-FLUOROURACIL (5-Fluoropyrimidine-2, 4-dione)

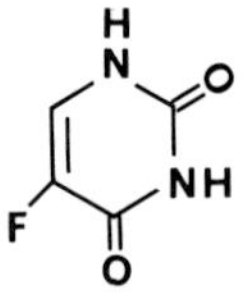

Local discomfort is frequent during the topical treatment of cutaneous neoplasms with 5-fluorouracil; occasionally an allergic contact dermatitis ensues. Sams (1968) reported sensitisation in two of 330 patients and Goette, Odom and Owens (1977) in two of their patients. Patch test reactions were elicited with fluorouracil 5 per cent in propylene glycol or hydrophilic ointment by Sams (1968) and with 0.5 per cent in water or 1 per cent in a cream base by Goette *et al.* (1977). Fifteen patients were tested intradermally with fluorouracil by Mansell *et al.* (1975) before and after therapy, and 11 converted from a negative to a positive response.

Patch testing

5-Fluorouracil ?1 per cent and 5 per cent in petrolatum.

NITROGEN MUSTARD (2,2'-Dichloro-*N*-methyldiethylamine; chlormethine; mechlorethamine)

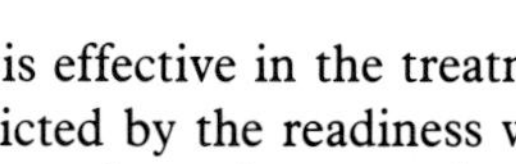

Topical nitrogen mustard is effective in the treatment of psoriasis and mycosis fungoides but its use is restricted by the readiness with which contact sensitivity is induced. Experimentally, guinea-pigs are also easily sensitised (Maguire, 1974).

Case reports

In 1970 Epstein and Ugel treated 12 psoriatic patients with weekly applications of a 0.05 per cent (50 mg per 100 ml) solution of nitrogen mustard and within seven weeks six had become sensitive. Intravenous injections of nitrogen mustard prior to topical application have failed to induce tolerance (Baer, Michaelides and Prestia, 1972).

Patients with mycosis fungoides may be less susceptible but they too are sensitised. Solutions of nitrogen mustard in concentrations of approximately 0.025–0.1 per cent (10–40 mg per 40 ml) were used to treat 21 patients and only six were sensitised (Van Scott and Winters, 1970). Desensitisation has been achieved by daily intravenous injections of minute amounts of nitrogen mustard, and immunological tolerance has been effected successfully by weekly injections prior to starting topical therapy (Van Scott and Kalmanson, 1973). The cross-reactivity of nitrogen mustard and its homologues has been investigated in patients sensitised by nitrogen mustard and several cross-reacted (Van Scott and Yu, 1974).

Urticaria and anaphylaxis induced by topical therapy were reported by Daughters, Zackheim and Maibach (1973). A challenge application of 0.02 ml of a 1:100 000 concentration to the forearm produced a local weal and flare with systemic symptoms which were terminated by adrenaline.

Patch testing
Nitrogen mustard ? concentration or base.

TRIAZIQUONE (2,3,5-Tris(1-aziridinyl)-p-benzoquinone; Trenimon)

This compound contains an alkylating ethyleneimino group and a benzoquinone ring.

Case report
A man with multiple basal cell carcinomas was treated with Trenimon ointment (containing 0.05 per cent triaziquone in eucerin) under occlusion and was sensitised. A patch test with the ointment was positive. Further lesions were treated and, though the intense inflammation was reduced by prednisolone 150 mg daily by mouth, the lesions ulcerated. The areas healed and biopsies showed no evidence of the carcinomas (Helm and Klein, 1965).

Patch testing
Triaziquone ?concentration or base.

BUSULPHAN (Myleran)

Pigmentation
Patients receiving busulphan (Myleran) orally for myeloid leukaemia have developed pigmentation of the skin, but not of the mucous membranes, as part of a syndrome resembling Addison's disease (Harrold, 1966; Sprunt and Rizza, 1966).

Another antitumour agent, BCNU (1,3-bis(2-chloroethyl)-1-nitrosourea; car-mustine), causes pigmentation but only when used topically. The effect was considered to be post-inflammatory by Frost and DeVita (1966).

Dyes — triphenylmethane

TRIPHENYLMETHANE (ROSANILINE) DYES

The triphenylmethane dyes form one group of the organic dyes. They are active against Gram-positive bacteria and have in the past been widely used in treatment, particularly of leg ulcers. They are extremely rare sensitisers.

BRILLIANT GREEN

Case report
Eleven patients with stasis eczema or ulcers reacted on routine patch testing with brilliant green 2 per cent in water. Eight of these reacted also to gentian violet (2 per cent aqueous), seven to crystal violet (2 per cent aqueous) and six to malachite green (2 per cent aqueous). Triphenylmethane 1 per cent in petrolatum elicited no positive reactions (Bielicky and Novák, 1969).

Patch testing
Brilliant green 2 per cent in water.

GENTIAN VIOLET

Gentian violet consists mainly of hexamethylpararosaniline chloride but has some admixture of pentamethyl and tetramethyl derivatives.
Crystal violet is almost pure hexamethylpararosaniline chloride.
Methyl violet is principally the pentamethyl compound.

Case reports
The first case of sensitivity reported was in a woman who developed dermatitis while being treated for vaginal candidiasis with a 3 per cent aqueous solution of gentian violet. A patch test with the solution was positive (Goldstein, 1940).
In 1958 Epstein described a woman with stasis eczema who reacted adversely to gentian violet and had a positive patch test to a 1 per cent solution of gentian violet. Two other patients had negative patch tests but positive intradermal tests.
Cross-reactions between brilliant green and gentian violet were reported by Bielicky and Novák (1969).

Irritant reactions. A 2 per cent aqueous solution of crystal violet (Pyoktanin) was applied to a child's gluteal fold and caused an area of necrosis (Meurer and Konz, 1977), and concentrations of 0.5 and 1 per cent have produced oral ulceration in neonates (Horsfield, Logan and Newey, 1976).

Immediate-type hypersensitivity. A woman who became cyanosed and then collapsed after the application of a 1 per cent solution of gentian violet and methyl green to a stasis ulcer was described by Michel, Buyer and Delorme (1958). An epicutaneous test with the solution was positive.

After a triphenylmethane dye (Alphazurine 2 G) had been injected intravenously into an ill man to determine the depth of burns, he went into profound shock and died. This was considered to be an anaphylactic reaction, the patient having been presensitised by a structurally related compound (Hepps and Dollinger, 1965).

Patch testing
Gentian violet 1 per cent in water.

PATENT BLUE VIOLET (Patent blue dye)

The technique of injecting patent blue dye intradermally to outline superficial lymphatics has been in use for many years. For lymphangiography of limbs it is injected into a web space to visualise the lymphatics prior to their cannulisation.

After an injection of dye for this purpose, three patients with malignant disease became shocked and one, a child, lost consciousness. Two had periorbital oedema and one had swollen lips and urticaria. Two of the patients had 'skin tests' to which they reacted (Mortazavi and Burrows, 1971). There was no mention that any of these patients had been injected with patent blue dye previously.

Ethylenediamine

ETHYLENEDIAMINE (1, 2-Diaminoethane)

$$H_2NCH_2CH_2NH_2$$

Ethylenediamine is used in medicaments and in industry.

PHARMACEUTICAL PREPARATIONS

Aminophylline
Aminophylline consists of two-thirds theophylline and one-third ethylenediamine and is prepared by dissolving theophylline in ethylenediamine hydrate, then evaporating to dryness. The ethylenediamine increases the solubility of theophylline.

CASE REPORTS — OCCUPATIONAL
Sensitisation by aminophylline was first reported from Israel in a pharmacist preparing aminophylline suppositories. Initially he developed eczema of his hands, arms and face and later became asthmatic. Patch tests: he reacted to aminophylline 1 per cent but not to theophylline 1 per cent; he refused to be

patch tested with ethylenediamine but agreed to inhalation tests. These had no immediate effect but 6 hours later precipitated status asthmaticus and a mild relapse of his eczema (Tas and Weissberg, 1958).

Similarly, a chemist in Vienna preparing theophylline-ethylenediamine suppositories was sensitised by the ethylenediamine. Patch tests: he reacted to ethylenediamine 1 per cent, but not to theophylline (Eberhartinger, 1964).

In the U.S.A. another pharmacist had had a severe widespread eczema for three years, when he was investigated by Baer, Cohen and Neidorff (1959). It was discovered that relapses coincided with his filling capsules with papavarine, amobarbital and aminophylline. Patch tests: he was tested with the three drugs and reacted only to aminophylline. On further testing he reacted to aminophylline 1 per cent aqueous and to ethylenediamine hydrochloride 1 per cent aqueous but not to theophylline. During the next four years he avoided aminophylline and remained well.

Sensitisation in the pharmaceutical industry was attributed by Eberhartinger (1964) to pharmacists being exposed to higher concentrations than are either patients or nurses.

Immediate-type hypersensitivity — aminophylline
In addition to the Israeli pharmacist described above, there has been another case report of immediate-type hypersensitivity to aminophylline, but the allergen was thought to be theophylline and not ethylenediamine (Wong, Lapappa and Haddad, 1971).

ETHYLENEDIAMINE AS A STABILISER
Tri-Adcortyl (Mycolog) cream (Squibb) contains triamcinolone acetonide, neomycin, gramicidin, nystatin, ethylenediamine and thiomersal. In the cream base, neomycin forms a complex with the nystatin unless prevented by adding ethylenediamine as a stabiliser. Ethylenediamine is not required in the ointment and in Great Britain it is present in only one other steroid cream and in a thiomersal preparation.

Case reports
In countries where this cream is a popular dermatological remedy sensitisation has become frequent; this is particularly so in the U.S.A.

In the University of California, from January 1967 to August 1970 inclusive, 523 patients were routinely patch tested and 44 (9 per cent) reacted to ethylenediamine, making it the commonest sensitiser in that department (Maibach and Epstein, 1971). Similarly, Fisher (1974) found it to be the most frequent contact allergen amongst his patients. In Copenhagen 1111 patients were routinely tested with this allergen and 2 per cent (23) reacted (Eriksen, 1975).

In 1967, Provost and Jillson reported the first 13 cases. Patch tests: each patient reacted to 1 per cent ethylenediamine dihydrochloride solution but only four of ten tested reacted to Mycolog cream. Following this paper Epstein and Maibach (1968) included ethylenediamine hydrochloride 1 per cent in petrolatum in their standard patch test series and detected 10 sensitised patients, although in only two did the history suggest an allergy to Mycolog cream. They confirmed false negative patch tests to Mycolog cream but showed them to be due to the low concentration of ethylenediamine (0.18 per cent) and not to suppression of the reaction by the steroid. By increasing the concentration of ethylenediamine in Mycolog cream to 1 per cent, three patients reacted to it while remaining negative to the standard formulation.

The importance of including ethylenediamine in a standard patch test series to detect unsuspected cases of sensitisation was confirmed by Crow (1972), but Hjorth (1969) did not find detection of ethylenediamine sensitivity to be so significant in Copenhagen. Among Hjorth's 1121 patients, 15 reacted to ethylenediamine hydrochloride 1 per cent in petrolatum; five had used Mycolog cream and of these, two reacted to neomycin and to ethylenediamine, and three to ethylenediamine alone. One reaction was considered to be irritant, and in nine no source for the sensitisation was traced.

St John's

Since 1972, ethylenediamine 1 per cent in petrolatum has been included in the standard patch test series; from 1972–1976, 0.7–2.8 per cent of all patients seen were found to be sensitive; 0.8–3.5 per cent of the men and 0.6–2.8 per cent of the women reacted (Table 6.9). There was no obvious explanation for the decrease in incidence in 1975 and 1976; according to the manufacturer the formulation of their cream containing ethylenediamine had not altered nor had its sales.

Table 6.9. Yearly incidence of ethylenediamine sensitivity (St John's, 1972–1976).

	Total			Males			Females		
	+ Ethd.	Tested	%	+ Ethd.	Tested	%	+ Ethd.	Tested	%
1972	36	1606	2.2	14	738	1.9	22	868	2.5
1973	43	1546	2.8	20	710	2.8	23	836	2.8
1974	38	1433	2.7	23	655	3.5	15	778	1.9
1975	13	1858	0.7	7	887	0.8	6	971	0.6
1976	16	1982	0.8	10	937	1.1	6	1045	0.6

The most likely source of contact in these patients was Tri-Adcortyl cream; however, some patients did deny ever having used it, but this may have been a faulty memory. Fifty-three patients were patch tested with Tri-Adcortyl cream and 31 (58 per cent) reacted.

Industrial uses

Ethylenediamine has many applications in industry. It is used as a solvent for albumin, casein and fibrin, as an additive in some electro-plating solutions and electrophoretic gels, as a corrosion inhibitor in antifreeze solutions, as a textile lubricant, as a stabiliser in rubber latex, for dehairing skins, in dyes, emulsifiers and polyamide resin adhesives, and for making ethylenediamine derivatives.

Despite this widespread use in industry, cases of occupational sensitisation are rarely reported.

Case reports — occupational

In 1951, Dernehl reported that in a Texan carbide and carbon chemical company, ethylene amines caused dermatitis, burns and occasionally asthma among the workers. Only some of the men with dermatitis had to change their job; patch tests were not done and there was no conclusion as to whether the dermatitis was irritant or allergic.

A mixture of ethylenediamine, diethylenetriamine and diethylenetetramine was used as an epoxy resin hardener in Bratislava and cases of sensitisation were seen by Hegyi (1960).

In Zurich, Burckhardt, Kaufmann and Brenn (1970) investigated a plastic factory worker who bottled ethylenediamine and was thereby exposed to its fumes. He developed a contact dermatitis of his face and reacted strongly to a patch test with 0.5 per cent ethylenediamine. A second man in this factory also had a positive patch test to 0.5 per cent ethylenediamine.

In the caprolactam polymerisation section, where ethylenediamine was used as a stabiliser of the synthetic fibre, a worker accidentally poured a mixture of ethylenediamine, acetic acid, benzylamine and dye on to his foot. This caused blisters and an abscess locally, and later eczema of his hands, arms, face and upper chest. His skin healed while he was away from work but relapsed on his return; but irritation of his throat and dyspnoea persisted for months. Patch tests: he reacted strongly to ethylenediamine 1 per cent in water; the tests with the following were negative: caprolactam 1 per cent (aqueous), benzylamine 1 per cent (aqueous), Mycolog, Phenergan and Benadryl ointments (Wüthrich, 1972).

Coolant oil dermatitis has been caused by ethylenediamine. In the first outbreak the concentrated soluble oil contained 3 per cent ethylenediamine base and a dilution of 1:10 was made for use. The men patch tested reacted to the neat oil and ethylenediamine, and 2 of 4 reacted to the 10 per cent dilution of the oil. In the second outbreak the biocide Panacide CA containing dichlorophen and ethylenediamine (p. 677) was added to the oil and men were sensitised to both compounds (Crow, Peachey and Adams, 1978).

Systemic absorption

Aminophylline

Two patients sensitised by ethylenediamine in topical applications were given aminophylline orally and developed a generalised eruption (Provost and Jillson, 1967). Another man similarily sensitised was treated with aminophylline suppositories; on the second day he had a diffuse erythema but as the cause was not recognised the aminophylline was continued and by the tenth day he had a generalised exfoliative dermatitis (Petrozzi and Shore, 1976). A similar patient was reported by Bernstein and Lorincz (1979).

The persistence of eczema in a woman, who was sensitised to triethylenetetramine when she worked with epoxy resin as a coil winder, was traced to ethylenediamine in the aminophylline she was taking; a patch test with ethylenediamine was positive (Rudzki, 1978).

Cross-reactions

Ethylenediamine tetracetic acid (EDTA)

Five patients sensitised by ethylenediamine in Mycolog cream did not react to

EDTA 1 per cent in water (Provost and Jillson, 1967). Six patients similarly sensitised were tested by Epstein (1974) with the disodium salt of EDTA 5 per cent in water and petrolatum; none of the six reacted. Another 30 ethylenediamine-sensitive patients were patch tested by Fisher (1975) with ethylenediamine tetra-acetate 1 per cent in petrolatum; none reacted.

In contrast to this lack of evidence of cross-reaction, Raymond and Gross (1969) reported that one man with no skin disease at the time but with a past history of poison ivy dermatitis and inguinal candidiasis reacted to 0.1 per cent EDTA and to 0.1 per cent ethylenediamine, both in water. The primary allergen in this case was unknown. A second patient may, however, have been sensitised separately by both allergens. A third patient had been sensitised definitely by EDTA in ophthalmic preparations but failed to react to ethylenediamine. In Copenhagen, in a series of routine patch tests, three patients reacted to ethylenediamine and to edetic acid, but the latter was thought likely to have been the primary allergen (Eriksen, 1975).

Conclusion: patients sensitive to ethylenediamine do not appear to cross-react with EDTA; patients sensitised by EDTA may cross-react with ethylenediamine.

Antihistamines
Fisher (1974) recommended that the following antihistamines, which are derivatives of ethylenediamine, should be avoided systemically and topically:

Tripelennamine citrate and hydrochloride	(Pyribenzamine)
Antazoline	(Antistin)
Chlorothen citrate	(Tagathen)
Methapyrilene hydrochloride	(Histadyl)
Pyrilamine maleate	(Pyma)

In addition (Fisher 1973)

Promethazine hydrochloride	(Phenergan)

In his series, Eriksen (1975) reported that several patients cross-reacted with promethazine hydrochloride.

However White (1978) patch tested 7 patients sensitive to ethylenediamine with many antihistamines and only 2 reacted, both to antazoline sulphate and one of these also to Anthisan (mepyramine maleate) cream.

Piperazine
Cross-reactions to piperazine have been reported (Calnan, 1975; Burry, 1978).

Diethylenetriamine
Cross-sensitisation was mentioned by Eriksen (1975).

Patch testing
Ethylenediamine 1 per cent in petrolatum.

Corticosteroids

Delayed and immediate-type hypersensitivity to corticosteroids do occur but are rare. The allergy may be quite specific without cross-reactions to other corticosteroids so that testing with the suspected compound is essential.

CORTICOTROPHIN (ACTH)

Immediate-type hypersensitivity, including anaphylaxis, was formerly a well recognised complication of treatment with extracts of porcine ACTH. The highly purified and synthetic preparations now available rarely induce allergy. However, there is a report of a patient sensitised by porcine ACTH, who reacted also to synthetic human ACTH (Forssman and Mulder, 1973). Allergic reactions to tetracosactrin have been reported; two patients subsequently received corticotrophin in carboxymethylcellulose without ill effect (Mohr, 1975).

Contact dermatitis has not been described.

HYDROCORTISONE

Contact dermatitis
In Copenhagen, from 1963 to 1964 hydrocortisone and hydrocortisone acetate were included in the routine patch test series; 0.3 per cent of all patients tested (i.e. six of 1835) were found to be sensitive (Alani and Alani, 1972).

Case reports
Since 1959, there has been a slow trickle of case reports of contact sensitivity to hydrocortisone. The first, by Burckhardt (1959), described a patient with eczema of an ear who had used a hydrocortisone-neomycin preparation for 2 years and had become sensitive to hydrocortisone acetate but not to neomycin. Then Kooij (1959) reported a patient whose eczema was exacerbated by a hydrocortisone ointment and who had positive patch tests to several hydrocortisone preparations (0.5–1 per cent) and to a pure solution of hydrocortisone succinate 6 per cent in water.

In 1960, five patients sensitised by one brand of hydrocortisone acetate ointment were investigated by Church (1960). The sensitiser, a 21-diol acetate, was a chemical impurity — a precursor of hydrocortisone acetate in the manufacturing process. Subsequent modification of the synthetic process eliminated the allergen. An impurity in hydrocortisone was also thought to be the sensitiser in the patient reported by Sönnichsen (1962). In another case, a patient with otitis externa was sensitised by a hydrocortisone cream; patch tests and intradermal tests with hydrocortisone acetate and succinate were positive (Wilkinson, McGarry and Solomon, 1967).

In a detailed study of contact sensitivity to topical steroids, Alani and Alani (1972) reported their investigation of 23 sensitised patients. Seventeen had leg eczema, three atopic eczema and three eczema of other sites. Patch tests with various hydrocortisone preparations were positive in 21 patients, and the authors concluded that the allergen was hydrocortisone, not an impurity.

Patch testing
Hydrocortisone 25 per cent in petrolatum (Alani and Alani, 1972).

Immediate type hypersensitivity
Anaphylactic reactions to injections of hydrocortisone have been reported (King, 1960; O'Garra, 1962).

PREDNISONE

Contact dermatitis

Case reports
A patient who reacted adversely to methylprednisolone acetate 0.25 per cent in Veriderm was reported by Coskey and Bryan (1967). Patch tests with this medicament, with methylprednisolone aqueous suspension and with methylprednisolone acetate powder 33 per cent in aqueous suspension, all were positive. A case of contact dermatitis due to prednisolone was described by Gutzwiller (1974): patch tests with prednisone and prednisolone, both 1 per cent in ethanol, were positive.

Patch testing
Prednisone ?5 per cent in petrolatum
Prednisolone ?5 per cent in petrolatum.

Immediate-type hypersensitivity
A woman developed a petechial eruption after taking prednisone by mouth and a widespread maculopapular rash after receiving an intra-articular injection of prednisolone acetate. When tested intradermally with prednisone, prednisolone and hydrocortisone, she consistently reacted (Comaish, 1969).

A young man with recurrent attacks of status asthmaticus developed urticaria, angio-oedema and increased bronchospasm after receiving methylprednisolone sodium succinate or hydrocortisone sodium succinate intravenously. When challenged with a large intravenous dose of methylprednisone sodium succinate, he reacted, but an intradermal test was negative; both oral challenge and skin tests with methylprednisolone were positive (Mendelson, Meltzer and Hamburger, 1974).

TRIAMCINOLONE ACETONIDE

Contact dermatitis

Case reports
Three patients sensitive to triamcinolone acetonide were reported by Bandmann, Huber-Riffeser and Woyton (1966), and in Alani and Alani's series (1972) three

patients had reacted to proprietary preparations containing this steroid. Coskey's (1978) patient reacted to the following four 16, 17 acetonides: halcinonide, fluocinonide, desonide and triamcinolone acetonide but not to others of the same group.

Patch testing
Triamcinolone acetonide ?5 per cent in petrolatum.

BETAMETHASONE 17-VALERATE

Contact dermatitis
Contact sensitivity to betamethasone valerate has been described in two patients by Alani and Alani (1976).

Patch testing
Betamethasone valerate 10 per cent in petrolatum.

Vitamins

Vitamin A acid: Retinoic acid

Case reports
Two men were found on patch testing to be sensitive to *trans*-retinoic acid, having reacted to 0.05 per cent in a petrolatum base and to 0.00625 per cent in the commercial lotion diluted with ethanol. The allergy was confirmed by leucocyte migration inhibition tests. A cross-sensitivity was presumed as neither man had previous exposure but the primary allergen was not identified (Jordan, Higgins and Dvorak, 1975). Following this report, Nordqvist and Mehr (1976) described a woman who had been sensitised by Retin-A liquid 0.05 per cent which she had used to treat a folliculitis of her legs. Patch tests: she reacted to the proprietary lotion diluted to 0.0065 per cent and to retinoic acid 0.01 per cent in ethanol and in acetone but she did not react to retinoic acid 0.05 per cent in petrolatum. Another patient used a cream containing 0.05 per cent alltrans-retinoic acid and was sensitised (Rudzki and Grzywa, 1978).

Patch testing
Retinoic acid 0.05 per cent in petrolatum and 0.01 per cent in ethanol.

VITAMIN B₁ (Thiamine)

Case reports
Two employees in a pharmaceutical firm, who were engaged in filling ampoules with thiamine, developed eczema of their hands and arms and, in one, also of the eyelids. Patch tests with pure thiamine hydrochloride were positive in both, and each relapsed on re-exposure (Combes and Groopman, 1950).

A very similar case, described in detail by Hjorth (1958), was that of a girl who filled vials with thamine at a pharmaceutical firm and developed eczema of her hands and wrists and around her mouth. She was patch tested and reacted to aqueous dilutions of thiamine down to 0.1 per cent and to co-carboxylase 1 per cent; none of the 100 controls reacted to 50 per cent thiamine or to 1 per cent co-carboxylase. An oral provocation test with 200 mg of thiamine caused a relapse of the girl's eczema. It was found that thiamine intracutaneously caused a weal and flare in normal subjects.

In a survey of pharmaceutical workers, Dalton and Pierce (1951) reported that one man developed eczema of exposed sites while working with thiamine hydrochloride and had a positive patch test to it. Nine other workers reacted on patch testing with this vitamin but whether or not they had eczema was not stated. All ten were given the vitamin orally (? dose) but none reacted.

During the synthesis of thiamine an intermediate product, ethoxymethyl-malodinitrile, has caused contact dermatitis among the workers (Rajka and Vincze, 1956).

Patch testing
Thiamine 10 per cent in petrolatum.

VITAMIN E (Tocopherol)

The eight tocopherols, which occur naturally, are all derivatives of dihydro-benzo-gamma-pyran. Chemically they act as antioxidants and structurally differ from each other in the number and position of the methyl groups. The alpha-form (vitamin E) is the most active biologically; it is a viscous oil obtained from plants, particularly wheat germ oil.

Vitamin E has been used for many years in medicaments and it has had a recent vogue as an ingredient of cosmetics. In Denmark and the U.S.A., where it has been included in a deodorant, it has caused dermatitis. In several of the cases reported, a striking feature of vitamin E sensitisation is the widespread dissemination of the eczema after the contact dermatitis has developed at the primary site.

Case reports
Synthetic vitamin E (α-tocopherol) was the allergen in a vitamin cream (containing vitamin E 5 mg/g) which had sensitised a girl who had applied it to her ear. A patch test with undiluted α-tocopherol was positive (Brodkin and Bleiberg, 1965).

A mother treated burns on her two sons aged 7 years and 4 years respectively with the contents of vitamin E capsules, and both developed at the burn site a confluent erythematous urticarial eruption which rapidly generalised. It cleared, with desquamation, in 7–10 days. Patch tests were considered inadvisable (Kassen and Mitchell, 1974).

A veterinary surgeon with fissured eczema of his fingers was patch tested with all the drugs he handled and he reacted to vitamin E (tocopherol acetate) 5 per cent and to Combelen (10-(3-dimethylaminopropyl)-2-propionylphenothiazine) 10 mg/ml (Hjorth, 1974).

In about 1972 a deodorant called Mennen E was marketed in the U.S.A. where it caused such a spate of cases of severe dermatitis that its distribution was stopped. In each of the three patients reported by Minkin, Cohen and Frank (1973) the axillae had become red and oedematous, and there followed a widespread, blotchy, morbilliform eruption. The dermatitis was sufficiently severe to require systemic steroids. The patients were not patch tested. A further three cases described by Aeling, Panagotacos and Andreozzi (1973) were males aged 16–22 years. Two patients had used the deodorant for 2–3 weeks before developing dermatitis, but in one the first application had caused axillary irritation and erythema which extended to his arms and thorax. A history of previous contact was not obtained. Four days later, having improved, he reapplied the deodorant and developed a spreading vesiculo-bullous eruption. In one of the other patients the eruption also spread to the arms and trunk. The aerosol deodorant contained *dl*-alpha-tocopherol, silicone, anhydrous alcohol and perfume. Patch tests: the tests with vitamin E oil 1 per cent were strongly positive; those with the other ingredients were negative. Two of the patients were tested with *dl*-α-tocopherol acetate from a capsule, but neither had reacted at two days.

Patch testing
dl-α-Tocopherol 20 per cent in petrolatum.

VITAMIN K

Case reports
Vitamin K_1 (phytomenadione) is an antidote to anticoagulants. A few patients receiving several drugs for liver disease have developed, at injection sites of vitamin K_1, red, tender infiltrated plaques, which may spread down the thigh, and are sometimes accompanied by a maculo-papular eruption. The erythematous plaques resolve but the sites may become sclerodermatous. Barnes and Sarkany (1976) reproduced the local lesion in one of their patients with an intradermal injection of vitamin K_1 and it was followed by a generalised eruption. The patient reported by Heydenreich (1977) responded to a patch test with the injection preparation of phytomenadione 1 per cent but six years later the same patch test elicited no reaction. Six patients who reacted only to oil-soluble vitamin K were described by Bullen *et al.* (1978); they considered that the pathogenesis was related to the large doses used in therapy rather than to immunological factors.

A synthetic form of vitamin K (2-methyl-1,4-naphthoquinone; menadione; vitamin K_3) is absorbed through normal skin, so Page and Bercovitz (1942) formulated it as a 1 per cent ointment and used it topically in the treatment of nine patients with ulcerative colitis. Five developed dermatitis. Patch tests were inconclusive and, as three controls gave irritant reactions to patch tests with the ointment, it was thought that the dermatitis had been an irritant effect. A similar ointment had been used on 24 newborn infants but none developed dermatitis. Watrous (1947) noticed that workers in the pharmaceutical industry who handled menadione developed dark brown staining of their skin, which in some became eczematous. There was no mention of patch testing.

A man working in a drug firm was found to be sensitive to 2-methyl-1,4-naphtho-hydroquinone (menadiol diacetate, vitamin K₄). Patch tests: he reacted to menadiol 0.1 per cent in olive oil and cross-reacted to menadione 0.1 per cent in olive oil (Jirásek and Schwank, 1965).

Patch testing
Appropriate vitamin K ? 0.1 per cent in petrolatum.

Other medicaments

APOMORPHINE

Two pharmacy workers, one a dispenser and the other a cleaner, developed dermatitis during the preparation of apomorphine capsules. One also had rhinitis and the other respiratory symptoms. Patch tests: both reacted to an aqueous solution of apomorphine 0.01 per cent. Prick tests with a 1 per cent concentration were negative (Dahlquist, 1977).

Patch testing
Apomorphine 0.01 per cent in water.

TINCTURE OF BENZOIN (Gum benzoin or benjamin)

Gum benzoin, a balsam obtained from *Styrax benzoin*, contains benzoic and cinnamic acids, vanillin and coniferyl benzoate. It is used in medicaments, cosmetics and perfumery and in preparing natural benzoic acid.

Tincture of benzoin is 10 per cent benzoin in alcohol. Compound tincture of benzoin contains 10 per cent benzoin, 2 per cent aloe, 8 per cent storax and 4 per cent Tolu balsam in alcohol.

Sensitisation in two patients was reported by Coskey (1978). One had used tincture of benzoin for pruritus ani and the other, a footballer, had applied it to his leg. Both patients developed a local and generalised eruption and both had positive patch test reactions to 10 per cent benzoin in alcohol, and these were also associated with a generalised flare.

Patch testing
Benzoin 10 per cent in alcohol.

BENZOPHENONES

Benzophenone (diphenyl ketone)

Sulisobenzone (5-benzoyl-4-hydroxy-
2-methoxybenzenesulfonic acid; Uval)

Mexenone (2-hydroxy-4-methoxy-
4'-methylbenzophenone; Uvistat)

Substituted benzophenones are effective ultraviolet light absorbers (Knox, Guin and Cockerwell, 1957) and have been widely used as topical sunscreens. They are also used in industry and may be present in textiles, plastics, rubber, paints and cosmetics.

Case reports
Ramsay, Cohen and Baer (1972) described a photosensitive man who developed immediate and delayed-type hypersensitivity when he used sulisobenzene (Sungold.) Scratch tests with sulisobenzone 1 per cent and with oxybenzone 1 per cent were positive. A patch test with sulisobenzone 5 per cent in water was positive, but that with oxybenzone was negative at one day. Scratch tests and patch tests in controls were negative.

Patch testing
Benzophenone 5 per cent in petrolatum.

BUFEXAMAC (2-(*p*-Butoxyphenyl)acetohydroxamic acid; Droxaryl)

Bufexamac is a non-steroid anti-inflammatory agent which has been used as a 5 per cent cream or ointment (Droxaryl) in the treatment of eczema. It is also formulated with neomycin and nystatin as Flogocid cream.

Case reports
Sensitisation has been reported from Belgium and Holland.

Two women with contact dermatitis from Flogocid cream were investigated by van Hecke (1973). Patch tests: both reacted to Flogocid cream, to Droxaryl cream and ointment and to bufexamac 1 per cent in petrolatum. One reacted to sodium lauryl sulphate 0.3 per cent in water.

Another woman used Droxaryl cream for pruritus vulvae and after one month developed such a severe spreading eczema that she required systemic steroids (Smeenk, 1973). Patch tests: she reacted to Droxaryl cream (5 per cent bufexamac), to bufexamac 5 per cent in petrolatum and to bufexamac 1 per cent in acetone. The reaction to bufexamac in acetone was stronger than to bufexamac in petrolatum. The positive patch tests persisted for several weeks. None of the 20 controls reacted to bufexamac 1 per cent in acetone.

Droxaryl cream also sensitised two women who applied it daily for several months to phlebitis of their legs. Patch tests: both reacted to Droxaryl cream and to bufexamac 5 per cent in petrolatum; neither reacted to the Droxaryl cream base (Lachapelle, 1975).

Patch testing
Bufexamac 5 per cent in petrolatum.

TRICYCLIC ANTIDEPRESSANT DRUGS

The irritant effect of this group of drugs applied undiluted for patch testing has been investigated by Pevny, Mahr and Schröpl (1974).

P-CHLOROBENZENESULPHONYLGLYCOLIC ACID NITRILE

$$Cl-\text{C}_6\text{H}_4-SO_2-O-CH_2-CN$$

Case report
During the development of a new method of synthesising a benzodiazepine tranquillizer, three people developed contact dermatitis from p-chlorobenzenesulphonylglycolic acid nitrile. It was considered to be a strong sensitiser, the allergen being the nitrile group. Patch tests: all three reacted to chlorobenzolsulphonylglycolic acid nitrile to a dilution of 0.001 per cent in acetone. None of the 10 controls reacted to this concentration but did to 0.1 per cent and 0.01 per cent (Richter and Scholz, 1970).

Patch testing
p-Chlorobenzenesulphonylglycolic acid nitrile 0.001 per cent in acetone.

CHROMONAR ([[3-[2-(Diethylamino]ethyl]-4-methyl-2-oxo-2H-1-benzopyran-7-yl]oxy]acetic acid ethyl ester)

$$C_2H_5OOCCH_2O-\cdots-CH_2CH_2N(C_2H_5)_2$$
$$CH_3$$

CHROMAR HYDROCHLORIDE (Carbocromène; Intensain)

Intensain is a coronary artery vasodilator which can be given intravenously, intramuscularly or orally.

Case reports

In Lille, three nurses working in a cardiac clinic developed a contact dermatitis after handling the drug for 4 months, 20 months and 3 years respectively. They had eczema of one or more of the following sites: eyelids, neck, hands and arms. Patch tests: all reacted to Intensain solution 0.8 per cent; two were tested with dihydro-streptomycin and one reacted. A patient, while on a course of Intensain by mouth, developed a widespread eruption which cleared when the drug was stopped. Intradermal tests with Intensain 0.08 per cent and 0.16 per cent were positive. A nurse in the clinic had an itchy eruption in her left antecubital fossa; she was patch tested and did not react, but intradermal tests were positive (Martin *et al.*, 1973; Huriez *et al.*, 1974).

Patch testing

Chromonar hydrochloride 0.8 per cent.

COUMARIN (1,2-Benzopyrone; Cumarin)

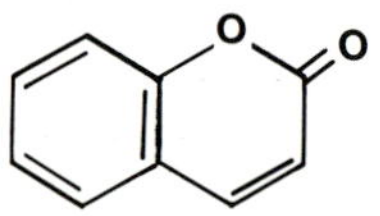

Coumarin is derived from plants and may be added as a perfume to topical preparations. Related compounds, bishydroxycoumarin (Dicumarol) and Warfarin, are anticoagulants.

Case report

A man used Jecovitol ointment (containing vanillin 0.11 per cent and coumarin 0.22 per cent as perfumes) on his ulcerated foot and developed a contact dermatitis with an ide reaction (van Ketel, 1973). Patch tests: he reacted to balsam of Peru 25 per cent, to vanillin 10 per cent, and to vanilla and coumarin 5 per cent in petrolatum. He was not challenged with an anticoagulant orally.

Patch testing

Coumarin ?5 per cent in petrolatum.

CROTAMITON (*N*-Ethyl-*o*-crotonotoluidide; crotonyl-*N*-ethyl-*o*-toluidine; Eurax.

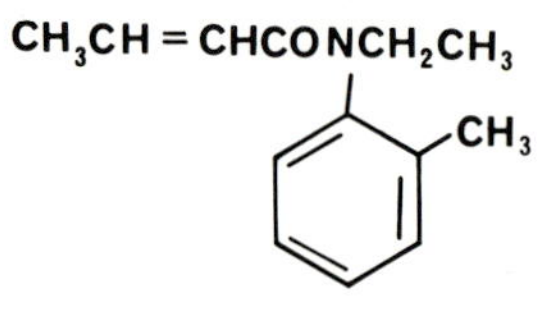

Eurax is used as an antipruritic and in the treatment of scabies; it is formulated as a 10 per cent cream or lotion.

Case reports
Eurax ointment causing contact dermatitis in a woman with otitis externa was reported by Bereston (1952). Patch tests: she reacted strongly to the Eurax ointment and to crotamiton, and responded weakly to the Eurax base.

Another woman developed a generalised eruption while using Eurax ointment on her stasis ulcer and dermatitis. Patch tests: Eurax ointment and crotamiton 5 per cent in petrolatum gave positive reactions; but those with each ingredient of the base were negative (Dijk and Marien, 1972).

St John's
> In Great Britain, Eurax (Geigy) is quite commonly used as a topical medicament; applied as a patch test it gives irritant reactions which are difficult to interpret. Several patients tested in the clinic have reacted initially to the ointment or lotion, but not when the test was repeated, or they have failed to react to each of the constituents.
>
> From 1971 to 1976 five women and one man were thought to have been sensitised by crotamiton in Eurax ointment. Two of the five women had noticed that it aggravated their eczema. The conditions for which the Eurax ointment had been used were: eczema (2), nylon stocking dermatitis (1), otitis externa and hand eczema (1), stasis eczema (1) and intertrigo of the groins (1). Patch tests: each patient reacted to Eurax ointment and to crotamiton 1 per cent in methyl ethyl ketone. Two patients were tested with each ingredient of the base but neither reacted.

Patch testing
Crotamiton 1 per cent in methyl ethyl ketone
(Eurax ointment, containing 10 per cent crotamiton, is mildly irritant.)

DIMERCAPROL (2,3-Dimercapto-1-propanol; British Anti-Lewisite BAL)

$$
\begin{array}{ccc}
\text{H} & \text{H} & \text{H} \\
| & | & | \\
\text{H}-\text{C}-\text{C}-\text{C}-\text{H} \\
| & | & | \\
\text{SH} & \text{SH} & \text{OH}
\end{array}
$$

Sensitising potential
BAL applied topically is a potent sensitiser. Its sensitising potential was studied by Sulzberger, Baer and Kanof (1946) who showed that 5 per cent BAL rubbed into normal skin sensitised 19 per cent of the subjects tested but when rubbed into burned skin it sensitised 77 per cent. Patch tests were done with BAL 5 per cent in an ointment base.

Patch testing
BAL 5 per cent in petrolatum.

EPHEDRINE (2-Methylamino-1-phenyl-1-propanol)

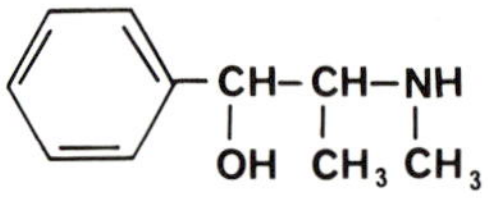

CH–CH–NH
| | |
OH CH$_3$ CH$_3$

Case report
Two days after using an oily inhalant containing ephedrine, a woman developed an acute eczema around her nostrils and a papular eruption scattered on her body. Patch tests: she reacted to the oily inhalant and, of the constituents, only to ephedrine 1 per cent in liquid petrolatum (Spencer, 1945).

Patch testing
Ephedrine ?1 per cent in petrolatum.

PHENYLEPHRINE HYDROCHLORIDE (*l-m*-Hydroxy-α-[(methylamino) methyl] benzyl alcohol hydrochloride; Fenox; Metaoxedrine; Neophryn)

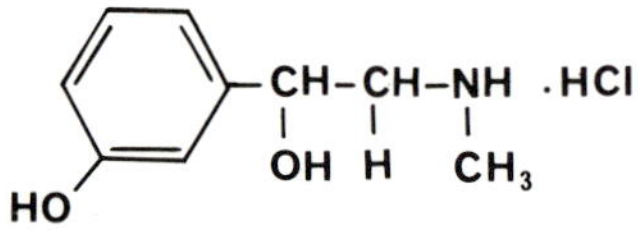

CH–CH–NH .HCl
| | |
OH H   CH$_3$
HO

   Phenylephrine hydrochloride (metaoxedrine chloride) 0.1 per cent is formulated with betamethasone 17-valerate 0.05 per cent and lignocaine hydrochloride 2.5 per cent as Betnovate Rectal Ointment (Glaxo). It is recommended for the treatment of haemorrhoids, anal fissures and pruritus ani.

Case report
Although this ointment is not intended for leg ulcers it was tried in the treatment of such a patient and the ulcer rapidly became larger and painful. Another man used it for his haemorrhoids and was sensitised. Patch tests: both patients were tested with metaoxedrine hydrochloride in water — the first man with 10 per cent and 5 per cent and he reacted, the second man with 1 per cent and 0.5 per cent and he reacted. Cross-sensitivity to related sympathomimetic amines was not demonstrated (Roed-Petersen, 1976).

Patch testing
Metaoxedrine hydrochloride 1 per cent and 5 per cent in water.

EPINEPHRINE (3,4-Dihydroxy-α-[(methylamino)methyl] benzyl alcohol; adrenaline)

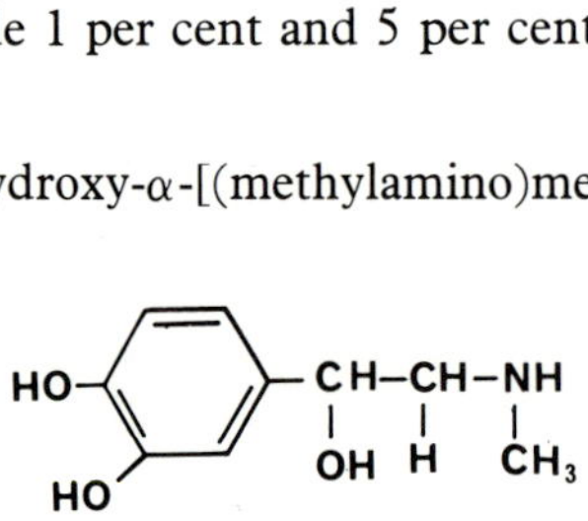

HO–
     CH–CH–NH
     | | |
     OH H   CH$_3$
HO

Case reports
Contact dermatitis to epinephrine has been described in two patients with

glaucoma using epinephrine bitartrate eye drops. Sensitisation in the first patient (Gibbs, 1970) was doubtful as the patch test reactions to epinephrine were not consistently positive. Although one year later a trial instillation of the drops into one eye reproduced the dermatitis, a patch test with the ophthalmic solution done at the same time was negative. The second patient (Alani and Alani, 1976) abandoned epinephrine bitartrate eye drops because of a contact dermatitis of the eyelids but subsequently had a severe relapse when treated with epinephrine borate drops. Patch tests: he reacted to epinephrine chloride 1 per cent and 0.1 per cent (a response to di-isopropyl fluorophosphate was unexplained).

Epinephrine bitartrate is recognised by ophthalmologists as being mildly irritant.

Patch testing

Epinephrine hydrochloride ⎫
Epinephrine chloride ⎬ 1 per cent and 0.1 per cent aqueous.

ICHTHAMMOL (Ichthyol)

Ichthammol, a sulphonated bitumen, is a brownish liquid derived from mineral deposits containing the remains of fishes. It consists of sulphur (about 10 per cent), ammonium sulphate (5–7 per cent), hydrocarbons, nitrogenous bases, acids and derivatives of thiophene. It has slight antiseptic properties.

Case reports

Two cases of sensitisation have been reported in England.

A man had previously used glycerine and ichthyol lotion to treat phlebitis, and when he subsequently applied it to a leg injury, he developed eczema at the site (Calnan, 1971). Patch tests: tests with glycerine and ichthyol solution and with ichthyol 5 per cent aqueous were positive; that with glycerine alone was negative. A woman with a stasis ulcer was found to be sensitive by Cooke and Hocken Robertson (1972). Patch tests: she reacted to ichthammol 5 per cent and 10 per cent in water. These authors pointed out that as ichthammol preparations sometimes irritate eczema, they are suspected of having caused sensitisation, but patch tests in such patients are negative.

Contact dermatitis from this medicament has also been reported by Bandmann (1971) from Munich. One woman applied pure ichtyhol to a boil and developed eczema; she reacted to a patch test with the pure ichthyol. Another woman used Ichthocortin cream on a leg ulcer and in consequence was sensitised; she was also allergic to the parabens it contained.

Patch testing

Ichthammol 5 per cent in water.

IODINE

Thirty years ago iodine was frequently used as a local antiseptic, and in 1938 iodine sensitivity was found in about 1 per cent of all the patients tested at the Finsen Institute in Copenhagen. By 1953, with the decline in its use, the incidence of iodine sensitivity had dropped to zero (Marcussen, 1962).

Patch testing
Iodine 0.5 per cent in ethanol.

Open test
Tincture of iodine painted on a small area and left uncovered.

Tincture of iodine contains iodine 2 per cent and sodium iodide (or potassium iodide) 2.4 per cent in ethanol.

1,3-Diiodo-2-hydroxypropane (Iothion)
In Denmark a White Tincture of Iodine containing diiodohydroxypropane is used as a topical antiseptic and sometimes causes a streaky bullous contact dermatitis. One such patient had a strong positive patch test to diiodohydroxypropane 0.05 per cent in ethanol. Tests in 20 controls were negative (Hjorth, 1972).

Patch testing
Diiodohydroxypropane 0.05 per cent in ethanol.

MECLOFENOXATE ((*p*-Chlorophenoxy)acetic acid 2-(dimethylamino)ethyl ester; centrophenoxine, Helfergin; Lucidril)

$$Cl-\text{\textcircled{}}-OCH_2COOCH_2CH_2N\begin{array}{c}CH_3\\CH_3\end{array}$$

Meclofenoxate 2.5 per cent is given parenterally to improve cerebral uptake of oxygen and glucose.

Case report
In France three nurses were sensitised. Patch tests were positive to 2.5 per cent meclofenoxate but negative to the following related compounds: *p*-chlorophenol, pentachlorophenol, *p*-chlorophenoxyacetic acid, trimethylamine chlorhydrate and dimethylamino-2-ethanol (Foussereau and Lantz, 1972).

Patch testing
Meclofenoxate ?2.5 per cent ?base.

NITROGLYCERIN

Case reports
Nitroglycerin is absorbed percutaneously but patients using such topical preparations have developed allergic contact dermatitis. The evidence was presumptive in the four cases reported by Chandraratna and O'Dell (1979) but the diag-

nosis was confirmed by positive patch test reactions to the medicament and to nitroglycerin 0.2 mg/ml (aqueous) in the patient described by Sausker and Frederick (1978).

Patch testing
Nitroglycerin 0.2 mg/ml in water.

PHENYLBUTAZONE (4-Butyl-1,2-diphenyl-3,5-pyrazolidinedione: Butazolidin)

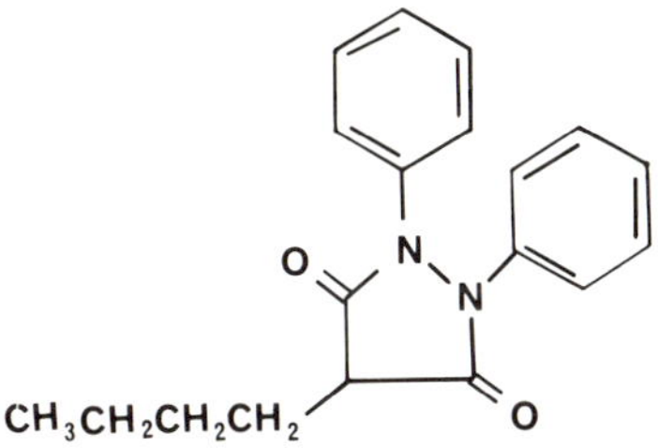

CH₃CH₂CH₂CH₂

Phenylbutazone is a pyrazolone compound used systemically in the treatment of rheumatic diseases. It has been formulated as a cream for phlebitis and inflammatory conditions of the muscles and connective tissues.

Case report
Two patients sensitised by phenylbutazone cream were reported by Krook (1975). Patch tests: both reacted to phenylbutazone 1 per cent but not to oxyphenbutazone 1 per cent. Another patient became febrile, with facial oedema and subsequently developed erythroderma following an injection of Tomonol containing phenylbutazone and isopropylaminophenazone (Vooys and van Ketel, 1977). Patch testing elicited reactions to phenylbutazone 1 per cent and 5 per cent and to oxyphenbutazone but not to isopropylaminophenazone or other pyrazolone compounds. Prior contact sensitisation was postulated but not established. The presence of skin lesions predisposes to sensitisation as occurred in the four patients reported by Thormann and Kaaber (1978).

Patch testing
Phenylbutazone 1 per cent in petrolatum.

p-HYDROXYPHENYLBUTAZONE (4-Butyl-2-(*p*-hydroxyphenyl)-1-phenyl-3, 5-pyrazolidinedione; oxyphenbutazone; Tanderil).

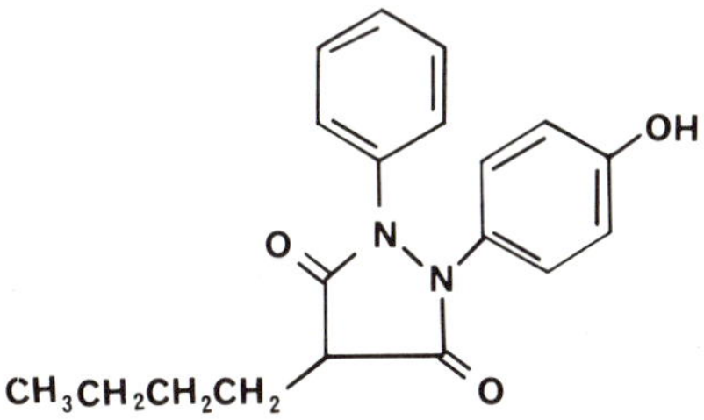

CH₃CH₂CH₂CH₂

Oxyphenbutazone is an anti-inflammatory pyrazolone compound given systemically for rheumatic conditions. It is also available as a 10 per cent eye ointment.

Case report
In a clinical trial, a 5 per cent oxyphenbutazone cream was used to treat a man's stasis dermatitis. After 2 weeks, the condition deteriorated, the eczema spreading to his legs and arms. Patch tests: he reacted to oxyphenbutazone 5 per cent in the cream base and 1 per cent in petrolatum; he cross-reacted to phenylbutazone 1 per cent in petrolatum (Krook, 1975).

Patch testing
Oxyphenbutazone 1 per cent in petrolatum.

PIPERAZINE (Diethylene diamine)

Piperazine
(diethylene diamine)

Hydroxyzine (1-(p-chloro-α- phenylbenzyl)-4-
(2-hydroxyethoxyethyl) piperazine; Atarax)

Piperazine is an anthelmintic effective against threadworms and roundworms; it is used also as a corrosion inhibitor and as a rubber accelerator.

Case reports
In France, nurses in a resuscitation unit became sensitive to piperazine through handling camphosulphonate of piperazine (Solucamphr) Foussereau and Benezra, 1967).

Occupational dermatitis in pharmaceutical workers has been reported (Calnan, 1975; Rudzki and Grzywa, 1977), and in a Swedish factory making piperazine as a vermifuge, over a period of years, several men were sensitised. One who developed dermatitis of his hands, arms and face, relapsed when he took Atarax (hydroxyzine dichloride). To explain this reaction it was suggested that hydroxyzine is metabolised to piperazine (Fregert, 1967). Another piperazine sensitive patient whose eczema was aggravated by taking Buclizine (Aphilan R, a piperazine derivative) and Atarax was reported by Calas *et al.* (1975).
Cross-reactions with ethylenediamine have been reported (Calnan, 1975; Burry, 1978).

Respiratory symptoms
In a report from Australia, McCullagh (1968) discussed the occupational hazards of piperazine and described the development of eczema and in one case of respiratory allergy in men preparing a sheep drench containing piperazine.

However, only one of four men with eczema reacted to a patch test with 1 per cent piperazine hexahydrate.

In a Swedish factory processing piperazine and ethylenediamine, 10 men had to stop work because of dermatitis or respiratory symptoms. One 55-year-old employee after two months in a dusty job developed eczema of exposed sites and genitalia and subsequently he also had respiratory symptoms. He did other work and remained well. Two years later he was patch tested with piperazine 1 per cent in water and the following day he had respiratory symptoms and at two days the patch test was strongly positive. Ethylene diamine gave no reaction (Fregert 1976).

Patch testing
Piperazine 5 and 1 per cent in water;
0.1 per cent in water if respiratory allergy is suspected.

PRACTOLOL (4'-(2-Hydroxy-3-isopropylaminopropoxy)acetanilide; Eraldin)

Skin eruptions and eye changes are well recognised complications of systemic treatment with practolol. An erythematous psoriasiform dermatitis with thickening of the palms and soles is particularly characteristic. Oral challenge causes a relapse (Felix, Ive and Dahl, 1974).

PROPRANOLOL (1-(Isopropylamino)-3-(1-naphthyloxy)-2-propanol; Inderal)

PHENOXYBENZAMINE (N-(2-Chloroethyl)-N-(1-methyl-2-phenoxyethyl)-benzylamine: Dibenyline; Dibenzyline)

Phenoxybenzamine hydrochloride is an alpha-adrenergic blocking agent.

Case report
A laboratory technician who prepared pharmacological compounds developed an acute eczema of her hands and face. Patch tests: she reacted to phenoxyben-zamine 1 per cent in water, but not to other compounds. Guinea-pigs were sensitised and reacted to related compounds possibly through the chlorethylamine part of the molecule; they did not react to dichloro-diethylamine (nitrogen mustard)(Mitchell and Maibach, 1975). Phenoxyben-zamine was reported as an irritant and sensitiser by Alexander and Spector (1975).

Patch testing
Phenoxybenzamine 1 per cent aqueous
Propranolol 1 per cent aqueous.

PROPANTHELINE BROMIDE ((2-Hydroxyethyl)diiosopropylmethylam-monium bromide xanthene-9-carboxylate; Pro-banthine; Prodixamon; Ercotina; Ketaman).

Propantheline bromide is anticholinergic with the peripheral, but not the central, actions of atropine. Topically it is used in the treatment of hyperhidrosis.

Case report
In Sweden a woman developed contact dermatitis of the axillae from the Ercotina Derm she had been using for one year to suppress axillary sweating. The eczema healed when she stopped using it, and relapsed when it was reap-plied. Patch tests: she reacted to Ercotina Derm, propantheline bromide and derivatives of xanthene-9-carboxylic acid; tests with phenothiazine and related substances were negative.

It was suggested that propantheline bromide and related chemicals are hydro-lysed on the skin surface to xanthene-9-carboxylic acid, this being the allergen (Fregert and Möller, 1967).

These results were not reproducible by Wereide (1968) in a woman with a similar acute contact dermatitis of the axillae from a month's use of Ercoril deodorant containing 5 per cent propantheline bromide. Patch tests: this woman reacted to propantheline bromide 1 per cent and 2 per cent aqueous, but not to sodium xanthene-9-carboxylate 1 per cent aqueous and β-diisopropyla-minoethanol 1 per cent aqueous.

Patch testing
Propantheline bromide ? per cent aqueous.

QUINIDINE (6-Methoxy-α-(5-vinyl-2-quinuclidinyl)-4-quinolinemethanol; β-quinine)

Quinidine sulphate, a dextrorotary stereoisomer of quinine, is used in the treatment of cardiac arrhythmias.

Contact dermatitis from quinidine is extremely uncommon; two cases reported from Stockholm were both from industrial exposure. Quinidine and quinine do not cross-react.

Case reports
After working for one year grinding drugs and medicaments in a pharmaceutical laboratory, a man developed an episodic dermatitis mainly on the exposed skin but also in the limb flexures. At the same time he complained of lacrimation and rhinorrhoea. Each attack was found to be preceded by exposure to quinidine sulphate. Patch tests: tests with crystals and a 0.5 per cent solution of quinidine sulphate were positive; he did not react to quinine (Fernström, 1965).

In a similar case described by Wahlberg and Forsback (1973), a man had been working in a pharmaceutical factory for two months when he developed dermatitis of his face, neck and upper chest. Shortly before this appeared, he had, in the process of scooping crystals of quinidine sulphate, raised large quantities of its dust. Patch tests: aqueous dilutions of quinidine sulphate from 0.5–0.0625 per cent elicited reactions. Testing with quinine hydrochloride 1 per cent was negative.

Patch testing
Quinidine sulphate 0.5 per cent aqueous.

QUININE

Quinine is an alkaloid obtained from the bark of various species of *Cinchona* trees. Quinine and quinidine are stereoisomers.

At one time quinine was quite widely used in scalp lotions, medications and contraceptives. It is still used by the pharmaceutical industry and also by food manufacturers, mainly for tonic water and bitter lemon.

Case reports
In the past, cases of sensitisation were recorded occasionally but are now rarely if ever seen. In reviewing the relevant literature, Calnan and Caron (1961) described five men with contact dermatitis from quinine. Four had been sensitised by contraceptive preparations, though one of them presented with acute dermatitis from a hair-restoring lotion containing quinine. The fifth man developed a generalised macular erythema each time he drank bitter lemon (containing 3 mg of quinine per 100 ml). One of the patients with contraceptive dermatitis had also developed a rash on his palms, soles and genitalia after ingesting quinine. Patch tests: all reacted to quinine sulphate 1–2 per cent.

Generalised eruptions following oral quinine in sensitised patients have been described by Klaschka (1964). However, the patient with generalised desquamation of the skin, caused possibly by quinine in tonic water, whom Callaway and Tate (1974) reported in a letter, had been neither challenged nor patch tested with quinine.

Occupational dermatitis. An outbreak of dermatitis in factory workers processing quinine was investigated by Hardie *et al.* (1978). Patch testing with a series of quinine and quinidine compounds established that in the majority the effect was irritant but one man was definitely sensitised and another man previously reported (p. 439) continued to have a severe photosensitive eczema and photopatch tests remained positive.

Patch testing
Quinine sulphate 1 per cent in water or petrolatum.

RESORCINOL (1,3-Benzenediol; *m*-dihydroxybenzene; Resorcin)

Resorcinol is keratolytic; it is also used in hair dyes, resins and tanning.

Therapeutically, it is widely used, particularly for acne, but sensitisation is infrequent. Patients sensitised by resorcinol were studied for cross-sensitivity to other hydroxybenzene chemicals by Caron and Calnan (1962) and Keil (1962).

Castellani's paint
Castellani's paint contains magenta, phenol, boric acid, resorcinol, acetone, ethanol and water. It is used extensively in Great Britain, but reactions to the resorcinol it contains occur occasionally. Two such cases of sensitisation from the resorcinol have been reported (Dave, 1973; Cronin, 1973), and another

patient who reacted to its use as a radiotherapy skin marker was described by Marks and West (1978).

St John's

During 1975 and 1976 a further 3 cases were seen. Two patients had used Castellani's paint on their feet and the third applied it to her stasis ulcer. Patch tests: each patient reacted to Castellani's paint and resorcinol 2 per cent in petrolatum.

Patch testing
Resorcinol 2 per cent in petrolatum.

SALICYLIC ACID (2-Hydroxybenzoic acid)

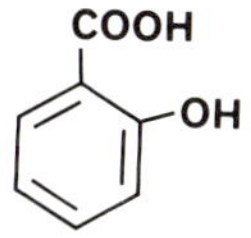

Salicylic acid

METHYL SALICYLATE

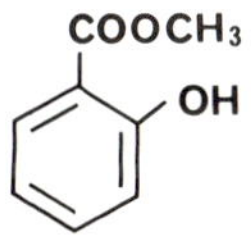

Methyl salicylate

Case report
Reactions to routine patch testing with 5 per cent salicylic acid in petrolatum detected five cases of sensitivity. Each had used salicylic acid preparations and four had noticed discomfort from them. Four of the patients had been sensitised by salicylic acid 2 per cent in spirit, which the men had used as an after-shave lotion and the woman had used as a cleanser. Each took aspirins but none reacted (Rudzki and Koslowska, 1976).

An analgesic ointment containing 12 per cent methyl salicylate sensitised a man and subsequently he relapsed when taking aspirin. Patch tests: he reacted to methyl salicylate 2 per cent (arachis oil) and sodium salicylate 2 per cent (aqueous) but not to an aqueous suspension of aspirin 5 per cent (Hindson, 1977).

SESAME OIL

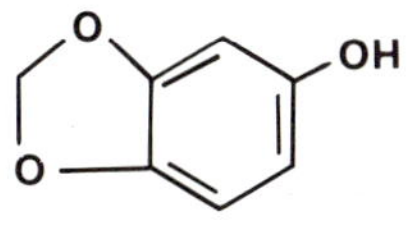

Sesamol (3,4-Methylenedioxyphenol)

Sesamolin   Sesamin

Sesame oil is derived from the seeds of cultivated *Sesamum indicum* L. [Pedaliceae]. It is used in the manufacture of cosmetic and pharmaceutical creams, margarine and iodised oil.

Case reports
In the Netherlands, Linimentum Zinci Oxydi Oleosum (Neth. P.) contains zinc oxide (60 parts), sesame oil (39.3 parts) and crude oleic acid (0.7 parts). This liniment is used in the treatment of stasis ulcers and eczema, and the sesame oil in it has caused contact dermatitis (Malten, 1972: Dijk, Neering and Vitányi, 1973). In an endeavour to isolate the allergens, the oil was fractionated by thin-layer and gas chromatography. The chromatograms were used to patch test 13 patients sensitive to sesame oil: twelve reacted to sesamin, twelve to sesamolin and eight to sesamol (Neering *et al.*, 1975).

Patch testing
Sesame Oil undiluted.

DIETHYLSTILBOESTROL (α,α^1-Diethylstilbenediol)

Case reports
Sensitivity to diethylstilboestrol was described by Fregert and Rorsman (1960) in a woman who developed dermatitis the first time she applied a hair lotion containing diethylstilboestrol 0.04 per cent in 70 per cent ethanol. The source of her sensitivity was not traced. Patch tests: she reacted to the hair lotion and to diethylstilboestrol 0.04 per cent, but not to other components of the lotion. Cross-reactions: there was cross-sensitivity to dienoestrol, hexoestrol, bisphenol A, *p*-benzyl-phenol, monobenzyl ether of hydroquinone and the benzyl ester of *p*-hydroxybenzoic acid. Other patients cross-reacted to benzoestrol (Fregert and Rorsman, 1962).

Patch testing
Diethylstilboestrol 1 per cent in ethanol.

STORAX

Storax is the purified balsam for the Turkish tree *Liquidambar orientalis*; it is a component both of Benzoin Inhalation and of Compound Benzoin Tincture. It has been used as a parasiticide.

Mastic (mastiche) is a resin derived from certain varieties of *Pistacia lentiscus* trees growing in Mediterranean countries. It is used in dentistry, to secure surgical dressings, and in lacquers, chewing gums and incense.

Case reports
Contact dermatitis from Mastisol (containing benzene, castor oil, methyl salicylate, prepared storax and mastic) was described by Mitchell and Dupuis (1972). Patch tests: their patient reacted to storax 2 per cent in petrolatum, benzoin 10 per cent in ethanol, and balsam of Peru 10 per cent in petrolatum.

A woman sensitive to diethylstilboestrol also reacted to storax and balsam of Peru (Fregert and Rorsman, 1960).

Patch testing
Storax 2 per cent in petrolatum.

THIOXOLONE (4-Hydroxy-1,3(2H)-benzoxathiol-2-one; tioxolone; Stepin; Acnosan; Camyna)

Thioxolone is used in the treatment of acne; it is formulated as a 0.1 per cent powder, a 0.2 per cent lotion and a 0.5 per cent solution or tincture.

Case reports
A girl treated her facial acne with Camyna powder for 10 days and then developed dermatitis of her face, hands and arms. Patch tests: she reacted to Camyna solution, lotion and powder, and to thioxolone in ethanol 0.5 per cent and dilutions to 0.005 per cent, but not to 0.001 per cent. Controls: twenty-five eczematous patients were tested with 0.5 per cent Camyna solution and none reacted (Wahlberg, 1971).

Another patient used Camyna solution (2 per cent) for facial acne and developed eczema of the face and widespread nummular patches (Blohm and Rajka, 1966). The solution was chromatographed and the paper strip used for patch testing: the patient reacted to thioxolone 0.005 per cent, but not to phenols.

Patch testing

Thioxolone ?0.5 per cent in ethanol.

TRIAFUR (Nitrofurylaminothiadiazole; 2-amino-5-(5-nitro-2-furyl)-1,3,
4-thiadiazole; Roinal; Furidiazina)

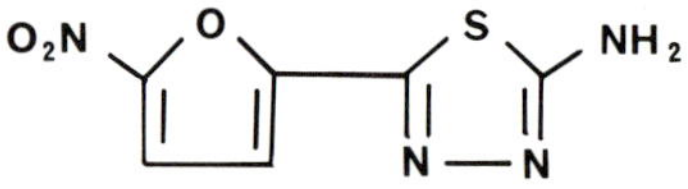

Case reports

In Sweden, five patients used either an ointment or suppositories containing this
thiadiazole compound (0.7 per cent) for haemorrhoids or pruritus ani and
developed contact dermatitis (Fregert, 1968). Patch tests: each reacted to the
medicament and to nitrofurylaminothiadiazole 1 per cent in petrolatum. By
studying the cross-sensitivity patterns it was established that the nitro group on
the furan ring and the close bonding of the furan and thiadiazole rings were
necessary to elicit a reaction.

Tests with nitrofurantoin (Furadantin) and nitrofurazone (Furacin), which
have no thiadiazole ring, were negative (Fregert, 1968).

Patch testing

Triafur 1 per cent in petrolatum.

TRITON X45 (*para*-Octyl phenol ethylene oxide)

This chemical is a wetting agent which has been widely used in cosmetics and
in pharmaceutical preparations. It is also used in textile processing, metal cleaning, and dry cleaning solvents, and as a solvent in inks for ball-point pens
(Comaish, 1970).

Case report

A woman used Nystaform ointment (Dome Laboratories) containing 5 per cent
Triton X45 on her genital skin and developed a contact dermatitis with a severe
secondary spread which required admission to hospital and treatment with systemic steroids. Patch tests: she reacted to Triton X45 0.1 per cent in water.
Controls: eleven were tested with Triton X45 1 per cent in water; two had irritant reactions, one a doubtful response and eight did not react (Comaish, 1970).

Patch testing

Triton X45 0.1 per cent in water.

XERUMENEX

Xerumenex (Napp Lab. Ltd.), containing 10 per cent triethanolamine polypeptide oleate condensate, is a solvent for ear wax.

Case reports

Sensitisation to Xerumenex causes severe reactions. A man put Xerumenex into both his ears and left it there overnight instead of flushing it out within 15–30 minutes as directed by the manufacturers. The next day he had acute eczema of his ears, face, neck and upper chest, and marked swelling of his eyelids. Patch tests: one drop of Xerumenex gave a reaction 8 cm in diameter, and of the ingredients he reacted strongly to triethanolamine polypeptide oleate-condensate 1 per cent; the other ingredients and triethanolamine 10 per cent elicited no reaction. Controls: of eight controls, three reacted slightly and one moderately to Xerumenex; and of six tested with 1 per cent triethanolamine polypeptide oleate-condensate one reacted weakly (Grice and Johnstone, 1972). A similar patient with a severe widespread eczema from Xerumenex was described by Boxley and Dawber (1976).

St John's

In 1975 and 1976, two patients, similar to those reported, were investigated. Patch tests: both reacted to Xerumenex strongly and to triethanolamine polypeptide oleate condensate.

Patch testing

Xerumenex 25 per cent

Triethanolamine polypeptide oleate-condensate 1 per cent.

Xerumenex undiluted is mildly irritant in patch tests, and several such reactions have been seen at St John's; these patients did not react when tested with the separate constituents.

References

Aeling, J.L., Panagotacos, P.J. & Andreozzi, R.J. (1973) Allergic contact dermatitis in vitamin E in aerosol deodorant. *Archives of Dermatology*, **108**, 579.

Agache, P. & Bidard De La Noë, A.M. (1972) Granulomes des fesses par pentazocine. *Bulletin de la Société Francaise de Dermatologie et de Syphilographie*, **79**, 37.

Alani, M.D. & Alani, S.D. (1972) Allergic contact dermatitis to corticosteroids. *Annals of Allergy*, **30**, 181.

Alani, S.D. & Alani, M.D. (1976a) Allergic contact dermatitis and conjunctivitis from epinephrine. *Contact Dermatitis*, **2**, 147.

Alani, S.D. & Alani, M.D. (1976b) Allergic contact dermatitis and conjunctivitis to corticosteroids. *Contact Dermatitis*,**2**, 301.

Alexander, S. & Spector, R.G. (1975) Phenoxybenzamine. *Contact Dermatitis*, **1**, 59.

Alleby, C.F. (1965) Skin sensitisation to remiderm and cross-sensitisation to hydroxy-quinoline compounds. *British Medical Journal*, **ii**, 208.

Amon, R.B., Lis, A.W. & Hanifin, J.M. (1975) Allergic contact dermatitis caused by idoxuridine. *Archives of Dermatology*, **111**, 1581.

Baer, R.L., Cohen, H.J. & Neidorff, A.H. (1959) Allergic eczematous sensitivity to aminophylline. *Archives of Dermatology*, **79**, 647.

Baer, R.L. & Ludwig J.S. (1952) Allergic eczematous sensitisation to neomycin. *Annals of Allergy*, **10**, 136.

Baer, R.L., Michaelides, P. & Prestia A.E. (1972) Failure to induce immune tolerance to nitrogen mustard. *Journal of Investigative Dermatology*, **58**, 1.

Baes, H. (1974) Allergic contact dermatitis to virginiamycin. *Dermatologica*, **149**, 231.

Bandmann, H.-J. (1971) Ichthyol dermatitis. *Contact Dermatitis Newsletter*, **10**, 224.

Bandmann, H.-J. (1972) Sind Chloramphenikolhaltige externa kontraindiziert. *Der Hautarzt*, **23**, 145.

Bandmann, H.-J.& Breit, R. (1974) Die medikamentöse allergische Kontaktdermatitis. *Internist*, **15**, 47.

Bandmann, H.-J., Breit, R. and Mutzeck, E. (1974) Allergic contact dermatitis from proxymetacaine. *Contact Dermatitis Newsletter*, **15**, 451.

Bandmann, H.-J. & Doenicke, A. (1970) Occupational dermatitis from propanidid. *Contact Dermatitis Newsletter*, **8**, 189.

Bandmann, H.-J., Hubert-Riffeser, G. & Woyton, A. (1966) Kontaktallergie gegen Triancinolonacetonid. *Hautarzt*, **17**, 183.

Bandmann, H.-J. & Mutzek, E. (1973) Contact allergy to gentamycin sulfate. *Contact Dermatitis Newsletter*, **13**, 371.

Barnes, H.M. & Sarkany, I. (1976) Adverse skin reaction from vitamin K_1. *British Journal of Dermatology*, **95**, 653.

Beare, J.M. (1947) Generalised skin sensitivity following local application of acriflavine: Report of case. *Lancet*, **1**, 410.

Behrbohm, P. & Lenzner, M. (1975) Sensitivity to falicain (Propoxypiperocainhydrochloride). *Contact Dermatitis*, **1**, 187.

Behrbohm, P. & Zschunke, E. (1965) Allergisches Ekzem durch das antimykotium 'Afungin' (Dibenzthion). *Dermatologische Wochenschrift*, **151**, 1447.

Bereston, E.S. (1952) Contact dermatitis due to N-ethyl-o-crotonotoluide ointment (Eurax). *Archives of Dermatology*, **65**, 100.

Berlin. A.R. & Miller, F. (1976) Allergic contact dermatitis from ethyl sebacate in haloprogin cream. *Archives of Dermatology*, **112**, 156.

Bernstein, J.E. & Lorincz, A.L. (1979) Ethylenediamine-induced exfoliative erythroderma. *Archives of Dermatology*, **115**, 360.

Bielicky, T. & Novák, M. (1969) Contact-group sensitisation to triphenylmethane dyes. *Archives of Dermatology*, **100**, 540.

Binnick, A.N. & Clendenning, W.E. (1978) Bacitracin contact dermatitis. *Contact Dermatitis*, **4**, 181.

Black, H. (1971) Allergy to cycloheximide (Actidione). *Contact Dermatitis Newsletter*, **10**, 243.

Black, H. (1972) *Contact Dermatitis Newsletter*, **12**, 323.

Bleumink, E., Lintum te J.C.A. & Nater J.P. (1974) Kontaktallergie durch Nitrofurazon (Furacin) und Nifurprazin (Carofur). *Hautarzt*, **25**, 403.

Bleumink, E. & Nater, J.P. (1972a) Allergic contact dermatitis to virginiamycin. *Dermatologica*, **144**, 253.

Bleumink, E. & Nater, J.P. (1972b) Allergic contact dermatitis to virginiamycin (Staphlomycin) and pristinamycin (Stapyocin). *Contact Dermatitis Newsletter*, **12**, 337.

Blohm, G. & Rajka, G. (1966) A simple method for combined chemical and dermatological analysis of chemical mixtures by paper chromatography. *Acta Dermato-venereologica*, **46**, 432.

Bojs, G. & Möller, H. (1974) Eczematous contact allergy to oxytetracycline with cross sensitivity to other tetracyclines. *Berufsdermatosen*, **22**, 202.

Boonen, W. & Waveren Hogervorst, van J.W. (1964) Hypersensitivity to antibiotics. *Dermatologica*, **128**, 394.

Bowyer, A. (1972) Tolnaftate *Contact Dermatitis Newsletter*, **12**, 339.

Boxley, J.D. & Dawber, R.P.R. (1976) Contact dermatitis to one ingredient of Xerumenex ear drops. *Contact Dermatitis*, **2**, 233.

Braun, W. & Schütz, R. (1968) Kontaktallergie gegen Nitrofurazon (Furacin) *Deutsche Medizinische Wochenschrift*, **93**, 1524.

Braun, W. & Schütz, R. (1969) Beitrag zur Gentamycin Allergie. *Hautarzt*, **20**, 108.

Breit, R. & Bandmann, H.-J. (1973) Contact dermatitis XXIV. The wide world of antimycotics. *British Journal of Dermatology*, **89**, 657.

Brodkin, R.H. & Bleiberg, J. (1965) Sensitivity to topically applied vitamin E. *Archives of Dermatology*, **92**, 76.

Brown, E.A. (1948) Reactions to penicillin. A review of the literature 1943– 1948. *Annals of Allergy*, **6**, 723.

Bullen, A.W., Miller, J.P., Cunliffe, W.J. & Losowsky, M.S. (1978) Skin reactions caused by vitamin K in patients with liver disease. *British Journal of Dermatology*, **98**, 561.

Burckhardt, W. (1959) Kontaktekzem durch Hydrocortison. *Hautarzt*, **10**, 42.

Burckhardt, W., Kaufmann, J. & Brenn, H. (1970) Ekzem durch Aethylendiaminin der kunst-Faserindustrie. *Dermatologica*, **141**, 154.

Burry, J.N. (1978) Ethylenediamine sensitivity with a systemic reaction to piperazine citrate. *Contact Dermatitis*, **4**, 380.

Burry, J.N. Kirk, J., Reid, J.G. & Turner, T. (1973) Environmental dermatitis: Patch test in 1000 cases of allergic contact dermatitis. *The Medical Journal of Australia*, **2**, 681.

Calas, E., Castelain, P.-Y., Blanc, A. & Campana, J.-M. (1975) Un nouveau cas de sensibilisation á la pipérazine. *Bulletin Société Francaise de dermatologie et de Syphiligraphie*, **82**, 41.

Callaway, J.L. & Tate, W.E. (1974) Toxic epidermal necrolysis caused by 'gin and tonic'. *Archives of Dermatology*, **109**, 909.

Calnan, C.D. (1967) Chlortetracycline sensitivity. *Contact Dermatitis Newsletter*, **1**, 16.

Calnan, C.D. (1971) Ichthyol. *Contact Dermatitis Newsletter*, **9**, 218.

Calnan, C.D. (1972) Contact dermatitis to mesulphen. *Contact Dermatitis Newsletter*, **11**, 283.

Calnan, C.D. (1975) Occupational piperazine dermatitis. *Contact Dermatitis*, **1**, 126.

Calnan, C.D. & Caron, G.A. (1961) Quinine sensitivity. *British Medical Journal*, **ii**, 1750.

Calnan, C.D. & Sarkany, I. (1958) Contact dermatitis from neomycin. *British Journal of Dermatology*, **70**, 435.

Caron, G.A. & Calnan, C.D. (1962) Studies in contact dermatitis. XIV resorcin. *Transactions of the St John's Hospital Dermatological Society*, **48**, 149.

Carruthers, J.A. & Cronin, E. (1976) Incidence of neomycin and framycetin sensitivity. *Contact Dermatitis*, **2**, 269.

Chandraratna, P.A.N. & O'Dell, R.E. (1979) Allergic reactions to nitroglycerin ointment: report of five cases. *Current Therapeutic Research*, **25**, 481.

Chung, C.W. & Carson, T.R. (1975) Sensitisation potentials and immunological specificities of neomycins. *Journal of Investigative Dermatology*, **64**, 158.

Church, R. (1960) Sensitivity to hydrocortisone acetate ointment. *British Journal of Dermatology*, **72**, 341.

Comaish, J.S. (1970) Reaction to triton X45. *Contact Dermatitis Newsletter*, **7**, 167.

Comaish, J.S. & Cunliffe, W.J. (1967) Absorption of drugs from varicose ulcers: A cause of anaphylaxis. *British Journal of Clinical Practice*, **21**, 97.

Comaish, S. (1969) A case of hypersensitivity to corticosteroids. *British Journal of Dermatology*, **81**, 919.

Combes, F.C. & Groopman, J. (1950) Contact dermatitis due to thiamine. *Archives of Dermatology*, **61**, 858.

Connor, B.L. (1973) Mesulphen in tineafax ointment. *Contact Dermatitis Newsletter*, **14**, 417.

Cooke, M.A. & Hocken Robertson, D.-E. (1972) Ichthammol dermatitis. *Contact Dermatitis Newsletter*, **11**, 299.

Coskey, R.J. (1971a) Contact dermatitis due to nystatin. *Archives of Dermatology*, **103**, 228.

Coskey, R.J. (1971b) Contact dermatitis due to nystatin: Reply. *Archives of Dermatology*, **104**, 438.

Coskey, R.J. (1978) Contact dermatitis due to multiple corticosteroid creams. *Archives of Dermatology*, **114**, 115.

Coskey, R.J. (1978) Contact dermatitis owing to tincture of benzoin. *Archives of Dermatology*. **114**, 128

Coskey, R.J. (1978) Contact dermatitis due to clindamycin. *Archives of Dermatology*, **114**, 446.

Coskey, R.J. & Bryan, H.G. (1967) Contact dermatitis due to methylprednisolone. *Journal of the American Medical Association*, **199**, 136.

Cronin, E. (1969) Genetris pessaries. *Contact Dermatitis Newsletter*, **6**, 134.

Cronin, E. (1973) Resorcin in castellani's paint. *Contact Dermatitis Newsletter*, **14**, 401.

Crow, K. (1972) Dermatitis from ethylenediamine. *Contact Dermatitis Newsletter*, **11**, 284.

Crow, K.D., Peachey, R.D.G. & Adams, J.E. (1978) Coolant oil dermatitis due to ethylenediamine. *Contact Dermatitis*, **4**, 359.

Dahlquist, I. (1977) Allergic reactions to apomorphine. *Contact Dermatitis*, **3**, 349.

Dalton, J.E. & Pierce, J.D. (1951) Dermatological problems among pharmaceutical workers. *Archives of Dermatology*, **64**, 667.

Daughters, D., Zackheim, H. & Maibach, H. (1973) Urticaria and anaphylactoid reactions. *Archives of Dermatology*, **107**, 429.

Dave, V.K. (1973) Contact dermatitis due to resorcin in Castellani's paint. *Contact Dermatitis Newsletter*, **13**, 384.

Dave, V.K. & Main, R.A. (1973) Contact sensitivity to sodium fusidate. *Contact Dermatitis Newsletter*, **14**, 398.

Davenport, P.M. & Wilheim, R.E. (1965) An unusual vasculitis due to diphenhydramine. *Archives of Dermatology*, **92**, 577.

Degreef, H. & Verhoeve, L. (1975) Contact dermatitis to miconazole nitrate. *Contact Dermatitis*, **1**, 269.

Dernehl, C.U. (1951) Clinical experiences with exposures to ethylene amines. *Industrial Medicine and Surgery*, **20**, 541.

Dijk, E. van., Neering, H. & Vitányi, B.E.J. (1973) Contact hypersensitivity to sesame oil in patients with leg ulcers and eczema. *Acta Dermato-venereologica*, **53**, 133.

Dijk, T.J.A. van & Marien, K. (1972) Allergic contact dermatitis from Eurax. *Contact Dermatitis Newsletter*, **12**, 344.

Dohn, W. (1960) Übersichten, Kontaktallergien gegen Antibiotica. *Hautarzt*, **11**, 433.

Douglas, W.W. (1975) Histamine and antihistamines; 5-Hydroxytryptamine and antagonists. In *Pharmacological Basis of Therapeutics* ed. Goodman L.S. and Gilman A. p. 636. London: Balliere Tindall.

Drake, T.E. (1974) Reaction to gentamicin sulfate cream. *Archives of Dermatology*, **110**, 638.

Eberhatinger, C. (1964) Kontaktallergie gegen Äthylendiamin. *Hautarzt*, **15**, 450.

Ekelund, A-G & Möller, H. (1969) Oral prevocation in eczematous contact allergy to Neomycin and Hydroxy-Quinolines. *Acta Dermato-venereologica*, **49**, 422.

Emmett, E.A. & Marrs, J.M. (1973) Allergic contact dermatitis from tolnaftate. *Archives of Dermatology*, **108**, 98.

Epstein, E. (1949) Dermatitis due to antihistaminic agents. *Journal of Investigative Dermatology*, **12**, 151.

Epstein, E. (1966) Allergic dermatitis from chlordantoin vaginal cream. *Obstetrics and Gynaecology*, **27**, 369.

Epstein, E. (1974) Negative patch tests to ethylenediamine tetra acetate in patients allergic to ethylenediamine. *Contact dermatitis Newsletter*, **16**, 475.

Epstein, E. & Maibach, H.I. (1968) Ethylenediamine. Allergic contact dermatitis. *Archives of Dermatology*, **98**, 476.

Epstein, E. Jr. & Ugel, A.R. (1970) Effects of topical mechlorethamine on skin lesions of psoriasis. *Archives of Dermatology*, **102**, 504.

Epstein, S. (1958) Dermal contact dermatitis. *Dermatologica*, **117**, 287.

Epstein, S. & Wenzel, F.J. (1962) Cross-sensitivity to various 'mycins'. *Archives of Dermatology*, **86**, 183.

Epstein, S. & Wenzel, F.J. (1963) Sensitivity to neomycin and bacitracin, cross-sensitisation or coincidence. *Acta Dermato-venereologica*, **43**, 1.

Eriksen, K. (1978) Cross allergy between paranitro compounds with special reference to DNCB and chloramphenicol. *Contact Dermatitis*, **4**, 29.

Eriksen, K.E. (1975) Allergy to ethylenediamine. *Archives of Dermatology*, **111**, 791.

Fanta, D. & Mischer, P. (1976) Contact dermatitis from tromantadine hydrochloride. *Contact Dermatitis*, **2**, 282.

Felix, R.H., Ive, A. & Dahl, M.G.C. (1974) Cutaneous and ocular reactions to practolol. *British Medical Journal*, **iv**, 321.

Fernström, A.I.B. (1959) Studies on procaine allergy with reference to urticaria due to procaine penicillin treatment. A. The most common types of reactions in penicillin treatment and a review of the literature on the incidence of reactions. *Acta Dermato-venereologica*, **39**, 433.

Fernström, A.I.B. (1960a) Studies on procaine allergy with reference to urticaria due to procaine penicillin treatment. B. The medical uses of procaine and reactions due to procaine penicillin. Reveiw of the literature. *Acta Dermato-venereologica*, **40**, 19.

Fernström, A.I.B. (1960b) Studies on procaine allergy with reference to urticaria due to procaine penicillin treatment. C. Reactions following procaine due to direct skin contact or injection; Hypersensitivity to procaine as an expression of cross-sensitisation; Effects of procaine penicillin in persons with clinically verified sensitivity to procaine or chemically related substances; Review of the literature. *Acta Dermato-venereologica*, **40**, 175.

Fernström, A.I.B. (1960c) Studies on procaine allergy with reference to urticaria due to procaine penicillin treatment. D. Serologic and skin tests and their clinical value in penicillin allergy; Review of the literature. *Acta Dermato-venereologica*, **40**, 273.

Fernström, A.I.B. (1962) Studies on procaine allergy with reference to urticaria due to procaine penicillin treatment. E. Original investigation. *Acta Dermato-venereologica*, **42**, 79.

Fernström, A.I.B. (1965) Occupational quinidine contact dermatitis, a concept apparently not yet described. *Acta Dermato-venereologica*, **45**, 129.

Fischer, T. & Hartvig, P. (1977) Absorption of 8-hydroxyquinolines. *Lancet*, **1**, 603.

Fish, A.J. & Freedman. S.O. (1964) Chemical groupings responsible for delayed-type intradermal reactions to procaine. *Journal of Investigative Dermatology*, **42**, 235.

Fisher, A.A. (1973) The broad implications of allergic sensitisation to ethylenediamine hydrochloride. *Contact Dermatitis Newsletter*, **14**, 418.

Fisher, A.A. (1974) Instructions for the ethylenediamine-sensitive patient. *Cutis*, **13**, 27.

Fisher, A.A. (1975) Does ethylenediamine hydrochloride cross-react with ethylenediamine tetraacetate? *Contact Dermatitis*, **1**, 267.

Fisher, A.A. (1976) The safety of topical erythromycin. *Contact Dermatitis*, **2**, 43.

Fisher, A.A. (1977) Erythromycin 'Free Base' — A nonsensitising topical antibiotic for infected, dermatoses and acne vulgaris. *Cutis*, **20**, 17.

Forssman, O & Mulder, J. (1973) Hypersensitivity to different ACTH peptides. *Acta Medica Scandinavica*, **193**, 557.

Förström, L., Hannuksela, M., Idänpään-Heikkilä, J. & Salo, O.P. (1977) Hypersensitivity reactions to gerovital®. *Dermatologica*, **154**, 367.

Förström, L. & Pirilä, V. (1978) Cross-sensitivity within the neomycin group of antibiotics. *Contact Dermatitis*, **4**, 312.

Foussereau, J. & Benezra, Cl (1967) Données nouvelles sur l'allergie de groupe á la pipérazine *Bulletin de la Société Francaise de dermatologie et de syphilographie*, **74**, 45.

Foussereau, J. & Lantz, J.P. (1972) Allergy to meclofenoxate. *Contact Dermatitis Newsletter*, **12**, 321.

Foussereau, J. Limam-Mestiri, S., Khochnevis, A. & Basset, A. (1971) L'allergie á l'association thérapeutique locale nystatine, néomycine et acetonide de triamcinolone. *Bulletin de la Société Francaise de Dermatologie et de Syphiligraphie*, **78**, 457.

Fregert, S. (1967) Exacerbation of dermatitis by perorally administered piperazine derivative in a piperazine-sensitised man. *Contact Dermatitis Newsletter*, **1**, 13.

Fregert, S. (1968) Cross-sensitisation among nitrofurylaminothiadiazoles. *Acta Dermato-venereologica*, **48**, 106.

Fregert, S. (1976) Respiratory symptoms with piperazine patch testing. *Contact Dermatitis*, **2**, 61.

Fregert, S., Hjorth, N., Magnusson, B., Bandmann, H.-J., Calnan, C.D. Cronin, E., Malten, K., Meneghini, C.L., Pirila, V. & Wilkinson, D.S. (1969) Epidemiology of contact dermatitis. *Transactions of the St John's Hospital Dermatological Society*, **55**, 17.

Fregert, S. & Möller, H. (1967) Allergic contact dermatitis from probantheline bromide. *Contact Dermatitis Newsletter*, **1**, 12.

Fregert, S. & Rorsman, H. (1960) Hypersensitivity to diethylstilboestrol. *Acta Dermato-venereologica*, **40**, 206.

Fregert, S. & Rorsman, H. (1962) Hypersensitivity to diethylstilboestrol with cross-sensitisation to Benzestrol. *Acta Dermato-venereologica*, **42**, 290.

Frost, P. & Devita, V.T. (1966) Pigmentation due to a new antitumour agent. *Archives of Dermatology*, **94**, 265.

Garcia-Perez, A. & Moran, M. (1975) Dermatitis from quinolines. *Contact Dermatitis*, **1**, 260.

Gellin, G.A., Maibach, H.I. & Wachs, G.N. (1972) Contact allergy to tolnaftate. *Archives of Dermatology*, **106**, 715.

Gibbs, R.C. (1970) Allergic contact dermatitis to epinephrine. *Archives of Dermatology*, **101**, 92.

Goette, D.K., Odom, R.B., & Owens, R. (1977) Allergic contact dermatitis from topical fluorouracil. *Archives of Dermatology*, **113**, 196.

Goldstein, M.B. (1940) Sensitivity to gentian violet. *Archives of Dermatology*, **41**, 122.

Goodman, M.H. (1939) Cutaneous hypersensitivity to the procaine anaesthetics. *Journal of Investigative Dermatology*, **2**, 53.

Göransson, K. (1976) Hypersensitivity to prilocaine. *Dermatologica*, **152**, 158.

Grice K & Johnstone, C.I. (1972) Contact dermatitis from xerumenex. *British Medical Journal*, **i**, 508.

Groen, J., Bleumink, E. & Nater, J.P. (1974) Variotin sensitivity. *Contact Dermatitis Newsletter*, **15**, 456.

Gutzwiller, P. (1974) Zum Problem der Kortikosteroid-allergie. *Dermatologica*, **148**, 253.

Hardie, R.A., Savin, J.A., White, D.A. & Pumford, S. (1978) Quinine dermatitis: Investigation of a factory outbreak. *Contact Dermatitis*, **4**, 121.

Harrold, B.P. (1966) Syndrome resembling Addison's disease following prolonged treatment with busulphan. *British Medical Journal*, **i**, 463.

Hecke, E. van (1973) Allergy to Bufexamac. *Archives Belges de Dermatologie*, **29**, 301.

Hegyi, E. (1960) Hautschäden durch Epoxydharze. *Lékařstvi*, **12**, 9. Abstract *Berufsdermatosen* (*1960*), **8**, 164.

Hegyi, E. (1969) Procain sensitivity 1948–1967. *Contact Dermatitis Newsletter*, **5**, 95.

Helm, F. & Klein, E. (1965) Effects of allergic contact dermatitis on basal cell epitheliomas. *Archives of Dermatology*, **91**, 142.

Hepps, S. & Dollinger, M. (1965) Anaphylactic death after administration of a triphenylmethane dye to determine burn depth. *New England Journal of Medicine*, **272**, 1281.

Heydenreich, G.(1977) A further case of adverse skin reaction from vitamin K₁. *British Journal of Dermatology*, **97**, 697.

Hindson, C. (1977) Contact eczema from methyl salicylate reproduced by oral aspirin (acetyl salicylic acid). *Contact Dermatitis*, **3**, 348.

Hjorth, N. (1958) Contact dermatitis from vitamin B₁ (Thiamine). *Journal of Investigative Dermatology*, **30**, 261.

Hjorth, N. (1969) Dermatitis from ethylenediamine. *Contact Dermatitis Newsletter*, **5**, 107.

Hjorth, N. (1972) Contact dermatitis from 1, 3-diiodo-2-hydroxypropane. *Contact Dermatitis Newsletter*, **12**, 322.

Hjorth, N. (1974) Contact dermatitis from vitamin E and from combelen (Bayer) in a veterinary surgeon. *Contact Dermatitis Newsletter*, 15, 434.

Hjorth, N. & Fregert, S. (1972) Textbook of Dermatology. ed. Rook A., Wilkinson, D.S. and Ebling, F.J. 2nd edition, p. 319. Oxford: Blackwell.

Hjorth, N. & Thomsen, K. (1968) Difference in the sensitising capacity of neomycin in creams and in ointments. *British Journal of Dermatology*, 80, 163.

Hofmann, H., Maibach, H.I., & Prout, E. (1975) Presumed generalised exfoliative dermatitis to Lidocaine. *Archives of Dermatology*, 111, 266.

Horsfield, P., Logan, F.A. & Newey, J.A. (1976) Oral irritation with gentian violet. *British Medical Journal*, ii, 529.

Hull, P.R. & Beer, H.A. De. (1977) Topical nitrofurazone, a potent sensitizer of the skin and mucosae. *South African Medical Journal*, 52, 189.

Huriez, Cl., Martin, P., & Bétourné, M. (1972) Allergic contact dermatitis from carbocroméne in nurses. *Contact Dermatitis Newsletter*, 12, 313.

Ippen, H. (1978) Kontaktekzem durch Isonicotinsaurehydrazid. *Dermatosen in Beruf und Umwelt*, 26, 57.

Jensen, O.C., Allen, H.J. & Nordecai, L.R. (1966) Neomycin contact dermatitis superimposed on otitis externa. *Journal of the American Medical Association*, 195, 131.

Jirásek, L. & Schwank, R. (1965) Berufskontaktekzem durch Vitamin K. *Hautarzt*, 16, 351.

Jordan, W.P., Higgins, M. & Dvorak, J. (1975) Allergic contact dermatitis to all-trans-retinoic acid; epicutaneous and leukocyte migration inhibition testing. *Contact Dermatitis*, 1, 306.

Kalveram, K., Günnewig, W., Wehling, K. & Forck, G. (1978) Tetracaine allergy: cross-reactions with para-compounds ? *Contact Dermatitis*, 4, 376.

Kassen, B. & Mitchell, J.C. (1974) Contact urticaria from a vitamin E preparation in two siblings. *Contact Dermatitis Newsletter*, 16, 482.

Keil, H. (1962) Group reactions in contact dermatitis due to resorcinol, *Archives of Dermatology*, 86, 212.

Kero, M., Hannuksela, M. & Sothman, A. (1979) Primary irritant dermatitis from topical clioquinol. *Contact Dermatitis*, 5, 115.

Ketel, van W.G. (1967) Allergic dermatitis caused by tineafax ointment. *Dermatologica*, 135, 121.

Ketel, van W.G. (1973) Allergy to cumarin and cumarin-derivatives. *Contact Dermatitis Newsletter*, 13, 355.

Ketel, van W.G. (1974) Allergy to miconazole nitrate (Daktarin). *Contact Dermatitis Newsletter*, 16, 517.

Ketel, van W.G. (1974) Polymixine B-sulphate and bacitracin. *Contact Dermatitis Newsletter*, 15, 445.

Ketel, van W.G. (1976) Immediate — and delayed — type allergy to erythromycin. *Contact Dermatitis*, 2, 363.

Kile, R.L. Rockwell, E.M. & Schwarz, J. (1952) Use of neomycin in dermatology. *Journal of the American Medical Association*, 148, 339.

King, R.A. (1960) A severe anaphylactoid reaction to hydrocortisone. *Lancet*, 2, 1093.

Kirton, V., & Munro-Ashman, D. (1965) Contact dermatitis from neomycin and framycetin. *Lancet*, 1, 138.

Klaschka, F. (1964) Zur Kasuistik hochgradiger Chinin-kontaktallergie. *Dermatologische Wochenschrift*, 149, 4.

Kligman, A.M. (1966) The identification of contact allergens by human assay. *Journal of Investigative Dermatology*, 47, 393.

Knisley, R.E., Settipane, G.A. & Albala, M.M. (1971) Unusual reaction to chlorambucil in a patient with chronic lymphatic leukaemia. *Archives of Dermatology*, 104, 77.

Knox, J.M., Guin, J., & Cockerell, E.G. (1957) Benzophenones: Ultraviolet light absorbing agents. *Journal of Investigative Dermatology*, 29, 435.

Kozákova, M. (1976) Sub-shock state brought on by epidermic skin test for chloramphenicol. *Ceskoslovenská dermatologie*, 51, 82.

Kooij, R. (1959) Hypersensitivity to hydrocortisone. *British Journal of Dermatology*, 71, 392.

Krook, G. (1975) Contact sensitivity to oxyphenbutazone (Tanderil) and cross-sensitivity to phenylbutazone (Butazolidin). *Contact Dermatitis*, 1, 262.

Lachapelle, J.M. (1975) Contact sensitivity to bufexamac. *Contact Dermatitis*, 1, 261.

Lachapelle, J.M. & Lamy, F. (1973) On allergic contact dermatitis to virginiamycin. *Dermatologica*, 146, 320.

Lane, C.G. (1921) Occupational dermatitis in dentists: Susceptibility to procaine. *Archives of Dermatology*, 3, 235.

Leifer, W. & Steiner, K. (1951) Studies in sensitisation to halogenated hydroxyquinolines and related compounds. *Journal of Investigative Dermatology*, 17, 233.

Lidén, S. & Goransson, K. (1975) Contact allergy to dibenzthion. *Contact Dermatitis*, 1, 258.

Magnusson, B., Blohm, S.-G., Fregert, S., Hjorth, N., Hovding, G., Pirilä, V. & Skog, E. (1968) Routine patch testing IV. *Acta Dermato-venereologica*, 48, 110.

Magnusson, B. & Kligman, A.M. (1969) The identification of contact allergens by animal assay: The guinea pig maximisation test. *Journal of Investigative Dermatology*, 52, 268.

Maquire, H.C. Jr. (1974) Induction of delayed hypersensitivity to nitrogen mustard in the guinea pig, *British Journal of Dermatology*, 91, 21.

Maibach, H. & Epstein, E. (1971) Ethylenediamine sensitivity: Incidence in San Francisco. *Contact Dermatitis Newsletter*, 9, 207.

Malten, K.E. (1972) Sesamoil contact hypersensitivity in leg ulcer patients. *Contact Dermatitis Newsletter*, 11, 251.

Mansell, P.W.A., Litwin, M.S., Ichinose, H. & Krementz, E.T. (1975) Delayed hypersensitivity to 5-fluorouracil following topical chemotherapy of cutaneous cancers. *Cancer Research*, 35, 1288.

March, C. & Greenwood, M.A. (1968) Allergic contact dermatitis to proparacaine. *Archives of Ophthalmology*, 79, 159.

Marks, J.G. & West, G.W. (1978) Allergic contact dermatitis to radiotherapy dye. *Contact Dermatitis*, 4, 1.

Marcussen, P.V. (1949) Professional streptomycin hypersensitiveness among hospital staffs. *Acta Dermato-venereologica*, 29, 410.

Marcussen, P.V. (1962) Variations in the incidence of contact hypersensitivities. *Transactions of the St John's Hospital Dermatological Society*, 48, 40.

Martin, P., Betourné, M., Martin, J.-J. & Huriez, Cl. (1973) Allergie au carbocroméne. *Bulletin de la Société Francaise de Dermatologie et de Syphiligraphie*, 80, 620.

Marzulli, F.N. & Maibach, H.I. (1973) Antimicrobials: Experimental contact sensitisation in man. *Journal of the Society of Cosmetic Chemists*, 24, 399.

McCullagh, S.F. (1968) Allergenicity of piperazine: A study in environmental aetiology. *British Journal of Industrial Medicine*, 25, 319.

Mendelson, L.M., Meltzer, E.O. and Hamburger, R.N. (1974) Anaphylaxis-like reactions to corticosteroid therapy. *Journal of Allergy and Clinical Immunology*, 54, 125.

Meneghini, C.L. & Angelini, G. (1975) Contact dermatitis from pyrrolnitrin (an antimycotic agent). *Contact Dermatitis*, 1, 288.

Meurer, M. & Konz, B. (1977) Hautnekrosen nach Anwendung 2 per cent iger Pyoktaninlösung. *Hautarzt*, 28, 94.

Michel, P.-J, Buyer, R. & Delorme. (1958) Accidents généraux (cyanose, collapsus cardio-vasculaire) par sensibilisation á une solution aqueuse de violet de genitiane et vert de méthyle en applications locales. *Bulletin de la Société Francaise de Dermatologie et de Syphiligraphie*, 65 183.

Michie, W. & Bailie, H.W.C. (1945) A case of penicillin reaction. *British Medical Journal*, i, 554.

Millard, L.G. & Rajah, S.M. (1977) Cutaneous reaction to chlorambucil. *Archives of Dermatology*, 113, 1298.

Minkin, W., Cohen, H.J. & Frank, S.B. (1973) Contact dermatitis from deodorants. *Archives of Dermatology*, 107, 774.

Mitchell, J.C. (1972) Contact dermatitis from proflavine dihydrochloride. *Archives of Dermatology*, 106, 924.

Mitchell, J.C. & Dupuis, G. (1972) Allergic contact dermatitis from storax (styrax). *Contact Dermatitis Newsletter*, 11, 274.

Mitchell, J.C. & Maibach, H.I. (1975) Allergic contact dermatitis from phenoxybenzamine hydrochloride. *Contact Dermatitis*, 1, 363.

Mohr, P.D. (1975) Allergic reactions to tetracosactrin. *British Medical Journal*, iv, 162.

Möller, H. (1970) Eczematous contact allergy to oxytetracycline and polymyxin B. *Contact Dermatitis*, 2, 289.

Mortazavi, S.H. & Burrows B.D. (1971) Allergic reaction to patent blue dye in lymphangiography. *Clinical Radiology*, 22, 389.

Moss, H.V. (1974) Allergic contact dermatitis due to halotex solution. *Archives of Dermatology*, 109, 572.

Nagreh, D.S. (1976) Contact dermatitis from proprietary preparations in Malaysia. *International Journal of Dermatology*, 15, 34.

Neering, H., Vitányi, B.E.J., Malten, K.E., Ketel, W.G. van & Dijk, E. van (1975) Allergens in sesame oil contact dermatitis *Acta Dermato-venereologica*, 55, 31.

Neldner, K.H. (1972) Contact dermatitis from animal feed additives. *Archives of Dermatology*, 106, 722.

Noble, D.S. & Pierce, G.F.M. (1961) Allergy to lignocaine. *Lancet*, 2, 1436.

Nordqvist, B.C. & Mehr, K. (1977) Allergic contact dermatitis to retinoic acid. *Contact Dermatitis*, 3, 55.

Norgaard, O. (1977) Pecilocinum-Allergie. *Hautarzt*, 25, 35.

North American Contact Dermatitis Group (1973) Epidemiology of contact dermatitis in North America: 1972. *Archives of Dermatology*, 108, 537.

O'Garra, J.A. (1962) Anaphylactic reactions to hydrocortisone injections. *British Medical Journal*, i, 615.

Osmundsen, P.E. (1975) Allergic contact dermatitis from idoxuridine. *Contact Dermatitis*, 1, 251.

Page, R.C. & Bercovitz, Z. (1942) Dermatitis from topical application of 2-Methyl-1, 4-naphthoquinone (synthetic vitamin K analogue). *American Journal of the Medical Sciences*, 203, 566.

Parks, D.L., Perry, H.O. & Muller, S.A. (1971) Cutaneous complications of pentazocine injections. *Archives of Dermatology*, 104, 231.

Petrozzi, J.W. & Shore, R.N. (1976) Generalised exfoliative dermatitis from ethylenediamine. *Archives of Dermatology*, 112, 525.

Pevny, I., Mahr, E. & Schropl, F. (1974) Toxische Hautreaktionem beim Epicutantest mit tricyclischen Psychopharmaka. *Hautarzt*, 25, 430.

Pirilä, V., Hirvonen, M.-L. & Rouhunkoski, S. (1968) The pattern of cross-sensitivity to neomycin secondary sensitisation to gentamicin. *Dermatologica*, 136, 321.

Pirilä, V. & Rouhunkoski, S. (1960) On cross-sensitisation between neomycin, bacitracin, kanamycin and framycetin. *Dermatologica*, 121, 335.

Poole, R.L., Griffith, J.F. & Macmillan, F.S.K. (1970) Experimental contact sensitisation with benzoyl peroxide. *Archives of Dermatology*, 102, 400.

Prisco, Di J., Soto, J.M. & Herrera, E. (1968) Phenergan sensitivity. *Contact Dermatitis Newsletter*, 4, 63.

Provost, T.T. & Jillson, O.F. (1967) Ethylenediamine contact dermatitis. *Archives of Dermatology*, 96, 231.

Pyle, H.D. & Rattner, H. (1944) Contact dermatitis from penicillin. *Journal of the American Medical Association*, 125, 903.

Rajka, G. & Pallin, O. (1964) Sensitisation to locally-applied antastene. *Acta Dermato-venereologica*, 44, 255.

Rajka, G. & Vincze, E. (1956) Erfahrungen uber Berufsekzeme in der Arzneimittelindustrie. *Berufsdermatosen*, 4, 124.

Ramsay, D.L., Cohen, H.J. & Baer, R.L. (1972) Allergic reaction to benzophenone. *Archives of Dermatology*, 105, 906.

Raymond, J.Z. & Gross, P.R. (1969) EDTA: Preservative dermatitis. *Archives of Dermatology*, 100, 436.

Richter, G. & Scholz, A. (1970) Kontaktekzem und makuloses Exanthem bei *p*-Chlor-benzolsufonyl-glykolsaurenitril-allergie. *Berufsdermatosen*, 18, 70.

Roed-Petersen, J. (1976) Contact sensitivity to metaoxedrine. *Contact Dermatitis*, 2, 235.

Roller, J.A. (1978) Contact allergy to clotrimazole. *British Medical Journal*, ii, 737.

Roupe, G. & Strannegard, O. (1969) Anaphylactic shock elicited by topical administration of bacitracin. *Archives of Dermatology*, 100, 450.

Rudolph, R.I. (1975) Allergic contact dermatitis caused by haloprogin. *Archives of Dermatology*, 111, 1487.

Rudzki, E. (1978) Dermatitis from epoxy resin, triethylenetetramine and ethylenediamine. *Contact Dermatitis*, 4, 53.

Rudzki, E. & Baranowska, E. (1974) Contact sensitivity in stasis dermatitis. *Dermatologica*, 148, 353.

Rudzki, E. & Grzywa, Z. (1977) Occupational piperazine dermatitis. *Contact Dermatitis*, 3, 216.

Rudzki, E. & Grzywa, Z. (1978) Dermatitis from retinoic acid. *Contact Dermatitis*, 4, 305.

Rudzki, E., Grzywa, Z. & Maciejowska, E. (1976) Drug reaction with positive patch test reaction to chloramphenicol. *Contact Dermatitis*, 2, 181.

Rudzki, E. & Kleniewska, D. (1970) The epidemiology of contact dermatitis in Poland. *British Journal of Dermatology*, 83, 543.

Rudzki, E. & Kloslowska (1976) Sensitivity to salicylic acid. *Contact Dermatitis*, 2, 178.

Sams, W.M. (1968) Untoward response with topical Fluorouracil. *Archives of Dermatology*, 97, 14.

Samsoen, M. & Jelen, G. (1977) Allergy to daktarin gel. *Contact Dermatitis*, 3, 351.

Sausker, W.F. & Frederick, F.D. (1978) Allergic contact dermatitis secondary to topical nitroglycerin. *Journal of the American Medical Association*, 239, 1743.

Schlicher, J.E., Zuehlke, R.L. & Lynch, P.J. (1971) Local changes at the site of pentazocine injection. *Archives of Dermatology*, 104, 90.

Scholz, A. von & Richter, G. (1977) Zur Allergie gegen Falicain (Propipokainhydrochlorid). *Dermatologische Monatsschrift*, 163, 966.

Schorr, W.F. & Ridgway, H.B. (1977) Tobramycin — neomycin cross-sensitivity. *Contact Dermatitis*, **3**, 133.

Schorr, W.F., Wenzel, F.J. & Hegedus, S.I. (1973) Cross-sensitivity and aminoglycoside antibiotics. *Archives of Dermatology*, **107**, 533.

Schreiber, M.M. & Naylor, L.Z. (1962) Antihistamine photosensitivity. *Archives of Dermatology*, **86**, 58.

Schulz, K.H., Schöpf, E. & Wex, O. (1970) Allergische Berufsekzeme durch Ampicillin. *Berufsdermatoscn*, **18**, 132.

Schwank, R. & Jirásek, L. (1963) Kontaktallergie gegen Chloramphenicol mit besonderer Berucksichtigung der Gruppensensibilisierung. *Hautarzt*, **14**, 24.

Seymour, R. & Raynor, C. (1974) Extensive leg ulceration from intravenous use of pentazocine. *The American Surgeon*, **40**, 671.

Sidi, E., Hincky, M. & Gervais, A. (1955) Allergic sensitisation and photosensitisation to Phenergan cream. *Journal of Investigative Dermatology*, **24**, 345.

Simpson, J.R. (1974) Reversed cross-sensitisation betwen quinine and iodochlorhydroxy-quinoline. *Contact Dermatitis Newsletter*, **15**, 431.

Skog, E. (1975) Systemic eczematous contact-type dermatitis induced by iodochlorhydroxyquin and chloroquine phosphate. *Contact Dermatitis*, **1**, 187.

Smeenk, G. (1973) Contact allergy to bufexamac. *Dermatologica*, **147**, 334.

Sneddon, I.B. and Glew, C.R. (1973) Contact dermatitis due to propanidid in an anaesthetist. *Practitioner*, **211**, 321.

Sönnichsen, N. (1962) Beitrag zur Hydrocortisone-uberempfindlichkeit. *Hautarzt*, **13**, 226.

Soto, J.M. (1968) Promethazine photosensitivity. *Contact Dermatitis Newsletter*, **3**, 53.

Spencer, G.A. (1945) Hypersensitivity to ephedrine. *Archives of Dermatology*, **51**, 48.

Sprunt, J.G. & Rizza, C.R. (1966) Pigmentation and busulphan therapy. *British Medical Journal*, i, 736.

Stoltze, R. (1966) Dermatitis medicamentosa in eczema of the leg. *Acta Dermato-venereologica*, **46**, 54.

Strauss, M.J. & Warring, F.C. (1947a) Contact dermatitis from streptomycin. *Journal of Investigative Dermatology*, **9**, 3.

Strauss, M.J. & Warring, F.C. (1947b) Epidermal sensitisation to streptomycin. *Journal of Investigative Dermatology*, **9**, 99.

Sulzberger, M.B., Baer, R.L. & Kanof, A. (1946) Clinical uses of 2, 3-dimercaptopropanol (BAL): V. skin sensitisation to BAL. *Journal of Clinical Investigation*, **25**, 488.

Sundararajan, V. (1970) Variotin sensitivity. *Contact Dermatitis Newsletter*, **8**, 188.

Suurmond, D. (1966) Patch test reactions to phenergan cream, promethazine and triethanolamine. *Dermatologica*, **133**, 503.

Tas, J. & Weissberg, D. (1958) Allergy to aminophylline. *Acta Allergologica*, **12**, 39.

Tharp, C.K. (1973) Contact urticaria to monoamylamine. *Contact Dermatitis Newsletter*, **14**, 391.

Thormann, J. & Kaaber, K. (1978) Contact sensitivity to phenylbutazone ointment (Butazolidine®). *Contact Dermatitis*, **4**, 235.

Van Scott, E.J. & Kalmanson, J.D. (1973) Complete remissions to mycosis fungoides lymphoma induced by topical nitrogen mustard (HN₂). *Cancer*, **32**, 18.

Van Scott, E.J. & Winters, P.L. (1970) Responses of mycosis fungoides to intensive external treatment with nitrogen mustard. *Archives of Dermatology*, **102**, 507.

Van Scott, E.J. & Yu, R.F. (1974) Antimitotic, antigenic and structural relationships of nitrogen mustard and its homologues. *Journal of Investigative Dermatology*, **62**, 378.

Velasco, J.E. & Africk, J.A. (1971) Contact dermatitis to mafenide acetate. *Archives of Dermatology*, **103**, 61.

Verbov, J.L. (1970) Sensitivity to sodium fusidate. *Contact Dermatitis Newsletter*, **7**, 153.

Vickers, H.R. (1946) Contact dermatitis caused by penicillin. *Lancet*, **1**, 307.

Vickers, H.R., Bagratuni, L. & Alexander, S. (1958) Dermatitis caused by penicillin in milk. *Lancet*, **1**, 351.

Vooys, S. Chr. & Ketel van W.G. (1977) Allergic drug eruption from pyrazolone compounds. *Contact Dermatitis*, **3**, 57.

Wahlberg, J.E. (1971) Sensitisation to thioxolone used for topical treatment of acne. *Contact Dermatitis Newsletter*, **10**, 222.

Wahlberg, J.E. & Forsbeck, M. (1973) Contact sensitivity to quinidine sulphate — an antiarrhythmic. *Contact Dermatitis Newsletter*, **14**, 412.

Wasilewski, C. (1970) Allergic contact dermatitis from nystatin. *Archives of Dermatology*, **102**, 216.

Watrous, R.M. (1947) Health hazards of the pharmaceutical industry. *British Journal of Industrial Medicine*, **4**, 111.

Wätzig, V. & Ruffert, K. (1977) Der Leukozyten-migrationshemmtest in der Hautkammer-eine invivo-methode zum Nachweis der Chloramphenikol — allergie. *Dermatologische Monatsschrift*, **163**, 5.

Wereide, K. (1968) Contact allergy to propantheline bromide. *Contact Dermatitis Newsletter*, **4**, 61.

Wereide, K. (1975) Sensitivity to azidamphenicol. *Contact Dermatitis*, **1**, 271.

White, M.I. (1978) Contact dermatitis from ethylenediamine. *Contact Dermatitis*, **4**, 291.

Wilkinson, R.D., Mcgarry, E.M. & Solomon, S. (1967) Allergic contact dermatitis to hydrocortisone. *Journal of Investigative Dermatology*, **48**, 295.

Wilson, H.T.H. (1958) Streptomycin dermatitis in nurses. *British Medical Journal*, i, 1378.

Wilson, H.T.H. (1966) Dermatitis from anaesthetic ointments. *Practitioner*, **197**, 673.

Wilson, H.T.H. (1971) Dermatitis from an acridine dye. *Contact Dermatitis Newsletter*, **9**, 212.

Wong, D., Lopapa, A.F. & Haddad, Z.H. (1971) Immediate hypersensitivity reaction to aminophylline. *Journal of Allergy and Clinical Immunology*, **48**, 165.

Wüthrich, B. (1972) Berufsekzem durch Aethylendiamin in der Kunstfaser-industrie. *Berufsdermatosen*, **20**, 200.

Yaffee, H.S. & Dressler, D.P. (1969) Topical application of mafenide acetate. *Archives of Dermatology*, **100**, 277.

7.

Metals

ANTIMONY	NICKEL
ARSENIC	NICKEL, CHROMATE AND COBALT
BERYLLIUM	PALLADIUM
CADMIUM	PLATINUM
CARBON	SELENIUM
CHROMIUM	SILICA
COBALT	SILVER
COPPER	TELLURIUM
GOLD	URANIUM
IRON	ZINC
LEAD	ZIRCONIUM

Antimony

Antimony is a hard and brittle metal, it is used to harden lead and is present in printer's type, lead bullets, shotgun ammunition and accumulator plates. Antimony salts have been used in the rubber industry and in the manufacture of glass and ceramics; antimony oxide is used for fireproofing fabrics, particularly military and special uniforms.

The few reports of antimony dermatitis have all been industrial.

Irritant dermatitis
In 1926 antimony sulphides were used extensively in the rubber industry and caused systemic toxicity and irritant dermatitis. Patch tests were not done (Quinby, 1926).

The manufacture of antimony trioxide carries some skin hazard. In 1965 a study of an antimony plant was reported (Stevenson, 1965). Of 150 men at risk, 17 furnace men and six others, working in hot conditions, developed skin lesions which in 11 began within three months of their starting work. The eruption, known as antimony spots, was extremely itchy and consisted of papules and pustules principally in the antecubital fossae and on the shins. It occurred mainly in the summer and required not only dust contamination but also heat and sweating for its development. If the men were transferred to a cool part of the factory, their skin healed in two weeks. Patch tests with antimony trioxide powder elicited no reactions.

Lichenoid eruption

Two cases of lichenoid eruptions from occupational contact with antimony tri-oxide have been described by Paschoud (1963, 1964). Both men developed the lesions after only a few weeks' exposure. They affected the bends of the elbows and knees and also the neck and wrists; the lesions subsided when the men were away from work and recurred when work was resumed. Patch tests: both men reacted to antimony trioxide and one also reacted to arsenic (p. 282).

Patch testing

Antimony trioxide powder

Antimony chloride 2 per cent in water.

Arsenic

Arsenic is not a true metal, it is a steel-grey crystalline semi-metal; it occurs in most soils and in many ores and minerals and is recovered as a by-product in the extraction of other metals. Its widespread distribution results in its absorption and traces are normally present in human tissue.

INORGANIC ARSENIC

Properties and uses

  (i) As an alloy arsenic enhances the heat resistance of copper and is used in boilers and it is present in shot to harden the lead.
 (ii) Lead, calcium and magnesium arsenates are used as weed-killers and insecticides; Paris green is cupric aceto-arsenite.
(iii) Coloured arsenical compounds (Scheele's green is copper arsenite) were widely used as pigments but nowadays rarely because of their toxicity.
 (iv) Arsenic is also used in the manufacture of glass.
  (v) As a medicament it is, or should be, obsolete: Fowler's solution contains potassium arsenite, and Asiatic pills contain arsenic trioxide.

Clinical features

In early industries skin lesions from arsenic were well recognised, dermatitis being known as 'smelter's itch'. The development of lesions is said to be dependent upon the circumstances, degree and duration of exposure, rather than the actual compound handled (Rossberg, 1967).

Systemic toxicity and carcinogenicity

Arsenic, in sufficient dose, is an acute lethal poison; in small amounts, absorbed over a prolonged period it is a carcinogen. Protracted poisoning by inorganic arsenicals produces, in the skin, raindrop pigmentation, keratoses and epitheliomata. Systemic neoplasms have also been recorded. Such chronic absorption and its effects have been described from medicaments (Sommers and McManus, 1953; Evans, 1977; Reymann, Møller and Nielsen, 1978), from therapy and occupational exposure (L'Epee *et al.*, 1973), from polluted well and drinking water (Degreef and Roelandts, 1974; Egyedi and Pataky, 1978) and in Singapore from Chinese herbal remedies (Tay, 1974). The benefit of constant medical supervision in vine dressers so exposed has been reported by Grobe (1977). The continuing hazard of arsenic absorption in steel bronze workers has been investigated by Clay, Dale and Cross (1977). In parts of the Argentine chronic arsenical poisoning is endemic and is a cause of lung cancer (Biagini *et al.*, 1978).

Irritant effect

Inorganic arsenicals are irritants and may cause folliculitis, pyoderma, ulceration of the skin and perforation of the nasal septum.

In 1962, in an American gold mine and smelter, an outbreak of irritant dermatitis occurred among the 100 workers and the 200–250 members of their families living in the adjacent camp (Birmingham *et al.*, 1965). To extract gold from the crude ore, the contaminant arsenic sulphides were oxidised to arsenic trioxide and sulphur dioxide; and in one day 40 tons of arsenic were burned off in the smelter. As the extraction system was inefficient, arsenic trioxide was discharged from the effluent stack on to the neighbourhood, settling on the ground as a yellow-grey dust. Within months of the process starting 32 of the 40 younger children attending the near-by school had developed skin lesions. These included an itchy eczema of the face and flexures mimicking atopic dermatitis, follicular and pustular lesions, usually of the face and neck and sometimes of the limbs, and ulcers of the palms, fingers and web spaces. Housewives and pre-school children were affected but not the older children who commuted to school and were thus out of the area for half the day. Of the 18 mill day workers, 9 had similar lesions and two had perforations of their nasal septa. Systemic toxicity did not occur and only one ore roaster had a raised urinary arsenic. The cats and dogs in the vicinity died, except for a surviving collie which had ulceration of its mouth and a paw.

The mill was temporarily closed and measures to improve hygiene were introduced: in three weeks there was marked healing of the dermatoses.

Six months later, 12 affected children and two mill workers were patch tested with 5 per cent arsenic trioxide in starch powder. Two children and one man reacted, but of these only one had had eczema and this did not recur despite continued exposure to small amounts of arsenic in the mill. It was concluded that most of the skin changes were irritant.

Arsenic trioxide applied experimentally to rabbits produced ulceration of moist, shaved neck folds but was harmless on dry open skin.

Sensitisation

The cutaneous effects of inorganic arsenic were investigated by Holmquist (1951) in a copper-ore smelting works in Sweden from 1932–1948. The study included 69 workmen and two female laboratory assistants with dermatitis; most of the cases were from the arsenic refinery where exposure was greatest. Exposed sites, particularly the face, were affected, although the hands were often spared due to wearing gloves; the scrotum and inner thighs were sometimes involved. All these patients reacted to patch tests with non-irritant concentrations of arsenic compounds. The irritancy of arsenicals was thought to predispose to sensitisation. Although removal from exposure was the most effective immediate therapy, continued contact did produce hardening.

Pseudo-atopic appearance
Atopic dermatitis can be mimicked by exposure to arsenic trioxide which can be either an irritant, as in the children described by Birmingham *et al.* (1965), or a sensitiser, as in Paschoud's (1964) report. A man working in a glass factory mixed powders, among which was arsenic trioxide. He developed a lichenoid, papular eruption in the bends of his elbows and knees, around the base of his neck and under his watch strap. The appearance of the eruption coincided with his doing this particular job. He was patch tested and reacted to Fowler's solution (1 per cent potassium arsenite) and to the arsenic trioxide powder. The tendency for the powder to fly about and to settle in moist body folds was thought to account for the misleading clinical distribution.

Patch testing
Patch testing with inorganic arsenic compounds was studied by Holmquist (1951) among the workers in the Swedish copper smelting works mentioned above, and in controls with other skin diseases. He found that:

(i) Arsenic compounds are irritants
(ii) False positive reactions to too high a concentration of test material may look exactly like an allergic response
(iii) Patch testing with too high a concentration causes active sensitisation
(iv) Arsenic trioxide, undiluted, was an irritant and a sensitiser; calcium and lead arsenate were found to be unreliable because of their insolubility
(v) Sodium arsenite 1 per cent solution was non-irritant and
(vi) Arsenic pentoxide 2.5 per cent solution was on the threshold of irritancy.

In the series reported by Eberhartinger, Ebner and Klotz (1969) a 1 per cent sodium salt of arsenic was reported as producing irritant follicular pustular reactions.

ORGANIC ARSENIC

Organic salts of arsenic, the arsphenamines, are used therapeutically and were prescribed particularly for syphilis. Other compounds such as Lewisite (dichloro(2-chlorovinyl)arsine) are highly toxic, vesicant gases; they were made but not used for chemical warfare.

Exfoliative dermatitis
This may occur as a complication of arsphenamine therapy.

Presensitisation by inorganic arsenic
A man and his wife were sensitised to inorganic arsenic when living in a mining camp. Thirteen years later they were given neoarsphenamine which provoked

systemic symptoms and an exudative eczema of such a severity that the course of treatment had to be stopped (Jones, 1940).

Contact dermatitis
In 1934, a physician and his assistant carried out a mass treatment of syphilis with arsphenamine and both developed eczema of their fingers. Patch tests with Salvarsan were positive initially but were not always reproducible. Patch testing with Fowler's solution (potassium arsenite 1 per cent) was negative (Vuletić, 1934).

Beryllium

Beryllium is a light, elastic, heat-stable grey metal with advantages offset by its brittleness. It exists chiefly as the ore beryl (beryllium aluminium silicate) and is found in the Argentine, Brazil, India, South Africa and parts of the United States of America.

Properties and uses
Valuable alloys are formed by beryllium, particularly the beryllium-copper alloy which is hard, strong, has a high tensile strength, withstands heat and corrosion and does not spark. It is used for making safety tools, precision and electrical equipment and special springs.

Beryllium disease
Those in contact with beryllium absorb and store the metal and excrete it slowly in the urine for years whether or not they ever develop symptoms. Lesions occur in only a few and may appear as a granulomatous disease years after exposure to beryllium has ceased. Exposure is an industrial hazard and either inhalation of beryllium or contact with it can result in disease. The majority of cases were reported in the 1940s from Russia, Europe and North America. Since then the disease has been intensively investigated in the U.S.A.; relatively few patients have been diagnosed in the U.K. A register of cases was started, in 1952, at the Massachusetts General Hospital and 616 cases had been indexed by 1960 (Tepper, Hardy and Chamberlain, 1961).

The risk was particularly great in plants extracting and processing beryllium and in the manufacture of fluorescent lights. The natural ore, beryl, is the only beryllium compound which can be handled with impunity and has never been implicated as a cause of disease.

Awareness of the hazard and effective preventive measures have now made this a rare condition.

The disease affects principally the skin and respiratory tract. Comprehensive reviews of the toxicology and clinical manifestations have been published (Tepper *et al.*, 1961; Browning, 1969).

Sensitisation
It has been shown that lymphocytes from guinea-pigs sensitised to beryllium

produce a macrophage migration inhibition factor when cultured with the soluble beryllium sulphosalicylate complex (Jones and Amos, 1974).

Skin

The cutaneous changes which occur are ulcers, irritant and allergic dermatitis and granulomas.

Beryllium ulcers

These ulcers, like chrome holes, are a toxic effect caused by crystals of a soluble beryllium salt contaminating a wound. Usually single and painless, they occur on the hands and arms and tend to persist until the crystals are removed by curettage. The histology shows an acute dermal inflammation (Tepper *et al.*, 1961; De Nardi *et al.*, 1953).

Irritant dermatitis

An irritant dermatitis, consisting of numerous small burns, may affect exposed sites such as the face, neck, hands and arms. Healing usually takes 1–2 weeks, but sometimes the lesions become beryllium ulcers (De Nardi *et al.*, 1953).

Allergic dermatitis

Thirteen patients working in two extraction plants were reported from Cleveland, Ohio, in 1951: ten furnace workers were sensitised by beryllium fluoride, two bottlers by ground metallic beryllium and a pipe fitter by the dust of various beryllium compounds. The men had frequently failed to use protective clothing. The dermatitis appeared within 7–14 days of starting work and affected exposed sites, principally the face, neck, hands and arms. Involvement of the eyelids and an associated conjunctivitis were common. The eruption subsided when they were away from beryllium and relapsed with re-exposure. On patch testing with beryllium fluoride, all 13 patients reacted to 1 per cent, 12 to 0.1 per cent and 5 to 0.01 per cent (Curtis, 1951).

Beryllium granulomas

Laceration by a broken fluorescent lamp can implant the beryllium phosphor (zinc beryllium silicate) in the skin and result in the formation of a cutaneous epithelioid granuloma. The wound may fail to heal, or it may close and then, about 1–4 months later, one or more nodules develop in the scar which may break down to form an ulcer. Treatment usually requires excision (Folesky, 1967) but a topical corticosteroid has been effective (Fisher, 1953).

These lesions caused by beryllium phosphors have not been associated with systemic disease (Tepper *et al.*, 1961).

A beryllium-copper alloy has caused skin and pulmonary granulomas. One patient worked for a firm of precious metal smelters and for over three years had operated a shearing machine to trim metal, including a 2 per cent beryllium-copper alloy. Fragments of metal often cut her skin and for one year she had developed multiple small papules at these traumatised sites. She also had small ulcers on her palms. She complained of a dry cough and increasing shortness of breath and although a miniature chest X-ray was normal further films showed fine stippling of both lung fields. Patch tests: she reacted to 2 per cent and 1 per cent beryllium sulphate and nitrate and the responses became granulomatous. These tests exacerbated her respiratory symptoms and signs (Sneddon, 1955).

Respiratory system

Acute disease
Acute respiratory disease occurs in conditions of relatively high atmospheric pollution; there may be nasopharyngitis, tracheobronchitis or pneumonitis. The disease is usually benign, resolving within 1–6 months, but it has been fatal; it may recur on exposure and it occasionally becomes chronic (Tepper *et al.*, 1961).

Chronic disease
This is a systemic granulomatous disease in which the pulmonary involvement is usually the presenting and the most disabling aspect of the condition, but the lymph nodes, liver, spleen, kidneys and other tissues may be affected. There is a latent period of a year or more before the onset of symptoms. The lung changes are very similar to those which occur in sarcoidosis. Patch tests with beryllium sulphate 1 per cent have elicited reactions in these patients (Norris and Peard, 1963).

Neighbourhood disease
Chronic respiratory disease has occurred in people living in the vicinity of beryllium plants and also in those at home handling the contaminated clothing of beryllium workers (Tepper *et al.*, 1961).

Diagnosis
The diagnosis is based on evidence of exposure to beryllium and a disease manifestation compatible with the diagnosis. In the granulomatous phase, the histology is that of an epithelioid granuloma, and the finding of beryllium in the tissue would be almost incontrovertible proof of the diagnosis. The patch test has not been considered diagnostic (Tepper *et al.*, 1961).

Patch testing
Patch tests with beryllium salts are:

(i) Positive in allergic contact dermatitis

(ii) Sometimes positive in the granulomatous disease, with (Sneddon, 1955) and without (Norris and Peard, 1963) skin lesions, and these positive reactions may, after 3–4 weeks, have the histology of a granuloma

(iii) Liable actively to sensitise the subject. In one series, 16 controls were tested with several beryllium salts and eight were sensitised by beryllium fluoride 2 per cent. Other but weaker sensitising salts were beryllium fluoride 1 per cent (one patient), beryllium chloride 2 per cent (two patients) and beryllium sulphate 2 per cent (one patient).

It would seem prudent to avoid concentrations of 2 per cent, and to patch test with:

Beryllium sulphate, chloride or nitrate 0.5–1.0 per cent in water.

Of these three salts, the sulphate, being the most soluble, may carry some risk of active sensitisation.

Cadmium

Cadmium is derived mainly from zinc and lead ores.

Properties and uses
This metal is electroplated on to iron and steel to form a rust-proof coating. It is also used in alloys, as an insecticide and as a pigment in glass, paints, and tattoos.

Causes of sensitivity
Cases of sensitivity to cadmium have been recorded but their validity is controversial (Fregert and Hjorth, 1972). Cadmium chloride 2 per cent (aqueous) was added to the standard series by Wahlberg (1977) and 25 of 1502 patients (1.7 per cent) reacted but none had a relevant history and only one patient reacted to a 1 per cent dilution. Cadmium sulphide is phototoxic (p. 832).

Suspenders and a pace-maker
Cadmium was reported as the sensitiser in some patients with suspender dermatitis (Mutter, 1962) and in a patient with eczema attributed to a pace-maker, although the composition of the metal was not ascertained. Patch tests: the patient reacted to cadmium chloride 2 per cent and potassium dichromate 0.5 per cent (Laugier *et al.*, 1975). It has been suggested by Hegyi *et al.* (1974) that the increase in nickel sensitivity among consumers may be explained by cadmium releasing nickel from the electro-plated layer covering the base metal.

Industrial — metal industry

(i) *Anti-corrosive.* Cadmium, used as an anti-corrosive, has caused dermatitis among metal workers (Borelli and Düngemann, 1964).

(ii) *Welders.* In a series of 256 metal workers, mainly welders, nine were sensitised to cadmium. The source of contact was the solid metal, its dust, or cadmium in solutions or in oils; it was not vapourised metal (Düngemann, Borelli and Wittman, 1972).

Patch testing
Cadmium sulphate 2 per cent in petrolatum (Mutter, 1962; Borelli and Düngemann, 1964)
and
Cadmium chloride 1 per cent in water (Wahlberg, 1977).

Carbon (graphite in 'lead' pencils)

Graphite is an allotropic form of carbon with a layered structure. To make 'lead' pencils graphite is cleansed, mixed with clay, forced through a die, baked and encased in wood. More clay and a higher temperature produce a harder pencil.

Case report
A clerk developed eczema affecting initially the region of his left breast; it cleared but then appeared on the right side and was associated with vesicles on his fingers. He suggested that the lead pencils he carried in his shirt pockets might be the cause. When patch tested he gave a bullous reaction to the lead of the pencil but did not react to the lacquer finish or to the wood. He removed his pencils from his pockets, handled them with care, and his skin healed (Friedman, 1956).

Chromium

Pure chromium is a steel grey metal; it derives its name from the Greek word colour because of the brightness of many of its salts. It occurs naturally as deposits of chrome iron ore or chromite, which are mixtures of iron and chromium oxides. It is mined in Russia, Turkey, Rhodesia and South Africa (Browning, 1969).

Trivalent chromium is present in soils and plants and is an essential trace element in man; the average intake in the U.S.A. is about 60 μg/ a day. Chromium is not stored in the body and is practically all excreted in the faeces (Schroeder, Balassa and Tipton, 1962) because the absorption of trivalent chromium from the gut is extremely small and the acidity of the gastric juice converts the better absorbed hexavalent chromium to the almost non-absorbable trivalent form (Donaldson and Barreras, 1966). Traces of chromium are absorbed; it affects carbohydrate metabolism, and work on rat tissue has shown that trivalent chromium is an essential cofactor for insulin (Mertz and Roginski, 1963). The importance of chromium in glucose metabolism has been reviewed by Mertz *et al* (1974). Chromium and its effects have been reviewed by Burrows (1978).

Industrial uses

1. As an alloy in steels, chromium confers hardness
2. It is electroplated over metal to give a hard, bright, durable finish
3. It is used in the manufacture of cutting tools
4. As a corrosion inhibitor
5. As a tanning agent
6. In the photographic and printing industries
7. As a mordant in dyeing
8. As a pigment
9. In the making of chromates.

Toxicity and carcinogenicity

Men making ferro-chrome alloys may develop metal fume fever which is a transient illness but it can go on to a chemical pneumonitis (Stoke, 1977). Another risk in these workers is pneumoconiosis (Taylor and Davies, 1977).

Chromate is implicated in causing lung and possibly nasal sinus tumours (Enterline, 1974) and it has been hypothesised that epoxyaldehyde released from tissue lipids by chromates are the carcinogens (Schoental, 1975).

Valencies

Chromium has valencies of two, three and six; the metal itself is non-sensitising, probably because of the monomolecular layer of insoluble chromium oxide (Cr_2O_4) on its surface (Fregert and Hjorth, 1968). The bivalent salts are unstable and therefore are not used commercially (Walsh, 1953). The trivalent compounds include chromic acid (Cr_2O_3), chromic sulphate ($Cr_2(SO_4)_3$) and chromium trichloride ($CrCl_3$), all of which are sensitisers. The hexavalent chromium compounds, or dichromates, are widely used in industry and are the most sensitising of the chrome compounds.

Sensitising capacity of trivalent (Cr_3) and hexavalent (Cr_6) chromium

A maximisation test was used by Kligman (1966) to assess the sensitising potential of trivalent and hexavalent chromium compounds. About half of a group of 23 human subjects were sensitised with the trivalent chrome salts, chromium trioxide and chromium sulphate, and graded as 3 on a sensitising scale of 1–5 in which grade 5 was the most potent allergen. The same technique was used with potassium dichromate and each one of 23 subjects was sensitised; potassium dichromate was graded as 5 on the same scale. A maximisation test was also used to sensitise guinea-pigs to potassium dichromate; 75 per cent of the animals were sensitised and it was graded as 4 on the same scale (Magnusson and Kligman, 1969). Three methods of inducing sensitisation to potassium dichromate in guinea-pigs were evaluated by Skog and Wahlberg (1970): each was effective but of the methods considered a combination of injections with painting of the skin (Polák and Turk, 1968) gave the best results and this finding was confirmed by Ziegler, Suss and Standau (1973). Experimental methods were further evaluated by Turk and Parker (1977, ii) and though the guinea-pigs could be made strongly reactive the effect was frequently transient.

Allergy to trivalent chromium compounds

For a chemical to become an allergen it must be capable of linking with protein by covalent bonds to form a stable conjugate (Eisen, 1959): Although the hexavalent dichromate (Cr_6) readily passes through the skin (Mali *et al.*, 1964), it does not link with protein (Samitz and Katz, 1964). In direct contrast, trivalent (Cr_3) chrome compounds hardly penetrate the epidermis (Spruit and Neer, 1966) but once through to the dermis readily combine with protein. This inability of chromate (Cr_6) to bind with protein has always made it unlikely that it could act as an antigen. However, it has been shown (Samitz and Katz, 1964) that constituents of the skin can reduce the hexavalent to the trivalent form and it has been demonstrated clinically that certain trivalent chromium compounds, if injected intracutaneously, will give positive reactions in patients sensitive to chromate (Fregert and Rorsman, 1964). Similarly with patch testing, by using a high concentration (0.1 M) of the trivalent salt, basic chromic sulphate, positive tests have been elicited in 75 per cent of 90 chromate (Cr_6) sensitive subjects (Fregert and Rorsman, 1965). Petrolatum releases trivalent chromium compounds and therefore is not a factor in the high patch concentrations required (Rudzki et al., 1978).

From studies in guinea-pigs Schneeberger and Forck (1974) also considered trivalent chromium to form the definitive antigen and they found the strength of its complexes with protein to be important in sensitisation.

These investigations make it likely that trivalent and not hexavalent chromium is the hapten in chromium sensitivity. Despite this, the hexavalent chromium compounds elicit stronger reactions both intracutaneously and epicutaneously (Fregert and Rorsman, 1966a). For this reason potassium dichromate continues to be used in the routine clinical investigation of patients.

Binding of chromium compounds by the skin

Neutron activation analysis has been used to estimate the chromium content of skin. No differences were found between skin taken from the lower arm and from the back of two patients with chromium eczema and control samples from similar sites in cadavers and the arm of a living subject (Kooten and Mali, 1967).

The binding of chromium to the skin, and its disappearance rate from an injection site have been estimated in chromate-sensitive subjects and in controls. No differences were found between them. When chromate was injected intracutaneously, after 10 minutes only 50 per cent remained at the test site; at two days there was 14–18 per cent and by two months 3–5 per cent of the original amount was still present (Bang Pedersen et al., 1969). The disappearance rate decreased with time; the greater part left the test site within the first few days, probably via the blood and lymphatics. The chemical properties of the chromium compound injected are important because it has been shown that sodium chromate (Cr_6) disappears more quickly from the skin than chromium trichloride (Cr_3) (Bang Pederson and Naversten, 1973). Trivalent chromium trichloride has been found by chemical analysis in the skin at sites of injections given 3–4 years previously. These deposits at test sites may cause repeated local flares in chromium-sensitive subjects (Fregert, 1971). At sites of dichromate patch tests the concentration of chromium is highest at the dermal-epidermal junction and in the upper mid-dermis (Lidén and Lundberg, 1979).

Isotope labelled sodium chromate has been applied as patch tests to study its absorption in two chromate-sensitive patients and in two normal controls. At the end of two days, approximately 10 per cent of the chromate was found in or on the skin at the patch test site and approximately 90 per cent was on the patch test. Absorption did occur as proved by a positive reaction in the sensitive subjects but the loss of these minute quantities was not detectable with the techniques employed. However, at one month a difference was observed; in the non-allergic controls 0.6–1 per cent of the labelled chromate remained in the skin at the patch test site, whereas in one sensitised subject none was found and in the other only 0.1 per cent of the amount originally applied remained (Bang Pedersen *et al*. 1970).

These investigations show that when chromium is injected intracutaneously similar amounts persist in the dermis in allergic and non-allergic subjects. In contrast, when the chromium is applied epicutaneously a smaller amount stays in the dermis of sensitive subjects than of controls, perhaps because the inflammation of the positive test causes shedding of the chromium from the epidermis and a more rapid clearance from the test site.

Incidence of chromate sensitivity

In industrialised countries, chromate is the commonest sensitiser in men, and the frequency of chromate sensitivity is therefore high in most recorded series. In contrast, a survey published by Nasution, Klokke and Nater (1973) of the causes of occupational dermatoses in Indonesia included no case of chromate sensitivity.

The following incidences have been reported:

Country	Patients tested	+ Chromate %	Report
Scandinavia	5558	7.4	Magnusson *et al*., 1968
Europe	4825	6.6	Fregert *et al*., 1969
Poland	1205	16.2	Rudzki *et al*., 1970
N. America	1200	8.0	N. American C.D. Group, 1973
New York	769	11.6	Baer and Ramsey, 1973
California	223	9.4	Epstein *et al*., 1968
New Zealand	216	8.3	Black, 1972
Patients with C.D.			
Australia	1000	13.5	Burry *et al*., 1973
Kuwait	389	57.0	Kanan, 1969

C.D. = Contact Dermatitis (Allergic).

The figures for sensitivity to chromate will be influenced by local factors such as the nature of the local industries, the degree of exposure to cement and other sources of chromate and the social and other factors which influence the proportion of men attending for patch testing. In the European study the numbers tested and the incidence of reactors were recorded for each centre (Table 7.1).

Table 7.1. Incidence of sensitivity to chromate in men and women in eight European centres (Fregert *et al*., 1969).

	Bari	Munich	Gothenburg	London	Wycombe	Nijmegen	Lund	Copenhagen
Pts. Tested	315	800	800	800	132	378	800	800
No. + Cr_6	65	64	51	50	8	20	35	27
%	21	8	6.4	6.3	6.1	5.3	4.4	3.4

The high incidence of chromate sensitivity in Bari, in Southern Italy, was due to the many men employed in building and construction work in that area, and to the selection of patients, there being twice as many men as women tested. In other centres the differences were not so striking, although chromate sensitivity was obviously commoner in Munich than Copenhagen. It is interesting that London and Wycombe had a similar incidence.

Similarly in the series reported from North America the incidence of sensitivity was shown to vary from city to city (Table 7.2.) but the local factors accounting for these differences were not discussed.

Table 7.2 Incidence of sensitivity to chromate in men and women in ten North American cities (North American C.D. Group, 1973).

	Bangor	Detroit	Hanover	Marsh-field	New Orleans	New York	Port-land	Rich-mond	San Francisco	Van-couver
No. Tested	59	20	197	129	24	44	229	207	126	165
No. + Cr₆	6	4	17	3	3	4	22	8	11	13
%	10	20	9	2	12	9	10	4	9	8

St John's

Every patient investigated in the Contact Clinic is tested with potassium dichromate 0.5 per cent in petrolatum; during the decade 1967–1976 a total of 16 571 patients were seen of whom 682 (4.1 per cent) gave positive reactions.

Changing incidence of chromate sensitivity

In those clinics which have reported their results there has been surprisingly little difference in the incidence of chromate sensitivity over the years:

Incidence of chromate sensitivity at varying intervals in five cities

Centre	Year	+ Chromate			
Copenhagen	1938	3%			
(Finsen Institute)	1945	1%			
	1955	3%			(Marcussen, 1962)
	1969	3%	M	F	(Fregert et al., 1969)
Stockholm	1948–'51	10.4%	(15.7	5.9)	
	1958–'61	8.8%	(14.6	4.9)	(Modée and Skog, 1962)
New York	1937	8.5%			(Rostenberg et al., 1937)
	1961	9.2%			(Baer et al., 1964)
Rome	1956–'59	23.9%			
	1959–'62	25.5%			
	1962–'65	17.4%★			(Scarpa et al., 1966)
Graz (Austria)	1952–'55	31%			
	1960–'63	40%			(Kresbach et al., 1965)

★(Concentration of chromate for testing was reduced from 1 per cent to 0.5 per cent which may have accounted for the fall in incidence)

St John's

There was remarkably little change from 1967 to 1976 in the yearly incidence of chromate sensitivity: the numbers ranged from 3.1–5.1 per cent of those tested, the average being 4.1 per cent (Table 7.3).

Table 7.3. Yearly incidence of chromate sensitivity (St John's 1967–1976).

	1967	1968	1969	1970	1971	1972	1973	1974	1975	1976	Total
No. Tested	1529	1604	1549	1906	1558	1606	1546	1433	1858	1982	16 571
No. +	47	70	65	72	73	70	79	60	63	83	682
%	3.1	4.4	4.2	3.7	4.7	4.4	5.1	4.2	3.4	4.2	4.1

Sex incidence

In the following series, where the sex incidence has been reported, chromate is a commoner sensitiser in men than women; the differences probably depend upon the selection of patients and pattern of employment in the industries of each area:

Table 7.4. Sex incidence of chromate sensitivity in five series

Country	+ Chromate M	F	Sex Ratio M:F	Report
Scandinavia	11.7%	3.0%	4:1	(Magnusson *et al.*, 1968)
Scandinavia	10.0%	2.0%	5:1	(Magnusson *et al.*, 1969)
Europe	10.7%	3.6%	3:1	(Fregert *et al.*, 1969)
N. America	10.0%	6.0%	2:1	(N. American C.D. Group, 1973)
Kuwait	218 pts	3 pts	73:1	(Kanan, 1969)

Even from city to city the sex ratio varies, as is shown in this Scandinavian series (Magnusson *et al.*, 1968). Possible reasons for these differences were not explored (Table 7.5):

Table 7.5. Sex ratio of chromate-sensitive patients in six Scandinavian centres (Magnusson *et al.*, 1968).

City	No. tested	+ Chromate M	F	Sex Ratio M : F
Bergen	307	13%	2%	6 : 1
Gothenberg	1000	13%	2%	6 : 1
Stockholm	510	12%	3%	4 : 1
Helsinki	500	23%	7%	3 : 1
Lund	1406	8%	3%	3 : 1
Copenhagen	1835	3%	2%	1.5 : 1

In the North American Series (North American C.D. Group, 1973) the numbers tested were too small to show valid differences between the various cities.

St John's

At St John's during the period 1967–1976 there was little change in the incidence of chromate sensitivity in either sex; it remained about 6.5 per cent for the men and 1.9 per cent for the women. The sex ratio was three males to one female, except for the anomalous incidence of 8:1 in 1968 for which there was no obvious reason (Table 7.6).

Table 7.6. Incidence of chromate sensitivity in men and women and the sex ratio (St John's, 1967–1976).

Year	Males No Tested	Cr_6 +	%	Females No Tested	Cr_6.+	%	M : F
1967	809	34	4.2	720	13	1.8	3 : 1
1968	812	62	7.6	792	8	1.0	8 : 1
1969	787	50	6.3	762	15	2.0	3 : 1
1970	916	55	6.0	990	17	1.7	3 : 1
1971	707	60	8.4	851	13	1.5	5 : 1
1972	738	55	7.4	868	15	1.7	4 : 1
1973	710	57	8.0	836	22	2.6	3 : 1
1974	655	36	5.5	778	24	3.1	2 : 1
1975	887	47	5.3	971	16	1.6	3 : 1
1976	937	63	6.7	1045	20	1.9	3 : 1
TOTAL	7958	519	6.5	8613	163	1.9	3 : 1

Associated metal sensitivities

It is more frequent, especially in men, for chromate sensitivity to occur alone than in association with reactions to cobalt or nickel. Among the patients seen between 1973–76 (inclusive) 70 per cent of the men and 57 per cent of the women reacted to chromate and not to the other two metals. The combination of chromate and nickel sensitivity was unusual in men (5 per cent) and women (11 per cent) (Table 7.7).

Table 7.7. Association of reactions to chromate, cobalt and nickel in men and women (St John's 1973–1976).

	Men		Women	
	No	%	No	%
Cr_6^+ Cob^- Ni^-	143	70	47	57
Cr_6^+ Cob^+ Ni^-	38	19	7	9
Cr_6^+ Cob^- Ni^+	10	5	9	11
Cr_6^+ Cob^+ Ni^+	12	6	19	23
Total Cr_6	203		82	

Causes of sensitivity to chromate

The causes of allergy to chromate vary from country to country and place to place depending upon local industry and the chemical environment. In some industries contact with chromate is a known hazard and it is easy to match the patient's chromate sensitivity to his job. In others it is possible with time and patience to trace a source of chromate contact at work or at home. However, there always remains a proportion of chromate sensitive patients, particularly women, in whom all attempts to discover the source of their allergy consistently fail.

Very few clinics have reported the incidence of causes of chromate allergy in their patients. Twenty-five years ago, in Finland, Pirilä (1954) listed the occupations of 140 chromate-sensitive patients as cement workers 57 per cent, lithographers and photographers 11 per cent, plating and metal workers 7 per cent, furriers 5 per cent, match factory workers 4 per cent, painters 3 per cent, miscellaneous 13 per cent. Another series from Austria (Kresbach, 1967), of 245 patients, gave the causes as cement 27 per cent, metal, car, railway and foundry workers and electricians 15 per cent, domestic work including cleaners and kitchen staff, publicans and brewery workers 13 per cent, carpenters, painters and textile workers and employees in the paper, shoe and porcelain industries 7 per cent, women with suspender dermatitis 5 per cent, dermatitis from medicaments 25 per cent and from rubber 8 per cent. In the last two neither the source nor the relevance of the allergy was known. In complete contrast, in Kuwait, of 221 patients sensitive to chromate the cause was cement in 82 per cent and footwear in 18 per cent (Kanan, 1969).

St John's

Men

The sources of exposure of the 519 chromate sensitive men, seen between 1967 and 1976, have been grouped in Table 7.8. Some were no longer employed in these jobs when they attended the clinic.

Nearly half (239) (46 per cent) had acquired the sensitivity from cement, usually as labourers, bricklayers or other workers on building sites and a few (19) were plasterers (plaster is finely divided cement). Between 1970 and 1976, 169 of the men with cement exposure attended the clinic and of these 32 (19 per cent) had used the cement at home for do-it-yourself construction work. The other occupations are listed in Table 7.8. The employment of the 48 men in the miscellaneous group comprised: tannery (5) tyre factory* (5) rubber factory* (1) painters and decorators (4) cleaners (4) diesel engines (4) glass workers (4) garages (3) French-polishers (3) paint factories (2) electricians (2) breweries (2) manufacture of television screens (2) laboratory assistants (2) paper mills (2) foundry (1) cable joiner (1) photography (1).

In 16 men the wearing of leather, usually shoes, may possibly have been the source of their sensitivity. In 83 men no source of exposure was found.

Table 7.8. Sources of chromate sensitivity in 519 men (St John's 1967–1976).

	No. Patients	%
Building	220 ⎫ 239	46
Plasterers	19 ⎭	
Engineering	104	20
Printers	17	3
Platers	12	2
Miscellaneous occupations*	48	9
??Leather	16	3
No source found	83	16
Total	519	

*In the miscellaneous group, although six of the men worked with rubber, chromate is not a recognised hazard of the rubber industry.

Women

In the women seen in this clinic it is usually very difficult to trace the source of exposure to chromate or to assess the relevance of the allergy. Between 1967 and 1976, 163 reacted to chromate. Their occupations have been listed (Table 7.9). Although leather was included as a possible source in 23 women, this was only on the basis of the patient having eczema of the feet. The miscellaneous group included a wide variety of apparently non-relevant occupations and, though women not at work were listed as housewives, the majority of those employed were also housewives.

Table 7.9. Sources of chromate sensitivity in 163 women (St John's, 1967–1976).

	No. Patients	%
Housewives	38	23
Domestic cleaners	13	8
Engineering	13	8
??Leather	23	14
Cement (DIY)	2	
Primer (DIY)	1	
Artists' paints	1	
Printing	1	
Miscellaneous (NSF)	71	44
Total	163	

(DIY = Do-it-yourself; NSF = No source found).

CLINICAL FEATURES

Chrome ulcers

It used to be thought that chrome ulcers or chrome holes were caused by the irritant effect of chromic acid or acid chrome salts until it was found that the alkaline hexavalent chromate solutions were much more caustic to the skin than the acidic chrome solutions (Meneghini, 1950). This was confirmed in guinea-pigs, in which ulcers were easily produced by chromates but not by trivalent chrome compounds (Samitz and Epstein, 1962). These holes occur particularly in men working in tanneries, electroplating and chrome chemical industries. In an Aktyubinsk chromium compound plant at one time chrome ulcers constituted 65 per cent of the cases of dermatitis, but with improvement in conditions the numbers were greatly reduced (Felker, Gaster and Pugina, 1974). The holes are punched-out ulcers and develop in broken skin on exposed sites such as the hands, feet, arms and face. On the hands they tend to develop over the knuckles or adjacent to the nails. Although they cause little pain they may be itchy. They have an inherent tendency to heal, they do not become malignant and do not result in sensitisation to chromates (Walsh, 1953). An ointment containing 10 per cent edathamil calcium as a chelating agent has been used for their treatment (Maloof, 1955) and in guinea-pigs ascorbic acid has reduced the healing time of such ulcers (Samitz, 1970).

A similar toxic necrosis affects the mucosa overlying the nasal cartilage; with destruction of the nasal mucous membrane the blood supply to the cartilage is impaired, leading to necrosis and perforation of the nasal septum. These perforations cause little discomfort; they do not cause deformity of the nose because the bone is unaffected and they are therefore usually discovered accidentally (Hunter, 1969).

Chromate sensitivity

Age distribution

St John's
At St John's no difference has been found between the ages of the chromate-sensitive men and women. In both, sensitisation corresponded with the working span of life.

The ages of 513 men and 162 women seen between 1967 and 1976 have been tabulated (Table 7.10). The ages of six men and one woman were not traced.

Table 7.10. Ages of 513 men and 162 women sensitive to chromate (St John's 1967–1976).

Years	0–10	11–20	21–30	31–40	41–50	51–60	61–70	71–90
Men	0	15	61	122	125	121	65	4
Women	0	13	35	23	29	41	15	6

Patterns of dermatitis

The distribution of the eczema has been studied in the patients seen at St John's. In about three-quarters of the men (83 per cent) and two-thirds of the women (69 per cent) the hands were affected with or without involvement of other sites. Involvement of the feet with sparing of the hands was rare in men (2 per cent) but not so infrequent among the women (10 per cent) and a discoid pattern was seen in a few men (4 per cent) but only one woman (Table 7.11). In five men and one woman the sites of the eczema were not recorded.

Table 7.11. Distribution of eczema in chromate-sensitive patients (St John's, 1967–1976).

	Men		Women	
Hands alone	150		44	
Hands + elsewhere	158	83%	31	69%
Hands + feet ± elsewhere	119		37	
Feet ± elsewhere	12	2%	17	10%
Discoid	19	4%	1	0.6%
Other sites	56		32	
Total	514		162	

Sources of chromate

Industrial sources of chromate include:

Cement	Galvanised sheets	Anti-corrosive in water systems
Anti-rust coatings	Oils	Ashes
Solvent (rare)	Foundry sand	Paper industry
Welding	Printing	Glues
Electroplating	Food laboratories	Paints
Milk testers	Primer paints	

also:

Glass polishes   Glass stains   and Glazing
Colour television screens and Magnetic tapes
Photographic chemicals and Wood preservatives.

Domestic sources of chromate include:

Bleaches and Detergents (variable)	Fabrics	Leather
Matches (safety)	Anti-emetic drug	Cardiac pace-maker (?)

CEMENT

Manufacture and chemical properties

The manufacture of cement and the sources of chromate in Portland cements have been studied by Johnston and Calnan (1958) and Fregert and Gruvberger (1972). Cement by the very nature of its ingredients does not have a constant chemical composition: its main natural constituents are chalk or limestone and clay or shale; coal, used as the fuel, becomes incorporated into it during manufacture and gypsum (calcium sulphate) is added to prolong the setting time of wet cement. Its approximate chemical composition is shown in Table 7.12:

Cement is irritant because it is alkaline, abrasive and hygroscopic. Dry cement powder consists mainly of fine particles called 'flour' and in this dry form it is relatively innocuous and men in cement factories, though exposed to

Table 7.12. Constituents of Portland cement (Johnston and Calnan, 1958)

Silica (SiO_2)	18–25%
Alumina (Al_2O_3)	3–10%
Oxide of iron (Fe_2O_3)	2–5%
Lime (CaO)	60–66%
Magnesia (MgO)	0.5–4%
Sulphuric anhydride (SO_3)	0.5–2.75%
Miscellaneous	1–4%

this dust hazard, rarely develop dermatitis (Calnan, 1960). Once cement is made wet either by slaking, which is the addition of water, or by absorption of water from the skin it liberates calcium hydroxide, making it alkaline and causing its most irritant dermatitic effect. As a powder, cement is not particularly abrasive but if the powder sets on the skin larger and more irritant particles form. When mixed with sand to make concrete, the mixture is very abrasive. The anhydrous compounds in cement make it hygroscopic and in both its dry and wet states it absorbs water from the skin. It has been suggested that the oxidising capacity of wet cement is partly responsible for its dermatitic properties (Rabito and Peserico, 1973).

Cement, because it often contains chromate and cobalt, also causes an allergic contact dermatitis; chromate is the principal allergen, whereas the cobalt is of much less importance. Sensitivity to chromate in cement workers was observed in 1939 but at that time it was attributed to the wearing of leather gloves (Bonnevie, 1939). It was not until 1950 when Jaeger and Pelloni (1950) obtained positive patch tests in 30 out of 32 men with cement eczema and found minute quantities of chromate in cement that the relevance and significance of this sensitivity was realised.

Chromate content of cements

The chromium in the raw materials is not in hexavalent form but is probably present as trivalent compounds. In 1958 it was found that 70 per cent came from the clay, 7 per cent from the chalk and 1 per cent from the gypsum (calcium sulphate) (Johnston and Calnan, 1958). An analysis of Belgian cement confirmed that the clay had the highest chromium content (Oleffe and Roosels, 1971).

In finished cement all the water-soluble chromium is in hexavalent form: it is derived from oxidation of chromium compounds in the intense heat of the kilns. In cement the total amount of chromium is not of great importance because this value can be high and yet the amount of water-soluble hexavalent chromate can be low (Fregert and Gruveberger, 1972). In the alkaline environment of cement, hexavalent chromate is water-soluble and is sensitising, therefore its concentration is of the greatest significance. Whereas trivalent chromium, being insoluble in alkali, is probably innocuous in cement, this is not absolutely certain as the skin may be capable of neutralising sufficient cement to solubilise some of the trivalent chromium. It has been verified (Fregert and Gruvberger, 1973i) that the concentration of water-soluble chromate is dependent upon the presence of water-soluble sulphate which for technical setting reasons is always added to cement as gypsum (calcium sulphate).

Twenty-four samples of British cement were examined for chromate and the content varied from 0–1200 µg per cent (Johnston and Calnan, 1958). Belgian cement was analysed by Brun (1963); he used sodium sulphate to estimate the free and absorbed chromate and obtained values of 0–35 mg/100 g. Another report from Belgium (Oleffe and Roosels, 1971) gave values for the chrome content of seven cements as 19–100 ppm. French cements were examined and the chromium content was between 30–250 ppm (Beurey et al., 1968). Eight cements from North and South Italy were analysed by Meneghini, Rantuccio and Petruzzellis (1969) and chromate was present in each one, the amount varying from 10–55 gamma Cr/g. Eight brands of Swedish cement were analysed by Wahlberg, Lindstedt and Einarsson (1977) and their chromate content was below 20 µg/g. Water-soluble chromate was estimated in 52 samples of Portland cement from nine countries by Fregert and Gruvberger (1972): the amounts ranged from 1–40 µg Cr/g, 50 samples contained 17 µg Cr/g or less and only two contained 37 and 40 µg Cr/g respectively. Forty-two samples of Portland cement made in the USA were examined by Perone et al. (1974) and all contained chromium ranging from 5–124 µg/g but of the filtrates from these 42 samples only 18 contained measurable quantities of chromate, the amounts varying from 0.1–5.4 µg/g.

It is not feasible to lower the chromate content of cement by changing the raw materials or by altering the manufacturing process but it has been found that the addition of ferrous sulphate reduces all the chromate to the trivalent form and it is precipitated despite the alkaline environment (Fregert and Gruvberger, 1973 ii; Fregert Gruvberger and Sandahl, 1979). Ferrous sulphate is inexpensive, the amount required completely to reduce the chromate is small and it does not affect the other properties of the cement. It is best added as a fresh 20 per cent solution at the time when the concrete or mortar is being mixed. If it is found to be a practical procedure thus to remove chromate from cement during its manufacture then the achievement of these investigators is very great.

Substances, some of which may be irritants or sensitisers, may be added to cement to give it special properties. These include:

1. *Air entraining agents*
    a. Soaps of wood rosin acids (e.g. sodium abietate)
    b. Alkylarylsulphonates
    c. Calcium lignosulphonate
    d. Proteins
    e. Other surface active agents

2. *Accelerators*
    a. Sodium silicate
    b. Calcium chloride
    c. Calcium formate
    d. Sodium or potassium carbonate
    e. Aluminium chloride
    f. Triethanolamine

3. *Retarders and water-reducing agents*

    a. Lignosulphonates (sulphite lyes, lignins) of Ca, Mg, Na, NH_4

    b. Hydroxy carbolyxic acids

    c. Carbohydrates

4. *Plasticisers*

    a. Lignosulphonate

    b. Surface active agents

    c. Calcium chloride

5. *Blowing agents*

    a. Aluminium

6. *Plastics*

    a. Polyvinyl acetate (PVA)

    b. Polyvinyl chloride (PVC)

    c. Polyvinyl propionate

    d. Polyesters

    e. Vinyl chloride

    f. Acrylic chloride

    g. Rubber latex (Natural and Synthetic)

    h. Epoxy resin

7. *Filler agents*

    a. Butyl stearate

8. *Colours*

    a. Cobalt aluminate and oxide

    b. Chromium oxide

    c. Iron oxide

    d. Cadmium sulphide

    e. Manganese oxides

    f. Monastral blue

    g. Carbon black

    h. Titanium dioxide

9. *Waterproofing agents*

    a. Ca, Al or Zn stearate

    b. Ca, Al or Zn oleate

    c. Butyl stearate

    d. Silicones

    e. Calcium palmitate

10. *Antifreezing agents*

    a. Calcium chloride
    b. Infusorial earth
    c. Methyl and ethyl alcohol
    d. Ethylene glycol
    e. Urea carbonate

11. *Fungicides*

    a. Copper sulphate

12. *Corrosion inhibitors*

    a. Sodium nitrate
    b. Sodium benzoate
    c. Sodium chromate   (Calnan, Fregert and Pirilä, 1969).

Occupations with exposure to cement
The greatest hazard from cement occurs on building and construction sites but men are also at risk in the manufacture of cement and there is an increasing number of men who use cement at home for do-it-yourself jobs. Occupations with cement contact include: bricklayers, labourers, plasterers, floor layers and tilers, carpenters, decorators and any worker on a building site. Lorry drivers for cement firms and plumbers are also at risk.

Quick lime
Eleven quick limes (calcium hydroxide) were analysed for chromate and they were found to contain 0.28–9.8 ppm (Weiler and Rüssel, 1974).

Incidence of cement dermatitis

Cement dermatitis as an occupational disease
In many countries cement dermatitis is an important cause of occupational dermatitis. In Germany cement eczema accounted for 10 per cent of the occupational dermatoses (Spier and Natzel, 1952). In Finland 1752 patients with occupational dermatoses were investigated and cement or lime was the cause in 12 per cent (Pirilä and Kilpiö, 1954). In France in 1957 bricklayers itch constituted 20–25 per cent of occupational skin diseases (Huriez, 1957); by 1966 the incidence of cement dermatitis had risen to 33 per cent of all occupational dermatoses (Huriez, Martin and Planque, 1969), and in 1973 it was the major cause of occupational dermatitis (Amphoux, Poli and Robin, 1973). In Switzerland, in parallel with the expansion of cement works and the building industry, there has been a gradual increase in the frequency of cement dermatitis from 30.8 per cent in 1951 to 40.3 per cent in 1959 and 34.8 per cent in 1960 (Gieser and Girard, 1965). In northern Italy, of 2272 patients with occupational eczema, 717 (32 per cent) were due to cement (Meneghini, Rantuccio and Riboldi, 1963). In Northern Ireland Burrows (1972) reported that 23 per cent of industrial injury benefits went to construction workers and in Great Britain it was estimated that

about 200 000 days were lost each year through 'eczema and dermatitis' in the building industry (Burrows and Calnan, 1965).

Incidence of cement dermatitis in men working with cement
It was reported by Meneghini and Petruzzellis (1968) in Bari, in southern Italy, that on a periodic examination of 980 men in a cement factory four (0.4 per cent) had an allergic contact dermatitis. In contrast, during a two-year observation period of 1500 men on a group of building sites 20 cases (1.3 per cent) developed an allergic dermatitis. They attributed the higher incidence in these men to contact with wet cement as opposed to the dry powder handled in the cement factory. In Kuwait, where rapid urbanisation led to many cases of cement dermatitis, the high humidity which occurs in that climate was considered by Kanan (1972) to be a crucial factor in facilitating chromate sensitisation and also to account for the periodicity of relapses. Men working on building sites have been investigated in Stockholm (1969) and it was found that 4.9 per cent of bricklayers and 5.9 per cent of concrete workers had eczema (Wahlberg, 1969). In Norway, around Bergen, 366 men on building sites were examined: 24 (7 per cent) showed on their hands the irritant traumatic effect of cement and 20 (5.5 per cent) had cement eczema (Høvding, 1970). In Northern Ireland it has been estimated that 3.5 per cent of those working in the building industry will develop a dermatitis severe enough to necessitate their being off work (Burrows, 1972).

Time of onset
It has been said that cement eczema is a disease of the older worker and in the Bergen study of men on building sites, of 24 men with eczema who were sensitive to dichromate, 14 had worked for 11 years or more before its onset (Høvding, 1970). In contrast, in the survey of building workers in Stockholm, of 34 men with eczema 14 had been in the trade for five years or less (Wahlberg, 1969).

Clinical features
There are two distinct types of cement dermatitis, one is the irritant effect of cement on the skin, the other is eczema. In some men these changes merge and in the early stages they may be difficult to differentiate.

Irritant effect
Many men working with cement for the first time notice this irritant effect as the skin of their hands becomes dry, hard, tight and uncomfortable. Hardening gradually ensues in most workers and their skin becomes resistant to these injurious effects but in a few the changes go on to painful fissuring and nail dystrophy (Calnan, 1960).

Cement burns
Severe alkali burns of the lower legs and feet from the calcium hydroxide in wet cement have been reported in four occupational construction workers and nine amateurs, two of whom were women. These extraordinary second to third degree burns followed kneeling in wet cement for 2–6 hours or the spilling of

wet cement down wellington boots. The immediate skin contamination was symptomless in some or produced smarting or burning in others, but in each patient within hours the affected skin became red or even black and in the majority this was followed by necrosis and ulceration which took weeks to heal and sometimes scarred. The alkali content of the cements was not known but where stated the patients had used pre-mixed concrete (Rowe and Williams, 1963; Vickers and Edwards, 1976; Hannuksela, Suhonen and Karvonen, 1976; Bandmann and Agathos, 1977; Flowers, 1978; Jünger and Witzani, 1978).

Eczema (dermatitis)

Some men develop eczema; in over half (57 per cent) the hands and arms are involved (Burrows and Calnan, 1965). The skin is red, scaly and thickened, usually with the appearances of a subacute or chronic eczema rather than those of an acute exudative dermatitis. When the eczema is severe it may spread to other areas of the body.

A clinical difficulty with cement dermatitis is its mimicry of constitutional patterns of eczema. This was first appreciated fifty years ago when men building the London Underground presented with eczema simulating seborrhoeic eczema, intertrigo, exfoliative dermatitis and erythroderma (O'Donovan, 1925). Since then these patterns have been well described and their frequency was reported by Burrows and Calnan (1965) in a group of 134 patients. Some (13 per cent) of the patients presented with discoid eczema which may affect the dorsa of the hands, arms, legs, and elsewhere. In others (10 per cent) the distribution was that of a seborrhoeic eczema with involvement of the scalp, face, ears, neck, axillae, waist and groins. This type of eczema occurs particularly in men who carry bags of cement and whose clothes become impregnated with dust which settles in the body folds and areas of sweat and friction, such as around the waist or under a belt. The dermatitis simulated stasis eczema in 7 per cent; it then affects the dorsa of the feet and spreads up over the ankles on to the lower legs. This is due to cement dust becoming trapped in boots and socks. In some of these patients there is an associated hand eczema. Eczema of the palms, often with the appearance of a constitutional pompholyx, may occur (9 per cent) and eczema of the knee and elbow flexures closely simulating atopic dermatitis has been described (Burrows and Calnan, 1965; Shannon, 1965).

A diagnosis of cement dermatitis must be considered in all patients working with cement or plaster either as a living or a hobby, regardless of the pattern of their eczema. In the group of 283 patients with a history of cement contact investigated by Burrows and Calnan (1965), 60 per cent were diagnosed as having cement dermatitis, 28 per cent had constitutional eczema or contact dermatitis from another cause, 9 per cent were doubtful cases of cement dermatitis and 3 per cent did not have eczema.

Incidence of chromate sensitivity in patients with cement dermatitis

There is usually a close correlation between cement eczema and sensitivity to chromate. Taking the average incidence of all reports available at that time Høvding (1970) found that 81 per cent of men with *eczema* from cement reacted to chromate. The figures recorded vary little; in two large series, one from Finland (Pirilä, 1954) of 90 patients, 82 per cent were sensitive and of 171 patients tested in London 78 per cent reacted (Burrows and Calnan, 1965). In a detailed study of men working on building sites in Norway, Høvding (1970) reported that of 20 men with cement eczema 17 (85 per cent) were allergic to chromate. Among construction workers with dermatitis in France (Duperrat and Lamberton, 1973) chromate is a significant allergen; this is also the case in Spain (Conde-Salazar Gomez and Gomez Urcuyo, 1976) and similarly in Kuwait (Kanan, 1969). In London (Burrows and Calnan, 1965) sensitivity was found to be as frequent (82 per cent) in those with eczema which mimicked a constitutional pattern as those with eczema of the hands and arms (74 per cent). However, countries do differ because in the U.S.A. (Perone et al., 1974) only one of 95 construction workers reacted to a patch test with 0.25 per cent dichromate despite 15 having an irritant dermatitis and 20 eczematous lesions at the time of patch testing.

In contrast to eczematous patients, 24 men with the *irritant* effect of cement on their hands (that is abrasions, dryness, cracks and fissures) were patch tested by Høvding (1970) and only two (8 per cent) reacted.

Incidence of chromate sensitivity in cement workers with normal skin (Latent allergy)

Healthy cement workers without a present or past history of skin trouble have been patch tested. Ninety-eight such men working in a factory making prefabricated concrete components were tested with dichromate (Burrows and Calnan, 1965) and three (3 per cent) reacted; six months later one had developed eczema of the hands. In Norway (Høvding, 1970) 366 men on building sites were investigated and nine (2.5 per cent) healthy workers were sensitive. In Switzerland two of 34 masons (6 per cent) gave positive patch tests (Hunziker and Musso, 1960).

Prognosis

It is usually thought that cement eczema carries a bad prognosis. Although there is an undoubted relationship between dermatitis from cement and sensitivity to chromate, the part this allergy plays in the initiation, severity or chronicity of the condition is unknown. Opinions differ: it has been suggested that the allergy precipitates and maintains the eczema (Høvding, 1970) but equally that it may be only a secondary factor and its existence is neither an aid to prognosis nor an influence on the course of the eczema (Burrows and Calnan, 1965).

In general changing work to avoid contact with cement does not seem to improve the prognosis very greatly; this has been studied in various centres. In London (Burrows and Calnan, 1965) the incidence of healing or great improvement was 30 per cent (11/37) among men who changed their jobs, and in Lausanne (Geiser and Girard, 1965) 24 per cent (14/59) of the men cleared. But in contrast in Zurich 81 per cent (17/21) of the men healed and in this report (Peter, 1968) and in Türk's (1975) opinion, change of employment was definitely beneficial. Pürschell and Fürst (1972) attributed relapses in new jobs to continued contact with the allergen through poor choice of alternative employment.

However, healing of the eczema also occurs if the men remain at their same cement jobs. In Geneva (Hunziker and Musso, 1960) 47 per cent (8/17) cleared and in Lausanne (Geiser and Girard, 1965) 9 per cent (4/46) recovered while still in contact with cement.

A special study was done in Bergen (Høvding, 1970) of masons and hodmen (bricklayers' labourers) while they were actually working on building sites. It was found that although 33 of the 366 men (9 per cent) gave positive reactions to chromate, only 17 of these had cement eczema. Of the 16 men with clear skins who were sensitive to chromate, seven had a past history of cement eczema but nine had never had eczema. Therefore in these men chromate sensitivity did not necessarily result in cement eczema and even if they did develop eczema the skin could heal completely and they were able to remain at work. Although the eczema in these men tended to be chronic and about 50 per cent of those with eczema had short periods off work, the eczema was not incapacitating and did not necessitate their changing jobs. On this basis the prognosis of cement eczema was thought not to be as gloomy as that usually given. A similar investigation was undertaken in Stockholm (Wahlberg, 1969) and there about 38 per cent of the men with eczema were off work for one or more periods. In France Duperrat and Lamberton (1973) supervised the men carefully and found they were able to remain at work.

Practically all these results indicate that it is inadvisable to make a cement worker change his job. Away from cement his eczema may heal but equally it may not and in new employment he is likely to lose status and money and if his eczema persists he has a double burden. If he remains at work his eczema may be manageable and his skin may even recover.

The cause of the chronicity of eczema, even when out of contact with cement, is unknown. It may be that the ubiquity of chromium makes avoidance of the allergen impossible or it is possible that the oral ingestion of chromium is a factor (p. 311).

OTHER SOURCES OF CHROMATE

Anti-rust coatings
The less-soluble salts of chromium — zinc, lead and barium chromate — are used as protective coatings on metal to prevent corrosion and rust formation. This use of chromate is widespread throughout the engineering industry and is easily overlooked as a source of chromate exposure.

In a car factory, chromate dermatitis was found to be most frequent among assembly workers and the source was traced to the steel nuts, bolts and screws which had been zinc plated and then, as is customary, treated with a chromate dip as a passivator to prevent oxidation and atmospheric erosion (Newhouse, 1963). Metal treated with chromate has caused dermatitis in ship workers and in others (Anderson, 1960) and labelling tins coated with anti-rust chromate solution resulted in dermatitis in two women factory workers (Hjorth, 1967).

Galvanised sheets
Hexavalent chromate is the only additive which inhibits oxidation in cast iron

and zinc (Hersch *et al.*, 1961). Iron sheets are best protected from rusting by galvanising them with zinc applied either by electroplating or by dipping them in molten zinc; to prevent the zinc corroding, oxidising or whitening with moisture, the metal is then coated with chromate. These sheets are used in the building industry and for ventilation ducts. This surface chromate can induce sensitisation or exacerbate a dermatitis in a previously sensitised person. Up to 2.5 mg of hexavalent chromate has been recovered from men's hands after four hours' work and although this accumulation of chromate is much greater than that which occurs with cement, the work is dry and the metal itself is not irritant (Foussereau and Benezra, 1970; Fregert, Gruvberger and Heijer, 1970). The deterioration of hand eczema in a chromate sensitive man working with galvanised sheet metal was investigated by Rycroft and Calnan (1977i). On the metal they found only trivalent chromium and its absorption through broken skin was thought to account for the relapse of his eczema.

Primer paints
Anti-rust primer paints are formulated with either:
Zinc potassium chromate, which contains insoluble zinc chromate and freely-soluble potassium dichromate, making this compound a considerable chromate hazard,
or:
Basic zinc chromate which yields little water-soluble chromate,
or:
Mixtures of the two types.

These compounds differ in their uses as do their paint bases; the common zinc chromate is usually in an alkyd base. To be effective against rust, paints require soluble chromate but the amount in the zinc potassium chromate approximates to that used for patch testing and it explains the sensitising and dermatitic potential of these primer paints (Adams *et al.*, 1976). Over 30 years ago Hall (1944) reported that primer paints caused dermatitis in aircraft workers. A similar primer paint produced an outbreak of dermatitis in 65 of 250 men (26 per cent) wet sandpapering car bodies. The eczema affected principally the hands and the arms: the appearances were variable, in some men the pattern was that of a discoid eczema, in others pompholyx and sometimes it was indistinguishable from atopic or seborrhoeic eczema (Engel and Calnan, 1963). A similar primer paint containing zinc chromate was used on a metal leg prosthesis and sensitised a cobbler on his amputation stump and he simultaneously developed eczema on his foot from his own shoe and on his hands from the shoes he mended (Bang Pedersen and Fregert, 1970).

Paints
Paints, particularly yellows and greens, may include chromium pigments and some contain chromate. The bright yellow paint on industrial equipment is likely to contain chromate.

Solvent
A degreasing solvent, containing 0.2 per cent sodium chromate as an anti-

corrosive, was used to remove paint and soot from diesel engine components requiring repair. After four years' exposure a mechanic developed hand eczema and was found to be allergic to chromate (Ros and Bang Pedersen, 1977).

Oils
Before use, lubricating and soluble cutting oils are very unlikely to contain chromate (Weiler, 1969; Oleffe *et al.*, 1971) although chromate has been found in an unused bore oil (Holz, Mappes and Weidmann, 1961) and it was thought to have sensitised previously unexposed workers. It may have been added as an anti-corrosive. In another instance a soluble oil was formulated with 0.8 per cent potassium dichromate and after dilution for use contained 0.01 per cent. This concentration sensitised a man working on a grinding machine (Calnan, 1978). The chromium content of unused oils is also low; Wahlberg *et al.* (1977) found 28 new mould oils to contain $< 0.19 \mu g/g$ and of 28 unused cutting fluids only one contained more than $1 \mu g/g$.

The possibility exists that after use oils may contain chromate derived from contact with steel or other metal. In such oils the chromium is present either as powdered metal, which can be removed by centrifugation, or as oil-soluble chromium salts (Rüssel and Weiler, 1971). Chromium was detected by atomic absorption in used cutting fluids by Einarsson *et al.* (1975) but not by Samitz and Katz (1975) using another method. Chromate in a contaminated oil caused a relapse of dermatitis in a previously-sensitised man (Weiler, 1969) and induced sensitisation in a man working with chromate-coated zinc galvanised iron sheeting (Fregert and Gruvberger, 1976).

Anti-corrosive in re-circulating and other water systems
Chromates are very effective anti-corrosives in re-circulating water systems. In the 1940s when diesel power began to replace steam power in railway engines, chromate was added to the radiator fluid of the engine for this purpose. Chromate dermatitis soon occurred among railway employees working on the maintenance of these diesel engines. Cases first occurred among those maintaining these diesel engines. The first cases were reported from the United States by Winston and Walsh (1951) and ten years later from England among fitters working for the Eastern Region of British Railways, which was the only section which used chromate as an anti-corrosive (Calnan and Harman, 1961). All these railwaymen were at particular risk because they handled both the chromate powder and the concentrated solutions prior to their dilution as radiator fluids. As with other types of chromate sensitivity the dermatitis persisted even after removal from the allergen (Calnan and Harman, 1961). Such cases have ceased because the chromate was such a hazard that it had to be replaced by other anti-corrosives.

Chromates may also be used in refrigeration, air conditioning and central heating systems. An electrician who added chromate powder to a central heating unit and a printer who used a machine with a water-cooling system were both sensitised to chromate and developed dermatitis (Calnan and Harman, 1961). Brine is used as a cooling agent in ice plants, and in breweries it is added to the yeast residues to lower the freezing point of the water. Chromate may be added residues, known as 'balm beer' (Wilson, 1971). Similarly chromate in the water coolant system of a gramophone record press sensitised a man (Calnan, 1978).

Welding

Chromium may be present in the core and coating of the electrode rods used in electric arc welding, in the rods used in other types of welding and also in the parent metal. Particularly when any of these metals are chromium alloys such as stainless steel containing 18 per cent chromium and 8 per cent nickel, the amount of hexavalent chromium formed is considerable. During welding, intense heat is generated to fuse the rod and parent metal and the chromium in the electrodes or rods is oxidised to the hexavalent form and is present in the fumes which surround the operation. Exposure to these gases containing chromate may cause an allergic contact dermatitis of the face (Fregert and Övrum, 1963) and sporadic inhalation of acetylene welding fumes by a man sensitive to chromate was the cause of his repeated episodes of hand eczema (Shelley, 1964). Inhalation of gases during acetylene welding caused asthma and urticaria in a railway worker but the allergen was not identified (Kaplan and Zeligman, 1963).

Metal fume fever complicated by pneumonia has been described in a welder (Ross, 1974); and an electro-welder, who after 18 years' work developed actinic keratoses and a metastasising squamous cell carcinoma, was reported by Haneke and Gutschmidt (1976). They implicated the UV-B radiation emitted during electro-welding.

Foundry sand

Men working in foundries with sand, or handling moulding sand (Hellier, 1962) may develop a chromate dermatitis of the hands. In Sweden the source of the chromate was found to be chromium magnesite bricks that had been discarded from a steel furnace and then ground and mixed with the foundry sand, which the men then handled (Fregert, 1963).

Boiler lining

In power house boilers the combustion chambers have a refractory lining containing trivalent chromium which is gradually converted to the hexavalent form by the heat and alkaline fuel ash. A fitter relining such a boiler developed chromate dermatitis (Rycroft and Calnan, 1977b).

Ashes

Obscure sources of contact with chromate have been sought to explain the persistence of chromate dermatitis in sensitised persons who are apparently removed from the source of the allergen. The fuels, wood, coal, coke and peat are derived from the soil and plants and contain trivalent chromium. After burning, wood ash is alkaline and contains sensitising chromate; coal and coke ash are not alkaline and the chromium remains in the relatively harmless trivalent form. Peat ash contains chromate only if combustion is complete (Fregert, 1962). In countries and districts where wood is a common form of fuel for fires and heating this source of chromate should not be overlooked.

Electroplating

Electroplating consists of coating one metal with a layer of another metal by means of an electric current. A tank is filled with a solution of the salt of the plating metal and the metal to be plated is immersed in the solution and acts as the cathode and another metal acts as the anode. These metals are connected to an electrical source and when a current passes the metallic ions of the plating solution are deposited on the cathode, which is the metal requiring plating. During plating a considerable mist arises from the solution in the plating tank. These metallic solutions are usually either acid or alkaline and are skin irritants. Before a metal can be plated it has to be thoroughly cleaned and polished, and this is done with solvents, soaps, alkalis and acids, all of which are irritants.

In chromium plating the bath contains chromic acid and sulphuric acid. During the passage of the electric current a large quantity of red-brown mist is given off which attacks the mucous membranes of the nose and causes ulceration and perforation of the septum. In 1969, 121 cases of chrome ulcerations were notified in Great Britain; of these 91 (75 per cent) occurred in the chromium plating industry (Henning, 1972). These workers are also at risk from the irritant effect of the cleansers and plating solutions on the skin and from the sensitising properties of hexavalent chromium which may cause allergic contact dermatitis.

In recent years these hazards have been reduced by exhaust ventilation over the baths, spray suppressants, protective clothing, adequate washing facilities and cleanliness of the working areas (Henning, 1972).

Printing

The printing industry has been considered to be one of the most dangerous as regards skin disease (Pirilä and Kilpio, 1954). Chromate, which is one of the hazards, is often present in the solutions used for cleaning plates. In Finland, of 149 patients with dermatitis working in this industry, 40 (27 per cent) were sensitive to chromium compounds (Pirilä and Kilpio, 1954). In an offset printing factory three men developed dermatitis and were found to be sensitive to chromate and cobalt. Spruit and Malten (1975) demonstrated that two of the materials they were handling contained 2000– 60 000 ppm of chromium.

Paper industry

Sensitivity to chromium compounds was the cause of dermatitis in one of 26 employees with occupational dermatitis in the paper industry in Finland (Pirilä and Kilpio, 1954). Men working in sulphate paper pulp factories are at risk in the sulphate recovery process, from chromium compounds present mainly in the sodium sulphate (Fregert, Gruvberger and Heijer, 1972). In the manufacture of paper, surface size gelatine, which may contain chromium, is applied to give a glossy finish to the paper. It was the cause of hand eczema in a machine operator rolling wood pulp in a paper factory (Connor, 1972).

Milk testers

Milk samples to be analysed for fat and protein are preserved with potassium dichromate. In the laboratory the chromate is added, either in solution by syringe or in tablets, which also contain mercuric chloride, to give a final 0.1 per cent concentration of dichromate in the milk samples. Principally the milk testers, but also the bottle cleaners, are at risk of being sensitised to the dichromate and cases of dermatitis of the hands, wrists, arms and other sites have been reported in France (Huriez, Martin and Lefèbvre, 1975), Northern Ireland (Rogers and Burrows, 1975) and Poland (Rudzki and Czerwinska-Dihnz, 1977). All the patients were patch tested with potassium dichromate and all reacted.

Food laboratory
A solution of potassium chromate 10 per cent is used as an indicator in the determination of the sodium chloride content of cooked food. A laboratory technician doing this estimation developed a vesicular eczema of the palms and fingers and was found on patch testing to be sensitised to dichromate (Bang Pedersen, 1977).

Glues
Glutin glues and gelatin may contain chromate. They are made from animal debris and if leather is the starting material then this is the source of the chromate. When skin, horns, hooves and bones are used the chromate is derived from the lime used in the initial stages of manufacture (Weiler and Rüssel, 1971).

Other industrial sources
Chromate dermatitis may also occur in glass polishers (Richter and Heidelbach, 1969), in stainers of glass and glaziers; in the making of colour television screens (Dower, Hill and Stevenson, 1973); from handling the magnetic tapes used for television recording (Krook, Fregert and Gruvberger, 1977); from photographic chemicals (p. 862); and wood preservatives.

Estimations have been made of the chromate content of 59 industrial products (Oleffe *et al.*, 1971).

Bleaches and detergents
Housewives' hand eczema is a frequent, recurring and probably universal problem and a specific aetiology is rarely found. In some countries chromate in bleaches and detergents is responsible.

Thirty-five years ago in France attention was focused on a popular liquid bleach (l'eau de Javel) to which chromate is added during production to stabilise and colour the solution. This bleach is still widely used in Belgium and France and it has been considered a significant cause of hand eczema in laundresses and those doing housework (Rabeau and Ukrainczyk, 1939). Cases were seen in Strasbourg and sensitivity to chromate was confirmed in these patients (Hilt, 1954). In 1963 in the Netherlands chromate was found in small quantities (0.3 μg/g–6.4 μg/g) in some but not all detergents; its source was the raw materials, since it was not added during manufacture. In contrast, chromate was present in each one of four liquid bleaches, the amounts varying between 9.8 μg/g–31.0 μg/g (Nater, 1963). These bleaches were considered the greater hazard because housewives change detergents but most of them use bleaches, sometimes even undiluted to clean vegetable stains from their hands. In Sweden, Wahlberg *et al.* (1977) estimated the total quantity of chromium (not chromate) in 19 detergents: 16 contained < 1.0 $\mu g/g$ and none exceeded 4 $\mu g/g$. In Israel in 1969, 50 women with typical housewives' hand eczema were patch tested and 47 (94 per cent) were found to be sensitive to chromate: the source was thought to be detergents and bleaches (Feuerman, 1969). A pitfall in the estimation of chromates in detergents is that perborates in the detergents may mask their presence and make them difficult to detect (Schuppli, 1967).

This source of chromate sensitivity does not seem to have been reported from other countries in recent years, either because it does not exist or because it is overlooked. An interesting study from Spain in 1973 (Garcia-Perez, Martin-Pascual and Sánchez-Misiego, 1973) reported that although in 1963 seven of nine bleaches and one of three liquid detergents had chromate added to them during manufacture, in 1972 only two of nine bleaches contained chromate and the detergents previously positive were then negative. This removal of chromate from the housewife's environment was reflected in a decrease in the number of housewives and domestic workers coming to the clinic with hand eczema. During the period 1963–1966 the average was 39 cases a year, of whom 30 per cent were sensitive to chromate, compared with 30 cases a year for the 1967–1972 period, of whom only 3 per cent were sensitive to chromate. There was no comparable fall in the incidence of chromate sensitivity in men.

Fabrics

Chromium compounds are used as mordants or fixing agents for dyes, and clothing dermatitis due to sensitivity to chromate has been reported from Germany. Of four women described, three were positive to dichromate and one to trivalent chromium, three reacted to their garments and chromate was found in the materials of each patient (Bockendahl, 1954; Ebner, 1967). Two Ceylonese nurses working in Nürnberg developed dermatitis of their necks. They were found to be sensitive to chromate and it was postulated that chromate might be present in the material of their uniform caps, either having been added during manufacture or from the caps having been washed in detergents (Roth, 1969). Chromate in green military textiles has caused dermatitis (p. 41) (Fregert *et al.*, 1978).

A powdered yellow dye containing 20 per cent zinc chromate was used in a machine for marking textiles and sensitised a woman working in an upholstery company. Although her own factory changed to titanium dioxide, the manufacturers of the machines and the dye refused to do so (Fregert and Gruvberger, 1976). Chromium salts are used also for dyeing the green felt of card tables and a chromium-sensitive Swedish patient thought his hand eczema relapsed when he played billiards. Felt from bridge tables was analysed and was found to contain nearly as much chromate as that present on galvanised metal sheets; a smaller amount was present in the worsted cloth of a billiard table but none was found in three green upholstery fabrics (Fregert, Hjorth and Gruvberger, 1970). Another patient suffered similarly from the green felt on card tables at Las Vegas. He too was sensitive to dichromate and reacted to a patch test with the green felt. Fisher (1976) designated the dermatitis as 'Blackjack Disease' after the card game and the patient solved his problem by playing in gloves.

Leather
(p. 70)

Matches
(p. 829)

Other sources of chromate
Chromate has even been added to an anti-emetic drug for alcoholics (Fregert, 1967) and dermatitis over a cardiac pacemaker may have been related to the patient's sensitivity to chromate or cadmium, but it was not proved (Laugier *et al.*, 1975).

Prognosis of chromate sensitivity
In men allergy to chromate carries a worse prognosis than does sensitisation to other allergens (Fregert, 1975; Czarnecki, 1979). The reason for this poor outlook is uncertain and it is not even known what part the chromate plays in the chronicity, or how important are constitutional factors. Continued contact with chromate may be the explanation or possibly the ingestion of chromate is significant.

Oral ingestion of chromate
Hexavalent but not trivalent chromium is well absorbed from the gut, but as the acidity of the gastric juices maintains the trivalent form it is likely that in a normal person little ingested chromate is absorbed (Donaldson and Barreras, 1966). However, some is absorbed as shown by Fregert (1965) who gave 50 μg of potassium dichromate to five chromate-sensitive patients and within two hours each had developed acute vesiculation of the palms and in one patient the eruption became generalised. Schleiff (1968) gave 1–10 mg of potassium dichromate orally to 20 chromate-sensitive patients and flared their previous eczema and in some there was a reactivation of positive patch test sites. In a double blind trial a tablet containing 7.1 mg of potassium dichromate (2.5 mg chromium) was compared with a placebo in 31 chromate-sensitive patients who currently had eczema. The chromate provoked a flare within 5–24 hours in 11 patients and the placebo aggravated two patients (Kaaber and Veien, 1977).

It is possible that the unwitting ingestion of chromate in food plays a part in the chronicity of the eczema in chromate-sensitive patients.

Photosensitivity
The photosensitising properties of chromium compounds are being investigated with increasing frequency. Tronnier and Turek (1969) reported the trivalent compounds to be the photosensitisers and suggested that reduction of hexavalent chromate to the trivalent form occurs in the skin. In Israel, Feuerman (1971) considered that the high incidence of chromate sensitivity in housewives with eczema may relate to the sunny climate and the photosensitising potential

of chromium. It has been shown by Wahlberg and Wennersten (1977) that subjects sensitive to dichromate will react to photopatch tests with weak concentrations of dichromate irradiated with short wave ultraviolet light (UVB). Long wave ultraviolet light (UVA) did not have this potentiating effect.

Patch testing

Routine diagnostic patch testing is done with the hexavalent salt of chromium.

Potassum dichromate ($K_2Cr_2O_7$) 0.5 per cent in petrolatum.

Many chromate-sensitive patients will also react to patch tests with trivalent salts; a suitable compound is

Basic chromic sulphate $A_5Cr(OH) SO_4$ 10 per cent in petrolatum
   (A = any uncharged group, usually H_2O).

Patch testing with cement is useless because its alkalinity makes it an irritant and neither a positive nor a negative reaction has any significance. Patch testing with other substances containing chromate is also often invalid, either because they are irritant or because their content of chromate is too low to elicit a positive response.

The suggestion (Spier and Natzel, 1953; Miescher, Amrein and Leder, 1955; Skog and Wahlberg, 1969) that patch testing with an alkaline buffered solution of dichromate (pH 10–12) to correspond with the alkalinity of cement increases the sensitivity of the test has not always been confirmed (Burrows and Calnan, 1965). The irritancy of alkaline solutions must make such patch tests difficult to evaluate and the results of somewhat doubtful significance. Emulsifiers have also been added to the dichromate-petrolatum patch test preparations and glycerol monostearate enhanced their sensitivity (Rudzki, 1976). Dichromate in petrolatum penetrates the skin better than as a solution in water (Liden and Lundberg, 1979).

An electron microscope study of allergic patch test reactions to chromate showed destructive cellular changes in skin which looked clinically normal and the effect of occlusion alone caused changes in the epidermal cells (Forslind and Wahlberg, 1977).

In vitro tests

The macrophage migration inhibition test was found to be a successful indicator of chromate sensitivity in guinea-pigs and migration was inhibited by hexavalent and trivalent chromium salts. However, migration inhibition factor was produced only by trivalent compounds (Polak and Frey, 1973). Leucocyte migration inhibition has been studied in man (Tio, 1976; Czernielewski, Libiszowski and Dudek, 1977) and trivalent salts have successfully inhibited migration.

These studies were thought to confirm that it is trivalent chromium which, conjugated with protein, is the 'true' antigen in this metal sensitivity (Polak and Frey 1973; Tio, 1976).

Anti-chrome barrier creams

It is so difficult to remove chromate from the environment that attempts have been made to formulate an anti-chrome barrier cream. The principle of such creams depends either upon reduction of hexavalent to trivalent chromium and chelation of the metal, or on chelation alone. A combination of sodium pyrosulphite as the reducing agent and tartaric acid as the chelating compound has been found to be effective (Samitz, Gross and Katz, 1962; Burrows and Calnan, 1965), as has ascorbic acid. The ascorbic acid acts both as a reducing and as a chelating agent (Samitz, 1970). Ointments containing anionic exchange resins which bind chromate ions are efficacious if used regularly (Schuppli, 1970). Ivosin cream was assessed by Amphoux and Robin (1975) and the men appeared to like it but for no obvious clinical reason.

Diphenylcarbazide test for chromate
This test detects chromate to a dilution of 10 parts per million.

1. The test material is shaken with hot water to extract the chromate and if necessary the solution is then filtered.
2. The filtrate is acidified by the addition of 10 per cent hydrochloric acid.
3. A few drops of a 1 per cent alcoholic solution of diphenylcarbazide are then added.

The development of a stable red colour is specific for hexavalent chromium salts (Newhouse, 1963).

Cobalt

Cobalt is a silver-grey, hard, magnetic metal which is usually found in association with nickel and often with arsenic. It is mainly derived as a by-product of copper and silver mining and comes principally from the copper mines of Zaire and Zambia and it is also mined with nickel in Canada and some is produced in the U.S.A. It was probably named by the 16th Century miners of Saxony, who thought of it as a kobold, or mischievious goblin, in the arsenic ore they worked.

When estimated by the sensitive technique of atomic absorption spectrophotometry traces of cobalt are shown to be ubiquitous and to be detectable in soil, water, plants and animal tissue. The only foods containing more than $1.0\,\mu g/g$ are sea foods (shrimps, scallops, smelt, blue gill and cod), cocoa, bran and molasses. Traces of cobalt were found in each of a series of human tissues examined, the greatest concentration being $1.2\,\mu g/g$ in fat; specimens from different countries showed geographic variations. On an average American hospital diet the cobalt intake was $166-436\,\mu g/day$; the metal is well absorbed through the jejunum, about 85 per cent is excreted in the urine and 15 per cent in the faeces: traces are found in the hair and sweat.

Cobalt is an essential trace metal but its functions other than as part of the vitamin B_{12} molecule are unknown. Man's daily requirement of vitamin B_{12} is $1\,\mu g$ containing $0.04\,\mu g$ of cobalt; although the daily intake of cobalt is greatly in excess of this, it is not stored in the tissues (Schroeder, Nason and Tipton, 1967).

Industrial properties

1. *Alloys*

The advantages of adding cobalt to alloys have been developed in the present century. Stellite is an important alloy, consisting of cobalt, chromium and tungsten, it remains hard even at high temperatures and is used for the high speed machining of hard metals. Tungsten carbide is bonded with about 10 per cent cobalt and is an excellent cutting metal (Alexander and Street, 1962). Cobalt alloys, because of their strength and heat resistance, are used in the making of jet engines and rockets. The alloy vitallium, which contains chromium, nickel, cobalt and molybdenum, is used in orthopaedic surgery for joint replacements.

2. *Magnets*

Nickel, aluminium and cobalt alloys are used in the making of powerful magnets.

3. *Pigments*

Cobalt blue has been used for centuries to colour glass and pottery.

4. *Paint driers*

The cobalt salts of organic acids, particularly cobalt naphthenate, are used as driers in paints and varnishes.

5. *Catalyst for benzoyl peroxide*

In the production and processing of unsaturated polyester resins.

6. *Electroplating*

Cobalt has been added to nickel solutions as a brightener, but this is probably no longer done.

Toxicity

Cobalt chloride was added to a particular brand of beer in order to improve its head of foam and caused a severe and sometimes fatal cardiomyopathy. Cases occurred in Quebec (Morin and Daniel, 1967) and in Belgium (Kesteloot *et al.*, 1968).

Sensitising properties

The metal itself sensitises as do its salts and oxides. To assess the sensitising potential of cobalt the maximisation test, using 25 per cent cobalt sulphate, was done on 25 human volunteers. Ten were sensitised giving the metal a grade of 3 on a 0–5 scale in which 1 contained the weakest sensitisers (Kligman, 1966). Cobalt chloride was used in a comparable study on animals by Wahlberg and Boman (1978) and all the animals were sensitised, classifying it as a Grade 5 allergen. The human study accords better with clinical experience.

Absorption of cobalt

The disappearance of the isotope ^{60}Co was measured from sites of intracutaneous injection in 3 cobalt-sensitive patients and in 3 controls. Measurements were taken over 48 hours; the absorption was found to be the same for the sensitised subjects and the controls (Haxthausen, 1954).

Incidence of cobalt sensitivity

Cobalt is sometimes considered to be an unimportant allergen and is often not included for routine testing. In New York it is a rare sensitiser (Fisher and Shapiro, 1956) and was omitted from the patch test series studied by the North American Contact Dermatitis Group (1973).

The following incidences have been reported:

Country	Patients Tested	Cobalt + %	Report
Scandinavia	5558	5	Magnusson *et al.*, 1968
Europe	4825	6.9	Fregert *et al.*, 1969
Munich, Germany	1660	5.4	Bandmann *et al.*, 1963
Warsaw, Poland	1205	12.3	Rudzki *et al.*, 1970
New Zealand	214	7.5	Black, 1972
California, U.S.A.	143	4.2	Epstein *et al.*, 1968

These figures will be greatly influenced by, and will reflect the incidence of, chromate and nickel sensitivity in the community because allergy to these metals is so often accompanied by reactions to cobalt.

St John's

From 1970–1976 (inclusive) 11 889 patients were routinely tested with cobalt chloride 1–2 per cent and a total of 487 (4 per cent) reacted, the majority in combination with sensitivity to chromate or nickel.

Sex incidence

In the series where the sex incidence has been reported there is a surprising unanimity of an almost 1:1 ratio (Table 7.13).

Table 7.13. Sex ratio of patients sensitive to cobalt in three different series.

Country	+ % Cobalt		Sex Ratio	Report
	M	F	M : F	
Scandinavia	5.2	4.8	1 : 1	Magnusson *et al.*, 1968
Europe	7.4	6.6	1 : 1	Fregert *et al.*, 1969
Poland	15.2	9.8	1.5 : 1	Rudzki *et al.*, 1970

Allergy to cobalt often accompanies chromate sensitivity in men and nickel sensitivity in women, and the 1:1 sex ratio in the Scandinavian and European series can be explained by the similarity of the numbers of men sensitised to chromate and women sensitised to nickel. However, in Poland women are more frequently sensitised to chromate than to nickel (p. 316).

St John's

At St John's from 1970–1976, 1.7–4.4 per cent of the males and 4.9–8.1 per cent of the females reacted to cobalt, a ratio of about one male to two to three females

(Table 7.14). This sex ratio closely reflected that of chromate: nickel sensitivity in men and women, which from 1970–1973 was 1:2 and from 1974–1976 was 1:3 (Tables 7.6 and 7.23).

Table 7.14. Incidence and ratio of cobalt sensitivity in men and women (St John's 1970–1976).

Year	No. Tested	M Cob. +	%	No. Tested	F Cob. +	%	M : F
1970	916	22	2.4	990	49	4.9	1:2
1971	707	31	4.4	851	59	6.9	1:2
1972	738	23	3.1	868	54	6.2	1:2
1973	710	28	3.9	836	57	6.8	1:2
1974	655	11	1.7	778	43	5.5	1:3
1975	887	17	1.9	971	64	6.6	1:3
1976	937	29	3.1	1045	85	8.1	1:3
TOTAL	5550	161	2.9	6339	411	6.5	1:2

A. COMBINED WITH NICKEL AND CHROMIUM

Most cases of cobalt sensitivity occur in association with nickel sensitivity in women and with chromate sensitivity in men. These allergies are often combined because the metals very often occur together. In particular, nickel and cobalt are so closely associated in the periodic table that one metal is practically always contaminated by the other (Marcussen, 1962).

In a study of eczematous patients in Munich by Bandmann and Fuchs (1963) 90/1660 (5.4 per cent) were sensitive to cobalt. Among these patients 14 reacted to cobalt only; 17 with suspender eczema reacted to nickel and cobalt; 41 reacted to chromate and cobalt, the principal contacts being cement and detergents; four patients were sensitive to nickel, chromate and cobalt. In 1963, at the Finsen Institute in Copenhagen, 300 consecutive patients were tested with cobalt chloride 2 per cent, nickel sulphate 5 per cent and potassium dichromate 0.5 per cent. Twelve patients (4 per cent) — eight women and four men — reacted to cobalt; three women and one man were sensitive to cobalt only, two women and three men reacted to cobalt and dichromate, and three women reacted to nickel and cobalt (Marcussen, 1963). In Warsaw 2225 patients were tested with the same concentrations of these three metals in water and 208 (9.3 per cent) reacted, of whom 87 were women and 121 were men, and of these, 33 women and 28 men reacted to cobalt only. In Poland (Rudzki and Kohutnicki, 1971) twice the number of women are sensitised to chromate and cobalt (36) as to nickel and cobalt (18). This reflects the high incidence of chromate sensitivity in Polish women (10.1 per cent) as compared with the number (5.5 per cent) sensitised to nickel (Rudzki and Kleniewska, 1970). In Warsaw, nickel and cobalt allergy could nearly always be traced to jewellery and clothing; chromate and cobalt allergy occurred particularly in construction workers and was found in 30/81 (37 per cent) of bricklayers. In 1966 in Lund in Sweden, 5416 patients, comprising 3087 women and 2329 men, were routinely tested with cobalt chloride 2.4 per cent, nickel sulphate 5.3 per cent and potassium dichromate

0.4 per cent. In this series 5 per cent (148) of the women and 4 per cent (97) of the men reacted to cobalt but only a minority, 14 women and 12 men, were sensitive to cobalt alone (Fregert and Rorsman, 1966).

Cobalt in cement

Insoluble cobalt oxide was found by Fregert and Gruvberger (1972) in samples of cement from several European countries in amounts varying from 17 to 63 μg of Co/g and 5–16 μg/g were the levels detected in eight samples of Swedish cement by Wahlberg, Lindstedt and Einarsson (1977). Cobalt was not detected in samples of American cement by Perone *et al.* (1974).

Insoluble compounds are thought not to be allergens but the clinical observation that cobalt in cement does sensitise indicates that the skin is capable of converting cobalt oxide to a soluble form (Fregert and Gruvberger, 1972). Although cobalt oxides are insoluble in water they form sparingly soluble complexes with amino acids such as cysteine and glutathione and the cobalt-cysteine complex has been shown to elicit patch test reactions in cobalt sensitive patients. Fregert and Gruvberger (1978) suggest that the formation of such complexes in the eczematous skin of chromate sensitive cement workers would explain their cobalt sensitivity.

In Spain Giménez-Camarasa (1967) found that of 126 patients with cement eczema, 86 per cent were sensitive to dichromate and 76 per cent to cobalt, whereas of 56 workers with other sources of occupational exposure to chromium salts none was sensitised to cobalt.

Cobalt and nickel

A combination of cobalt and nickel allergy was shown by Pirilä and Förström (1966) to occur with some sources of exposure and not with others. Whereas in suspender eczema 63 per cent (55/87) were sensitive to nickel and cobalt, the incidence was only 16 per cent among both nickel platers (15/93) and pottery workers (7/44).

St John's

As in other reported series, reactions to cobalt in men are associated with chromate sensitivity and in women with nickel sensitivity. Only a small proportion of the men (22 per cent) and women (7 per cent) reacted to cobalt and not to either of the other metals (Table 7.15).

Table 7.15. Association of reactions to cobalt, chromate and nickel in men and women (St John's, 1973–1976).

	Men		Women	
	No.	%	No.	%
$Cob^+ Cr_6^+ Ni^-$	38	(45)	7	(3)
$Cob^+ Cr_6^- Ni^+$	16	(19)	205	(82)
$Cob^+ Cr_6^+ Ni^+$	12	(14)	19	(8)
$Cob^+ Cr_6^- Ni^-$	19	(22)	18	(7)
TOTAL Cob^+	85		249	

Sources of combined metal sensitivity

Men

Cobalt and chromate. During the 1973–76 period, 50 men reacted to both cobalt and chromate. Their source of exposure was:

cement 28 (56 per cent) engineering 8 (16 per cent) miscellaneous 14 (28 per cent).

In contrast to the patients seen in Spain the combination of chromate and cobalt sensitivity did not relate specifically to contact with cement but occurred in about 25 per cent of the 203 chromate-sensitive men seen during this period regardless of the source of exposure:

	Source		$+Cob$ $+Cr_6$	%
203 Men + Cr_6	Cement	102	28	27
	Engineering	41	8	20
	Miscellaneous	60	14	23
	Total	203	50	25

Cobalt and nickel. In the 1973–76 period 16 men reacted to cobalt and nickel and 12 to cobalt, nickel and chromate. The sources of exposure were principally jewellery and clothing:

16 $(cob^+ ni^+)$
Watches (7): neck chains and pins (4): unknown (5).
The occupations of these last five patients were: an engineer, a mailing clerk, a cleaner, an architect and a veneer worker.

12 $(cob^+ ni^+ Cr_6^+)$
Watches (6): keys etc. (1): unknown (5).
Of the five patients in the 'unknown' group, three worked on building sites, one was a chemist and one was unemployed.

Women

Cobalt and Nickel. During the four years 1973–76, 224 women reacted to cobalt and nickel, of whom 19 were also sensitive to dichromate. The source of sensitisation was:

Jewellery and clothing 220 (98 per cent): source not found 3 (1 per cent): no information 1.

Cobalt and Chromate. In this same period only 7 women reacted to cobalt and dichromate but not to nickel.

The dichromate sensitivity and possibly the cobalt allergy may have related to wearing leather shoes in one patient and to detergents in another. No source for the combined allergy was found in four women and none was sought in another.

B. COBALT AS THE PRINCIPAL OR ONLY METAL ALLERGEN

Incidence

Contact dermatitis due entirely to cobalt is unusual and in this respect cobalt is a rare allergen. In the study in Lund (Fregert and Rorsman, 1966) the incidence was 0.5 per cent for both women (14/3087) and men (12/2329).

St John's

During the period 1970–1976 the incidence of patients who reacted to cobalt and were negative to both nickel and chromate was 0.7 per cent for both the men (37/5550) and the women (45/6339) (Table 7.16).

It is interesting that the yearly incidence of independent cobalt allergy remained so steady over those seven years and the rise in nickel sensitivity in women was not paralleled by an increase in sensitivity to cobalt when cobalt was the only metal allergen.

Table 7.16. Incidence of sensitivity to cobalt 'only' in men and women (St John's 1970–1976).

	Males			Females		
	No. Tested	Cob +	%	No. Tested	Cob +	%
1970	916	7	0.8	990	6	0.6
1971	707	6	0.8	851	18	2.1
1972	738	5	0.7	868	3	0.3
1973	710	6	0.8	836	5	0.6
1974	655	3	0.5	778	2	0.3
1975	887	7	0.8	971	5	0.5
1976	937	3	0.3	1045	6	0.6
Total	5550	37	0.7%	6339	45	0.7%

('Only' = the patients not reacting to either dichromate or nickel)

SOURCES OF EXPOSURE

Non-occupational

Sensitivity to cobalt may relate to:

Jewellery or metal on clothing	Plastic	Vitamin B_{12}
Dental plates	Shell splinters	Prostheses.

Detergents contain practically no cobalt. Nineteen Swedish detergents were analysed by Wahlberg *et al.* (1977): 16 contained $< 1 \mu g/g$ of cobalt and in none did the level exceed $4 \mu g/g$.

Jewellery and metal on clothing

A few patients with typical dermatitis from fashion jewellery or metal on clothing react to cobalt and not to nickel. Three such cases were reported from the Finsen Institute in 1962, but it was considered a very unusual occurrence (Marcussen, 1962). Unless both metals are routinely used for patch testing these cases will be missed, the clinical picture will seem bizzarre and the patient will be wrongly reassured that he or she is not sensitive to metal.

A case of cobalt sensitivity has been attributed to a lipstick case (Marcussen, 1963).

St John's

Jewellery and clothing were thought to have sensitised 16 of the 45 women and one of the 37 men seen between 1970 and 1976.

Plastic (pp. 322 and 631)

Vitamin B_{12}:

A most unusual patient was reported from New York who became sensitive to the cobalt in vitamin B_{12}. A dermatitis developed at the site of injection which flared when the vitamin was given orally; patch tests were positive to vitamin B_{12} and cobalt (Fisher, 1972). A cobalt-sensitive patient, injected intradermally with crystalline vitamin B_{12}, gave a tuberculin-type response (Rostenberg and Perkins, 1952).

Dental plates

Chrome-cobalt pegs, used to fasten false teeth to a dental plate, produced a stomatitis mimicking pemphigus in a cobalt-sensitive patient (Fisher, 1972). Another patient developed eczema of the thenar and hypothenar eminences and on patch testing reacted only and strongly to 2 per cent cobalt sulphate. For one year she had worn a dental plate made of vitallium which contains nickel, chromium and cobalt; she removed this plate and her hands healed in three weeks (Clendenning, 1971).

Shell splinters

A man with recurrent oedema of the face developed periorbital swelling after an injection of iron and cobalt. On patch testing he was found to be sensitive to cobalt, which was then found in shell splinters buried in his left arm. Release of cobalt from this metal was thought to account for his facial oedema (Nürnberger and Arnold, 1969).

Prostheses

Cobalt chromium molybdenum alloys (e.g. vitallium) have been used successfully for orthopaedic joint replacements and for other prostheses including heart valves. These alloys are suitable for weight-bearing prostheses because the metal is electrolytically inert, it has little tendency to self-welding and usually it is well tolerated by the tissues. It is also advantageous that the metal can be cast and the cost of these joints is not prohibitive. The disadvantage of the alloy is the release of wear products such as cobalt which are both toxic to the tissues and sensitisers. Stainless steel is sometimes used for prostheses but not only does it require to be forged, which is difficult, but it also corrodes. A new non-toxic, non-sensitising alloy suitable for prostheses has yet to be developed.

	Cob Cr alloy %	Stainless steel %
Nickel	0–2.5	10–14
Chromium	27–30	16–19
Cobalt	60–65	Trace
Carbon	0.2–0.35	0.03–0.08
Molybdenum	5–7	2–3.5
Iron	0.7–1	Balance
Silicon	0–1	1.0
Manganese	0–1	2.0
Tungsten	0	
Copper		0.25

It was shown by Coleman, Harrington and Scales (1973) that when a cobalt-chrome alloy was used in a total hip replacement so that metal articulated against metal, raised levels of cobalt and chromium could be found in the blood and urine of the patients. When polythene was used for one of the hip components the release of metal was much less. Samitz and Katz (1975) soaked stainless steel screws, wires and prostheses, either entire or cut to a suitable size, in body fluids and demonstrated that nickel was released.

The cobalt-chrome alloy has been widely used for total hip and other joint replacement surgery and there have been several reports that unsatisfactory arthroplasties are associated with metal sensitivity, in particular with cobalt sensitivity usually occurring alone and not in association with allergy to nickel or chromate. The results of patch tests in various series are listed:

	Failed				Prostheses Satisfactory				
No	Metal +	Cob	Ni	Cr₆	No	Metal +	Cob	Ni	Cr₆
14	9	8	1	1	24	0				(Evans et al., 1974)
7	6	6								(Jones et al., 1975)
23	15	10	6	2	27	4	4	3		(Elves et al., 1975)
35	16	13	4	2						(Munro-Ashman et al., 1976)

Approximately two-thirds of the patients with unsatisfactory arthroplasties are sensitive to metal; the fact that cobalt is the usual allergen is explained by the high content of cobalt in the alloy. The relationship of the metal sensitivity to the failure of the joint is not established and it is not known whether the loosening causes or follows the metal sensitivity. In one centre (Jones and Lucas, 1975) about a third of patients with metal to metal prostheses are sensitive to metal and yet such patients may have perfect hip function.

Dermatitis was recorded in some of these patients but it was not severe and occurred irrespective of a metal allergy (Elves et al., 1975). Two of the patients investigated by Munro-Ashman and Miller (1976) had dermatitis: one who was sensitive to nickel had a bullous eruption around a metal to metal knee prosthesis, and the other, who was allergic to cobalt, developed a diffuse eruption resembling a vasculitis after his hip prosthesis was removed. Foussereau and Laugier (1966) described a nickel sensitive woman whose eczema cleared when an orthopaedic plate and screws were removed, and a man, also sensitive to nickel, who had an acute episode of eczema and purpura on his legs following the removal of an orthopaedic nail.

The acquisition of metal sensitivity in 66 patients undergoing a total hip replacement with a metal to plastic prosthesis was studied by patch testing them before and 6–12 months after the operation (Nater *et al.*, 1976). In 62 the reactions to the tests were negative before and after the arthroplasty. Three patients reacted to nickel and one to cobalt postoperatively; one of them had a previous history of metal allergy but testing prior to the operation had elicited no reaction.

Occupational causes
In industry sensitivity to cobalt has been acquired from:

Pigments for pottery and china	Printing inks	Pigments in plastic
Driers in paints	Polyester manufacture	Paper making
Magnetic tapes	Cattle food	

(Lubricating oils may contain cobalt).

Pigments in pottery and china
In the pottery industry cobalt pigments are added to the clay to neutralise the yellow colour of the iron oxides. The cobalt is added as an insoluble carbonate but traces of soluble cobalt remain in the slightly alkaline clay. Cobalt compounds are also used in coloured glazes and for decorating pottery.

A pottery factory was investigated in Finland and it was found that the clay shop workers were at particular risk, whereas dermatitis was rare in those decorating the fired clay or handling finished articles. A total of 436 employees were tested with a series of selected allergens including 5 per cent cobalt nitrate; 277 worked in the clay shops handling wet clay and of these 9 reacted strongly to cobalt; 159 workers from other sections were tested and only one in the glazing shop was positive to cobalt.

In the clay workers the dermatitis affected mainly the forearms and backs of the hands; it improved at weekends, on holiday and in three men who were given cobalt-free clay. The patient doing the glazing had the dermatitis only in the summer when sweating was more profuse (Pirilä, 1953).

Cobalt dyes are also used in the making of china, and of 56 cases sensitised to cobalt in this job, 12 also reacted to nickel (Pirilä and Geier, 1964).

Printing inks
In one factory three offset printers developed dermatitis and each was found on patch testing to be sensitive to potassium dichromate (0.5 per cent) and cobalt chloride (1 per cent). An analysis of their working materials demonstrated the source of the cobalt sensitivity to be the inks which contained 11–1400 ppm of cobalt (Spruit and Malten, 1975).

Pigments in plastic

St John's
In 1969, at St John's, a man aged 21 years was seen with a five-month history of

eczema of the hands and chest which cleared when he was away from work. He worked for a firm making sheets of PVC plastic and he handled the hot plastic as it went into the machine. On patch testing he reacted to cobalt and dichromate and it was ascertained that a cobalt dye was used in the plastic. He changed to being a milkman and when seen two months later he was completely clear.

In the 1970–'76 series cobalt sensitivity in two women was attributed, though not proven, to contact with finished plastic in the homes, one from PVC covering on chairs and the other from her spectacle frames.

Humidity indicator

The hydration of paper sacks, used to line tyre containers, was monitored by discs containing a hygroscopic salt of cobalt sulphate which was blue when moist and pink when dry. These discs sensitised a man handling the sacks (Sertoli *et al.*, 1978).

Drier in paints

Cobalt salts, particularly cobalt naphthenate, are used as driers in oil paints and in varnishes. Two men with cobalt dermatitis from this source have been reported from Finland: one worked in a paint factory (Pirilä, 1947), the other, a painter, had dermatitis of the hands and arms and was shown at a meeting of the Finnish Dermatological Society (Pirilä, 1954). In Czechoslovakia 24 subjects working with polyester paints were examined by Kadlec, Hanslian and Folprechtová (1974) and of 10 with dermatitis, six were found to be sensitised to cobalt.

St John's

Two painters and decorators, one aged 59 years and the other 43 years, complained of cracking and peeling of the fingers and hands which in the older man was initially intermittent but then became worse and spread to his arms and neck. On patch testing both men reacted to cobalt but not to nickel or chromate. It was ascertained from one of the paint manufacturers that the oil paints contained a lead cobalt drier and that a drier containing 6 per cent cobalt naphthenate was sold for use when mixing paints. They suggested the use of other paint driers based on lead.

Cobalt sensitivity was attributed to paint thinners in two further patients; one was a paint sprayer and the other had worked embossing glass.

Cobalt in polyesters

Cobalt naphthenate is also used as an accelerator in the manufacture of polyester resins. Two industrial cases of sensitivity have been reported from Holland (Malten and Zielhuis, 1964) and a doubtful one from England (Bourne and Milner, 1963).

A boy aged 11 years with eczema under his spectacles, wrist-watch and around the mouth was found to be sensitive to cobalt. The dermatitis was attributed to cobalt in the metal and in the polyester ball point pen and fountain pen which he was in the habit of sucking (Grimm, 1971).

Sulphate recovery process

This process in a paper factory sensitised one man to cobalt (Fregert, Gruvberger and Heijer, 1972).

Magnetic tapes

Magnetic tapes used for television or sound recording contain chromium dioxide and cobalt or nickel oxides. A man handling such tapes at work was sensitised to chromium, cobalt and nickel and had a positive patch test to the coated side of the magnetic tape (Krook, Fregert and Gruvberger, 1977).

Cattle food

Cobalt salts may be added to the fodder mixture for cattle; a man working in a chemical factory preparing animal foodstuff became sensitised to cobalt (Breucker, 1966).

Lubricating oils

Organic cobalt compounds may be added to lubricating oils (Fregert and Hjorth, 1972).

St John's

From 1970–1976 a total of 37 men and 45 women reacted to cobalt but not to chromate or nickel. Not even a possible source of exposure was traced in about 80 per cent of the men and 55 per cent of the women, those sources that were known or probable are listed:

	Men	Women
Jewellery and clothing	1	16 (35%)
Plastic		2
Hip replacement		1
Paint driers	4	
Cement	3	
Inspecting cadmium-nickel batteries		1
No source found	29 (80% approx)	25 (55%)
Total	37	45

HARD METAL DUST

Hard metal consists of tungsten combined with carbon to form tungsten carbide which is then bound with metal cobalt powder; other metallic carbides are added to achieve particular grades of metal. The dried carbide and cobalt powders are mixed with wax and a solvent, pressed into shape and fused and set by heat. The metal is then ground to its final shape by carborundum and diamond wheels. The metal dust is valuable and much is recovered by local extraction but workers are exposed to some hard metal dust during all stages of the manufacturing process (Bech, Kipling and Heather, 1962).

This extremely hard alloy is used for rock drills, the cutting edges of tools, in armaments, for dyes and radiotherapy screens.

Dermatitis

Dermatitis from hard metal dust may be an irritant effect or an allergic reaction to cobalt.

In Sweden, the 360 employees of a hard metal works were investigated and 34 (9.4 per cent) were diagnosed as having skin changes due to their occupation.

(i) Sixteen had eczema affecting the elbow flexures, wrists, eyelids and between the fingers; of the 14 patch tested to metals and other allergens only three had significant reactions and in each it was to cobalt chloride 2 per cent in water. In the majority the eczema was considered to be an irritant effect of the metal dust aggravated by prolonged cleansing, necessitated by the difficulty of removing the dust from the skin.

(ii) Pruritus, particularly of the lower leg, occurred in eight patients; patch tests were negative in the seven tested and this discomfort was also attributed to the irritant effect of the dust.

(iii) Folliculitis occurred in six patients of whom three had acne.

(iv) Neurodermatitis was found in four or five workers (Skog, 1963).

An English tool grinder had hard metal disease and dermatitis of the backs of the hands, face and eyelids, which cleared away from work. A patch test with cobalt was negative (Calnan, 1967).

In contrast to these findings is the report from the United States (Schwartz *et al.*, 1945) of a plant which began manufacturing cemented tungsten carbides into cutting tools and dyes and found an increasing incidence of dermatitis among the 1200 workers. The cemented carbide was made by mixing powders of tungsten, tantalum, titanium carbides, carbon and metallic cobalt, pressing them into moulds, shaped as cutting edges and then fusing them in an electric furnace. The dust count was high throughout the plant but particularly in the metal room where the unfused powders were handled. Twenty patients were examined, most of whom worked in the metal room. The distribution of the dermatitis was that caused by a dust and affected the antecubital fossae, sides of the neck, eyelids, flexor arms, hands and in a few was generalised. In two sweepers the eczema was localised to their advancing foot and ankle, which were the sites most exposed to the floor dust. Six workers were patch tested to each ingredient of the alloy and to the final mixture of powders. All six reacted to the cobalt powder and to the powder mixture; two controls were negative. Some of the employees affected at one time appeared to have hardened and recovered.

Hard metal disease

Workers making hard metal and those using hard metal tipped tools in engineering shops are exposed to hard metal dust and are at risk of developing respiratory disease from the cobalt. The acute form is an allergic asthma which may go on to a chemical pneumonitis, but it clears when exposure ceases. Some develop chronic progressive pulmonary fibrosis which may cause death. Electronmicroscopy has shown crystals to be present in the fibrotic areas but cobalt has not been demonstrated, probably due to its solubility in the tissue fluids (Payne, 1977). Twelve cases of hard metal disease have been described in tool room grinders (Bech, 1974).

Patch testing

To separate cobalt and nickel sensitivity it is important that a pure cobalt salt be used for patch testing. Cobalt salts are mild irritants and a concentration of 2 per cent applied as a patch test sometimes causes a punctate erythema which may become purpuric. This speckled reaction is probably follicular.

A suitable patch test concentration is:

Cobalt chloride 1 per cent in petrolatum.

Occasionally the slight punctate effect is seen with this concentration but it is easily discernable from an allergic response.

In vitro tests
Specific transformation of lymphocytes has been detected in some cobalt sensitive patients (Veien and Svejgaard, 1978).

Copper

Copper has been known since pre-historic times. It is a red-brown, malleable metal which is widely distributed throughout the world both as the metal and as ores. In moist air it becomes covered with a green film of basic copper salts.

Properties and uses
Copper has a higher conductivity for electricity and heat than any other metal except silver. It is used mainly in the electrical industry and for pipes conveying water or gas. Its principal alloys are:

Brass: consisting of two parts copper and one part zinc with trace amounts of antimony, arsenic, lead, nickel and tin.

Bronze: is an alloy of copper and tin, and may also contain lead, phosphorus, nickel and zinc. Gunmetal is bronze with a high zinc content.

Toxicity
Workers exposed to an excess of copper dust may develop symptoms similar to those of the common cold; ulceration and perforation of the nasal septum have also been described, as has metal fume fever. These and other toxic effects have been reviewed by Cohen (1974).

Sensitising potential
This is extremely low. From 1963–1973, only three patients sensitised to copper or its salts were seen in the Allergy Department of the New York Skin and Cancer Unit (Fisher, 1973).

St John's
From 1960–1976, one case of sensitivity has been seen.

Causes of sensitivity
Sensitivity is usually acquired from contact with the metal itself.

Emblem, coins, watch band and copper beating

A woman aged 20 years, who had an acute vesicular eczema of her left palm and adjacent fingers, reacted to a patch test with 1 per cent copper sulphate. She had been in the habit of sleeping with a copper emblem in her left hand, and when she stopped this practice her hand healed (Gaul, 1954). Another patient, who handled coins at work, developed hand eczema and reacted on patch testing with copper sulphate 1 per cent (Russell, 1968).

A patient, who presented with a band of eczema on her left wrist, said that, for the past five years, her metal watch band, a ring and her spectacle ear pieces had all caused irritation. On patch testing she gave no response to nickel and chromium but reacted to copper-containing coins, metallic copper and copper sulphate 5 per cent, 2.5 per cent and 1.25 per cent. A biopsy of the reaction to metallic copper showed spongiosis and an infiltrate with eosinophils (Saltzer and Wilson, 1968).

St John's

In 1961, a left-handed housewife was seen with a one year's history of eczema affecting predominantly her left hand. Her hobby was copper-beating. On patch testing she reacted only to copper sulphate 1 per cent and 0.5 per cent; when re-tested four months later with 0.5 per cent she still reacted. She was advised to stop handling copper and, although her hands improved during the next nine months, they did not heal completely.

Associated with lichen planus

In Stockholm, a woman was investigated for pain in her face and lichen planus of her buccal mucosa and tongue. Considerable electropotential differences were found between her dental gold alloys and amalgam fillings, all of which contained copper. When patch tested, she consistently reacted to metallic copper, but the reactions to copper hydroxide and oxides, which initially were positive, later became negative; testing with copper sulphate 1 per cent also was negative. Replacement of all the copper-containing metal eliminated the electropotential differences and was followed by cure of the patient's symptoms including disappearance of the lesions on her mucosae and tongue (Frykholm *et al.*, 1969).

An intra-uterine contraceptive containing copper

Two weeks after the insertion of a copper-containing intra-uterine contraceptive device, a woman developed widespread eczema, which was not controlled by systemic steroids. Within two days of removal of the contraceptive the eczema had faded, and within two weeks it had cleared completely. Patch testing with 5 per cent copper sulphate elicited a 4+ response (Barranco, 1972).

Occupational dermatitis

A definite case of sensitivity was that of a welder who developed dermatitis of his palms and fingers corresponding to sites of contact with the welding mouthpiece made of brass (copper and zinc) and the copper welding wire. Patch tests: he reacted to copper suphate 0.1 per cent in petrolatum (Förström, Kiistala and Tarvainen, 1977).

Dermatitis of the hands in 10 furniture polishers was attributed to copper sulphate added as a colouring agent to commercial alcohol. Patch tests: each patient reacted to the commercial blue spirit and copper sulphate 5 per cent in water and 15 controls were negative (Dhir, Rao and Mehrotra, 1977). Another report in 1952 described five patients who developed eczema while working with brass in the following occupations: dismantling brass electrical fixtures, operating a machine cutting out brass watch balances, assembling brass toys, and work in a plating room and in a brass foundry. Although all the patients reacted to patch tests with brass, testing with pieces of metal can be misleading. Three were tested with copper and zinc and each reacted to copper only (Morris, 1952). A metal worker who was sensitised to several metals also reacted to a patch test with copper oxide (Bockendahl, Remy and Masuch, 1974).

Patch testing

Copper is a rare allergen and experience of patch testing with copper salts is limited. Being irritants, their use in high concentrations gives misleading toxic reactions, as may testing with pieces of the metal. Pure copper, applied as a patch test, is corroded by the skin and the addition of sodium chloride increases the corrosion and promotes an irritant reaction (Gaul, 1958 i). These corrosion products have caused an irritant dermatitis under the nose pads and ear pieces of a spectacle frame (Gaul 1958 ii).

Copper sulphate 1 per cent in water and
                 0.1 per cent in petrolatum.

Gold

Gold occurs naturally both as an ore and as a free metal and has been found in the rocks and rivers of many countries. As a precious metal it has been prized and treasured for centuries; deposits of gold are now found and mined mainly in South Africa.

Properties of gold

Gold is a soft yellow metal which is extremely malleable and ductile, and unlike base metals it does not corrode. Chemically it is very unreactive, resisting attack by air and oxygen, and it is insoluble in most acids. It is, however, attacked by aqua regia (kingly water), which is a mixture of nitric and hydrochloric acids and was so called because it dissolved the noble metals gold and platinum.

A. Alloys

Gold forms alloys with such metals as silver, copper, nickel, platinum, palladium, manganese, zinc and mercury.

Composition of some jewellery alloys

Pure gold is alloyed with metals to counteract its softness and give it hardness and strength. A carat is a 24th part; the carat number indicates the proportion of gold in an alloy — the higher the carat number the greater the quantity of gold.

Yellow gold rings

In Britain most wedding rings are made of 22, 18 or 9 carat gold; the alloys in the 22 and 18 carat gold rings contain copper and silver but no nickel or zinc. A 9 carat ring contains only 37.5 per cent gold, the other constituents being copper, silver and zinc and occasionally a small amount of nickel.

White gold rings

Gold was originally whitened to mimic platinum: this is usually done by adding either palladium or nickel. Palladium gives the better colour but is expensive and softer than nickel. Although nickel has the desirable qualities of hardness, cheapness and durability, jewellers prefer not to add it to the alloy because it does not improve the colour. Gold of 22 carats cannot be whitened but an 18-carat gold can be bleached and may contain up to 17 per cent nickel. Lower carats are similarly decolourised, and a 9-carat gold, in which 37.5 per cent gold is alloyed with 62.5 per cent silver, is also white but is relatively soft. White gold is frequently plated with rhodium to increase its brilliance.

Nickel in other yellow gold jewellery

A small amount of nickel does not decolourise gold. Up to 5 per cent nickel is occasionally added to yellow gold to increase its hardness and resilience and to make it suitable for the spring clips on earrings and the pins on brooches. This alloy is not used for rings because they do not require these properties.

Canadian jewellers gold

The following gold alloys are used in Canada for jewellery (Table 7.17):

Table 7.17. Percentage composition of Canadian gold jewellery alloys (Mitchell, 1972).

Yellow Gold	Carat	Gold	Silver	Copper	Zinc	Nickel
	10	41.6	17.0	41.0	3.0	
	14	58.3	12.0	28.0	3.0	
	18	75.0	15.0	10.0	0.5	
White Gold	10	41.6		30.8	12.3	15.2
	14	58.6		22.2	8.7	10.8
	18	75.0		3.5	5.0	16.5

B. Complex compounds

Complex compounds of gold with other chemicals such as potassium cyanide are easily formed; this is the basis of a method for extracting gold from ores.

Uses of gold

1. As a reserve of wealth.
2. In jewellery, either as an alloy or as gold plating for cheaper jewellery in which a base metal such as copper is first electroplated with an anti-corrosive layer of nickel and then with gold of varying thickness. Rolled gold is a thin layer of gold applied by mechanical pressure to a metal base.
3. As gold leaf, which is gold beaten to a thickness of less than 0.00002 cm, and used for lettering, the decoration of books and other adornment.

4. In dentistry as alloys.
5. A colloidal solution of gold in stannic acid, known as Purple of Cassius, may be used to make ruby glass and to colour enamel and porcelain.
6. Complex gold salts are used for toning in photography.
7. Rarely, pieces of chemically resistant apparatus are made of a gold-platinum alloy.

Sensitising potential
Metallic gold and its soluble salts sensitise. The maximisation test on humans showed that gold chloride is a potentially strong allergen; it sensitised 16 of 23 subjects, making it grade 4 on a 0–5 scale, in which grade 5 comprised the strongest allergens. The discrepancy between this result and the clinical rarity of sensitisation was attributed to the inertness of gold and its insolubility in skin secretions (Kligman, 1966).

Incidence of sensitivity
Allergy to gold is rare and incidences of sensitivity have not been recorded; only isolated cases have been reported.

St John's
It is possible to give only an approximate estimate of the incidence of gold sensitivity in this clinic because patients are not routinely tested with a gold salt and the difficulty in interpreting patch test results sometimes makes the diagnosis uncertain. From 1967 to 1976, 0–5 cases were diagnosed each year (Table 7.18).

Table 7.18. Yearly incidence of gold sensitivity in women and men (St John's, 1967–1976).

Year	1967	1968	1969	1970	1971	1972	1973	1974	1975	1976
No. of women	1	0	1	0	4	4	1	2	1	1
No. of men	0	0	0	0	0	1	0	0	0	0

Sex incidence
The allergy is much commoner in women than men; of the 16 patients seen between 1967 and 1976, 15 were women and one was a man.

Causes of sensitivity and the clinical features
Sensitivity is acquired from metallic gold and from gold salts.

A. Metallic gold
Metallic gold objects which have been reported as causing dermatitis include rings, earrings, other jewellery, dental crowns and an orbital implant.

St John's
During the decade 1967 to 1976, 15 women and one man were diagnosed as being sensitive to gold. Metallic gold sensitised the women, the sources being rings (11), earrings (2) and a dental crown (1). One woman had no history of gold dermatitis and no relevance was found for her patch test reactions to gold salts. The man was an electroplater and had had an occupational dermatitis.

Rings

Although rings are the most frequent cause of allergy to metallic gold, only about 12 cases have been reported in the literature (Gaul, 1954; Chenoweth, 1957; Cowan, 1960; Fox, Kennedy and Rostenberg, 1961; Malten and Mali, 1966; Bowyer, 1967; Comaish, 1969; Rytter and Schubert, 1971; Nava and Briatico-Vangosa, 1971; Cooke and Hocken Robertson, 1973), one of which was not patch tested (Chenoweth, 1957). Nine were women: five had developed the dermatitis from their wedding rings (Cowan, 1960; Cooke and Hocken Robertson, 1973; Chenoweth, 1957) but a sixth, who presented with wedding ring dermatitis, had been pre-sensitised by gold earrings and a gold watch (Comaish, 1969). Of the three men (Fox *et al.*, 1961; Malten and Mali, 1966; Nava and Briatico-Vangosa, 1971), one also had dermatitis from a gold medallion. This patient noticed that in winter he could tolerate gold for four days but that in summer the eczema reappeared within two days (Fox *et al.*, 1961).

Eczema, sometimes vesicular (Cowan, 1960), was the usual change under the ring but in one woman the appearance was pseudogranulomatous, with erythema and nodules (Comaish, 1969). A biopsy in this patient showed, in the epidermis, hyperkeratosis, acanthosis, some follicular plugging and very slight spongiosis; in the dermis there was an infiltrate of histiocytes and lymphocytes which was mainly perivascular but was in some areas confluent. There were few plasma cells or eosionophils.

The time interval between first wearing the rings and the onset of the dermatitis varied from three months in two women to 18 months in a third. Two women transferred their rings to their right hands, and it took seven weeks of continuous wear in one case and three weeks of wear during warm weather in the other to reproduce the dermatitis.

Clinical details were given for eight patients: the eczema was confined to the area under the ring in three, hand eczema, which had begun under a gold ring, was present in two and a further spread to the arms had occurred in three. In two of these the trunk was affected and in one the face also, and in another patient the eczema, which began on her hands, had become generalised within one month and was particularly severe under her wedding ring.

St John's

Women with hand eczema are patch tested with gold salts if they give a present or past history of an eczema beginning under a gold ring or because their eczema is worse under their rings. This is particularly likely with a wide band gold ring, or if many rings are worn together on one finger. In the great majority the eczema is due to irritation from detergents, soap and water and very few of these patients are sensitive to gold.

From 1967 to 1976, 15 women were diagnosed as being allergic to gold. Wedding rings had sensitised 10 women and an ornamented ring another. Of these, five described dermatitis from other gold jewellery including a watch, watchstrap, earrings and neck chains. The time interval between starting to wear the ring and developing dermatitis was recorded as 2–3 months in two patients and 8–20 years in four women.

Other jewellery

The initiation of sensitivity by other gold jewellery seems to be extremely rare.

Earrings have been reported to do so (Comaish, 1969; Elgart and Higdon, 1971; Young, 1974; Fisher, 1974) and a gold watch sensitised one of Fisher's (1974) patients.

St John's

Two women were sensitised by earrings. One, aged 58 years, had had pierced ears for 25 years when new 18-carat gold earrings caused dermatitis of her ear lobes which recurred every time she wore them. No other sites were affected. The second patient was aged 19 years when she had her ears pierced; the gold studs caused dermatitis which healed when she removed the earrings. Subsequently her wedding ring and a gold watch caused dermatitis.

A gold orbital implant

Possibly the first recognised case of allergy to metallic gold was in a woman aged 34 years who had her left eye enucleated and a 14-carat gold ball implanted into the orbital capsule. Five years later she developed a seropurulent discharge from her left orbit and an itchy vesicular eczema on her left eyelids and adjacent skin. The patient endured much discomfort for three years until the diagnosis was suspected and then confirmed by patch tests which were positive to gold sodium thiosulphate 0.5 per cent, gold leaf and the gold ball. The gold ball was removed and replaced by a plastic prosthesis; one week later the orbit was dry and was still normal two years later (Forster and Dickey, 1949).

Dental crowns

Four cases have been reported. One woman, sensitised by earrings, subsequently developed dermatitis from gold rings and a watch but the eczema subsided within a few days if she removed this gold jewellery. She noticed that the dermatitis was worse in the summer. Two years later a gold crown was put on one of her teeth and within days the adjacent gum became inflamed and the eczema re-appeared under her ring and persisted despite taking off the ring. Both the eczema and gingivitis resisted treatment. Patch tests: undiluted gold sodium thiosulphate elicited a severe reaction and subsequently 0.5 per cent gold trichloride gave a strongly positive response. Ten months later the crown was removed and within one month her gums and hands had healed (Elgart and Higdon, 1971). Another woman had gold crowns put on both lower canines and within four months she developed inflammation of the oral mucosa in contact with the gold. She was able to continue to wear her gold wedding ring and watch without trouble. Patch tests: she reacted to gold trichloride 1 per cent and 0.1 per cent. The gold crowns were replaced with acrylic ones and her mouth healed completely (Schöpf, Wex and Schulz, 1970). A similar case, described by Klaschka (1975), tolerated a gold crown for 15 years and then developed an erosion of the adjacent mucosa. Patch tests with gold chloride 0.5 per cent (aqueous) confirmed her sensitivity to gold despite which she continued to wear her gold jewellery without discomfort. A fourth patient who preferred to retain the gold in her mouth was described by Young (1974).

A denture made of gold platinum alloy sensitised and caused erythema of the palate in a woman who subsequently wore a plastic plate without trouble. In another woman a gold-china-metal bridge caused a burning discomfort and redness of her tongue. Both patients reacted to patch tests with gold dicyanoaurate

0.001 per cent; 126 controls were negative (Fregert, Kollander and Poulsen, 1979).

St John's

A woman aged 34 years had had painful erosions of the inner side of her left lip for five years. At about the time they had first appeared, she had had a gold filling put in her second left upper incisor. This tooth was removed two years later and replaced by a false one which was attached to a gold crown on the adjacent canine. She then developed reddening and slight erosion of the mucosa exactly opposite the crown and she noticed a slight rash under her wedding ring. On patch testing she reacted to gold chloride 0.5 per cent but not to 0.1 per cent; she developed an erosion from sodium chloroaurate 2 per cent. Open tests with these salts were positive. The crown was removed and replaced by a porcelain one; when she was seen four months later the mucosa was normal.

B. Gold salts

A man who rested his arm on crystals of gold trichloride lying on a laboratory bench developed an irritant dermatitis and subsequently an allergic papular eruption at the site of contact. A biopsy showed features simulating a lymphoma or an insect bite reaction: in the dermis there was a dense infiltrate composed of lymphocytes, plasma cells and large cells, and there was also clumping of nuclei; the epidermis showed hyperkeratosis and follicular plugging. Patch tests with gold trichloride 1 per cent and with gold potassium chloride 1 per cent were both positive, as were intradermal tests with 0.01 per cent of these salts (Shelley and Epstein, 1963). The lesions took six months to disappear.

Industrial gold dermatitis

Soluble gold salts, including gold trichloride ($AuCl_3.2H_2O$), are used in gold plating, gilding glass and porcelain (Fregert and Hjorth, 1972) and in the manufacture of ruby glass. Gold trichloride and complex gold salts such as sodium tetrachloroaurate dihydrate ($Na[AuCl_4].2H_2O$) are used in photography.

Gold plating

There are a few scattered reports of dermatitis from gold plating. Gold cyanide has sensitised Russian workers gilding watches; of 37 employees with dermatitis, 35 were patch tested and of them, 28 reacted to 1 per cent gold cyanide. By care, protection and local treatment, 31 patients were healed or greatly improved and only six had to be removed from all contact with gold cyanide (Somov and Khaimovsky, 1964). In Germany, in 1967, a gold plating factory was opened and calcium gold cyanide was used in it. After four months one employee had been sensitised and after about one year three of the ten workers handling the compound had developed eczema of their hands and face and one had an acute conjunctivitis. As potassium gold cyanide was considered to be a potent allergen, aqueous dilutions of 0.1 per cent and 0.2 per cent were advised for patch testing (Schmollack, 1971). In 1971, four men employed as gilders in Italy developed eczema on exposed sites and were found to be sensitive to gold salts (Nava and Briatico-Vangosa, 1971). In France, a woman who prepared gold and chrome baths for plating fountain pens became sensitised to the gold and developed asthma and hand eczema (Sidi and Hincky, 1965).

Gold potassium cyanide (KAu (CN$_2$) — Irritant
A man working in an electronics firm cleaned gold electrodes with gold potassium cyanide and inadvertently contaminated his right hand. He developed pustules and necrotic erosions on the fingers and a purple brown discolouration and partial onycholysis of the free ends of some finger nails. Within six weeks the skin and nails had returned to normal (Budden and Wilkinson, 1978).

St John's

Allergic dermatitis
A man aged 31 years, who worked as a gold electroplater, gave a five months' history of dermatitis beginning on the fingers of his right hand, spreading to his left hand and then to his arms and face. Remissions and relapses coincided exactly with avoiding and with handling gold solutions. He also mixed and used epoxy resins. On patch testing he reacted to gold chloride 0.1 per cent, potassium bromoaurate 0.1 per cent and epoxy resin but not to sodium chloroaurate 0.1 per cent.

Irritant dermatitis
Both the gold salts and the acids used in plating are irritants. A woman aged 23 years had been making up solutions of potassium gold cyanide for one year when she developed eczema on the palmar surfaces and sides of her fingers, worse on the right than the left. It persisted for one year, during which she continued to work. Patch testing with gold salts gave irritant responses only.

A man aged 37 years had been a gold plater for five months when he developed dermatitis on his hands, arms and face and conjunctivitis in his left eye. His symptoms improved when he stayed off work. On patch testing he gave weak reactions to persulphates, which he handled, but failed to react to gold salts and 1 per cent tetraethylenepentamine, an organic gold brightener. He avoided persulphates for two months without any benefit.

Patch Testing
A considerable difficulty in the diagnosis of gold sensitivity is the lack of a reliable chemical for patch testing. Tests with gold leaf are usually negative but have twice been reported as positive (Forster and Dickey, 1949; Cowan, 1960).

Irritancy. Most gold salts seem to be irritant, some because they are acidic; this irritancy makes the interpretation of positive patch tests difficult. It is not unusual for a patient to react to one gold salt and not to others, and to wear gold jewellery without trouble. Such a patient is almost certainly not sensitive to gold. Patch testing with gold salts, particularly gold chloride, may cause a purple discolouration of the skin.

Acantholysis. Patch testing with gold chloride (Fox *et al.*, 1961) and gold trichloride (Malten and Mali, 1966) has been reported as causing acantholysis.

Persistence of allergic positive patch tests
In the same way that the clinical lesions are sometimes persistent (Shelley and Epstein, 1963) or pseudogranulomatous (Comaish, 1969) so may the patch tests be infiltrated and long lasting. This type of response has been elicited by 1 per

cent and 2 per cent gold chloride and appeared as a deep dermal reaction (Bowyer, 1967) and as red non-eczematous papules which remained for three to six months (Shelley and Epstein, 1963; Comaish, 1969). The histology showed only slight spongiosis but a striking dermal infiltrate composed of lymphocytes and histiocytes around vessels (Bowyer, 1967; Comaish, 1969) and also round appendages (Bowyer, 1967).

Urticaria
The patient sensitised by a gold ball orbital implant (Forster and Dickey, 1949) was patch tested twice with the gold ball, and each time she developed eczema at the test site and a widespread urticaria.

St John's
Several gold salts in various dilutions and gold leaf have been used without finding a completely reliable test substance. There have been no positive reactions to gold leaf.

In sensitised patients a thickened, red response, localised to the patch test, occurs quite frequently and in some patients it has persisted for longer than six weeks.

Infiltration and thickening of the patch test site cannot be used as a criterion for differentiating an allergic from an irritant reaction because this dermal response occurs and looks identical in both. As an irritant effect it is usually seen with too high a patch test concentration. In a series of 102 patients patch tested with gold sodium thiosulphate 5 per cent in petrolatum, 18 gave irritant reactions, many of which were of this thickened type.

Patients suspected of being allergic to gold are tested with:

	%	Diluent
Gold sodium thiosulphate	1.0 and 0.5	petrolatum
Gold chloride	0.5 and 0.1	water
Potassium bromoaurate	0.1	water
Sodium chloroaurate	0.1	water
Potassium dicyanoaurate	0.001	ethanol

A patient is diagnosed as sensitive to gold if there is a definite reaction to at least two of these salts coupled with a relevant clinical history.

BLACK DERMOGRAPHISM

Black dermographism refers to the black marks caused by metal rubbing on skin; the same discolouration can be produced on the rough surface of linen, wood or coarse paper. The effect is mechanical and depends upon friction between a metal and a hard mineral powder, which abrades the metal surface and forms a dust of extremely finely divided metal. This is always black and stains the skin or fabric. Many metals produce this discolouration, but gold, being soft, is relatively easily abraded. Many inorganic powders are effective, particularly titanium dioxide and calcium carbonate, and such powders are present in face powders, talcum powder and other cosmetics. The zinc oxide in ointments and the dust from the street or factories will also cause staining. These black marks occur more readily on the thick keratin of the palm than on other sites (Urbach and Pillsbury, 1943).

RADIODERMATITIS FROM RADIOACTIVE RINGS

The mishap of gold-containing radon seeds which escaped into the jewellery market and by being made into rings caused radiodermatitis of the fingers, has been reported from the U.S.A. This hazard can be avoided by refining gold or by testing each new batch for radioactivity.

In each of the following reports, radioactivity of the rings was confirmed.

The first patients were a husband and wife who had been married for 26 years and had worn rings for the first five years. They both developed on their ring fingers a dermatitis which was attributed to soap and detergents but which failed to heal when the rings were removed. When recognised as radiodermatitis the areas were excised and grafted (Simon and Harley, 1967). Another man developed a squamous cell carcinoma under a ring he had worn for 30 years and had to have the finger amputated (Gerwig, 1968). A second woman had developed dermatitis under her wedding ring after wearing it for two years but she continued to wear it for a further 42 years. The skin under the ring had by then become red, scaly and atrophic and its histology showed the changes of a radiation keratosis (Leone, 1968).

Iron

Most metals exist in the earth's crust as minerals or ores, in which they are chemically combined with other elements. Just as rust does not resemble iron, nor verdigris copper, so are ores dissimilar to the metals they contain. Ores deep in the earth are mined: superficial ones are quarried. The recovery of metals from ores by fire or by chemicals is known as smelting.

Iron compounds

Iron and moderate heat produce a spongy mass of *forged iron* which can be hammered into shape. Iron ore and blast furnace heat form *pig iron* which can be remelted to give *cast iron*; this can be poured into shapes when molten but when set it is brittle because of its 3.5 per cent carbon content. Cast iron was used to construct the first European metal bridge at Ironbridge in 1799. *Steel*, the most important ferrous metal, is an iron-carbon alloy to which other elements such as chromium, nickel, molybdenum and tungsten may be added. Steel is made *stainless* by the addition of up to 20 per cent chromium, and the addition of nickel enhances its resistance to corrosion and heat. *Wrought iron*, still used for gates, is made by melting and moulding pig iron (Alexander and Street, 1965).

Iron tattooing of the skin of the arms in ten car workers occurred during spot welding of the components (Jirásek, 1978).

Sensitisation

Only 2 cases, both industrial, have been reported.

Steel and cast iron particles

The first report from Rotterdam (Nater, 1960) described a man aged 44 years who had been employed in a steel plant for 2½ years, and then suddenly developed an acute vesicular eczema on his soles and legs. He worked with streams of steel particles under high pressure, and these contaminated his clothing, particularly his socks and trousers. When patch tested he reacted to ferric sulphate 10 per cent, ferric chloride 1 per cent and 2 per cent, but not to ferric chloride 0.1 per cent, ferrous sulphate 10 per cent or to other metals.

The second patient, investigated in New York (Baer, 1973), was a 66-year-old tool-maker with a 5 year history of a papulo-vesicular eczema which began on his ankles and legs, and later spread to his hands, arms and trunk. He machined and cut metal and operated a lathe; among the metals he used were cast iron and steel. The metal dust impregnated his shoes and socks. Patch tests: he reacted to ferric chloride 2 per cent in water and not to other metals. Topical medicaments and greater cleanliness of his working clothes were effective treatment, despite his remaining at his job.

Patch-testing

These two patients reacted to ferric chloride 2 per cent in water.

Rusters

Rusters are workers in precision engineering who by handling metal make it rust. Within days of their touching metal the surface is blemished and rusts causing corrosion of the component. Such workers are a hazard and may lose their jobs.

Rusters have been described by Collins (1957), Buckley and Lewis (1960) and Burton, Pye and Brookes (1976). This undesirable facility occurs in both men and women and has been thought to be related to the high chloride content of their sweat and usually to an increased rate of palmar sweating. In one patient, Burton *et al*. (1976) reported the sodium chloride content of the axillary sweat to be 190 mmol/1 and his palmar sweat to contain 1000 mmol/1, whereas in controls the level was 80 mmol/1. Jensen (1979) found the composition of their sweat to be normal and the crucial factor was hyperhidrosis. Corrosion increased with higher sweating rates. A high copper content protects the metal (Jensen & Nielsen, 1979). Rusters are healthy and do not have fibrocystic disease of the pancreas.

The management of rusters is difficult; Burton *et al*. (1976) suggested cool clothes, a cool environment, low salt intake, frequent hand washing and cleansing the metal of sweat with a solvent. A most effective remedy was found by Bang Pederson (1977) to be the reduction of palmar sweating by the method Shelley and Hurley (1975) described for axillary hyperhidrosis (p. 107).

Lead

Lead is soft enough to be cut with a knife and to leave a mark on paper, and it is sufficiently malleable to be moulded into pipes or rolled into sheets of foil.

Although lead is water resistant it is sufficiently weak for the expansion of water as it becomes ice to burst lead pipes.

Lead poisoning is well known, whereas dermatitis from lead is practically unknown.

Case reports

One case possibly sensitised to lead has been reported by Fregert (1973). A truck driver, who developed eczema on the distal parts of his fingers, blamed the lead electrodes and hydrochloric acid which he handled when changing batteries. On patch testing he reacted to 0.2 per cent aqueous lead chloride and to 0.5 per cent aqueous lead acetate; lead metal induced no reaction. He subsequently wore gloves at work and his fingers remained healed.

A painter, who had used lead paints for 20 years, presented with a bullous dermatitis from a lead oxide ointment. Patch tests with lead oxide and lead acetate elicited strong reactions. He was then found to have labyrinthine and neurological disease due to chronic lead poisoning (Czarnecki and Fritsch, 1978).

Nickel

Nickel was given its name by the early copper miners in Germany who found that copper ore contaminated with nickel was difficult to work. Thinking that this must be a machination of the devil, they called the ore Kupfernickel, or devil's copper.

The first isolation of nickel was in 1751, and now the richest source of it in the world is Ontario. The metal is mined as ores in combination with sulphur, copper, iron and arsenic. It is refined either by fusion with sodium sulphide followed by electrolytic extraction (Orford process), or by combination with carbon monoxide to form nickel carbonyl and subsequent purification by dissociation (Mond process). Current methods of refining nickel are outlined by Morgan (1979). Nickel salts are green in colour.

A comprehensive report on the biological effects of nickel was published by the National Academy of Sciences (1975) and the metabolism and toxicology of nickel was reviewed by Sunderman (1977).

Nickel is naturally present in food, but the concentration may be increased during processing or cooking by contamination from equipment made of nickel alloy. The highest concentration of nickel is in green leafy vegetables, whereas there is little or none in animal products such as meat, milk and eggs. The daily intake varies: a normal American diet contains about 300–600 μg or less (Schroeder, Balassa and Tipton, 1962), and in Canada the intake was estimated as 347 and 576 μg daily (Kirkpatrick and Coffin, 1974).

Most of the ingested nickel is excreted in the faeces, and only about 5 per cent appears in the urine (Schroeder *et al.*, 1962). Measurements of serum and urinary nickel in normal subjects reflect the environmental exposure, and levels vary with the geographical location. In Florida, Sunderman (1967) found the mean concentration of nickel in serum to be 2.2 μg/100ml, whereas in a similar study in central Connecticut, Nomoto and Sunderman (1972) estimated the mean serum level as $0.26 \mu g/100ml$ and they attributed the difference to a variation in the populations studied. The populations of Sudbury, Ontario and Hartford, Connecticut, were compared by McNeely, Nechay and Sunderman (1972). In Sudbury, where the tap water contained $200 \mu g$ of nickel/1, the average serum nickel was $4.6 \mu g/1$, and the urinary nickel output was $7.9 \mu g/day$, whereas in Hartford, where the tap water contained only $1.1 \mu g$ of nickel/1, the average serum nickel was $2.6 \mu g/1$, and the urinary nickel excretion was $2.5 \mu g/day$. In a further study in Holland, Spruit and Bongaarts (1977) found that those occupationally exposed to nickel had considerably higher levels of nickel in their plasma and urine than were found in a group of volunteers; and in these workers, the concentrations fell after they had been on holiday. The results were as follows:

No. of subjects	Plasma $\mu g/1$	Urine $\mu g/1$	Scalp hair $\mu g/g$
Volunteers			
10–24	1.8	0.6	0.8
Occupationally exposed			
7–15	10.6	18.0	14.5
After holidays			
8	5.3	1.8	

Sensitisation to nickel did not influence the results in either group. Menné, Mikkelsen and Solgaard (1978) gave single doses of nickel sulphate (5.6 mg) to 13 subjects and found their urinary nickel excretion to be raised for the following two to three days.

The serum level rises after an acute myocardial infarction, acute stroke, and acute burns, whereas the levels are low in hepatic cirrhosis and chronic uraemaia (McNeely, Sunderman and Nechay, 1971).

It is difficult to detect nickel in tissues, but in a study in the United States it was found in 87 per cent of the specimens of intestines and skins which were examined (Schroeder *et al.*, 1962).

Measurements of trace amounts of nickel in body fluids and tissues have been bedevilled by the difficulty of the analyses and results have varied. Atomic absorption is the preferred method for nickel analysis (Spruit, 1979).

Industrial properties of nickel

The metal is hard, strong and silver-white in colour; it resists corrosion and can be polished to give a bright gloss. Nickel has two principal industrial uses: the formation of alloys, and electroplating.

1. *Alloys.* Nickel forms alloys with many metals including iron, copper, manganese, zinc, and chromium. It is added to some stainless steel to give it strength and toughness, and a widely used variety of steel contains 18 per cent chromium and 8 per cent nickel.

2. *Electroplating.* As it resists corrosion better than iron, nickel is plated onto the base metal as a protective layer. It may or may not be over-plated with

another metal such as chromium (which gives a hard, bright coating), or silver or gold. Nickel maintains the adhesion of other metals plated onto its surface, and so prevents their peeling off, as they are prone to do when plated directly onto the base metal.

3. Nickel acts as a *catalyst* in the production of solid fats from hydrogenated oils.

4. It is used in the *manufacture* of enamels and glass.

Toxicity and carcinogenicity
The toxicology of nickel concerns mainly the noxious gas nickel carbonyl; poisoning is effectively treated with sodium diethyldithiocarbamate (Sunderman, 1971). Exposure to nickel dust and fumes increases the risk of neoplasms of the lungs (Konetzke, 1974; Kreyberg, 1978) and of the nose (Torjussen and Solberg, 1976).

Sensitising potential of nickel
It is usually the metal itself that sensitises, but its water-soluble salts nickel chloride ($NiCl_2$) and nickel sulphate ($NiSO_4$) are also strong sensitisers. Some nickel oxides (e.g. Ni_2O_3) and nickel hydroxide ($Ni(OH)_2$) can elicit contact dermatitis, but heated nickel oxide (NiO) does not do so because of its extreme insolubility (Fregert and Hjorth, 1972).

The facility with which nickel sensitises has been investigated. In 1963, the skin of 172 male volunteers was damaged by freezing, and a 25 per cent aqueous solution of nickel chloride, containing 0.1 per cent sodium lauryl sulphate, was applied to the site under occlusion on three occasions at five day intervals. Sixteen (9 per cent) were sensitised (Vandenberg and Epstein, 1963). A much higher incidence of sensitisation was achieved with the maximisation technique: nickel sulphate 10 per cent was used for the induction in 25 subjects, and 12 were sensitised. The metal was graded as 3 (a moderate sensitiser) on a 1–5 scale in which grade 1 contained the weakest allergens (Kligman, 1966). These results correlated well with a maximisation test carried out on guinea-pigs; half the animals were sensitised by nickel sulphate, and nickel had the same moderate grade 3 rating (Magnusson and Kligman, 1969).

Using a different technique, Turk and Parker (1977ii) successfully sensitised guinea-pigs to nickel sulphate, but with another method Samitz *et al.* (1975) failed to induce sensitisation with either the same salt, or nickel-amino acid complexes or nickel-guinea-pig skin complexes. One difficulty in working with guinea-pigs is that nickel elicits a reaction even in normal animals, and Wahlberg (1976) also found that testing the animals with nickel prior to sensitisation reduced the reactivity induced.

Heat, moisture, sweating and friction aggravate nickel dermatitis clinically, and probably facilitate sensitisation by increasing the amount of nickel dissolved in the sweat and absorbed by the skin (Fisher and Shapiro, 1956; Calnan, 1956).

Absorption and localisation in skin and nails
The penetration of nickel sulphate through skin from the arch of the foot and through the great toe nails of cadavers was investigated by Kolpakov (1964),

using histochemical techniques. In the epidermis the barrier to penetration was found to be the stratum corneum, whereas other layers were freely permeable. When applied to the hypodermis, nickel tended to accumulate in the Malpighian layer, in the sweat glands including their efferent ducts, and in the walls of blood vessels. Nickel solution applied to the internal or external surfaces of nails penetrated only the superficial layers, and in neither instance did it pass through the thickness of the nail.

Colorimetric, spectrophotometric and histochemical studies, carried out later on skin from the abdominal wall and arch of the foot, confirmed that the horny layer is the epidermal barrier to nickel absorption. This barrier effect was found throughout its thickness (Kolpakov et al., 1972). Similar results were obtained using histochemical stains on skin sections soaked in 1 per cent nickel sulphate for 15 minutes. Nickel was found in the deeper part of the horny layer and in the inner root sheaths of the hairs. The carboxyl groups of the keratin were found to be important in the binding of nickel (Wells, 1956). Diffusion of ^{63}Ni through the epidermis was found by Samitz and Katz (1970) to be slight, and they observed little enhancement by sweat or detergents. They confirmed also that nickel is bound to the epidermis by carboxyl groups rather than by amino acids.

Skin to which a patch test with nickel sulphate has been applied was examined also by Wells (1956), and again the nickel was seen to be held in the keratin scales. Nickel that penetrated the epidermis went through the sweat ducts and hair follicles; it passed directly through the epidermis only if the latter was damaged. The irritant, pustular patch test reactions to nickel, which occur occasionally, are due to the accumulation of nickel in the parakeratotic plugs at the mouths of sweat ducts. This causes acute inflammation and the formation of an intraepidermal pustule (Wells, 1956).

The absorption of radioactive ^{57}Ni through the skin in normal and nickel-sensitive subjects has been measured. It was found that two-thirds of the nickel penetrated through the skin in 24 hours, equally in normal and nickel-sensitive persons. At the time when a patch test became positive, only 10–15 per cent of the 'resorbed' nickel remained on the skin (Nørgaard, 1955).

Incidence of nickel sensitivity

In many countries nickel is the commonest sensitiser in women, causing its incidence to be high in series of reported patch tests:

Country or city	Patients tested	+ Nickel	Report
Scandinavia	5558	5.9%	Magnusson et al., 1968
Europe	4825	6.7%	Fregert et al., 1969
Poland	1205	4.9%	Rudzki et al., 1970
N. America	1200	11.0%	N. Am. C.D. Group, 1973
New York	769	10.7%	Baer et al., 1973
California	224	8.5%	Epstein et al., 1968
New Zealand	214	5.6%	Black, 1972
	Patients with C.D.		
Australia	1000	4.7%	Burry et al., 1973
Kuwait	389	9.0%	Kanan, 1969

C.D. = Contact Dermatitis (Allergic)

In the European series of Fregert *et al.* (1969) the numbers tested and the incidence of reactors was recorded for each centre (Table 7.19):

Table 7.19. Incidence of sensitivity to nickel (men and women) in eight European countries (Fregert *et al.*, 1969).

City	London	Wycombe	Goth.	Nijmegen	Lund	Copenhagen	Munich	Bari
Total No. Tested	800	132	800	378	800	800	800	315
No. +	80	14	71	34	48	39	31	6
%+	10	10	9	9	6	5	4	2

England had the highest incidence of sensitivity, being 10 per cent for both Wycombe and London. The low figure of 2 per cent for Bari in Southern Italy was partly influenced by the preponderence of males who were tested there, whereas in other clinics more females were included.

In the American series (North American Contact Dermatitis Group, 1973), the various cities participating in the study also recorded their incidence of nickel sensitivity (Table 7.20).

Table 7.20. Incidence of sensitivity to nickel (men and women) in ten North American Cities (North American Contact Dermatitis Group, 1973).

City	Bangor	Detroit	Hanover	Marshfield	New Orleans	New York	Portland	Richmond	San Fran.	Vancouver
No. Tested	59	20	197	129	24	44	229	207	126	165
No. +	12	2	18	12	5	3	19	20	10	30
% +	20	10	9	9	21	7	8	10	8	18

In contrast to Europe, nickel sensitivity was frequent throughout North America.

St John's
Every patient who attended the contact clinic from 1967–1976 was routinely patch tested with nickel sulphate 5 per cent or 2.5 per cent in petrolatum. During this ten year period a total of 16 571 were tested, of whom 1506 (9 per cent) reacted to nickel (Table 7.21).

The variations in the figures between individual European cities and between them and the American cities suggest that there is a real difference in the incidence of nickel sensitivity in various communities. These differences may simply reflect the popularity of cheap metal jewellery. In Finland 980 members of the general population were patch tested with 5 per cent nickel sulphate and 4.5 per cent reacted (Peltonen, 1979).

Changing incidence of nickel sensitivity
In 1959, a report was published on the changing incidence of nickel sensitivity in patients investigated in the Finsen Institute in Copenhagen from 1936–1955 (Marcussen, 1959). Over this 20 year period the incidence increased from 1.8 per cent to 3.2 per cent, except for a sharp drop (0.8 per cent) in 1945 due to cessation of nickel imports but the numbers rose again when the metal was once more brought into the country. This illustrates well that the incidence of sensitivity parallels the presence of an allergen in the environment.

Other centres have reported their frequency of nickel sensitivity at different time intervals:

	Year	+ Nickel %	Report
Copenhagen (Finsen Institute)	1936	1.8	
	1945	0.8	
	1955	3.2	Marcussen, 1959
	1969	4.9	Fregert et al., 1969
Stockholm	1948–51	(M 7.9) 8.8 (F 9.4)	
	1958–61	(M 1.5) 6.9 (F10.5)	Modée et al., 1962
New York	1937	12.3 (definite +)	Rostenberg et al., 1937
	1961	11.2	Baer et al., 1964
	1972	7.0	N. Am. C.D. Grp. 1973
Rome	1956–59	2.6	
	1959–62	4.8	
	1962–65	5.2	Scarpa et al., 1966
Essen (Germany)	1967	0.5	
	1975	5.0	Reichenberger et al., 1976
Graz (Austria)	1952–55	12	
	1960–63	20	Kresbach et al., 1965
Bratislava (Czechoslovakia)	1948	4 pts. +	
	1963	3 pts. +	
	1966	31 pts. +	Hegyi, 1967

These figures show that there is a general trend towards increased nickel sensitivity. In Stockholm the fall in incidence was due to the decrease in this allergy among the men tested. In the early series, the sensitised men were chiefly building workers or shop assistants, but in the second series particular occupations were not involved. In New York there was little difference between 12 per cent in 1937 and 11 per cent in 1961 but in the 1972 study the reported incidence had dropped to 7 per cent. In Bratislava (Hegyi, 1967), nickel sensitivity was to be combatted by forbidding the sale of nickel-plated clips on brassières, suspender belts and men's sock suspenders.

St John's

At St John's, from 1967–1975, the yearly incidence of nickel sensitivity overall remained about 9 per cent until 1976 when the figure rose to 13 per cent (Table 7.21).

Table 7.21. Yearly incidence of nickel sensitivity (St John's 1967–1976).

Year	1967	1968	1969	1970	1971	1972	1973	1974	1975	1976	Total
No. tested	1529	1604	1549	1906	1558	1606	1546	1433	1858	1982	16 571
No. +	95	131	110	148	129	148	169	140	173	263	1 506
%	6	8	7	8	8	9	11	9	9	13	9

Sex incidence

In Europe and North America nickel sensitivity is more common in women than in men, although in Poland this predominance is slight. In contrast, in Kuwait more men than women are sensitised. This was explained by the greater exposure of men to nickel from watch straps and metal on clothing, chiefly press-studs on underpants, and by the fact that women in Kuwait do not wear suspenders (Kanan, 1969). It may also be inferred that at least up to 1969 few women in Kuwait wore cheap metal jewellery.

Sex incidence of nickel sensitivity in five series.

Country	+ Ni F%	M%	Sex ratio F:M	Report
Scandinavia	9.3	2.5	4:1	Magnusson et al., 1968
Scandinavia	8	4	2:1	Magnusson et al., 1969
Europe	10.2	1.8	6:1	Fregert et al., 1969
Czechoslovakia	4.3	1.1	4:1	Hegyi et al., 1974
Poland	5.5	4.3	1:1	Rudzki et al., 1970
N. America	15	5.5	3:1	N. Am. C.D. Group, 1973
Kuwait	10 pts.	24 pts.	1:3	Kanan, 1969

In the Scandinavian series (Magnusson et al., 1968) the sex incidence was recorded for each of the six cities and there were very marked variations.

Sex ratio of nickel sensitive patients in six Scandinavian centres (Magnusson et al., 1968).

City	No. Tested	+ Nickel% F:M	Sex ratio F:M
Helsinki	500	15:1	15:1
Lund	1406	9:1	9:1
Copenhagen	1835	6:1	6:1
Gothenburg	1000	11:4	3:1
Stockholm	510	7:3	2:1
Bergen	307	9:5	2:1

These differences may have been due to the selection of patients or to variation in the exposure of patients to nickel in their environment. It is notable that the sex incidences in Gothenburg (3:1) and Stockholm (2:1) are similar, and this is in complete contrast to the 9:1 ratio in Lund in the south of Sweden. Finland's 15:1 ratio is also in striking contrast to that of Norway where it was 2:1. In Peltonen's (1979) study of the general population in Turku, Finland, 8 per cent of the women and 0.8 per cent of the men were sensitive. These differences remain unexplained.

Modée and Skog (1962) reported from Stockholm that from 1948–1951, 8.8 per cent of the patients were nickel sensitive and the sex ratio was 1:1. The corresponding figures for the years 1958–1961, was 6.9 per cent and the sex ratio had changed to seven females to one male.

St John's

At St John's during the decade 1967–1976 the incidence of nickel sensitivity gradually rose in both sexes. In 1967, 12 per cent of the women were sensitive and by 1976 the figure had increased to 21 per cent; during this same period the incidence among the men changed from 1 per cent to 4 per cent (Table 7.23). During this decade the sex ratio of those sensitised averaged seven females to one male.

Table 7.23. Incidence of nickel sensitivity in women and men and the sex ratio (St John's 1967–1976).

Year	Females			Males			F:M
	No. Tested	Ni +	%	No. Tested	Ni +	%	
1967	720	85	12	809	10	1	9:1
1968	792	117	15	812	14	2	8:1
1969	762	97	13	787	13	2	7:1
1970	990	123	12	916	25	3	5:1
1971	851	124	15	707	5	1	25:1
1972	868	133	15	738	15	2	9:1
1973	836	142	17	710	27	4	5:1
1974	778	121	16	655	19	3	6:1
1975	971	155	16	887	18	2	9:1
1976	1045	224	21	937	39	4	6:1

Associated metal sensitivities

In a proportion of patients nickel sensitivity is associated with allergy to cobalt and chromate. The incidence of such combined reactions has been calculated for the patients seen in the four year period 1973–1976. Nearly two-thirds of both the women and the men reacted to nickel and not to either of the other two metals, a third of the women but a sixth of the men responded to nickel and cobalt, and a combination of nickel and chromate sensitivity was particularly uncommon (1 per cent) in women (Table 7.24).

Table 7.24. Association of reactions to nickel, cobalt and chromate in women and men (St John's 1973–1976).

	Women		Men	
	Nos.	%	Nos.	%
$Ni^+ Cob^- Cr_6^-$	409	64	65	63
$Ni^+ Cob^+ Cr_6^-$	205	32	16	15
$Ni^+ Cob^- Cr_6^+$	9	1	10	10
$Ni^+ Cob^+ Cr_6^+$	19	3	12	12
Total Ni^+	642		103	

Causes of nickel sensitivity

Up to 1930 nickel dermatitis was an occupational disease and occurred particularly in the plating industry. Since then the emphasis has shifted from sensitisation at work to sensitisation in the home by nickel plated metal and objects made of nickel alloy. The early case reports were summarised by Wilson (1956) and Marcussen (1960).

In a Danish survey of 621 nickel-sensitive patients seen between 1936 and 1955 only 4 per cent were due to nickel plating, 9.5 per cent were sensitised by handling nickel-containing objects at work and 86.5 per cent were sensitised by similar articles at home. It was thought that after primary sensitisation by domestic contact with nickel some patients subsequently developed dermatitis of the hands from handling nickel-containing objects at work. High risk occupations were listed as hairdressers, nickel platers, restaurant workers and kitchen staff, metal industries, seamstresses, tailors, nurses, doctors, dentists, cashiers and shop assistants (Marcussen, 1960).

In less industrialised countries the elimination of occupational dermatitis has probably been slower. In Calcutta in 1957 electroplating was still the cause of nickel dermatitis in 120/184 (65 per cent) of nickel-sensitive patients (Lahari, 1957).

St John's

Women

In 1956 Calnan emphasised the increased incidence of nickel dermatitis among women and the source of their sensitivity which, at that time, was nickel plated suspenders. Since then at St John's Hospital nickel has remained the commonest sensitiser in women, but nowadays the allergy is more often acquired from cheap metal jewellery than from clothing. During the quinquennium 1972–1976, 775 women were found on patch testing to be sensitive to nickel. In 674 (86 per cent) the allergy related to jewellery, clothing and domestic objects and in only 45 (6 per cent) was the allergy thought to have occupational significance. These women were working with duplicating machines (3), putting metal eyelets into shoes (1), handling coins as a bus conductress (1), assembling electric meters (1), moving bread trays and baskets in a bakery (1) and the other 38 were currently hairdressers, all with hand eczema, in whom the nickel sensitivity was presumed but not proved to be significant. In other women occupational exposure to nickel may have been important but the relationship was too tenuous to be certain. No source was found for the allergy in 41 women (5 per cent) and no information regarding it was recorded in 15 (2 per cent).

Men

Allergy to nickel in men has been infrequent. During the five years 1972–1976 118 nickel sensitive men were seen. In the majority (65) (55 per cent) watches or watch straps had caused the dermatitis usually alone, but occasionally in conjunction with other nickel contacts. In 11, jewellery, rings, neckchains, clothing fasteners or miscellaneous objects were responsible; in 3 it was spectacle frames and in one a wheel chair (13 per cent). In only 3 (2.5 per cent) was the allergy occupational; 2 were electroplaters and one used a duplicating machine. In 16 patients no source for the sensitivity was found and in 19 no relevant information was recorded (30 per cent).

Domestic sources of nickel contact

In industrial and probably also in non-industrial countries, nickel is ubiquitous and everyone is in daily contact with it in the home. Nickel is present in:

1. Electroplated metal
2. Nickel alloys.

Electroplated metal is almost certainly the more frequent sensitiser. It has been suggested by Hegyi *et al.* (1974) that the addition in recent years of cadmium to nickel plating solutions has facilitated corrosion of the plated layer, thereby releasing nickel and making it available to induce sensitisation. They consider this to be a factor in the increased incidence of nickel allergy.

Electroplated metal

Clothing

In the 1950s suspenders were made of iron, plated with nickel, and this close contact of the skin with nickel caused many cases of allergic dermatitis. Cheap metal jewellery has now replaced suspenders as the most frequent cause of nickel dermatitis.

There are several reasons for this eclipse of suspender dermatitis. By the early 1960s the metal parts of underclothes were painted and this protected the skin from contact with nickel; women bought new roll-ons and brassières more frequently, giving less time for the paint to chip off, whereas the old-fashioned corset, kept for years, was rarely worn. Sensitivity to nickel had become widely recognised by both general practitioners and the public so that when dermatitis occurred women often changed from metal to nylon suspenders without consulting a dermatologist. Many found that they remained free from trouble simply by ensuring that their metal clips were painted. Nickel-sensitive women challenged by a doctor as to what type of suspenders they wear usually reply nylon, but if the suspenders are examined they are nearly always found to be painted metal. With the introduction of the mini-skirt in 1966 suspenders became unfashionable and were replaced by tights or panty hose. Girls now grow up never having worn suspenders, and as young and middle aged women have also adopted tights, suspender dermatitis has become a clinical rarity.

There is an increasing use of white or coloured plastic coatings over the hooks and eyes used for brassières and the metal rings on brassière straps may be similarly covered. This helps nickel-sensitive women to avoid eczema due to their brassière clips and fastenings.

Silver-coloured snap fasteners, press fasteners and hooks and eyes are all nickel plated. When black, they are covered with a black lacquer. Some of these fasteners are made of nylon as are many zips.

Jewellery

Few women can afford to wear only the precious metals and a vast amount of so-called costume or gear jewellery is worn and silver coloured ornaments, particularly those made of cheaper metals, may contain nickel.

Already by 1956 earrings had become the commonest sensitiser in the United States and even then earring dermatitis was regarded as a cardinal sign of nickel sensitivity. Among a group of 40 nickel-sensitive women, 32 had earring dermatitis and 18 suspender dermatitis (Fisher and Shapiro, 1956). In 1967, in the U.S.A. nickel dermatitis was prevalent in adolescent girls following ear piercing, possibly with nickel-containing needles and the subsequent wearing of nickel containing earrings for pierced ears (Gaul, 1967; Watt and Baumann, 1968). Since men have adopted this fashion, they too are being sensitised (Fisher, 1974).

In Britain, among cheaper earrings, the clip-on type are still frequently worn but pierced ears are becoming increasingly popular among adolescents. The facility of clip-on earrings to sensitise may be explained by their pressure on the ear-lobes, the prolonged exposure, and possibly by sweating under the metal. In pierced ears there is also extremely close contact between the metal and the skin.

Neck chains, necklace clasps, rings, brooches, bracelets, watches and watch straps are all possible sources of nickel contact.

Costume jewellery is made by electroplating a base metal first with copper and then with nickel. Some of the ornaments are sold with only this nickel finish, others are finally plated with gilt, gold, rhodium or silver. Very cheap jewellery has an aluminium coating which is dyed to mimic gold. The ear-wires of earrings for pierced ears are frequently finished with a plating of gold or rhodium. In plated articles the gold finish is often incomplete and the underlying nickel is exposed to cause dermatitis and give a positive dimethylglyoxime test (Yoshikawa, Hadame and Hijikata, 1978).

Watch cases and straps
The majority of silver-coloured watches sold in the United Kingdom have stainless steel case backs and they do not cause nickel dermatitis. The backs of cheaper watches are made of a brass and plated with nickel or copper in order to maintain the adhesion of the final chrome finish. The bezel (grooved side part) of the watch is often made in the same way. In many watches the winding wheel, the shank or the bar to hold the strap are nickel plated and are unsuspected sources of nickel contact.

Metal watch bands may be stainless steel or a base metal, plated with nickel or silver to prevent the final chromium or gold-plating peeling off from friction and sweating during wear.

Spectacles
Silver coloured metal spectacle frames are likely to have a composition similar to that of watches. The limbs of a celluloid spectacle frame were reinforced with metal struts made of an alloy containing 30 per cent nickel, 1–3 per cent manganese and 65–68 per cent copper. As the plastic aged the nickel was leached out and caused a retro-auricular dermatitis. On patch testing the patient showed reactions to nickel and corroded plastic, but not to the undamaged celluloid or its components (Jirásek, Kobikova and Jirásková, 1976).

Needles and pins
Hand sewing needles are practically all made from nickel-plated steel. Pins may be nickel-plated, stainless steel or brass. Cheilitis from holding pins in the mouth has been reported (Calnan, 1956). Knitting needles and crochet hooks are made of anodised aluminium or plastic; no nickel-plated ones have been made in Britain for 30 years.

Kitchen equipment
Cutlery may be made of electroplated nickel silver (E.P.N.S.), stainless steel, or the cheaper types of nickel-plated base metal.

Taps, door handles and knobs may be chromium-plated over nickel; once the chromium wears off the nickel is exposed.

Other metal articles
Metal lipstick cases have caused cheilitis (Wilson, 1956) and irritation of the scalp from hair grips has been described (Calnan, 1956). Hair slides may have metal clasps and would certainly contain nickel as do many other everyday objects such as silver-coloured metal thimbles.

Systemic reactions

Nickel-plated cannulae used for intravenous infusions were thought to be the cause of post-operative eruptions in two nickel-sensitive women. One developed a generalised erythema with vesicles on the fingers and toes, and the other had urticaria. This patient was tested with 1 per cent nickel sulphate; a prick test elicited a weal and a patch test was positive (Stoddart, 1960). Similarly there was a previous history of nickel sensitivity in six women who developed anaphylactoid reactions, urticaria or angio-oedema after intravenous infusions through nickel plated cannulae. Histologically the lesions showed vasculitis not eczema. All six women reacted to a patch test and a prick test with 1 per cent nickel sulphate. In addition passive transfer with the sera of five of the patients was positive. A nickel plated cannula was left in distilled water for two days and released 20 mg of nickel (Holti, 1974). Nickel plated retractors, in contact with the peritoneum and the wall of an abdominal incision but not touching the skin, caused post-operative dermatitis in several nickel sensitive women (Kvorning, 1975).

Plastics plated with nickel

A new hazard derives from the method which has been devised of plating plastics with nickel, apparently designed to enhance the appearance of the article and to make it more saleable. It is used on transistor radios, cameras, microphones, car accessories, kitchen equipment, clothing accessories and jewellery (Fregert, 1972).

Nickel alloys

Nickel combines with other metals to form alloys; as the whiteness of nickel bleaches the colour of other metals, alloys containing nickel are usually silver in colour. It is difficult to assess how often they sensitise, some alloys certainly release nickel, others appear not to do so.

Stainless steel

Steel is an iron-carbon alloy made stainless or corrosion-resistant by the addition of chromium or nickel. It has been said (Fisher, 1972) that stainless steel is harmless to nickel-sensitive subjects because the nickel is so firmly bound that it cannot be leached out by sweat or body fluids and is unable to initiate or elicit a nickel dermatitis. However, under certain conditions nickel is released (see below).

Prostheses

Prostheses are occasionally made of stainless steels containing 10–14 per cent nickel (with up to 35 per cent in a pacemaker wire and probe) or of cobalt chromium alloys containing 2.5 per cent nickel (Samitz and Katz, 1975). It has been shown by these authors that metals of the type used for prostheses if immersed in physiological saline, sweat or blood release nickel, detectable as parts per million, into the leaching fluids.

Sensitisation by the nickel in this type of buried metal has been reported. Barranco and Solomon (1972) reported that nickel in stainless steel orthopaedic screws in a woman's knees was thought to have caused her widespread eczema. She was sensitive to nickel and recovered when the screws were removed. Another woman (Pegum, 1974), known to be sensitive to white metal, tolerated a steel osteotomy plate containing 8–12 per cent nickel and 17–20 per cent chromium for three years before developing dermatitis and suppuration round the plate. Both resolved after the plate was removed. Patch tests: she reacted to nickel, chrome and the plate. Such adverse reactions may be delayed. A patient of Lyell and Bain (1974) with a confirmed nickel allergy had her mitral valve replaced by a metal prosthesis containing nickel and at follow-up nearly two years later she was well. Subsequently this valve leaked and had to be replaced, as did a second similar nickel valve, whereas a third nickel-free valve worked satisfactorily (Lyell, 1978). A fractured jaw wired with stainless steel in a nickel sensitive woman failed to heal until the wire was removed (Roed-Petersen, Roed-Petersen and Jørgensen, 1979).

Domestic metal articles
A large amount of kitchen equipment is made of metal, commonly stainless steel which is also used for cutlery and scissors. It has been shown by Katz and Samitz (1975) that significant amounts of nickel are leached from such metals by sweat and detergents. Stainless steels shown to release nickel have had negative dimethylglyoxime tests.

Coins
So-called silver coins rarely contain silver and its presence is simulated by a cupro-nickel alloy.

	Copper %	Nickel %	Tin %	Zinc %	Silver %
British decimal coins					
Silver (5p, 10p, 50p,)	75	25	—	—	—
Nickel brass (old 3d)	79	1	—	20	
Bronze (½p, 1p, 2p)	97	—	½	2½	—
United States					
Silver Cents 5	75	25	—	—	—
10 and 25	92	8	—	—	—
50	60	—	—	—	40
Bronze Cent 1	95	—	—	5	—
Sweden					
Crown		25			

Silver coloured coins readily release nickel when soaked in human sweat, sweat and sodium lauryl sulphate (Samitz and Pomerantz, 1958), ethylic ether and synthetic sweat and water (Bang Pedersen *et al.*, 1974). The release is increased by raising the temperature (Menné and Solgaard, 1978). Such coins contaminate other copper coins, bank notes and similarly the hands of subjects counting or handling silver coins. This degree of nickel contamination was thought by Bang Pedersen *et al.* (1974) not to elicit dermatitis in a nickel sensitive subject if the skin of the hands was healthy but to be a significant factor in the chronicity of an already existent hand eczema. However, nickel sensitive women with pompholyx type hand eczema failed to react to Christensen and

Moller's (1975) provocation test in which for six minutes their hands were immersed in a bowl containing coins and other nickel objects.

Cases have been reported of coins causing hand eczema. A nickel sensitive cashier developed palmar eczema and her relapses exactly paralleled the intermittent occasions on which she did this work (Bettley, 1971). Palmar eczema ascribed to coins has also been described by Husain (1977). A housewife developed eczema of the fingers and was found to be sensitive to nickel and copper: the eczema was attributed to the handling of coins (Black, 1972). Two other patients developed eczema of the fingers from coins; one carried them in the fingers of her gloves, while the other used them to scratch her nose, causing the eczema of her fingers and patches on the nose which resembled seborrhoeic eczema. The dermatitis cleared in both patients once they avoided nickel coins (Fisher, 1973).

Jewellery

White gold may contain nickel, palladium or silver, but nickel is unlikely to be present in yellow gold because its bleaching action masks the yellow of the gold and produces a silver coloured alloy. This statement, though generally correct, is not strictly accurate because a yellow rolled gold wire on a spectacle frame was found to contain 0.7 per cent nickel which was insufficient to whiten the metal. This wire was wrapped around a core of silver containing 12 per cent nickel. A patient seen at St John's developed nickel dermatitis from his spectacle frame. Although the metal core did not seem to be exposed, it, rather than the yellow gold-nickel wire, may have been the source of his dermatitis.

Tin-nickel alloy

An alloy in which the nickel does not dissociate is a tin-nickel compound containing approximately 65 per cent tin and 35 per cent nickel. It was used to plate the base metal of suspenders for nickel-sensitive women and it effectively prevented dermatitis (Calnan, 1962).

Silver-nickel surgical clips

Following a thyroidectomy, a patient developed an acute eczema under nickel silver clips, which had been used to close the wound. She had a previous history of nickel dermatitis, but was not patch tested (Booth, 1971).

Systemic Reaction

Immediate Type Hypersensitivity

A woman with a fractured neck of femur was treated by the insertion of a Smith-Petersen vitallium nail and on the following day developed generalised pruritus and widespread urticaria. A patch test and a prick test with nickel sulphate 2 per cent were positive. Exactly one year later the nail was removed; the urticaria disappeared within a day but the patient remained dermographic. The alloy vitallium consists of chromium 27–30 per cent, molybdenum 5–7 per cent, iron 0.75 per cent, carbon 0.5 per cent, nickel 1 per cent, silicon 1 per cent, manganese 1 per cent and cobalt balance (McKenzie, Aitken and Ridsdill-Smith, 1967).

Detergents

In Holland in 1969, the role of nickel in detergents as a possible source of nickel exposure was investigated by Malten, Schutter, van Senden and Spruit (1969) and Malten and Spruit (1969). In 1965, EDTA (ethylenediaminetetraacetic acid) had been added to all detergents in amounts sufficient to chelate the nickel and render it inert, but this procedure did not reduce the number of nickel-sensitive women attending hospital. Using the cup test method, a solution containing 10 μmNi/l failed to elicit a reaction in a highly sensitised subject. It was therefore considered that 1 μmNi/l was a safe environmental concentration for those sensitive to nickel, and it was thought unlikely that this concentration could induce sensitisation. The concentration of nickel in detergent suds was estimated as 0.2–0.9 μmNi/l (2–9 ppm) which is too small to elicit a response even in those sensitised. The addition of EDTA to detergents is a further protection. It was concluded that nickel in detergents is not a particular hazard.

The concentration of nickel in six detergent powders in England was estimated spectrographically in 1956, and as it was found to be less than 10 parts per million it was not considered to be significant in the cause of hand eczema (Wells, 1956). In 1971 a large manufacturer of detergent products in England was maintaining a standard of no more nickel than 1 part per million in the end product principally by screening the raw materials. The incorporation of chelating agents was an additional safeguard.

In Sweden, Wahlberg, Lindstedt and Einarsson (1977) used an atomic absorption spectrophotometer to estimate the nickel content of detergents and found that 12 of 19 products contained $> 1.0 \mu$g/g and the highest value was 5.7 μg Ni/g.

In France a series of detergents were examined and the concentrations of nickel varied from a trace to 430 ppm. The levels were higher in powders than liquids. The presence of this nickel was considered a significant hazard for nickel sensitive patients with hand eczema (Barrière et al., 1979).

Tap water

A nickel sensitive woman, who noticed that her hand eczema was worse in her own flat than when she was staying in her parents' home, was investigated in Sweden (Fregert, 1971). Nickel in the tap water was estimated by the atomic absorption method. It was found that the first hot water which came out of the taps in the patient's flat in the morning contained 140–1300 μg Ni/l and the cold water 50–1100 μg Ni/l. After running the water for five minutes the amounts fell to 0–2 μg Ni/l.

Clinical features

Over the past 20 years the clinical features of nickel sensitivity in women have changed. Nowadays fewer patients present with obvious nickel dermatitis and the allergy, particularly in older women, is often found in the investigation of another pattern of eczema. The age of onset has altered from a wide range to the teenager and young woman, and the source is no longer the suspender but cheap metal jewellery, and fasteners on clothing such as jeans studs. A secondary spread, so striking a pattern in Britain in the 1950s, is now rarely seen.

Age of onset

Sensitisation in infancy has been reported. A baby aged seven months developed patches of eczema on his abdomen and back which corresponded with the press-studs on his rubber pants. He was patch tested and reacted strongly to nickel 3 per cent (Reiffers *et al.*, 1974). Another baby aged 15 months, with no previous history of nickel dermatitis, developed eczema from a metal clip within 16 hours of its being applied. On patch testing he reacted strongly to nickel sulphate 2.5 per cent in petrolatum (Finn, 1974). A boy in whom sensitivity to nickel was confirmed by patch testing when he was 13 years old had had dermatitis from zips even when he was a baby and at school he had continued to have trouble from nickel plated objects (Tegner and Fregert, 1973).

St John's

The youngest children seen in this clinic have been an Asian girl aged four years who attended with nickel dermatitis on her arms from a bangle, and a boy aged eight years who initially had dermatitis, caused by snap fasteners on his napkins, when he was three to four months old.

Women

In the 1956 study of 400 women with nickel dermatitis (Calnan, 1956), the age of onset was fairly evenly distributed through the decades from 11–60 years. Since then the age at which this sensitivity is acquired has gradually decreased until now it is usually an acquisition of the teenager. From 1967–1972, 679 nickel sensitive women attended the clinic and in 356 the age of onset of their sensitivity could be estimated from the patient's recollection of her age when she first developed nickel dermatitis. This same assessment could be made for 423 of the 642 nickel sensitive women who were seen in the four years 1973–1976. In the 1967–1972 period 43 per cent of the patients had been sensitised during the ages of 11–20 years and in the 1972–1976 span 53 per cent had been sensitised in this decade (Table 7.25).

Table 7.25 Ages of onset of nickel sensitivity in women (St John's 1956–1976).

Age years	0–10 %	11–20 %	21–30 %	31–40 %	41–50 %	51–60 %	61–70 %	71–80 %	Total No. Patients
1956	—	18	27	24	20	9	2	—	380
1967–72	2	43	26	11	10	6	2	—	356
1973–76	0.5	53	26	9	8	3	—	—	423

Men

Between 1967–1972, 82 men were found to be sensitive to nickel but in only 26 was the age of onset of symptoms recorded; this information was given for 54 of the 103 men seen from 1973–1976. The numbers are small but unlike those for women, they show no grouping into particular ages (Table 7.26).

Table 7.26. Ages of onset of nickel sensitivity in men (St John's 1967–1976).

Age years	0–10	11–20	21–30	31–40	41–50	51–60	61–70	71–80	Total No. Patients
1967–72	1	5	8	5	4	2	1		26
1973–76	2	10	11	11	10	7	2	1	54

Patients presenting with nickel dermatitis

In the late 1950s, contact dermatitis from nickel, particularly on clothing, became readily recognised by general practitioners and even by patients themselves, and it gradually became unusual for patients to present to the dermatologist with this contact dermatitis. In the 1960s most cases were diagnosed on routine patch testing of patients with other types of eczema and a relevant past history was generally obtained. In the 1970s this trend began to reverse as it has become not at all unusual for teenagers and patients in their twenties to be referred to the dermatologist with an undiagnosed nickel dermatitis from jewellery. This is still infrequent in the older woman, but occurs occasionally.

St John's

Women

In the 1950s, as the era of suspender dermatitis waned, active nickel dermatitis became uncommon until the 1970s when it reappeared in young women in the jewellery phase of sensitisation. During the decade 1967–1976 the proportion of the nickel sensitive women who had presented with nickel dermatitis, from readily identifiable sources such as jewellery and clothing, rose from 14 per cent in 1967–71 to 24 per cent in 1972–74 and to 37 per cent by 1975–76 (Table 7.27). In many of these patients the nickel dermatitis co-existed with an eczema not explained by nickel contact. In the four years 1973–1976, 209 women were seen with a contact dermatitis from nickel, but only in 61 (30 per cent) was the allergy the entire cause of their eczema while in 148 (70 per cent) its relevance was partial.

Table 7.27. Numbers of women in each decade presenting with active nickel dermatitis (St John's 1967–1976).

Age — years	1967–71 Total + Ni	C.D.	1972–74 Total + Ni	C.D.	1975 and 76 Total + Ni	C.D.
0–10	0	0	1	1	0	0
11–20	85	24	91	49	106	55
21–30	138	21	135	25	131	53
31–40	99	4	54	5	41	12
41–50	95	11	42	6	43	10
51–60	87	8	53	6	33	6
61–70	39	6	16	3	22	3
71–80	3	0	4	0	3	1
Total	546	74	396	95	379	140
		14%		24%		37%

Men

Of the 185 nickel-sensitive men seen from 1967–1976, 44 (24 per cent) had nickel dermatitis when they came to the clinic. The majority (32) of these patients were seen in the last four years, 1973–1976, and the proportion in whom the allergy was the sole cause of their eczema was the same 30 per cent (9 of 32) as in the women; the relevance was partial in 70 per cent (23 of 32).

Clinical patterns
Nickel-sensitive patients do not necessarily develop eczema at every site of nickel contact. The production of a reaction is determined by sweating, pressure and friction under each piece of metal, and the ease with which the metal releases nickel.

Jewellery
The enthusiasm of young women for fancy jewellery is the usual source of their sensitisation to nickel. In Britain the commonest cause is clip-on ear rings and young women present with well-defined patches of eczema on each ear-lobe. It is surprising how often girls will continue to wear ear rings and tolerate the discomfort of the eczema they know they produce. Murno-Ashman, MacDonald and Feiwel (1975) reported that three nickel sensitive women with pierced ears continued to wear their ear rings until they dropped out leaving them with ear lobes permanently split in two. Fissured granuloma of the ear has also occurred in association with nickel dermatitis (Ayala, 1976). Hooped ear rings may cause dermatitis of the neck while sparing the ears (Shore and Berger, 1974).

Rings cause eczema of the fingers and may precipitate hand eczema. Neck chains sometimes produce symmetrical patches of eczema on either side of the base of the neck. The localisation is probably due to friction and pressure of the chains at these sites but the clinical pattern is not immediately obvious as a nickel dermatitis. Necklace clasps produce patches on the back of the neck which might be mistaken for lichen simplex. More easily recognisable are bands of eczema on the arms from bracelets, or watches. A unilateral dermatitis is often made symmetrical by moving the metal from one side to the other. A striking feature in some of these young women is the persistence of the eczema on their neck or arms despite the removal of all nickel jewellery. The original contact dermatitis is perpetuated by rubbing and scratching and it can be difficult to break the patients of this habit and heal their skin.

Watches and watch straps
Watches and watch straps cause dermatitis in both sexes and are the commonest source of sensitivity to nickel in men seen at St John's. The back of the watch causes an eczematous patch on the extensor surface of the lower forearm. The metal bracelet may give a band of eczema encircling the area round to the watch, or the eczema may be patchy, occurring at the sites of maximum friction. The buckle on the strap is often responsible for a patch of eczema on the flexor surface of the wrist.

Spectacles
Metal spectacle frames cause eczema at the sites of contact on the nose, temples and ears.

Clothing

The features of suspender dermatitis were described by Calnan (1956) and Wilson (1956) over twenty years ago. At that time the suspender area was the primary site of nickel dermatitis in 95 per cent of the women. The suspenders produced localised areas of eczema on the fronts and backs of the thighs, corresponding to some or all of the four suspenders. The back ones produced dermatitis more commonly than those in front because of the greater pressure on and friction from back suspenders.

As yet, brassières have not been discarded and dermatitis is still seen on women's backs from unpainted metal hook fasteners. The metal rings on the fronts of shoulder straps are generally painted and so rarely cause trouble.

Any type of nickel plated hook, press-stud fastener or metal zip may cause dermatitis if in contact with the skin. The current fashion for jeans has produced from the stud fastener a clinically distinctive patch of eczema on the central abdomen of many young patients. This has been dubbed a Jeanodermatosis by a wag in our clinic.

Vasculitis

It has been suggested by Hjorth (1976) that the ingestion of nickel by sensitised women may produce lesions on the back which mimic excoriations and have the histological features of an allergic vasculitis.

Secondary spread

A secondary spread was a very characteristic feature in women with suspender dermatitis and occurred in 75 per cent of the patients seen at St John's Hospital (Calnan, 1956). When the primary site was the ears or elsewhere the incidence was only 35 per cent. This secondary eruption was not related to nickel contact; it was usually eczematous, and in the elbow flexures it was often papular. In most patients the spread was symmetrical and affected the antecubital fossae, eyelids, sides of the neck, inner thighs, and it sometimes became generalised. Not all these sites were involved in any one patient, and its severity varied. Non-eczematous patterns occurred very occasionally, and included erythema multiforme, urticaria, generalised pruritus and generalised prurigo. The clear description of this pattern of eczema was most important because previously its connection with nickel dermatitis had largely gone unrecognised, and these patients were often labelled as having 'flexural eczema'. It was suggested that the spread was haematogenous and resembled the 'id' of a fungus infection.

Features of the secondary spread were: it often brought the patient to the dermatologist; the patients rarely connected it with their suspender dermatitis; and they often failed to mention the latter or even denied its existence. A most striking feature was that it recurred without a flare of the primary site and it was even described as occurring before the onset of the primary eruption (Calnan, 1956; Wilson, 1956).

Scepticism about this secondary eruption has been expressed. Fisher (1973) thinks that all these sites can be explained by inadvertent nickel contact and Marcussen (1957) considered that all except the elbow flexures are due to contamination.

St John's

Women
The disappearance of suspender dermatitis has meant that a secondary eruption has become rare, but it still does occur and clinically the sites do not appear to be areas of nickel contact. In all the patients seen from 1967–1976 the secondary spread was eczematous, and the incidence was 2 per cent (28 of 1321) (Table 7.28).

Table 7.28. Numbers of women with a secondary spread (St John's 1967–1976).

Age years	0–10	11–20	21–30	31–40	41–50	51–60	61–70	71–80	Total
No. of Patients	0/1	17/282	4/404	3/194	2/180	0/173	2/77	0/10	28/1321 2%

Men
From 1967–1976, no man was seen with a secondary spread from nickel dermatitis probably because in men this eczema is localised and usually comparatively mild.

ASSOCIATED PATTERNS OF ECZEMA
Of the 400 nickel-sensitive women reported from St John's in 1956, 43 (11 per cent) had in addition the following patterns of eczema: seborrhoeic (13), exogenous (12), unclassified (10), atopic (4), nummular (3) and hypostatic (1) (Calnan, 1956). In none of these eczemas is an association with nickel sensitivity obvious.

Incidence of hand eczema in nickel-sensitive patients
In Calnan's (1956) series a striking association was that of hand eczema which occurred in 81 (20 per cent) of the patients. Another report from London (Wilson, 1956) described 85 women of whom 14 (17 per cent) had hand eczema. In Copenhagen 350 women were studied and 100 (29 per cent) had involvement of the hands, either as a primary site or as a spread from nickel dermatitis of the thighs or face and neck (Marcussen, 1957). In the south of Sweden of 165 patients sensitive to nickel 86 (52 per cent) had hand eczema (Christensen and Möller, 1975). In the Finnish study (Peltonen, 1979) 20 per cent of the nickel sensitive subjects in the general population had hand eczema compared with over 50 per cent among nickel sensitive clinic patients.

St John's
During the decade 1967–1976, about half the nickel-sensitive patients had hand eczema, either alone or in association with eczema of other sites. However, as many of the patients who attend this clinic have hand eczema it is not possible to deduce from these figures alone that there is a significant relationship between this common pattern of eczema and this common allergen.

Women
The incidence of hand eczema in nickel sensitive women did not change between 1967 and 1976. From 1967–1971, there were 546 nickel sensitive women of whom 316 (58 per cent) had hand eczema, and from 1972–1976 there were 775 of whom 420 (54 per cent) had hand eczema. This proportion was not influenced by the ages of the patients (Table 7.29).

Table 7.29. Incidence of hand eczema in nickel sensitive women of various ages (St John's 1967–1976).

		1967–1971				1972–1976	
	Ni+	Hand Ecz.	%	Ni+	Hand Ecz.	%
0–10	0	41		1	0	
11–20	85	41	48	197	98	50
21–30	138	81	59	266	140	53
31–40	99	62	63	95	55	58
41–50	95	58	61	85	45	53
51–60	87	54	62	86	56	65
61–70	39	20	51	38	22	58
71–80	3	0		7	4	57
Total	546	316	58	775	420	54

Men

Throughout the decade 1967–1976 about two thirds of the men who were nickel sensitive had hand eczema:

	Ni+	Hand Eczema	%
1967–1971	67	44	66
1972–1976	118	74	63

Incidence of nickel sensitivity in patients with Hand Eczema

Of greater significance is the incidence of nickel sensitivity in patients with hand eczema. Patients with hand eczema were studied in the south of Sweden (Agrup, 1969) and nickel sulphate 5.4 per cent in water was included in the patch test series: 12 per cent of the women (56 of 462) were sensitive but none of the 250 men. Nickel was the commonest sensitiser among these women and was thought to be the main or a contributory cause of the hand eczema in 11 per cent (49) of them.

A thousand patients, seen in the contact clinic at St John's Hospital in 1971–1972, were analysed in detail. Of 238 women *with* hand eczema, 50 (21 per cent) were sensitive to nickel whereas of 285 women *without* hand eczema 34 (12 per cent) were nickel-sensitive. Among the 50 patients with hand eczema and nickel sensitivity, the sequence was as follows: in 23 the allergy preceded the hand eczema by six months to 40 years; in seven the hand eczema came first by a few weeks to ten years; and in six patients the sensitivity and the hand eczema occurred simultaneously. Eight women gave no history of nickel dermatitis and for six this information was not recorded (Cronin, 1972). In many of the patients seen since that time there has been a striking gap, often of many years, between the onset of nickel sensitivity and the development of the hand eczema.

In contrast were the findings in a European investigation of 2383 females and 1035 males, all of whom were patch tested with nickel sulphate 5 per cent in petrolatum. Of the women with hand eczema 11 per cent reacted to nickel and of those without hand eczema 9 per cent were sensitive. Two per cent of the men with hand eczema were allergic to nickel, but only 1 per cent of the men without hand eczema were sensitive (Wilkinson *et al.*, 1970).

Practically all the studies suggest that in women there is a definite relationship between hand eczema and nickel sensitivity. In some, the connection was established (Bettley, 1971; Black, 1972; Fregert, 1971), but in the majority it is far from obvious.

Oral ingestion of nickel

Christensen and Möller (1975) studied the clinical pattern of the hand eczema in nickel sensitive women and established that the majority (77 per cent) had a symmetrical, vesicular eruption of the palms and palmar aspects and sides of the fingers — so-called pompholyx — and that it was often episodic. Twelve women with this pompholyx type of eczema were studied, while their hands were in a quiescent phase, by Christensen and Möller (1975 ii). External exposure by covering their hands with nickel-containing objects had no effect. They were then given orally 25 mg of nickel sulphate containing 5.6 mg of nickel, and after 30 hours nine of the twelve women had a considerable increase in the number of vesicles on their palms and in seven of the patients there was an eczematous flare at sites of previous nickel patch tests or nickel eczema. Further confirmation that the ingestion of nickel is significant is the finding by Menné and Thorboe (1976) that in four nickel sensitive women the urinary excretion of nickel rose immediately after a flare of the vesicular eczema of the palms.

Each of 28 women with pompholyx hand eczema was given a tablet containing 2.5 mg of nickel; within hours four developed urticaria and after two to three days the eczema was definitely worse in 13 and possibly so in four. These 17 patients were given a low nickel diet for six weeks, three cleared and six improved. After two to four weeks on a normal diet, seven of the nine relapsed. Urinary levels of nickel fell during the diet period but did not correlate with improvement. The diet consisted of:

Permitted foods
All meats, poultry, fish (except herring), eggs, milk, yoghurt, butter, margarine, cheese, 1 medium-sized potato per day. Small amounts of the following: cauliflower, cabbage, carrots, cucumber, lettuce. Polished rice, flour (except whole-grain), fresh fruits (except pears), marmalade, jam. Coffee, wine and beer.

Prohibited foods
Canned foods and acid foods cooked in stainless steel utensils, herring, oysters, asparagus, beans, mushrooms, onions, corn (maize), spinach, tomatoes, peas, whole-grain flour, fresh and cooked pears, rhubarb. Tea, cocoa and chocolate. Baking powder (Kaaber, Veien and Tjell, 1978).

However such diets should be checked as there are likely to be regional differences in the nickel content of foods. For instance in Poland (Rudzki and Grzywa, 1977) margarine may contain nickel up to 0.2 mg per kg, and 250 g of margarine (0.05 mg Ni) caused a flare of eczema in a nickel sensitive woman including sites of previous nickel dermatitis. Her hands were not affected.

Saucepans made of aluminium, teflon and enamel do not release nickel into boiling water whereas those of stainless steel do so if the pH of the water is acid, as would occur in cooking rhubarb or apples (Christensen and Möller, 1978). Oxalic acid in food is particularly active in this release of nickel and canned food is another source (Brun, 1979).

In a woman who was very sensitive to nickel only a limited correlation was found between the clinical activity of her eczema, over periods of more than a month, and the concentration of nickel in her urine and plasma. It was concluded that factors influencing the nickel concentration in body fluids required further study (de Jongh et al., 1978; de Jongh and Spruit, 1978).

Chelation of nickel
Chelation of ingested nickel has been tried therapeutically. Diethyldithiocarbamate (DDC) 400 mg daily for 20 days and later tetraethylthiuramdisulphide (TETD) 300 mg daily for two months were given with improvement to one woman by Menné and Kaaber (1978). Another patient received 1 g DDC a day for two months; her urinary nickel excretion increased tenfold and she too appeared to benefit (Spruit, Bongaarts and de Jongh, 1978).

These chelators may cause an initial transient flare of the eczema and as TETD is Antabuse, alcohol must be avoided.

Industrial dermatitis
Nowadays nickel is an infrequent overt cause of occupational dermatitis. In Essen the cases of nickel allergy seen from 1967–1975 were reviewed. The sensitisation was thought to have originated at work and to be responsible for the dermatitis in most of the 26 men but of the 213 women this diagnosis was made in only 20, of whom one was a photographer and 19 were metal workers (Reichenberger, Ebke and Patiri, 1976).

Hairdressing is a popular occupation among young women but it exposes them to the risk of developing hand eczema and of those who are seen by a dermatologist and are referred for patch testing nearly half have been found to be sensitive to nickel. In Wahlberg's (1975) series, 14 of 35 (40 per cent) hairdressers were allergic to nickel, and at St John's Hospital the incidence was 22 of 50 (44 per cent) female hairdressers (Marks and Cronin, 1977).

Reichenberger et al. (1976) did not attribute this sensitisation among hairdressers to occupational contacts, nevertheless Wahlbert (1975) considered that the leaching of nickel from metal hairdressing equipment was significant in the causation of these hairdressers' hand eczema.

Metal food containers, handled at work, were incriminated as causing eczema on the pulps of the fingers of a nickel sensitive woman (Serrano Ortego and Sanchez Muros, 1976).

Twenty-eight unused mould oils were analysed by Wahlberg et al. (1977) and although nickel was detected in some it did not exceed $1 \mu g/g$. Similarly 28 unused cutting fluids were examined and 27 contained $< 0.3 \mu g$ Ni/g but one contained $19.4 \mu g/g$. Despite the theoretical risk of nickel being leached from metals into grinding oils during engineering work this does not, in practice, seem to be a hazard (Samitz and Katz, 1975).

Eight brands of Swedish cement were examined for nickel and they were found to contain between 5 and 59 $\mu g/g$ (Wahlberg et al., 1977).

St John's

Men
From 1967–1976, five men were seen with an occupational dermatitis due to nickel; four were electroplaters and one used a duplicating machine.

Electroplating industry
Since the improvement of conditions in the electroplating industry, occupational dermatitis among these workers has become unusual. Four electroplaters with dermatitis were seen between 1967 and 1976, and each was sensitive to nickel.

In 1966, a small nickel-plating factory was visited where over the years several men had developed dermatitis. At the time of the visit three of five men had on the backs of their hands an eczema which came and went, and one also had involvement of the eyes. The metal to be plated was first cleaned in sulphuric acid then plated in a tank with solutions of nickel chloride and nickel sulphate at a pH of 4–5. The men wore gloves. The room was hot and humid. Each man was patch tested with nickel and all the tests were negative. It was concluded that the dermatitis was an irritant effect of the cleaning and plating solutions, aggravated by the heat and humidity of the working area.

Diallylamine, an additive used to make the metal surface shiny, was reported as a sensitiser by Fregert (1973). His patient reacted to a patch test with diallylamine 0.001 per cent in water; 12 controls did not respond to 0.1 per cent.

Women
During the decade 1967–1976, six women and one man were seen with an occupational nickel dermatitis of the hands from working on duplicating machines. Six other women had hand dermatitis due to various types of occupational exposure to nickel.

Offset duplicating
Offset duplicating or printing is an easy and rapid method of replicating many copies from an original master. The master copy is typed and then swabbed, often by hand, with an ink-repellant solution, which protects the image-free paper and allows only the ink to be taken up by the printed letters. The master is then placed on a chrome cylinder in the machine where it is kept constantly wet by another ink-repellant liquid. These solutions may contain nickel but it is not essential and is only used in the formulation by some manufacturers. After use the machine is cleaned with a solvent called a blanket wash. The operatives may or may not wear gloves.

Six women and one man have been seen with hand eczema due to the nickel in the ink-repellant solutions; all the patients had used one particular make of machine and did the work as a full-time job, so that they had daily contact with the solutions.

Five were young women aged 17–24 years; the sixth woman was 50 years old and the man 40 years of age. The eczema began at varying times: in three patients it was 2, 6 and 18 months respectively after starting work. The 50-year-old woman had used the machine for ten years without trouble, and then after a break of nine months returned to it, and within three months she developed hand eczema. One patient thought that the eczema and the job coincided and although the 17-year-old girl had had hand eczema before she began work, it subsequently deteriorated. This information was not recorded for one patient. The eczema usually affected the fingers first and then spread to the hands, and in one patient the arms were also affected. Five of the patients had involvement of other nickel sites; in three the hand eczema came first; and two had already been sensitised by nickel, in clothing or jewellery, by the time they started work. Of these two, one's hands remained clear for six months, while the other already had hand eczema which worsened when she began this job.

All the patients were patch tested with nickel sulphate 5 per cent or 2.5 per cent, and each reacted. One of the women was also sensitive to a thiuram from rubber gloves.

Four patients changed their jobs and their hands healed or greatly improved; one then returned to the work and her hand eczema relapsed. Three patients were not followed up.

Miscellaneous occupations
The jobs of six other women with an occupational hand eczema due to nickel were as follows:

1. Sewing covers on to the metal frames of umbrellas.
2. Making paint brushes during which the patient pushed bristle heads into metal clips.
3. Working in a shoe factory manually inserting metal eyelets into leather.
4. A bus conductress handling coins.
5. Making electric meters.
6. Handling bakery trays and baskets.

A bizarre dermatitis, hardly classifiable as occupational, was that of a 23-year-old dancer who had been sensitised by nickel in jewellery five years previously. During her dancing she had to wear a metal brassière, necklaces and bracelets, and she developed a dermatitis from all of them.

Hairdressers
During the quinquennium 1972–1976, 38 hairdressers were seen with hand eczema who were sensitive to nickel. However, the role of nickel in the aetiology of the hand eczema, in these predominantly young girls, is not clear.

Patch testing
Nickel sulphate is the salt used for patch testing and the most suitable diluent is petrolatum.

Nickel salts are irritant, particularly to the pores of sweat ducts; a 5 per cent concentration is a mild irritant, but 2.5 per cent is practically non-irritant.

St John's
The efficacy of patch testing with 5 per cent and 2.5 per cent nickel sulphate in petrolatum was evaluated by applying them concurrently to two series of routine patients, first in 1968 and again in 1973. In the first group there were 75 nickel-sensitive patients and in the second group 64 nickel-sensitive patients. In both series the weaker concentration failed to detect 20 per cent of those sensitised (Table 7.30). In the two groups a few patients (8/139, 6 per cent) had positive tests to the 2.5 per cent and were negative to the 5 per cent concentration. This anomalous result was probably due either to a fault in the technique or to greater pressure or occlusion of the weaker patch test. In none of these patients was the 5 per cent concentration re-applied (Cronin, 1975).

Table 7.30. Results of patch testing with 5 per cent and 2.5 per cent nickel sulphate in petrolatum (St John's 1968 and 1973).

Year	Total +ve Ni	Positive 5% only	Positive 5% and 2.5%	Negative 5%	Negative 2.5%
1968	75	71	56	4	15 (20%)
1973	64	60	47	4	13 (20%)
Total	139	131	103	8	28 (20%)

Conclusion

The most suitable concentration for routine patch testing is:

5 per cent nickel sulphate in petrolatum.

This concentration is a mild irritant in some patients: a purely poral or follicular reaction should be checked by repeating the 5 per cent test, applying 2.5 per cent and checking the history. Reactions to 5 per cent are rarely severe and do not preclude its use.

The non-specific pressure effect makes patch testing with coins and other metal objects unreliable and it should be avoided.

Pustular patch tests to nickel

Nearly 50 years ago it was observed that the salts of heavy metals gave pustular patch test reactions particularly in atopics (Steiner, 1929). This was confirmed in the 1940s and it was emphasised that nickel sulphate produces this effect (Sulzberger and Goodman, 1936; Sulzberger, 1940). In London in 1955, 50 atopics were patch tested with four metal salts and they gave a higher incidence of 'follicular' or irritant responses than did subjects with discoid eczema or controls. Nickel sulphate 5 per cent in water was used for testing and produced a strong pustular reaction in one atopic who subsequently had a negative test to a 2.5 per cent dilution (Wilson, 1955). This reaction of atopics was studied more recently by Uehara, Takahashi and Ofuji (1975) and they found that 5 per cent nickel sulphate elicited pustular patch test reactions when applied to dermatitic or traumatised skin but not if applied to the normal skin of these patients. They concluded that the effect was irritant.

Positive patch test and negative history

It is not infrequent for a patient with a positive nickel patch test to give and maintain, despite detailed questioning, a completely negative history of nickel dermatitis from jewellery, clothing or other obvious source. This may be explained by sensitisation occurring without further challenge or by the dermatitis being so mild as to have been unnoticed or forgotten by the patient, or again the level of sensitivity may be so low that dermatitis is not elicited by the usual nickel contacts. Another possibility is the failure of the physician to recognise the patient's existing eczema as a nickel dermatitis.

St John's

Information on this point has not always been recorded in the notes, but from those in which it was given it can be estimated that between 1967 and 1971 the incidence of nickel sensitive women in whom no source for the allergy could be traced was 11 per cent and in the next period 1972–1976 it was 5 per cent (Table 7.31). Comparable figures for the men were 29 per cent and 14 per cent (Table 7.32). The reduced incidences in the second period probably reflect the greater number of patients who attended the clinic with obvious nickel dermatitis and more careful history taking.

Table 7.31. Incidence of women with a positive patch test to nickel and a negative history (St John's 1967–1976).

	Total + Ni	Source found	Source not found	No. Inform.
1967–1971	546	441	59 (11%)	45
1972–1976	775	719	41 (5%)	15

Table 7.32. Incidence of men with a positive patch test to nickel and a negative history (St John's 1967–1976).

	Total + Ni	Source found	Source not found	No. Inform.
1967–1971	67	33	18 (29%)	16
1972–1976	118	83	16 (14%)	19

In vitro tests for nickel sensitivity

Laboratory techniques have been used in an attempt to devise a reliable *in vitro* test for the diagnosis of nickel sensitivity but reports of the success of these methods have varied.

In 1962, Aspern and Rorsman added dilutions of nickel to cultures of lymphocytes from normal and nickel-sensitive subjects, but there was no inhibition of mitoses in the cell cultures from the nickel sensitive patients.

The lymphocyte transformation test was used initially by Grosfeld *et al.* (1966) with equivocal results and then by Pappas, Orfanos and Bertram (1970) who concluded that the effects obtained were non-specific. However, success with this method was reported by Macleod, Hutchinson and Raffle (1970) who observed a significantly increased thymidine uptake in all cultures from seven of twelve nickel sensitive subjects; the failure of uptake in five was attributed to the toxic effect of the nickel on the cells. They reported later an increased thymidine uptake ratio (TUR) in six of eight nickel sensitive patients (Hutchinson, Raffle and Macleod, 1972). Similar good results have been obtained with this test by Millikan, Conway and Foote (1973), Gimenez-Camarasa *et al.* (1975) and Svejgaard *et al.* (1978). The TUR has been found to be decreased in atopic, compared with non-atopic, nickel-sensitive subjects (Kim and Schöpf, 1976). To elucidate the nature of the protein-nickel conjugates which effect this transformation autoradiographic studies were carried out on the cell cultures using [63]Ni. These showed that 20 per cent of the lymphocytes bound the nickel salts to their cell surfaces, but this was not the stimulating factor as the proportion of bound cells was the same from both sensitised and control subjects (Hutchinson, Mcleod and Raffle, 1975).

The leucocyte migration inhibition test has been used, but reports of the results conflict. The method was found ineffective, with nickel salts as the antigen, by Macleod, Hutchinson and Raffle (1976) but by using nickel protein complexes significant inhibition of leucocyte migration was obtained by Mirza *et al*. (1975) and Thulin (1976).

Leucocyte aggregation was studied by Macleod, Hutchinson and Raffle (1976). They observed that the number of aggregates was increased when nickel sulphate was added to blood from nickel-sensitive donors as compared with blood from controls.

Dermal sensitivity

The possibility of distinct epidermal and dermal types of sensitivity was postulated in 1956, on the basis that some clinical and patch test reactions appeared to be predominantly epidermal and others to be dermal. This dual allergy was reported for both drugs and metals and particularly for nickel (Epstein, 1956: Epstein 1962a). The characteristics of dermal sensitivity were given as:

1. The clinical appearances are those of a papular eruption rather than a vesicular eczema.
2. Patch tests with nickel are either papular or negative.
3. Intradermal tests with nickel sulphate (1/10 000) give a delayed reaction which can be persistent.
4. Histologically the infiltrate is in the dermis with little or no involvement of the epidermis (Epstein, 1962b).

This concept of a dual sensitivity is not generally accepted (Rostenberg, 1962).

Treatment

The best treatment for nickel dermatitis is to avoid contact with the metal, but, although this is quite practicable for jewellery, it may be difficult to discard every piece of metal. Direct skin contact can be prevented by covering or backing the metal with material, or painting, varnishing or covering it with plastic. A clear liquid polyurethane plastic material painted on to a cleaned, polished, slightly abraded metal was found to be effective as long as the coating remained intact over the metal without peeling off (Moseley and Allen, 1971).

Spraying both the skin and a metal-plated object with a steroid aerosol before contact has also prevented dermatitis (Fisher, 1964).

The dimethylglyoxime (DMG) spot test for nickel

This test detects nickel to a concentration of 1 in 100 000. It is performed by adding:

1. One drop of a 1 per cent alcoholic solution of dimethylglyoxime
2. One drop of a 10 per cent ammonium hydroxide solution

to the suspected material or to a metal surface. If the solution turns pink or red the test is positive. If the metal surface is irregular, the test solutions may be applied to cotton wool which is then rubbed over the suspected metal (Fisher, 1977). This is a useful method for detecting nickel in cracks and crevices.

It has been stressed by Fisher (1972) that the nickel in stainless steel does not give a positive dimethylglyoxime test. This is because the metal does not dissociate from the alloy, and so is not available either to give a positive DMG test or to produce dermatitis. Although generally true, stainless steel has been shown to release nickel and to cause dermatitis (p. 350).

ALLERGY TO NICKEL, CHROMATE AND COBALT

It is not uncommon for patients to be sensitive to more than one of the metals nickel, chromate or cobalt. These combined allergies arise not as cross-reactions, but because exposure to these metals occurs from the same sources (Fregert and Rorsman, 1966).

Both a series from Lund (Fregert and Rorsman, 1966) and the patients seen at St John's illustrate that these combined allergies fall into definite patterns which are relatively frequent or very infrequent.

Frequent associations
  (i) Nickel and cobalt in women from electroplated jewellery and metal on clothing.
 (ii) Chromate and cobalt in men from occupational sources such as cement, which contains traces of both these metals.

Infrequent associations
  (i) Chromate and nickel. It has been shown that the nickel oxide in cement is insoluble and therefore non-sensitising, so that a combined sensitivity to nickel and chromate does not relate to cement (Fregert and Gruvberger, 1972).
 (ii) Association of sensitivity to nickel, chromate and cobalt is not common in either sex.

In 1966 a report was published from Lund (Fregert and Rorsman, 1966) on the investigation of a series of 277 women and 261 men demonstrating the co-existence of sensitivity to these metals. The patients were patch tested with aqueous solutions of nickel sulphate 5.25 per cent, cobalt chloride 2.38 per cent and potassium dichromate 0.44 per cent. The results are tabulated below and are compared with the results in patients seen at St John's during the four years 1973–1976 (Table 7.33).

St John's
   From 1973 to 1976, 714 women and 303 men have been seen with sensitivity to one or more of these metals. The patients were tested with nickel sulphate 2.5–5 per cent, cobalt chloride 1 per cent and potassium dichromate 0.5 per cent, each diluted in vaseline. The number of women is more than double the number of men because in this clinic nickel sensitivity in women is more than twice as common as chromate allergy in men.
   The results from London and Lund show similar trends in the incidences of combined sensitivity; they are dissimilar in the higher incidences of nickel sensitivity in male and female patients seen at St John's but the gap of 10 years between the investigation of the two series may partly explain this disparity.

Table 7.33. Allergy to nickel, chromium and cobalt alone or combined in Lund (Fregert and Rorsman, 1966) and St John's (1973–1976).

	F				M			
	Lund		St John's		Lund		St John's	
	No	%	No	%	No	%	No	%
Ni only	89	32	409	57	8	3	65	22
Cr only	35	13	47	7	146	56	143	47
Cob only	14	5	18	2.5	12	4.5	19	6
Ni Cob	103	37	205	29	12	4.5	16	5
Cr Cob	13	5	7	1	46	18	38	13
Cr Ni	5	2	9	1	10	4	10	3
Cr Ni Cob	18	6	19	2.5	27	10	12	4
Total Patients	277	100	714	100	261	100	303	100

Palladium

Palladium is the cheapest and lightest of the platinum group of metals; it is less resistant to corrosion than is platinum. It is used as a catalyst in jewellery, in dental alloys and in telecommunication systems.

Sensitisation
One definite case of sensitivity has been reported. A research chemist, after working with precious metals for 6 months, developed eczema on his hands, arms and face, which improved when he was away from work. When patch tested with all the metals he used, he reacted to nickel-free sodium palladium dichloride 1 per cent and 0.1 per cent, and to nickel sulphate 1 per cent and 0.1 per cent. He did not react to platinum or to other metals of the group. He continued his work but avoided palladium and nickel, and his skin healed (Murno-Ashman, Munro and Hughes, 1969).

A patient who had possibly been sensitised to platinum by a ring also reacted on patch testing with a palladium ring, but she was not tested with a palladium salt (Sheard, 1955).

Patch-testing
The patient described reacted to sodium palladium dichloride 1 per cent and 0.1 per cent (? diluent).

Platinum

Platinum is a grey-white, ductile metal which is softer than silver; it is found as grains or nuggets in alluvial deposits in Alaska, Colombia and Russia and in nickel and copper ores in Canada, South Africa and Russia. It is hardened when alloyed with copper, silver or other metals of the platinum group, which includes palladium, iridium, osmium, rhodium and ruthenium (Browning, 1969).

Properties and uses

Platinum usually has a valency of 2 or 4, and it readily forms complex salts; it resists corrosion even better than gold. It has many industrial uses, including the following:

(i) For electrical and similar equipment
(ii) In the chemical industry, particularly as a catalyst
(iii) In the manufacture of glass and ceramics
(iv) For electroplating
(v) In jewellery
(vi) For sensitised paper used in photography.

Sensitising potential

Complex platinum salts seem to be potent allergens in the platinum refining industry. Metallic platinum is almost non-sensitising.

Causes of sensitivity

All reported cases of sensitivity, except one, have been due to industrial exposure, and they showed both immediate- and delayed-type hypersensitivity. The exception is a patient who was sensitised by a platinum ring (Sheard, 1955).

Metallic platinum

Ring

One patient has been reported. A woman, after being married for 7 years, developed dermatitis on her right and left ring fingers on which she had worn her wedding and engagement rings. The rings were cleaned; she wore them again and had a severe exacerbation. She was then patch tested and reacted to her wedding ring (palladium 90 per cent, ruthenium 10 per cent), her engagement ring (platinum 90 per cent, iridium 10 per cent), a commercial grade of pure platinum and a specimen of 90 per cent platinum with 10 per cent iridium. She did not react to a rhodium ring. Her rings were then heavily plated with rhodium and although she wore them for 5 weeks without trouble the eczema then recurred (Sheard, 1955).

The clinical description of this patient suggests a sensitivity to this group of metals, but patch testing with pieces of metal is inconclusive as false positive responses may be produced by pressure alone.

Platinum salts — occupational

Sensitivity seems to be reported only from inhalation or contact with chloroplatinic acid or its complex soluble salts — sodium and ammonium chloroplatinates, ammonium hexachloroplatinate and ammonium tetrachloroplatinate. The handling of metallic platinum is harmless.

Platinum refinery works

The hazard from complex platinum salts occurs predominantly in refinery workers among whom a high incidence of sensitivity has been reported. Four English refineries were investigated in 1945 and it was found that, of 91 men exposed to chloroplatinate salts, 52 (57 per cent) had asthma and 13 (14 per cent) had dermatitis. The greatest risk was from the salts in a dry dusty form but there was also some hazard from the wet processes causing droplets in the atmosphere (Hunter, Milton and Perry, 1945). A platinum refinery and laboratory in Pennsylvania were studied by Roberts (1951) for 5 years, and he reported that of thcir 21 employees, 60 per cent had definite symptoms and 40 per cent had minor symptoms. In 1969, a study from France of 51 refinery workers reported major symptoms in half and minor symptoms in one fifth of the employees (Parrot et al., 1969). The same high incidence of sensitisation causing eczema, urticaria, rhinitis and asthma has been reported from a refinery in Prague, where 28 of the 30 employees were sensitised to platinum and 6 to rhodium (Jirásek and Kalenský, 1975).

Clinical features
The latent period for sensitisation varied from months to years; in some the sensitivity was so acute that even the slightest exposure, such as just entering the workshop or meeting men from the refinery, caused a relapse.

The symptoms have been called platinosis (Roberts, 1951) and involve either the respiratory system or the skin or both. The discomfort may be mild or the symptoms severe and disabling.

Respiratory tract and eyes. Those affected develop sneezing, coryza and a burning, itching discomfort of the eyes with lacrimation and conjunctivitis. They may have a dry cough, tightness of the chest, shortness of breath, wheezing and asthma, which can be very severe.

Skin. The changes described are those of eczema, pruritus and urticaria. The clinical pattern is very variable. The eczema affects the exposed sites, principally the wrists, forearms, antecubital fossae and hands and there may be a further spread to the face and neck. The thigh has been involved from a contaminated pocket (Parrot et al., 1969). Some patients complain of generalised pruritus but have no visible skin lesions (Poole, 1974).

Patients also develop urticaria, which can be severe.

The condition of those sensitised tends to become progressively worse, forcing them to transfer to another department or to change their jobs completely. Once exposure ceases the symptoms practically always disappear, although persistent asthma has been reported in one man (Parrot et al., 1969).

St John's
In 1968, a man aged 38 years, after working in a platinum refinery for 6 months, developed asthma and urticaria which continued despite his leaving the firm. A year later, bronchial inhalation tests provoked asthma and urticaria. His symptoms persisted, and when seen in 1973 he had chronic hand eczema. It was then impossible to be certain if there was any relationship between his present eczema and his original platinum eruption. Patch testing with ammonium tetrachloroplatinate in water elicited a reaction at 1 per cent but not at 0.25 per cent. He also reacted to ammonium hexachloroplatinate 0.1 per cent in water. In addition he reacted to balsam of Peru 25 per cent and to potassium dichromate 0.5 per cent.

Laboratory workers

Two cases, both men, have been described. One, from South Africa, had for 1 year been preparing a platinum catalyst, during which he evaporated chloroplatinic acid. Initially he developed coryza, lacrimation and asthma, and 3 months later a contaminated handkerchief evoked an irritant dermatitis on one thigh. This was followed 2 weeks later by a more widespread eczema (Marshall, 1952). The second patient, seen at St John's, was an analytical chemist who used ammonium hexachloroplatinate in assaying the purity of platinum. For 7 years, exposure to hexachloroplatinate or tetrachloroplatinate salts had caused respiratory symptoms which often necessitated his taking time off work, and on contact with the skin, they produced weals within a few minutes (Levene and Calnan, 1971).

Photography

Perhaps the first series of cases reported was in 1911 from Chicago, where the workers in 40 photographic studios were examined and 8 were found to have respiratory and skin symptoms from handling a paper containing potassium chloroplatinite (Karasek and Karasek, 1911).

Other reports

A report from France in 1965 described the same respiratory and cutaneous symptoms in men working with chloroplatinic acid in the precious metal industry (Sidi and Hincky, 1965). The allergy was so acute in some that merely the presence of overalls from the workshop was sufficient to precipitate an eruption on the face and eyelids.

Skin testing

Immediate-type hypersensitivity

The concentrations of allergen and the techniques for prick, nasal and inhalation tests with complex platinum salts have been described by Pickering (1972).

Patch testing

Platinum chloride 1 per cent aqueous (Fregert and Hjorth, 1972).
Chloroplatinic acid 1 per cent was used by Marshall (1952) and his patient developed a bullous reaction.
Ammonium tetrachloroplatinate 0.25 per cent and 1.0 per cent in water $\left.\begin{array}{l} \\ \\ \end{array}\right\}$ St John's.
Ammonium hexachloroplatinate 0.1 per cent in water

Hyposensitisation

Hyposensitisation by repeated intradermal injections of increasing strengths of sodium chloroplatinate was effective in a woman with dermatitis. The hyposensitivity was maintained by weekly injections of 0.05 ml of 1×10^{-8} sodium chloroplatinate; after 2 years, scratch testing, which had initially been positive with a 1×10^{-8} dilution, became positive only at 1×10^{-4}. After the injections were stopped, she remained well and continued to work during the subsequent

3 years. This treatment was recommended only for exceptional cases (Roberts, 1951).

A laboratory worker with respiratory symptoms and urticaria was similarly hyposensitised by intradermal injections of ammonium hexachloroplatinate but, during the course, he developed symptoms of serum sickness. Although he was able to work with ammonium hexachloroplatinate, contact with ammonium tetrachloroplatinate still produced sneezing, lacrimation and urticaria (Levene and Calnan, 1971).

Platinum salts cause histamine release
It has been shown in the guinea-pig that platinum salts also act as histamine-releasing agents (Roberts, 1951).

Selenium

Selenium is a semi-metal found in rocks and soils throughout the world, but there are no true deposits. It is obtained as a by-product from the copper refining industries of Canada and Rhodesia.

Properties and uses
Chemically selenium is similar to sulphur. Its principal use is in the electrical and electronics industry for making rectifiers which convert alternating to direct current. The glass industry uses it to remove the green tinge from inferior glass and to make red glass. It is also used as a pigment in orange and red paints, to assist the vulcanisation of rubber, as a corrosion inhibitor, as a catalyst and in some insecticides.

Toxicity and dermatitis
Compounds of selenium are severe irritants, and they are readily absorbed through the lungs, gastro-intestinal tract and damaged skin. The most characteristic sign of absorption is the smell of garlic from the breath. Selenium dioxide, which is important in industry, is a light powder, which dissolves in water or sweat to form noxious selenious acid. Inhaled, selenium dioxide causes pulmonary oedema, in the eyes conjunctivitis, and on the exposed skin burns or dermatitis. If it penetrates under the nails, the nail beds become extremely painful (Glover, 1954).

In a selenium refinery plant, 11 employees developed dermatitis, conjunctivitis and inflammation of the upper respiratory tract. Investigation showed no evidence of sensitisation and it was concluded that all the effects were due to irritation (Jirásek and Kalensky, 1975).

Silica

Silica granulomas are a non-allergic foreign body epithelioid reaction to silica in the colloidal form (Shelley and Hurley, 1960).

Direct sensitisation to a silicon compound has not been reported, but 4 patients sensitised to 2,2-bis(4-hydroxyphenyl) propane (Bisphenol A) cross-reacted to dimethyldi(4-hydroxyphenyl) silane (Fregert and Rorsman, 1961).

Silver

Silver is a white, shining, malleable metal with a high electrical and thermal conductivity. Its ores are found in Mexico and in parts of North and South America; it occurs in plant humus and is present in wheat flour, bran and mushrooms (Browning, 1969).

Properties and uses
The softness of silver is counteracted by alloying it with other metals: it then has a variety of industrial applications. Sterling silver contains at least 92.5 per cent pure silver and 7.5 per cent alloy, usually copper.

Silver jewellery
Silver jewellery or wire is usually made of a silver-copper alloy; small amounts of zinc and cadmium may be added to give special properties.

In silver-plated jewellery the base metal is a nickel-copper alloy.

Incidences of sensitivity
Allergy to silver is now most rare but in the 1940s, when silver nitrate was a popular remedy, patients were sometimes sensitised. At the Finsen Institute in 1948, the incidence was about 0.3 per cent of all patients tested; since then, the numbers have gradually decreased, and none was seen in 1953 (Marcussen, 1962).

Causes of sensitivity

Silver Alloys

Coins
In 1954, after working as a postmaster for 10 months, a man aged 55 years developed a dry, scaly fissured eczema on his finger tips and left palm. These sites corresponded with those used to handle coins. A patch test with silver nitrate 1 per cent evoked a vesicular response, and pure silver caused erythema (Gaul, 1954).

Silver salts

Silver nitrate
In 1948, Gaul and Underwood described a man who developed a vesicular reaction to the 10 per cent silver nitrate used for marking patch tests. He recalled having applied in the past a solution of silver nitrate to an area of eczema on his heel and having to stop it after 2 weeks because the eczema suddenly worsened and spread. On patch testing he reacted to 5 per cent and 10 per cent aged

silver nitrate but not to 10 per cent fresh silver nitrate; a test with silver foil was positive but with silver chloride powder was negative.

Silver nitrate is kept in an amber bottle because on exposure to air and light it decomposes, forming small amounts of nitric acid, silver nitrite and colloidal silver, which liberates silver ions. The ionised silver was thought to be the sensitiser in this patient and explained the discrepancy between the results of testing with old and with fresh solutions.

In the 1940s, silver nitrate, used therapeutically, occasionally sensitised (Marcussen, 1962).

A silver chloride complex
A radiographer, who processed films by hand, developed a papular eczema under her watch strap. Patch tests were positive to 1 per cent silver chloride complexed with sodium thiosulphate, to 1 per cent silver nitrate and to the fixing fluid. Although silver chloride is very insoluble, it was suggested that in the fixing tank, it formed a soluble complex with sodium thiosulphate and that this contaminated the patient's wristwatch strap. Ionic silver was postulated as the sensitiser (Marks, 1966).

Patch testing
Silver nitrate 1 per cent in water is probably reliable.

Immediate-type hypersensitivity
Argyrol is a colloidal solution of silver or silver oxide in alkaline proteins. Immediate-type hypersensitivity has been reported following its use in the nose and as a pharyngeal spray; scratch testing with 1 per cent argyrol was positive and intradermal testing gave a severe local reaction and constitutional symptoms (Criep, 1943).

Tellurium

Tellurium is used in the vulcanisation of rubber, in alloys, as a colour for glass, as a catalyst and in a diagnostic test for diphtheria.

Posioning in two research workers was reported by Blackadder and Manderson (1975); both had the characteristic smell of sour garlic in their breath, sweat and urine. An unusual feature was a bluish-black discolouration of the skin in streaks on the face and neck and in patches in the finger webs. This was thought to be due to the absorption of tellurium esters through the skin and the deposition of tellurium in the dermis and subcutaneous tissues. They recovered without treatment.

Uranium

Two men preparing uranium for an atomic energy plant developed hand eczema. They were patch tested with 2 per cent sodium and calcium salts of uranium, to which they reacted (Thiers et al., 1961).

Zinc

Zinc oxide — irritant
Workers handling zinc oxide powder may develop so-called zinc pox: these acne-like lesions are caused by follicular occlusion and occur in moist areas such as the axillae and groins (Schwartz, Tulipan and Birmingham, 1957).

Metal fume fever
Metal is galvanised by dipping it into molten zinc at a temperature of 475°C. During subsequent welding some of the surface zinc is vaporised and if the fine metal particles are inhaled into the lungs then galvaniser's poisoning or welder's ague ensues. The illness, which lasts one to two days, begins with nausea, thirst, headache and pains in the limbs and this phase is followed by malaria-like shivering and fever. Symptoms occur with an air concentration of 5–10 mg Zn/m^3 and during the welding of galvanised metal the air level may rise to 100 mg Zn/m^3. Adequate ventilation and airline masks prevent the condition (Calnan, 1979).

Sensitisation
One possible case of sensitivity has been reported. A telephone engineer who worked with zinc and copper developed inflammation under a zinc ointment dressing. Patch tests with a piece of metallic zinc and with zinc sulphate 1 per cent were positive; he reacted to metallic copper strongly and also to 0.01 per cent copper sulphate. Contamination of the zinc by copper was not completely excluded (Meer, 1957).

Zirconium

Zirconium is a non-toxic metal and has never caused systemic disease; it has been used surgically in clips, plates and screws without trouble. Occasionally it causes cutaneous granulomas.

Properties and uses
Zirconium is used in nuclear reactors, in the steel industry as an alloy, in radio valves, in photographic flash bulbs and as a lining for electric furnaces and crucibles. Basic zirconium salts tan leather well but are expensive.

Sensitising potential
In guinea-pigs, the intradermal injection of zirconium carbonate induced no measurable granuloma formation and though zirconium aluminium glycine complex produced a granuloma it was as a consequence of damage to collagen (Turk and Parker, 1977 i). Sensitisation was effected with sodium zirconium lactate (Turk and Parker, 1977 ii) and an ultrastructural study confirmed the presence of epithelioid cells and giant cells similar to those found in zirconium granulomas in man (Turk and Parker, 1978). In man the sensitising potential of zirconium is very low (Shelley and Hurley, 1958).

Causes of sensitivity
Applied topically, zirconium may sensitise and produce localised skin granulomas. This has occurred with deodorant sticks containing soluble sodium zirconium lactate and from preparations containing insoluble zirconium oxide which are used to treat poison ivy dermatitis. The number of cases reported is relatively small, as these deodorant sticks were used by millions of people without causing harm (Shelley and Hurley, 1958).

Clinical features

Deodorant granulomas
The water-soluble salt, sodium zirconium lactate, acts as a deodorant by combining with offensive fatty acids and possibly by having anti-bacterial properties; it reduces sweating by poral occlusion. It was first added as the active ingredient to deodorant sticks in 1955 in the U.S.A.

By 1958, there had been reports of 70 cases with a chronic papular eruption, confined to the axillae, sometimes itchy but usually without epidermal change. Habitual shaving, which caused small cuts, and the irritancy of the zirconium combined to facilitate its penetration; and although the majority had used the deodorant stick for many months before the granulomas first appeared, in a few they followed the first application. Spontaneous involution usually occurred within months but could take 2 years. The histology was of an epithelioid granuloma (Shelley and Hurley, 1958).

To study the formation of these granulomas, 30 male volunteers rubbed a 5 per cent zirconium stick onto one shaved axilla for 5 minutes every day for 8 weeks. One man was sensitised and at 4 weeks developed numerous axillary papules, some of which were in the line of scratch marks. The histology at 10 weeks was a typical epithelioid granuloma. The papules involuted slowly and had almost disappeared by 5 months. Three men developed a transient irritant dermatitis. A further 20 men applied 0.5 per cent and 10 per cent zirconium sticks; irritation was more frequent with the 10 per cent stick which caused a papular eruption in 4 men but in only one was this granulomatous.

Patch tests with the zirconium deodorant were negative in the 2 sensitised men and in 20 controls. Intradermal tests with sodium zirconium lactate 0.02 ml were positive in the 2 sensitised men; both reacted to 1/100 and 1/1000 and one to 1/10 000. A very sensitive subject reacted to $0.2 \mu g$. Controls were negative (Shelley and Hurley, 1958).

Topical preparations for poison ivy dermatitis. The rationale for using zirconium oxide to treat poison ivy dermatitis is based on *in vitro* evidence that it absorbs the *Rhus* allergens (Blumenthal, 1953); clinically, however, it has been found to be ineffective (Epstein and Allen, 1964). Despite this, preparations containing insoluble zirconium oxide are marketed in the U.S.A. and are bought and used by many for the prophylaxis and treatment of poison ivy dermatitis. Eczematous skin is permeable to this insoluble compound.

The first report of a patient with allergic granulomas was that of Williams and Skipworth (1959) since when occasional cases have been reported. One patient was sensitised by an ointment containing 4 per cent zirconium oxide (Baler, 1965) and 2 others by a 2 per cent suspension (Epstein and Allen 1964; Lopresti and Hambrick, 1965). About 6 weeks to a few months after the application, red-brown papules appear at the sites of previous dermatitis, usually on the face, neck and arms. The lesions can be suppressed by local or systemic steroids but reform and are very persistent; they may last for 18 months or longer. The insolubility of the zirconium oxide, which has been found in a nodule present for 18 months (Baler, 1965), explains their chronicity. The histology of the lesions is an epithelioid granuloma. Abraded tests or intradermal tests produce granulomas in a few weeks.

Patch testing
Patch testing on normal skin is negative. Testing on traumatised skin produces in about 4 weeks papules which histologically are epithelioid granulomas.

Zirconium oxide 2 per cent and 4 per cent in a lotion or ointment base on abraded skin have been effective (William and Skipworth, 1959; Baler, 1965; LoPresti and Hambrick, 1965). Zirconium lactate 1 per cent has been applied to skin denuded of epidermis (Epstein and Allen, 1964).

Intradermal testing
In all subjects, concentrations of zirconium salts higher than 1/1000 produce visible foreign body reactions; in controls these regress but in those sensitised they progress to form epithelioid granulomas. Zirconium is found in the macrophages of the foreign body reaction but not in the epithelioid cells of the allergic response (Epstein, Skahen, Krasnobrod, 1962).

To avoid this non-specific effect, only dilutions of 1/1000 or greater should be used for testing.

Suitable concentrations are:

Sodium zirconium lactate 1/1000, 1/10 000, aqueous (Shelley and Hurley, 1959).

References

Adams, R.M., Fregert, S., Gruvberger, B. & Maibach, H.I. (1976) Water solubility of zinc chromate primer paints used as antirust agents. *Contact Dermatitis*, **2**, 357.
Agrup, G. (1969) Hand eczema. *Acta Dermato-venereologica*, Vol. 49, Suppl. 61, p. 44.
Alexander, W. & Street, A. (1965) Metals in the Service of Man. 4th ed. pp. 123, 159, 162 Harmondsworth: Penguin.
Amphoux, M., Poli, J.P. & Robin, J. (1973) Bilan des travaux récents sur les dermatoses professionnelles dans l'industrie du batiment et des travaux publies. *Archives des Maladies Professionnelles de Médicine du Travail et de Sécurité Sociale*, **34**, 238.
Amphoux, M & Robin, J. (1975) Doppleblindversuch mit einer Schutzsalbe (Invosin) an den Handen von Zementarbeitern. *Berufsdermatosen*, **23**, 214.
Anderson, F.E. (1960) Cement and oil dermatitis. The part played by chromate sensitivity. *British Journal of Dermatology*, **72**, 108.
Aspegren, N. & Rorsman, H. (1962) Short-term culture of leucocytes in nickel hypersensitivity. *Acta Dermato-venereologica*, **42**, 412.
Ayala, F. (1976) Granuloma fissurato dell 'orecchio associato a dermatite da contatto da nichel. *Giornale Italiano di Dermatologia Minerva Dermatologica*, **111**, 581.

Baer, R. (1973) Allergic contact sensitisation to iron. *Journal of Allergy and Clinical Immunology*, 51, 35.

Baer, R.L., Lipkin, G., Kanof, N.B. & Biondi, E. (1964) Changing pattern's of sensitivity to common contact allergens. *Archives of Dermatology*, 89, 3.

Baer, R.L., Ramsey, D.L. & Biondi, E. (1973) The most common contact allergens. *Archives of Dermatology*, 108, 74.

Baler, G.R. (1965) Granulomas from topical zirconium in poison ivy dermatitis. *Archives of Dermatology*, 91, 145.

Bandmann, H.J. & Agathos, M. (1977) Toxische ulcerose Kontaktdermatitis durch vorgefertigten Beton (cement burns). *Berufsdermatosen*, 25, 108.

Bandmann, H.-J. & Fuchs, G. (1963) Uber die Kobaltkontaktallergie, ihre Beziehung zur Bichromat und Nickelkontaktallergie, sowie ihre gewerbedermatologische Bedetung. *Hautarzt*, 14, 207.

Bang Pedersen, N. (1977) Chromate in a food laboratory. *Contact Dermatitis*, 3, 105.

Bang Pedersen, N. (1977) Topical treatment of a 'ruster'. *British Journal of Dermatology*, 96, 332.

Bang Pedersen, N., Bertilsson, G., Fregert, S., Lidén, K. & Rorsman, H. (1968) Disappearance of chromium injected intracutaneously. *Archives of Allergy*, 36, 82.

Bang Pedersen, N. & Fregert, S. (1970) Primer on a leg prosthesis as a source of chromate. *Contact Dermatitis Newsletter*, 8, 191.

Bang Pedersen, N., Fregert, S., Brodelius, P. & Gruvberger, B. (1974) Release of nickel from silver coins. *Acta Dermato-venereologica*, 54, 231.

Bang Pedersen, N., Fregert, S., Naversten, Y. & Rorsman, H. (1970) Patch testing and absorption of chromium. *Acta Dermato-venereologica*, 50, 431.

Bang Pedersen, N. & Naversten, Y. (1973) Disappearance of chromium (III) trichloride injected intracutaneously. *Acta Dermato-venereologica*, 53, 127.

Barranco, V.P. (1972) Eczematous dermatitis caused by internal exposure to copper. *Archives of Dermatology*, 106, 386.

Barranco, V.P. & Soloman, H. (1972) Eczematous dermatitis from nickel. *Journal of the American Medical Association*, 220, 1244.

Barrière, H., Boiteau, H.-L., Géraut, C. & Métayer, C. (1979) Allergie aux détergents et allergie au nickel. *Annales de Dermatologie et de Venereologie*, 106, 33.

Bech, A.O. (1974) Hard metal disease and tool room grinding. *Journal of the Society of Occupational Medicine*, 24, 11.

Bech, A.O., Kipling, M.D. & Heather, J.C. (1962) Hard metal disease. *British Journal of Industrial Medicine*, 19, 239.

Bettley, F.R. (1971) Nickel coin dermatitis. *Contact Dermatitis Newsletter*, 9, 198.

Beurey, J., Barbier, J.-M., Pernot, Cl., & Weber, M. (1969) Enquete allergologique chez des sujets travaillant en cimenterie ou sur des chantiers. *Annals de Dermatologie et de Syphiligraphie*, 96, 481.

Biagini, R., Rivero, M., Salvador, M. & Cordoba, S. (1978) Hidroarsenicismo cronico y cancer de pulmon. *Archivos Argentinos de Dermatologia*, 28, 151.

Birmingham, D.J., Key, M.M., Holaday, D.A. & Perone, V.B. (1965) An outbreak of arsenical dermatoses in a mining community. *Archives of Dermatology*, 91, 457.

Black, H. (1972) *Contact Dermatitis Newsletter*, 12, 323.

Black, H. (1972) Dermatitis from nickel and copper in coins. *Contact Dermatitis Newsletter*, 12, 326.

Blackadder, E.S. & Manderson, W.G. (1975) Occupational absorption of tellurium: a report of two cases. *British Journal of Industrial Medicine*, 32, 59.

Bluementhal, W.B. (1953) Some properties of zirconium compounds significant to cosmetic technologist. *Journal of the Society of Cosmetic Chemists*, 4, 69.

Bockendahl, H. (1954) Chromnachweis und Chromgehalt gefärbter Kleiderstoffe. *Dermatologische Wochenschrift*, 130, 987.

Bockendahl, H., Remy, W. & Masuch, E. (1974) Untersuchungen zum Mechanismus des Kontaktekzens gegen Kupfer. *Archiv für Dermatologische Forschung*, 250, 167.

Bonnevie, P. (1939) Aetiologie und Pathogenese der Ekzemkrankheiten. Nyt Nordisk Forlag Arnold Busck Kopenhagen. p. 327.

Booth, R.P. (1971) Possible allergie skin reaction to nickel clips. *Medical Journal of Australia*, 2, 546.

Borelli, S. & Düngemann, H. (1964) Aktuelle Kontaktekzem-ursachen in der Metallindustrie. *Berufsdermatosen*, 12, 1.

Bourne, L.B. & Milner, F.J.M. (1963) Polyester resin hazards. *British Journal of Industrial Medicine*, 20, 100.

Bowyer, A. (1967) Epidermal reactions and prolonged dermal reactions to patch testing with gold salts. *Acta Dermato-venereologica*, 47, 9.

Breucker, G. & Höfs, W. (1966) Kobalthaltiges Futtermittel für Wiederkaüer als berufliches Ekzematogen. *Dermatologische Wochenschrift*, 152, 218.

Browning, E. (1969) *Toxicity of Industrial Metals.* 2nd ed., pp. 67, 119, 255, 256, 270, 296. London: Butterworths.

Brun, R.M. (1963) Contribution á l'étude des chromates du ciment. Nouvelle technique pour le tests epicutané au ciment. *Dermatologica*, **129**, 79.

Brun, R. (1979) Nickel in food: the role of stainless-steel utensils. *Contact Dermatitis*, 5, 43.

Buckley, W.R. & Lewis, C.E. (1960) The 'ruster' in Industry. *Journal of Occupational Medicine*, 2, 23.

Budden, M.G. & Wilkinson, D.S. (1978) Skin lesions and nail lesions from gold potassium cyanide. *Contact Dermatitis*, 4, 172.

Burrows, D. (1972) Prognosis in industrial dermatitis. *British Journal of Dermatology*, **87**, 145.

Burrows, D. (1978) Chromium and the skin. *British Journal of Dermatology*, **99**, 587.

Burrows, D. & Calnan, C.D. (1965) Cement dermatitis. II. Clinical aspects. *Transactions of the St John's Hospital Dermatological Society*, **51**, 27.

Burrows, D. & Calnan, C.D. (1965) Cement dermatitis. II Clinical aspects. *Transactions St John's Hospital Dermatological Society*, **51**, 27.

Burry, J.N., Kirk, J., Reid, J.G. & Turner, T. (1973) Environmental dermatitis: Patch test in 1000 cases of allergic contact dermatitis. *Medical Journal of Australia*, 2, 681.

Burton, J.L., Pye, R.J. & Brookes, D.B. (1976) Metal corrosion by chloride in sweat. *British Journal of Dermatology*, **95**, 417.

Calnan, C.D. (1956) Nickel dermatitis. *British Journal of Dermatology*, **68**, 229.

Calnan, C.D. (1960) Cement dermatitis. *Journal of Occupational Medicine*, 2, 15.

Calnan, C.D. (1962) Observations on dermatoses due to metals. Proceedings of the XII international congress of dermatology. p. 453. *Excerpta Medica Foundation*.

Calnan, C.D. (1967) Case report. *British Journal of Dermatology*, **79**, 60.

Calnan, C.D. (1978) Chromate in coolant water of gramophone record presses. *Contact Dermatitis*, **4**, 246.

Calnan, C.D. (1979) Metal Fume fever. *Contact Dermatitis*, 5, 125.

Calnan, C.D., Fregert, S. & Pirillä, V. (1969) Cement additives. *Contact Dermatitis Newsletter*, **6**, 112.

Calnan, C.D. & Harman, R.R.M. (1961) Studies in contact dermatitis. XIII Diesel coolant chromate dermatitis. *Transactions of the St John's Hospital Dermatological Society*, **46** 13.

Chenoweth, E. (1957) Contact dermatitis from 18-carat gold. *Medical Journal of Australia*, ii, 20.

Christensen, O.B. & Möller, H. (1975)i Nickel allergy and hand eczema. *Contact dermatitis*, 1, 129.

Christensen, O.B. & Möller, H. (1975)ii External and internal exposure to the antigen in the hand eczema of nickel allergy. *Contact Dermatitis*, 1, 136.

Christensen, O.B. & Möller, H. (1978) Release of nickel from cooking utensils. *Contact Dermatitis*, **4**, 343.

Clay, J.E., Dale, I. & Cross, J.D. (1977) Arsenic absorption in steel bronze workers. *Journal of the Society of Occupational Medicine*, **27**, 102.

Clendenning, W.E. (1971) Allergy to cobalt in metal denture as cause of hand dermatitis. *Contact Dermatitis Newsletter*, **10**, 225.

Cohen, S.R. (1974) A review of the health hazards from copper exposure. *Journal of Occupational Medicine*, **16**, 621.

Coleman, R.F., Herrington, J. & Scales, J.T. (1973) Concentration of wear products in hair, blood and urine after total hip replacement. *British Medical Journal*, i, 527.

Collins, K.J. (1957) The corrosion of metal by palmar sweat. *British Journal of Industrial Medicine*, **14**, 191.

Comaish, S. (1969) A case of contact hypersensitivity to metallic gold. *Archives of Dermatology*, **99**, 720.

Conde-Salazar Gomez, L. & Gomez Urcuyo, J.F. (1976) Sensibilidad a los componentes de la goma en obreros de la construcción. *Actas Dermo-Sifiliograficas*, **67**, 297.

Connor, B. (1972) Chromate dermatitis and paper manufacture. *Contact Dermatitis Newsletter*, **11**, 265.

Cooke, M.A. & Hocken Robertson, D.E. (1973) Gold sensitivity. *Contact Dermatitis Newsletter*, **13**, 382.

Cowan, M.A. (1960) Contact dermatitis due to gold. *British Journal of Dermatology*, **72**, 348.

Criep, L.H. (1943) Allergy to argyrol. *Journal of the American Medical Association*, **121**, 421.

Cronin, E. (1972) Clinical prediction of patch test results. *Transactions of the St. John's Hospital Dermatological Society*, **58**, 153.

Cronin, E. (1975) Patch testing with nickel. *Contact Dermatitis*, 1, 56.

Curtis, G.H. (1951) Cutaneous hypersensitivity due to beryllium. *Archives of Dermatology*, **64**, 470.

Czarnecki, N. (1979) Die Persistenz der Chromatallergie beim Zementekzem. *Hautarzt*, **30**, 80.

Czarnecki, N. & Fritsch, P. (1978) Kontaktallergie auf Blei. *Hautarzt*, **29**, 445.

Czernielewski, A., Libiszowski, T. & Dudek, H. (1977) Die Anwendung des Leukozyten-migrationshemmtestes (LMH) bei der Diagnostik der Chromatsensibilisierung. *Dermatologische Monatsschrift*, **163**, 399.

Degreef, H. & Roelandts, R. (1974) Arsenical intoxication due to pollution. *Archives Belges de Dermatologie*, **30**, 35.

DeNardi, J.M., van Ordstrand, H.S., Curtis, G.H. & Zielinski, J. (1953) Berylliosis. *Archives of Industrial Hygiene and Occupational Medicine*, **8**, 1.

Dhir, G.G., Rao, D.S. & Mehrotra, M.P. (1977) Contact dermatitis caused by copper sulphate used as colouring material in commercial alcohol. *Annals of Allergy*, **39**, 204.

Donaldson, R.M. & Barrcras, R.F. (1966) Intestinal absorption of trace quantities of chromium. *Journal of Laboratory and Clinical Medicine*, **68**, 484.

Dower, F.H., Hill, R.N. & Stevenson, C.J. (1973) Chromate dermatitis in colour television manufacture. *Contact Dermatitis Newsletter*, **14**, 395.

Düngemann, H., Borelli, S. & Wittman, J. (1972) Kupfer und Kadmium Kontaktekzeme bei schweissern, schleifern, galvaniseuren und ahnlichen Berufsgruppen. *Arbeitsmedizin, Sozialmedizin, Arbeitshygience*, **7**, 85.

Duperrat, B. & Lamberton, J.N. (1973) A propos des dermites du ciment peut-on prévoir l'avenir du cimentier allergique? *Archives des Maladies Professionnelles de Medicine du Travail et de Sécurité Sociale*, **34**, 242.

Eberhartinger, Chr., Ebner, H. & Klotz, L. (1969) Zur Kenntnis und Interpretation follikulärer, papulo-pustulöser Reaktionen im Epikutantest. *Berufsdermatosen*, **17**, 241.

Ebner, H. (1967) Chromatkontakt Allergie als Ursache von Bekleidungsekzemen. *Dermatologica*, **135**, 355.

Egyedi, K. & Pataky, E. (1978) Dermatologische Aspekte der Arsenintoxikation durch Trinkswasser. *Dermatosen in Beruf und Umwelt*, **26**, 54.

Einarsson, O., Kylin, B., Lindstedt, G. & Wahlberg, J.E. (1975) Chromium cobalt and nickel in used cutting fluids, *Contact Dermatitis*, **1**, 182.

Eisen, H.N. (1959) Cellular and Humoral Aspects of the Hypersensitive State. ed. Lawrence, H.S. p. 89, London: Cassell.

Elgart, M.L. & Higdon, R.S. (1971) Allergic contact dermatitis to gold. *Archives of Dermatology*, **103**, 649.

Elves, M.W. Wilson, J.N., Scales. J.T. & Kemp, H.B.S. (1975) Incidence of metal sensitivity in patients with total joint replacements. *British Medical Journal*, **1**, 376.

Engel, H.O. & Calnan, C.D. (1963) Chromate dermatitis from paint. *British Journal of Industrial Medicine*, **20**, 192.

Enterline, P.E. (1974) Respiratory cancer among chromate workers. *Journal of Occupational Medicine*, **16**, 523.

Epstein, S. (1956) Contact dermatitis due to nickel and chromate. *Archives of Dermatology*, **73**, 236.

Epstein, S. (1962a) Epidermal and dermal reactions in a case of sensitivity to nickel. *Journal of Investigative Dermatology*, **38**, 37.

Epstein, S. (1962b) Newer contact sensitisers in the home. Dermatoses due to environmental and physical factors. Ed. Rees, Rees B. p. 244 Springfield, Illinois: Thomas.

Epstein, W.L. & Allen, J.R. (1964) Granulomatous hypersensitivity after use of zirconium-containing poison oak lotions. *Journal of the American Medical Association*, **190**, 940.

Epstein, E., Rees, W.J. & Maibach, H.I. (1968) Recent experiences with routine patch test screening. *Archives of Dermatology*, **98**, 18.

Epstein, W.L., Skahen, J.R. & Krasnobrod, H. (1962) Granulomatous hypersensitivity to zirconium: Localization of allergen in tissue and its role in formation of epithelioid cells. *Journal of Investigative Dermatology*, **38**, 223.

Evans, S. (1977) Arsenic and cancer. *British Journal of Dermatology*. 97, Suppl. 15. p. 13.

Evans, M.E., Freeman, M.A.R., Miller, A.J. & Vernon Roberts, B. (1974) Metal sensitivity as a cause of bone necrosis and loosening of the prosthesis in total joint replacement. *Journal of Bone and Joint Surgery*, **56-B**, 626.

Felker, A. Ya., Gaster, E.I. & Pugina, E.G. (1974) The dynamics of occupational skin diseases in workers of the aktyubinsk chromium compounds plant. *Vestnik Dermatology*, **6**, 30.

Feuerman, E.J. (1969) Housewives eczema and the role of chromates. *Acta Dermato-venereologica*, **49**, 288.

Feuerman, E.J. (1971) Chromates as the cause of contact dermatitis in housewives. *Dermatologica*, **143**, 292.

Finn, O.A. (1974) Nickel sensitivity in infancy. *Contact Dermatitis Newsletter*, **16**, 512.

Fisher, A.A. (1953) Nonsurgical treatment of cutaneous beryllium granuloma. *Archives of Dermatology*, **68**, 214.

Fisher, A.A. (1964) Steroid aerosol spray in contact dermatitis. *Archives of Dermatology*, **89**, 841.

Fisher, A.A. (1972) Contact dermatitis: At home and abroad. *Cutis*, **10**, 719.

Fisher, A.A. (1972) Safety of stainless steel in nickel sensitivity. *Journal of the American Medical association*, **221**, 1279.

Fisher, A.A. (1973) *Contact Dermatitis*. 2nd ed. pp. 100, 102, 115 Philadelphia: Lea and Febiger.

Fisher A.A. (1974) Ear piercing hazard of nickel-gold sensitisation. *Journal of the American Medical Association*, **228**, 1226.

Fisher, A.A. (1974) Metallic gold: The cause of a persistent allergic 'dermal' contact dermatitis. *Cutis*, **14**, 177.

Fisher, A.A. (1976) 'Blackjack disease' and other chromate puzzles. *Cutis*, **18**, 21.

Fisher, A.A. (1977) Metal dermatitis — some questions and answers. *Cutis*, **19**, 156.

Fisher, A.A. & Shapiro, A. (1956) Allergic eczematous contact dermatitis due to metallic nickel. *Journal of the American Medical Association*, **161**, 717.

Flowers, M.W. (1978) Burn hazard with cement. *British Medical Journal*, i, 1250.

Folesky, H. (1967) Bemerkungen zum Beryllium-granulom. *Berufsdermatosen*, **15**, 93.

Forslind, B. & Wahlberg, J.E. (1977) Assessment of chromium allergy: Features of patch test reactions at electron microscopic resolution. *Acta Dermato-venereologica*, **57**, 29.

Forster, H.W. & Dickey, R.F. (1949) A case of sensitivity to gold-ball orbital implant. *American Journal of Ophthalmology*, **32**, 659.

Förström, L., Kiistala, R. & Tarvainen K. (1977) Hypersensitivity to copper verified by test with 0.1 per cent Cu SO₄. *Contact Dermatitis*, **3**, 280.

Foussereau, J. & Benezra, Cl. (1970) Les Eczemas Allergiques Professionnels, p. 225. Paris: Masson et Cie.

Foussereau, J. & Laugier, P. (1966) Allergic eczemas from metallic foreign bodies. *Transactions of the St John's Hospital Dermatological Society*, **52**, 220.

Fox, J.M., Kennedy, R. & Rostenberg, A. Jr. (1961) Eczematous contact sensitivity to gold. *Archives of Dermatology*, **83**, 956.

Fregret, S. (1962) The chromium content of fuel ashes with reference to contact dermatitis. *Acta Dermato-venereologica*, **42**, 476.

Fregret, S. (1963) Contact dermatitis due to chromate in foundry sand. *Acta Dermato-venereologica*, **43**, 477.

Fregert, S. (1965) Sensitisation to hexa- and trivalent chromium. *Proceedings of the Congress of the Hungarian Dermatological Society*. April. p. 50.

Fregert, S. (1967) An odd use of potassium dichromate. *Contact Dermatitis Newsletter*, **1**, 5.

Fregert, S. (1971) Nickel in tap water. *Contact Dermatitis Newsletter*, **9**, 202.

Fregert, S. (1971) Remaining chromium in intracutaneous test sites. *Contact Dermatitis Newsletter*, **10**, 233.

Fregert, S. (1972) 'Plastics and metal — a combination that stimulates the sale'. *Contact Dermatitis Newsletter*, **12**, 329.

Fregert, S. (1973) Allergic contact dermatitis from diallylamine in a nickel plating solution. *Contact Dermatitis Newsletter*, **14**, 415.

Fregert, S. (1973) 'Allergic contact dermatitis from lead?' *Contact Dermatitis Newsletter*, **13**, 352.

Fregert, S. (1975) Occupational dermatitis in a 10 year material. *Contact Dermatitis*, **1**, 96.

Fregert, S. & Gruvberger, B. (1972) Chemical properties of cement. *Berufsdermatosen*, **20**, 238.

Fregert, S. & Gruvberger, B. (1973 i) Correlation between alkali sulphate and water-soluble chromate in cement. *Acta Dermato-venereologica*, **53**, 225.

Fregert, S. & Gruvberger, B. (1973 ii) Factors decreasing the content of water-soluble chromate in cement. *Acta Dermato-venereologica*, **53**, 267.

Fregert, S. & Gruvberger, S. (1976) Chromate dermatitis from oil emulsion contaminated from zinc-galvanised iron plate. *Contact Dermatitis*, **2**, 121.

Fregert, S. & Gruvberger, B. (1976) Chromate dermatitis from zinc chromate used for marking textiles. *Contact Dermatitis*, **2**, 124.

Fregert, S. & Gruvberger, B. (1978) Solubility of cobalt in cement. *Contact Dermatitis*, **4**, 14.

Fregert, S., Gruvberger, B., Göransson, K. & Normark, S. (1978) Allergic contact dermatitis from chromate in military textiles. *Contact Dermatitis*, **4**, 223.

Fregert, S., Gruvberger, B. & Heijer, A. (1970) Chromium dermatitis from galvanised sheets. *Berufsdermatosen*, **18**, 254.

Fregert, S., Gruvberger, B & Heijer, A. (1972) Sensitisation to chromium and cobalt in processing of sulphate pulp. *Acta Dermato-venereologica*, **52**, 221.

Fregert, S., Gruvberger, B. & Sandahl, E. (1979) Reduction of chromate in cement by iron sulfate. *Contact Dermatitis*, **5**, 39.

Fregert, S. & Hjorth, N. (1968) In *Textbook of Dermatology*. Ed. Rook, A.J., Wilkinson, S.D., Ebling, F.J.G. 1st ed. p. 1880 Oxford: Blackwell Scientific Publications.

Fregert, S. & Hjorth, N. (1972) In *Textbook of Dermatology*. Ed. Rook, A.J. Wilkinson, D.S. Ebling, F.J.G. 2nd ed. pp. 395, 397, 418. Oxford: Blackwell Scientific Publications.

Fregert, S., Hjorth, N. & Gruvberger, B. (1970) Chromate in bridgetable felt. *Contact Dermatitis Newsletter*, 8, 173.

Fregert, S., Hjorth, N., Magnusson, B., Bandmann, H.-J., Calnan, C.D., Cronin, E., Malten, K., Meneghini, C.L., Pirilä, V. & Wilkinson, D.S. (1969) Epidemiology of contact dermatitis. *Transactions of the St John's Hospital Dermatological Society*, 55, 17.

Fregert, S. Kollander, M. & Poulsen, J. (1979) Allergic contact stomatitis from gold dentures. *Contact Dermatitis*, 5, 63.

Fregert, S. & Ovrum, P. (1963) Chromate in welding fumes with special reference to contact dermatitis. *Acta Dermato-venereologica*, 43, 119.

Fregert, S. & Rorsman, H. (1961) Allergy to a carbon-functional organic silicon compound, dimethyldi-(4-hydroxy-phenyl)-silane. *Nature*, 192, 989.

Fregert, S. & Rorsman, H. (1964) Allergy to trivalent chromium. *Archives of Dermatology*, 90, 4.

Fregert, S. & Rorsman, H. (1965) Patch test reactions to basic chromium (III) sulphate. *Archives of Dermatology*, 91, 233.

Fregert, S. & Rorsman, H. (1966) Allergic reactions to trivalent chromium compounds. *Archives of Dermatology*, 93, 711.

Fregert, S. & Rorsman, H. (1966) Allergy to chromium, nickel and cobalt. *Acta Dermato-venereologica*, 46, 144.

Friedman, A.A. (1956) Dermatitis of the breast from 'lead' pencils. *Archives of Dermatology*, 73, 384.

Frykholm, K.O., Frithiof, L., Fernström, Å.I.B., Moberger, G., Blohm, S.G. & Björn, E. (1969) Allergy to copper derived from dental alloys as a possible cause of oral lesions of lichen planus. *Acta Dermato-venereologica*, 49, 268.

Garcia-Perez, A., Martin-Pascual, A. & Sánchez-Misiego, A. (1973) Chrome content in bleaches and detergents. Its relationship to hand eczema in women. *Acta Dermato-venereologica*, 53, 353.

Gaul, L.E. (1954) Incidence of sensitivity to chromium, nickel, gold, silver and copper compared to reactions to their aqueous salts including cobalt sulphate. *Annals of Allergy*, 12, 429.

Gaul, L.E. (1958i) Ring dermatitis. *Archives of Dermatology*, 77, 526.

Gaul, L.E. (1958ii) Dermatitis from metal spectacles. *Archives of Dermatology*, 78, 475.

Gaul, L.E. (1967) Development of allergic nickel dermatitis from earrings. *Journal of the American Medical Association*, 200, 176.

Gaul, L.E. & Underwood, G.B. (1948) The effect of aging a solution of silver nitrate on its cutaneous reaction. *Journal of Investigative Dermatology*, 11, 7.

Geiser, J.D. & Girard, J. (1965) Remarques sur les cas d'eczema au ciment observés á la clinique de dermato-vénéréologie de Lausanne de 1947 á 1961. *Dermatologica*, 131, 93.

Gerwig, T. (1968) Radioactive jewellery as cause of cutaneous tumour. *Journal of the American Medical Association*, 205, 595.

Giménez-Camarasa, J.M. (1967) Cobalt contact dermatitis. *Acta Dermato-venereologica*, 47, 287.

Giménez-Camarasa, J.M., Garcia-Calderon, P., Asensio, J. & Moragas, De J.M. (1975) Lymphocyte transformation test in allergic contact nickel dermatitis. *British Journal of Dermatology*, 92, 9.

Glover, J.R. (1954-55) Some medical problems concerning selenium in industry. *Transactions of the Association of Industrial Medical Officers*, 4, 94.

Grimm, I. (1971) Ungewöhnliche form einer Kontaktdermatitis durch Kobalt beieinem 11 jahrigen Kind. *Berufsdermatosen*, 19, 39.

Grobe, J.-W. (1977) Gutachterliche und therapeutische Befunde und Beobachtungen bei Moselwinzern mit Arsenintoxikationspatfolgeschadigung. *Berufsdermatosen*, 25, 124.

Grosfeld, J.C.M., Penders, A.J.M., de Grood, R. & Verwilghen, L. (1966) *In vitro* investigations of chromium and nickel hypersensitivity with culture of skin and peripheral lymphocytes. *Dermatologica*, 132, 189.

Hall, A.F. (1944) Occupational contact dermatitis among aircraft workers. *Journal of the American Medical Association*, 125, 179.

Haneke, E. & Gutschmidt, E. (1976) Plattenepithelkarzinom bei einem Elektroschweisser. *Berufsdermatosen*, 24, 119.

Hannuksela, M., Suhonen, R. & Karvonen, J. (1976) Caustic ulcers caused by cement. *British Journal of Dermatology*, 95, 547.

Haxthausen, H. (1954) Allergic cobalt eczema. *Acta Dermato-venereologica*, 34, 57.

Hegyi, E. (1967) Increasing incidence of nickel sensitivity. *Contact Dermatitis Newsletter*, 2, 32.

Hegyi, E. Doležalová, A., Búthová, D. & Husár, I. (1974) On epidemiology of the contact eczema caused by nickel. *Berufsdermatosen*, 22, 193.

Hellier, F.F. (1962) Current Problems in Occupational Dermatitis. Proceedings of the XII International Congress of Dermatology. Washington: Excerpta Medica Foundation. p. 471.

Henning, H.F. (1972) Chromium plating. *Annals of Occupational Hygiene*, 15, 93.

Hersch, P., Hare, J.B., Robertson, A. & Sutherland, S.M. (1961) An experimental survey of rust preventives in water. II. The screening of organic inhibitors. *Journal of Applied Chemistry*, 11, 251.

Hilt, J. (1954) La dermite du chrome hexavalent dans le cadre des dermites eczémateuses par sensibilisation aux métaux, *Dermatologica*, 109, 143.

Hjorth, N. (1967) New source of contact with chromate. *Contact Dermatitis Newsletter*, 1, 14.

Hjorth, N. (1976) Nickel vasculitis. *Contact Dermatitis*, 2, 356.

Holti, G. (1974) Immediate and Arthus-type hypersensitivity to nickel. *Clinical Allergy*, 4, 437.

Holz, H., Mappes, R. & Weidmann, G. (1961) Chromatallergie bei Bohrolekzem. *Berufsdermatosen*, 9, 113.

Holmquist, I. (1951) Occupational arsenical dermatitis. *Acta Dermato-venereologica*. 31, Suppl. 26.

Høvding, G. (1970) Cement Eczema and Chromium Allergy. An Epidemiological Investigation. Thesis. University of Bergen.

Hunter, D. (1969) *The Diseases of Occupations*, p. 423, London: English Universities Press.

Hunter, D., Milton, R. & Perry, K.M.A. (1945) Asthma caused by the complex salts of platinum. *British Journal of Industrial Medicine*, 2, 92.

Hunziker, N. & Musso, E. (1960) A propos de l'eczéma au ciment. *Dermatologica*, 121, 204.

Husain, S.L. (1977) Nickel coin dermatitis. *British Medical Journal*, ii, 998.

Hutchinson, F., Macleod, T.M. & Raffle, E.J. (1975) Nickel hypersensitivity nickel binding to amino acids and lymphocytes. *British Journal of Dermatology*, 93, 557.

Hutchinson, F., Raffle, E.J. & Macleod, T.M. (1972) The specificity of lymphocyte transformation *in vitro* by nickel salts in nickel sensitive subjects. *Journal of Investigative Dermatology*, 58, 362.

Huriez, C. (1957) Occupational Skin Diseases. Acta Dermato-venereologica. Proceedings 11th International Congress of Dermatology. Vol. II, p. 245.

Huriez, Cl., Martin, P. & Lefebvre, M. (1975) Sensitivity to dichromate in a milk analysis laboratory. *Contact Dermatitis*, 1, 247.

Huriez, C., Martin, P. & Planque, Mme. (1969) Dermites des Cimentiers. *Annales de Dermatologie et de Syphiligraphie*, 96, 375.

Jaeger, H. & Pelloni, E. (1950) Tests epicutanés aux bichromates, postifs dans l'eczema aux ciment. *Dermatologica*, 100, 207.

Jensen, O. (1979) 'Rusters'. The corrosive action of palmar sweat: 1. Sodium chloride in sweat. *Acta Dermato-venereologica*, 59, 135.

Jensen, O. Nielsen, E. (1979) 'Rusters'. The corrosive action of palmar sweat: 11. Physical and chemical factors in palmar hyperhidrosis. *Acta Dermato-venereologica*, 59, 139.

Jirásek, L. (1978) Occupational exogenous siderosis of the skin. *Československá Dermatologie*, 53, 249.

Jirásek, L. & Kalenský, J. (1975) Hypersensitivity to platinum, rhodium, gold, copper, antimony and other precious metals and occupational dermatitis caused by selenium. *Československá Dermatologie*, 50, 361.

Jirásek, L., Kobiková, M. & Jiráskova, M. (1976) Retroauricular eczema caused by the nickel of celluloid-rimmed spectacles. *Československá Dermatologie*, 51, 369.

Johnston, A.J.M. & Calnan, C.D. (1958) Cement dermatitis. I. Chemical aspects. *Transactions of the St John's Hospital Dermatological Society*, 41, 11.

Jones, D.A., Lucas, K.H., O'Driscoll, M., Price, C.H.G. & Wibberley, B. (1975) Cobalt toxicity after McKee hip arthroplasty. *Journal of Bone and Joint Surgery*, 57-B, 289.

Jones, J.M. & Amos, H.E. (1974) Contact sensitivity *in vitro*: Activation of actively allergized lymphocytes by a beryllium complex. *International Archives of Allergy and Applied Immunology*, 46, 161.

Jones, W.R. (1940) Arsenical sensitisation, induced previous to arsphenamine therapy. *The Urologic and Cutaneous Review*, 44, 452.

Jongh, G.J. de, Spruit, D., Bongaarts, P.J.M. & Duller, P. (1978) Factors influencing nickel dermatitis. 1. *Contact Dermatitis*, 4, 142.

Jongh, G.J. de & Spruit, D. (1978) Factors influencing nickel dermatitis. 11. *Contact Dermatitis*, 4, 149.

Jünger, H. & Witzani, R. (1978) Zement-ulcera. *Dermatosen in Beruf und Umwelt*, 26, 120.

Kaaber, K. & Veien, N.K. (1977) The significance of chromate ingestion in patients allergic to chromate. *Acta Dermato-venereologica*, 57, 321.

Kaaber, K., Veien, N.K. & Tjell, J.C. (1978) Low nickel diet in the treatment of patients with chronic nickel dermatitis. *British Journal of Dermatology*, 98, 197.

Kadlec, K., Hanslian, L. & Folprechtová, A. (1974) Incidence of skin diseases as a result of work with polyester paints. *Československá Dermatologie*, 49, 281.

Kanan, M.W. (1969) Contact dermatitis in Kuwait. *Journal of the Kuwait Medical Association*, 3, 129.

Kanan, M.W. (1972) Cement dermatitis & atmospheric parameters in Kuwait. *British Journal of Dermatology*, **86**, 155.

Kaplan, I. & Zeligman, I. (1963) Urticaria and asthma from acetylene welding. *Archives of Dermatology*, **88**, 188.

Karasek, S.R. & Karasek, M. (1911) Report Illinois State Commission Occupational Disease p. 97. Quoted by Hunter, D., Milton, R. and Perry, K.M.A. (1945) Asthma caused by the complex salts of platinum. *British Journal of Industrial Medicine*, **2**, 92.

Katz, S.A. & Samitz, M.H. (1975) Leaching of nickel from stainless steel consumer commodities. *Acta Dermato-venereologica*, **55**, 113.

Kesteloot, H., Roelandt, J., Willems, J., Claes, J.H. & Joossens, J.V. (1968) An enquiry into the role of cobalt in the heart disease of chronic beer drinkers. *Circulation*, **37**, 854.

Kim, C.W. & Schöpf, E. (1976) A comparative study of nickel hypersensitivity by the lymphocyte transformation test in atopic and non-atopic dermatitis. *Archives for Dermatological Research*, **257**, 57.

Kirkpatrick, D.C. & Coffin, D.E. (1974) The trace metal content of representative Canadian diets in 1970 and 1971. *Canadian Institute of Food Science and Technology Journal*, **7**, 56.

Klaschka, F. (1975) Contact allergy to gold. *Contact dermatitis*, **1**, 264.

Kligman, A.M. (1966) The identification of contact allergens by human assay. III. The maximisation test: A procedure for screening and rating contact sensitisers. *Journal of Investigative Dermatology*, **47**, 393.

Kolpakov, F.I. (1964) Permeability of skin to nickel compounds. *Federation Proceedings*, **23**, T475.

Kolpakov, F.I., Guzei, T.N., Koplakova, A.F. & Momot, V.M. (1972) The skin barrier. *Vestnik dermatologii i venerologii*, **46**, 13.

Konetzke, G.W. (1974) Die kanzerogene Wirkung von Arsen und Nickel. *Archiv für Geschwulstforschung*, **44**, 16.

Kooten, van W.J. & Mali, J.W.H. (1967) Determination of chromium content in human skin by means of neutron activation analysis. *Proceedings Symposium Nuclear Activation Technique in the Life Sciences, Amsterdam.* p. 567.

Kresbach, H. (1967) Untersuchungen zur Aetiopatahogenese der Kontaktekzeme. *Berufsdermatosen*, **15**, 317.

Kresbach, H. & Willingshofer, H. (1965) Untersuchungen zur Aetiopathogenese der Kontaktekzeme. *Berufsdermatosen*, **13**, 321.

Kreyberg, L. (1978) Lung cancer in workers in a nickel refinery. *British Journal of Industrial Medicine*, **35**, 109.

Krook, G., Fregert, S. & Gruvberger, B. (1977) Chromate and cobalt eczema due to magnetic tapes. *Contact Dermatitis*, **3**, 60.

Kvorning, S.A. (1975) Post-operative dermatitis following non-epidermal nickel contact. *Contact Dermatitis*, **1**, 327.

Lahari, K.D. (1956–1957) Nickel dermatitis. *Indian Journal of Dermatology*, **2**, 110.

Laugier, P., Hunziker, N., Orusco, M., Brun, R., Reiffers, J. & Posternak, F. (1975) Dermite de contact par 'pace-maker'. *Dermatologica*, **150**, 219.

L'Épée, P., Texier, L., Lazarini, H.J., Ducombs, G., Doignon, J., Larcebau, S. & Miegeville, M.J. (1973) L'arsenicisme cutané d'évolution tardive. Les cancers arsenicaux. *Archives de Maladies Professionnelles de Médecine du Travail et de Sécurité Sociale*, **34**, 475.

Leone, R.A. (1968) Radiodermatitis caused by a radioactive gold ring. *Journal of the American Medical Association*, **206**, 2113.

Levene, G.M. & Calnan, C.D. (1971) Platinum sensitivity: treatment by specific hyposensitisation. *Clinical Allergy*, **1**, 75.

Lidén, S. & Lundberg, E. (1979) Penetration of chromium in intact human skin *in vivo*. *Journal of Investigative Dermatology*, **72**, 42.

LoPresti, P.J. & Hambrick, G.W. Jr. (1965) Zirconium granuloma following treatment of Rhus Dermatitis. *Archives of Dermatology*, **92**, 188.

Lyell, A. & Bain, W.H. (1974) Nickel allergy and valve replacement, *Lancet*, **1**, 408.

Lyell, A. (1978) To be published.

Macleod, T.M., Hutchinson, F. & Raffle, E.J. (1970) The uptake of labelled thymidine by leucocytes of nickel sensitive patients. *British Journal of Dermatology*, **82**, 487.

Macleod, T.M., Hutchinson, F. & Raffle, E.J. (1976) The leukocyte migration inhibition test in allergic nickel contact dermatitis. *British Journal of Dermatology*, **94**, 63.

Macleod, T.M., Hutchinson, F. & Raffle, E.J. (1976) Leucocyte aggregation in subjects with nickel dermatitis. *Clinical and Experimental Immunology*, **26**, 528.

Magnusson, B., Blohm, S-G., Fregert, S., Hjorth, N., Høvding, G., Pirilä, V. & Skog, E. (1968) Routine patch testing IV. *Acta Dermato-venereologica*, **48**, 110.

Magnusson, B., Fregert, S., Hjorth, N., Høvding, G., Pirilä, V. & Skog, E. (1969) Routine patch testing V. *Acta Dermato-venereologica*, **49**, 556.

Magnusson, B. & Kligman, A.M. (1969) The identification of contact allergens by animal assay. The guinea pig maximisation test. *Journal of Investigative Dermatology*, **52**, 268.

Mali, J.W.H., Kooten, van W.J., Neer, van F.C.J. & Spruit, D. (1964) Quantitative aspects of chromium sensitisation. *Acta Dermato-venereologica*, **44**, 44.

Maloof, C.C. (1955) Use of edathamil calcium in treatment of chrome ulcers of the skin. *Archives of Industrial Health*, **11**, 123.

Malten, K.E. & Mali, J.W.H. (1966) Kontakt-ekzem durch Goldverbindungen. *Allergie und Asthma*, **12**, 31.

Malten, K.E., Schutter, K., van Senden, K.G. & Spruit, D. (1969) Nickel sensitisation and detergents. *Acta Dermato-venereologica*, **49**, 10.

Malten, K.E. & Spruit, D. (1969) The relative importance of various environmental exposures to nickel in causing contact hypersensitivity. *Acta Dermato-venereologica*, **49**, 14.

Malten, K.E. & Zielhuis, R.L. (1964) Industrial Toxicology and Dermatology in the Production and Processing of Plastics, p. 79 Amsterdam: Elsevier.

Marcussen, P.V. (1957) Spread of nickel dermatitis. *Dermatologica*, **115**, 596.

Marcussen, P.V. (1959) The rise in incidence of nickel sensitivity. *British Journal of Dermatology*, **71**, 97.

Marcussen, P.V. (1960) Ecological considerations on nickel dermatitis. *British Journal of Industrial Medicine*, **17**, 65.

Marcussen, P.V. (1962) Variations in the incidence of contact hypersensitivities. *Transactions of the St John's Hospital Dermatological Society*, **48**, 40.

Marcussen, P.V. (1962) Eczematous allergy to metals. *Acta Allergologica*, **17**, 311.

Marcussen, P.V. (1963) Cobalt dermatitis. Clinical picture. *Acta Dermato-venereologica*, **43**, 231.

Marks, R. (1966) Contact dermatitis due to silver. Case report. *British Journal of Dermatology*, **78**, 606.

Marks, R. & Cronin, E. (1977) Hand eczema in hairdressers. *Australian Journal of Dermatology*, **18**, 123.

Marshall, J. (1952) Asthma and dermatitis caused by chloroplatinic acid. *South African Medical Journal*, **26**, 8.

McKenzie, A.W., Aitken, C.V.E. & Ridsdill-Smith, R. (1967) Urticaria after insertion of Smith-Petersen, vitallium nail. *British Medical Journal*, **iv**, 36.

McNeely, M.D., Nechay, M.W. & Sunderman, F.W. (1972) Measurements of nickel in serum and urine as indices of environmental exposure to nickel. *Clinical Chemistry*, **18**, 992.

McNeely, M.D., Sunderman, F.W. & Nechay, M.W. (1971) Abnormal concentrations of nickel in serum in cases of myocardial infarction, stroke, burns, hepatic cirrhosis and uraemia. *Clinical Chemistry*, **17**, 1123.

Meer, B.J. van der (1957) Een geval van contactallergie voor koper en zink. *Nederlands Tijdschrift voor Geneeskunde*, **101**, 2166.

Meneghini, C.L. (1950) Cutaneous ulcers in workers exposed to chromium. *Rassegna di medicina industriale*, **19**, 161.

Meneghini, C.L. & Petruzzellis, V. (1968) Incidence of dermatitis in cement workers. *Contact Dermatitis Newsletter*, **3**, 55.

Meneghini, C.L., Rantuccio, F. & Petruzzellis, V. (1969) Cr6 content in cements. *Contact Dermatitis Newsletter*, **5**, 108.

Meneghini, C.L., Rantuccio, F. & Riboldi, A. (1963) Klinisch-allergologische Beobachtungen bei beruflichen ekzematösen Kontakt-dermatosen. *Berufsdermatosen*, **11**, 181.

Menné, T. & Kaaber, K. (1978) Treatment of pompholyx due to nickel allergy with chelating agents. *Contact Dermatitis*, **4**, 289.

Menné, T., Mikkelsen, H.I. & Solgaard P. (1978) Nickel excretion in urine after oral administration. *Contact Dermatitis*, **4**, 106.

Menné, T. & Solgaard, P. (1979) Temperature-dependent nickel release from nickel alloys. *Contact Dermatitis*, **5**, 82.

Menné, T. & Thorboe, A. (1976) Nickel dermatitis — nickel excretion. *Contact Dermatitis*, **2**, 353.

Mertz, W. & Roginski, E. (1963) The effect of trivalent chromium on galactose entry in rat epididymal fat tissue. *Journal of Biological Chemistry*, **238**, 868.

Mertz, W., Toepfer, E.W., Roginski, E.E. & Polansky, M.M. (1974) Present knowledge of the role of chromium. *Federation Proceedings*, **33**, 2275.

Miescher, G., Amrein, H.P. & Leder, M. (1955) Chromatüberempfindlichkeit und Zementekzem. *Dermatologica*, **110**, 266.

Milikan, L.E., Conway, F. & Foote, J.E. (1973) *In Viro* studies of contact hypersensitivity: Lymphocyte transformation in nickel sentivity. *Journal of Investigative Dermatology*, **60**, 88.

Mirza, A.M., Perera, M.G., Maecia, C.A., Dziubynskyj, O.G. & Bernstein, I.L. (1975) Leukocyte migration inhibition in nickel dermatitis. *International Archives of Allergy and Applied Immunology*, 49, 782.

Mitchell, J.C. (1972) Metallic content of some jeweller's gold. *Contact Dermatitis Newsletter*, 11, 255.

Modeé, J. & Skog, E. (1962) A comparison of results of patch testing in 1951 and 1961. *Acta Dermato-venereologica*, 42, 280.

Morgan, L.G. (1979) Manufacturing processes: refining of nickel. *Journal of the Society of Occupational Medicine*, 29, 33.

Morin, Y. & Daniel, P. (1967) Quebec beer drinkers' cardiomyopathy: Etiological considerations. *Canadian Medical Association Journal*, 97, 926.

Morris, G.E. (1952) Industrial dermatitis due to contact with brass. *New England Journal of Medicine*, 246, 366.

Moseley, J.C. & Allen, H.J. (1971) Polyurethane coating in the prevention of nickel dermatitis. *Archives of Dermatology*, 103, 58.

Munro-Ashman, D., MacDonald, A. & Feiwel, M. (1975) Split earlobe syndrome. *Contact Dermatitis*, 1, 393.

Munro-Ashman, D. & Miller, A.J. (1976) Rejection of metal to metal prosthesis and skin sensitivity to cobalt. *Contact Dermatitis*, 2, 65.

Munro-Ashman, D., Munro, D.D. & Hughes, T.H. (1969) Contact dermatitis from palladium. *Transactions of the St John's Hospital Dermatological Society*, 55, 196.

Mutter, M. (1962) Vorschläge für die epikutane Testanalyse zur Klarung der Kontaktallergie bei der klinischen Diagnose 'Strumpfbandekzem'. *Allergie und Asthma*, 8, 117.

Nasution, D., Klokke, A.H. & Nater, J.P. (1973) A survey of occupational dermatoses in Indonesia. *Berufsdermatosen*, 21, 215.

Nater, J.P. (1960) Epidermale Überempfindlichkeit gegen Eisen. *Hautarzt*, 11, 223.

Nater, J.P. (1963) Possible causes of chromate eczema. *Dermatologica*, 126, 160.

Nater, J.P., Brian, R.G., Deutman, R. & Mulder, Th.J. (1976) The development of metal hypersensitivity in patients with metal-to-plastic hip arthroplasties. *Contact Dermatitis*, 2, 259.

National Academy of Sciences (1975) Medical and biologic effects of environmental pollutants. Nickel. Washington, D.C: National Academy of Sciences.

Nava, C. & Briatico-Vangosa, G. (1971) Allergia da sali di oro. *Medicina del Lavoro*, 62, 572.

Newhouse, M.L. (1963) A cause of chromate dermatitis among assemblers in an automobile factory. *British Journal of Industrial Medicine*, 20, 199.

Nomoto, S. & Sunderman, F.W. (1970) Atomic absorption spectrometry of nickel in serum, urine and other biological materials. *Clinical Chemistry*, 16, 477.

Nørgaard, O. (1955) Investigation with radioactive Ni 57 into the resorption of nickel through the skin in normal and in nickel-hypersensitive persons. *Acta Dermato-venereologica*, 35, 111.

Norris, G.F. & Peard, M.C. (1963) Berylliosis: Report of two cases, with special reference to the patch test. *British Medical Journal*, i, 378.

North American Contact Dermatitis Group (1973) Epidemiology of contact dermatitis in North America: 1972. *Archives of Dermatology*, 108, 537.

Nürnberger, F. & Arnold. W. (1969) Quincke-Ödem als Ausdruck einer Kobaltallergie infolge Sensibilierung durch kobalthaltige Granatsplitter. *Berufsdermatosen*, 17, 21.

O'Donovan, W.J. (1925) Lime dermatitis. *Lancet*, i, 599.

Oleffe, J. & Roosels, D. (1971) Chrome et environnement de travail en fonction de la reparation des dermatoses professionelles. *Archives Belges de Dermatologie et de Syphiligraphie*, 27, 259.

Oleffe, J., Roosels, D., Vanderkeel, J. & Groetenbriel, Cl. (1971) Presence du chrome dans l'environnement de travail. *Berufsdermatosen*, 19, 57.

Pappas, A., Orfanos, C.E. & Bertram, R. (1970) Non-specific lymphocyte transformation *in vitro* by nickel acetate. *Journal of Investigative Dermatology*, 55, 198.

Parrot, J.-L., Hébert, R., Saindelle, A. & Ruff, F. (1969) Platinum and platinosis. *Archives of Environmental Health*, 19, 685.

Paschoud, J.-M. (1963) Deux cas d'eczéma de contact lichénoide rappelant de trés prés le lichen plan. *Dermatologica*, 127, 99.

Paschoud, J.-M. (1964) Notes cliniques au sujet des eczémas de contact professionnels par l'arsenic et l'antimoine. *Dermatologica*, 129, 410.

Payne, L.R. (1977) The hazards of cobalt. *Journal of the Society of Occupational Medicine*, 27, 20.

Pegum, J.S. (1974) Nickel allergy. *Lancet*, 1, 674.

Peltonen, L. (1979) Nickel sensitivity in the general population. *Contact Dermatitis*, 5, 27.

Perone, V.B., Mofitt, A.E., Possick, P.A., Key, M.M., Danziger, S. & Gellin, G.A. (1974) The chromium, cobalt and nickel contents of American cement and their relationship to cement dermatitis. *American Industrial Hygiene Association Journal*, 35, 301.

Peter, K. (1968) Uber das Schicksal der Patienten mit Gewerbeekzem. *Dermatologica*, 136, 236.

Pickering, C.A.C. (1972) Inhalation tests with chemical allergens: Complex salts of platinum. *Proceedings of the Royal Society of Medicine*, **65**, 273.

Pirilä, V. (1947) On occupational diseases of the skin among paint factory workers, painters, polishers and varnishers in Finland. *Acta Dermato-venereologica*, 27, Suppl. 16. p. 75.

Pirilä, V. (1953) Sensitisation to cobalt in pottery workers, *Acta Dermato-venereologica*, **33**, 193.

Pirilä, V. (1954) On the role of chrome and other trace elements in cement eczema. *Acta Dermato-venereologica*, **34**, 136.

Pirilä, V. (1954) Case report. *Acta Dermato-venereologica*, **34**, 375.

Pirilä, V. & Förström, L. (1966) Pseudo-cross-sensitivity between cobalt and nickel. *Acta Dermato-venereologica*, **46**, 40.

Pirilä, V. & Geier, L. (1964) Über Kobaltallergie bei Porzellanarbeitern. *Hautarzt*, **15**, 491.

Pirilä, V. & Kilpio, O. (1954) On occupational dermatoses in Finland. A report of 1752 cases. *Acta Dermato-venereologica*, **34**, 395.

Polák, L. & Frey, J.R. (1973) Studies on contact hypersensitivity to chromium in the guinea pig. *International Archives of Allergy and Applied Immunology*, **44**, 51.

Polák, L. & Turk, J.L. (1968) Studies on the effect of systemic administration of sensitisers in guinea pigs with contact sensitivity to inorganic metal compounds. *Clinical and Experimental Immunology*, **3**, 245.

Purschel, W. & Furst, G. (1972) Berufsbedingtes Kontaktekzem-katamnesen und Rehabilitation. *Berufsdermatosen*, **20**, 174.

Quinby, R.S. (1926) Health hazards in the rubber industry. *Journal of Industrial Hygiene*, **8**, 103.

Rabeau, H. & Ukrainczyk, Mlle. (1939) Dermites des 'blanchisseuses'. Role du chrome et du chlore (en France). *Annales de Dermatologie et de Syphiligraphie*, **10**, 656.

Rabito, C., Peserico, A. (1973) Sull'etiologia della sensibilizziono nell'eczema da cemento. Giornale Italiano di dermatologica. *Minerva Dermatologica*, **108**, 287.

Reichenberger, M., Ebke, M. & Patiri, C. (1976) Zur Nickelsensibilisierung bei Frauen und ihre Relevanz zur beruflichen Tatigkeit. *Berufsdermatosen*, **24**, 91.

Reiffers, J., Hunziker, N., Brun, R. & Vidmar, B. (1974) Sensibilisationes cutanées allergiques peu communes. *Dermatologica*, **148**, 285.

Reymann, F., Møller, R. & Nielsen, A. (1978) Relationship between arsenic intake and internal malignant neoplasms. *Archives of Dermatology*, **114**, 378.

Richter, G. & Heidelbach, U. (1969) Chromatekzem nach Glasmattierung mit einem Korund. *Berufsdermatosen*, **17**, 8.

Roberts, A.E. (1951) Platinosis. *Archives of Industrial Hygiene and Occupational Medicine*, **4**, 549.

Roed-Petersen, B., Roed-Petersen, J. & Jørgensen, K.D. (1979) Nickel allergy and osteomyelitis in a patient with metal osteosynthesis of a jaw fracture. *Contact Dermatitis*, **5**, 108.

Rogers, S. & Burrows, D. (1975) Contact dermatitis to chrome in milk testers. *Contact Dermatitis*, **1**, 387.

Rook, A.J. (1974) Personal communication.

Ros, A.M. & Bang Pedersen, N. (1977) Chromate in a defatting solvent. *Contact Dermatitis*, **3**, 105.

Ross, D.S. (1974) Welders' metal fume fever. *Journal of the Society of Occupational Medicine*, **24**, 125.

Rossberg, J. (1967) Berusbedingte Arsen-schädigungen der Haut. *Dermatologische Wochenschrift*, **153**, 977.

Rostenberg, A. (1962) Dermatoses due to Environmental and Physical Factors. Ed. Rees, Rees B. Discussion p. 281 Springfield, Illinois: Thomas.

Rostenberg, A. & Perkins, A.J. (1952) Nickel and cobalt dermatitis. *Journal of Allergy*, **22**, 466.

Rostenberg, A. & Sulzberger, M.B. (1937) Some results of patch tests. *Archives of Dermatology*, **35**, 433.

Roth, W.G. (1969) Beitrag zur perifocalen Ausbreitung der Chromatsensibilisierung. *Berufsdermatosen*, **17**, 107.

Rowe, R.J. & Williams, G.H. (1963) Severe reactions to cement. *Archives of Environmental Health*, **7**, 709.

Rudzki, E. & Czerwinska-Dihnz, I. (1977) Sensitivity to dichromate in milk testers. *Contact Dermatitis*, **3**, 107.

Rudzki, E. & Grzywa, Z. (1977) Exacerbation of nickel dermatitis by margarine. *Contact Dermatitis*, **3**, 344.

Rudzki, E. & Kleniewska, D. (1970) The epidemiology of contact dermatitis in Poland. *British Journal of Dermatology*, **83**, 543.

Rudzki, E. & Kohutnicki, Z. (1971) Sensitisation to cobalt and chromium and to cobalt and nickel in men and women. *Contact Dermatitis Newsletter*, **9**, 196.

Rudzki, E., Zakrzewski, Z., Prokopczyk, G. & Kozlowska, A. (1976) Application of emulsifiers for the patch test. *Dermatologica*, **153**, 333.

Rudzki, E., Zakrzewski, Z., Prokopczyk, Q. & Kozlowska, A. (1978) Contact sensitivity to trivalent chromium compounds. *Dermatosen in Beruf und umwelt*, **26**, 83.

Russell, B.F. (1968) Dermatitis from handling coins. *Contact Dermatitis Newsletter*, **4**, 67.

Rüssel, H.A. & Weiler, K.-J. (1971) Über das Workommen von Chrom in gebrauchten Mineralolen. *Berufsdermatosen*, **19**, 23.

Rycroft, R.J.G. & Calnan, C.D. (1977 i) Relapse of chromate dermatitis from sheet metal. *Contact Dermatitis*, **3**, 177.

Rycroft, R.J.G. & Calnan, C.D. (1977ii) Chromate dermatitis from a boiler lining. *Contact Dermatitis*, **3**, 198.

Rytter, M. & Schubert, H. (1971) Gold Allergie infolge einer primär epikutanen Sensibilisierung durch einen Goldring. *Dermatologica*, **142**, 209.

Saltzer, E.I. & Wilson, J.W. (1968) Allergic contact dermatitis due to copper. *Archives of Dermatology*, **98**, 375.

Samitz, M.H. (1970) Ascorbic acid in the prevention and treatment of toxic effects from chromate. *Acta Dermato-venereologica*, **50**, 59.

Samitz, M.H. & Epstein, E. (1962) Experimental cutaneous chromate ulcers in guinea pigs. *Archives of Environmental Health*, **5**, 463.

Samitz, M.H., Gross, S. & Katz, S. (1962) Inactivation of chromium ion in allergic eczematous dermatitis. *Journal of Investigative Dermatology*, **38**, 5.

Samitz, M.H. & Katz, S. (1964) A study of the chemical reactions between chromium and skin. *Journal of Investigative Dermatology*, **43**, 35.

Samitz, M.H. & Katz, S.A. (1975) Skin hazards from nickel and chromium salts in association with cutting oil operations. *Contact Dermatitis*, **1**, 158.

Samitz, M.H. & Katz, S.A. (1975) Nickel dermatitis hazards from prostheses. *British Journal of Dermatology*, **92**, 287.

Samitz, M.H. & Katz, S.A. (1976) Nickel-epidermal interactions: Diffusion and binding. *Environmental Research*, **11**, 34.

Samitz, M.H., Katz, S.A., Scheiner, D.M. & Lewis, J.E. (1975) Attempts to induce sensitisation in guinea pigs with nickel complexes. *Acta Dermato-venereologica*, **55**, 475.

Samitz, M.H. & Pomerantz, H. (1958) Studies of the effects on the skin of nickel and chromium salts. *Archives of Industrial Health*, **18**, 473.

Scarpa, C. & Ferrea, E. (1966) Group variations in reactivity to common contact allergens. *Archives of Dermatology*, **94**, 589.

Schleiff, P. (1968) Provokation des Chromatekzems zu Testzwecken durch interne Chromzufuhr. *Hautarzt*, **19**, 209.

Schmollack, E. (1971) Berufliche Kontaktekzeme durch Kaliumgoldzyanid. *Dermatologische Monatsschrift*, **157**, 821.

Schneeberger, H.W. & Forck, G. (1974) Tierexperimentelle Chromallergie. *Archiv für Dermatologische Forschung*, **249**, 71.

Schoental, R. (1975) Chromium carcinogenesis, formation of epoxyaldehydes and tanning. *British Journal of Cancer*, **32**, 403.

Schopf, E., Wex, O. & Schulz, K.H. (1970) Allergische Kontaktstomatitis mit spezifischer Lymphocytenstimulation durch Gold. *Hautarzt*, **21**, 422.

Schroeder, H.A., Balassa, J.J. & Tipton, I.H. (1962) Abnormal trace metals in man — chromium. *Journal of Chronic Diseases*, **15**, 941.

Schroeder, H.A., Balassa, J.J. & Tipton, I.H. (1962) Abnormal trace metals in man — nickel. *Journal of Chronic Diseases*, **15**, 51.

Schroeder, H.A., Nason, A.P. & Tipton, I.H. (1967) Essential trace metals in man: cobalt. *Journal of Chronic Diseases*, **20**, 869.

Schuppli, R. (1967) Synthetische Waschmittel und Metallionen. *Dermatologica*, **135**, 403.

Schuppli, R. (1970) Über einem neuen Typus von Schutzsalben gegen Chromatekzeme. *Berufsdermatosen*, **18**, 350.

Schwartz, L., Peck, S.M., Blair, K.E. & Markuson, K.E. (1945) Allergic dermatitis due to metallic cobalt. *Journal of Allergy*, **16**, 51.

Schwartz, L., Tulipan, L. & Birmingham, D.J. (1957) *Occupational Diseases of the Skin*. 3rd ed., pp. 889, 287 London: Henry Kimpton.

Serrano Ortega, S. & Sanchez Muros, J. (1976) Pulpitis profesional por niquel. *Actas Dermo-Sifiliograficas*, **67**, 767.

Sertoli, A., Fabri, P., Spallanzani, P. & Giannotti, B. (1978) Unusual contact dermatitis to a cobalt salt. *Contact Dermatitis*, **4**, 314.

Shannon, J. (1965) Pseudo-atopic dermatitis. *Dermatologica*, **131**, 176.

Sheard, C. (1955) Contact dermatitis from platinum and related metals. *Archives of Dermatology*, **71**, 357.

Shelley, W.B. (1964) Chromium in welding fumes as cause of eczematous hand eruption. *Journal American Medical Association*, **189**, 772.

Shelley, W.B. & Epstein, E. (1963) Contact sensitivity to gold as a chronic papular eruption. *Archives of Dermatology*, **87**, 388.

Shelley, W.B. & Hurley, H.J. (1958) The allergie origin of zirconium deodorant granulomas. *British journal of Dermatology*, **70**, 75.

Shelley, W.B. & Hurley, H.J. (1960) The pathogenesis of silica granulomas in man: A non-allergic colloidal phenomenon. *Journal of Investigative Dermatology*, **34**, 107.

Shelley, W.B. & Hurley, H.J. (1975) Studies on topical antiperspirant control of axillary hyperhidrosis. *Acta Dermato-venereologica*, **55**, 241.

Shore, R.N. & Berger, B.J. (1974) Earring dermatitis sparing the ears. *Archives of Dermatology*, **109**, 95.

Sidi, E. & Hincky, M. (1965) Problémes d'actualité concernant les dermatoses professionnelles. *Revue Francaise D'Allergie*, **5**, 198.

Simon, N. & Harley, J. (1967) Skin reactions from gold jewellery contaminated with radon deposit. *Journal of the American Medical Association*, **200**, 254.

Skog, E. (1963) Skin affections caused by hard metal dust. *Industrial Medicine and Surgery*, **32**, 266.

Skog, E. & Wahlberg, J.E. (1969) Patch testing with potassium dichromate in different vehicles. *Archives of Dermatology*, **99**, 697.

Skog, E. & Wahlberg, J.E. (1970) Sensitisation and testing of guinea-pigs with potassium bichromate. *Acta Dermato-venereologica*, **50**, 103.

Sneddon, I.B. (1955) Berylliosis: A case report. *British Medical Journal*, i, 1448.

Sommers, S.C. & McManus, R.G. (1953) Multiple arsenical cancers of skin and internal organs. *Cancer*, **6**, 347.

Somov, B.A. & Khaimovsky, G.D. (1964) Allergic dermatitis caused by aurum compounds in watch industry. *Vestnik Dermatologii i Venerologii*, No. 10, 33.

Spier, H.W. & Natzel, R. (1952) Zur Pathogenese des Zementekzems. *Archiv für Dermatologie und Syphilis*, **193**, 537.

Spier, H.W. & Natzel, R. (1953) Chromatallergie und Zementekzem. *Hautarzt*, **4**, 63.

Spruit, D. (1979) The reliability of the analyses of Co, Cr and Ni in biological liquids. *British Journal of Dermatology*, **100**, 601.

Spruit, D. & Bongaarts, P.J.M. (1977) Nickel content of plasma, urine and hair in contact dermatitis. *Dermatologica*, **154**, 291.

Spruit, D., Bongaarts, P.J.M. & de Jongh, G.J. (1978) Dithiocarbamate therapy for nickel dermatitis. *Contact Dermatitis*, **4**, 350.

Spruit, D. & Malten, K.E. (1975) Occupational cobalt and chromium dermatitis in an offset printing factory. *Dermatologica*, **151**, 34.

Spruit, D. & Neer, van F.C.J. (1966) Penetration rate of Cr(iii) and Cr(vi). *Dermatologica*, **132**, 179.

Steiner, K. (1929) Uber die Ergebnisse und den Wert der funktionellen Hautprufung mittels der Lappchenprobe bei Hautkranken und bei Haut Gesunden. *Archiv für Dermatologie und Syphilis*, **157**, 600.

Stevenson, C.J. (1965) Antimony spots. *Transactions of the St John's Hospital Dermatological Society*, **51**, 40.

Stoddart, J.C. (1960) Nickel sensitivity as a cause of infusion reactions. *Lancet*, **2**, 741.

Stoke, J. (1977) Metal fume fever in ferro-chrome workers. *Central African Journal of Medicine*, **23**, 25.

Sulzberger, M.B. (1940) Dermatologic Allergy, p. 175. Springfield, Illinois: Thomas.

Sulzberger, M.B. & Goodman, J. (1936) The relative importance of specific skin hypersensitivity in adult atopic dermatitis. *Journal of the American Medical Association*, **106**, 1000.

Sunderman, F.W. (1967) Spectrophotometric measurements of serum nickel. *Clinical Chemistry*, **13**, 115.

Sunderman, F.W. (1971) The treatment of acute nickel carbonyl poisoning with sodium diethyldithiocarbamate. *Annals of Clinical Research*, **3**, 182.

Sunderman, F.W. (1977) A review of the metabolism and toxicology of nickel. *Annals of Clinical and Laboratory Science*, **7**, 377.

Svejgaard, E., Morling, N., Svejgaard, A. & Veien, N.K. (1978) Lymphocyte transformation induced by nickel and sulphate: an *in vitro* study of subjects with and without a positive nickel patch test. *Acta Dermato-venereologica*, **58**, 245.

Tay, C.H. (1974) Cutaneous manifestations of arsenic poisoning due to certain Chinese herbal medicine. *Australian Journal of Dermatology*, **15**, 121.

Taylor, D.M. & Davies, J.C.A. (1977) Ferro-alloy workers' disease a report of a recent case against the background of twelve years experience. *Central African Journal of Medicine*, 23, 28.

Tegner, E. & Fregert, S. (1973) A case of sensitisation to nickel in infancy. *Contact Dermatitis Newsletter*, 14, 424.

Tepper, L.B., Hardy, H.L. & Chamberlain, R.I. (1961) *Toxicity of Beryllium Compounds*, pp. 13, 32, 80, 35, 63 Amsterdam: Elsevier.

Thiers, M.M., Chanial, G., Rivoire, J. & Muller, F. (1961) Dermites professionnelles par sensibilisation aux urantes de sodium et de calcium. *Archieves Des Malades Prodessionnelles de Medécine du Travail et de Sécurité Sociale*, 22, 168.

Thulin, H. (1976) The leucocyte migration test in nickel contact dermatitis. *Acta Dermatovenereologica*, 56, 377.

Tio, D. (1976) A study on the clinical application of a direct leucocyte migration test in chromium contact allergy. *British Journal of Dermatology*, 94, 65.

Torjussen, W. & Solberg, L.A. (1976) Histological findings in the nasal mucosa of nickel workers. *Acta Oto-laryngologica*, 82, 266.

Tronnier, H. & Turek, B. (1969) Licht und Chromekzem. *Berufsdermatosen*, 17, 1.

Turk, B.M. (1975) Katamnestische Untersuchungen bei Berufsekzematikern unter besonderer Berucksichtigung der Sensibilisierung gegenuber Dichromat-Ionen. Inaugural dissertation, Munchen. Quoted by Breit, R. and Turk, R.B.M. (1976) *British Journal of Dermatology*, 94, 349.

Turk, J.L. & Parker, D. (1977 i) Granuloma formation in normal guinea pigs injected intradermally with aluminium and zirconium compounds. *Journal of Investigative Dermatology*, 68, 336.

Turk, J.L. & Parker, D. (1977 ii) Sensitisation with Cr, Ni and Zr salts and allergic type granuloma formation in the guinea pig. *Journal of Investigative Dermatology*, 68, 341.

Turk, J.L., Badenoch-Jones, P. & Parker, D. (1978) Ultrastructural observations on epithelioid cell granulomas induced by zirconium in the guinea-pig. *Journal of Pathology*, 124, 45.

Uehara, M., Takahashi, C. & Ofuji, S. (1975) Pustular patch test reactions in atopic dermatitis. *Archives of Dermatology*, 111, 1154.

Urbach, E. & Pillsbury, D.M. (1943) The phenomenon of 'Black dermographism'. *Journal of the American Medical Association*, 121, 485.

Vandenberg, J.J. & Epstein, W.L. (1963) Experimental nickel contact sensitisation in man. *Journal of Investigative Dermatology*, 41, 413.

Veien, N.K. & Svejgaard, E. (1978) Lymphocyte transformation in patients with cobalt dermatitis. *British Journal of Dermatology*, 99, 191.

Vickers, H.R. & Edwards, D.H. (1976) Cement burns. *Contact Dermatitis*, 2, 73.

Vuletić, A. (1934) Über Salvarsanuberempfindlichkeit und akute Salvarsanintoxikation infolge beruflicher Benetzungen der Finger mit Salvarsanlösungen. *Archiv für Dermatologie und syphilis*, 169, 436.

Wahlberg, J.E. (1969) Health-screening for occupational skin diseases in building workers. *Berufsdermatosen*, 17, 184.

Wahlberg, J.E. (1975) Nickel allergy and atopy in hairdressers. *Contact Dermatitis*, 1, 161.

Wahlberg, J.E. (1976) Sensitisation and testing of guinea pigs with nickel sulphate. *Dermatologica*, 152, 321.

Wahlberg, J.E. (1977) Routine patch testing with cadmium chloride. *Contact Dermatitis*, 3, 293.

Wahlberg, J.E. & Boman, A. (1978) Sensitisation and testing of guinea pigs with cobalt chloride. *Contact Dermatitis*, 4, 128.

Wahlberg, J.E. Lindstedt, G. & Einarsson, Ö. (1977) Chromium, cobalt and nickel in Swedish cement, detergents, mould and cutting oils. *Berufsdermatosen*, 25, 220.

Wahlberg, J.E. & Wennersten, G. (1977) Light sensitivity and chromium dermatitis. *British Journal of Dermatology*, 97, 411.

Walsh, E.N. (1953) Chromate hazards in industry. *Journal of the American Medical Association*, 153, 1305.

Watt, T.L. & Baumann, R.R. (1968) Nickel earlobe dermatitis. *Archives of Dermatology*, 98, 155.

Weiler, K.-J (1969) Rezidivierendes Chromkontaktekzem durch Umgang mit Chromstahl. *Berufsdermatosen*, 17, 316.

Weiler, K.-J. & Russel, H.A. (1971) Das Chromekzem durch Glutineleim und Kalk. *Berufsdermatosen*, 19, 292.

Weiler, K.-J. & Russell, H.A. (1974) Das Chromekzem durch Branntkalk. *Berufsdermatosen*, 22, 116.

Wells, G.C. (1956) Effects of nickel on the skin. *British Journal of Dermatology*, 68, 237.

Wilkinson, D.S., Bandmann, H.-J., Calnan, C.D., Cronin, E., Fregert, S., Hjorth, N., Magnusson, B., Maibach, H.I., Malten, K.E., Meneghini, C.L. & Pirilä, V. (1970) The Role of contact allergy in hand eczema. *Transactions of the St John's Hospital Dermatological Society*, 56, 19.

Williams, R.M. & Skipworth, G.B. (1959) Zirconium granulomas of the glabrous skin following treatment of Rhus dermatitis. *Archives of Dermatology*, 80, 273.

Wilson, H.T.H. (1955) Standard patch tests in eczema and dermatitis. *British Journal of Dermatology*, **67**, 291.

Wilson, H.T.H. (1956) Nickel dermatitis. *Practioner*, **177**, 303.

Wilson, H.T.H. (1971) Chrome dermatitis in a brewery. *Contact Dermatitis Newsletter*, **10**, 228.

Winston, J.R. & Walsh, E.N. (1951) Chromate dermatitis in railroad employees working with diesel locomotives. *Journal of the American Medical Association*, **147**, 1133.

Yoshikawa, K., Hadame, K. & Hijikata, T. (1978) Nickel underneath gold plating. *Contact Dermatitis*, **4**, 371.

Young, E. (1974) Contact hypersensitivity to metallic gold. *Dermatologica*, **149**, 294.

Ziegler, V., Suss, E. & Standau, H. (1973) Bemerkungen zum tierexperimentellen Chromatekzem. *Allergie und Immunologie*, **19**, 29.

8.

Pesticides

FUNGICIDES
PHENOLS
  Pentachlorophenol
  p-Chloro-o-cresol
  Tetrachlorodihydroxydiphenyl
  sulphide (Vanicide BL)
  o-Benzyl-p-chlorophenol
  (Chlorophene; Santophen 1)
NITROPHENOLS
  4,6-Dinitro-o-cresol
  Dinobuton
  Nitrofen
  Dinocap
QUINONES
  Chloranil
  Dichlone
  Dithianone
DITHIOCARBAMATES and THIURAMS
  Ziram
  Zineb
  Maneb
  Benomyl
  Thiram
CAPTAN and SIMILAR CHEMICALS
  Captan
  Phaltan
  Difolatan
CHLORONITROBENZENES
  Pentachloronitrobenzene
  DNCB
MERCURY COMPOUNDS

ORGANO-TIN COMPOUNDS
MERCAPTOBENZOTHIAZOLE
PHOSPHOTHIOATE
  Plondrel
HERBICIDES
AMIDES
  Randox
BIPYRIDYLIUMS
  Diquat
  Paraquat
INSECTICIDES
PYRETHROIDS
ORGANOTHIOCYANATES
  Rodannitrobenzene
DDT
DD
LINDANE
  Gamma benzene hexachloride
CYCLODIENES
  Dieldrin
ORGANOPHOSPHORUS COMPOUNDS
  Parathion
  Malathion
  Naled
CARBAMATES
OMITE
DAZOMET
RODENTICIDES
WARFARIN
ANTU

The use of pesticides has greatly increased during the past 30 years and they are now an accepted part of our environment. Greater specificity of action is being achieved to ensure that only one particular class of organism is killed; this reduces their hazard but increases their number. Their toxicity is carefully assessed and is under continual review, but reports on their dermatological effects are comparatively few. Agricultural and horticultural chemicals tend to be handled by amateurs working alone or by men working in small groups on farms, often some distance from a dermatological clinic. Cases of dermatitis in such workers are much less likely to find their way to hospital, or even to be recognised for what they are, than dermatitis in workers in large groups in industry. It is likely that many of these chemicals cause more dermatitis than is reported.

The following classification is based on that in *Pesticides in the Environment* (Ed. White-Stevens, 1971), which is an informative account of the chemistry and activity of these agents. Their efficacy and use has also been summarised comprehensively by Marderosian (1970).

In the account that follows, the chief consideration is the importance of these chemicals in dermatology, not in agriculture. When familiar, the common names are used in preference to recommended chemical nomenclature, and where the appropriate concentration for use in patch testing seems uncertain a ? is put before the recommended dilution.

Fungicides

A. INORGANIC

Sulphur, free or combined as lime-sulphur, is still used extensively as a fungicide, and for the same purpose copper salts have, for two hundred years, been utilised for spraying fruit and vegetable crops. Bordeaux mixture, consisting of copper sulphate and lime, controls mildew disease of grapes.

B. ORGANIC

1. PHENOLS

Chlorinated phenols have enhanced fungicidal activity but, as they are toxic, they can be used only for soil and fabrics or as a wood preservative.

Pentachlorophenol (Santophen 20; Penta)

This chemical is used particularly as a wood preservative.

Patch testing
Pentachlorophenol 1 per cent in water.

4-Chloro-2-hydroxytoluene (*p*-Chloro-*o*-cresol)

4-Chloro-2-hydroxytoluene
(*p*-chloro-*o*-cresol)

(4-Chloro-*o*-toloxy)acetic acid
(4-chloro-2-methylphenoxyacetic acid)

A man reported by Fregert (1968) developed dermatitis of exposed sites on two occasions, each after using a spray containing chloromethylphenoxyacetic acid. Although patch testing with 1 per cent of this chemical was negative, the patient reacted to 0.1 per cent *p*-chloro-*o*-cresol in alcohol, which is used in the manufacture of the pesticide.

Patch testing
p-Chloro-*o*-cresol 0.1 per cent in alcohol
Chloromethylphenoxyacetic acid 1 per cent in petrolatum.

Dichlorphene: 2,2'-Methylenebis(4-chlorophenol) (see p. 677)

Vanicide BL (3,3',5,5'-Tetrachloro-2,2'-dihydroxydiphenyl sulphide)

This fungicide and germicide is used to control algae.

Patch testing
? concentration.

o-**Benzyl-*p*-chlorophenol** (Chlorophene; Santophen 1; 4-chloro-*d*-phenyl-*o*-cresol; 2-benzyl-4-chlorophenol)

o-Phenylphenol (page 00)

These two compounds have similar actions; orthophenylphenol (p. 681) is used to protect fruit and vegetables.

Patch testing
Santophen ? concentration
o-Phenylphenol 1 per cent ? aqueous.

2. NITROPHENOLS

All are powerful fungicides and some are insecticides.

4,6-Dinitro-*o*-cresol (DNOC; 2-Methyl-4,6-dinitrophenol)

A man inadvertently used this chemical in its concentrated form to treat fruit trees. After 15 days he noticed that his proximal nail plates were yellow; within two months this was marked and was associated with a slight and painless paronychia (Baran, 1974).

Patch testing
? concentration.

Dinobuton (Acrex)

Picric acid (2,4,6-trinitrophenol)

Dinobuton is employed principally as an insecticide and is used to kill red spider mites; however, it is also effective against mildew.

When a chemical works in Sweden began manufacturing Acrex, which contains 50 per cent dinobuton, it was found that, as a result of grinding the ingredient, a yellow dust settled throughout the whole factory. Within weeks, workers began to complain of yellow staining of their hair and nails and of irritation of their face, neck and arms.

It was thought that, as dinobuton and picric acid have a similar chemical structure, and both cause comparable staining, there might be a causal relationship between these two features.

Patch testing of controls with dinobuton in petrolatum established that concentrations of up to 40 per cent are non-irritant but that this concentration actively sensitises. Of six workers patch tested, two reacted to 30 per cent and to 40 per cent (Wahlberg, 1974).

Patch testing
Dinobuton 1–10 per cent in petrolatum.

Nitrofen: (2,4-Dichlorophenyl 4'-nitrophenyl ether)

A farmer came into contact with nitrofen when cutting a hedge which had been sprayed with this pesticide. Following his second exposure he developed an eruption on his forehead, face, neck, forearms and hands.

A patch test with nitrofen 0.5 per cent in olive oil was positive (Solomons, 1972).

Patch testing
Nitrofen 0.5 per cent in petrolatum or olive oil.

Dinocap: (Crotonic acid 2-(1-methylheptyl)-4,6-dinitrophenyl ester; Karathane)

Dinocap prevents mildew on fruit, vegetables and flowers.

Patch testing
Dinocap ? 1 per cent in petrolatum.

QUINONES

These are oxidation products of phenol.

Tetrachloro-*p*-benzoquinone (Chloranil)

Dichlone (2,3-Dichloro-1,4-naphthoquinone)

Dithianone (5,10-Dihydro-5,10-dioxonaphtho(2,3-b)-1,4-dithiin-2,3-dicarbonitrile)

This chemical sensitised a woman horticulturist. She developed an eruption on her hands, arms, face and ears which was directly related to her work. When patch tested, she reacted to 1 per cent Dithianone (Calnan, 1969).

Patch testing
Dithianone 1 per cent in petrolatum.

4. DITHIOCARBAMATES AND THIURAMS

This group of chemicals is extensively used for seeds, plants and fruits. When used as fungicides they seem rarely to sensitise.

Dithiocarbamates
In guinea-pigs, the dithiocarbamates, maneb, mancozeb and zineb have been found to be strong sensitisers (Matsushita, Arimatsu and Nomura, 1976).

Ziram (Bis(dimethyldithiocarbamato)zinc; zinc dimethyldithiocarbamate)

$$H_3C \diagdown N-C \diagup{S} \diagdown Zn \diagup{S} \diagdown C-N \diagup{CH_3}$$

Patch testing
Ziram 1 per cent in petrolatum.

Zineb ([Ethylenebis(dithiocarbamato)]zinc; zinc ethylenebis(dithiocarbamate))

$$NH-CH_2-CH_2-NH$$

Six patients with dermatitis from Zineb were described by Scarpa and Ippolito (1959). Another three men developed dermatitis of their hands as a result of working with tobacco treated with Zineb and Maneb; each was found to react to both these chemicals on patch testing (Laborie and Dedieu, 1964).

Members of the International Contact Dermatitis Research Group tested 655 eczematous patients with Zineb 1 per cent in petrolatum; three patients gave positive reactions but none was thought relevant.

Patch testing
Zineb 1 per cent in petrolatum.

Maneb (Ethylenebis(dithiocarbamato)manganese; manganous ethylenebis(dithiocarbamate))

$$CH_2NHC-S \diagdown Mn \diagup CH_2NHC-S$$

Three cases of Maneb and Zineb sensitivity in tobacco workers have been described (Laborie and Dedieu, 1964). Dermatitis has also been reported (Nater, Terpstra and Bleumink, 1979) in a draftsman from inadvertent contact with Maneb used to spray the office flowers and in a florist.

Members of the International Contact Dermatitis Research Group routinely patch tested 655 patients with Maneb 1 per cent in petrolatum; 35 reacted, but in only one of these, a florist with hand eczema, was the reaction thought possibly to be clinically relevant. These results suggest that Maneb 1 per cent in petrolatum is an irritant concentration for patch testing.

St John's

A man aged 57 years grew roses as a hobby and was sensitised by a Maneb rose spray. In addition he had an unrelated photodermatitis. On patch testing he was strongly positive to the spray and he reacted also to Zineb 1 per cent; he was not tested with Maneb. Avoiding this spray had little influence on his dermatitis.

Patch testing
Maneb 0.5 per cent in petrolatum.

Mancozeb
Mancozeb is a combination of zinc and manganese ethylene bisdithiocarbamate; its use as a fungicide on wheat and barley seeds has caused dermatitis in south Australia (Burry, 1976).

Benomyl: (Methyl-1-butylcarbamoyl-2-benzimidazole carbamate)

This fungicide is effective against a wide range of fungi and is used to prevent scab and mildew on apples.

Benomyl was used by a flower grower to spray carnations; after the second spraying, seven women, who were either budding or cutting the flowers, developed an eruption on the skin of exposed sites. Patch tests with Benomyl 10 per cent were positive in all the patients, whereas three controls were negative to this concentration; one control, however, reacted to Benomyl 20 per cent coupled with ultraviolet light exposure (Savitt, 1972).

A nurseryman, who worked with roses, developed a mild irritant dermatitis of his hands in the summer only (Fregert, 1973). The eruption became worse and spread to his face and neck. On patch testing he reacted to wool alcohols and to two pesticides, one of which was Benomyl 0.1 per cent in water. Fregert wondered whether the sparcity of similar reports might be due to these attacks of dermatitis being so transient that the patients are not referred for investigation. van Ketel (1976) reported a case and stressed that picking plants containing residues of the fungicide was an important source of sensitisation.

Patch testing
Benomyl 0.1–per cent in water or petrolatum.

Barban: (Chloro-butynyl-chlorophenyl-carbamate); Carbyne

$$\text{NHCOOCH}_2\text{C} \equiv \text{CCH}_2\text{Cl}$$

Dermatitis in an agricultural sprayer was caused by Carbyne and its degradation product 2-chloro-4-aminophenol was suggested as the cause of his associated depigmentation (Brancaccio and Chamales, 1977).

THIURAMS
Thiurams are members of the group of dithiocarbamates. In rubber they commonly act as sensitisers, but when used as fungicides their contact with the skin
is minimal and they rarely seem to cause dermatitis.

Thiram: Bis(dimethylthiocarbamoyl) disulphide; tetramethylthiuramdisulphide;
TMDT)

Thiram is widely used on grass, lawns, farmland and fruit and vegetable
crops; as a herbicide it rarely sensitises.

In 1958, Schulz and Herrmann described five dock labourers who had
developed dermatitis after contact with thiram which had been sprinkled on
bananas to prevent them rotting. Another patient, reported by Shelley (1964),
developed a widespread dermatitis after contact with thiram used as a fungicide
on a golf course. This chemical was applied to the man's arm for 15 minutes
and it produced a large eczematous reaction and a generalised flare, despite the
patient being on systemic steroids.

St John's
A retired man, aged 68 years, used a thiuram insecticide in his garden and subsequently developed a rash on his hands, arms and face. When patch tested, he
reacted to TMTD 2 per cent and to three related thiurams. He discarded the spray
and his skin healed.

Patch testing
Tetramethylthiuramdisulphide 1 per cent in petrolatum.

Tetmosol: (tetraethylthiurammonosulphide; bis(diethylthiocarbamoyl)sulphide)

This chemical may be used as a fungicide, but it is also effective against fleas, lice and other parasites on cats and dogs. Tetmosol is a standard treatment for human scabies and does not appear to cause trouble from sensitisation.

St John's
A woman, aged 58 years, had had hand eczema for eight years; this relapsed after she treated her cat with Tetmosol, and again at a later date when she wore rubber gloves to clean her house. She had positive patch tests to the Tetmosol solution and to the two thiurams tested; these were tetramethylthiuramdisulphide and tetraethylthiuramdisulphide, both 1 per cent in petrolatum.

Patch testing
Tetmosol 1 per cent in petrolatum.

5. CAPTAN AND SIMILAR CHEMICALS

Captan: (*N*-(Trichloromethylthio)-4-cyclohexene-1,2-dicarboximide)

This fungicide is in extensive use on fruit, vegetables and plants of all types.

Its sensitising potential was assessed in 205 human subjects by Marzulli and Maibach (1973); using a concentration of 1 per cent, both for induction and for challenge, they sensitised nine (4.4 per cent). Captan 1 per cent in petrolatum was tested on 509 patients by members of the International Contact Dermatitis Research Group. Sixteen (3 per cent) of these patients reacted, but in none was it considered to be clinically relevant and the reactions were thought to be mild irritant responses.

After three weeks' exposure to Captan, a fruit farmer developed dermatitis of his hands and face. Patch tests with Captan 1 per cent in vaseline and with the related chemical Phaltan 1 per cent in petrolatum were both positive (Fregert, 1967).

Patch testing
Captan 1 per cent and 0.5 per cent in petrolatum.

Phaltan: (*N*-(Trichloromethythio)phthalimide; Folpet)

Phaltan 1 per cent in petrolatum was tested on 509 routine eczematous patients by the International Contact Dermatitis Research Group; 50 (10 per cent) reacted, indicating that this is an irritant concentration for patch testing. In only one patient, a florist, was the reaction thought likely to be significant. When 107 patients were tested using a reduced concentration, 0.1 per cent in petrolatum, only three (3 per cent) reacted, but in none was the reaction considered to be relevant.

Patch testing
Phaltan 0.05 per cent and 0.1 per cent in petrolatum.

Difolatan: (N-(1,1,2,2-Tetrachloroethylthio)-4-cyclohexene-1,2-dicarboximide)

This chemical is used to prevent blight on potatoes and is also sprayed on fruit and farm crops.

Sensitivity is probably not uncommon among farmers and other workers who handle difolatan frequently. Cottel (1972) reported that the manufacturers recognised it as a potent sensitiser following trouble with it in their industrial plant. He also described farmers with an airborne type of acute contact dermatitis, in which the eruption was incapacitating and relapsed when they came into contact with residual fungicide on crops or in orchards. Patch tests with difolatan 0.1 per cent in water were positive in these cases.

A similar outbreak has been described in Japanese farmers who used difolatan to spray tangerine orchards. In 1966, 264 men (25 per cent) were found to have dermatitis, and in the following year the number had increased to 356 (38 per cent). The eruption resembled a slight to severe sunburn and affected the face, neck and arms. It usually cleared within a week of stopping spraying (Takamatsu et al., 1968). Urticarial, mobilliform and eczematous eruptions and asthma occurred in workers packing difolatan (Camarasa, 1975) and dermatitis with wheezing developed in a difolatan plant maintainance worker (Groundwater, 1977).

Patch testing
Difolatan 0.1 per cent in petrolatum.

6. CHLORONITROBENZENES

These compounds are effective fungistatics in soil and on stored potatoes.

Pentachloronitrobenzene: (PCNB; Brassicol)

St John's

Within weeks of starting work as a packer of pesticide powders, a man, aged 46 years, developed eczema of his arms, legs, forehead, trunk and scrotum. The condition cleared while he was off work for two weeks and relapsed on his return.

When patch tested, he reacted to thiram 2 per cent (TMTD) and to one of the chemicals he packed, namely PCNB 1 per cent in petrolatum. He also reacted to parts of his shoes, this being attributed to contamination by PCNB dust. Although he did not pack thiram, it was handled in the firm.

Patch testing
PCNB ? 0.5 per cent and 1 per cent in petrolatum.

DNCB: (1-Chloro-2,4-dinitrobenzene; dinitrochlorobenzene; DNCB)

This chemical is such a potent sensitiser that it has been used for many years to induce contact sensitivity experimentally.

It was reported to be an occupational hazard by Bernstein in 1912; he cited nine men who came into contact with it possibly in the manufacture of dyes. He emphasised the yellow discolouration, particularly of the face, and the violent dermatitis which occurred.

It is now being sold as an algicide for use in recirculating water cooling systems in many countries, including the U.S.A., Canada, Italy, the U.K. and Holland.

Sensitisation by contact with DNCB in this occupation has been reported from California where it occurred in two men described by Zimmerman (1970) and in four air-conditioning repair men recorded by Adams *et al.* (1971). Clinically characteristic was a vesiculo-bullous eruption, delineating splashes on the skin. Two of the repair men were patch tested with, and reacted to, DNCB 10^{-6}. Another patient, seen in Holland, was a chemistry technician trained in testing industrial water equipment. He experienced attacks of hand eczema each time he handled recirculating cooling water. He reacted when patch tested with DNCB 0.25 per cent in water (Malten, 1974).

Patch testing
DNCB ? 0.01 per cent and 0.1 per cent in water.

7. MERCURY COMPOUNDS

Phenyl mercuric nitrate (p. 688)

8. ORGANO-TIN COMPOUNDS

Organic tin compounds are used to prevent mildew in wood, textiles and paints.

$$(C_4H_9)_3 SnOH \qquad\qquad CH_3COO Sn (C_6H_5)_3$$

Tributyl tin hydroxide   Triphenyl tin acetate

Tributyltin oxide (TBTO) is used mainly to protect wood and is applied as a one per cent paint; in marine paints it is combined with copper oxide or tributyltin fluoride in concentrations of 3–6 per cent. During use protective clothing should be worn. Unless washed off, skin contamination causes an acute burn and soiled clothing produces an itching erythema. TBTO is an irritant but not a sensitiser (Gammeltoft, 1978). Cuprinol, a wood preservative widely used in Britain, contains tributyltin oxide.

Patch testing
Tributyltin oxide 0.01 and 0.001 per cent in water.

9. 2-MERCAPTOBENZOTHIAZOLE: (MBT; 2-Benzothiazolethiol)

Salts of this weak acid prevent mildew in fabrics and control slime and algae. When used for this purpose it has not been reported as causing dermatitis, although it is a well known sensitiser in rubber.

Patch testing
Mercaptobenzothiazole 1 per cent in petrolatum.

10. PHOSPHOTHIOATE

Phosphothioate compounds are fungicides; chemically they are related to the organophosphorus group.

Plondrel: (*o-o*-Diethyl-phthalimido-phosphothioate)

Plondrel is sprayed on roses to protect them from mildew and it is left as a deposit particularly on the leaves. Sprayers are probably protected by adequate clothing but florists and those who cultivate roses are exposed to the Plondrel which remains on the plants. Four patients with hand eczema who were sensitised through such contact were reported by van Ketel (1975). Patch tests: each was positive to Plondrel 0.1 per cent in petrolatum; 20 controls were negative. Three patients reacted to roses sprayed with Plondrel and two to roses which had not been sprayed.

St John's
In 1977, a foreman in a chemical works was sensitised to Plondrel despite wearing full protective clothing. His job included adding Plondrel and other chemicals to a

mixer but also he repaired protective suits which might have been incompletely cleaned. Patch tests: he reacted strongly to Plondrel 1 per cent in MEK.

Patch testing
Plondrel 0.01 per cent in petrolatum.

Active sensitisation with Plondrel 0.1 per cent has been reported (van Ketel, 1977).

Herbicides

1. AMIDE HERBICIDES

Randox: *N,N*-Diallyl-2-chloroacetamide; (Randox; CDAA)

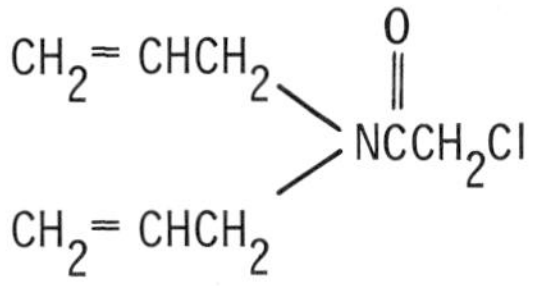

$$CH_2 = CHCH_2$$
$$CH_2 = CHCH_2$$
$$NCCH_2Cl$$

Three farmers were sensitised by Randox as a result of spilling it on their shoes and continuing to wear them. After 10–21 days, each developed swelling and a striking violaceous discoloration of their feet. The parts of their thighs under their trouser pockets were affected in two, the hands in one and the wrists in another. Two of the patients, when patch tested, developed bullous reactions to 1 per cent Randox; it was found that a more suitable dilution for patch testing was 0.1 per cent, although even this acted as a mild irritant in controls (Spencer, 1966).

Chloroacetamide, the preservative, also is a sensitiser (p. 698).

Patch testing
Randox ? 0.01 per cent and 0.1 per cent in petrolatum.

2. BIPYRIDYLIUM HERBICIDES

These chemicals, in the presence of light, chlorophyll and oxygen, rapidly kill all types of foliage, but they are absorbed and inactivated by soil. Their defoliant action facilitates the harvesting of crops such as potatoes and cotton, and they are frequently used as weed killers by gardeners and farmers.

Their toxicity on ingestion has made them notorious. The gut, liver and kidney are particularly susceptible to injury, as are the alveolar walls which react in repair by producing excessive pulmonary fibrosis.

Chemically they are quaternary salts of certain dipyridyls and were developed following the observation that quaternary ammonium compounds destroy young plants.

Diquat: (6,7-Dihydrodipyrido[1,2-a:2′,1′-c]pyrazidiinium dibromide; Reglone)

Patch testing
? concentration.

Paraquat: (4,4-Dipyridylium-1,1-dimethyl dichloride; Gramoxone; Weedol)

Sensitisation by these chemicals has not been reported. The advice of the manufacturers to avoid skin contamination, and wash immediately if this occurs, is designed to prevent toxicity and not because the chemicals are particular irritants. Death from percutaneous absorption of paraquat has occurred in a fruit farmer's wife through scratches acquired while pruning trees (Newhouse, McEvoy and Rosenthal, 1978) and in a spray operator whose skin was excessively contaminated with a concentrated solution (Jaroš, 1978).

Sharvill (1971) described a boy whose trousers became contaminated with a paraquat solution as a result of which he developed a necrotic ulcer on the undersurface of his scrotum. The paraquat had been diluted as recommended, but the facts that he had worn the wet trousers for more than an hour in the heat of a summer day and that his clothes caused a certain amount of chafing, were thought to have contributed to the reaction.

Patch testing
? concentration.

Damage with softening and discolouration of the finger nails, particularly at the base, was described in three patients by Samman and Johnston (1969). Each man handled the weed killer as part of his work, one being a forester, one a farmer and the other a market gardener. The damage occurred only when there was contact with the concentrated chemical. A more recent paper (Hearn and Keir, 1971) described similar damage to 55 of 296 spray operators who used diluted paraquat on a sugar estate in Trinidad. It was stressed that the degree of contamination of the nails had been gross, and that simple precautions could have prevented it. On cessation of contact, the nails returned to normal.

Insecticides

Inorganic arsenicals are amongst the oldest insecticides but are being replaced by newer chemicals. Sodium fluoride may be used when insects become resistant to chlordane and DDT. Nicotinoids are powerful insecticides, but their use is limited by their toxicity to the nervous system of man and animals.

It has been shown that some insecticides, such as chlordane and dieldrin, may persist on the skin for months or even years after the last exposure (Kazen *et al.*, 1974).

1. PYRETHROIDS

Pyrethrums, which are derived from *Chrysanthemum cinerariaefolium* and *Chrysanthemum coccineum*, act by paralysing insects. Their properties as insecticides depend upon the presence of five esters: pyrethrins I and II, cinerins I and II and jasmoline II, the concentrations of which vary in different strains. Similar chemicals, such as Allethrin, have been prepared synthetically.

When R = CH₃ and R¹ = CH₂CH = CH₂, this becomes
Allethrin ≡ (2,2-dimethyl-3-(2-methylpropenyl)cyclopropane carboxylic acid ester with 2-allyl-4-hydroxy-3-methyl-2-cyclopenten-1-one.

Pyrethrum is widely used in household sprays, in which it is often combined with other chemicals to potentiate its insecticidal properties. The pyrethrums are effective against many household pests including flies and mosquitoes; their low mammalian toxicity makes them safe for use in the home.

Episodes of dermatitis among growers of pyrethrum flowers and those who came into contact with the powdered plants were reported from Kenya by Sequeira (1936). Pyrethrum was used in Copenhagen and Lund to test routinely eczematous patients; it was reported that between 1–2 per cent reacted (Magnusson, 1968). However, it was subsequently omitted from their standard series as there were no reactions in 120 patients (Fregert and Hjorth, 1969).

Patch testing
Pyrethrum 2 per cent in petrolatum.

2. ORGANOTHIOCYANATES

Rodannitrobenzene: 1-Rodan-2,4-dinitrobenzene

These chemicals are sometimes used in preference to pyrethrum in household insecticides.

A man, who a year previously had had a mild dermatitis from this chemical, handled it for just one day and developed a severe contact dermatitis of his hands, arms and face. On patch testing he reacted to rodannitrobenzene 1 per cent in petrolatum, PPD, *p*-aminobenzene and his rubber gloves (Fregert, 1967).

Patch testing
Rodannitrobenzene 1 per cent in petrolatum.

3. DDT (1,1,1-Trichloro-2,2-bis(*p*-chlorophenyl)ethane; dichlorodiphenyl-trichloroethane)

$$Cl-\langle\bigcirc\rangle-\underset{\underset{CCl_3}{|}}{CH}-\langle\bigcirc\rangle-Cl$$

For years DDT has been used as an insecticide particularly in the control of malaria, but it is not easily broken down and persists in the soil and on foliage. DDT is a peripheral nerve poison, which is soluble in fat and is stored in the fat depots of the body; normally exposure is from eating contaminated food, principally animal foods. Absorption from the skin only occurs when it is in an oily base, not when it is applied topically in powder form as in the control of lice. Once absorbed it is metabolised in the liver to less harmful derivatives. In general, toxic side effects have not occurred in workers handling DDT nor have they been reported from the usual environmental exposure (Upholt and Kearney, 1966). However, resistant strains of insects are beginning to emerge, and recent reports of its possible carcinogenic effects in animals have received much publicity, although they have not yet been substantiated. Concern is felt about the persistence of DDT in the environment and its use may be restricted.

Sensitisation has been reported in cotton workers in whom it caused dermatitis of the face, neck, chest and hands. The allergy was diagnosed on the basis of positive patch tests to 3 per cent DDT. These workers were also handling benzene hexachloride (Mirakhmedov and Karimov, 1972).

DDT 1 per cent in petrolatum was used by members of the International Contact Dermatitis Research Group to patch test 655 routine eczematous patients; there were no positive reactions.

Patch testing
DDT 1 per cent in petrolatum.

4. DD

$$Cl\ CH_2\ CH = CHCl$$

1,3-Dichloropropene

DD is a highly toxic mixture of chlorinated 3C hydrocarbons including 1,3-dichloropropene, 1,2-dichloropropane and related compounds. It also contains 1 per cent epichlorhydrin. It is ploughed into the soil to control worms and is used extensively in Holland to protect potato crops. If farmers inadvertently drip it onto their shoes during spraying it causes a vesicular dermatitis of the feet. Two farmers who started with an eruption on their feet and then with subsequent contact with DD developed a more widespread eruption were investigated by Nater and Gooskens (1976); they also had a third patient, who sprayed pesticides and each year developed a rash when exposed to DD. Patch tests with DD 1 per cent in acetone and 1,3-dichloropropene 1 per cent in acetone were positive in one farmer and negative in the other two patients; all three were negative to 1,2-dichloropropane. They concluded that DD, although usually causing an irritant dermatitis, can also occasionally sensitise.

Patch testing
DD 1 per cent in acetone
1,3-dichloropropene 1 per cent in acetone
1,2-dichloropropane 1 per cent in acetone.

5. LINDANE: (1,2,3,4,5,6-Hexachlorocyclohexane; HCC)

This is the active constituent of γ-benzene hexachloride (BHC; Gammexane; Lorexane) and is effective against mites and insects. The toxoicity of γ-benzene hexachloride has been reviewed by Solomon, Fahrner and West (1977), and by Solomon *et al.* (1977) who studied its deposition in the brains of guinea-pigs after topical application.

An allergic contact dermatitis affecting a plant protection guard, a pest controller and 12 workers in a factory making pesticides containing hexachlorocyclohexane (HCH) was investigated by Behrbohm and Brandt (1960). The dermatitis was attributed to contaminants present in both technical and purified HCH. Sensitisation of those exposed to HCH was confirmed by Hegyi and St'ota (1965), who found that delta-heptachlorocyclohexane had the most marked sensitising potential and elicited the most severe reactions.

Lindane 1 per cent in petrolatum was tested on 655 routine eczematous patients by members of the International Contact Dermatitis Research Group; there were no positive reactions.

Patch testing
Lindane 1 per cent in petrolatum.

6. CYCLODIENES

Aldrin and dieldrin belong to this group; they act on the ganglia of the central nervous system and cause death with violent convulsions.

Dieldrin: 1,2,3,4,10,10-Hexachloro-6,7-epoxy-1,4,4a,5,6,7,8,8a-octahydro-endo-exo 1,4:5,8-dimethanonaphthalene)

Despite its potency, the use of this chemical is limited by its toxicity; like DDT it accumulates in animal fat and is excreted in milk.

Patch testing
? concentration.

7. ORGANOPHOSPHORUS COMPOUNDS

About forty of these highly successful insecticides are commercially available. They inactivate cholinesterase at the myoneural junctions and also in the parasympathetic system and as a result cause death from respiratory failure. They are readily absorbed from the gut, respiratory tract and skin and are extremely toxic to warm-blooded animals and to man (Upholt and Kearney, 1966). The incidence of poisoning and injury from pesticides, including organophosphates, has been analysed by Hearn (1973), and their potential for causing dermatitis has been reviewed by Rycroft (1977).

Other metabolic effects of the organophosphorus compounds have made them effective herbicides and fungicides (e.g. Plondrel p. 402).

Parathion: (*O,O*-Diethyl *O-p*-nitrophenyl phosphorothioate)

This is an extremely toxic chemical. When using it the greatest care must be taken, including the wearing of protective clothing, as it is absorbed through the skin. A woman used a methyl parathion spray to kill bed bugs and a few hours later developed erythema multiforme. A nasal challenge reproduced the lesions (Bhargava, Singh and Soni (1977).

Patch testing
? concentration.

(Open test 1 per cent in alcohol.)

Malathion: (S-(1,2-Dicarbethoxyethyl)O,O-dimethyldithiophosphate)

$$
\begin{array}{c}
CH_3O \\
 \searrow \overset{\displaystyle S}{\underset{}{\parallel}} \\
\quad P-SCHCOOC_2H_5 \\
CH_3O \nearrow \qquad \mid \\
CH_2COOC_2H_5
\end{array}
$$

This compound inhibits cholinesterase in insects, but, being rapidly detoxified in man and vertebrates, it is much less toxic than other members of the group (Upholt and Kearney, 1966). It is safe for use in the home and garden.

Cases presenting with contact dermatitis have not been reported, but its sensitising potential has been investigated in human volunteers. Milby and Epstein (1964) found that 10 per cent Malathion sensitised half their subjects, whereas at a concentration of 1 per cent or less it sensitised only a third. Using 1 per cent technical Malathion, they patch tested 200 workers exposed occupationally to the chemical; six (3 per cent) reacted. Five of these six gave histories of unexplained episodes of dermatitis, but in none had the Malathion been suspected as the cause and none had had to change his job. Kligman (1966) confirmed that it was a potent sensitiser and he accounted for the lack of clinical cases of dermatitis by the low concentration (usually about 1 per cent) which is used, and by the transient skin contact.

It was suggested to Milby and Epstein (1964) that a contaminant, diethyl fumarate, might be the sensitiser, and when tested their subjects reacted to this chemical, as did those of Kligman (1966). This finding led to a reduction in the concentration of diethyl fumarate in technical Malathion, and lessened the allergenic hazard of this pesticide.

Malathion 0.5 per cent in petrolatum was used to test 455 routine eczematous patients by members of the International Contact Dermatitis Research Group; there was one (unexplained) positive reaction.

Patch testing
Malathion 0.5 per cent in petrolatum.

Naled: (Dimethyl-1,2-dibromo-2,2-dichloroethyl phosphate; Dibrom)

$$
\begin{array}{c}
CH_3O \\
\searrow \quad \nearrow^{\displaystyle O} \qquad Br\ Br \\
P \qquad \qquad \mid\ \ \mid \\
\nearrow \quad \searrow O-C-C-Cl \\
CH_3O \qquad\qquad\qquad \mid\ \ \mid \\
H\ \ H
\end{array}
$$

This is a less frequently used member of the organo-phosphorus group of insecticides; the bromine in the molecule makes it less toxic than parathion, but it is not as safe as Malathion.

In the United States of America, four women employed in the cutting of unflowered chrysanthemum plants developed dermatitis mainly of the face, neck, hands and arms. The plants had been sprayed, two hours prior to cutting, with a mixture of Naled, Captan and Dicofal and were probably still wet; this mixture had been used many times previously. All four women were tested with each ingredient of the spray; the tests with Naled 60 per cent in xylene were positive in three cases, but those with the other constituents were negative in all four cases. Naled is broken down by hydrolysis, and, provided several hours were allowed to elapse between using this spray and handling the plants, the women could continue working (Edmundson and Davies, 1967).

Patch testing
? concentration.

8. CARBAMATES

Methyl carbamates are weak cholinesterase inhibitors; they are more toxic than the phenyl carbamates which are used as herbicides. Carbaryl (1-naphthyl *N*-methylcarbamate) is considered one of the safest pesticides; it is known to contaminate the skin of spraymen and plant workers without apparent hazard (Comer *et al.*, 1975).

9. OMITE: (2-(*p-tert*-Butylphenoxy)-cyclohexyl 2-propynyl sulphite; BPPS)

This miticide was used on orange trees by 47 Japanese farmers; forty developed an irritant dermatitis and 43 had symptoms of systemic toxicity. In one man an allergic contact dermatitis was suspected because his rash flared up ten days after the initial eruption. Three control subjects gave irritant patch test responses to 0.05 per cent BPPS (Nishioka, Kozuka and Tashiro, 1970).

Patch testing
? concentration.

10. DAZOMET: (3, 5-Dimethyl-1,3,5,2H-tetrahydrothiadiazine-2-thione; Mylone®)

This compound is used as a nematocide, soil fumigant and weed-killer.

While preparing a diluted solution of Dazomet for flushing through water pipes as an algicide, a factory worker spilt the concentrated chemical on his arm. Despite washing immediately, he developed, two to three days later, an acute vesicular dermatitis. He had a positive patch test to 0.25 per cent Dazomet in water (Black, 1973).

A tomato grower repeatedly spread granules of Dazomet onto the soil and then hoed them in. On the last occasion he also injected chloropicrin and while doing so one foot began to burn. As he found granules of Dazomet in his boots, he washed his feet and legs. Two days later he had a livid, bullous dermatitis of his feet, legs and hands, which spread to other areas. Patch tests with Dazomet in approximate concentrations of 0.25 per cent and 0.125 per cent and an open test with 0.5 per cent were all positive.

It is relevant that the patient had a past history of a reaction to formalin, because Dazomet hydrolyses to formalin.

Positive patch tests to chloropicrin 0.5 per cent and 0.25 per cent in water may have been false positives and sensitisation to this chemical was not established. (Chloropicrin is trichloronitromethane (nitrochloroform; CCl_3NO_3).)

Patch testing
Dazomet ? 0.25 per cent in water
Chloropicrin ? 0.25 per cent in water.

Rodenticides

These compounds are used to kill mice, rats and squirrels, and many, such as thallium sulphate, strychnine and arsenic, are extremely toxic.

Warfarin: (3-(α-Acetonylbenzyl)-4-hydroxycoumarin)

This anticoagulant prevents the formation of prothrombin, and it is widely used as a rodenticide; the animals die of exhaustion from widespread haemorrhages.

Patch testing
Warfarin ? 0.05 per cent in petrolatum.

Antu: (1-(1-Naphthyl)-2-thiourea)

This compound is widely used in the control of rats.

An occupational contact dermatitis from this chemical as an ingredient of a rat poison was reported by Laubstein (1962). The patient reacted when patch tested with Antirax A 10 per cent in vaseline.

Patch testing
Naphthyl thiourea 1 per cent and 2 per cent in petrolatum.

References

Adams, R.M., Zimmerman, M.C., Bartlett, J.B. & Preston J.F. (1971) 1-chloro-2,4-dinitrobenzene as an algicide. *Archives of Dermatology*, **103**, 191.

Baran, R.L. (1974) Nail damage caused by weed killers and insecticides. *Archives of Dermatology*, **110**, 467.

Behrbohm, P. & Brandt, B. (1960) Allergisches Kontaktekzem durch technische und gereinigte Hexachlorcyclohexanpräparate bei der Anwendung im Pflanzenschutz und in der Schädlingsbekämpfung. *Berufsdermatosen*, **8**, 95.

Bernstein, M.J. (1912) A dermatitis caused by 'di-nitro-chlorbenzole'. *Lancet*, **1**, 1534.

Bhargava, R.K., Singh, V. & Soni, V. (1977) Erythema multiforme resulting from insecticide spray. *Archives of Dermatology*, **113**, 686.

Black, H. (1973) Dazomet and chloropicrin. *Contact Dermatitis Newsletter*, **14**, 410.

Brancaccio, R.R. & Chamales, M.H. (1977) Contact dermatitis and depigmentation produced by the herbicide Carbyne®. *Contact Dermatitis*, **3**, 108.

Burry, J.N. (1976) Contact dermatitis from agricultural fungicide in South Australia. *Contact Dermatitis*, **2**, 289.

Calnan, C.D. (1969) Dithianone sensitivity. *Contact Dermatitis Newsletter*, **6**, 119.

Camarasa, G. (1975) Difolatan dermatitis. *Contact Dermatitis*, **1**, 127.

Comer, S.W., Staiff, D.C., Armstrong, J.F. & Wolfe, H.R. (1975) Exposure of workers to carbaryl. *Bulletin of Environmental Contamination and Toxicology*, **13**, 385.

Cottel, W.I. (1972) Difolatan. *Contact Dermatitis Newsletter*, **11**, 252.

Edmundson, W.F. & Davies, J.E. (1967) Occupational dermatitis from naled. *Archives of Environmental Health*, **15**, 89.

Fregert, S. (1967) Allergic contact dermatitis from the pesticide rodannitrobenzene. *Contact Dermatitis Newsletter*, **2**, 4.

Fregert, S. (1967) Allergic contact dermatitis from the pesticides captan and phaltan. *Contact Dermatitis Newsletter*, **2**, 28.

Fregert, S. (1968) Allergic contact dermatitis from p-chloro-o-cresol in a pesticide. *Contact Dermatitis Newsletter*, **3**, 46.

Fregert, S. (1973) Allergic contact dermatitis from two pesticides. *Contact Dermatitis Newsletter*, **13**, 367.

Fregert, S. & Hjorth, N. (1969) Results of standard patch test with substances abandoned. *Contact Dermatitis Newsletter*, **5**, 85.

Gammeltoft, M. (1978) Tributyltinoxide is not allergenic. *Contact Dermatitis*, **4**, 238.

Groundwater, J.R. (1977) Difolatan dermatitis in a welder: non-agricultural exposure. *Contact Dermatitis*, **3**, 104.

Hearn, C.E.D. (1973) A review of agricultural pesticide incidents in man in England and Wales, 1952–71. *British Journal of Industrial Medicine*, **30**, 253.

Hearn, C.E.D. & Keir, W. (1971) Nail damage in spray operators exposed to paraquat. *British Journal of Industrial Medicine*, **28**, 399.

Hegyi, E. & St'ota, Z. (1965) Zur Frage der Allergen-spezifizitat der Komponenten des technischen Hexachlorzyklohexans. *Berufsdermatosen*, **13**, 193.

Jaroš, F. (1978) Acute percutaneous paraquat poisoning. *Lancet*, **i**, 275.

Kazen, C., Bloomer, A., Welch, R., Oudbier, A. & Price, H. (1974) Persistence of pesticides on the hands of some occupationally exposed people. *Archives of Environmental Health*, **29**, 315.

Ketel, W.G. van (1975) Allergic dermatitis from a new pesticide. *Contact Dermatitis*, **1**, 297.

Ketel, W.G. van (1976) Sensitivity to the pesticide benomyl. *Contact Dermatitis*, **2**, 290.

Ketel, W.G. van (1977) Active sensitisation by o.o.diethyl-phtalimido-phosphotioate (Plondrel). *Contact Dermatitis*, **3**, 51.

Kligman, A. (1966) The identification of contact allergens by human assay: III. The maximisation test: A procedure for screening and rating contact sensitisers. *Journal of Investigative Dermatology*, **47**, 393.

Laborie, F. & Laborie, R. & Dedieu, E.H. (1964) Allergie aux fongicides de la gamme due menébe et du zinébe. *Archives des Maladies Professionnelles de Médecine du Travail et de Sécurité Sociale*, **25**, 419.

Laubstein, H. (1962) Kontaktekzem durch ein Rodentizid. *Berfusdermatosen*, **10**, 154.

Magnusson, B., Blohm, S.-V., Fregert, S., Hjorth, N., Høvding, G., Pirilä, V. & Skog, E. (1968) Routine patch testing IV. *Acta Dermato-venereologica*, **48**, 110.

Malten, K.E. (1974) DNCB in cooling water. *Contact Dermatitis Newsletter*, **15**, 466.

Marderosian, A.H. (1970) *Pesticides in Remington's Pharmaceutical Sciences*. Pennsylvania: Mack Publishing.

Marzulli, F.N. & Maibach, H.I. (1973) Antimicrobials: Experimental contact sensitisation in man. *Journal of the Society of Cosmetic Chemists*, **24**, 399.

Matsushita, T., Arimatsu, Y. & Nomura, S. (1976) Experimental study on contact dermatitis caused by dithiocarbamates maneb, mancozeb, zineb and their related compounds. *International Archives of Occupational and Environmental Health*, **37**, 169.

Milby, T.H. & Epstein, W.L. (1964) Allergic contact sensitivity to malathion. *Archives of Environmental Health*, **9**, 434.

Mirakhmedov, U.M. & Karimov, A.M. (1972) The effect of pesticides on the skin of agricultural workers. *Vestnik dermatologii i venereologii*, **46**, 50.

Nater, J.P. & Gooskens, V.H.J. (1976) Occupational dermatitis due to a soil fumigant. *Contact Dermatoses*, **2**, 227.

Nater, J.P., Terpstra, H. & Bleumink E. (1979) Allergic contact sensitisation to the fungicide Maneb. *Contact Dermatitis*, **5**, 24.

Newhouse, M., McEvoy, D. & Rosenthal, D. (1978) Percutaneous paraquat absorption. *Archives of Dermatology*, **114**, 1516.

Nishioka, K., Kozuka, T. & Tashiro, M. (1970) Agricultural miticide (BPPS) dermatitis. *Skin Research*, **12**, 15.

Rycroft, R.J.G. (1977) Contact dermatitis from organophosphorus pesticides. *British Journal of Dermatology*, **97**, 693.

Samman, P.D. & Johnston, E.N.M. (1969) Nail damage associated with handling paraquat and diquat. *British Medical Journal*, **1**, 818.

Savitt, L.E. (1972) Contact dermatitis due to benomyl insecticide. *Archives of Dermatology*, **105**, 926.

Scarpa, C. & Ippolito, F. (1959) La dermatite da ditiocarbammati, nuova entitá clinica. *Dermatologica*, *Napoli*, **10**, 257.

Schulz, K.H. & Herrmann, W.P. (1958) Tetramethylthiuramdisulphide, ein Thioharnstoffderivat als Ekzemnoxe bei Hafenarbeitern. *Berufsdermatosen*, **6**, 130.

Sequeira, J.H. (1936) Pyrethrum dermatitis. *British Journal of Dermatology*, **48**, 473.

Sharvill, D.E. (1971) Reaction to paraquat. *Contact Dermatitis Newsletter*, **9**, 210.

Shelley, W.B. (1964) Golf course dermatitis due to thiram fungicide. *Journal of the American Medical Association*, **188**, 415.

Solomon, L.M., Fahrner, L. & West, D.P. (1977) Gamma benzene hexachloride toxicity. *Archives of Dermatology*, **113**, 353.

Solomon, L.M., West, D.P., Fitzloff, J.F. & Becker, A.M. (1977) Gamma benzene hexachloride in guinea pig brain after topical application. *Journal of Investigative Dermatology*, **68**, 310.

Solomons, B. (1972) Sensitisation to nitrofen. *Contact Dermatitis Newsletter*, **12**, 336.

Spencer, M.C. (1966) Herbicide dermatitis. *Journal of the American Medical Association*, **198**, 1307.

Takamatsu, M., Futatsuka, M., Arimatsu, Y., Maeda, H., Inuzuka, T. & Takamatsu, S. (1968) Epidemiologic survey on dermatitis from a new fungicide used in tangerine orchards in kumamoto prefecture. *Journal of the Kumamato Medical Society*, **42**, 854.

Upholt, W.M. & Kearney, P.C. (1966) Pesticides. *New England Journal of Medicine*, **275**, 1419.

Wahlberg, J.E. (1974) Yellow staining of hair and nails and contact sensitivity to dinobuton. *Contact Dermatitis Newsletter*, **16**, 481.

White-stevens, R. (ed.) (1971) *Pesticides in the Environment*, vol. 1, part 1. New York: Marcel Dekker.

Zimmerman, M.C. (1970) Dinitrochlorobenzene in water systems. *Contact Dermatitis Newsletter*, **7**, 165.

9.

Photosensitisers

PHOTOTOXIC

TOPICAL
  Pitch and coal tar
  Furocoumarins
    Dermatitis bullosa striata pratensis
    Berloque dermatitis
  Dyes
    Neutral Red
    Disperse Blue 35
  Various chemicals — experimental
    Bithionol
    Tetrachlorosalicylanilide
    Tribromosalicylanilide
    8-Methoxypsoralen
SYSTEMIC
  Drugs
    Tetracyclines
    Demethylchlortetracycline (Declomycin;
    Ledermycin)
    Chlortetracycline (Aureomycin)
    Doxycycline (Vibramycin)
    Oxytetracycline (Terramycin)
    Tetracycline (Achromycin)
      Photo-onycholysis
    Chlorpromazine (Largactil)
    Contraceptives — oral — oestrogens
    Frusemide (Lasix)
    Griseofulvin (Grisovin)
    Nalidixic Acid (Negram)
    Vinblastine
  Porphyrins
  Furocoumarins

PHOTOALLERGIC

TOPICAL
  Halogenated Phenols
    Tetrachlorosalicylanilide (TCS)
    Tribomosalicylanilide (TBS)
    Dibromosalicylanilide (DBS)
    Bromochlorosalicylanilide (Multifungin)
    Trichlorcarbanilide (TCC)
    Bithionol
    Fentichlor
    Hexachlorophene
      Buclosamide (Jadit)
    Chlorophenylphenol

Drugs
  Phenothiazines
    Promethazine hydrochloride (Phenergan)
    Chlorpromazine hydrochloride (Largactil)
  Sulphonamides
  Diphenhydramine hydrochloride (Benadryl)
  Quinine

Various chemicals
  Moquizone
  Quindoxin (Grofas)
  Thiourea
  Perfumes

Results of Photopatch testing

SYSTEMIC
  Drugs
    Promethazine hydrochloride (Phenergan)
    Thioridazine (Melleril)
    Trimeprazine tartrate (Vallergan)
    Chlorothiazide (Saluric)
    Hydrochlorothiazide (Hydrosaluric)
    Frusemide (Lasix)
    Quinethazone (Aquamox)
    Chlorpropamide (Diabinese)
    Carbutamide (Nadisan)
    Tolbutamide (Orinase; Rastinon)
    Amantadine hydrochloride (Symmetrel)
    Chlordiazepoxide hydrochloride (Librium)
    Cyclamate sodium
    Pyrithioxin (Encephabol)
    Triacetyldiphenolisation (Laxagen)
    8-Methoxypsoralen

PHOTOTOXIC AND PHOTOALLERGIC

SYSTEMIC
  Drugs
    Quinidine
    Sulphanilamide

SUNSCREENS
  Short wave ultraviolet light
  Long wage ultraviolet light
  Adverse reactions
    Para-aminobenzoic acid — contact
                                dermatitis

SUNSCREENS (ctd)

Isoamyl-*p-N,N*-dimethylaminobenzoate
(Spectraban)

      — immediate
        discomfort
      — contact
        dermatitis

α-Glyceryl *p*-aminobenzoate (Escalol 106)
      — photoallergy

Mexenone   — contact
             dermatitis

Sulisobenzone — contact
             dermatitis

Cinnamate   — contact
             dermatitis

Introduction

The term photosensitivity is a general one, used to describe any eruption caused by light: it does not inply an allergic mechanism. When the pathogenesis of the reaction is known the dermatitis can be identified as phototoxic, or photoallergic.

It is often difficult to deduce from the literature whether reactions to a compound should be designated as phototoxic or photoallergic. In the following account, chemicals have been classified according to what seems to be the general consensus of opinion. Many chemicals are probably both phototoxins and photoallergens.

The pathogenesis of drug-induced photosensitivity has been reviewed by Levene and Magnus (1969), Harber and Baer (1972), Jarratt (1976) and Magnus (1976). Photoallergy was reviewed by Epstein (1977 and Frain-Bell, 1979).

The light spectrum can be divided simply as follows:

UV-C	UV-B	UV-A		
	Short wave ultraviolet	Long wave ultraviolet	Visible light	Infra red
	Sunburn spectrum			
280 nm	290–320 nm	320–400 nm	380–770 nm	700$^+$ nm

The action spectrum of a photosensitiser consists of those wavelenght(s) which elicit the clinical reaction *in vivo*; it usually but not always coincides with the absorption spectrum of the compound, which is an *in vitro* estimation. The photosensitisers whose action spectra have been determined are listed below. The details of the investigations from which these data have been culled are given in the following chapters.

	Action spectrum (nm)
Phototoxic — Topical	
Pitch and coal tar	340–430
Furocoumarins	330–360
Neutral red	?
Disperse blue 35	400–700
Halogenated phenols	LUV*

*LUV = long wave ultraviolet (320–400 nm)

	Action spectrum (nm)
Phototoxic — Systemic	
Demethylchlortetracycline	290–320
Lichenoid eruption	310$^+$
Oxytetracycline	290–320
	340–380
Oestrogen	320$^+$
Nalidixic acid	LUV
Experimental intradermal tests	320–400
Porphyrins	400–410
Furocoumarins	LUV
Photoallergic — Topical	
Halogenated phenols	LUV
Quindoxin	LUV
Diphenhydramine (Benadryl)	290–320
Quinine	300–400
Photoallergic — Systemic	
Chlorothiazide	275–310
Quinethazone	290–320
Amantadine hydrochloride	320–400
Cyclamate	?295–400$^+$
Promethazine hydrochloride (Phenergan)	LUV
Quinidine	LUV

It is of interest to compare the action spectra of the following photodermatoses (Magnus, 1974) in which the sunburn spectrum rather than light of longer wave lengths is the critical factor.

Polymorphic light eruption:	290–310 nm (occasionally LUV*)
Hutchinson's summer prurigo:	50 per cent = 290–310 nm (occasionally LUV)
	50 per cent = have normal light tests
Photosensitive eczema:	290–310 nm (occasionally LUV)
Hydroa vacciniforme:	290–310 nm (occasionally LUV)
	some have normal light tests
Actinic reticuloid:	250–400 or up to 500 nm

*LUV = long wave ultraviolet (320–400 nm)

Persistent light reactor
The term persistent light reactor refers to the distressing clinical condition in which there is continued light sensitivity after all known contact with the precipitating factors has ceased.

It appears to be triggered by an episode of allergic photocontact dermatitis induced by a topical photosensitiser. Halogenated phenols have been principally responsible, but promethazine and quinoxaline (Quindoxin) have had the same effect.

Systemically administered drugs such as nalidixic acid may induce light sensitivity lasting as long as a year, but not indefinitely.

Photosensitive eczema
Photosensitivity, often unrecognised, may be superimposed on an established eczema. In Ramsay and Kobza Black's series (1973), the 16 patients were men,

and most were over 50 years old. All were sensitive to the sunburn spectrum and three also to 340 nm. No cause was found, but the use of sunscreens was therapeutically helpful.

Methods of phototesting

The methods of demonstrating photosensitivity differ fundamentally for phototoxic and photoallergic reactions. Basically they can be summarised as:

Phototoxicity
  (i) may require intradermal injection, stripping or occlusion of the skin
 (ii) light exposure must be immediate (i.e. within 0–2 hours of effective skin absorption)
(iii) read early (within several hours)
(iv) oral challenge — large does for several days.

Photoallergy
  (i) epicutaneous, as for a patch test
 (ii) light exposure after 1–2 days
(iii) read after another 1–2 days
(iv) oral challenge — ? single dose.

Phototoxic

1. TOPICAL

Certain compounds are phototoxic on topical application; they can be divided into four groups:
1. Pitch and coal tar
2. Furocoumarins
3. Dyes
4. Various Chemicals.

1. Pitch and coal tar

White workers exposed to pitch may develop an abnormal susceptibility to sunlight which is popularly known as the 'smarts. A parallel photophobia may be present. There is a latent period of two or more weeks between the first exposure to pitch and the onset of symptoms. The summer sun then causes smarting and burning of the exposed skin which is usually, but not always, followed by erythema. The discomfort begins 15 minutes after sun exposure and disappears after one to four hours in the shade. Glass does not protect against it. In most cases the symptoms clear in the winter. Pitch impregnates and darkens the skin of those who work with it, but once contact ceases the skin gradually lightens and the susceptibility to sunburn is lost.

This photodermatitis has been well described and was investigated with a monochromator by Crow *et al.* (1961). In one worker and three controls the action spectrum of pitch was found to be 340–430 nm. The photoreaction caused smarting and was followed generally by an urticarial weal but sometimes by erythema; occasionally there was no visible change. The reaction was thought to be photodynamic ($\equiv$ phototoxic).

Coal tar

The phototoxicity of coal tars was found by Kaidbey and Kligman (1977) to diminish with their refinement and the least active of the tars studied was liquor carbonis detergens. Long ultraviolet light (UV-A) elicited the reaction which occurred in two stages, an immediate weal and burning being followed in one to two days by a red infiltrated plaque. Post inflammatory pigmentation was quite persistent. Tar photosensitisers include anthracene, fluoranthene, phenanthrene, benzpyrine and acridine. Vegetable and bituminous tars are not phototoxic.

2. Furocoumarins

Furocoumarins increase the skin's susceptibility to sunlight, causing an exaggerated sunburn reaction and subsequent pigmentation. They can be applied topically or given systemically. Certain isomers of the furocoumarins are called psoralens. Interesting accounts of these compounds are given by Pathak, Krämer and Fitzpatrick (1974), and Musajo *et al.* (1974).

Furocoumarins occur naturally in some plant families and they are also synthesised. They are condensation products of a furan ring and a coumarin.

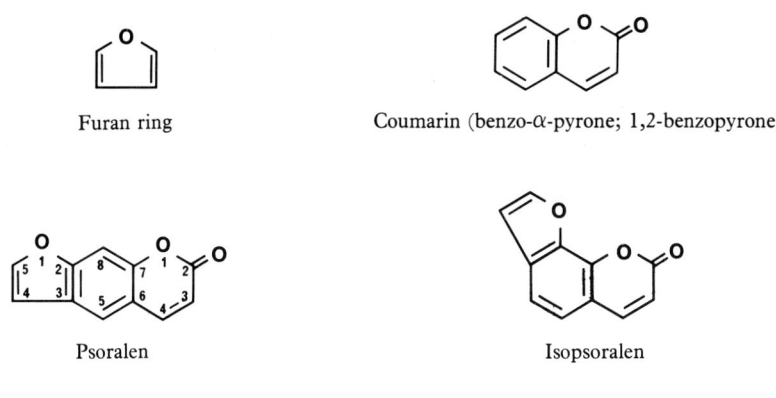

Furan ring   Coumarin (benzo-α-pyrone; 1,2-benzopyrone)

Psoralen   Isopsoralen

There are many isomers of the furocoumarins but only those with a linear structure resembling psoralen are photoactive. An angular configuration, as in isopsoralen, or substitution at the 3 position, destroys the photoactivity of the compound, probably by interfering with the binding sites of the molecule.

Twenty-eight different furocoumarins are known to occur naturally and of these psoralen, 8-methoxypsoralen (xanthotoxin, methoxsalen) and 5-methoxypsoralen are particularly photoactive in the skin.

8-Methoxypsoralen   5-Methoxypsoralen

Trisoralen (4, 5′, 8-trimethylpsoralen) is made synthetically and is very photoactive.

4,5′,8-Trimethylpsoralen

It has been shown that, on exposure to long wave ultraviolet light, active psoralens form photoadducts with the pyrimidine bases, cytosine, uracil and thymine, of the DNA molecule. The energy emitted by the complex damages the DNA segment. The reaction does not require oxygen.

The absorption spectrum of psoralens is 210–330 nm, but it changes, as does the action spectrum, to the long wave ultraviolet range, with a peak at 330–350 nm once the drug is complexed with DNA.

Normal skin burns when exposed to short wave ultraviolet light (290–320 nm) but is unharmed by environmental long wave (320–360 nm); the presence of psoralens makes the skin susceptible to these longer wavelengths. The inflammatory photoreaction caused by these compounds in the skin comprises erythema and scaling, followed by acanthosis, hyperpigmentation and an increase in the number and activity of the melanocytes. The severity of the reaction depends upon the concentration of psoralen in the skin, its potency, and the dose of active irradiction. Without light, psoralens in the skin are harmless.

Phytophotodermatitis

Phytophotodermatitis occurs from plants containing psoralens, most of these naturally occurring psoralens are found in the following four plant families:

1. Umbelliferae (*Ammi majus* L., carrot, celery, dill, fennel, parsley, parsnip)
2. Rutaceae   (bergamot, citrus fruit, gas plant, lime, rue, *Xanthoxylum flavum*)
3. Leguminosae (Bavachi or *Psoralea corylifolia*, *Coronilla* species)
4. Moraceae   (figs, other *Ficus* species).

There are two clinical patterns of plant photodermatitis:

1. Dermatitis bullosa striata pratensis from direct contact with plants
2. Berloque (berlock) dermatitis from bergamot perfumes.

Dermatitis bullosa striata pratensis

The name dermatitis bullosa striata pratensis was coined by Oppenheim in the 1920s to describe an eruption which occurred after sunbathing on grass. The patient presents with an acute red streaky eruption, which is often bullous, on sites where there has been contact with plants and exposure to the sun. The skin heals with a marked pigmentation which reproduces the pattern of the original dermatitis.

The common plants reputed to cause phytophotodermatitis have been listed by Pathak, Daniels and Fitzpatrick (1962), Pathak (1974) and Woods (1962). In an historical review of irritant plants, Woods (1962) also described those plants which are direct skin irritants and discussed the extraneous factors which can simulate a plant dermatitis.

The causes of phytophotodermatitis will vary with the local flora. In Britain, frequently responsible, are the wild parsnip and *Anthriscus*, and the *Heracleum* species are also quite common causes in much of the country when the weather conditions are appropriate. Rue (*Ruta graveolens*) is a very popular garden shrub, particularly in the variety known as 'Jackmans' blue' and it too causes phytophotodermatitis. Giant hogweed (*Heracleum mantegazzianum*) (Umbelliferae) grows throughout the northern temperate zone, and dermatitis has been reported in Scotland, especially amongst children (Drever and Hunter, 1970), and in Vancouver, after seeing five children and a man who had developed dermatitis from cutting this plant down, Camm, Buck and Mitchell (1976) wrote an interesting and comprehensive account of *H. mantegazzianum*. They photopatch tested three normal controls by applying juice from the plant's stem to two sites on their backs and after two hours one site was occluded with black plastic and the other irradiated with long wave ultraviolet light for 20 minutes. At two days the irradiated sites were red and indurated while the control areas remained normal. In Germany, a common source is cow parsnip (*Heracleum sphondylium*) (Umbelliferae), where it caused dermatitis in 58 soldiers after they did exercises in an open field (Quadripur and Gründer, 1975). In the New England States, the gas plant (*Dicatamnus albus*) (Rutaceae), or wild parsnip, (*Pastinaca sativa*) (Umbelliferae) are likely to be responsible (Sommer and Jillson, 1967).

A thesis on celery dermatitis has been written by Riboulleau (1970).

Table 9.1. Common plants implicated in causing phytophotodermatitis (adapted from Pathak, 1974)

Common name	Botanical name	Family
Lime	*Citrus aurantiifolia*	Rutaceae
Citron	*Citrus medica (C. acida)*	Rutaceae
Sour (Seville) orange	*Citrus aurantium*	Rutaceae
Bergamot	*Citrus aurantium* var. *bergamia*	Rutaceae
Lemon	*Citrus limon*	Rutaceae
Gas plant, burning bush	*Dictamnus alba (D. fraxinella)*	Rutaceae
Common rue	*Ruta graveolens*	Rutaceae
	Phebalium argenteum	Rutaceae
Wild beaked parsley (wild chervil)	*Anthriscus sylvestris*	Umbelliferae
Common beaked parsley	*Anthriscus vulgaris*	Umbelliferae
Celery	*Apium graveolens*	Umbelliferae
Giant hogweed	*Heracleum mantegazzianum*	Umbelliferae
	Heracleum maximum (*H. dulce*)	Umbelliferae
Parsnip (wild variety)	*Pastinaca sativa* (*P. urens*)	Umbelliferae
Cow parsnip; hogweed	*Heracleum sphondylium*	Umbelliferae
Fennel	*Foeniculum vulgare*	Umbelliferae
Dill	*Anethum graveolens*	Umbelliferae
	Peucedanum oreoselium	Umbelliferae

Common name	Botanical name	Family
Wild carrot, (garden carrot)	*Daucus carota (sativa)*	Umbelliferae
Masterwort	*Peucedanum ostruthium*	Umbelliferae
	Ammi majus	Umbelliferae
Angelica	*Angelica archangelica*	Umbelliferae
Fig	*Ficus carica*	Moraceae
Bindweed	*Convolvulus arvensis*	Convolvulaceae
Argimony	*Agricmonia eupatoria*	Rosaceae
Goosefoot	*Chenopodium* spp.	Chenopodiaceae[a]
Scurfy pea, bavchi	*Psoralea corylifolia*	Leguminosae
St John's wort	*Hypericum perforatum*	Hypericaceae[b]
	Hypericum crispum	Hypericaceae

[a]Chenopodiaceae have caused phototoxity when they have been eaten in quantity as might occur in a famine
[b]Hypericaceae cause photodermatitis after ingestion, but only in domestic animals

Polyacetylenic compounds. Compositae plants contain polyacetylenic compounds, one of which, alpha-terthienyl, a thiophene, has been identified as being phototoxic (Chan *et al.*, 1977). Pain and erythema occurs within minutes of irradiating the site of application.

Berloque dermatitis

Berloque dermatitis is a bizarre pigmentation occurring on light-exposed skin after the application of eau de Cologne or other perfumes containing oil of bergamot. The name berloque (French) or berlock (German) refers to the pendant or drop-like shape of the patches.

Clinically the initial phase of erythema may be so insignificant as to pass unnoticed, or it may be intense with oedema of the skin. It is followed by a conspicuous and unsightly pigmentation of the perfumed sites exposed to the sun. The sides of the neck and arms are most frequently affected. The brown patterns reflect the way in which the perfume runs down the skin, and the discolouration persists for several months. The infrequency of this condition nowadays was attributed by Marzulli and Maibach (1970) to the lowered concentration of natural bergamot oils added to perfumes and to the use of either furocoumarin-free or artificial bergamot.

Crude bergamot contains 0.3–4 per cent bergapten (5-methoxypsoralen) and the much less active bergamottin (5-geranyloxypsoralen). Bergapten, by intensifying the skin's reaction to long wave ultraviolet radiation (320–440 nm), causes the pigmentation.

The effect was reproduced by Harber *et al.* (1964) in subjects who had had a previous history of berloque dermatitis, but not in controls without such a history. The perfume was applied under Saran wrap, and after 24 hours the sites were irradiated with light of the 320–450 nm waveband. That absorption is the crucial factor was established by Burdick (1966) when he demonstrated that all subjects reacted if the perfume was applied to stripped skin. This phototoxic reaction was studied in detail by Marzulli and Maibach (1970) in man and animals; they also found it easy to reproduce the effect in man by applying the psoralens to stripped skin.

Frain-Bell and Zaynoun (1975) used 10 per cent oil of bergamot in petrolatum and a suberythema dose of long wave ultraviolet light for photopatch
testing 30 normal controls and 147 patients with various photodermatoses: 17
per cent of the controls and 27 per cent of the patients reacted. When testing
for phototoxic reactions it is essential to ensure that the bergamot oil contains
the active psoralen, bergapten. A method for quantifying the amount of bergapten in an oil is described by Zaynoun, Johnson and Frain-Bell (1977a). They
found the photoxicity of bergapten (5-MOP) almost to equal that of xanthotoxin
(8-MOP) and studied in detail the factors which affect the elicitation of the
phototoxic reaction (Zaynoun, Johnson and Frain-Bell), 1977b).

3. Dyes

Some dyes such as eosin, methylene blue, toluidine blue, acridine orange and
acriflavine have long been known to be phototoxic. Their action is photodynamic and dependent on oxygen. Neutral red and disperse blue 35 have similar properties. The phototoxic effects of eosin, rose bengal and dibromofluores-
cein have been studied in detail by Morikawa *et al.* (1976).

Neutral red

C.I. Basic Red 5. C.I. No. 50040;
3-amino-7-dimethylamino-2-methylphenazine hydrochloride;
toluylene red; neutral red chloride.

Dyes which photo-inactivate viruses are thought to act by either splitting off
or altering residues of the purine base guanine in the viral deoxyribonucleic
acid. When the resulting complex is exposed to light, the molecule is damaged
(Sastry and Gordon, 1966).

This principle was found by Felber *et al.* (1973) to be effective in the treatment of recurrent herpes simplex infections. In practice, the herpetic vesicles
are ruptured, painted with an 0.1 per cent aqueous solution of neutral red and
then exposed to fluorescent light for two consecutive periods of 15 minutes.
However, in a detailed study of 96 patients, Myers *et al.* (1975) found that
neutral red and light neither hastened resolution in attackes of herpes simplex,
nor reduced the recurrence rate.

Neutral red is also a contact allergen. In 1973, Mitchell and Stewart described
a woman who developed a severe contact dermatitis while treating her herpes
simplex with a 3 per cent aqueous solution of neutral red. She was patch tested
and reacted strongly to the 3 per cent solution she had been using and also to a
dilution of 0.05 per cent. Patients similarly sensitised by this treatment have
been seen by Conant and Maibach (1974); they patch tested one patient and she
reacted to aqueous neutral 0.1 per cent. Two patients seen by Dahlquist and
Fregert (1967) had been sensitised by a surgical preoperative disinfectant containing 0.1 per cent benzethonium chloride and 0.05 per cent neutral red, added

as a pH indicator. When patch tested, both patients reacted to neutral red 0.05 per cent in alcohol and to *p*-aminobenzene (? concentration).

Carcinogenicity. Bowen's disease of the penis has followed photodye therapy for herpes progenitatlis (Berger and Papa, 1977).

Disperse Blue 35 (a mixture)

Disperse blue 35 is a mixture of intermediates. Workers employed in its manufacture noticed a transient burning and erythema of their exposed skin when leaving the factory on sunny days, and they reacted similarly to sunlight through window glass. This photodermatitis was investigated by Gardiner *et al.* (1972) by photopatch testing. As irradiation with the 400–700 nm waveband elicited the reaction on the first exposure to the dye, the mechanism was demonstrably a phototoxic response to long wave light.

A phototoxic textile dermatitis from bikinis has been reported in two women by Hjorth and Möller (1976). The first woman complained that after sunbathing in a new brown bikini she developed a burning erythema on her back under the brassière strap. She washed the suit but wearing it again produced the same effect. The skin pigmented to form a brown band across her back and the shape of the bow fastening was visible. The second patient had brown triangles on her chest corresponding with the shoulder straps of her black and white bikini. Patch tests, performed only in the first patient, elicited no reaction. The dyes in the fabrics of the two suits, both of which were made of polyester and cotton, were extracted with ethanol and separated by thin layer chromatography; the whole extracts and certain fractions elicited photopatch test reactions in healthy volunteers. A chromatogram of Disperse Blue 35 gave fractions similar to those obtained from the extracts of the brown bikini, but not of the black one.

Disperse blue 35 is known to be a contact allergen and as a textile dye it has caused allergic contact dermatitis (Cronin, 1968).

4. Various chemicals
The phototoxicity of seven compounds was evaluated *in vitro* by their photo-killing effect on suspensions of *Escherichia coli*, and *in vivo* by their alteration of the median erythema dose of long wave ultraviolet radiation for guinea pig skin (Kobayashi, Wada and Mizino, 1974). Their results were as follows:

Photokilled *E. coli*		Phototoxic guinea pig skin	
Yes	*No*	*Yes*	*No*
Bithionol	Hexacholorphane	Bithionol	Tribromosalicylanilide
Tetrachlorosalicylanilide	Irgasan CF₃	Tetrachlorosalicylanilide	Hexachlorophane
Tribromosalicylanilide	Trichlorocarbanilide	8-Methoxypsoralen	Irgasan CF₃
8-Methoxypsoralen			Trichlorocarbanilide

The results of the two methods corresponded except for tribromosalicylanilide which was not phototoxic on the guinea pig skin; failure of absorption was suggested as a possible reason for this.

Phototesting

Topical application. The skin may require stripping or occlusion.

Light exposure. Approximately 2 hours after application, expose to long wave UVR for about 20 minutes.

Reading. Immediately, 7 hours, 1 day, 2 days and longer

Vehicles. The choice of vehicle has been found by Kaidbey and Kligman (1974) to have a profound influence on the demonstration of phototoxic reactions. The optimum base for coal tar was vanishing cream, although eucerin and hydrophilic ointment were also effective. If, however, petrolatum was used the response was less, and almost nil with lanolin or carbowax. For chlorpromazine, cold cream was a better base than hydrophilic ointment, whereas petrolatum and carbowax greatly diminished the reactions. Methoxsalen elicited maximum responses when formulated in hydrophilic ointment or lanolin, both being better than petrolatum or carbowax. Suhonen (1976) studied the phototoxicity of methoxsalen in different vehicles and found it to be most readily released from aqueous bases, and the reactions were augmented by the addition of ethanol.

Identification of topical photosensitisers

The following method of identifying topical phototoxic compounds in man was devised by Kaidbey and Kligman (1978a) and found to be reliable. The test material was diluted to 2.5 per cent in ethanol, methanol or, if insoluble, in Hydrophilic Ointment U.S.P.; 50 μ1 was applied to the untanned skin of the midback and spread over 3–2 cm square and covered with an occlusive dressing for six hours. It was then irradiated with UV-A and visible wavelengths from a Xenon arc lamp with a Schott WG-345 filter. The initial exposure was 8.5 min and, if there was no response, it was increased to 14 min. Materials causing no reactions were then tested on scarified skin using the same exposures. The readings were done immediately after irradiation and at 24 and 48 hours. Controls were an irradiated vehicle site and an unirradiated drug site.

2. SYSTEMIC

Phototoxicity can be induced systemically by:
1. Drugs
2. Porphyrins
3. Furocoumarins

1. **Drugs**

Phototoxicity induced by a drug depends largely on its dose and the amount of light administered. However, it is also influenced by the degree of skin pigmentation, as dark negroes are less responsive than fair-skinned subjects with a low tolerance to the sunburn spectrum. Phototoxic reactions can be elicited on the first exposure to the drug. Clinically, the phenothiazines and demethylchlortetracycline have caused the most trouble.

Experimental

In experimental animals, phototoxic reactions have been demonstrated to chlorpromazine, prochlorperazine, demethylchlortetracycline, tetracycline, chlorothiazide, chlordiazepoxide and quinoline methanols, and it has been shown that the reaction is elicited by the long wave ultraviolet light (Sams and Epstein, 1967; Sams 1966; Ison and Blank, 1967; Ison and Davis, 1969). The mouse tail technique is a satisfactory method for studying the phototoxicity of various groups of drugs (Ljunggren and Möller, 1978).

In man, intradermal injection of the drug, followed by irradiation with long wave ultraviolet light (320–400 nm), was found by Kligman and Breit (1968) to be a satisfactory method of demonstrating phototoxicity from the following drugs:

Demethylchlortetracycline	Sulphanilamide
Chlortetracycline	Sulphisoxazole
Tetracycline hydrochloride	Chlorothiazide
Chlorpromazine	Tolbutamide
Promethazine	Griseofulvin.

The optimum time for reading the results was 2 and 6 hours after irradiation. Oral administration or simple topical application of the drugs was unreliable, but stripping the skin, to promote absorption, greatly increased the effectiveness of the topical method. With this method the reactions were most intense at 4–8 hours, but the best time for comparing the phototoxic response with that in non-irradiated stripped skin of controls was at 24 hours. These authors stressed the disparity between the experimental demonstration of phototoxicity and the clinical safety of most of these drugs.

Clinical

The following drugs taken systemically may cause phototoxicity:

Tetracyclines

Demethylchlortetracycline	(Declomycin)
Chlortetracycline	(Aureomycin)
Doxycycline	(Vibramycin)
Oxytetracycline	(Terramycin)
Tetracycline	(Achromycin)

Photo-onycholysis

Chlorpromazine hydrochloride
Contraceptives — oral — oestrogens
Frusemide
Nalidixic Acid
Vinblastine

Demethylchlortetracycline 7-chloro-6-demethyltetracycline; Declomycin; Ledermycin

Demethylchlortetracycline (DMCT) is the most phototoxic of the tretracyclines. The reaction is dose-dependent. Cahn, Levy and McMillen (1961) showed that white men taking 600 mg daily became photosensitive, but they could tolerate the sun if the dose was 450 mg daily. This phototoxic effect was minimal in coloured men. As the sunburn spectrum (280–320 nm) was responsible, the effect was stopped by window glass. Ten volunteers were given 600 mg of DMCT daily by Blank, Cullen and Catalano (1968), and after one week they were taken sailing on a sunny day. Seven developed an abnormal reaction within five hours of exposure, and two more within two days. In seven the reaction was sufficiently severe to require systemic steroids. Both phototoxicity and photo-onycholoysis from DMCT have been described by Orentreich, Harber and Tromovitch (1961) and Bethell (1977).

A lichenoid eruption, lasting only a few days, appeared two weeks after the sunburn effect in three patients described by Jones, Lewis and Reisner (1971). They were unable to reproduce the response by challenging the patients with DMCT and exposing them to sunlight. In a letter, Maibach, Epstein and Sams (1974) reported the same lichenoid eruption in three of 200 experimental subjects receiving 600 mg of DMCT daily for four days followed by exposure to sunlight through a film of plastic which excluded rays shorter than 310 nm. In these three subjects the lichenoid rash lasted for several weeks to two months. They too were unable to reproduce the effect at will.

Chlortetracycline Aureomycin; Biomycin

Chlortetracycline given in large doses can cause phototoxicity of the exaggerated sunburn type. In New York, 135 patients with brucellosis were given chlortetracycline 2.5–4 g daily, and in the summer two men developed a severe phototoxicity requiring withdrawal of the antibiotic (Harris, 1950). Thirteen patients with chronic liver disease were given 2 g of chlortetracycline daily, and four became photosensitive (Shaffer *et al.*, 1950). Similarly, 10 out of 63 children given 15 mg per kilo body weight daily developed an increased susceptibility to sunburn during bright sunny weather (Verhagen, 1965).

Doxycycline 6-deoxy-5-hydroxytetracycline; Vibramycin

Fifteen volunteers were given doxycycline 200 mg daily for one week, and while on a day's sea trip 11 developed a reaction; this took the form either of an exaggerated but transient sunburn, or of paraesthesiae principally of the hands, feet or nose (Frost, Weinstein and Gomez, 1972). In another similar experiment, two out of ten subjects reacted (Blank, Cullen and Catalano, 1968). A more severe blistering sunburn of the hands, and onycholysis of all 20 nails, occurred in a fair-skinned boy taking doxycycline for his acne (Frank, Cohen and Minkin, 1971).

Oxytetracycline Biostat; Imperacin; Terramycin

A 20-year-old man became photosensitive after taking oxytetracycline 2 g daily for three days, and he remained intolerant of the sun for six months. Phototesting showed that he reacted to the sunburn spectrum (290–320 nm). After the episode his light tests became normal, but on receiving 500 mg of oxytetracycline as a single oral dose they were again abnormal (Tromovitch and Jacobs, 1963). However the patient reported by Ramsay (1977) reacted to long wave UVR (340–380 nm).

Tetracycline Achromycin

A 60-year-old man has been taking 2 g of tetracycline hydrochloride daily for a week when he went on a fishing trip and developed severe sunburn. The dose was reduced to 1 g a day, but ten days later he developed pain in his finger tips, followed by onycholysis (Segal, 1963). A similar exaggerated sunburn reaction and onycholysis in a woman and a boy was reported by Frank, Cohen and Minkin (1971) and onycholysis without sunburn by Rothstein (1977). Porphyria-like cutaneous changes occurred in five patients, who were exposed to strong sun, while taking tetracycline hydrochloride for acne vulgaris. Once the drug was stopped four recovered and one improved (Epstein et al., 1976).

Photo-onycholysis

A phototoxic onycholysis of the finger-nails and toe-nails may develop in patients taking tetracyclines and who are exposed to strong sunlight. Pain in the tip of the digit may be the first symptom, followed by intense erythema and separation of the distal nail plate from the nail bed. A few or all of the nails may be affected. The condition heals when the antibiotic is stopped, but even if the drug is continued the nails will grow normally provided the dosage is moderate and the patient avoids strong sunlight.

These nail changes are almost invariably associated with an exaggerated sunburn effect, although it was not mentioned in the case due to chlortetracycline reported by Harris (1950) or in another due to tetracycline described by Dombros (1973). There was no accompanying skin phototoxicity in Rothstein's (1977) patient.

The following tetracyclines have been reported as causing photo-onycholysis:

Chlortetracycline (Aureomycin): (Harris, 1950; Shaffer et al., 1950)
Demethylchlortetracycline (Declomycin): (Orentreich et al., 1961; Veber, 1962; Bethel, 1977)
Doxycycline (Vibramycin): (Frank et al., 1971)
Tetracycline (Achromycin): (Segal, 1963; Frank et al., 1971; Domonkos, 1973; Rothstein, 1977).

Photo-onycholysis has also been reported in patients receiving photo-chemotherapy with 8-methoxypsoralen and sun exposure for vitiligo (Zala, Omar and Krebs, 1977) and with 8-methoxypsoralen and long wave UVL for mycosis fungoides (Briffa and Warin, 1977). Once protected from light the nails grow normally.

Chlorpromazine hydrochloride Largactil

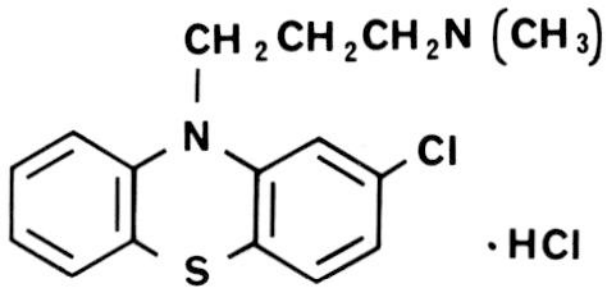

$$CH_2CH_2CH_2N\,(CH_3)_2$$

· HCl

Chlorpromazine given systemically photosensitises, and the incidence of reactions rises as the dose exceeds 100 mg daily. Patients may develop a mild to severe sunburn reaction, an erythematous blotchy maculo-papular eruption, or, in those previously sensitised by skin contact, an eczematous rash (Calnan, 1958).

Photocontact dermatitis to chlorpromazine is an allergic reaction usually cell mediated but immediate-type hypersensitivity has been described in a nurse (Horio, 1975).

Photosensitivity from systemic administration of chlorpromazine is generally a phototoxic reaction. It has been investigated experimentally by Ljunggren and Möller (1976, 1977a,b) and Ljunggren (1977) and the cellular mechanism involved has been studied by Johnson (1974). The urticarial reaction which occurs in some patients may be explained by the experiments of Lam and Tomlinson (1976) in which they demonstrated that *in vitro* chlorpromazine releases histamine from guinea pig skin. Patients photosensitised by receiving the drug and nurses by handling it were investigated by Raffle *et al.* (1975) but, using the lymphocyte transformation test, they were unable to distinguish between a phototoxic and a photoallergic reaction.

ORAL CONTRACEPTIVES (Oestrogen)

Ethinyloestradiol Ethynylestradiol; 17-ethinylestradiol

Oral contraceptives may precipitate prophyria through the hepatotoxic effect of their oestrogen content. A photodermatitis resembling polymorphic light eruption was first described by Erickson and Peterka (1968); it was provoked by various types of oral contraceptive and also by oestrogen alone. As light filtered by window glass elicited the reaction it was concluded that wavelengths longer than 320 nm were responsible. A rash similar to polymorphic light eruption in four women, and porphyria cutanea tarda in two other women was attributed by Horkay *et al.* (1975) to liver damage from oestrogens in contraceptive pills. Once the pill was stopped, the rash cleared and the liver function tests returned to normal in all four patients with the condition resembling polymorphic light eruption, but the clinical remission was only partial in the two patients with porphyria cutanea tarda. Both required further treatment, and in only one did the liver function tests become normal.

Frusemide 4-Chloro-*N*-furfuryl-5-sulfamoylanthranilic acid; Frusemide

In south Australia, four patients with chronic renal failure developed blisters on the dorsa of the hands, shins and feet while taking high doses of frusemide (240–1.500 mg daily). Some of the bullae were haemorrhagic, but they healed without scarring and there was no associated skin fragility. Subsequently, three of these patients were given high doses of frusemide intravenously without relapse. The high dosage was considered to be of greater importance than the amount of sunlight, which is always plentiful in south Australia (Burry and Lawrence, 1976).

Griseofulvin (7-chloro-2'4, 6-trimethoxy-6' β -methylspiro (benzofuran-2(3H), 1'(2)cyclohexene)-3,4'-dione; Grisovin

Listing the side effects of griseofulvin, Goldfarb and Sulzberger (1960) included one patient with photosensitivity and Calnan (1960) mentioned three hearsay cases but none had been under his own care. Two men with an increased sunburn reaction, while taking griseofulvin 1 g daily, were described by Lamb *et al.* (1961); when investigated they both reacted to unfiltered ultraviolet light.

In mice griseofulvin causes increased excretion of porphyrins but in man porphyrin metabolism is not significantly disturbed (Rimington *et al.*, 1963; Watson *et al.*, 1968).

A case of cold urticaria from griseofulvin has been described by Chang (1965); this patient also reacted when tested with ultraviolet light, but he had no clinical photosensitivity, possibly because he avoided direct sun exposure.

Griseofulvin may be an occasional photosensitiser but clinically this rarely seems to be the problem.

Nalidixic Acid 1-ethyl-7-methyl-4-oxo-1, 8-naphthyridine-3-carboxylic acid; Negram

Nalidixic acid, an antibacterial compound introduced in 1962, is particularly effective in urinary tract infections.

It causes photosensitivity, but whether the mechanism is phototoxic or photo-allergic is uncertain.

The majority of cases reported have been in women because, being prone to urinary infections, they are more likely to be given the drug. The eruption characteristically is bullous and involves exposed sites, especially the feet and lower legs. Blisters develop on the dorsa of the feet and hands, and on the lower legs. There may be facial erythema with small blisters on the forehead, and petechiae on the legs have been described. Neither the dose of the drug nor the duration of its administration is crucial but strong sunlight is essential to elicit the eruption. Patients tolerant of nalidixic acid in a dull climate may blister within days of going on a sunny holiday. The bullae can appear six weeks after stopping the drug, and although they generally continue to erupt for 1–3 months, this can continue for a year. The skin is fragile, and mild trauma causes blistering. The drug can be given again without relapse provided strong sunlight is avoided (Ramsay and Obreshkova, 1974; Brauner, 1975; Baes, 1968).

Seven patients were investigated by Ramsay and Obreshkova (1974), who photopatch tested three of them, with negative results. They showed that long wave ultraviolet radiation was responsible, and demonstrated photosensitivity experimentally in three controls who took nalidixic acid 4 g daily for one week.

Vinblastine sulphate Velbe

A case of phototoxicity from vinblastine sulphate has been reported by Breza, Halprin and Taylor (1975). A 34-year-old man with Hodgkin's disease became photosensitive after two months' treatment with vinblastine sulphate, 10 mg intravenously every three weeks. The sunburn spectrum was responsible, as light through window glass caused no reaction. The effect was reproduced locally in five control subjects by injecting intradermally 0.2 μg of vinblastine sulphate, and then irradiating the site with a suberythema dose of ultraviolet light. Each produced the same response as the patient.

2. Prophyrins
In the porphyrias the endogenous circulating porphyrins cause the abnormal reaction to sunlight. The action spectrum is long wave ultraviolet light, in the waveband 400–410 nm.

3. Furocoumarins
Furocoumarins, or psoralens, given orally augment the skin's reaction to long wave ultraviolet light. In the treatment of vitiligo they are given two hours before irradiation.

Phototesting

(i) Intradermal injection, or stripping or occlusion of the skin
Immediate light exposure
Long wave ultraviolet irradiation for 3–16 minutes
Read at 2–6 hours, except when taking psoralens which cause peak reactions at 2–3 days (Kligman and Breit, 1968)

(ii) Oral administration
     Drug given for several days
     Light exposure
       Monochromator
       Short wave ultraviolet irradiation
       Long wave ultraviolet irradiation
       (A day's sailing in sunny weather has been used)
     Read at approximately 5 hours and about 2 days.

Photoallergic

1. TOPICAL

Topical photoallergens have been grouped into:

1. Halogenated phenols
2. Drugs
3. Various chemicals

The results of photopatch testing at St John's have been summarised (p. 442).

1. **Halogenated phenols**
Halogenated phenols have been widely used as antibacterial compounds in soaps, antiseptic preparations, toiletries and cosmetics. They have now been reported from many parts of the world as causing allergic photocontact dermatitis. Men particularly are affected (Freeman and Knox, 1968; Epstein, Wuepper and Maibach, 1968; Osmundsen, 1970), and skin pigments afford no protection as Negroes are as vulnerable as Caucasians (Freeman and Knox, 1968; O'Quinn, Kennedy and Isbell, 1967).

The majority of patients are photosensitised for only a transient period but in a few the intolerance of light persists and they pass into the awful stage of being persistent light reactors.

Trichlorocarbanilide and hexachlorophane have been widely used for many years and there are few reports of their being primary photosensitisers. The sensitising potential of these two chemicals is very low, but on photopatch testing they may cross-react with related compounds.

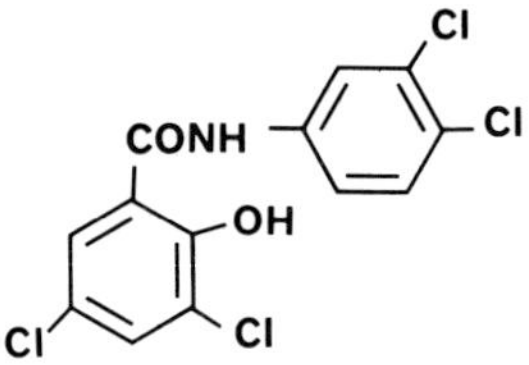

3,3′,4,5′-Tetrachlorosalicylanilide; Irgasan BS200

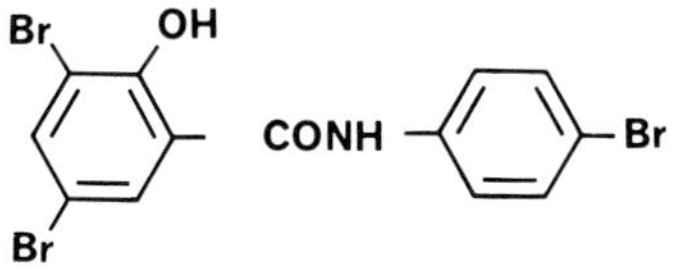

3,4',5-Tribromosalicylanilide; Tribromsalan

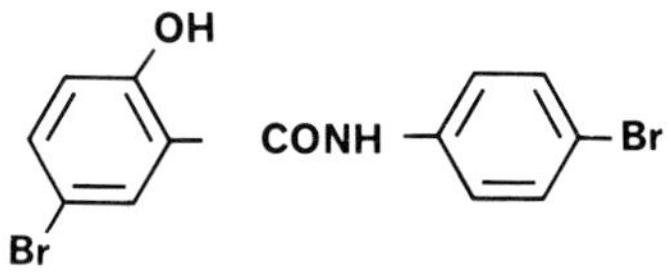

5,4'-Dibromosalicylanilide; Dibromsalan

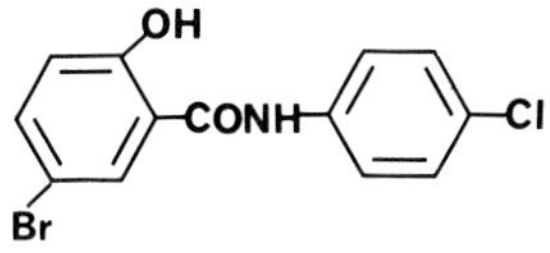

5-Bromo-4'-chlorosalicylanilide;
bromochlorosalicylanilide; Multifungin.

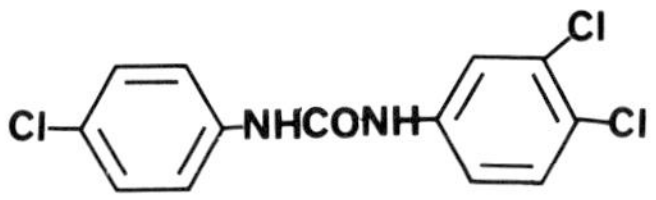

3,4,4'-Trichlorocarbanilide; Triclocarban.

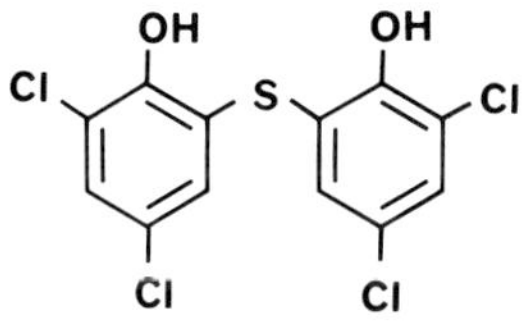

2,2'-Thiobis (4,6-dichlorophenol); Bithionol

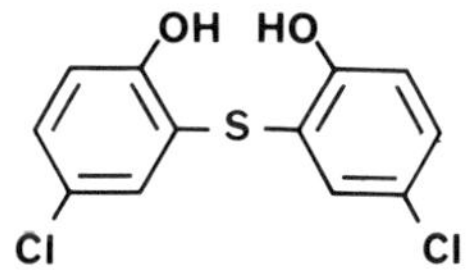

2,2'-Thiobis[4-chlorophenol]; Fentichlor; S7

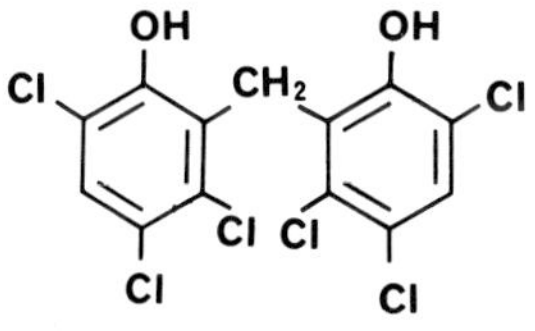

2,2'-Methylenebis [3,4,6-trichlorophenol];
Hexachlorophane.

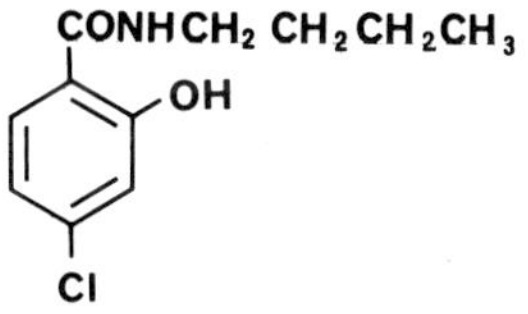

N-Butyl-4-chlorosalicylamide; Buclosamide
Jadit

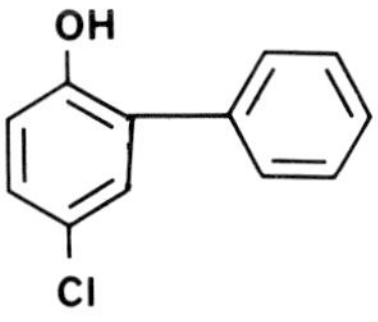

4-Chloro-2-phenylphenol

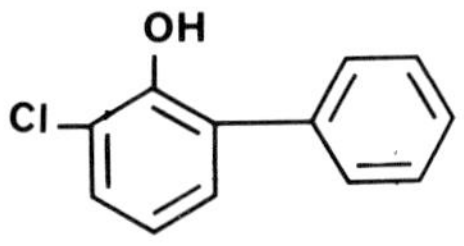

6-Chloro-2-phenylphenol

Tetrachlorsalicylanilide; 3,3',4,5'-tetrachlorosalicylanilide; TCS; Irgasan BS200

In England, in July 1960, two popular brands of soap were marketed containing 0.2 per cent tetrachlorosalicylanilide (TCSA) as a germicide. They caused an epidermic of photodermatitis and were withdrawn in October 1960. Wilkinson (1961) was the first to recognise the condition when he investigated an outbreak of dermatitis in the foundry section of a factory where 29 men out of 106 at risk were affected. With perspicacity, he realised that their daily use of 30 bars of a germicide soap could be significant. This factory episode has been described in detail by Wynn Jones (1962).

The dermatitis affected men more than women and it began acutely after unaccustomed light-exposure. The exposed skin became red, scaly and oedematous and there was usually marked swelling of the eyelids. The initial phase was followed by pigmentation and lichenification.

Patch tests: in a series described by Calnan, Harman and Wells (1961), 102 patients, 87 men and 15 women, were patch tested with TCSA 1 per cent or less in a solvent, and 90 reacted. Of 74 patients, 26 had positive patch tests without light-irradiation, but in 48 the tests required irradiation with ultraviolet light before they became positive.

The majority of patients healed rapidly, once contact with TCSA had ceased; a few remained light-sensitive for a short time and a very few patients contined to be photosensitive (Wilkinson, 1962).

In the United States, a soap containing 0.5 per cent tetrachlorosalicylanilide was marketed in a small test area and caused photosensitisation. Vinson and Flatt.(1962) confirmed the diagnosis by photopatch tests in eight subjects who had recovered from the eruption.

Experimentally in guinea pigs, Horio (1976) effected photosensitisation to TCSA, TBS and bithionol by irradiation with UV-A and it was shown by Horio and Ofujui (1976) that in photosensitised guinea pigs non-irradiated TCSA (prohapten) remained longer in the skin than did irradiated TCSA (hapten). They also demonstrated that TCSA was eliminated more quickly from the irradiated skin of photosensitised guinea pigs than it was from control animals. Only some skin proteins are capable of being the carrier protein in photoallergy to TCSA (Kochevar and Harber, 1977).

Tribromosalicylanilide; 3,4'5-Tribromosalicylanilide; TBS; Tribromsalan

In England, in November 1960, tribromosalicylanilide (TBS) was substituted for tetrachlorosalicylanilide (TCSA) in the germicidal soaps, but in 1961 it, too, was withdrawn and replaced by trichlorocarbanilide (TCC) (Wilkinson, 1962). Positive patch test reactions to TBS were usually cross-reactions to TCSA but Wilkinson (1962) thought that TBS was probably the primary sensitiser in two patients.

In the United States, soaps containing TBS (0.75 per cent or less, Osmundsen, 1968) were reported by Epstein and Enta (1965) to have photosensitised one and one woman, both of whom recovered when they stopped using the soap. Three men sensitised by soaps were described in detail by Harber, Harris and Baer (1966) and in one of these the dermatitis persisted. Harber, Targonvik and Baer (1967) then reported the investigation of 32 photosensitive patients (27 men and five women) of whom 12 had become persistent light reactors. On photopatch testing, all 32 patients reacted to a halogenated salicylanilide and 25 reacted to TBS.

In Denmark, in 1965, a toilet soap containing 2 per cent TBS caused a sharp outbreak of photodermatitis. On a surmise of the incidence of cases, Osmundsen (1968) considered TBS to be as potent a photoallergen as TCS. He investigated 39 cases (32 men and seven women). Each recovered on withdrawal of the soap, and within three weeks their tolerance of sunlight had returned to normal. Photopatch tests with long wave ultraviolet light were positive in all 39 patients. The TBS-compound in the responsible soap contained 95 per cent TBS; this, and not an impurity, was thought to be the sensitiser.

In Japan, TBS is occasionally a primary photosensitiser (Masuda et al., 1971).

From south Australia, Burry and Donald (1968) reported their photopatch test results in three men and two women with transient reactions to light, and in one man with a persistent light-reaction from TBS. They ascertained that since 1964 one popular brand of toilet soap had contained TBS; they thought it very probable that other cases had occurred but had gone unrecognised.

Dibromosalicylanilide (4',5-Dibromosalicylanilide; DBS; Dibromsalan)
A man and a woman, photosensitised by a particular brand of soap containing dibromosalicylanilide, were reported from the United States by Molloy and Mayer (1966). Both had positive photopatch tests.

Thirty-two patients with a photocontact dermatitis from a halogenated chemical were investigated by Harber, Targovnik and Bacr (1967) and many (25/30) had positive photopatch tests to DBS in association with reactions to TCSA and TBS. A similar pattern of reactions was seen in the series reported by Epstein, Wuepper and Maibach (1968).

In Germany, DBS used to be added to shampoos, hair lotions and an antiseborrhoeic agent but as it sensitised five hairdressers its use was discontinued (Behrbohm and Zschunke, 1966).

Multifungin (5-Bromo-4'-chlorosalicylanilide; BCSA)
Multifungin is used in Australia as an antifungal application. In four cases of photosensitisation described by Burry (1967) the treated areas of skin remained particularly susceptible to subsequent sun exposure.

Trichlorocarbanilide (3,4,4'-Trichlorocarbanilide; TCC; Triclocarban)
Trichlorocarbanilide (TCC) is widely used as a germicide in soaps and toiletries. Its sensitising potential was investigated by Maibach et al. (1978) and its use in soap was considered to be practically without hazard. Only one case report of primary photosensitisation has been traced (Freeman and Knox, 1968). This patient has been sensitised by a soap and, when photopatch tested, reacted to TCC only.

A deodorant marketed in Scandinavia and Finland has caused contact sensitivity principally to propantheline bromide but also to TCC. There have been three relevant reports: Hannuksela (1975) described two patients with positive patch tests to 5 per cent TCC; Osmundsen (1975) reported one man with a positive patch to 1 per cent TCC in petrolatum; and Ågren-Jonsson and Magnusson (1976) recorded three patients with positive patch tests to 2 per cent TCC in ethanol. These latter authors suggested that the irritant effect of the propylene glycol base facilitated contact sensitisation to both propantheline bromide and TCC.

Bithionol (2,2'-Thiobis[4,6-dichlorophenol])
Bithionol has been added to soaps, shampoos, cosmetics and antiseptic creams. Primary photosensitisation was reported in the United States by Jillson and Baughman (1963). Of their eight patients, three recovered but five became persistent light reactors. Plain patch tests with bithionol were usually negative in their patients, whereas photopatch tests were positive. However, 20 patients with photocontact dermatitis from bithionol were investigated by O'Quinn, Kennedy and Isbell (1967) and the majority reacted to both the occluded and the light-exposed bithionol patch tests.

In Japan, bithionol became the principal photosensitiser (Masuda *et al.*, 1971) and its use was therefore banned. It is also prohibited in cosmetic and antibacterial preparations in the United States.

Fentichlor; 2,2'-thiobis(4-chlorophenol);2,2'-dihydroxy-5,5'-dichlorodiphenyl sulfide; S7; Fenticlor
Fentichlor is used as an antibacterial and antifungal agent. In south Australia, three patients developed transient photosensitivity after using fentichlor on exposed sites, and another two were photosensitised by systemic absorption from covered areas (Burry, 1967; 1968). Cross-sensitivity has been reported between fentichlor and bithionol (Burry, 1967).

A patient in Wales was photosensitised by a proprietary hair cream containing fentichlor (Beer, 1970), and in Dublin a man developed a localised contact dermatitis of the feet after using S7 jelly. A patch test with the whole jelly was positive, but the base alone elicited no reaction (Dupont, 1972). Actinic reticuloid supervening on fentichlor sensitivity has been reported in one man (Clayton and Feiwell, 1976).

Four patients who became persistent light reactors after being sensitised to fentichlor, three by hair creams and one through industrial exposure, have been described in detail by Ramsay (1979).

Hexachlorophane (2,2'-Methylenebis (3,4,6,-trichlorophenol); pHisohex; G-11)
Hexachlorophane was a popular germicide in soap and toiletries until awareness of its toxicity greatly restricted its use.

Reports of hexahclorophane causing contact dermatitis or primary photosensitisation are rare. Three men, who had positive patch tests to hexachlorophane but not to bithionol and the halogenated salicylanilides, were reported by O'Quninn, Kennedy and Isbell (1967). It was confirmed that each had been using a soap, a shampoo or a shaving preparation containing hexachlorphane. This was stopped and their dermatitis cleared.

A man described by Burry and Donald (1968) used a soap containing hexachlorophane and developed a transient photodermatitis. He had positive photopatch tests to hexachlorophane and to fentichlor.

In Tokyo, six of 48 patients with a photocontact dermatitis had positive photopatch tests to hexachlorophane. Despite their cross-reactions to other halogenated phenols, it was thought that some of these patients may have been primarily sensitised by hexachlorophane (Masuda *et al.*, 1971).

Buclosamide (*N*-butyl-chlorosalicylamide; Jadit)
Buclosamide is a topical antimycotic agent. Occasional cases of photosensitivity to it have been reported. Five were described by Jung and Schwarz (1964), and two by Burry (1970), in the latter, the sites of application remained particularly sensitive to sunlight, a phenomenon he described as 'localised persistent light reactions'. Photodermatitis is frequent in Malaysia, where Jadit is widely used, and was the most frequent topical photosensitiser (15 cases) among the patients investigated by Nagreh (1975).

Chloro-2-phenylphenol
Dowicide 32 is the trade name for a mixture of 4-chloro-2-phenylphenol and 6-chloro-2-phenylphenol. It is a germicide which is used industrially in disinfectants of the pine oil type, detergents, textiles, adhesives based on starch or protein, and as a fungicide in the construction and automobile industries. It is irritant in concentrations above 2 per cent, and it is not intended for use in domestic soaps (Adams, 1972).

Four workers in one school district suddenly became photosensitive, and it was only through Adams' (1972) pertinacity that he discovered the cause to be Dowicide 32 in a recently introduced liquid soap which contained 1.8 per cent of this germicide. Each patient had positive photopatch tests to 1 per cent aqueous, 4,6-dichloro-2-phenylphenol and 4,chloro-2-phenylphenol; and one of them also reacted to 6-chloro-2-phenylphenol. None reacted to bithionol, carbanilide-mix, dichlorphene, hexachlorophane or salicylanilide-mix.

Cross-reactions
Halogenated phenols frequently cross-react. Patients sensitised by tribromosalicylanilide were found by Osmundsen (1970) to photocross-react to salicylanilide, hexachlorphane, trichlorocarbanilide, fentichlor and Jadit. Baughman (1964) reported patients sensitised by bithionol who cross-reacted to tetrachlorosalicylanilide, tribromosalicylanilide and hexachlorophane, but not to trichlorocarbanilide.

It is to be noted that tetrachlorosalicylanilide, although not the primary allergen, may give a stronger photopatch test reaction than the primary sensitiser, with which it is cross-reacting (Epstein and Enta, 1965; Harber, Harris and Barr, 1966).

2. Drugs

PHENOTHIAZINE DERIVATIVES

Promethazine hydrochloride (Phenergan)

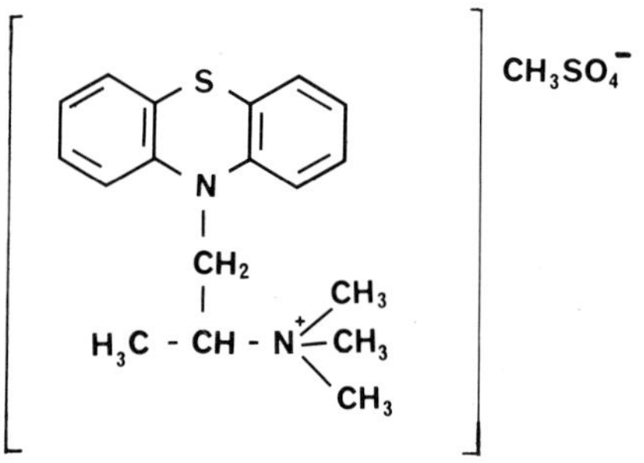

Multergan

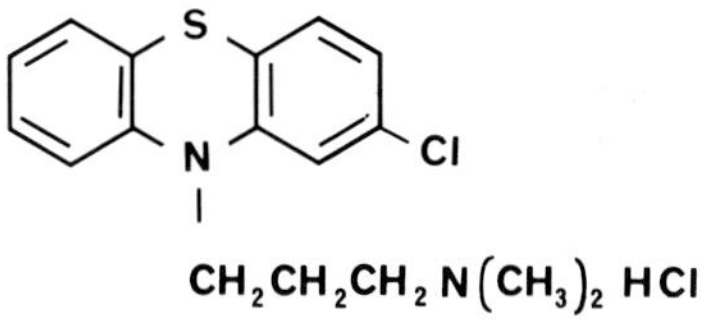

Chlorpromazine hydrochloride

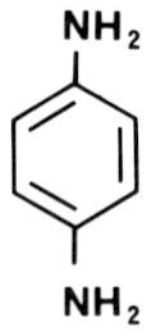

p-Phenylenediamine

In France, in the 1950s, Phenergan cream was a popular remedy and it caused many adverse reactions (Sidi, Hincky and Gervais, 1955). Mostly, the reaction was an irritant effect of the cream base, but patch testing confirmed that some patients had been sensitised by the promethazine. The majority developed a photodermatitis which was often severe, and in some the photosensitivity persisted for years. Ingestion of Phenergan caused recurrences. Patch testing demonstrated cross-reactions to p-phenylenediamine and to Multergan (an antihistamine with a similar chemical structure). Of 11 promethazine-sensitive patients patch tested with chlorpromazine, three reacted, and two relapsed after taking a Largactil tablet. Epstein (1960) reported a case of allergic photocontact dermatitis from promethazine, but the evidence is doubtful because patch tests and photopatch tests with promethazine, though positive in the acute stage, were negative when repeated five months later.

In the series reported from Malaysia by Nagreh (1975), promethazine hydrochloride was a quite frequent cause (12 cases) of photosensitivity.

Chlorpromazine hydrochloride

Chlorpromazine photosensitises patients who receive it parenterally, and personnel who handle it. The later include nurses, pharmacists, hospital workers and relatives administering the drug, and workers in pharmaceutical factories who process it or just casually come into contact with it. In the early days of chlorpromazine manufacture, occupational dermatitis was a considerable problem (Calnan, 1958),but it has been solved by stringent precautions to prevent exposure.

In Calnan's (1958) series, hospital workers presented with one of four patterns of dermatitis: (i) a photo-dermatitis, (ii) an eruption on the face simulating seborrhoeic eczema, (iii) a chronic fissured eczema of the fingers, (iv) or a dermatitis of the eyelids, elbow flexures and fingers.

The factory workers developed a red scaly eczema of light-exposed skin including the eyelids. The relationship to sunlight was striking in only some patients but those most severely affected were greatly aggravated by sun. The photosensitivity sometimes persisted for months or for one to two years.

Patients were patch tested in duplicate with chlorpromazine, but only one patch was irradiated with ultraviolet light at two days. However, as both patch tests were left uncovered, each was in fact exposed to light. Practically all the patients with chlorpromazine dermatitis had a positive patch test, a third becoming positive after the UVR exposure. Late reactions may have been due to inadvertent light exposure (Calnan, 1958).

SULPHONAMIDES

Sulphapyridine (N'-2-pyridylsulphanilamide; 2-sulphanilamidopyridine)

$$H_2N-\langle\bigcirc\rangle- SO_2NH -\langle\bigcirc\rangle$$

Topical sulphonamides were used in the Armed Forces during World War II in the treatment of all types of infected skin conditions. Many men were photosensitised and some developed severe eruptions. The majority healed completely but a few remained intolerant of the sun for long periods (Peterkin, 1945).

DIPHENHYDRAMINE (2-diphenylmethoxy-*N*,*N*-dimethylethylamine; Benadryl)

$$\begin{array}{c} C_6H_5 \\ \\ C_6H_5 \end{array} \!\! > \!\! CHO\,CH_2CH_2\,N \!\! < \!\! \begin{array}{c} CH_3 \\ \\ CH_3 \end{array}$$

A photo-allergic reaction to topically applied diphenhydramine was described by Emmett (1974). Photopatch tests irradiated with the sunburn range of ultraviolet light (UV-B) (290–320 nm) were positive, while long wave ultraviolet light (UV-A) had no effect and covered patch tests were negative. Similar tests in ten controls were negative. A second patient reported by Horio (1976) had received diphenhydramine topically, orally and by injection. He reacted to a patch test and a photopatch test with diphenhydramine 1 per cent in petrolatum, the eliciting ultraviolet light being long wave UV-A (300–420 nm) and not the UV-B spectrum to which Emmett's (1974) patient had responded.

QUININE (formula p. 263)

An industrial chemist, who was a persistent light reactor, was shown by Johnson *et al.* (1975) to be photosensitive to quinine. The positive photopatch test was elicited by long wave UVR (300–400 nm). This photo-allergy was thought to be significant in the aetiology of his light sensitivity.

3. VARIOUS CHEMICALS

Moquizone; 1-morpholinoacetyl,3-phenyl,4-oxo-1,2,3,4,tetrahydro quinoxaline hydrochloride

This drug, which is a derivative of quinoxaline, is used as a choleretic in Italy and South America. Photosensitisation in patients receiving it has been reported in Italy (Leoni *et al.*, 1976).

Quindoxin; Quinoxaline *N,N*-dioxide; Grofas

Quindoxin has been added to pig and chicken food as a growth promoting factor, the concentration in the final feed being 20–50 mg/kg. Imperial Chemical Industries Ltd have now withdrawn quindoxin from their market because it was shown experimentally to produce nasal, liver and kidney tumours in rats. It is possible that the carcinogenic effect on the nasal mucosa is due to its selective uptake of quinoxaline 1,4-dioxide or its metabolites (Tucker, 1975).

In Northern Ireland, a pig meal containing quindoxin caused a spate of dermatitis among pig breeders. Both men and women were affected. The dermatitis was scaly with a tendency to fissure, and was most severe in the light-exposed areas. Photopatch tests with quindoxin 0.1 per cent in petrolatum were positive. Plain patch tests remained negative if kept completely protected from light, but once the opaque covering was removed, they became positive. None of the patients was positive to ethoxyquin (Dawson and Scott, 1972; Scott and Dawson, 1974). Quindoxin was sold throughout Ireland and Great Britain and the prevalence of cases in Northern Ireland was unexplained.

Further cases occurred; five were seen in the Cambridge area (Editor's note, Scott and Dawson, 1974) and two male pig farmers in Scotland became persistent light reactors (Frain-Bell and Gardiner, 1975; Johnson *et al.*, 1975). Seven patients were investigated in detail by Zaynoun, Johnson and Frain-Bell (1976). Four remained light sensitive, all reacted to a photopatch test with quinoxaline dioxide 0.01 per cent, but none responded to a non-irradiated patch test. It was concluded that the parent compound, and not a contaminant or a photoproduct, was the allergen.

A man employed in a factory mixing and compounding animal foodstuffs developed an eruption on his hands, face and legs. Unexposed patch tests with Grofas 5 per cent (pet.) and quinoxaline dioxide 5 per cent (pet.) gave reactions but the response was intensified in the tests exposed to long wave ultraviolet light. The patient left the factory and made a complete recovery (Calnan, 1975).

Thiourea (Thiocarbamide. CH_4N_2S)

Thiourea is used in photography as a fixing agent and to remove stains from negatives; in photocopy paper it is present as an antioxidant to prevent yellow discolouration. It is also used in the manufacturer of resins and as an accelerator in the vulcanisation of rubber.

Photosensitivity from thiourea in photocopy paper has been reported in two men by Leun *et al.* (1977). The first had a positive photopatch test to the paper and reacted to UV-A; he ceased contact with the paper and during the next three years his photosensitivity diminished. The second reacted to UV-B; it was recommended that he use a particular British paper which does not contain thiourea.

Perfumes

Musk ambrette (2-methoxy-3,5-dinitro-4 methyl-tertiary butylbenzene) was the photosensitiser in the after-shave lotions and colognes used by the three men investigated by Raugi, Storrs and Larsen (1979). (Similar patients have been seen at St John's.)

The synthetic fragrance 6-methylcoumarin is related to the psoralens. In concentrations of 0.001 per cent to 0.4 per cent it is used in cosmetics, toiletries and soaps. It is not phototoxic but it has induced photoallergy and the photomaximisation test has shown it to be a potent photocontact allergen (Kaidbey and Kligman, 1978c).

Results of photopatch testing

In Toronto, Wasserman and Haberman (1975) reviewed their investigations of 250 patients referred with possible photosensitivity. The diagnosis was confirmed or accepted in 140, of whom 14 had an allergic photocontact dermatitis. Four reacted to tribrominated salicylanilide only; six reacted to one or more of the following five bacteriostatic compounds — tribrominated salicylanilide, hexachlorphane, dichlorophene, bithionol and polybrominated salicylanilide; one reacted to *para*-phenylenediamine; another reacted to *para*-aminobenzoic acid, benzocaine and *para*-phenylenediamine; and two reacted to soaps. Ten had become persistent light reactors. Systemic phototoxicity to hydrochlorothiazide and tetracycline was diagnosed in these patients. Topical phototoxicity from oil of bergamot occurred in three patients and from chlorpromazine in one.

In the clinic of the University of California, San Francisco, from 1967 to 1975 there was a reduction in the number of patients with postive photopatch tests to halogenated salicylanilides and related compounds. This was attributed to the removal of potent photosensitisers from soaps and deodorants but the figures were also influenced by fewer patients being referred for photopatch testing in the later years of the study (Smith and Epstein, 1977).

St John's

Photosensitive patients referred to the Contact Clinic for investigation are tested with a standard series of photosensitising chemicals, applied twice:

1. As a series of plain patch tests
2. A duplicate series which, after removal at two days, is irradiated with long wave ultraviolet light. (Technique p. 8)

The following chemicals constituted the standard series:

Bithionol	1 per cent in petrolatum
Buclosamide (Jadit)	10 per cent in water
Fentichlor	1 per cent in petrolatum
Hexcahlorophane	1 per cent in petrolatum
Tetrachlorosalicylanilide	1 per cent in petrolatum
Tribromosalicylanilide	1 per cent in petrolatum
Trichlorocarbanilide	1 per cent in petrolatum
Chlorpromazine	1 per cent in petrolatum
Promethazine	2 per cent in petrolatum
Sulphapyridine	5 per cent in petrolatum
Quinine	1 per cent in petrolatum
Trimeprazine (from 1973)	1 per cent in petrolatum
Sunscreens	
para-aminobenzoic acid	1 per cent in petrolatum
2-Ethoxyethyl p-methoxycinnamate	1 per cent in petrolatum
Isoamyl dimethylaminobenzoate (from 1975)	5 per cent in petrolatum

The results in the patients tested from 1970–1976 have been analysed. As the plain patch tests are not routinely occluded with black material, many are inadvertently exposed to light, invalidating a distinction between plain and photopatch tests.

Each year since 1971 about 25 per cent of the patients tested have reacted to one or more of the chemicals in this series (Table 9.2). From 1970–1976, a total of 56 patients gave positive reactions; 47 were men and nine were women.

Table 9.2. Number of patients with positive reactions to the photopatch test series (St John's, 1970–1976).

Year	Number of patients tested	Number of patients with positive reactions	%
1970	60	4	7
1971	44	13	29
1972	28	8	29
1973	34	13	38
1974	18	4	22
1975	18	6	33
1976	32	8	25

The incidence of reactions varies among the chemicals. It is often impossible to establish with certainty the source and therefore it is frequently difficult to assess the significance of the reactions in the aetiology of the photosensitivity. Twenty-two of the 56 patients had more than one reaction.

The number of responses elicited by each chemical has been listed below together with the frequency with which a sensitising exposure was definitely established:

Chemical	+ reactions	source certain
Fentichlor	16	6
Bithionol	11	0
TCS	9	3
TCC	4	0
Jadit	3	1
Hexachlorophane	2	0
TBS	2	0
Chlorpromazine	17	2 (had taken related drugs)
Promethazine	13	5
Trimeprazine	4	1
Sulphapyridine	1	0
Quinine	1	0
Sunscreens — Contact Allergy		
Cinnamate	4	
Isoamyldimethylaminobenzoate	2	
PABA	3	

Unrecognised plant dermatitis

Sensitisation to airborne pollens and some plants such as chrysanthemum can cause a diffuse eczema of the face, neck, hands and arms which closely resembles a photosensitivity (p. 504). To guard against this misdiagnosis, patients should be additionally tested with plants and oleoresins (Frain-Bell, 1979) appropriate for the area; when sensitivity to the Compositae is suspected patch testing should include sesquiterpene lactones. A combination of contact dermatitis and photocontact dermatitis from lichens has been reported from Norway (Thune, 1977). The allergens are thought to be atranorin, physodalic and pysodic acids.

At St John's the patients are routinely tested with chrysanthemum leaf and unsuspected cases of chrysanthemum dermatitis are continually being rescued from the melée of photodermatitis. Plant oleoresins are used in selected cases.

Photopatch tests

Duplicate patch tests are applied. After two days they are removed and read; then one set is immediately covered with black material and the other irradiated with long wave ultraviolet light for an appropriate period, usually about 30 minutes. Both tests are read again at four days (see p. 8). Photosensitisers and their concentrations for photopatch testing are listed:

	Concentration	Diluent
Bithionol	1%	petrolatum
Chloro-2-phenylphenol	1%	petrolatum
Chlorpromazine	1%	petrolatum
Dibromosalicylanilide	1%	petrolatum
Diphenylhydramine	1%	petrolatum
Fentichlor	1%	petrolatum
Hexachlorophane	1%	petrolatum
Jadit	1%	petrolatum
Multifungin	1%	petrolatum
Promethazine	1%	petrolatum
Quindoxin	0.1, 0.05, 0.01%	petrolatum
Quinine	0.1, 0.05, 0.01%	petrolatum
Sulphapyridine	5%	petrolatum
Tribromosalicylanilide	1%	petrolatum
Tetrachlorosalicylanilide	0.1%	petrolatum
Trichlorocarbanilide	1%	petrolatum

St John's

The Current photopatch test series includes a chrysanthemum leaf and Sunscreens (1,5,6,7) to avoid missing an unsuspected contact dermatitis.

		concentration %
1	Mexenone	4
2	Trichlorocarbanilide	1
3	Chlorpromazine	1
4	Promethazine	2
5	PABA	1
6	2-ethoxyethyl-p-methoxycinnamate	5
7	Isoamyl dimethylaminobenzoate	5
8	Musk ambrette	5
9	Potassium dichromate	0.5
10	Sulpha-mix	5
	Sulphamylon	
	Sulphadiazine	
	Sulphathiazide } EACH	1
	Sulphamerazine	
	Sulphacetamide	
11	Chrysanthemum leaf	

Each in petrolatum except
PABA in ethanol

2. SYSTEMIC

Drugs

Promethazine hydrochloride (10-(2-Dimethylaminopropyl)phenothiazine hydrochloride; Phenergan)

A patient who became photosensitive while taking promethazine orally was investigated by Epstein and Rowe (1957). Although there was no history of topical contact with the drug, a patch test with Phenergan was positive and the reaction was accentuated by irradiation with long wave ultraviolet light. There was photocross-sensitivity to chlorpromazine. In Venezuela, Phenergan cream is a popular remedy and is a frequent cause of photosensitivity. Many of the patients require admission to hospital; the course of the photodermatitis is often prolonged and exacerbations by light-exposure are frequent. Soto (1968) reported 50 cases: in each a patch test with the cream elicited a reaction; 36 were photopatch tested and all responded.

Thioridazine (10-[2-(1-methyl-2-piperidyl)ethyl]-2-(methylthio)phenothiazine; Mellaril; Meleril; Melleril)

A case in which thioridazine was possibly the primary photoallergen was described by Suhonen (1976). The patient initially developed a photodermatitis while taking both thioridazine and chlorpromazine; the drugs were stopped and she remained well until 14 years later when she was given 200 mg of thioridazine and the next day she had a severe recurrence. Photopatch tests: she reacted to thioridazine, chlorpromazine and promethazine (each 1 per cent), whereas ten controls similarly tested with thioridazine gave no reaction, and only irritant responses to it when the dose of UV-A was increased ten-fold.

Trimeprazine (10-[3-(dimethylamino)-2-methylpropyl phenothiazine; Vallergan)

Two patients with a dermatitis of light-exposed areas had positive patch tests to trimeprazine (?concentration) as well as to other phenothiazines. Photopatch tests were not done (Duperrat and Lamberton, 1960).

Chlorothiazide (6-chloro-2H-1,2,4-benzothiadiazine-7-sulfonamide 1, 1-dioxide; Diuril; Saluric)

Hydrochlorothiazide (6-chloro-3,4-dihydro-7-sulfamoyl-2H-1,2,4-benzothiadiazine 1,1-dioxide; Hydrosaluric; Hydro-Diuril)

Chlorothiazide and hydrochlorothiazide are sulphonamide derivatives. An eczematous photodermatitis has been reported in two patients taking chlorothiazide 500 mg daily, and a lichen planus-like eruption affected the exposed areas of two women, one taking chlorothiazide, and the other taking hydrochlorothiazide 50 mg daily. The eruptions cleared when the drugs were discontinued. Patch tests and photopatch tests with tablets crushed in saline were negative, but after ingestion of the drugs phototests with the sunburn spectrum (275–310 mm) elicited reactions. The effect was thought to be photo-allergic (Harber, Lashinsky and Baer, 1959a and 1959b). A similar lichenoid dermatitis has been described in two patients by Kennedy *et al.* (1961). In other cases there has been an exaggerated sunburn reaction which faded to leave marked pigmentation of the dorsa of the hands. Photo-allergic reactions from chlorothiazide have also been seen in south Australia (Burry and Lawrence, 1976).

Frusemide (see p. 429)
In south Australia patients on average doses of frusemide occasionally develop a photodermatitis which, clinically, was thought to be photo-allergic (Burry and Lawrence, 1976).

Quinethazone (7-chloro-2-ethyl-1,2,3,4-tetrahydro-
4-oxo-6-quinazolinesulfonamide; Hydromox; Aquamox)

Quinethazone, an oral diuretic, caused a photodermatitis in a woman who had been taking 100 mg daily for one week. She had previously had similar eruptions from chlorothiazide and hydrochlorothiazide. Phototesting confirmed that the sunburn spectrum was responsbile (Miller and Beltrani, 1966).

Chlorpropamide (1-(*p*-chlorophenylsulfonyl)-3-propylurea; Diabinese)

A woman in Detroit, after taking chlorpropamide 500 mg daily for three months, spent a July afternoon in the sun and developed an eczematous photo-dermatitis. She remained in the dark and her skin cleared. Her drug therapy was then changed to phenformin and she again became tolerant of the sun. It was probably significant that prior to this episode she had had eczema of the hands and face whilst receiving the related drug tolbutamide. While she was taking chlorpropamide, phototests with a hot quartz light were positive; patch tests and photopatch tests were negative (Hitselberger and Fosnaugh, 1962). A patient with a photodermatitis from chlorpropamide was included in the report by Kennedy *et al.* (1961).

Carbutamide (1-butyl-3-sulfanilylurea; Nadisan)

$$H_2N - \langle \text{benzene ring} \rangle - SO_2NHCONH(CH_2)_3CH_3$$

Carbutamide caused a photodermatitis in two patients, one of whom was subsequently given tolbutamide without ill-effects (Burchkhardt, Burckhardt and Schwarz-Speck, 1957). Another patient taking carbutamide developed a bullous eruption of the face, arms and legs after sun exposure (Schreus and Ippen, 1958).

Tolbutamide (1-butyl-3-(*p*-tolylsulfonyl)urea; Orinase)

$$H_3C - \langle \text{benzene ring} \rangle - SO_2NHCONH(CH_2)_3CH_3$$

Tolbutamide is included in lists of oral hypoglycaemic drugs which cause photosensitivity, but no reports incriminating it specifically have been traced.

Amantadine (1-adamantanamine; Symmetrel)

$$\text{adamantane} - NH_2$$

Livedo reticularis is a well-recognised complication of amantadine therapy (Shealy, Weeth and Mercier, 1970; Vollum, Parkes and Doyle, 1971). A woman with Parkinson's disease, who developed a photodermatitis, was described by Ketel and Goedhart-van Dijk (1974). She had been taking orphenadrine hydrochloride (Disipal) 150 mg daily for three years, amantadine 100 mg daily for three months and amitryptilene hydrochloride (Tryptizol) 30 mg daily when she developed eczema of the light-exposed areas. Photopatch tests using these drugs undiluted, and irradiation with long wave ultraviolet light (320–400 nm) were positive only where amantadine had been applied. Similar tests in five controls were negative.

Chlordiazepoxide (7-chloro-2-methylamino-5-phenyl-3H-1,4-benzodiazepine 4-oxide; Librium)

$$\text{structure: chlorobenzodiazepine with } NHCH_3, C_6H_5, O$$

Chlordiazepoxide was reported by Luton and Finchum (1965) as causing a photoallergic reaction in a man who was taking 25–75 mg daily for two weeks. The eruption began on the soles and spread widely to include light-exposed sites and the mouth. Phototesting with the sunburn spectrum was positive only while the patient was taking the drug.

Cyclamate, sodium (Sodium cyclohexylsulfamate)

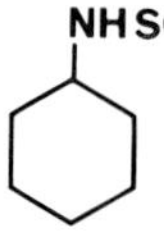

NHSO₃Na — rendered: $NHSO_3Na$

In Philadelphia, a Negro woman trying to lose weight consumed 3600 mg of cyclamate a day in a low-calorie drink during mid-summer. After two months she developed a photodermatitis which was directly related to taking the cyclamates. Phototesting with a light source emitting the 295–420 nm waveband was abnormal when the patient was taking cyclamates as she had done previously, and reverted to normal when she stopped them (Lamberg, 1967).

Pyrithioxin (3,3'-(dithiodimethylene)bis[5-hydroxy-6-methyl-4-pyridinemethanol]; pyritinol; Encephabol)

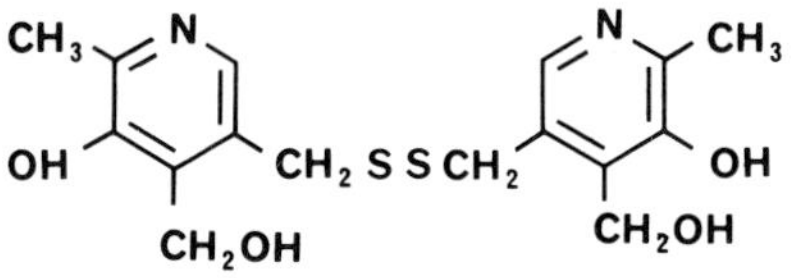

CH₃   N   N   CH₃
OH   CH₂ S S CH₂   OH
   CH₂OH   CH₂OH

A lichenoid eruption affecting the exposed skin, associated with erosive lesions in the mouth, developed in a man aged 62 years with cerebral arteriosclerosis who had been taking, amongst other drugs, pyritinol for six weeks. A photopatch test with 20 per cent pyritinol in petrolatum, irradiated with ?long wave ultraviolet light, was positive. The reaction was considered to be photoallergic (Ishibashi, Hirano and Nishiyama, 1973).

Triacetyldiphenylisatin (1-acetyl-3,3bis(*p*-hydroxyphenyl)oxindole diacetate; TDI; Laxagen; Unilax)

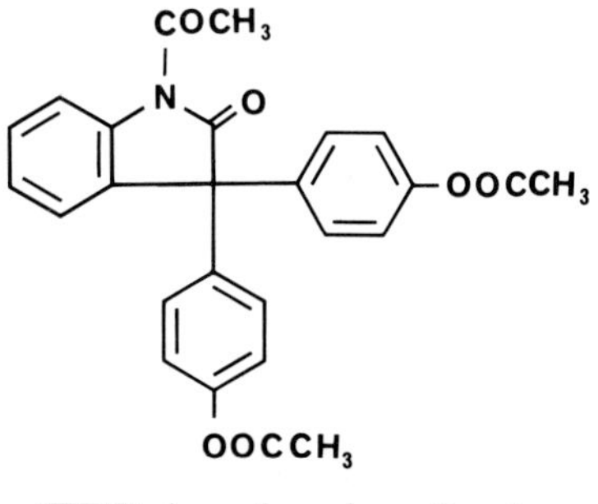

COCH₃
N   O
OOCCH₃
OOCCH₃

Triacetyldiphenylisatin (TDI) is a laxative. It photosensitised two patients, both of whom had positive photopatch tests to TDI 0.1 per cent in ethanol (Jung, 1967).

8-Methoxypsoralen
A psoriatic patient who developed a photoallergic dermatitis from oral 8-methoxpsoralen reacted to UVA but not to UVB or UVC (Plewig, Hofmann and Braun-Falco, 1978).

Phototoxic and photoallergic

SYSTEMIC DRUGS

Quindine sulphate

Quinidine (6-methoxy- α -(5-vinyl-2-quinuclidinyl)-4-quinolinemethanol)
(formula p. 263)

Livedo reticularis — ?phototoxic. Three patients taking quinidine sulphate or
bisulphate developed a livedo reticularis type of eruption after sun exposure.
The changes began after two hours in one patient and after two days in the
other two. The arms and legs were mainly affected and in each patient the network became purpuric. One patient (Marion and Terrien, 1973) was taking
quinidine sulphate 300 mg three times a day, and when the drug was stopped
the eruption regressed. The other two patients (de Groot and Wuite, 1974) were
taking quinidine durettes, formulated to maintain a constant level of
quinidine — they contain 250 mg quinidine bisulphate and 12–13 per cent
dihydroquinidine in a spongy base consisting of polyvinyl chloride, polyvinyl
acetate, polyethylene glycol 6000, magnesium stearate and talcum venetum. One
patient was taking 3–5 daily; his patch tests and photopatch tests were negative
but while he was on the drug, sun exposure caused a relapse. He was able to
continue to take the durettes provided he avoided the sun. The second patient
was taking three durettes three times a day and when they were stopped the
rash cleared. She was neither photopatch tested nor challenged with the drug.

Dermatitis — ?idiosyncrasy ?photoallergy. Three elderly men developed photodermatitis while taking quinidine sulphate. Two were taking the extended-release
form. The rash cleared when the drug was stopped,,but it relapsed in both
when challenged with quinidine sulphate 300 mg four times a day. One of the
patients remained in hospital and relapsed within a week, and the second
relapsed on the fourth day, having spent the previous afternoon in the sun. The
third patient was kept in a dark room but on the fourth day phototesting
showed him still to be light-sensitive. Each of the patients reacted to long wave
ultraviolet light (UV-A: 320–400 nm). Three patients taking quinidine sulphate,
who were not photosensitive, had normal light tests, and two controls given
quinidine sulphate intradermally did not develop local photosensitivity (Pariser
and Taylor, 1975). This same photosensitivity occurred in a black man after a
year's treatment with quinidine gulconate 648 mg daily; he, too, reacted to
UV-A while taking the drug but he required a long period of exposure (Pariser
and Pariser, 1977).

A similar patient was reported by Gammer and Gross (1976). Aged 82 years,
she developed an eczematous photodermatitis after taking quinidine for one
month. Eleven months later all her drugs were stopped, she was treated in a
dark room and the eruption cleared. She was challenged with quinidine 400 mg
every six hours and relapsed severely within a day.

Sulphanilamide (*p*-aminobenzenesulphonamide; Prontosil album)

$$H_2N \text{—} \langle \rangle \text{—} SO_2NH_2$$

Sulphanilamide injected intradermally, and the site irradiated with light, produced phototoxic reactions in each of six volunteers. Two were sensitised by the injections and became photo-allergic to sulphanilamide (Epstein, 1939). The photosensitising properties of sulphanilamide were also studied by Burckhardt (1941) and experimentally in guinea pigs by Schwarz and Speck (1957).

Phototesting

Photopatch tests
If the drug is absorbed topically.

Oral administration
Relatively small amount, one or several doses

Light exposure. Monochomator, Short wave ultraviolet light, Long wave ultraviolet light

Reading. One day, two days and longer.

Sunscreens

The function of a sunscreen is to absorb light and thus to protect the skin from injurious radiation. Several chemicals will, with varying degrees of efficacy, screen the short wave ultraviolet light of the sunburn spectrum, but so far there are no comparable compounds which absorb long wave ultraviolet light. In a study of several light screening agents, Macleod and Frain-Bell (1971; Frain-Bell, 1979) emphasised the importance of using a sunscreen appropriate for the spectrum to which the patient is sensitive. The many sunscreen preparations available in Australia have been classified by Robertson and Groves (1977) according to their percentage transmission of various wavelengths.

It was emphasised by Thompson, Maibach and Epstein (1977) that it is easy to overlook a contact dermatitis from a sunscreen as responsible for the deterioration in a photosensitive patient.

Short wave ultraviolet light
The principal chemicals used topically to screen short wave ultraviolet light are *para*-aminobenzoic acid (PABA) and its esters, benzophenones (mexenone) and cinnamates. The benzophenones also absorb some long wave ultraviolet light. Both 5 per cent PABA in ethanol and 2.5 per cent amyl *p*-dimethyl-aminobenzoate (isoamyl-*p*-*N*,*N*-dimethyl aminobenzoate; Escalol 506; padimate) in ethanol were shown by Pathak, Fitzpatrick and Frenk (1969) to be effective

against the sunburn spectrum. In a later study, Langner and Kligman (1972) found 5 per cent aminobenzoic acid in a hydroalcoholic solution to be the most protective sunscreen and its effect was enhanced by repeated applications and by hydration of the skin prior to application. To maintain protection, two hours should elapse between topical application and immersion in water. However, the practical feasibility of using such large quantities of a solution, as suggested in this study, was queried in a letter by Bergstresser (1974). Macleod and Frain-Bell (1975) reported that the most efficacious sunscreen is a mixture of 5 per cent *para*-aminobenzoic acid and 2.5 per cent of the ester amyl dimethyl-aminobenzoate in 70 per cent ethanol. To maintain adequate protection they advised re-application after sunbathing or swimming.

A thin film of red veterinary petrolatum was found by MacEachern and Jillson (1964) to be an effective screen against both the sunburn spectrum and longer wavelengths, and they pooh-poohed the idea that it was cosmetically unacceptable. Yellow petrolatum had some sunscreeing effect but white petrolatum had none.

Long wave ultraviolet light
Titanium dioxide scatters light and thereby acts as a physical barrier to its penetrating the skin. Macleod and Frain-Bell (1975) found it to be a satisfactory screen for long wave ultraviolet light and that it was cosmetically acceptable if formulated with colouring agents.

Adverse reactions
The esters of PABA are well known contact sensitisers, and cases of sensitisation by the benzophenones and cinnamates occasionally occur. There have been reports of adverse reactions to the aminobenzoates, associated directly with light exposure.

p-Aminobenzoic Acid (PABA)
Contact sensitivity to *p*-aminobenzoic acid (PABA) is occasionally reported. Horio and Higuchi (1978) described a six-year-old girl with xeroderma pigmentosum who developed both a contact and a photocontact sensitivity to PABA; the latter reaction was elicited by long wave ultraviolet light. The importance of an alcohol base was emphasised by Mathias, Maibach and Epstein (1978) in their report of a case of allergic photocontact dermatitis from a 5 per cent PABA lotion.

St John's
Since 1970, only two patients, both men, have been found to be sensitive to PABA. One had had a photosenstive eczema for two years, the other a polymorphic light eruption for 10 years. In both patients the allergy was detected on routine patch testing. Patch tests: each patient reacted to PABA 1 per cent in petrolatum.

Patch testing
PABA 1 per cent in alcohol (petrolatum gives false negative reactions (Mathias Maibach and Epstein 1978).

Isoamyl-p-N,N-dimethylaminobenzoate
(Amyl *p*-dimethylaminobenzoate; Padimate A; Escalol 506; Spectraban

Immediate discomfort. Immediate burning and discomfort of the skin has followed light exposure after the application of 2.5 per cent isoamyl-*p*-N,N-dimethylaminobenzoate (Escalol 506; Spectraban) in 65 per cent ethanol, whereas 5 per cent PABA in 70 per cent ethanol did not have this effect (Katz, 1970). Some months later an attempt to reproduce this reaction in the same subjects was unsuccessful (Blank, 1971). A similar burning effect on the face from an alcoholic solution containing two esters of aminobenzoic acid was described in a letter by Parrish, Pathak and Fitzpatrick (1975). Exposure to sunlight and swimming in chlorinated water evoked the reaction.

Phototoxicity. Kaidbey and Kligman (1978b) have found padimate A to be phototoxic with an action spectrum in the UV-A region. They concluded that it is ineffective as a sunscreen.

Contact dermatitis

St John's
A woman, aged 33 years, with a polymorphic light eruption since the age of 6 years, noticed aggravation of her skin eruption when she used Spectraban. Patch tests: isoamyl dimethylaminobenzoate 5 per cent in butane was positive. Spectraban was negative (?false negative); PPD and PABA were also negative. An open test with Spectraban was positive.

Another photosensitive patient, who repeatedly had positive patch tests to Spectraban, did not react to the individual constituents, including isoamyl dimethylaminobenzoate 5 per cent in butane.

Glyceryl p-aminobenzoate (Escalol 106)

A woman with both contact allergy and photocontact allergy to glyceryl *p*-aminobenzoate was described by Goldman and Epstein (1969). She applied a sunscreen lotion containing glyceryl *p*-aminobenzoate to her legs, sunbathed for 30 minutes, and two hours later began to develop on her legs a dermatitis which became vesiculo-bullous. A plain patch test with glyceryl *p*-aminobenzoate 2.5 per cent in ethanol was positive. Photopatch tests with unfiltered light and light filtered through window glass were positive and of much greater intensity than the plain patch test. This increased reaction was thought not to be a simple augmentation of the photopatch test reaction by light.

Many patients reported as sensitised to glyceryl PABA have also reacted to benzocaine. Fisher (1977), suspecting an explanation other than cross-sensitivity, found that, in the manufacture of glyceryl PABA, benzocaine is also produced and that 1–18 per cent is present in these Escalol 106 sunscreens. Amyl *para*-dimethyl PABA (Escalol 506; Padimate A) and octyl dimethyl PABA (Escalol 507; Padimate 0) did not contain benzocaine.

Alpha-glycerol ester of ortho-amino-meta-(2,3 dihydroxypropoxy) benzoic acid
This aminobenzoic acid compound, present in a sunscreen as a UV-A filter, sensitised a man with a chronic polymorphous light eruption. On patch testing he reacted to it (5 per cent in pet.) but not to PABA or iso-butyl-*p*-aminobenzoate (van Ketel, 1977).

BENZOPHENONES

Mexenone (2-hydroxy-4-methoxy-4'-methylbenzophenone; Uvistat)

The value of benzophenones as ultraviolet light absorbers was investigated by Knox, Guin and Cockerell (1957). They rarely sensitise.

Oxybenzone and deoxybenzone
A patient with a polymorphic light eruption became sensitive to his benzophenone sunscreen and was found to react to both active ingredients, oxybenzone and deoxybenzone (Thompson, Maibach and Epstein, 1977). Solbar,®, which contains dioxybenzone 3 per cent oxybenzone 3 per cent sensitised another patient and on patch testing he reacted strongly to dioxybenzone (2 per cent pet.) and weakly to oxybenzone (2 per cent pet.) (Pariser, 1977).

St John's
From 1967–1975 sensitisation by benzophenone has been confirmed in only one patient. A 12-year-old girl with a polymorphic light eruption had used Uvistat (which contains 4 per cent mexenone) for a year when it suddenly caused acute oedema of her face. Patch tests: she reacted to Uvistat and to mexenone 5 per cent in petrolatum, but not to the ingredients of the cream base.

Two other patients who reacted to Uvistat itself were subsequently patch tested with mexenone 5 per cent and each constituent of the base, and all the tests were negative.

Sulisobenzone (5-benzoyl-4-hydroxy-2-methoxybenzenesulphonic acid; Spectra-Sorb UV 284; Uval; Uvinal MS-40)

A photosensitive patient with an urticarial and a contact sensitivity to sulisobenzone has been reported by Ramsay, Cohen and Baer (1972).

Cinnamate (2-ethoxyethyl *p*-methoxycinnamate; *p*-methoxycinnamic acid 2-ethoxy-ethyl ester; Giv-Tan)

St John's
From 1970–1976, two men and two women seen had been sensitised by this cinnamate compound in sunscreens. One man was frequently abroad and for six years had attributed his eruption solely to sun exposure. His light-tests were normal and his dermatitis appeared to be entirely due to a contact sensitivity to cinnamates. The second patient was mildly photo-sensitive- she had used several sunscreens, but could not identify one as making her worse. In the third and fourth patients, neither of whom was photosensitive, the cause and effect was obvious and the contact allergy had been recognised by both. [One has been previously reported (Cronin, 1971).]

Patch tests: each of the patients reacted to ethoxyethyl methoxycinnamate 1 per cent in petrolatum and patients one, three and four to their various suntan preparations. They all reacted to balsam of Peru. Cross-reactions: one patient was tested with other cinnamates and she responded to benzyl cinnamate, methyl cinnamate and cinnamyl alcohol (each 5 per cent in pet.), but not to cinnamic acid (5 per cent in pet.), or to cinnamaldehyde (1 per cent in pet.) She did not knowingly eat cinnamates, and her skin remained normal by simply avoiding cinnamate sunscreens.

Homomenthyl salicylate
Two patients, who developed a follicular eruption from homonenthyl salicylate in a suntan lotion (Coppertone), were described by Rietschel and Lewis (1978). Patch tests: both patients reacted to 2 per cent homomenthyl salicylate; one was tested with the lotion and was positive.

References

Adams, R.M. (1972) Photoallergic Contact Dermatitis to Chloro-2-phenylphenol. *Archives of Dermatology*, **106**, 711.

Ågren-Jonsson, S & Magnusson, B. (1976) Sensitisation to propantheline bromide, trichlorocarbanilide and propylene glycol in an antiperspirant. *Contact Dermatitis*, **2**, 79.

Baes, H. (1968) Photosensitivity caused by nalidixic acid. *Dermatologica*, **136**, 61.

Baughman, R.D. (1964) Contact photodermatitis from bithionol. *Archives of Dermatology*, **90**, 153.

Beer, W.E. (1970) Sensitivity to fentichlor. *Contact Dermatitis Newsletter*, **8**, 188.

Behrbohm, P. & Zschunke, E. (1966) Arbeitsbedingtes Ekzem durch 5,4'-Dibrom-salicylanilid in haarkosmetischen Praparaten. *Berufsdermatosen*, **14**, 169.

Berger, R.P. & Papa, C.M. (1977) Photodye herpes therapy — cassandra confirmed? *Journal of the American Medical Association*, **238**, 133.

Bergstresser, P.R. (1974) Comment on sunscreen studies by Langner and Kligman. *Archives of Dermatology*, **109**, 96.

Bethell, H.J.N. (1977) Photo-onycholysis caused by demethylchlortetracycline. *British Medical Journal*, **2**, 96.

Blank, H. (1971) Immediate cutaneous reaction to a sunscreen. *Archives of Dermatology*, **103**, 461.

Blank, H., Cullen, S.I. & Catalano, P.M. (1968) Photosensitivity studies with demethylchlortetracycline and doxycycline. *Archives of Dermatology*, **97**, 1.

Brauner, G.J. (1975) Bullous photoreaction to nalidixic acid. *American Journal of Medicine*, **58**, 576.

Breza, T.S., Halprin, K.M. & Taylor, R. (1975) Photosensitivity reaction to vinblastine. *Archives of Dermatology*, **111**, 1168.

Briffa, D.V. & Warin, A.P. (1977) Photo-onycholysis caused by photochemotherapy. *British Medical Journal*, **2**, 1150.

Burchkhardt, W. (1941) Untersuchungen uber die Photoaktivitat einiger Sulfaniliamide. *Dermatologica*, **83**, 63.

Burckhardt, W., Burckhardt, K. & Schwarz-Speck, M. (1957) *Schweizerische Medizinische Wochenschrift*, **87**, 954.

Burdick, K.H. (1966) Phototoxicity of shalimar perfume. *Archives of Dermatology*, **93**, 424.

Burry, J.N. (1967) Photoallergies to fentichlor and multifungin. *Archives of Dermatology*, **95**, 287.

Burry, J.N. (1968) Cross-sensitivity between fentichlor and bithionol. *Archives of Dermatology*, **97**, 497.

Burry, J.N. (1970) Persistent light reactions from buclosamide. *Archives of Dermatology*, **101**, 95.

Burry, J.N. & Donald, G.F. (1968) Photo-contact dermatitis from soap. *British Journal of Dermatology*, **80**, 711.

Burry, J.N. & Lawrence, J.R. (1976) Phototoxic blisters from high frusemide dosage. *British Journal of Dermatology*, **94**, 495.

Cahn, M.M., Levy, E.J. & Mcmillen, J.A. (1961) Nature and incidence of photosensitivity reactions to demethylchlortetracycline. *Archives of Dermatology*, **84**, 485.

Calnan, C.D. (1958) Studies in contact dermatitis. V. Photosensitivity from chlorpromazine. *Transactions of the St John's Hospital Dermatological Society*, **41**, 26.

Calnan, C.D. (1960) Drug reactions with griseofulvin. *Transactions of the St John's Hospital Dermatological Society*, **45**, 54.

Calnan, C.D. (1975) Dermatitis from quinoxaline dioxide. *Contact Dermatitis*, **1**, 384.

Calnan, C.D., Harman, R.R.M. & Wells, G.C. (1961) Photodermatitis from soaps. *British Medical Journal*, **2**, 1266.

Camm, E., Buck, H.W.L. & Mitchell, J.C. (1976) Phytophotodermatitis from *Heracleum mantegazzianum*. *Contact Dermatitis*, **2**, 68.

Chan, G.F.Q., Prihoda, M., Towers, G.H.N. & Mitchell, J.C. (1977) Phototoxicity evoked by alpha-terthienyl. *Contact Dermatitis*, **3**, 215.

Chang, T.-W. (1965) Cold urticaria and photosensitivity due to griseofulvin. *Journal of the American Medical Association*, **193**, 848.

Clayton, R. & Feiwel, M. (1976) From fentichlor sensitivity to actinic reticuloid. *Proceedings of the Royal Society of Medicine*, **69**, 379.

Conant, M. & Maibach, H.I. (1974) Allergic contact dermatitis due to neutral red. *Archives of Dermatology*, **109**, 735.

Cronin, E. (1968) Studies in contact dermatitis. XVIII. Dyes in clothing. *Transactions of the St John's Hospital Dermatological Society*, **54**, 156.

Cronin, E. (1971) Contact dermatitis from cinnamate. *Contact Dermatitis Newsletter*, **9**, 216.

Crow, K.D., Alexander, E., Buck, W.H.L., Johnson, B.E., Magnus, I.A. & Porter, A.D. (1961) Photosensitivity due to pitch. *British Journal of Dermatology*, **73**, 220.

Dahlquist, I. & Fregert, S. (1967) Allergic contact dermatitis from Neutral Red in quaternary ammonium salt solution. *Contact Dermatitis Newsletter*, **2**, 16.

Dawson, T.A.J. & Scott, K.W. (1972) Contact eczema in agricultural workers. *British Medical Journal*, **3**, 469.

Domonkos, A.N. (1973) Phototoxic onycholysis (case report). *Archives of Dermatology*, **108**, 733.

Drever, J.C. & Hunter, J.A.A. (1970) Giant hogweed dermatitis. *Scottish Medical Journal*, **15**, 315.

Duperrat, B. & Lamberton, J.N. (1960) Allergie á la phenothiazine. *Bulletin de Dermatologie et de Syphiligraphie*, **67**, 941.

Dupont, C. (1972) Sensitivity to fentichlor. *Contact Dermatitis Newsletter*, **12**, 327.

Emmett, E.A. (1974) Diphenydramine photoallergy. *Archives of Dermatology*, **110**, 249.

Epstein, J.H. (1977) Photoallergy. *The Australian Journal of Dermatology*, **18**, 51.

Epstein, J.H., Tuffanelli, D.L., Seibert, J.S. & Epstein, W.L. (1976) Porphyria-like cutaneous changes induced by tetracycline hydrochloride photosensitisation. *Archives of Dermatology*, **112**, 661.

Epstein, J.H., Wuepper, K.D. & Maibach, H.I. (1968) Photocontact dermatitis to halogenated salicylanilides and related compounds. *Archives of Dermatology*, **97**, 236.

Epstein, S. (1939) Photoallergy and primary photosensitivity to sulfanilamide. *Journal of Investigative Dermatology*, **2**, 43.

Epstein, S. (1960) Allergic photocontact dermatitis from promethazine. *Archives of Dermatology*, **81**, 175.

Epstein, S. & Enta, T. (1965) Photoallergic contact dermatitis. *Journal of the American Medical Association*, **194**, 1016.

Epstein, S. & Rowe, R.J. (1957) Photoallergy and photocross-sensitivity to phenergan. *Journal of Investigative Dermatology*, **29**, 319.

Erickson, LR. & Peterka, E.S. (1968) Sunligh sensitivity from oral contraceptives. *Journal of the American Medical Association*, **203**, 980.

Felber, T.D., Smith, E.B., Knox, J.M., Wallis, C. & Melnick, J.L. (1973) Photodynamic inactivation of herpes simplex. *Journal of the American Medical Association*, **223**, 289.

Fisher, A.A. (1977) The presence of benzocaine in sunscreens containing glyceryl PABA (Escalol 106). *Archives of Dermatology*, **113**, 1299.

Frain-Bell, W. (1979) What is that thing called light? *Clinical and Experimental Dermatology*, **4**, 1.

Frain-Bell, W. & Gardiner, J. (1975) Photocontact dermatitis due to quindoxin. *Contact Dermatitis*, **1**, 256.

Frain-Bell, W. & Zaynoun, S. (1975) The oil of bergamot photopatch test. *Contact Dermatitis*, **1**, 245.

Frank, S.B., Cohen, H.J. & Minkin, W. (1971) Phthoto-oncholysis due to tetracycline hydrochloride and doxycycline. *Archives of Dermatology*, **103**, 520.

Freeman, R.G. & Knox, J.M. (1968) The action spectrum of photocontact dermatitis. *Archives of Dermatology*, **97**, 130.

Frost, P., Weinstein, G.D. & Gomez, E.C. (1972) Phototoxic potential of minocycline and doxycycline. *Archives of Dermatology*, **105**, 681.

Gammer, S. & Gross, P.R. (1976) Photoallergy induced by quinidine. *Cutis*, **17**, 72.

Gardiner, J.S., Dickson, A., Macleod, T.M. & Frain-Bell, W. (1972) The investigation of photocontact dermatitis in a dye manufacturing process. *British Journal of Dermatology*, **86**, 264.

Goldfarb, N.J. & Sulzberger, M.B. (1960) Experiences in one hundred thirty-seven patients treated with oral griseofulvin. *Archives of Dermatology*, **81**,859.

Goldman, G.C. & Epstein, E. (1969) Contact photosensitivity dermatitis from sun-protective agent. *Archives of Dermatology*, **100**, 447.

Groot, W.P., de & Wuite, J. (1974) Livedo racemosa-like photosensitivity reaction during quinidine durettes medication. *Dermatologica*, **148**, 371.

Hannuksela, M. (1975) Allergy to propantheline in an antiperspirant (Ercoril® lotion). *Contact Dermatitis*, **1**, 244.

Harber, L.C. & Baer, R.L. (1972) Pathogenic mechanisms of drug-induced photosensitivity. *Journal of Investigative Dermatology*, **58**, 327.

Harber, L.C., Harris, H. & Baer, R.L. (1966) Photoallergic contact dermatitis. *Archives of Dermatology*, **94**, 255.

Harber, L.C., Harris, H., Leider, M. & Baer, R.L. (1964) Berloque dermatitis. *Archives of Dermatology*, **90**, 572.

Harber, L.C., Lashinsky, A.M. & Baer, R.L. (1959a) Skin manifestations of photosensitivity due to chlorothiazide and hydrochlorothiazide. *Journal of Investigative Dermatology*, **33**, 83.

Harber, L.C., Lashinsky, A.M. & Baer, R.L. (1959b) Photosensitivity due to chlorothiazide and hydrochlorothiazide. *New England Journal of Medicine*, **261**, 1378.

Harber, L.C., Targovnik, S.E. & Baer, R.L. (1967) Contact photosensitivity patterns to halogenated salicylanilides. *Archives of Dermatology*, **96**, 646.

Harris, H.J. (1950) Aureomycin and chloramphenicol in brucellosis. *Journal of the American Medical Association*, **142**, 161.

Hitselberger, J.F. & Fosnaugh, R.P. (1962) Photosensitivity due to chlorpropamide. *Journal of the American Medical Association*, **180**, 62.

Hjorth, N. & Moller, H. (1976) Phototoxic textile dermatitis ('Bikini Dermatitis'). *Archives of Dermatology*, **112**, 1445.

Horio, T. (1975) Chlorpromazine photoallergy: co-existence of immediate and delayed type. *Archives of Dermatology*, **111**, 1469.

Horio, T. (1976a) Allergic and photoallergic dermatitis from diphenhydramine. *Archives of Dermatology*, **112**, 1124.

Horio, T. (1976b) The induction of photocontact sensitivity in guinea pigs without UVB radiation. *Journal of Investigative Dermatology*, **67**, 591.

Horio, T. & Higuchi, T. (1978) Photocontact dermatitis from P-aminobenzoic acid. *Dermatologica*, **156**, 124.

Horio, T. & Ofuji, P. (1976) The fate of tetrachlorosalicylanilide in photosensitised guinea pigs. *Acta Dermato-Venereologica*, **56**, 367.

Horkay, I., Tamási, P., Prékopa, A. & Daimy, L. (1975) Photodermatoses induced by oral contraceptives. *Archiv fur Dermatologische Forschung*, **253**, 53.

Ishibashi, A., Hirano, K. & Nishiyama, Y. (1973) Photosensitive dermatitis due to pyritinol. *Archives of Dermatology*, **107**, 427.

Ison, A. & Blank, H. (1967) Testing drug phototoxicity in mice. *Journal of Investigative Dermatology*, **49**, 508.

Ison, A.E. & Davis, C.M. (1969) Phototoxicity of quinoline methanols and other drugs in mice and yeast. *Journal of Investigative Dermatology*, **52**, 193.

Jarratt, M. (1976) Drug photosensitisation. *International Journal of Dermatology*, **15**, 317.

Jillson, O.F. & Baughman, R.D. (1963) Contact Photodermatitis from bithionol. *Archives of Dermatology*, **88**, 409.

Johnson, B.E. (1974) Cellular mechanism of chlorpromazine photosensitivity. *Proceedings of the Royal Society of Medicine*, **67**, 871.

Johnson, B.E., Zaynoun, S. Gardiner, J.M. & Frain-Bell, W. (1975) A study of persistent light reaction in quindozin and quinine photosensitivity. *British Journal of Dermatology*, **93**, (suppl. 11) 21.

Jones, H.E., Lewis, C.W. & Reisner, J.E. (1972) Photosensitive lichenoid eruption associated with demeclocycline. *Archives of Dermatology*, **106**, 58.

Jung, E.G. (1967) Photoallergic durch Triacetyldiphenylisatin (TDI). *Archiv fur Klinische und Experimentelle Dermatologie*, **229**, 170.

Jung, E.G. & Schwarz, K. (1964) Photoallergisches Jadit-Ekzem. *Dermatologica*, **129**, 401.

Kaidbey, K.H. & Kligman, A.M. (1974) Topical photosensitisers: influence of vehicles on penetration. *Archives of Dermatology*, **110**, 868.

Kaidbey, K.H. & Kligman, A.M. (1977) Clinical and histological study of coal tar phototoxicity in humans. *Archives of Dermatology*, **113**, 592.

Kaidbey, K.H. & Kligman, A.M. (1978a) Identification of topical photosensitising agents in humans. *Journal of Investigative Dermatology*, **70**, 149.

Kaidbey, K.H. & Kligman, A.M. (1978b) Phototoxicity to a sunscreen ingredient. Padimate A. *Archives of Dermatology*, **114**, 547.

Kaidbey, K.H. & Kligman, A.M. (1978c) Photocontact allergy to 6-methylcoumarin. *Contact Dermatitis*, **4**, 277.

Katz, S.I. (1970) Relative effectiveness of selected sunscreens. *Archives of Dermatology*, **101**, 467.

Kennedy, B., O'Quinn, S., Perret, W.J., Tilley, J.C. & Henington, V.M. (1961) Phototoxic and photoallergic skin reactions resulting from modern drug therapy. *Journal of the Louisiana State Medical Society*, **113**, 365.

Ketel, W.G. van (1977) Allergic contact dermatitis from an aminobenzoic acid compound used in sunscreens. *Contact Dermatitis*, **3**, 283.

Ketel, W.G. van & Goedhart-van Dijk, B. (1974) Fotosensitisation by Amantadine (Symmetrel). *Dermatologica*, **148**, 124.

Kligman, A.M. & Breit, R. (1968) The identification of phototoxic drugs by human assay. *Journal of Investigative Dermatology*, **51**, 90.

Knox, J.M., Guin, J. & Cockerell, E.G. (1957) Benzophones: ultraviolet light absorbing agents. *Journal of Investigative Dermatology*, **29**, 435.

Kobayashi, F., Wada, Y. & Mizuno, N. (1974) Comparative studies on phototoxicity of chemicals. *Journal of Dermatology*, **1**, 93.

Kochevar, I.E. & Harber, L.C. (1977) Photoreactions of 3,3'4', 5-tetrachlorosalicylanilide with proteins. *Journal of Investigative Dermatoloy*, **68**, 151.

Lam, S.K. & Tomlinson, D.R. (1976) Chlorpromazine-induced histamine release from guinea pig skin *in vitro* — a photosensitive reaction. *Archives for Dermatological Research*, **255**, 219.

Lamb, J.H., Jones, P.E., Morgan, R.J., Everett, M.A. & Penrod, J.N. (1961) Further studies in light-sensitive eruptions. *Archives of Dermatology*, **83**, 568.

Lamberg, S.I. (1967) A new photosensitiser: the artificial sweetner cyclamate. *Journal of the American Medical Association*, **201**, 747.

Langner, A. & Kligman, A.M. (1972) Further sunscreen studies of aminobenzoic acid. *Archives of Dermatology*, **105**, 851.

Leoni, A., Cogo, R., Schettin, D., Piccoli, L. (1976) Una nuova dermatosi jatrogena. *Giornale Italiano di Dermatologia*, **111**, 182.

Leun, J.C. van der, Kreek, E.J. de, Leeuwen M.D. van, & Weelden, H. van (1977) Photosensitivity owing to thiourea. *Archives of Dermatology*, **113**, 1611.

Levene, G.M. & Magnus, I.A. (1969) Drug reactions. VII. Photosensitivity to systemically administered drugs. *British Journal of Dermatology*, **81**, 712.

Ljunggren, B. (1977) Phenothiazine phototoxicity: toxic chlorpromazine photoproducts. *Journal of Investigative Dermatology*, **69**, 383.

Ljunggren, B. & Moller, H. (1976) Phototoxic reaction to chlorpromazine as studied with the quantitative mouse tail technique. *Acta Dermato-venereologica*, **56**, 373.

Ljunggren, B. & Moller, H. (1977a) Phenothiazine phototoxicity: an experimental study on chlorpromazine and related tricyclic drugs. *Acta Dermato-venereologica*, **57**, 325.

Ljunggren, B. & Moller, H. (1977b) Phenothiazine phototoxicuty: an experimental study on chlorpromazine and its metabolites. *Journal of Investigative Dermatology*, **68**, 313.

Ljunggren, B. & Moller, H. (1978) Drug phototoxicity in mice. *Acta Dermato-venereologica*, **58**, 125.

Luton, E.F. & Finchum, R.N. (1965) Photosensitivity reaction to chlordiazepoxide. *Archives of Dermatology*, **91**, 362.

MacEachern, W.N. & Jillson, O.F. (1964) A practical sunscreen — red vet pet. *Archives of Dermatology*, **89**, 147.

Macleod, T.M. & Frain-Bell, W. (1971) The study of the efficacy of some agents used for the protection of the skin from exposure to light. *British Journal of Dermatology*, **84**, 266.

Macleod, T.M. & Frain-Bell, W. (1975a) A study of chemical light screening agents. *British Journal of Dermatology*, **92**, 417.

Macleod, T.M. & Frain-Bell, W. (1975b) A study of physical light screening agents. *British Journal of Dermatology*, **92**, 149.

Magnus, I.A. (1974) Action spectra of actinic reticuloid and various uncommon photodermatoses. *Sunlight and Man*. Eds. Fitzpatrick, T.B. Pathak, M.A., Harber, L.C., Seiji, M. and Kukita, A. p. 720. Tokyo: University of Tokyo Press.

Magnus, I.A. (1976) *Dermatological Photobiology*. p. 211. Publications, Blackwell Scientific Oxford: London.

Maibach, H., Bandmann, H.–J., Calnan, C.D., Cronin, E., Fregert, S., Hjorth, N., Magnusson, B., Malten, K.E., Meneghini, C.L., Pirilä, V., Wilkinson, D.S. & Johannsen, F.R. (1978) Triclocarban: evaluation of contact dermatitis potential in man. *Contact Dermatitis*, **4**, 283.

Maibach, H.I., Epstein, J. & Sams, M. (1974) Photosensitive lichenoid eruption associated with demecylocycline. *Archives of Dermatology*, **109**, 97.

Marion, D.F. & Terrien, C.M. (1973) Photosensitive livedo reticularis. *Archives of Dermatology*, **108**, 100.

Marzulli, F.N. & Maibach, H.I. (1970) Perfume phototoxicity. *Journal of the Society of Cosmetic Chemist*, **21**, 695.

Masuda, T., Honda, S., Nakauchi, Y., Ito, H., Kinoshita, M., Harada, S., Yaoita, H. & Mizoguchi, M. (1971) Photocontact dermatitis due to bithionol, TBS, diaphene and hexachlorophene. *Japanese Journal of Dermatology*, **81**, 238.

Mathias, C.G.T., Maibach, H.I. & Epstein, J. (1978) Allergic contact photodermatitis to para-aminobenzoic acid. *Archives of Dermatology*, **114**, 1665.

Miller, R.C. & Beltrani, V.S. (1966) Quinethazone photosensitivity dermatitis. *Archives of Dermatology*, **93**, 346.

Mitchell, J.C. & Stewart, W.D. (1973) Allergic contact dermatitis from neutral red applied for herpes simplex. *Archives of Dermatology*, **108**, 689.

Molloy, J.F. & Mayer, J.A. (1966) Photodermatitis from dibromsalen. *Archives of Dermatology*, **93**, 329.

Morikawa, F., Fukuda, M., Naganuma, M. & Nakayama, Y. (1976) Phototoxic reaction to xanthine dyes induced by visible light. *Journal of Dermatology*, **3**, 59.

Musajo, L., Rodighiero, G., Caporale, G., Dall'acqua, F., Marciani, S., Bordin, F., Baccichetti, F. & Bevilacqua, R. (1974) Photoreactions between skin-photosensitisng furocoumarins and nucleic acids. *Sunlight and Man*. Eds. Fitzpatrick, T.B., Pathak, M.A., Harber, L.C., Seiji, M. and Kukita, A. p. 369. Tokyo: University of Tokyo Press.

Myers, M.G., Oxman, M.N., Clark, J.E. & Arndt, K.A. (1975) Failure of neutral-red photoinactivation in recurrent herpes simplex cirus infections. *New England Journal of Medicine*, 293, 945.

Nagreh, D.S. (1975) Photodermatitis — study of the condition in Kuantan, Malaysia: *Contact Dermatitis*, 1, 27.

O'Quinn, S.E., Kennedy, B.C. & Isbell, K.H. (1967) Contact photodermatitis due to bithionol and related compounds. *Journal of the American Medical Association*, 199, 89.

Orentreich, N., Harber, L.C. & Tromovitch T.A. (1961) Photosensitivity and photo-onycholysis due to demethylchlortetracycline. *Archives of Dermatoloy*, 83, 730.

Osmundsen, P.E. (1968) Contact photodermatitis due to tribromsalicylanilide. *British Journal of Dermatology*, 80, 228.

Osmundsen, P.E. (1970) Contact photodermatitis due to tribromsalicylanilide (cross-reaction pattern). *Dermatologica*, 140, 65.

Osmundsen, P.E. (1975) Concomitant contact allergy to propantheline bromide and TCC. *Contact Dermatitis*, 1, 251.

Pariser, D.M. & Taylor, J.R. (1975) Quinidine photosensitivity. *Archives of Dermatology*, 111, 1440.

Pariser, R.J. (1977) Contact dermatitis do dioxybenzone. *Contact Dermatitis*, 3, 172.

Pariser, R.J. & Pariser, D.M. (1976) Quinidine photosensitivity. *Archives of Dermatology*, 112, 1610.

Parrish, J.A., Pathak, M.A. & Fitzpatrick, T.B. (1975) Facial irritation due to sunscreen products. *Archives of Dermatology*, 111, 525.

Pathak, M.A. (1974) Phytophotodermatis. *Sunlight and Man*. Eds. Fitzpatrick, T.B., Pathak, M.A., Harber, L.C., Seiji, M. and Kukita, A. p. 502 Tokyo: University of Tokyo Press.

Pathak, M.A., Daniels, F. & Fitzpatrick, T.B. (1962) The presently known distribution of furocoumarins (Psoralens) in plants. *Journal of Investigative Dermatology*, 39, 225.

Pathak, M.A., Fitzpatrick, T.B. & Frenk, E. (1969) Evaluation of topical agents that prevent sunburn — superiority of para-animobenzoic acid and its ester in ethyl alcohol. *New England Journal of Medicine*, 280, 1459.

Pathak, M.A., Kramer, D.M. & Fitzpatrick, T.B. (1974) Photobiology and photochemistry of furocoumarins (psoralens). *Sunlight and Man*. Eds. Fitzpatrick, T.B., Pathak, M.A., Harber, L.A., Seiji, M. and Kukita, A. p. 335 Tokyo: University of Tokyo Press.

Peterkin, G.A.G. (1945) Skin eruptions due to the local application of sulphonamides. *British Journal of Dermatology*, 57, 1.

Plewig, G., Hofmann, C. & Braun-Falco, O. (1978) Photoallergic dermatitis from 8-methoxypsoralen. *Archives of Dermatological Research*, 261, 201.

Quadripur, S.A. & Grunder, K. (1975) Kasuistischer beitrag uber eine Gruppenerkrankung mit Photodermatitis Bullosa Striata Pratensis (Oppenheim). *Hautarzt*, 26, 495.

Raffle, E.J., Macloed, T.M. Hutchinson, F. & Ballinger, B. (1975) Chlorpromazine photosensitivity. *Archives of Dermatology*, 111, 1364.

Ramsay, C.A. (1977) Long wave ultraviolet radiation sensitivity induced by oxytetracycline: a case report. *Clinical and Experimental Dermatology*, 2, 255.

Ramsay, C.A. (1979) Skin responses to ultraviolet radiation in contact photodermatitis due to fentichlor. *Journal of Investigative Dermatology*, 72, 99.

Ramsay, C.A. & Kobza Black, A. (1973) Photosensitive Eczema. *Transactions of the St John's Hospital Dermatological Society*, 59, 152.

Ramsay, C.A. & Obreshkova, E. (1974) Photosensitivity from nalidixic acid. *British Journal of Dermatology*, 91, 523.

Ramsay, D.L., Cohen, H.J. & Baer, R.L. (1972) Allergic reaction nto benzophenone. *Archives of Dermatology*, 105, 906.

Raugi, G.J., Storrs. F.J. & Larsen, W.G. (1979) Photoallergic contact dermatitis to men's perfumes. *Contact Dermatitis*; 5, 251.

Riboulleau, M. (1970) Les dermites provoquées par le céleri. *Thèse de Tours*.

Rietschel, R.L. & Lewis, C.W. (1978) Contact dermatitis to homomenthyl salicylate. *Archives of Dermatology*, 114, 442.

Rimington, C., Morgan, P.N. Nicholls, K., Everall, J.D. & Davies, R.R. (1963) Griseofulvin administration and porphyrin metabolism. *Lancet*, 2, 318.

Robertson, D.F. & Groves, G.A. (1977) Classification of sunscreens preparations. *Australasian Journal of Dermatology*, 18, 109.

Rothstein, M.S. (1977) Onycholysis through phototoxicity. *Archives of Dermatology*, 113, 520.

Sams, W.M. (1966) The experimental production of drug phototoxicity in guinea pigs. II. Using artificial light sources. *Archives of Dermatology*, 94, 773.

Sams, W.M. & Epstein, J.H. (1967) The experimental production of drug phototoxicity in guinea pigs. I. Using sunlight. *Journal of Investigative Dermatology*, **48**, 89.

Sastry, K.S. & Gordon, M.P. (1966) The photodynamic inactivation of tobacco mosaic virus and its ribonucleic acid by acridine orange. *Biochimica and Biophysica Acta*, **129**, 32.

Schreus, H.Th. & Ippen, H. (1958) Photoallergic, Hervogerufen durch ein orales Antidiabetikum, **83**, 98.

Schwarz, K. & Speck, M. (1957) Experimentelle Untersuchungen zur Frage der Photoallergie der Sulfonamide. *Dermatologica*, **14**, 232.

Scott, K.W. & Dawson, T.A.J. (1974) Photo-contact dermatitis arising from the presence of quindoxin in animal feeding stuffs. *British Journal of Dermatology*, **90**, 543.

Segal, B.M. (1963) Photosensitivity, nail discolouration and onycholysis. *Archives of Internal Medicine*, **112**, 165.

Shaffer, J.M., Bluemle, L.W., Sborov, V.M. & Neefe, J.R. (1950) Studies on the use of aureomycin in hepatic disease. IV. Aureomycin therapy in chronic liver disease. *American Journal of the Medical Sciences*, **220**, 173.

Shealy, C.N., Weeth, J.B. & Mercier, D. (1970) Livedo reticularis in patients with parkinsonism receiving amantadine. *Journal of the American Medical Association*, **212**, 1522.

Smith, S.Z. & Epstein, J.H. (1977) Photocontact dermatitis to halogenated salicylanilides and related compounds. *Archives of Dermatology*, **113**, 1372.

Sidi, E. Hincky, M. & Gervais, A. (1955) Allergic sensitisation and photosensitisation to phenergan cream. *Journal of Investigative Dermatology*, **24**, 345.

Soto, J.M. (1968) Promethazine photosensitivity. *Contact Dermatitis Newsletter*, **3**, 53.

Sommer, R.G. & Jillson, O.F. (1967) Phytophotodermatitis (solar dermatitis from plants). *New England Journal of Medicine*, **276**, 1484.

Suhonen, R. (1976) Thioridazine photosensitivity. *Contact Dermatitis*, 2 179.

Suhonen, R. (1976) Phototoxicity of methoxsalen in various vehicles. *Contact Dermatitis*, **2**, 264.

Thompson, G., Maibach, H & Epstein, J. (1977) Allergic contact dermatitis from sunscreen preparations complicating photodermatitis. *Archives of Dermatology*, **113**, 1252.

Thune, P. (1977) Contact allergy due to lichens in patients with a history of photosensitivity. *Contact Dermatitis*, **3**, 267.

Tromovitch, T.A. & Jacobs, P.H. (1963) Photosensitivity to oxytetracycline. *Annals of Internal Medicine*, **58**, 529.

Tucker, M.J. (1975) Carcinogenic action of quinoxaline 1, 4-dioxide in rats. *Journal of the National Cancer Institute*, **55**, 137.

Veber, L.L. de (1962) Photosensitivity, loosening of the nails and teetch in association with demethylchlortetracycline (declomycin). *Canadian Medical Association Journal*, **86**, 168.

Verhagen, A.R.H.B. (1965) Photosensitivity due to chlortetracycline. *Dermatologica*, **130**, 439.

Vinson, L.I. & Flatt, R.S. (1962) Photosensitisation by tetrachlorosalicylanilide. *Journal of Investigative Dermatology*, **38**, 327.

Vollum, D.I., Parkes, J.D. & Doyle, D. (1971) Livedo reticularis during amantadine treatment. *British Medical Journal*, **2**, 627.

Wasserman, G.A. & Haberman, H.F. (1975) Photosensitivity: results of investigation in 250 patients. *Canadian Medical Association Journal*, **113**, 1055.

Watson, C.J., Lynch, F., Bossenmaier, I. & Cardinal, R. (1968) Griseofulvin and porphyrin metabolism. *Archives of Dermatology*, **98**, 451.

Wilkinson, D.S. (1961; Photodermatitis due to Tetrachlorsalicylanilide. *British Journal of Dermatology*, **73**, 213.

Wilkinson, D.S. (1962) Further experiences with halogenated salicylanilides. *British Journal of Dermatology*, **74**, 295.

Woods, B. (1962) Irritant plants. *Transactions of the St John's Hospital Dermatological Society*, **48**, 75.

Wynn Jones, D.W. (1962) Investigation of an outbreak of photodermatitis confined to one shop in a large factory. *British Journal of Industrial Medicine*, **19**, 100.

Zala, L., Omar, A. & Krebs, A.. (1977) Photo-onycholysis induced by 8-methoxypsoralen. *Dermatologica*, **154**, 203.

Zaynoun, S. Johnson, B.E. & Frain-Bell, W. (1976) The investigation of quindoxin photosensitivity. *Contact Dermatitis*, **2**, 343.

Zaynoun, S.T., Johnson, B.E. & Frain-Bell, W. (1977a) A study of oil of bergamot and its important as a phototoxic agent. I. Characterisation and quantification of the photoactive component. *British Journal of Dermatology*, **96**, 475.

Zaynoun, S.T., Johnson, B.E. & Frain-Bell, W. (1977b) A study of oil of bergamot and its importance as a phototoxic agent. II. Factors which affect the phototoxic reaction induced by bergamot oil and psoralen derivatives. *Contact Dermatitis*, **3**, 225.

10.

Plants

J.N.S. Mitchell.*

GENERAL CONSIDERATIONS
  Nomenclature identification
  and selection for testing
  Physiology and biochemistry
THE PLANT FAMILIES
  Alliaceae
  Alstroemeriaceae
  Amaryllidaceae
  Anacardiaceae
  Araceae
  Araliaceae
  Aspidiaceae
  Begoniaceae
  Boraginaceae
  Bromeliaceae
  Cactaceae
  Cannabidaceae
  Capparidaceae
  Chenopodiaceae
  Compositae
  Cruciferae
  Euphorbiaceae
  Geraniaceae
  Gesneriaceae
  Ginkgoaceae
  Gramineae
  Hydrophyllaceae

Allergens
Patch testing
Clinical features

Iridaceae
Labiatae
Lauraceae
Leguminosae
Liliaceae
Moraceae
Myrtaceae
Orchidaceae
Polygonaceae
Primulaceae
Ranunculaceae
Rosaceae
Rubiaceae
Rutaceae
Saxifragaceae
Solanaceae
Umbelliferae
Urticaceae
Zingiberaceae

Plant dermatitis

Phytodermatitis is commanding an increasing amount of attention in the world of contact dermatitis and although its importance has never been underrated, it is only now beginning to receive the intensive study which has been lacking in the past. The subject is huge and the relevant botany and phytochemistry daunting to those who have no horticultural bent.

This chapter attempts no more than to introduce the reader gently to the subject and to offer an overview of plant dermatitis, with selected references. There is a brief general introductory section followed by a discussion of plants known to cause dermatitis, arranged under the various plant families.

*Consultant Dermatologist, Western Infirmary, Glasgow.

For the student requiring an exhaustive account, the treatise on *Botanical Dermatology* by Mitchell and Rook (1979) is recommended without reserve as the definitive work.

General considerations

PLANT NAMES (Chicheley Plowden, 1972)

Common names for plants have no place in scientific writing; at best confusing, they can seriously mislead. All ambiguity is removed if botanical names are used (Rook, 1961a). These are based on the well known binomial system, with added refinements to indicate different varieties (Rook, 1961b), hybrids and the like (Porter, 1967). The authority (e.g. L. for Linnaeus) can be omitted in dermatological writing, otherwise the full scientific name of a plant must appear in any valid report. Examples of correct usage are:

Lactuca sativa var. *longifolia*	: A natural variety
Primula malacoides 'Jubilee'	: A cultivated variety
x *Solidaster*	: A new generic name for an intergeneric hybrid from crossing *Solidago* with *Aster*
Syringa x *josiflexa* (*reflexa* x *josikaea*)	: An interspecific hybrid from crossing *Syringa reflexa* with *S. josikaea*

Name endings for some of the higher divisions are useful to know, thus: -aceae (Family); -oideae (Subfamily); -eae (Tribe); -inae (Subtribe).

PLANT IDENTIFICATION

For a scientific report, precision in identifying a plant is mandatory. The only sure way for a dermatologist untrained in botany is to approach the nearest University Department of Botany, or Botanical Gardens, who will recommend a taxonomist willing to help; otherwise Kew Gardens are invariably helpful (Rook, 1977).

SELECTION OF PLANTS FOR TESTING

Once a plant causing contact allergy in a patient has been identified, it is commonly necessary to patch test him with other species to which he may cross-react. In general, these are likely to belong to the same genus, less to related genera in the same tribe or family, and less again to more distantly related species (Rook, 1961a).

The best approach is, by consulting Willis (1973), to find a plant's family, then to refer to a text such as Hutchinson (1973) where an appropriate selection of related genera and species will be found. Where favourite cultivated plants are concerned, the problem should be tackled along the lines discussed by Rook (1961b).

PLANT PHYSIOLOGY AND BIOCHEMISTRY

Despite the voluminous literature, these subjects have little to offer the dermatologist. The few known plant allergens belong to the so-called 'secondary plant products', and this is assumed to be a general rule.

Secondary products are chemically diverse metabolites accessory rather than central to the chemistry of life processes. Seemingly manifestations of an unplanned biosynthetic prodigality of plants, they probably have an as yet unidentified role in primary metabolism. They contain a variety of chemicals: the alkaloids are well known, but the terpenes and phenolic compounds interest the dermatologist most. Terpenes are known allergens in e.g. *Citrus* spp. and celery (*Apium graveolens*), whereas the phenols are basically derivatives of catechol, resorcinol and hydroquinone, which number several proven and notorious sensitisers (p. 476).

These chemicals, the allergens included, are present to a varying degree in certain plant extracts including essential oils, ethereal oils, resins, balsams and oleoresins. These terms are scattered widely throughout the literature on plant dermatitis, but convey only vague concepts, basically because they originated in commerce. It is useful to know that *ethereal oils* are extracted by organic solvents and are likely to be more allergenic than *essential oils*, the product of harsher steam distillation. Various plant parts can yield them e.g. roots (ginger), bark (cinnamon), fruit (*Citrus* spp.). *Resins* can be exemplified by pine resin which, on distillation, yields turpentine and the hard resinous residue colophonium. *Balsams* are best considered to be pathological secretions of an injured plant. *Oleoresins* are natural mixtures of resins and essential oils.

THE ALLERGENS

Few plant allergens have been isolated and identified, the techniques being complex; they were neatly reviewed by Benezra (1973). Each known allergen is discussed in the appropriate plant family in this chapter, and the chemical structural formulae can be found there. Most allergens belong to the oleoresin (e.g. in *Primula obconica* and in 'poison ivy' and other *Toxicodendron* spp.); but a few are water-soluble (e.g. in *Allium* spp. — garlic etc.), possibly being glycosides (Rook, 1960; Cairns, 1964).

The *clinical allergenicity* of a plant depends on botanical factors. Thus, the antigen may be sequestered in resin canals and released only if the plant is bruised; this applies to *Toxicodendron* spp. It may, however, be readily released by fragile glandular hairs (in *Primula obconica*), or be excreted onto the leaf, or coat the pollen (some *Ambrosia* — 'ragweed'– spp.), or be disseminated widely by wind on trichomes and tiny fragments of powdered dried plants (especially *Parthenium hysterophorus*). The amount of allergen synthesised varies not only among different populations of the same species (chemovars) but also in the same specimen, being influenced by the stage of growth, state of health, cultural conditions and geographical location of the plant.

The inter-relationships between allergens and cross-reactions are discussed on page 466.

PATCH TESTING

The following routine is adapted from Rook (1961a) and Mitchell & Rook (1977):

1. Patch test whenever possible with the actual plants to which the patient has been exposed, but if not practicable, use well-grown healthy specimens of the same species or horticultural variety.

   Ask the patient to bring flowers and leaves from *all* suspect plants, including 'weeds'. Divide the plants into 3 parts: one for testing; one for identification; one for possible extraction later. Specimens can be stored in the freezer.

   Start testing with plants known to cause dermatitis, and if negative test with the others.

2. Test initially with the leaf, then, if positive, test with the flower-head, stalk and petal, and pollen of the same species or variety.

3. Test with botanically related species of any plant eliciting a positive reaction and, in the case of horticultural varieties, with other varieties of the same species or hybrid. Gardeners must be tested with all varieties of *Chrysanthemum*, *Tulipa* or *Narcissus* they grow.

4. Test routinely with terpenes found widely among plants and often available in pure form e.g. α-pinene, limonene and geraniol. If this is not possible use turpentine. Routine testing with alantolactone is not recommended (p. 505); it can miss contact allergy to Compositae plants and it can sensitise.

5. Control patch tests on 5–20 normal subjects are essential when testing plants of unknown irritancy. Special care is needed when testing plants of families known to have irritant species e.g. Capparidaceae, Cruciferae, Euphorbiaceae, Papaveraceae, Ranunculaceae.

Techniques

a. *The leaf* (Rook, 1962): Gently bruise a piece 1 cm square; apply to previously normal skin under occlusion for 48 hours; read at 20 minutes and 24 hours later. Weeds may give irritant reactions in up to 40 per cent of cases (Shelmire, 1940), but if applied for only 1 hour the leaf causes no irritation yet elicits reactions in sensitive subjects. House plants, however, are not irritant (Lynne-Davies and Mitchell, 1974).

b. *Oleoresins*, especially for weeds, were preferred by Shelmire (1940); he described in detail how to prepare them, and used a dilution of 1:50 in acetone as an open test. Commercial preparations are available (Hollister-Stier Lab., Spokane, Washington, U.S.A.). For use, they have been pipetted directly onto filter paper and occluded (Bergh, 1975) but to be reliable they should be applied, in petrolatum, as closed tests (Roed-Petersen and Hjorth, 1976), As the shelf-life is not known, replace these extracts once or twice a year.

c. *Other plant parts*: Testing with bulbs, carrots, citrus fruit etc. is described where appropriate in the text. To test irritant plants for allergenicty, aqueous or ethanolic extracts can be used, starting with 10 per cent and gradually increasing the concentration to 20 per cent or more.

d. *Photopatch tests* are discussed in Chapter 1.

There is a limited place for 'batteries' of plant allergens in the investigation of phytodermatitis. A list for use in testing chefs and other kitchen workers (Hjorth, 1975) is given on page 172; others, applicable to horticulturists, forestry workers and the like, can be found in Foussereau and Benezra (1970). For convenience, the allergens relevant to plant dermatitis have been taken from Fregert and Bandmann (1975) and listed in Table 10.1.

Table 10.1. Plant derivative test substances (From Fregert and Bandmann, 1975)

Test substance	Conc. & Vehicle	Test Substance	Conc. & Vehicle
Abietic acid	5% pet.	Laurel, oil of[a]	2% pet.
Alantolactone	0.1% pet.	Lavender, oil of	2% pet.
Balsam of Peru[a]	10% pet.[b]	Lemon, oil of	2% pet.
Balsam of Canada	25% pet.	Lemon grass, oil of	2% pet.
Balsam of Pine	20% MEK	d-Limonene	2% pet.
Balsam of Spruce	20% MEK	Mirbane oil	10% 0.0
Balsam of Tolu	10% alc.	Neroli, oil of	2% pet.
Beeswax	30% pet. & 0.0 ana	Orange, oil of	2% pet.
		Pentadecylcatechol	0.1-1% MEK
Benzyl cinnamate	5% pet. or 10% alc.	Peppermint, oil of	2% pet.
Bergamot oil	2% pet.	α-Pinene	15% 0.0
Bitter almonds, oil of	10% 0.0	Primin (synthetic)[a]	1 μg: prepared unit
Cassia, oil of	2% pet.		
Cedarwood oil	10% pet.	Pyrethrum	2% pet. or 5% MEK
Cinnamic acid	10% pet.		
Cinamic alcohol	10% pet.	Spearmint, oil of	2% pet.
Cinnamic aldehyde	1% alc.	Storax, oil of	2% pet.
Cinnamon, oil of[a]	0.5% pet.	Tobacco	as is
Citral	2% pet.	Turpentine[a]	10% pet.
Citronella, oil of	2% pet.	Turpentine peroxides[a]	0.3% prepared
Cloves, oil of	2% pet.		
Colophony[a]	10% pet.[c]	Usnic acid	1% pet.
Coniferyl benzoate	2% pet.	Vanilla	as is
Dammar resin	20% alc. or pet.	Vanillin	10% pet.
		Venice turpentine (larch turpentine)	20% pet.
Dipentene, *see* Limonene		Fruit (orange, citrus peel)	as is
Essential oils	1% pet.	Plant, leaf, flower, pollen, bulb	as is
Eucalyptus, oil of	2% pet.	Spice	as is
Eugenol	5% pet.	Spice, oils of	5% ethanol
Geraniol	5% pet.	Wood, exotic	dry sawdust
		Wood, pine and spruce	balsams of pine & spruce

[a]Marketed   [b]also as 25% pet.   [c]also as 20% pet.

Cross-reactions

The complexity of cross-reactions in plant dermatitis reflects the somewhat random distribution of chemically identical or very similar allergens throughout the plant kingdom. Sesquiterpene lactones, quinones and substituted phenols are all at the back of many of these reactions, and they tend to be clustered among species of the same or related genera. Spectacular exceptions occur, such as cross-reactions to sesquiterpene lactones in plants as different as liverworts (*Frullania*) and chrysanthemums (Mitchell, 1975a), and in plant families as diverse as Lauraceae, Compositae, Magnoliaceae and Jubilaceae (Mitchell, 1974a). The breadth of cross-reaction patterns is illustrated in the useful list of those met in contact allergy to Balsam of Peru, given by Mitchell (1975a). Added complexities include: the unpredictable allergen content of individual species (p. 463); the well-known phenomena of variety-specific sensitivity (Rook, 1961b) and of patients developing their own spectrum of cross-sensitivities, which tends to widen as sensitivity increases; and the important role played by the order of sensitisation. Patients sensitised by *Primula obconica* may cross-react to *Dalbergia* ('rosewood'), but the converse does not hold. Inevitably, cross-reactions are unlikely to yield their secrets quickly, and their value and predictability in practice will in general long remain empirical.

CLASSIFICATION (Mitchell, 1975a, b)

The principal varieties of phytodermatitis are:

1. **Irritant phytodermatitis** (Woods, 1962)

   a. *Chemical*
   Families notorious for their irritant species include the Euphorbiaceae, Cruciferae and Ranunculaceae. The chemical responsible is peculiar to each e.g. protoanemonin in Ranunculaceae plants.

   b. *Physical*
   Plant parts responsible range from trichomes and spicules, coase hairs, raphides (p. 473), to spines which usually cause mechanical injury.

   c. *Physical and chemical*
   Examples are stinging hairs with histamine and acetylcholine in nettles (*Urtica*), and trichomes with an endopeptidase in cowhage (*Mucuna pruriens*).

2. **Allergic contact phytodermatitis**

   a. *Immediate hypersensitivity* — contact urticaria (p. 24).

   b. *Delayed contact hypersensitivity*
   Only a few of the allergens are known (p. 463).

c. *Physical and allergic reactions in concert*
This may occur in reactions to glochids of the prickly pear (*Opuntia*).

3. **Phytophotodermatitis** (pp. 419 and 535)
Furocoumarins and long wave ultraviolet light are involved. Notable families with species responsible are: Umbelliferae, Rutaceae and Moraceae.

4. **Pseudophytophotodermatitis**
These reactions resemble Group 3 morphologically but are due to irritant or allergic reactions on a background of sunburn. They gave some Ranunculaceae plants a false notoriety as photosensitisers.

The following are closely allied to phytodermatitis and may seem to be reactions to plants:

i. *Parasitophytophotodermatitis*: due to fungi parasitic on plants such as reeds (*Arundo*).
ii. *Epiphytodermatitis*: Lichens and liverworts growing on trees can cause contact allergy blamed on the tree.
iii. *Parasitophytophotodermatitis*: celery (*Apium graveolens*) produces furocoumarins, and is thus a photosensitiser, *only* when parasitised by the fungus *Sclerotina*.
iv. *Pseudophytodermatitis*: due to plant contamination by e.g. fungicides, pesticides, dyes, mites.

INCIDENCE

The true incidence of plant dermatitis is unknown, as it varies geographically with the local flora, as does the substantial occupational element. Thus estimates tend to have a regional relevance. The several published lists of plants known to cause dermatitis (e.g. Shelmire, 1940; Dorsey, 1962; Hjorth, 1969; Whiting, 1971; Nasution *et al.*, 1973) carry these limitations.

Phytodermatitis seems not to be rare, is frequently not seen by dermatologists and often remains unrecognised. Weed dermatitis in particular, at least in Europe, seems to be neglected (Roed-Petersen and Hjorth, 1976). There are, however, some incontrovertible facts:

The commonest causes
In North America, most adults are contact allergic to poision ivy and other *Toxicodendron* spp., but in Europe *Primula obconica* is the commonest cause of non-occupational plant dermatitis. Roed-Petersen and Hjorth (1976) cast doubt on this being still the case, but confirmation is lacking (Rook, 1977). In North America and Europe, chrysanthemum of florists is a significant sensitiser, especially occupationally, and in parts of the subcontinent of India (p. 494) there is an epidemic of contact dermatitis from *Parthenium hysterophorus*.

The type of plant

Flowers and vegetation cause dermatitis on quite a wide scale, but mainly among horticulturists, florists and, in the U.S.A., where *Ambrosia* (ragweed) and *Toxicodendron* ('poison ivy' etc.) species abound, among outdoor workers. Fruit and vegetables cause trouble on a restricted scale, usually among growers and handlers, rarely consumers. Common sensitising plants are listed in Table 10.2, fruit and vegetables in Table 10.3.

Table 10.2. Some commoner sensitising plants ([a] USA esp., [b] India esp., [c] Europe esp.)

Family	Genus	Common name	Family	Genus	Common name
Amaryllidaceae	*Narcissus*	Daffodil, narcissus	Compositae	*Iva*[a]	Marshelder
Anacardiaceae	*Toxicodendron*[a]	Poison ivy and oak		*Parthenium*[b]	Feverfew
Araliaceae	*Hedera*	Ivy		*Tanacetum*	Tansy
Compositae	*Ambrosia*[b]	Ragweed		*Xanthium*	
	Chrysanthemum	of florists & species	Liliaceae	*Tulipa*	Tulip
	Helenium	Sneezeweed	Primulaceae	*Primula*[c]	Primula

Table 10.3. Some sensitising vegetables and fruit

Family	Genus	Common name	Family	Genus	Common name
Alliaceae	*Allium*	Chive, leek, onion, garlic	Liliaceae	*Asparagus*	
Bromeliaceae	*Ananas*	Pineapple	Rutaceae	*Citrus*	Orange, lemon, lime
Compositae	*Cichorium*	Chicory, endive	Umbelliferae	*Apium*	Celery
	Cynara	Artichoke		*Daucus*	Carrot
	Lactuca	Lettuce		*Pastinaca*	Parsnip
Cruciferae	*Armoracia*	Horseradish		*Petroselinum*	Parsley
	Brassica	Brussels sprouts, cabbage			

Sex

Primula obconica causes dermatitis mainly in women, *Ambrosia* spp. almost exclusively in older men.

Age

Contact allergy to *Toxicodendron* species is mainly a disease of adults, whereas the violent irritant reactions to some plants (e.g. of Ranunculaceae) are a childhood phenomenon.

CLINICAL FEATURES

The clinical picture is diverse and reflects mainly the differences between irritant, allergic and photocontact reactions. Modifying factors include the mode and amount of exposure, the site of contact, the patient's age and sex, and the climate.

Generally, phytodermatitis is seasonal, except where evergreens, hot-house or pot plants are concerned. With chronicity, however, it may become perennial with seasonal exacerbations. Sites of predilection are exposed skin, particularly the lids and periorbital regions, which are often itchy and swollen, and the fingers and hands, where the dermatitis tends to be patchy or well marginated.

Typically, the rash is streaky, rectilinear and blotchy, with papules that often aggregate. Distributed more or less at random, the characteristic asymmetry may be lost with repeated exposure. In diversity, it ranges from a nondescript scaly or vesicular fissured hand eczema, or a flexural dermatitis, to a lichenoid reaction, on all exposed sites, that looks deceptively chronic and imparts a falsely aged and weather-beaten appearance to the skin (p. 502). Overall, the lack of vesiculation, unless exposure is dense, is remarkable.

Each type of plant tends to elicit its own brand of reaction. As a rule, *weeds* cause an itchy erythema and lichenification of the face, neck, forearms, hands, flexures, legs and ankles of outdoor workers, whereas reactions to *flowers and shrubs* tend to occur in housewives and florists, and spare the flexures and lower limbs. *Bulb* handling, especially of tulips, can cause a highly characteristic dry, scaly, fissuring and very irritable rash on the fingertips (p. 521). However, dermatitis from *fruit and vegetables* affects only those who frequently handle culinary products; it is often very localised to just a few fingertips which hold the produce, although reactions to citrus fruit and juice can be more widespread on the face and upper limbs. However, some (e.g. apple, potato, carrot, parsnip) can cause immediate reactions in certain atopic subjects, especially those allergic to birch pollen (Hannuksela and Lahti, 1977) — tingling, itch, even oedema of lips and mouth, and hand dermatitis. Alimentary and laryngeal symptoms can also occur.

Irritant dermatitis

Irritant dermatitis can occur after the first exposure to a plant. Hairs and bristles elicit papules or punctate erythema, and irritant chemicals may cause leaf-like or linear vesicles or bullae. In general, the severity is greater in the young, in hot and humid weather, and where the stratum corneum is thin. Young children often develop a papular and bullous reaction which can resemble a phytophotodermatitis, but appears more rapidly and leaves less pigmentation. Children under 5 years old frequently react with close-set red papules scattered across all exposed sites, whereas the older child often quickly responds with itch, burning, even pain, as well as erythema. Repeated exposure can elicit dermatitis. Very irritant plants, usually tropical ones, can provoke intense reactions with haemorrhagic bullae, even necrosis.

Allergic contact dermatitis

Allergic contact dermatitis deserves no special mention here. It is less common in children and usually affects gardeners, florists, regular food handlers and outdoor workers. However contact with the allergens in essential oils used in perfume has to be borne in mind (Rudzki *et al.*, 1976) (p. 159).

Phytophotodermatitis (p. 419)
Phytophotodermatitis classically comprises striate erythema and irregular linear bullae, arising 12–24 hours after exposure to the plant and sun; it quickly heals to leave pigmentation lasting many months.

The *diagnosis* of phytodermatitis can be difficult. The resemblance of irritant reactions with sunburn to phytophotodermatitis is close (see above). Greater trouble arises in distinguishing a phytodermatitis on exposed sites, caused by an airborne allergen (p. 502), from a pollen dermatitis, atopic dermatitis or a photodermatitis (Hjorth *et al.*, 1976). This is discussed on page 503. A useful diagnostic sign is involvement of the triangle of skin behind the earlobe in phytodermatitis, not in photodermatitis (Wilkinson, 1976).

Plant dermatitis may be suggested by the patient's occupation or the effect of season, but a history of contact with plants can be elusive. Plants at home, on the way to work, in the office or at friends' homes commonly pass unnoticed (British Medical Journal, 1965). Patients must be told to look for them. Moreover, suspected plants have to be seen in the clinic or where they grow before they can be identified and assessed as possible causes of dermatitis, although competent gardeners and florists should be able to produce an accurate list. The inability of the general population, dermatologists included, to recognise *Primula obconica* is, however, remarkable (Hjorth, 1970a); the same probably applies to most other plants.

TREATMENT

Acute reactions
Acute reactions are managed along conventional lines. Applications should be bland and soothing: saline compresses until exudation is controlled, when simple creams are suitable. Heavy sedation may be needed if irritation is intense, and bed-rest is indicated for widespread reactions with malaise or secondary infection. Infection is best treated with systemic antibiotics. Only in the severest cases are systemic corticosteroids indicated, and even then they may be of limited value (p. 484).

Chronic dermatitis
More chronic dermatitis may respond to topical steroids, but long term management hinges on strict avoidance of further contact with the offending plants. This applies to the sensitising and cross-reactive species, which must be sought, recognised and accurately identified.

Housewives and amateur gardeners can be persuaded to dispose of all plants to which they are sensitive and then avoid contact. Keen gardeners, however, may need help in restocking the garden or hot-house with acceptable substitutes, while horticulturists and florists, with a livelihood at stake, must be given comprehensive lists of harmful and safe varieties before it can be decided whether there is a commercially profitable range that they can handle. This is commonly possible where chrysanthemums, tulips, hyacinths and *Narcissus* are involved. If, however, no suitable range can be found, or if outdoor workers cannot avoid weeds, hyposensitisation has to be considered. This has been used with considerable difficulty and a modicum of success in patients sensitive to 'poison ivy' (p. 484) and 'ragweed' (p. 506). With few exceptions, it is scarcely worthwhile.

The plant families

ALLIACEAE

Allium is the best known genus. Cultivated species include:

Allium ascalonicum:	shallot	*A. sativum*:	garlic
A. cepa:	onion	*A. schoenoprasum*:	chive
A. porrum:	leek		

The characteristic odour of onion is due to allylpropyl disulphide, and although garlic contains the same substance, its smell is mainly that of diallyl disulphide (Burks, 1954).

Allergens

The allergens are mostly in the outer part of the bulbs (Rook, 1962), but none has been isolated or identified. Those of onion and garlic are soluble in water, ethanol and acetone, and are heat and acid labile (Burks, 1954; Bleumink *et al.*, 1972; Bleumink and Nater, 1973).

Whether the species share allergens is undecided. Burks (1954) thought that onion and garlic might, but Bleumink and Nater (1973) found no cross-reactions to these two species, and considered their antigens to be different. Moreover, the case of contact hypersensitivity to onion, garlic and tulip reported by Bleumink *et al.* (1972) shed no light on the matter, for tulip alone had the only known allergen, tuliposide A. Support for the view that onion, garlic and tulip may have no common or cross-reacting allergens came from the study by van Ketel and de Haan (1978) of three cases of onion and garlic contact hypersensitivity in cooks. Their patch tests with garlic extracts were positive, whereas onion extracts (except for the ethanol extract in one case) and α-methylene- δ -butyrolactone elicited no reaction. Allyl disulphide, however, might be an allergen common to garlic, leek and chive (Hjorth and Roed-Petersen, 1976).

The *incidence* of contact allergy to *Allium* spp. is unknown; they infrequently cause irritant dermatitis, possibly photosensitivity. Onion and garlic in a standard patch test series elicited reactions in 6 per cent and of the 13 cases discovered only two had been suspected clinically (Bleumink and Nater, 1973). Among food handlers studied by Hjorth and Roed-Petersen (1976), garlic was the commonest sensitiser; of 28 tested, 10 reacted to garlic, and of the latter seven reacted also to onion, and four to both leek and chive.

Clinical features

Clinically, a predominantly unilateral hand eczema is usual (Rook, 1960),

Like 'Tulip Finger' (p. 521) it tends to start on the finger tips (Bleumink and Nater, 1973). The 37-year-old housewife reported by Burks (1954) was typical. Precise sites of contact with garlic cloves held during chopping were affected; these were the ends of both thumbs and the left index and middle fingers. Patch tests with onion and garlic were both positive and caused a flare-up of the dermatitis. Eating garlic had the same effect.

The first case to be reported (Edelstein, 1950) was unusual. It was in a 56-year-old meat grinder who developed an itchy, erythematous, scaly and vesicular eruption on the forearm that he habitually used to wipe garlic-contaminated meat off his machine. The rash cleared provided he avoided contact with garlic. A patch test with garlic (?as is) was positive, and the reaction lasted a month. The interest in the case reported by Bleumink et al. (1972) lay in the fact that the 30-year-old restauranteur, who developed hand eczema on being sensitised by garlic, had positive patch tests to onion and tulips as well as to garlic.

Patch tests

As the cut surface of raw onion or garlic can be irritant, the degree varying between specimens, aqueous and ether extracts have been used (Burks, 1954; Bleumink and Nater, 1973). (Five ounces of solvent are poured onto 15 g of chopped and macerated bulbs: the filtrate is used full strength.) For garlic, an aqueous extract has been preferred (10 g peeled garlic cloves crushed in 10 ml distilled water, kept at room temperature overnight, then filtered) (Pasricha and Guru, 1979).

Other species

Allium triquetrum (Onion weed plant), native to the Mediterranean, is common in south-west England, south Wales and the Channel Islands. Grown for ornament in New Zealand, it escaped and is now widespread.

A representative case was in a man, described by Black (1972), who, within an hour of handling the plant, developed a rash on his face, especially the lids. It began with marked swelling and resolved over 3–4 days passing through a crusted, scaly phase. Itch was not outstanding, but at the height of the reaction be coughed, wheezed and his eyes watered. He had hay fever when the plant was in flower. Patch tests with stalk sap, flowers and the leaf all were positive. Before sensitisation, he had handled onions and eaten pickled onions with impunity, but subsequently sudden wheezing and tightness of the throat occurred if he ate pickled onions.

ALSTROEMERIACEAE

This new family was once included in the Amaryllidaceae. Both belong to the order Liliiflorae.

Alstroemeria (Peruvian lily) species have irregularly trumpet-shaped flowers on slender leafy stems. They bloom from June to September and are long-lasting when cut.

A number of the Liliiflorae contain tulip allergens (p. 520) (Slob, 1973) and as all species of *Alstroemeria*, *Erythronium* and *Tulipa* yield tulipaline-A, they are potentially allergenic (Slob, 1973). This could be just an extraction artefact

(Mitchell, 1974b), but the substantial amounts of tuliposide-A in many *Alstroemeria* species makes it unlikely.

Predictably, *Alstroemeria* can cause a 'Tulip Finger'-like reaction, and cases of contact hypersensitivity to both *Alstroemeria* and *Tulipa* have been reported (Rook, 1961b, 1970a; Cronin, 1972).

Many employees in a large floriculture centre, where cultivars and species of *Alstroemeria* were bred and grown, developed a contact-like dermatitis through handling stems and leaves of the plants (van Ketel *et al.*, 1975). Ten workers, four with and six without dermatitis, were patch tested with several parts of a number of the plants, and also with tulip allergen and tulip bulb. The four with dermatitis had had frequent contact with *Alstroemeria* and all reacted to some part of the plant and to tulip bulb and tulipaline-A. None of the dermatitis-free patients reacted. These results are consistent with tulipaline-A being the allergen and account for reciprocal cross-sensitivity to *Tulipa* and *Alstroemeria*.

AMARYLLIDACEAE

The Amaryllis family is closely allied to the Liliaceae and Iridaceae. Many species have lily-like flowers and possess 'lily' names. *Galanthus* (Snowdrop) and *Narcissus* are representative genera.

Narcissus is the botanically correct generic name for all species classed as narcissi, but those with a central trumpet at least as large as the surrounding petals are commonly known as daffodils.

Many naturalised, wild species are grown as pot or garden plants and their equally numerous naturalised, large hybrids are produced for market and show. The selection of wild species is so wide that, depending on their derivation, all degrees of allergenicity are met among their hybrids (Rook, 1961b, 1962).

Botanical aspects

Narcissus bulbs have several layers of abrasive *tecta* (outer coat) (Overton, 1926). They contain bundles of highly irritant needle-shaped clacium oxalate crystals (*raphides*) (Hjorth and Wilkinson, 1968) which, together with alkaloids and mucus, are also distributed widely throughout the plant within slime vessels. When the flower is twisted off, these canals are ruptured and the irritant contents escape, being expressed by the surrounding cells (van der Werff, 1959). The number of raphide producing cells and the proportion of oxalic acid to calcium oxalate vary considerably among species.

Allergens

Allergens are probably produced by *Narcissus*, *Galanthus* and possibly *Hippeastrum*, but none has yet been isolated or identified (Mitchell, 1974b). The opinion that reactions to *Narcissus* are allergic (Hjorth and Wilkinson, 1968) was supported by patch test studies indicating that aqueous, ether and acetone extracts of the plant's leaves and flowers contain allergen (Bleumink and Nater, 1974). However, only the aqueous leaf extract of *Galanthus* seems to be allergenic. *Narcissus*, unlike several other members of the Liliiflorae (Slob, 1973), does not produce tulipaline-A (Rook, 1970a).

Irritants

Penetration of the skin by raphides causes most of the irritant reactions, which are intensely pruritic and involve exposed areas and sites of friction. Several genera other than *Narcissus* are irritant (Mitchell, 1974b) and still others are thought to be (Bleumink and Nater, 1974).

Clinical features

The incidence is unknown. Of the many workers in the narcissus industry few complain; van der Werff (1959) thought that they either change their job, are just temporary workers, or accept their lot as irremediable. He found that, depending on the varieties of *Narcissus* handled, dermatitis occurs in between 20 and 100 per cent of workers.

Narcissus dermatitis ('Lily Rash'; 'Narcissus Rot') was first reported among 'lily' packers in the Scilly Islands (Walsh, 1910). It is caused mainly by heavy and industrial exposure to the juice rather than by casual contact (Mitchell, 1975a). Those who cut, bunch and pack narcissi or daffodils are most at risk, but workers who pick off flower heads or pack bulbs (van der Werff, 1959), or florists who handle the flowers (Bleumink and Nater, 1974) also can develop dermatitis. It occurs particularly in Jersey and the Scilly Islands, where 'Actaea' and 'Princeps' are notorious hybrids, although Palmer (1934) found 'trumpet daffodils' and 'jonquil narcissi' troublesome.

The dermatitis may be limited to the finger sides (Hjorth and Wilkinson, 1968), but can be widespread and very severe (Rook, 1961b). Usually the hands and forearms are affected, but other exposed areas such as the face, lids and neck, and friction sites, particularly the waist and anogenital region, are quite commonly involved.

Characteristically, the rash is papular, the pruritus notorious and the eyelids often red and swollen (Rook, 1960a, 1962). However, a scaly erythema can be the only visible manifestation, and vesicles are remarkably rare (van der Werff, 1959). Despite their vicissitudes, these patients seem able to continue at work.

Patch Testing

The leaf or stem can be used (p. 464).

Management

Pruritus due to raphides is relieved by washing with weak acid (Hjorth and Wilkinson, 1968). When necessary, it may be possible to find a commercially acceptable selection of *Narcissus* varieties that the patient can handle (Rook, 1962).

Other genera

Irritant dermatitis has been caused by *Crinium* (Cape lily), *Haemanthus* (Blood lily), *Pancratum* (Mediterranean lily) and *Hippeastrum* (Barbados lily), the last possibly being also allergenic (Mitchell, 1975a). Suspected species were listed by Bleumink and Nater (1974).

ANACARDIACEAE (THE CASHEW FAMILY)

Tropical trees and shrubs with resinous bark characterise the Anacardiaceae. Potentially allergenic plants are more numerous in this family than in any other (Maibach and Hjorth, 1973), and genera of dermatological interest include: *Anacardium*, *Mangifera*, *Rhus* (including *Toxicodendron*), *Semecarpus* and *Smodingium*.

Botanical features

Morphologically, Anacardiaceae plants range from climbers and shrubs to trees, but the commonest by far, at least in North America, are the so-called 'poison ivy' and 'poison oak'. These names are merely descriptive of the overall aspect of a trifoliate plant which could be one of many *Toxicondendron* species. (*Toxicodendron* is a section of *Rhus* (Fernald, 1950).) These species show a remarkable adaptability to the environment (Shelmire, 1941a), and when grown under identical conditions they can look very much alike (Shelmire, 1941b). In North America, the commonest species, *Toxicondendron radicans*, is very inconsistent and can grow as a short vine in the east and south, and as a small shrub in the west.

Toxicodendron species

Toxicondendron species are numerous, but conservative botanists agree to three, viz. *T. radicans*, *T. querquifolium* and *T. diversilobum*, while some add several varieties (Shelmire, 1941a, b) such as *T.r. microcarpa* and *T.r. rydbergii*. Inevitably, however, dermatologists will adhere to the vague and botanically reprehensible common names, using 'poison ivy' for the climbers and 'poison oak' for a shrub, expecting the latter to have a more oak-shaped leaf. Four species, with synonyms, are listed in Table 10.4. For further details see Kingsbury (1964) or Fernald (1950).

Table 10.4. Four common *Toxicodendron* species

Species	Morphology	Leaf	Locality	Synonyms
T. radicans	Woody rope-like vine, shrub or sub-shrub	Groups of 3 leaflets. Top-hairy; under smooth	Ubiquitous	*Rhus toxicodendron*, *R. radicans*, Poison ivy, Poison vine or creeper, Mark weed
T. diversilobum	Upright shrub. Spreading	Trifoliate (can be 5). Both sides hairy. More oak-like	Dry barren areas	*Rhus toxicodendron*, *R. diversiloba*, Western poison oak
T. querquifolium	Never climbs	Densely pubescent	Poor sandy soils where *T. radicans* does not grow	*Rhus toxicodendron*, *R. querquifolia*, Eastern poison oak
T. vernix	Tall rangy shrub up to 15' or tree. Never a vine	7–13 leaflets	Damp, woody swampy areas only	*Rhus vernix*, Poison dogwood, elder or sumac

The *plant sap*, which is milky white, irritant (but see below) and contains the allergens, is confined to a system of canals which ramifies throughout the bark, stems and leaves. In air, the sap blackens to form a varnish-like substance which, on extraction by organic solvents, yields a viscous, allergenic oleoresin termed urushiol. *T. verniciferum* yields the most toxic oleoresin (Woods and Calnan, 1976).

Other dermatologically important plants are listed in Table 10.5, which also contains references.

Anarcadium occidentale yields an edible fruit, the cashew apple (Orris, 1958), which envelops the cashew nut. The roasted kernel of the latter is a great delicacy (Ratner *et al.*, 1974), but cells within the two layers of the nut's hull secrete the allergenic resin which is extracted commercially as cashew nut shell oil for use in industry.

The allergens

Anacardiaceae plants produce some of the most potent allergens known; even brief contact can sensitise a considerable proportion of those exposed. In the U.S.A. they account for more allergic contact dermatitis than is caused by all other allergens together. Whether the sap of *Toxicodendron* spp. is also irritant (Shelmire, 1941a; Howell, 1959) or not (Kligman, 1958a) has not been settled, but cashew nut shell oil indubitably is to a high degree (Kligman, 1958c). However, the sequestration of the allergens within resin canals (see above) means that the plant is innocuous unless bruised (Kligman, 1958a).

Fruit of *Mangifera indica* (Keil *et al.*, 1946) and of *Anacardium occidentale* contains no allergen, but the former may be contaminated by stem sap and the latter by cashew nut shell oil.

Most allergen in *Toxicodendron* spp. is found in the root, which can cause dermatitis all year round (Shelmire, 1941a). The amount produced varies with the plant's variety, habitat and stage of growth (Shelmire, 1941a, b). This is, however, unlikely to be of clinical importantce for, irrespective of the source, age or stage of growth, the leaves, stems and roots all differ little in their potency as patch test material (Kligman, 1958a). Seasonal variations in reactions could equally well be due to the ease with which young leaves are bruised, to the attraction of the countryside in spring and to the increasing respect for the plants as the year advances.

Chemically, the allergens belong to the phenolic moiety of the oleoresin, and are catechol and resorcinol derivatives with a long aliphatic side chain (R in the basic formula below), *meta* to at least one hydroxyl group (Keil *et al.*, 1946):

Catechol   Resorcinol   Basic Formula

The side-chain usually has 15 carbon atoms, sometimes 17, and it can contain up to three double bonds; thus there are saturated, mono-, di- or tri-olefinic

Table 10.5. Other allergenic members of the Anacardiaceae

Species	Principal features	Growth	Site of allergen	Geography	Synonyms
Anacardium occidentale (Orris, 1958; Ratner *et al.*, 1974)	Edible fruit and nut. Cashew nut shell oil of commercial value	Largely cultivated (for oil)	Shell oil, possibly wood	India, Africa, C. America, Brazil, E. Indies	Cashew nut
Gluta renghas (Fasal, 1945)	Yields a good varnish	Tree	Sap	Indo-Malaysia	Rengas
Mangifera indica (Brown and Brown, 1941; Keil *et al.*, 1946)	Edible fruit	Tree up to 40 ft high. Cultivated for fruit	Sap, e.g. on fruit peel from stem	Indo-Malaysia; cultivated in India, Australia, Phillipines, Hawaii, Brazil, C. America, Mediterranean, Florida, California	Mango, King of Fruits, Apple of the Tropics
Rhus succedanea (Findlay *et al.*, 1974)	Wax from crushed berries	Tree	Sap	Japan	Wax Tree
Rhus typhinia (Maibach & Hjorth, 1973)	Hardy ornamental tree or shrub	Tree. New brown shoots hairy	Leaf sap	E. North America, Danish & Swedish gardens	Antler tree, Staghorn sumac, Velvet sumac
Semecarpus anacardium	Heat-resistant oleoresin for marking ink	Tree	Sap (& ink)	India, Malaya	Marking nut tree Indian marking nut
Smodingium arguum (Findlay *et al.*, 1974)	Popular cultivated shrub in gardens, home and school	Small tree	Sap	Southern Africa	Rainbow leaf tree, Um-tovane Tovana
Toxicodendron striatum (de Hurtado, 1970)	Related to *T. verniciferum*	Tropical tree	Sap; also irritant	S. America, C. & N. South America	*Rhus striata*
T. verniciferum	Lacquer & wood used commercially	Tree	Sap. the most toxic urushiol containing plant	Japan, China, India	*Rhus verniciferum* Japanese lacquer tree

compounds. For greater detail see Johnson *et al.* (1972) and Dawson *et al.* (1946).

The urushiols from 'poison ivy' and 'poison sumac' and lobinol from 'poison oak' are probably identical, but Japanese lacquer urushiol differs in its triolefin and in the relative proportions of the catechols. All, however, yield only 3-n-pentadecylcatechol (PDC) on dehydrogenation.

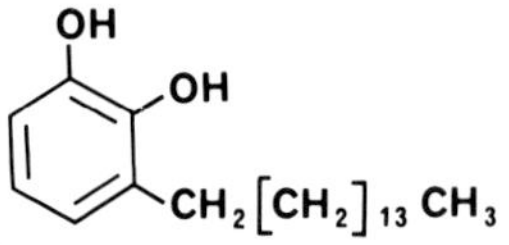

$$\text{OH} \atop \text{OH}$$
$$CH_2[CH_2]_{13}CH_3$$

3-n-Pentadecylcatechol (PDC)

Smodingium argutum produces catechols related to the above, but some have C-17 side-chains; two of these heptadecylcatechols were identified by Findlay *et al.* (1974).

Cashew nut shell oil has 12 allergens. These are combinations of 3 basic structures with either unsaturated, mono-, di- or tri-olefinic pentadecyl side-chains (R) (Fig. 10.1). In the oil, 10 per cent is cardol and 70 per cent cardanol; most of the anacardic acid is converted to cardanol in the heating process (Kligman, 1958c).

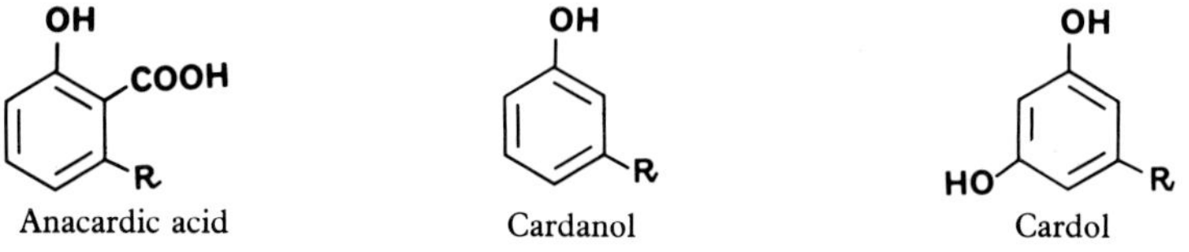

| Anacardic acid | Cardanol | Cardol |

R: $C_{15}H_{31}$, $C_{15}H_{29}$, $C_{15}H_{27}$ or $C_{15}H_{25}$

Cashew nut shell oil allergens

The relative allergenicity of the oleoresins and the individual chemicals is not known precisely, although gas chromatography is a useful guide (Baer *et al.*, 1963). Oleoresins from *T. radicans*, *T. diversilobum* and *T. vernix* are equipotent (Epstein, 1958), but *T. verniciferum* yields the most reactive, and *Anacardium occidentale* the most unstable (a problem in antigen preparation).

Chemical structure influences allergenicity (Dawson, 1956; Baer *et al.*, 1966, 1967, 1968). Two hydroxyl groups on the benzene ring are optimal, and, in general, side-chain unsaturation and instability parallel allergenic potency, although the most potent *Toxicodendron* antigen is the diolefin (Johnson *et al.*, 1972). Not unexpectedly, the natural allergens are the most effective of all (Kligman, 1958a), but their inherent instability renders comparisons at best approximate.

Cross-reactions

Cross reactions depend in part on allergen stereochemistry (Baer *et al.*, 1968). As a rule, those sensitive to 'poision ivy' will tend to react to similarly structured simple chemicals such as resorcinol, hexylresorcinol, hydroquinone and its monobenzyl ether. Fortunately, however, a long side chain is necessary to elicit strong reactions, otherwise biological compounds such as adrenalin could be brought into the cross-reacting net (Kligman, 1958a).

There is almost complete cross-reactivity among *Toxicodendron* allergens; quite frequently cross-reactions occur between them and mango skin sap, cashew nut shell oil and the marking nut (*Semecarpus anacardium*) (Livingood *et al.*, 1943; Epstein, 1958; Kligman, 1958c; Howell, 1959). They also occur to the sap of *Gluta rhengas* (p. 482) and other urushiol plants (Goldstein, 1968), and to *Ginkgo biloba* allergens (p. 515).

Incidence

The overall incidence of contact allergy to *Toxicodendron* spp. is unknown, but in the U.S.A. they account for most plant dermatitis and the larger part of allergic contact dermatitis. Thus, Epstein (1958, 1959) found that about 85 per cent of a large number of adults, there, reacted to patch tests with PDC 1:100. However, only about half of these are clinically sensitive and react to the leaf rubbed on the skin. It is curious that only 50 per cent or so of sensitive patients are aware of it, whereas 15 per cent of persons mistakenly believe themselves to be allergic to the plants (Greenberg and Mallozzi, 1940). Probably about one person in four living in a 'poison ivy' area is sensitive to the vine or shrub (Shelmire, 1941a). Cases have also been seen in Victoria, Australia (Apted, 1978).

Sex
The *sexes* are affected equally.

Age
Although neonates can be sensitised (Strauss, 1931) clinical sensitivity is rare before age 5 years and uncommon before 8 (Epstein, 1959), probably through lack of exposure. After the third decade, the incidence drops (Kligman, 1958a), yet some persons are sensitised in their eighth decade. Some, however, remain tolerant for life.

Race
Susceptibility is less in dark skinned people (30–40 per cent) than in white (50 per cent) (Kligman, 1958a), possibly because Negroes are more tolerant of contact allergens. However, American Indians are as susceptible as Whites. From a study of racial and environmental factors Epstein and Claiborne (1957) concluded that the only valid differences are between Orientals born 'abroad' (in the Orient or Hawaii) and all other people. To attribute this to Anacardiaceae allergen exposure in childhood (e.g. in Japanese lacquer or mango) is speculative.

Season and *degree of exposure* are minor factors; most people are sensitised by casual contact.

Clinical features

Dermatitis from *Toxicodendron* spp., especially 'poison ivy', 'poison oak' and 'poison sumac', is usually seen in persons 10–40 years old (Epstein, 1973), the age when opportunity for contact is greatest. Unless exposure maintains a high degree of sensitivity, those who had mild or moderate attacks in childhood, or many years previously, are tolerant of casual contact in adult life, even if exposure is severe. Nevertheless, a moderate stimulus can awaken a dormant sensitivity.

In eastern North America, most cases occur in spring and summer, but in the western U.S.A., there is no seasonal trend. Roots are a hazard throughout the year (p. 476).

Sap from bruised stems or leaves is the usual source of allergen, but oleoresin-contaminated smoke from burning leaves can affect the very sensitive (Epstein, 1958). Contact is not exclusively rural (e.g. in city cemeteries) and can be hard to trace. Easily overlooked are poison ivy at the roadside, even cultivated in a garden (Laur et al., 1978), and allergen contaminated clothing, pets, cows' udders, tools, garden implements (Stanton and Wilson, 1971), outdoor sport equipment and even insects. Such contaminating allergen is stable for long periods if dry; warmth and moisture, as in washing clothes, inactivates it.

Sources of cross-reactions to other Anacardiaceae plants can be even more covert (Etter 1951; Goldstein, 1968) e.g. Japanese lacquer on a variety of items of furniture, table-ware or ornaments; Chinese Ningpo varnish; handling mangos; laundry marking ink (p. 482). Ginkgo tree allergens also cross-react (p. 515).

Just a few seconds' contact with sap may elicit dermatitis in the very sensitive, but usually an attack can be aborted by washing off the allergen within an hour. The latent period is usually 24–48 hours, but it can range from 5 or 6 hours to 8 or 10 days (Brown, 1922; Epstein, 1959). It is rarely longer than 10 days and tends to be abbreviated by denser exposure, heat and humidity, and greater individual susceptibility.

Itch and erythema precede a streaky erythema, papules and vesicles. In severe attacks, oedema and characteristically voluminous (allergen-free) bullae occur, and in the worst cases there can be a widespread eruption with marked facial, neck and limb oedema and constitutional upset. Attacks of this magnitude in the already ill, or when secondarily infected, can be fatal (Epstein, 1958).

The severity of an attack cannot be predicted, even if the degree of exposure and of the patient's patch test sensitivity are known. The more sensitive tend to react more acutely, yet persons with comparable sensitivity may show quite disparate reactions (Kligman, 1958a).

Rate of healing depends in part on clinical severity, but individual variation is considerable and attacks can be protracted by allergen-contaminated finger-nails, fomites or clothing.

Mucosal involvement is not rare, but is limited to areas near the skin, e.g. the mouth after chewing leaves, or the anus during oral hyposensitization.

Systemic symptoms are met in the severest attacks if sufficient allergen is absorbed; the accompanying eruption is urticarial, scarlatiniform, morbilliform or, rarely, erythema multiforme-like.

Unusual features and sequelae include:

a. Leukocytosis of 10 000–18 000/mm³ (5–22 per cent eosinophils);
b. Renal tubule disease (a sequel to secondary infection);
c. Wealing within 12 hours of exposure, indicating immune complex formation from absorbed allergen and circulating antibody. It is met mostly in hyposensitisation;
d. Pompholyx and id reactions to circulating allergen; and
e. Hyperpigmentation or late leukoderma.

Differential diagnosis includes causes of a streaky dermatitis, particularly those of plant origin or closely resembling them (Mitchell, 1975a). Reactions to very irritant plants and phytophotodermatitis (p. 419) cause most difficulty.

Reactions to Anacardiaceae plants other than *Toxicodendron* spp. (Merrill, 1944):

1. *Mangifera indica* (Mango)

Fruit and stems affect the picker rather than the consumer, but there is individual susceptibility. Pickers experience an extensive reaction on the fingers, backs of the forearms and hands, and the genitals. Eating mango produces erythema, swelling and vesicles on the lips (especially the upper) and a vesicular rash on the face, mostly around the mouth and on the chin. Starting 6–24 hours after exposure, it takes 1–2 weeks to settle. In severe cases bullae and eyelid oedema are seen, and ingestion causes stomatitis, acute gastrointestinal symptoms (Brown and Brown, 1941) and urticaria with shock (Goldstein, 1968) even anaphylaxis (Dang and Bell, 1967).

Mango and *Toxicodendron* dermatitis are analagous and those sensitive to the latter react to the former, given enough exposure.

2. *Anacardium occidentale*

After extraction of the cashew nut shell oil from the hull of the nut, residual resin is removed from the kernel. However, as this process may be abbreviated to secure a raw-looking nut which health stores prefer, the kernel may carry a residue of allergen (see below).

The oil is used in phenol formaldehyde resin synthesis, cold-setting cement, printers' ink, insulating varnish, floor tiles, brake linings and typewriter rolls, all of which are sources of allergen.

The nut and wood are used to make voodoo dolls and swizzle sticks, and a curious outbreak of facial dermatitis in children was traced to toys made of cashew nut shells (Orris, 1958).

Five patients, very sensitive to 'poison ivy', ate large numbers of allergen contaminated nuts supplied by a health store (Ratner *et al.*, 1974) and all developed widespread dermatitis. This demonstrated combined contact allergy and a systemic drug-type of reaction, analogous to some responses to penicillin or antihistamines.

3. *Semercarpus anacardium*

Semecarpus anacardium yields black tarry resin used as laundry marking ink (bhilwanol). On clothing (Livingood *et al.*, 1943) and accidentally contaminating mail (Goldsmith, 1943), it has caused dermatitis in 'poison ivy' sensitive patients.

4. *Gluta renghas*

Gluta renghas produces a mahogany-like wood with an irritant sap. If varnished before fully dry, and used for furniture or carvings, the wood can elicit dermatitis (Fasal, 1945).

5. *Smodingium argutum* ('Rainbow leaf' tree)

Smodingium argutum can cause a streaky allergic contact dermatitis resembling a 'poison ivy' reaction (Findlay *et al.*, 1974; Hindson and Oliver, 1975). In a third of Findlay's cases, the attacks were severe, with erythema, oedema and bullae in a streaky angular pattern. A mild localised eruption characterised the others, and all tended to recur. The plant is a potent sensitiser, and cross-sensitivity to *Toxicodendron* species is usual.

Ginkgo biloba [Ginkgoaceae] (p. 515)

Allergens cause cross-reactions in persons contact sensitive to Anacardiaceae plants. They are encountered in oriental lacquer ware, soaps and varnishes, as well as the edible fruit.

Patch testing

1. *Toxicodendron* spp.

a. The *leaf* contains all the allergens and is sometimes the only effective test material (Auerbach and Baer, 1964), but it varies in potency, is a bother to collect, and can cause severe reactions. A fresh, mature, crushed 'poison ivy' leaf can be firmly applied to the back with the thumb; or the 'finger-leaf' test (Kligman, 1958b) can be used — the index of a non-sensitive person, contaminated by leaf sap, is applied firmly to the skin for 5 seconds without rubbing or twisting. Leaves stored in a moist jar in a refrigerator keep for at least 2 months.

b. *Oleoresin*, prepared commercially or in the laboratory, is easier to use than the leaf and is more allergenic than PDC. However, it is less antigenic than the leaf, and its potency is variable and falls off with time. It is applied in a concentration of 10^{-1} and clinical sensitivity is represented by a reaction to 2 g at this dilution (Epstein *et al.*, 1974).

c. *PDC* is pure, stable and gives reproducible results (Epstein, 1958), but is a minor allergen, expensive and in short supply. Although sensitized patients occasionally fail to react to it (Auerbach and Baer, 1964), it was used in preference to crude oleoresin by Kligman (1958a). Synthetic PDC 0.1 per cent in acetone is satisfactory, read at 96 hours at least. Concentrations as high as 1.0 per cent may be needed to elicit reactions in some cases, but irritation can occur at even weaker dilutions. Fregert and Bandmann (1975) recommended 0.1–1.0 per cent in MEK (Table 10.1 p. 465).

2. *Anacardium occidentale*

Cashew nut shell oil is cheap, readily available, stable, potent and of reasonably constant composition (p. 485). However, suitable test material is fresh, raw cashew nut, crushed and moistened with water, applied under occlusion (Ratner *et al.*, 1974).

3. *Mangifera indica*

PDC is adequate.

The *relative potency* of some of these allergens, in terms of the equivalent concentration of PDC, is: Leaf = 10^{-4} (Epstein, 1958): active extract of leaf = 10^{-1}; commercial oleoresin = 10^{-1} (Auerbach and Baer, 1964); mango stem sap = 10^{-1} (Keil *et al.*, 1946).

Routine patch testing with oleoresin or PDC is undesirable. It can sensitize (5–10 per cent) and if repeated it can render overt a subclinical sensitivity (Epstein, 1958). In undoubted clinical sensitivity it is contraindicated, as intense, even bullous reactions can result.

The value of patch tests with these allergens lies in assessing changes in sensitivity during hyposensitization (p. 484), and in eliciting dermatitis for trials of topical corticosteroids (Kaidby and Kligman, 1976). They have also shown that avoidance of contact with the allergen for long periods reduces the degree of sensitivity (Kanof and Rostenberg, 1941).

Cross-reactions

In sensitivity to 'poison ivy', cross-reactions to mango stem sap (Keil *et al.*, 1945), to phenolic extracts of cashew nut shell oil, *Semecarpus anacardium*, *Gluta renghas*, *Ginkgo biloba* fruit pulp and *Toxicodendron verniciferum* commonly occur (Ratner *et al.*, 1974) and sometimes also to iodoform, quinidine and resorcinol (Stanton and Wilson, 1971). On the other hand, significant sensitivity to PDC is met in patients sensitised by resorcinol and 4-phenylcatechol (Caron and Calnan, 1962).

Prophylaxis

The patient must learn to recognise and avoid the relevant plants. Barrier creams are of no practical value, and chemical detoxicants, such as chelators, couplers or oxidisers, are useless (Kligman, 1958a).

Any allergen on the skin must be washed off with strong laundry soap and water, and clothing changed and washed to oxidise the allergen. For full protection, this must be carried out immediately, but 5 minutes' delay may not be critical for the moderately sensitive, and even after half an hour all is not lost. However, after 1 hour, washing at best reduces self-contamination. A 10 per cent aqueous solution of potassium permanganate, applied within 5 minutes of exposure, may help the moderately sensitive (Howell, 1943) but is scarcely practicable.

Guinea-pigs given PDC coupled to human serum albumin parenterally could not be contact sensitised subsequently by PDC (Mason and Lada, 1954); this is, however, of only theoretical interest.

Treatment

a. *General*

Mild attacks. Topical calamine lotion, with or without added phenol 1 per cent or menthol 0.1 per cent, may suffice. Very cold or moderately warm water soothes pruritus, but topical corticosteroids are of doubtful value.

Moderate attacks. Bullae should be opened, the roof left in place and the site dried with potassium permanganate baths. For oedematous areas, Burow's solution 1:10 is helpful, and for eyelid oedema, cold saline wet dressings are suitable. Once facial lesions have dried, a simple ointment (such as zinc oxide) can be used, and for resolving dermatitis topical corticosteroids become useful (Epstein, 1973). Oral antihistamines can alleviate pruritus.

Severe attacks. Topical therapy is the same as for moderate attacks, but sometimes systemic corticosteroids are indicated.

If the situation is desperate, 4 mg of dexamethasone can be injected intramuscularly immediately, and oral prednisolone started in a dose tailored to the individual requirements (Epstein, 1973). On average, a starting dose of 70–100 mg is gradually reduced by 10 mg per day until the daily dose is 10 mg, when the drug is stopped. A single daily dose is given unless it exceeds 100 mg, when it is divided into two equal doses. These higher doses are reduced by 20–40 mg daily, but once 80–100 mg is reached, further reduction is as above. A representative course would be:

Day	1	2	3	4	5	6	7	8	9	10	11	12
Prednisolone (mg)	80	70	60	50	45	40	35	30	25	20	15	10

Diphenhydramine (Benadryl) 50 mg or hydroxyzine HCl (Atarax) 25 mg orally are useful sedatives and antipruritics.

The use of '*Rhus*' extracts for acute attacks is to be condemned as hazardous, even lethal (Shaffer and Burgoon, 1951), and irrational.

b. *Hyposensitisation*

With rare exceptions (Kligman, 1958b), only hyposensitisation, not desensitisation, can be achieved in '*Rhus*' dermatitis. It requires a stoical patient as the course is long and arduous, and followed by maintenance therapy indefinitely. Consequently it is undertaken only when the need is great, as in unavoidable heavy occupational exposure (e.g. telephone repair work; forestry) or in susceptibility to very severe attacks.

Astonishing success claimed in the past, using tiny doses of allergen, was probably a placebo response, a renowned effect of this potent allergen (Rovito, 1956). Patch test sensitivity was unaffected (Greenberg and Mallozzi, 1940). Shelmire (1941a, c) estimated that, to produce hyposensitisation with the then available allergens, would have taken up to 200 injections over 3½–60 years.

In his exhausitive reviews of hyposensitisation in '*Rhus*' dermatitis, Kligman

(1958b, c) discussed topical, parenteral and oral allergen administration, and compared PDC, oleoresin and cashew nut shell oil. He considered the oral route to be effective, the easiest and the least troublesome. He preferred the pure but expensive PDC to the equally effective but less stable and more variably potent oleoresin, but his final choice was cashew nut shell oil (Kligman, 1958c). It is readily available, cheap and effective as an allergen for oral use. The relative activity of the three allergens given orally, and parenterally, can be seen in Table 10.6, which gives for each the total dose required to initiate, and then to produce peak hyposensitisation, as judged by changes in patch test sensitivity (Kligman, 1958 b, c):

Table 10.6. Total dose (g) of allergen to initiate and give peak hyposensitisation

| Route | Oral | | Intramuscular | |
Degree of hyposensitisation	Initiating	Maximum	Initiating	Maximum
Oleoresin	1.0–1.2	2.5–3.0	0.6–0.8	2.0–2.5
PDC	1.5–1.8	3.5–4.0	0.8–1.0	2.5–3.0
Cashew nut shell oil		3.5–4.0		

None of the allergens is toxic; any side-effects are allergic. All are dispensed for use to the same prescription:

Allergen	10.0
Aerosol OT	2.5
Tenox 11	0.1
Ethanol	90.0

and stored in a dropper bottle (30 drops $\simeq 1$ ml). Aerosol OT [bis(2-ethylhexyl) sodium sulphosuccinate] is a wetting agent (see below); Tenox 11 is an antioxidant containing butylated hydroxyanisole.

Cashew nut shell oil should be pre-washed with dilute sulphuric acid to remove amines and to precipitate out mineral salts.

Courses are started 4 months before the season begins i.e. no later than February in north-east U.S.A. Gradually increasing amounts of allergen are given each day, and when the largest practicable and tolerated dose is reached it is continued until the 'total dose' for peak hyposensitisation has been taken. Maintenance therapy then follows. A practical dosage schedule is given at the end of this section (p. 486).

The 'total dose' is all important. Average figures are given in Table 10.6; less is insufficient and more imparts no added benefit. The time taken is irrelevant except in terms of convenience. Results are not brilliant (see below).

The course tends to progress with fits and starts, for side-effects, met usually early on and as the dose is being increased, call for temporary dose reduction and slower progress. Sometimes it seems impossible to overcome allergic reactions, even at modest dosages, but a short course of systemic corticosteroids may breach these barriers. Intractably and severely intolerant patients have to settle for a protracted, often stormy, course.

If at any stage exposure to the wild allergen occurs, the course should be suspended temporarily.

Side-effects. Pruritus and erythema are the commonest cutaneous reactions and can be local or generalised. About 50 per cent of the more sensitive patients experience them, especially with oral courses. Flares-up at old sites of dermatitis, often long since healed, are seen, unpredictably, in under 10 per cent of patients. Urticaria is dose-dependent and uncommon, while pompholyx and erythema multiforme-like reactions are rare. Pruritus ani can be maddening, but Aerosol OT in the formulation has reduced its frequency to only 1/150.

If the allergen is administered as recommended below, oral mucosal reactions occur in only 5 per cent or so of patients. Parenteral hyposensitisation is not recommended, for reactions, either local or systemic, range from mild to intense and mirror the sensitivity and the vigour of the course.

Maintenance therapy. Hyposensitisation starts to wane about 4–6 weeks after an oral course (8–10 weeks if parenteral), and by 6–8 months patch test sensitivity has returned to pre-treatment levels. Some benefit, however, remains, for reactions seem to be less violent than previously.

Repeated doses of allergen taken throughout the year will maintain hyposensitisation, although peak protection when the leaves are out can be achieved by seasonal administration. Such maintenance therapy is taken indefinitely or until the need no longer exists.

Results. Clinical improvement is appreciated as milder, briefer and more localised attacks. Objective assessment is complicated by the placebo effect (Epstein, 1958) and the inability to standardise environmental exposure. Quantitative patch tests give the best guide and have been discussed in great depth by Kligman (1958b).

In general, a one-hundred-fold reduction in patch test sensitivity can be expected; i.e. a 2+ reaction to PDC 10^{-6} becomes a 2+ reaction to PDC 10^{-4}. This small reward can, however, represent a considerable clinical improvement and make an intolerable sensitivity bearable. An interesting feature is that reactions to the weakest concentration are lost first and, as hyposensitisation wears off, they are the last to return.

Hyposensitisation in practice. For a conservative course with oral cashew nut shell oil (Kligman, 1958c), the allergen is dispensed as on page 485. The prescribed dose is stirred thoroughly into a full glass of tepid water then drunk through a disposable or glass straw. The recommended dosage schedule (30 drops ≏ 1 ml) is:

Week 1:	1 drop daily
Week 2:	2 drops daily
Week 3:	3 drops daily
Week 4:	4 drops daily

Then add one drop every four days to a maximum of 20 drops per day, and continue that until a total of 35 ml has been taken. Maintenance therapy is then begun, the dose being 5 drops daily.

Some bold patients may accelerate the course, the timid slow it down. In general, the pace should not be forced.

Intolerance of less than 5 drops per day may be overcome by giving 15–20 mg of prednisolone daily while the dose of allergen is increased by 1 drop every 3 days. Once 10 drops per day is tolerated, prednisolone is stopped, the allergen dose reduced to 5 drops daily, and the course advanced again in standard fashion.

In the main, the early stages cause most difficulty. Half the patients experience some trouble and have to stop temporarily to let things settle and then proceed once more at a lower dose, and increase it by no more than one drop per week. A lower dose merely protracts a course, which may take 3½–8 months to complete.

The corresponding details for a conservative course using PDC or oleoresin by mouth are detailed by Kligman (1958b). The alternative approach, with the parenteral administration of alum-precipitated pyridine extract of *Rhus toxicodendron* had been reported by Passenger (1963) to be effective.

ARACEAE (ARUM FAMILY)

The floral characteristic of this mostly tropical family consists of a central fleshy column (spadix) subtended by a large bract (spathe). Many species are cultivated for their attractive foliage, some as foods. *Dieffenbachia*, *Philodendron* and *Scindapsus* are familiar genera.

Philodendron scandens (*P. cordatum* is a common misnomer) is the most popular foliage house plant in the U.S.A., and has small glossy heart-shaped leaves. The related *P. sellosum*, a warm climate outdoor plant with large divided leaves, is grown on patios and in roof gardens, often as a mound.

Nusery men recognise *Philodendron* as a common sensitiser, especially of those who cultivate it. Most cases, however, remain undiagnosed. The plant at home or in the office is a definite hazard. Contact may be accidental or result from plucking (Dorsey, 1962) or polishing the leaves, or from watering it. Moisture seems to facilitate allergen transfer. Housewives are exposed far less than nurserymen as they water the plant with greater care and handle it less.

Dermatitis
Dermatitis from *P. scandens* and related species was reviewed by Ayres and Ayres (1958) who thought it might not be rare. Their 12 cases resembled mild 'poison ivy' reactions. There was a streaky, blotchy erythema with vesicles and exudation, particularly on the hands and forearms, less often on the abdomen and lower limbs. The eyelids may be affected alone (Harris, 1942), but severe lid oedema and pruritus may be part of a more widespread reaction (Dorsey, 1958). The condition is also met in Denmark (Hjorth, 1962).

Patch testing
Moist, not dry, crushed leaves or stems are suitable.

All species of the related *Monstera* have an acrid caustic juice. *M. deliciosa* yields an edible fruit, and has a large attractive perforated leaf, but causes contact dermatitis.

Scindapsus aureus (syn. *Pothos aureus*; *Rhaphodophora aurea*; Hunter's robe; Taro vine) is a popular indoor climber in Scandinavia. It is thought to sensitise nurserymen commonly. Biting the stem causes intense irritation, and all parts of the plant bear needle-like hairs.

Mobacken (1975) reported a case of acute hand dermatitis in a florist, caused by *S. aureus* and confirmed by patch testing with the plant's leaf. He queried the rarity of the condition, and in response Mitchell and Rook (1976) drew attention to the confused nomenclature (see synonyms) and remarked that the plant, as *Pothos*, is a well recognised cause of dermatitis, being, on an annual basis, the commonest cause of contact dermatitis in Honolulu.

Arisaemia triphyllum (Jack in the Pulpit) is toxic if eaten, and its leaves and corms can cause dermatitis (McCord, 1962).

Arum maculatum (Cuckoo pint) is irritant when crushed as the sap contains raphides (Woods, 1962).

Dieffenbachia seguina, if chewed, irritates the oral mucosa intensely and can swell the throat alarmingly; the plant also causes dermatitis (Dorsey, 1962).

The irritant genera are listed by Mitchell (1975a).

ARALIACEAE (IVY FAMILY)

Hedera (Ivy), the best known genus, comprises 15 species of evergreen climbers popular as house plants and in the garden. The species of dermatological interest are *H. helix* (English ivy) and the closely related *H. canariensis* (Algerian or Canary Island ivy); both have numerous varieties. *H. helix* is the smaller with a 5-pointed leaf, whereas that of *H. canariensis* is 3-pointed with a red stem and may be variegated.

a. *Hedera canariensis* causes more dermatitis, possibly because it has a larger leaf with more allergen, and because it grows faster and needs more frequent pruning. The seasonal nature of reactions coincides with the pruning which becomes necessary as growth slows down after the rainy season. Like 'poison ivy', plant parts have to be bruised to release the allergenic sap. The nature of the allergen is unknown.

Occupational dermatitis is rare because there are few supplying nurseries where the plant is cut and propagated, but in them dermatitis is common among the staff. Retailers are trouble-free.

The overall incidence is unknown, but it may not be rare (Dorsey, 1959). Clinically, reactions resemble acute 'poison ivy' dermatitis (Dorsey, 1957, 1959) but on a lesser scale. Symptoms appear 24–48 hours or less (Hambly and Wilkinson, 1978) after exposure, especially on the backs of the hands and forearms, the flexor surfaces of the wrists, the face and periorbital region. Urticario-papular lesions with a tendency to form plaques and surrounded by linear streaks, characterise mild or moderately severe attacks. In severer cases, pruritus is considerable, and the eruption is vesiculo-bullous with prominent striate and streaky markings. Episodes take a couple of weeks to subside.

Widespread involvement is unusual, probably because contact is generally domestic, the subject well protected, and the water-soluble allergen quickly washed off. Moreover, contamination of clothing is minimal.

Patch tests: sap from crushed stems and leaves, kept moist under occlusion. Cross-reactions to other *Hedera* species are the rule.

Treatment

Response to topical applications is minimal, but systemic corticosteroids and ACTH, if indicated, are effective.

b. *H. helix* also is allergenic, but reports of its causing dermatitis are few (Goldman *et al.*, 1956; Roed-Petersen, 1975). Nevertheless, it may not be as rare (Roed-Petersen, 1975) as Hjorth (1965) suspected.

The clinical picture is similar to dermatitis from *H. canariensis* and thus to a mild 'poison ivy' reaction.

Papular urticaria from *Bryobia* mites on *Hedera* is a curiosity (Woods, 1962). Irritant genera are listed by Mitchell (1975a).

ASPIDIACEAE

Arachnoides adiantiformis (Leather-leaf fern) is being increasingly imported to Europe from the U.S.A., Honduras and Puerto Rico for background use in floral arrangements. Long-term contact led to allergic contact dermatitis on the palms and fingers of a florist (Hausen & Schulz, 1978). The allergen, present only during sporogenesis, has been isolated, but not identified.

BEGONIACEAE (BEGONIA FAMILY)

Begonia can cause dermatitis (Hjorth, 1969) but information is scanty and imprecise. *Begonia rex* is irritant, whereas *B semperflorens* has elicited allergic patch test reactions (Agrup, 1969).

BORAGINACEAE (BORAGE FAMILY)

Most are blue-flowered, and many are garden plants. The stiff hairs on the following species give irritant, confusing patch test reactions (Woods, 1962):

Borago officinalis (Borage)
Echium vulgare (Blue weed; Viper's bugloss)
Lycopsis arvensis (Bugloss)
Pentaglottis sempervirens (Alkanet)
Pulmonaria officinalis★ (Lungwort)
Symphytum officinale (Comfrey)

★(*Pulmonaria* may also be allergenic)

BROMELIACEAE (PINEAPPLE FAMILY)

Ananas comosus (Pineapple) is cultivated for food, other species for ornament.

Pineapple contains known skin irritants: the proteolytic enzyme bromelin, raphides and acid, mostly citric acid. Bromelin in the juice, rubbed into the skin, causes considerable damage; pressure is essential for this effect which seems to be purely physicochemical, not allergic. Although somewhat thermostable, the enzyme is destroyed by heating the canned fruit. The irritant raphides, however, neither damage nor alter the permeability of the skin.

Eating too much raw pineapple causes a burning sensation in the mouth and lips — a reminder that the juice can be used as a meat softener [a property shared with *Bromelia pingrum* (Maya) and *Carica papaya* (Pawpaw)].

In the pineapple canning industry, in the absence of mechanisation and protective clothing, pineapple handlers, to a man, get dermatitis. In 1951 Polunin reported that it was a considerable problem in Malaysia, not in Hawaii or Queensland.

After a few days at work, especially with fresh 'Mauritius Pine', skin exposed to juice and pressure develops painful, raw areas. The epidermis separates from the dermis at the tips of the finger pad ridges, and deep fissures form. It is the hand used to hold the pineapple that is affected. Subsequently the pressure sites turn white and are painless at work, and in time the fingerprints lose their clarity. Although slow to heal, the hands never go septic, and at the end of the season the skin reverts to normal. The overall effect has been attributed to bromelin, as the raphides and citric acid only cause very rapid irritation on contact.

CACTACEAE (CACTUS FAMILY)

These leafless, fleshy plants produce showy flowers. Cactus species are characteristically barbed. The awl-shaped, larger and sometimes sheathed spines arise from areolae; they inspire caution. However, if tempted to pick the blossom or fruit, the individual may encounter the tufts of short fuzzy barbed bristles (glochids), five to eight on each of the 25–30 aerolae per cactus (*Opuntia*) leaf. The bristles have retrorse, hook-like bristles which prevent their extraction once in the skin. Most reactions are irritant, but some may be allergic (Schreiber *et al.*, 1971).

Opuntia lingularis (Cholla cactus) glochids cause immediate pain on entering the skin. Erythema and swelling develop in 72 hours, and subside after 1–3 days, only if the spines are removed. Retained spines produce papules and plaques, sometimes like granuloma annulare, with a central punctum and bristle. It may take 3–4 months for these to resolve once the bristles have been rejected. During extrusion the epidermis may become warty.

Other effects include (Winer and Zeilenga, 1955): suppuration, interphalangeal ankylosis, nerve paralysis and cystic osteolysis.

The cholla and prickly pear varieties of *Opuntia* are responsible for the rare allergic reactions. Clinically they consist of flesh-coloured, domed, 2–4 mm papules with a central black dot. They are restricted to the limbs, usually occur in groups of 3–6, and last for 2–8 months. Positive skin tests with glochid extracts evidence their allergic nature (Schreiber *et al.*, 1971). Immediate hypersensitivity is necessary for subsequent granuloma formation, but delayed hypersensitivity is also involved.

Opuntia ficus indica (Prickly pear) grows in North and South America, Mexico and around the Mediterranean. There are two main varieties in Israel: the common or yellow sabra (*O.f. indica*); and the red sabra (*O. cochinillufera*). Dermatitis occurs in the fruit handlers; viz. pickers, distributors and sellers (Shanon and Sagher, 1956). The glochids readily break off, get into the clothes, and cause '*sabra dermatitis*', an occupational hazard disconcertingly like scabies. It is seasonal, from July to October.

The sites of predilection are: the hands and finger webs, and to a lesser extent the wrists, arms, buttocks, genitals and trunk. Nasal furuncles and irritation of the mouth and eyes may occur. The eruption comprises vesicles, pinhead and pea-sized papules, pustules, crusts and some ulceration. Burning and itch are particularly troublesome at night. Involvement of an isolated area can, however, give a reaction clinically not unlike a comedo naevus (Banerjee, 1977).

The palpable embedded glochids are diagnostic. These cause the reaction, for if the barbs are rubbed onto the skin experimentally, a stabbing sensation is experienced within half an hour, followed 1½ hours later by widespread pruritus which lasts for 10 days. At the sites of contact, round pointed papules with an urticarial halo appear.

Treatment consists of removing the spines. An easy method is to layer on wax, let it set, then pull it off. Emollients may be soothing.

CANNABIDACEAE (HEMP FAMILY)

Cannabis and *Humulus* are well known genera of controversial value.

Humulus lupulus (Brewer's or European hop) has, for well over four centuries, been used to flavour beer. Its female inflorescence (hop cone) is aromatic with hop-oil and sticky with resin which contains humulone and lupulone. Hop allergen may belong to the oil or resin.

Hop pickers' dermatitis occurs only in September. Its incidence is unknown, partly due to the casual nature of the workforce. Possibly 1:30 pickers are affected to some degree, but only 1:3 000 severely (Cookson and Lawton, 1953).

Clinically, there is a more papular and oedematous than exudative facial reaction. As sensitivity increases, itchy erythematous papules appear on sites of contact, and in severe cases there is considerable oedema of the lids, lips, nose, fingers, backs of the hands and flexor surfaces of the forearms. The milder cases may clear or become hardened, but the severer ones tend to get worse.

Patch tests. The cut surface of a hop cone; fresh hop oil; or hop resin including humulone and lupulone.

CAPPARIDACEAE (CAPER FAMILY)

This is the tropical counterpart of the Cruciferae (Mustard family). Capers (pickled flower buds of *Capparis* spp.) are used in sauces.

Many genera, *Capparis* included, cause cutaneous reactions and they all have irritant species. All species studied to-date contain thioglucosides of the 'mustard oil' type (p. 511), which, with their isothiocyanate derivatives, are also found in species of the Cruciferae and a few other plant families. A detailed list is included in a comprehensive account of this family (Mitchell, 1974c).

A characteristic glucoside is glucocapparin, which is hydrolysed enzymatically:

$$\text{Glucocapparin} \xrightarrow[\text{(enzyme)}]{\text{myrosinase}} \text{Hydrogen, sulphate, D-glucose and isothiocyanate}$$

The isothiocynate (CH_3NCS), not the thioglucoside, is the skin irritant, and the reaction is comparable to enzymatic hydrolysis of sinigrine (p. 511). The 'mustard oils' were so named because they were originally derived from mustard plants, but isothiocyanates is the preferred term. All have the same irritant, even vesicant effect.

Exposure to *Capparidaceae* spp. can occur in home gardening where spider flowers are the most likely source; *Cleome spinosa* is a popular garden annual.

CHENOPODIACEAE

Salsola kali (Russian thistle) is a widespread weed native to Russia but common in arid regions of the U.S.A. where it can cause irritant dermatitis or contact urticaria (Powell and Smith, 1978). The latter reaction is akin to a prick test as sharp floral bracts penetrate the skin, seemingly introducing an as yet unidentified allergen. The eruption affects exposed skin and comprises papules and weals lasting a day or two. Prick tests not patch tests may be positive.

COMPOSITAE (COMPOSITE OR DAISY FAMILY)

The Compositae is one of the largest families of flowering plants. Its members are mostly herbaceous and grown for ornament, although some are cultivated as vegetables. Being so vast, it has two subfamilies and 12 Tribes (Clapham, Tutin and Warburg, 1962; Willis, 1973).

Asteroideae (Tubuliflorae)
This subfamily has 11 Tribes, of which the Heliantheae (including the obsolete Helenieae), Asterae and Anthemideae contain most of the plants responsible for contact allergy (Rook, 1960; Mitchell, 1969; Mitchell and Dupuis, 1971). Members of this subfamily often have resin canals, but latex is rare. Heliantheae are found mainly on the American continent, Anthemideae mostly in the Old World.

Lactucoïdeae (Ligulifloreae)
This, the other subfamily, has only one tribe, the Lactuceae (Cichoriëae). All

species have latex, but no resin canals; *Cichorium* and *Lactuca* are familiar genera in the tribe.

Botanical considerations

The family characteristic is a uniform inflorescence comprising many tiny flowers (florets) each at the apex of a stem and clustered to form a flower head (capitulum). The plants commonly have resin canals or latex, rarely both, and accurate identification of the genera and species can be very difficult, especially in the Lactucoïdeae, as all have latex and usually are yellow flowered.

Pollination is by insects in most species, but in some it is by wind, and these latter species are more commonly associated with oleoresin dermatitis. The pollen has a protein core, and an outer coat that may contain or be contaminated by oleoresin. In the wind-pollinated species, the grains are tiny, about 15μ (Sutton, 1919), and clearly oleoresin on such pollen will disseminate far further than on the larger sticky pollen of the insect pollinated species. (*Ambrosia elatior* and *Artemisia* spp. exemplify the former.)

Trichomes have been seen electron microscopically on the leaf of *Parthenium hysterophorus* and are probably present on those of other species. They and other tiny particles of powdered dried plants are disseminated widely by wind (Hjorth et al., 1976.)

The Compositae plants produce a wide range of secondary products in amounts determined by the plant's maturity and health, as well as the soil (Mitchell, 1969, 1975a); the allergens belong to this group of compounds and are mostly in the oleoresin. The latter, at least in *Ambrosia* spp., flows through oil passages to the leaf surface (Mitchell, 1975a) where it is visible on close inspection as tiny sticky globules (Shelmire, 1939); it may also be seen on flowers and stems.

All Compositae plants known to have caused allergic contact dermatitis were listed, with relevant references, by Mitchell (1969, 1975a), and those genera and species known to contain either proven or potentially allergenic sesquiterpene lactones (see below) were tabulated by Mitchell and Dupuis (1971) and Mitchell et al. (1972a). They are invaluable sources of information. Table 10.7 gives the genera known to have caused allergic contact dermatitis, the allergens being sesquiterpene lactones in the oleoresin.

Table 10.7. Compositae Genera with Sesquiterpene Lactones Causing Contact Allergy (after Mitchell and Dupuis, 1971).

Genus	Common name	Genus	Common name
Ambrosia	Ragweed	*Franseria*	Poverty weed
Anthemis	Chamomile	*Gaillardia*	
Arctium	Burdock	*Helenium*	Sneezeweed
Artemisia	Sage brush/Wormwood	*Iva*	Marshelder
Chrysanthemum spp.	Pyrethrum, tansy	*Parthenium*	Feverfew
Cynara	Artichoke	*Xanthium*	Cocklebur
Eupatorium	Boneset		

The bulk of sensitising weeds belong to the Compositae (Mackoff and Dahl, 1951) especially the Heliantheae and Anthemideae tribes, but it seems that each of these tribes has some species with, and others without, a high allergenic potential. Thus, in the former, the wind pollinated genera are the more trouble-some.

Grater (1975) drew up a useful list of weeds to indicate their frequency as sensitisers:

a. Frequent: *Ambrosia, Helenium microcephalum, H. tenuifolium, Iva, Parthe-nium hysterophorus*
b. Moderate: *Xanthium, Amphiachyris dracunculoides*
c. Infrequent: *Aster elixis, A. multiflorus, Achillea millefolium*

Because of the wide geographical variation in the commoner sensitising species, the dermatologist has to know those responsible in his area. The follow-ing are simply illustrative:

USA and Canada: *Ambrosia* spp., and to a lesser extent *Xanthium, Erigeron* and *Iva* (Mitchell, 1969); *Ambrosia elatior, A. psilostachya* and *Iva xanth-ifolia* (Brunsting and Anderson, 1934).
Texas: *Helenium tenuifolium, H. microcephalum, Iva angustifolia, Parthenium hysterophorus, Xanthium speciosum* and *Ambrosia elatior* (Shelmire, 1939).
Australia: *Cryptostemma* (Capeweed) (Mitchell, 1969)
Europe: Chrysanthemum of florists.
India: *Parthenium hysterophorus* (Lonkar et al., 1974)

Four genera merit separate mention:

1. *Ambrosia* (Ragweed) (Sutton, 1919)
The species are widespread in North America, but not in south British Colum-bia. *Ambrosia elatior* and *A. trifida*, which replaces it in southern and eastern U.S.A., are the most important and are illustrated in Sutton (1919). *A. psilos-tachya* and *A. cumanensis* are interesting in their chemical diversity in different populations and localities (Mitchell and Lynne-Davies, 1974). The allergens are easily spread without bruising the plant as the oleoresin is on the leaf surface and pollen (see above).

2. *Helenium* (Sneezeweed) (Balyeat et al., 1932)
Species are found throughout the U.S.A., especially the south-west, at road-sides and in waste sites. Livestock refuse to eat them. They vary geographically, and all carry bitter aromatic resinous globules on their leaves, stems and yellow flowers. *H. microcephalum* is illustrated in Balyeat et al. (1932).

3. *Parthenium hysterophorus* (Feverfew) (Kahn and Grothaus, 1936; Lonkar et al., 1974)
Thriving on waste ground, particularly in southern U.S.A. (Ogden, 1957), this plant is adventive in India where it was accidentally introduced into the Maharashtea State on the West Coast with some grain. Initially very local, it spread especially along railways, roads and canal banks, helped along by floods. This sometime perennial weed is so vigorous that it swamped the local weeds and created havoc in the agricultural and dairy industries by crowding out use-ful plants and vegetables (Lonkar et al., 1976). Ironically its only competitor in

India is *Xanthium strumarium*, itself allergenic. *Parthenium hysterophorus* blooms in spring and autumn and produces sticky pollen in adhesive clumps. In the dry season it becomes powdered and the tiny fragments are disseminated by the wind.

Curiously, this species is common in Argentina, Mexico and the West Indies, but has caused no major outbreaks of dermatitis there, and although it is a major cause of weed dermatitis in Texas and Minnesota (Shelmire, 1940; Mackoff and Dahl, 1951), epidemics have not been a feature.

4. *Chrysanthemum* consists of three groups:

    a. *Species*: *C. parthenium*, *C. coccineum* (*Pyrethrum rosum*), *C. maximum* etc.
    b. *Indoor varieties*: A vast range, hybridised for cutting and show.
    c. *Highly hybridised derivatives* of the original Chinese and Japanese wild species (Rook, 1961 b; Hausen and Schulz, 1973) classified in detail according to type of bloom (Hay, 1971).

Terminology is confused. Schulz *et al.* (1975) regarded chrysanthemum of florists, *C.x morifolium* and *C. indicum* as synonymous, but Hausen and Schulz (1973) considered that Chrysantheme of the German literature is *C. indicum*, whereas in Britain, France and the U.S.A. *C.x morifolium* is implied. To remove ambiguity they proposed, for standard usage, either 'Chrysanthemum of the *C. indicum* group' or 'Florists' Chrysanthemum'. Here, chrysanthemum of florists will be used, or is implied by the term chrysanthemum.

Over 500 cultivars are in existence for the garden and hothouse (Bleumink *et al.*, 1973), and new varieties from crossing or mutation continually replace the old. Nowadays, mature chrysanthemums are available all year round (Malten, 1973), a facility provided by 5 main varieties (75 per cent of it by only two of them). Some of these varieties are more allergenic than others, and patients need not react to all.

The history of chrysanthemum cultivation, the plant's composition, and the manifestations of chrysanthemum dermatitis were surveyed by Hausen and Schulz (1973). Most cases were due to *C.x morifolium*, some to *C. indicum* and a few to *C. leucanthemum*, *C. maximum*, pyrethrum etc.

The allergens

The allergens reside in the rich content of secondary products, especially essential oils and terpenoids, of Compositae species (Herout and Sorm, 1969). They are mostly sesquiterpene lactones (Mitchell, 1975a), a large group of related compounds which are not only being isolated and identified in increasing numbers from this and other plant family members (Mitchell and Dupuis, 1971; Mitchell *et al.*, 1972a; Stampf *et al.*, 1978), but also being synthesised and studied experimentally on humans and guinea-pigs (Stampf *et al.*, 1978). The chemotaxonomy is complex and knowledge empirical, for although individual genera and species tend to produce their own selection of these lactones, it can vary even between populations of the same species (Mitchell, 1969), and possibly between cultivars, as may be the case with chrysanthemums which seem to show allergenic specificity.

The most prolific producers of allergenic sesquiterpene lactones among Compositae plants belong to *Ambrosia*, *Artemisia* and *Chrysanthemum* (Mitchell et al., 1972a), but some tribes have yet to be shown to make them, while many species contain the same lactones. Species of other plant families producing these compounds have been discussed by Mitchell *et al.* (1970, 1972a) and listed by Storrs *et al.* (1976). Families listed include Jubilaceae, Lauraceae and Magnoliaceae.

There are 5 basic groups of sesquiterpene lactones:

I

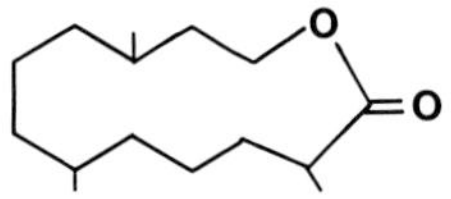

Germacranolide

II

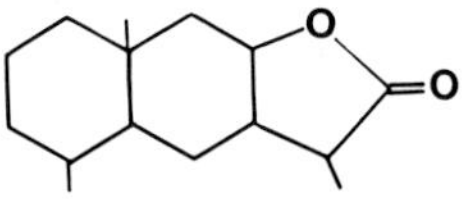

Eudesmanolide (Santanolide)

III

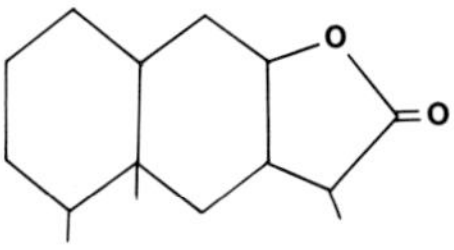

Eremophilanolide

IV

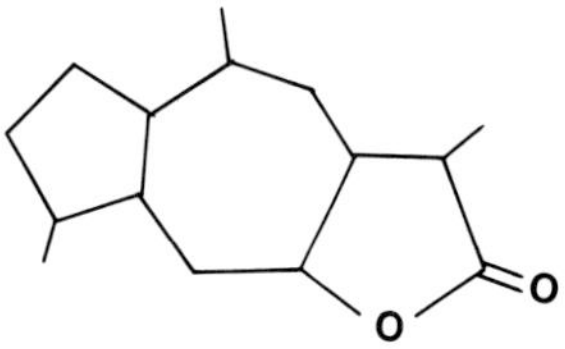

Guaianolide

V

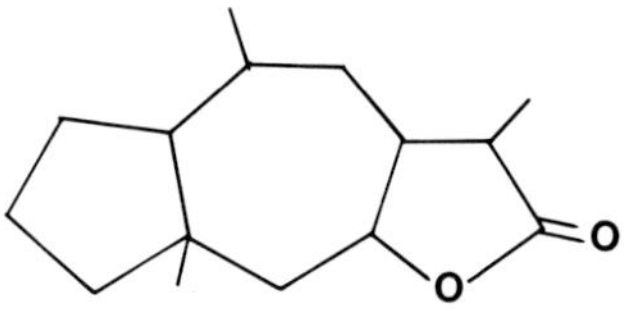

Pseudoguaianolide

All contain potential allergens as judged by molecular configuration (see below), and all suspected allergens have belonged to one or other of them except group III. Allergens from different groups can cross-react (Mitchell *et al.*, 1971a).

Evidence to date suggests, but has not proved, that these lactones are the actual allergens in contact hypersensitivity to Compositae (Mitchell, 1975b). Proof is difficult when so many similar chemicals are involved for already more than 210, isolated and identified, satisfy the minimal criteria for allergenicity (Mitchell and Dupuis, 1971; Mitchell *et al.* 1972a).

On a molecular basis, the fundamental requirement for a sesquiterpene lactone to be allergenic is the presence of an α-methylene ($=CH_2$) group (Mitchell and Shabata, 1969; Mitchell and Dupuis, 1971) exocyclic to a γ-lactone ring. Alantolactone exemplifies this (Mitchell, 1975b):

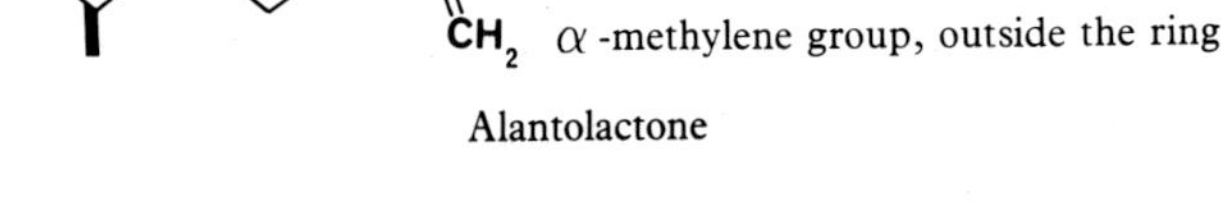

γ-butyrolactone ring $\Rightarrow$

$C = O$

$C = O$

CH_2 α-methylene group, outside the ring

Alantolactone

If the α-methylene group is reduced (R= CH$_2$ → R — CH$_3$), allergenicity is lost (Mitchell *et al.*, 1970); thus the C = C grouping conjugated to the lactone is an immunological requisite. The necessary stereochemistry may be involved in protein-allergen interaction (Mitchell, 1975a). However, the above criteria are necessary, *not* sufficient, for allergenicity. This is readily evidenced by the failure of tulip allergen, α-methylene-γ-butyrolactone (p. 520), to cross-react with Compositae sesquiterpene lactone allergens (Benezra, 1973; Stampf *et al.* 1978). Other, as yet obscure, requirements in molecular structure are necessary for allergenicity and cross-reactivity (Rodriguez *et al.*, 1977).

The principal allergenic sesquiterpene lactones in *Ambrosia* and other Heliantheae species (Mitchell and Lynne-Davies, 1974) are: Ambrosin, Ambrosiol, Coronopilin, Cumanin, Damsin, Isabelin, Parthenin and Psilostachyin, but most characteristic of the Heliantheae are Ambrosin, Parthenin and above all Coronopilin (Fig. 10.2).

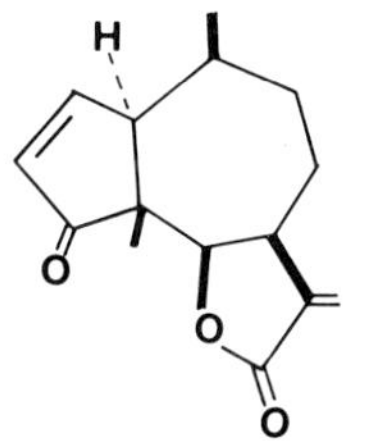

Ambrosin 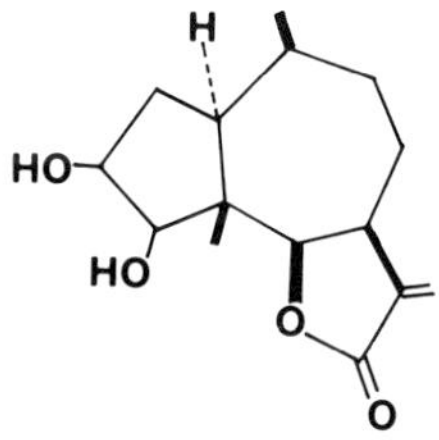   Ambrosiol 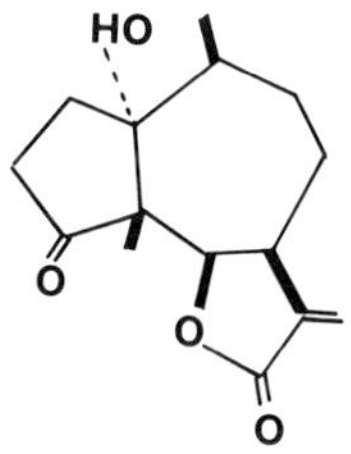   Coronopilin

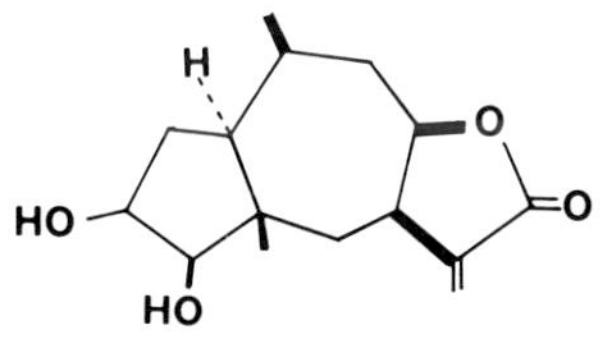

Cumanin 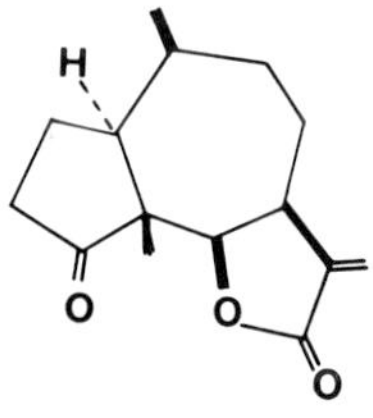   Damsin

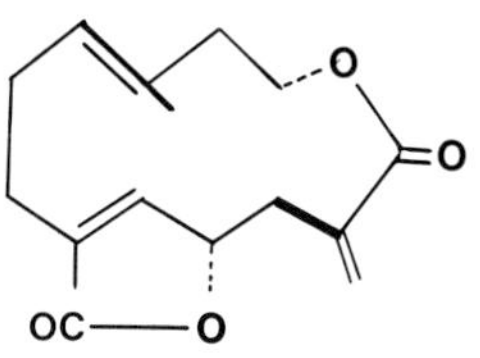

Isabelin 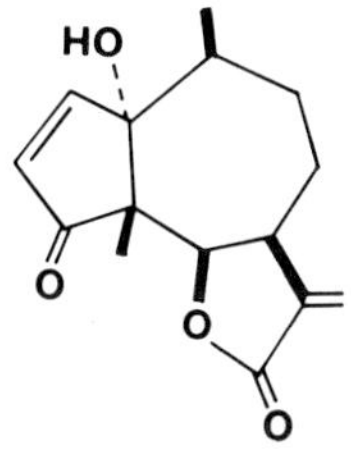   Parthenin 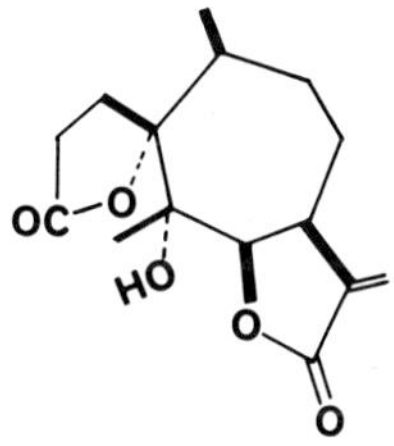   Psilostachyin

Principal Heliantheae Allergenic Sesquiterpene Lactones.

Similar data are available for other Compositae species and tribes, and give some insight into the complexities of cross-reactions met in this family (p. 499). There is, however, no exhaustive account of the allergens in sensitising Compositae plants. The following representative selection deals with some of those met in *Ambrosia*, chrysanthemum of florists, *Parthenium hysterophorus* and pyrethrum.

a. *Ambrosia* allergy exemplifies the difficulty in assessing the roles of allergens in the pollen and the rest of the plant (p. 502).

Pollen has been said to contain 6 antigens (Cohen and Michelini, 1958) and to be a common cause of 'ragweed' dermatitis (Shelmire, 1940), the pollen oil being blamed (Brown. *et al.*, 1931), but it is probably of only minor importance (Shelmire, 1939). If the dermatitis is worst in the pollen season, it is probably because the plant has more allergen then (Cohen, 1959). Moreover, it is as yet undecided whether pollen protein and oleoresin share any allergens (Milford, 1930).

Ambrosia spp. are known to synthesise at least 13 allergenic sesquiterpene lactones, but $\triangle$-3-carene and α-pinene also occur (Mitchell and Lynne-Davies, 1974), explaining, possibly, cross-reactions to turpentine in some cases of 'ragweed' oleoresin dermatitis. It is the rule for these species to produce lactones, but the constituents of their oleoresin vary considerably among the varieties, and this may account for Brunsting and Anderson (1934) finding that, although most of their cases reacted to 3 different species, 4 reacted to just one.

The *mechanism of allergy* to these plants is complex. The oleoresin either on the living plant, on wind-borne powdered parts or on pollen can elicit allergic contact dermatitis (Grater, 1975). Alternatively, inhaled pollen can be absorbed and react with reaginic antibody to cause wealing. However, both can occur in the same patient (Cohen, 1959).

b. *Chrysanthemum*. The species, but not florists' chrysanthemum, contain parthenolide which has elicited positive patch tests in patients contact allergic to *Chrysanthemum* spp. (Mitchell *et al.*, 1971a).

The allergens in chrysanthemum of florists have caused major difficulties in isolation and identification, and resolution remains incomplete. Originally there were grounds for incriminating sesquiterpene lactones, as an ethanolic extract of flowers and leaves (not stems) is allergenic, and because patients hypersensitive to the plant react to alantolactone or cumambrin A (Bleumink *et al.*, 1976). More than three were thought to be involved (Hausen and Schulz, 1975), and since then four have been isolated and one identified as arteglasin A by Hausen and Schulz (1976). The other three elicit positive patch tests and are likely to be guaianolides. In addition Campolmi *et al.* (1978) have demonstrated large amounts of alantolactone in the flowers, less in the leaves. Bleumink *et al.* (1976) thought there may be *no* variety specificity and that cross-reactions could well be based on other chemicals abundant in the oleoresin and shared with other plants. Nevertheless, arteglasin A explains cross-reactions to e.g. *Artemesia douglasiana*, *Achillea millefolium*, *Matricaria chamomilla* and possibly *Arnica montana* (Paschoud, 1965). The cross-sensitivity pattern can be wide, as in a florist who reacted to florists' chrysanthemum (and primula) and to arnica, sunflower, chamomile, yarrow, *Frullania*, tansy and mugwort (Hausen and Schulz, 1978a).

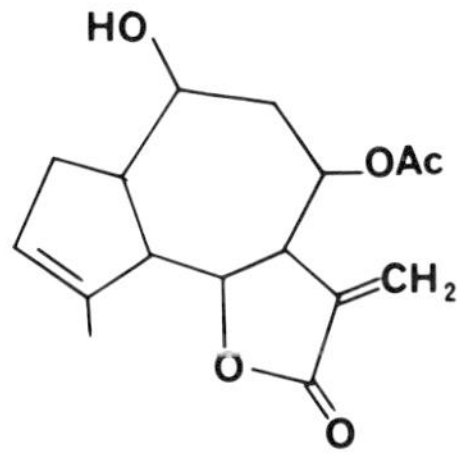

Cumambrin A 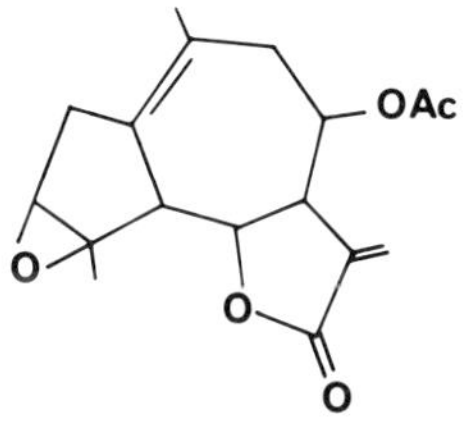   Arteglasin A

c. *Parthenium hysterophorus*. The highest concentration of allergen is in glandular trichomes on both leaf surfaces, phyllaries and achenes (Rodriguez *et al.*, 1976). Parthenin is probably the principal allergen (Lonkar and Jog, 1972; Lonker *et al.*, 1976), but ambrosin is present, too, in the capitulum and leaves (Hjorth *et al.*, 1976). Patch testing 24 cases (Singh and Sharma, 1978) showed 17 to react to the stem, 11 to the flower, 9 to pollen and only 7 to an extract: all 11 tested with parthenin reacted. Much work remains to be done on the allergenicity of this species (Rao *et al.*, 1978).

Not all patients hypersensitive to the plant react to alantolactone (Lonkar *et al.*, 1974) which therefore is unsatisfactory as a screening allergen for Compositae plant allergy. Cross-reactions occur to *Helenium, Dahlia, Iva, Chrysanthemum* (Lonkar *et al.*, 1974), and to other *Parthenium* spp. (Rodriguez *et al.*, 1977), with the usual highly individualistic patterns.

d. *Pyrethrum* (Mitchell *et al.*, 1972b) consists of dried flower heads of *Chrysanthemum cinerariifolium* and *C. coccineum*. The principal allergen is the non-insecticidal sesquiterpene lactone pyrethrosin; a minor allergen is the insecticidal pyrethrin II:

OCOCH$_3$

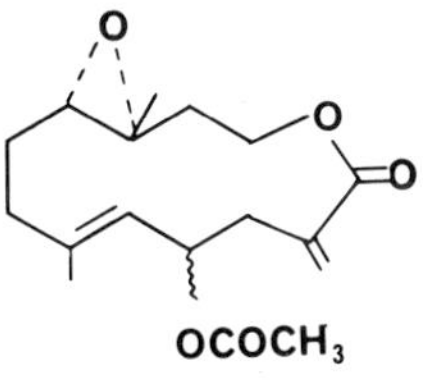

Pyrethrosin

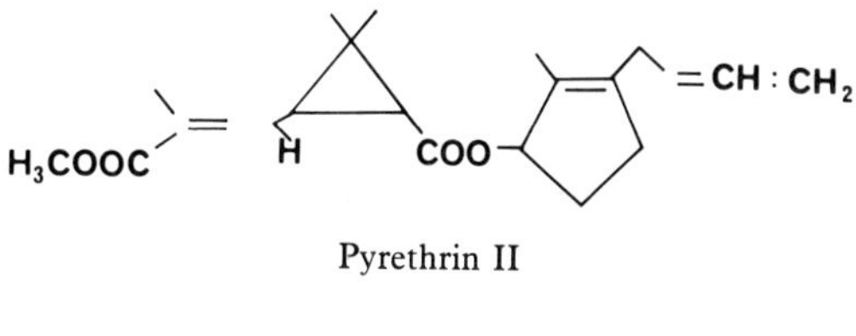

Pyrethrin II

Cross-reactions

The Compositae family is renowned for the frequency of cross-reactions (Mitchell, 1972) not only between its members but also with plants of other families. The topic was discussed by Mitchell (1975b) and is mentioned on page 496.

The dicta of Rook (1960) are illustrated well by this family, and the complexity and empiricism of the cross-reactions stem from many variables. These include:

1. Different species produce the same or related allergens.
2. Species may have some populations that do, and others that do not, produce an allergen, and geographical variation in this respect is well documented (Miller *et al.*, 1968).
3. The output of an allergen by a single specimen can vary widely.
4. The primary sensitivity determines cross-reactivity, e.g. a person sensitised by tulip may cross-react to chrysanthemum, but not vice-versa (Benezra, 1973).
5. Patients have their own cross-sensitivity pattern (Mitchell *et al.*, 1971a; Grater, 1975; Mitchell, 1975a).

There is no guarantee that sensitivity to one species will carry any specific cross-sensitivity. Although *Ambrosia artemisiifolia* is antigenically the most polyvalent of that genus (Brunsting and Williams, 1936), no plant or allergen will reliably screen for contact hypersensitivity to Compositae species. Thus Mitchell (1972) dismissed *Ambrosia*, whereas alantolactone is unsatisfactory (see above). A suitable sesquiterpene lactone 'mix' is awaited, and meanwhile commercial oleoresin preparations can be used (Roed-Petersen and Hjorth, 1976), or alternatively a crude sesquiterpene lactone extract made (Hausen, 1977).

Reports mentioning cross-reactions are numerous (e.g. Brunsting and Anderson, 1934; Brunsting and Williams, 1936; Shelmire, 1940; Jordan *et al.*, 1942; Fisher, 1952; Hjorth *et al.*, 1976; Stampf *et al.*, 1978), and their clinical importance has been discussed by Rodriguez *et al.* (1977), but the subject is beyond the scope of this chapter.

Incidence

The incidence of allergic contact dermatitis from Compositae plants is not known. However, general impressions have been expressed e.g.

a. Weeds occasionally cause (seasonal) dermatitis (Brunsting and Anderson, 1934; Shelmire, 1939).
b. Plants and flowers other than *Rhus* spp. form a small fraction of causes of contact dermatitis in the U.S.A. (Maibach and Epstein, 1964).
c. Weed dermatitis is now rare in Texas (Howell, 1971).
d. Hypersensitivity dermatitis from American weeds other than 'poison ivy' is not common (Grater, 1975). The latter listed the better known sensitising weeds (p. 494).

Parthenium hysterophorus is causing epidemic allergic contact phytodermatitis in parts of India (Lonkar and Jog, 1972) (p. 494), and chrysanthemum of florists, a recognised and not infrequent sensitiser (Hausen and Schulz, 1973), is one of the commonest causes of occupational dermatitis among florists in northern West Germany (Hausen and Schulz, 1975). 'Ragweed' dermatitis, judging by the number of reports in the literature, would seem to be a problem of some consequence, and *Helenium microcephalum* appears to be a rather common cause of dermatitis (Balyeat *et al.*, 1932). Otherwise, reports of phytodermatitis from other Compositae plants, and weeds in general throughout the world, are sparse, probably unjustifiably so.

Sex and age influence the incidence especially of dermatitis from *Ambrosia* spp. and *Parthenium hysterophorus*. Males outnumber females 20:1 and for obscure reasons most cases are in older men. Thus, Brunsting and Anderson's (1934) youngest patient was 24 years old, and the average age at onset is around 40 years (Brunsting and Williams, 1936).

Occupation is important, for most 'ragweed' dermatitis affects farmers and other outdoor workers who daily come into contact with vegetation (Shelmire, 1939). However, the type of work and clothing are not the only factors involved (Lonkar *et al.*, 1974; Mitchell, 1975a).

Seasonal variation reflects the plant's growth cycle, and most cases occur during pollination when the plant's growth is most vigorous (p. 498). In the U.S.A. 'ragweed' dermatitis is a problem mainly from August to the first killing frost, but patients with long-term sensitivity tend to be troubled from June to December.

Clinical features
There is wide geographical variation in the Compositae species responsible for dermatitis. A representative selection is given on page 494.

In most instances, sensitivity is the result of heavy and protracted exposure, for example to chrysanthemum of florists in horticulture or floristry, or to weeds in outdoor occupations and sports. The latter include farm employees and other field workers, telephone linesmen, golf-green keepers, cemetry workers, anglers and hunters. Flour and grain handlers are also at risk (Jordon *et al.*, 1942).

The number of sensitising species is vast, and the following are discussed as representative: *Ambrosia* spp., *Parthenium hysterophorus* and chrysanthemum of florists. Some genera, less frequently responsible, are outlined on page 507. Those used as foods (e.g. lettuce, endive), in perfumery (e.g. *Saussurea lappa*) or medicaments (*Matricaria chamomilla*, *Anthemis nobilis*) are discussed in the appropriate chapters.

a. *Ambrosia species*:
Farming in the U.S.A., especially in the great farm belt (Fromer and Burrage, 1953), entails chronic direct exposure to these weeds. Indirect contact occurs when oleoresin adheres to clothing, cows' udders, winter feed (Mitchell, 1969), grain (Mitchell, 1975a), and can sometimes account for perennial dermatitis (Brunsting and Anderson, 1934). Since the introduction of mechanisation, however, the problem is said to be rare in Texas (Howell, 1971).

In northern U.S.A., the season usually starts in early summer, often one particular week in July or August; it is established by August, reaches a peak in September (Brunsting and Anderson, 1934) and quickly ends after the first killing frost. With chronicity or secondary infection, symptoms are more continuous with seasonal exacerbations.

In southern U.S.A. it is more perennial (Grater, 1975). In seasonal cases, exposure to the allergen out of season leads to only mild and brief flares-up. In the season, however, dust storms exacerbate the condition, and rain damps it down, probably by altering the amount of airborne allergen (Brunsting and Anderson, 1934).

Pollen (Fromer and Burrage, 1953; Sutton, 1919) (p. 498) oleoresin may aggravate existing 'ragweed' dermatitis (Shelmire, 1940); it is, however, a minor factor (Howell, 1971) and probably trivial compared with allergen on tiny airborne particles from powdered plants (Lonkar *et al.*, 1974; Hjorth *et al.*, 1976). Its protein can cause localised patches of lichenified dermatitis on the lids, neck or antecubital fossae, as well as Type I allergic reactions (Epstein, 1960), and, if inhaled, it may flare up the eczema in sensitive patients. This dual role of *Ambrosia* in allergy was mentioned by Hjorth *et al.* (1976) in discussing classical 'ragweed' oleoresin dermatitis due to several Compositae species, and seasonal aggravation of atopic dermatitis in adolescents sensitive to intradermal pollen tests.

The *distribution* resembles a pollen dermatitis. The face, lids, periorbital region and neck are almost invariably affected; the backs of the hands, wrists and arms frequently; the ankles and legs sometimes, and the trunk and groins, patchily, occasionally. The skin of the penis and front of the scrotum can become thickened and erythematous (Shelmire, 1939). The extent of the dermatitis can range from just the lids to universal (Brunsting and Anderson, 1934); from an isolated hand eczema due to milking resin-contaminated udders, to widespread involvement of the face, neck, ankles and moist flexural regions in grain handlers (Jordon *et al.*, 1942). It is rarely generalised.

The picture characteristically is that of elderly unwashed men whose wrinkled skin makes them look even older and weather-beaten (Grater, 1975).

The *morphology* is almost pathognomonic (Brunsting and Anderson, 1935). It looks very chronic (Mitchell, 1969), vesicles are rare (Epstein, 1960), but severity varies with sensitivity and density of exposure. Moderately severe erythema, thickening and pruritus lead to lichenification, scaling and fissuring. Lichenification appears in sites easily rubbed, such as the face, front and sides of the neck, and the flexures (Shelmire, 1939). Vesicles do occur if particles of allergen adhere to the skin, or as part of a major reaction to massive exposure, when bullae and oozing can also result (Shelmire, 1939). Irrespective of the severity, pruritus is intense.

In winter, perennial cases have residual lichenification which hospitalisation alone will clear, and takes 3–6 weeks to do so. Outpatients probably retain the eruption on account of intermediate contact with allergen.

Symptoms in the first year are minimal and clear quickly as the 'season' ends. Subsequently they start earlier, last longer and eventually become perennial, and meanwhile the eruption becomes more widespread and multiple sensitivities tend to be added (Fromer and Burrage, 1953).

Cross-reactions (p. 499), which are the rule, are usually to *Iva* (Mitchell, 1969) and sometimes to turpentine and pyrethrum (Brunsting and Anderson, 1934) and *Chrysanthemum* (Fisher, 1952).

Differential diagnosis

1. *Photodermatitis*: Hjorth *et al.* (1976) showed how closely contact allergy to Compositae plants can masquerade as photodermatitis, and although involvement of shaded areas is helpful in diagnosis, modern fabrics may transmit sufficient light to make this sign unreliable. A useful sign, however, is sparing of the skin behind the earlobes in true photodermatitis (p. 470). Nevertheless, sunscreens have been used for suspected photosensitisation by pollen, with beneficial results in two cases (Fromer and Burrage, 1953).
2. *Atopic dermatitis*: may resemble 'ragweed' dermatitis in its chronic form (Mitchell, 1969), but the former is flexural and the latter usually affects extensor surfaces (Fromer and Burrage, 1953). However, Grater (1975) stated that flexural lichenification is characteristic of 'ragweed' reactions. An association between the two conditions (Epstein, 1960) is a moot point. Mitchell (1969) quoted three reports in which 13 of 47 patients had both conditions. It may be a casual relationship (Brunsting and Anderson, 1934) or be significant, as when atopic dermatitis, in patients with positive intra-dermal tests to ragweed allergens, is seasonal or is seasonally exacerbated and flares up with inhalation tests (Tuft and Heck, 1952).
3. *Neurodermatitis*: lacks a past history of seasonal dermatitis.
4. *Seborrhoeic dermatitis*: can be emulated by less severe cases with a scaly scalp, mild lichenification, scaly lids and nasolabial folds, and spread down the V of the neck (Fromer and Burrage, 1953).

b. *Parthenium hysterophorus*:
First described as a cause of severe dermatitis by French (1930), this weed and the extensive and most pruritic reactions it causes, were discussed by Kahn and Grothaus (1936) who stated that it, 'ragweed' and 'pyrethrum' are the worst weeds for causing phytodermatitis.

Dermatitis from this weed is epidemic in parts of India (p. 494) and in the New World it is a common sensitising species. Most patients are adult agricul-tural men in the age range 40–60 years but the weed in wasteland and kitchen gardens can be responsible for cases amongst others. Initially restricted to the growing season (in India the plant blooms thrice yearly and its season lasts 6–8 months), the dermatitis becomes perennial with seasonal exacerbations. The allergen seems to be airborne as the condition clears only in weed-free areas, and takes 5 weeks to do so (see also Hjorth *et al.*, 1976).

At the onset (Lonkar and Jog, 1972), itch and rash occur symmetrically on the face, round the eyes and over the V of the neck. Faintly erythematous excoriated papules appear on the back of the neck, followed by papulo-vesicles which coalesce and involve the entire face and anterior abdomen, the wrists, forearms and upper back. Phases of acute oedema and oozing alternate with more chronic lichenification and hyperpigmentation. At its peak, all uncovered sites are involved, which in the Indian usually means everywhere except palms, soles, axillae and under a loin-cloth. Some cases may be photocontact hypersensitive to an allergen, other than parthenin, in the plant (Bhutani and Lao, 1978).

Lichenification, sometimes nearly universal, is the cardinal sign in later stages; it is associated with secondary infection, fissuring and hyper- or hypopigmentation. Polished, ridged nails and alopecia are evidence of the intense pruritus. The lack of response to topical or systemic corticosteroids is notorious (Lonkar and Jog. 1972; Lonkar *et al.*, 1974), but some cases respond to ACTH (Ogden, 1957). The condition can be so severe that exudation and secondary infection lead to considerable disability. Death has followed skin or respiratory infection, but spontaneous resolution has been reported in only one case (Lonkar *et al.*, 1974).

Differential diagnosis includes:

1. *Atopic dermatitis*, even with white dermographism. However, the upper lids and dorsa of the hands are always affected, the fronts of the wrists are relatively spared and a more or less localised patch of inframammary dermatitis is characteristic.
2. *'Seborrhoeic neurodermatitis'* (Atopic dermatitis in seborrhoeic areas) resembles cases with scalp involvement and lichenification of the face, neck, upper trunk and antecubital fossae.
3. *Lichenoid polymorphic light eruption or actinic reticuloid.* Involvement of the lids and of the extensor rather than flexor limb surfaces are helpful signs; moreover, the forehead is not spared. In such cases, it seems that the sun is aggravating the phytodermatitis and lowers the skin's resistance to the allergens.

c. *Chrysanthemum*

Chrysanthemum of florists is not only one of the commonest plant sensitisers in floristry and horticulture (Campolmi *et al.*, 1978), but is probably a commoner cause of dermatitis than is recognised (Hausen and Schulz, 1973). From the review by Hausen and Schulz (1973) of the relevant literature, it can be estimated that chrysanthemum of florists had caused the dermatitis in 8–10 of 14 gardeners, 7 of 18 florists, but only one of five housewives. The other 6 gardeners and 7 florists had been sensitised by several *Chrysanthemum* spp., especially *C. parthenium* and *C. maximum*.

The dermatitis is seasonal in gardeners, but perennial in florists in whom it is usually due to chrysanthemum of florists (Mitchell, 1975a). Although sensitivity to a single horticultural variety can occur (Rook, 1961b), this may be unusual (Bleumink *et al.*, 1973). The reaction can be acute with considerable swelling and exudation (Paschoud, 1965), but commonly it rapidly becomes subacute or chronic in appearance and consists of a chronic, thickened dermatitis of the face, neck, hands and arms (Hjorth and Fregert, 1972), so typical of contact allergy to many Compositae species. The distribution accounts for Calnan's (1978b) recommendation that chrysanthemum leaf should be included in photoallergy patch test series. A case progressing to actinic reticuloid, typical both clinically and histologically and augmented by UV-A and UV-B irradiation, has been reported by Schmedekampf *et al.* (1978).

The data tabulated by Hausen and Schulz (1973) show that the face and hands are almost invariably affected, whereas the neck, forearms and genitals are much less often involved.

As with all Compositae plant sensitisation, there is a wide, but individual, spectrum of cross-sensitivity. These have been well illustrated in reports by Paschoud (1965), Mitchell (1969), Mitchell et al. (1971b) and Bleumink et al. (1976). Clearly the history is all important when interpreting such test results.

Patch tests

(a) *Pollen, stem or leaf* of the suspected plant can be used (Fromer and Burrage, 1953). Apply a piece of leaf (p. 464) for one hour (Shelmire, 1940), as at least 40 per cent of relevant, succulent weeds irritate if applied for longer, especially to moist skin. Controls are necessary. Ground dried leaves, occluded for 24 hours, do not irritate but frequently elicit clinically irrelevant reactions in weed-sensitive cases (Shelmire, 1939).

(b) *Oleoresin* (Shelmire, 1939, 1940; Shelmire and Black, 1937) in open tests is less irritant than in closed and is more suited for use in large test batteries; Grater (1975) used a dilution of 1:10 for general use and 1:20 for *Ambrosia* spp., read at 48–72 hours. Serial dilutions can be used to quantify sensitivity. A dye (e.g. D & C green 6) may be added (Fromer and Burrage, 1956) (FD & C Yellow 3, a sensitiser, is unsuitable). Unfortunately, Hjorth et al. (1976) found acetone and ethanolic solutions of oleoresin prone to give false negative open tests, and in preference used commercially prepared (Hollister-Stier) oleoresins in petrolatum as closed patch tests. They acknowledged that the then available extracts varied in potency (see also Shelmire, 1940) and that active sensitisation could occur. For closed tests, Fisher (1952) recommended oleoresin 1:10 in acetone, but Fromer and Burrage (1953) started with 1:10³ to avoid flares-up, and increased the concentration to 1:10 if there was no reaction.

Closed patch testing with oleoresin, used with discretion and caution, seems to be the *preferred technique*. However, studies on the use of diethyl ether extracts of Compositae plants, 1 per cent in petrolatum (Hausen, 1977), which contain the sesquiterpene lactones of the species extracted, may well show this to be a preferred test substance.

(c) *Pure sesquiterpene lactones*, alantolactone excepted, are not readily available. The use of alantolactone 0.25 per cent in petrolatum as a routine screening test (Mitchell and Dupuis, 1971) has failed to detect chrysanthemum allergy (Hjorth, 1970b), can actively sensitise, and is unsatisfactory as a test substance for Compositae plant allergy (Grater, 1975; Hjorth et al., 1976). It has been likened to using PPD as a screening test substance for dye contact hypersensitivity (Grater, 1975).

In tests with many weeds, the commoner sensitisers must be segregated (Shelmire, 1940). Reactions may take more than 48 hours, and rarely 5–7 days, to reach a peak, and they tend to be prolonged, lasting 6 weeks or more (Mitchell and Dupuis, 1971). Not only can they vary in the same person, but the degree of sensitivity to 'ragweed' is itself vary variable (Mitchell, 1969).

Little has been written about testing with individual species. *Parthenium hysterophorus* flower heads are the most allergenic parts, and reactions tend to be vesicular and exudative. Chrysanthemum can be tested by using an ethanolic extract of flowers and leaves of chrysanthemum varieties (Bleumink *et al.*, 1973).

Cross-reaction (see p. 499)

Treatment
For *acute attacks*, astringents, baths and lotions (Brunsting and Anderson, 1934) are little bettered by more modern applications.

Established cases of Compositae dermatitis tend to be corticosteroid resistant, even to systemic steroids (Lonkar and Jog, 1972). The use of oleoresin phylactically is illogical and hazardous (Shelmire, 1940).
Complete control is attained only by avoiding direct and intermediate contact with the plant allergens. Insect-pollinated genera such as *Chrysanthemum* (Shelmire, 1940) present few problems, but wind-pollinated plants or those which powder when dry and become airborne can create insuperable difficulties. Only admission to hospital or moving to a weed-free area may provide relief.

Occupational chrysanthemum dermatitis requires the grower or florist to eliminate offending varieties from stock. Patch testing with a wide range may show which are safe to handle (Mitchell, 1975a) and whether there are sufficient to sustain a viable livelihood. The value of topical hyposensitisation with alcoholic extracts of the plant (Campolmi *et al.*, 1978) remains to be determined.

Prophylaxis has not been studied so extensively as in 'poison ivy' dermatitis (p. 484). Unfavourable (Brunsting and Williams, 1936) and favourable (Sulzberger and Wise, 1930; Shelmire, 1939) reports were noted by Fisher (1952) whose own four cases, and others, had improved clinically and in patch test sensitivity.

Parenteral oleoresin (Brunsting and Williams, 1936; Fromer and Burrage, 1953) or pollen (Sutton, 1919) have been used, but they entail too many injections, for too long and with too many side-effects.

Oral hyposensitisation is effective (Shelmire, 1939; Fisher, 1952; Fromer and Burrage, 1953); but it entails taking oleoresin daily for many months or years. A course is started once the skin has cleared after the first frost, or as early as possible and at least a month or more before the spring weeds appear, and never in the 'ragweed' season. The dose is increased regularly unless reactions such a pruritus, rashes or urticaria occur, when it is reduced or the course temporarily suspended.
The oleoresin is supplied in three concentrations, 1:100, 1:50 and 1:25 in corn oil and the patient is given a 28.5 ml bottle-full of each to take in turn, as below. The prescribed dose is dispensed by hand into gelatin capsules, care being taken not to contaminate the fingers. The dosage is:

Week 1 = 1 drop daily immediately after food; Week 2 = 2 drops daily.

Subsequently the dose is increased as rapidly as possible — by 3 or more drops per week. Some patients manage a full capsule (12 drops) daily within a month; with time, it usually become easier to raise the dose. On starting the next bottle, the number of drops is halved, but increased as quickly as possible. Pruritus ani or dermatitis are rate-limiting symptoms.

Maintenance therapy with 12 drops daily of the 1:25 oleoresin in corn oil is started as soon as the third bottle is finished.

Side effects: Pruritus ani is worst, especially in the earlier stages. Rashes, including urticaria, signify too rapid dose increases and require the course to be suspended until things settle, when smaller increments are introduced. Antacids palliate dyspepsia.

Contact with the plants must be avoided until the course is completed; inadvertent exposure requires temporary suspension of the hyposensitisation.

Whether or not there is any practical value in adding chrysanthemum, pyrethrum or even turpentine allergens to the hyposensitising mixture for patients who also have positive patch tests to them has not been reported.

As with 'poison ivy' hyposensitisation, the principal benefit from the procedure comprises briefer, milder and more localised attacks.

Control of the weeds is scarcely feasible, although it has been reported that the arsenic containing weed-killer, Ansar 529®, is effective against *Parthenium hysterophorus* (Hausen, 1978c).

Other genera and species

The following selection is representative of other Compositae genera and species reported as having caused contact dermatitis.

1. *Anthemis cotula* (Stinking mayweed) and *Arctium lappa* (Giant or great burdock) are both irritant weeds (Woods, 1962); the latter is 'used herbally for skin diseases and for purifying the blood' (Polunin, 1969). *Artemisa ludoviciana* (Prairie sage) is listed as *A. stellerana* (Dusty miller) in Clapham, Tutin and Warburg (1962). It is an escaped garden plant, and it produces sesquiterpene lactones, ludovicins included, which have caused contact hypersensitivity (Mitchell *et al.*, 1971b).

2. *Arnica montana*, a yellow-orange, daisy-like flower, contains an active principle, arnicine. Flores arnicae, used in folk medicine in Poland, sensitised a woman who subsequently reacted to the plant in her garden (Rudzki and Grzywa, 1977). In a study of three patients with occupational dermatitis due to contact with *A. longifolia* and *A. montana*, during their cultivation, harvesting and phytochemical analysis, Hausen *et al.* (1978) were able to show by patch tests that the allergens are sesquiterpene lactones. In *A. longifolia* these included carabron, helenalin and an acetyl derivative of the latter; in *A. montana* helenalin acetate and probably arnifolin were responsible. They pointed out that handling drugs derived from Compositae plants carries the risk of contact sensitisation. Hausen (1978b) subsequently reported that the principal suspected allergens in *A. montana* are helenalin and its methacryl acid ester.

3. *Chrysanthemum species* (p. 495) include the familiar *C. maximum* (Shasta daisy) and *C. carinatum*. Of special interest are *C. cinerariifolium* (Dalmatian pyrethrum) and *C. coccineum* (Common pyrethrum), as pyrethrum insect powder (p. 499) is made from their dried flower heads. This is the major cause of dermatitis from *Chrysanthemum* spp. Most is produced in Japan, Yugoslavia and Kenya. In Kenya, *C. cinerariifolium* flowers all year round, produces larger and brighter yellow blooms than varieties in the other two countries, and has caused epidemic contact dermatitis (Sequeira, 1936). The flowers are irritant and more allergenic than the extract (Martin and Hester, 1941); the principal allergens are mentioned on page 499. The pollen also can be allergenic (Feinberg, 1934), whereas acetic acid and chrycinnerol in the plant are irritants (Mitchell *et al.*, 1972b). The insectidal moiety consists of esters of pyrethrins I and II.

According to Feinberg (1934), pyrethrum causes trouble in three ways: the insecticidal element is toxic if ingested; the oleoresin causes contact hypersensitivity; and the pollen elicits type I reactions.

Occupational dermatitis occurs mainly among those grinding and weighing the crude material, which elicits erythema, vesicles and papules, especially in moist sites, aggravated by sweating in summer. Once sensitised, patients suffer extreme pruritus of the face and hands, eyelid oedema, and attacks which can be triggered by the presence of dry flowers in the same room (Martin and Hester, 1941).

In the Kenyan epidemic, prominent features were: papules and vesicles especially on the forehead, a scarlatiniform reaction with oedema, fissuring in the flexures, aggravation by sunlight, and coryzal symptoms. The insecticide can sensitise gardeners (Feinberg, 1934). Cross-reactions are the rule.

4. *Cichorium* species (p. 182): *Cichorium endiva* (Cultivated endive) is widely grown as a salad plant, often in varieties with strongly crisped leaves, and *C. intybus* (Chicory: Wild succory) roots yield the chicory of commerce. Both species cause allergic contact dermatitis in those occupationally exposed. Apart from workers in the chicory industry (p. 182), reported cases have been in salad makers only, due probably to the low allergen content of the immature plants used for salads (Mitchell, 1975a) and the necessity for intense exposure to sensitise and to elicit reactions. Patients with occupational contact dermatitis from *Lactuca sativa* commonly cross-react to *C. endiva* (Krook, 1977).

Two patients, contact allergic to *Cichorium*, were reported by Friis *et al.* (1975). Both had hand eczema spreading onto the forearms. One, a greengrocer, reacted to patch tests with *C. intybus* var. *foliosum* leaf, *C. intybus* root and ether extracts of leaves of both; tests with *Lactuca sativa* (lettuce) and alantolactone 1 per cent in petrolatum were negative. The other, a produce manager, reacted to fresh leaf of *C. endiva*, fresh root of *C. intybus*, fresh leaf of lettuce and to alantolactone 1 per cent in petrolatum.

One of the food handlers studied by Hjorth and Roed-Petersen (1976) reacted to 'chicory salad' (? *C. endiva*) and to *Allium cepa* (Onion), *A. sativum* (Garlic) and allylisothiocyanate (p. 512). Such reactions may be based on sesquiterpene lactones, for *C. intybus* and *Lactuca virosa* yield lactucin and *C. intybus* lactopicrin, both of which are potentially allergenic (p. 510).

5. *Cryptostemma calendulacea* (Capeweed) is native to South Africa and resembles Australian dandelion weed. The pollen from its yellow spring blossom can cause hay fever, or eczema of the face, neck and limb flexures. Localised dermatitis and photosensitivity on the forehead, ears and eyes have been attributed to its oleoresin (Hand, 1944).

6. *Dahlia* species: Huge numbers of hybrids of this originally Mexican genus are grown as garden plants, but contact sensitivity to *Dahlia* seems to be rare. Calnan has described two cases: one (1973a) in a woman who had had finger eczema since childhood worse in summer, and who had noticed that contact with the plant irritated her hand; on being patch tested, she reacted only to *Dahlia* leaf. The other (Calnan, 1978a) was in a market gardener who had recurrent dermatitis on her hands, forearms, lids and round her mouth.

7. *Gaillardia* species (Blanket flower): are garden plants in the U.K., but in the U.S.A. most of the 28 species there are wild and ubiquitous. Depending on the climate, they bloom between March and August.
   Three cases of seasonal dermatitis due to *Gaillardia* were reported by Rostenberg and Good (1935). Two were in women — a florist with hand eczema and a housewife with dermatitis of her lips, arms and legs. The man had eyelid dermatitis and lichenification on his neck: he reacted to patch tests with *Gaillardia*, *Ambrosia* and pyrethrum.

8. *Humea elegans* (Amaranth feathers) is a tall graceful plant with a red spiky flower and aromatic leaves. The genus, with 5 species, is Australian, especially in the south. Greenhouses and conservatories in Europe may harbour it, and it can cause a most violent dermatitis, particularly in gardeners. Cronin (1968) reported such a case in a gardener who, through handling the plant in a pot, developed an acute vesicular dermatitis of his forearms and chin. Rook (1970b) reported another case in a gardener. Both patients reacted to patch tests with the leaf.

9. *Inula brittanica*: a Central and Southern European weed, caused dermatitis in a horse-boy who handled hay containing it (Hegyi, 1967). Patch tests with the plant were strongly positive, but, apart from a moderate reaction to *I. germanica* (the nearest species phylogenetically), tests with five related species were negative.

10. *Iva microcephala*, one of 15 known species of 'marsh elder' native to North and South America, but common only in the Gulf Coast area, was described and illustrated by Williams *et al.* (1960) in a report of contact allergy to it. The clinical features comprised weeping eczema on the backs of the hands and forearms, the V of the neck, the chest and face. Only by careful history-taking and relevant patch testing was the diagnosis made.

11. *Lactuca sativa* (Garden lettuce) is cultivated as a vegetable in several varieties: *L. sativa* var. *longifolia* (Romaine), *L. s.* var. *foliosa* (Cabbage lettuce) and *L. s.* var. *capitata* (Iceberg). *Lactuca* as a cause of contact *dermatitis* was reviewed by Friis *et al.* (1975). Their patient, a produce manager, had hand and forearm dermatitis and reacted to patch tests with fresh leaf of cabbage lettuce. Krook (1973) described a more widespread dermatitis on the hands, face, arms and legs of a gardener who reacted to a patch test with *L. sativa* stalk. He also described in detail (Krook, 1977) simultaneous immediate and delayed contact dermatitis in persons with occupational dermatitis from *L. sativa* and *Cichorium endiva*. All four patients reacted to patch tests with fresh *fully grown* leaf of both species, cross-reacted to other Compositae allergens, and had predominantly hand dermatitis; two developed vesicles within 5 minutes of applying crushed lettuce leaf to previously affected sites. Moreover, one patient had contact urticaria from the species and had experienced alarming throat swelling on eating endive. Rinkel and Balyeat (1932) reported the case of a salad maker with widespread dermatitis on her hands, forearms, neck and around her nose and mouth. The eruption was chronic with acute exacerbations, and comprised erythema, papules and vesicles, and if she ate lettuce the dermatitis flared and she developed urticaria. Once she avoided lettuce the dermatitis cleared completely. The allergen may be lactucin (Friis *et al.*, 1975) and cross-reaction to *Cichorium* is very common.

12. *Saussurea lappa* [Cynareae] root yields costus root oil (Costus absolute) used in some perfumes (Mitchell and Epstein, 1974) prepared particularly in India. The Cynareae has few sensitising plants e.g. *Cynarea scolymus* (Globe artichoke). Costus root oil, however, is a potent sensitiser (Mitchell, 1975a) and contains several sesquiterpene lactones (Mitchell, 1974d) which are probably allergens. Cross-reacting genera include *Chrysanthemum*, *Lactuca* and *Cichorium*, but the relationship between plant and perfume dermatitis is an open question, even for those derived from Compositae plants (Rodriguez & Mitchell, 1977).

13. *Tagetes minuta* (Mexican marigold) is a rapidly spreading common weed in south east Africa, especially in the Kenyan Highlands, and in subtropical America. It is toxic to animals, irritant, even vesicant, on intact skin and can cause protracted allergic contact dermatitis (Verhagen *et al.*, 1968).

Skin reactions to it resemble those to the related *Helenium* (Verhagen and Nyaga, 1974). Contact allergy starts on the hands, spreads to other exposed sites, and encroaches onto covered parts, especially the perineum and genitals. Hallmarks are chronicity with lichenifications, scaling and pigmentation; pruritus is intense. Acute exudative exacerbations occur especially in the rainy season, but the severity usually reflects the vigour of the plant's growth.

The flower head contains most of the allergen, but some is secreted by glands onto the leaf surface. It probably is a sesquiterpene lactone as cross-reactions occur to *Chrysanthemum x morifolium* and pyrethrum (but not to the related *T. erecta*). Once sensitised, the patient inevitably has to change his job, residence or both (Verhagen and Nyaga, 1974).

14. *Taraxacum* spp. (Dandelion) contain potentially allergenic sesquiterpene lactones and can sensitise (Mitchell, 1975c).

15. *'Australian Bush Dermatitis'* refers to a chronic incapacitating dermatitis of exposed skin of men in the Australian Bush.

At least 28 Compositae species, known sensitisers, occur in South Australia: these are listed by Burry *et al.* (1973) who tabulated the more common Compositae genera found in that part of the world.

This condition is thought to be due to wind-borne pollen, dust or both, released from Compositae plants in the dry summer conditions. Of the 13 cases patch tested by Burry *et al.* (1975), 11 reacted to 'ragweed' [according to Ford (1963), *Ambrosia psilostachya* grows in Australia], 9 to *Chrysanthemum* (?species or variety), 7 to pyrethrum, 4 each to 'wild artichoke' and *Olearia axillaris*. There were a few reactions to several other genera.

Eleven of these 13 patients were male outdoor workers aged 42–76 years and showed the typical seasonal lichenoid dermatitis of exposed sites. (Two exceptions, one sensitive to *Chrysanthemum maximum*, the other to *Cynara scolymus*, had linear bullous reactions.) Recently, Burry (1979) reported a case, closely resembling Australian Bush Dermatitis, due to 'fleabane', reputedly either *Conyza alba* or *C. bonariensis*.

16. *Miscellaneous wild flowers*: Hjorth (1974a) studied the case of a woman with vesicular hand eczema who kept wild flowers in a vase indoors. He patch tested her with Hollister-Stier's oleoresins and she reacted to *Tanacetum vulgare* (tansy), *Artemisia absinthum* and *Achillea millefolium* (yarrow). He wondered how common contact allergy to wild flowers really is. Hausen (1978a) is undertaking a detailed study of the sensitising capacity of some weeds common in Germany and Denmark, and has found 70 of those tested so far to be allergenic — the allergens being on the plant surface are likely to promote airborne spread.

CRUCIFERAE (CRUCIFER, MUSTARD OR WALLFLOWER FAMILY)

Familiar members of this family are wallflowers, cabbage, turnips and Shepherd's purse. A family characteristic, shared with the Capparidaceae in particular (p. 492), is the ability to produce a wide range of thioglucosides; these vary in type among the species, and in amount with the stage of the plant's growth. Harmless thioglucoside is broken down enzymatically in the presence of water into irritant isothiocyanates (p. 492).

Thus:

$$\underset{\text{(Thioglucoside)}}{\text{Sinigrin}} \xrightarrow[\text{(Enzyme)}]{\text{myrosinase}} \text{Allylisothiocyanate}$$

The isothiocyanates can be allergenic or irritant. Phenolics tend to be more irritant, and those with unsaturation β, γ to the nitrogen molecule are immunologically active:

Phenyl isothiocyanate (irritant)   Allylisothiocyanate (allergenic)

This subject has been covered in detail by Mitchell and Jordan (1974), who gave a complete list of Cruciferae plants that yield allyl- or benzyl isothiocyanates. Examples are:

(i) Salad plants = *Lipidum sativum* (Garden cress);
(ii) Vegetables = *Brassica oleracia* Capitata (Cabbage), *B.o.* var. *hort* (Brussels sprouts, cauliflower, broccoli etc);
(iii) Condiments = *Armoracia lapathifolia* (Horse radish), *Brassica nigra* (Black mustard);
(iv) Garden plants = *Tropaeolum majus* (Nasturtium);
(v) Weeds = *Alliaria officinalis* (Wild garlic), *Capsella bursapastoris* (Shepherd's purse).

Brassica oleracia 'Botrytis' (Cauliflower) allergy caused hand dermatitis in a plant grower with multiple cutaneous allergies (van Ketel, 1975). *Patch tests*: ethanolic and aqueous extracts of leaves and edible parts of cauliflower, other cultivars of *B. oleracia* (Red cabbage and Brussels sprouts) and *B. campestris* (Rape seed) were positive. The allergen is unknown, the allergy is rare and reports are few.

Raphanus sativus (Radish), used in salads, caused allergic contact dermatitis in a waitress (Mitchell and Jordan, 1974). She developed an acute vesiculo-bullous eruption on both palms, and especially the finger sides, three weeks after starting work involving chopping radish and other vegetables for salads.

Patch tests
Radish root (as is), allyl and benzyl isothiocyanate (each 0.1 per cent in petrolatum), and a week-old mixture of sinigrin and myrosinase all elicited positive reactions. The latter test was informative: the freshly prepared mixture is inert so the positive reaction was, by implication, due to enzymatically released allylisothiocyanate.

EUPHORBIACEAE (SPURGE FAMILY)

Some members are cactus-like, many, such as Poinsettia, are ornamental, and others yield food or medicines. Copious milky latex in stems and other parts is characteristic and contains a caustic resin 'euphorbin', which is probably a complex chemical euphorbiosteroid (Calnan, 1975). British spurges are small weeds, but tropical species (see below) are trees capable of causing grievous inflammation (Woods and Calnan, 1976). Other species have stinging hairs like nettles (Woods, 1962.)

Euphorbia flowers are small, often with petal-like bracts (e.g. Poinsettia). Succulents are cactus-like.

Arabis albida (Snow on the mountain), a pink or white flowered cushion-like plant, has juice which causes dermatitis. If ingested, systemic poisoning, conjunctivitis and inflammation of the throat and perioral region result.

Codiaeum variegatum is a popular decorative potted evergreen plant. It caused an allergic, hyperkeratotic eczema on the tips of the thumbs and index fingers of a gardener. There was some onycholysis. Patch tests: the leaf and flower stalk elicited positive reactions in the patient, not controls (Tafel Kruger and van Ketel, 1976). Hybrids, used as indoor plants, commonly cause a progressive widespread eczema in gardeners who nip off leaf stems when preparing cuttings. They react to patch tests with an aqueous extract of the sap (Schmidt and Ølholm-Larsen, 1977).

Hausen and Schulz (1977) studied a gardener contact hypersensitive to the plant, and were able to sensitise guinea-pigs with a methanolic extract of the leaves. They found the latex to be allergenic, not irritant; the allergen remains unidentified.

Euphorbia peplus (Petty spurge) is a small, light green, wild or garden plant, branching on short stems from the base, and with broadly ovate leaves. Patch tests: a piece of leaf caused in controls an irritant type of response comprising erythematous papules, vesicles or bullae (Calnan, 1975).

E. pulcherrina (Poinsettia), a native of Mexico, is a popular house plant for Christmas. It has elliptical bright green leaves and flowers surrounded by coloured (usually deep crimson) bracts. A man, who cut and bunched red varieties, would develop, within half an hour of every exposure, intense pruritus then painful erythema often with papules and vesicles. As the pain subsided, pruritus returned and the skin crusted (D'Arcy, 1974).

Hippomane mancinella is a large, branching, poisonous tree with apple-like fruit. It grows in dense thickets or on beaches in the Caribbean and Central American coastland. The extremely irritant latex, in its branches, leaves and fruit, causes a 'poison-ivy'-like dermatitis; the results of swallowing it are disastrous (Satulsky, 1943a).

Sixty cases of dermatitis caused by this plant were described by Satulski and Wirts (1943). There were extreme burning and pain, with discrete and confluent erythematous macules and sometimes vesicles, on the face and neck. Conjunctivitis and intense lid oedema featured in some. The latex is so irritant that even indirect contact, as from dew dripping off the leaves, causes intense reactions.

Synadenium grantii, a succulent shrub native to the Zambesi but found also in greenhouses, has leaves tinged with red, and clustered deep red flowers.

A gardener let some of the irritant latex drip onto his forearm whilst pruning one of the shrubs. Within four hours he experienced burning of his face and neck, and by eight hours erythematous streaks studded with bullae had appeared on the dorsa of his hands and forearms. Resolution was rapid. Latex placed on his forearm caused intense irritation within six hours and a bulla appeared overnight: the reaction is irritant, not phototoxic (Rook, 1965).

Ricinus communis (Castor oil plant) is used for landscaping, or runs wild. Its coloured beans attract children who eat them and suffer the effects of the notorious phytotoxin ricin. Merely holding its stems, leaves or beans can lead to dermatitis (Dorsey, 1962).

GERANIACEAE (GERANIUM FAMILY)

Pelargonium includes common favourite species which are tender evergreen plants found in the greenhouse, house or garden. The common zonal pelargoniums, often referred to as 'geraniums', are an hybrid race, known also as *P. x hortorum*, derived largely from *P. zonale*. These zonal and scented varieties can cause dermatitis (Rook, 1961b) and, although varietal differences in allergenicity have yet to be reported, they probably will be.

Anderson (1923) described the case of a youth who developed vesicular dermatitis, with some thick-walled bullae, on the dorsa and sides of his fingers, spreading to the backs of his hands. The patient attributed it to removing dead leaves from a 'geranium' (unidentified); a crude patch test was positive.

Pelargonium graveolens and *P. domestica* (*P. x hortorum*) were significant causes of plant dermatitis in Hjorth's (1969) series.

Geranium maculatum, like many related species, has hairy leaves which cause dermatitis (McCord, 1962).

GESNERIACEAE (GESNERIA FAMILY)

The large flowers of some species are a popular feature.

Streptocarpus (Cape primrose (in Britain); Trumpet flower (in Sweden)) species often have foxglove-like flowers. Some are unique in having only one leaf throughout their life. Most European varieties have the South African species *S. rexei* as a parent, and are blue, violet or red, hairy-leaved house plants (van Ketel, 1973). Some are grown in greenhouses.

Streptocarpus tends to elicit in the sensitive acute reactions resembling primula dermatitis (Rook, 1968) (p. 527). A streaky erythema, commonly with vesicles, erupts on the hands, forearms and sometimes the face and neck. However, in van Ketel's (1973) cases, the pattern was nummular.

Patch tests
The leaf elicited positive reactions in the seven cases (all female) of the combined series of Agrup and Fregert (1968), van Ketel (1973) and Rook (1968). Controls were always tested; only one reacted (an irritant response). Hjorth (1974b), however, cautioned against testing with *Streptocarpus* leaf as 10 per cent

of the 33 persons he tested had irritant reactions. An ether extract (10 per cent w/w) and a dried extract 10 per cent in petrolatum were not irritant; but no mention was made about their value as test allergens.

Van Ketel (1973) studied the cross-reactions in his two patients as they had reacted to balsam of Peru. Caffeic acid (present in *Streptocarpus*) and cinnamic acid (in balsam of Peru) both elicited positive patch tests, and would account for the cross-reactions. However, members of this family vary in the amount of cinnamic acid derivatives they produce, so cross-reactions between its members are unpredictable. Agrup and Fregert (1968) also studied these cross-reactions and found one patient reacted to plants from five different families.

Sinningia speciosa (Gloxinia) has irritant hairy leaves (Rook, 1968).

GINKGOACEAE (GINKGO FAMILY)

There is only one genus and one species, *Ginkgo biloba* (Maidenhair tree), in this family. A deciduous tree with fern-shaped leaves, it is unknown in the wild state but has remarkable longevity (1000 years) and resistance to disease. The fruit pulp is irritant, offensively pungent and always toxic, but the roasted nut is always safe. The tree's products are used in cosmetics, soaps and fine oriental lacquer ware.

The pulp contains a saturated fatty acid, ginkgoic acid, which on reduction becomes ginkgol and hydroginkgol; it also yields bilobol which can be reduced to hydrobilobol. Ginkgol and hydroginkgol are identical to cardanol and hydrocardanol (p. 478) respectively, whereas bilobol closely resembles cardol (p. 478), hence the cross-reactions between components of *Ginkgo* and members of the Anacardiaceae (Sowers *et al.*, 1965) (p. 476).

An outbreak of contact dermatitis among preparatory schoolgirls was traced, by Sowers *et al.* (1965), to their having walked through *Ginkgo* fruit on the ground under the tree. Squashing the pods underfoot splattered the juicy pulp onto their legs; other sites were slightly affected. Most girls developed a reaction, and it ranged from erythematous papules to an often streaky, oedematous, papulo-vesicular erythema. Itch was usually intense. The distribution apart, it resembled 'poison ivy' dermatitis.

Patch tests
The pulp invariably caused irritant reactions; an acetone extract elicited no response in controls except some who were 'poison ivy' sensitive.

GRAMINEAE (GRASS FAMILY)

Grasses, grains such as maize, oats and wheat, sugar cane and bamboo belong to the Gramineae. Many species cause mechanical irritation: sharp trichomes from barley (*Hordeum vulgare*) and other cereal awns are a well-recognised cause of cereal dust dermatitis; spicules on millet (*Panicum*), rice (*Zizania*) and bamboo (*Bambusa*) elicit dermatitis in workers handling crops or litter straw (Woods, 1962).

Schuff (1951) reported what seemed to be an allergic occupational dermatitis among tennis racquet makers caused by bark- and hair-free bamboo (no botanical data were given).

Dermatitis from flour and grain is discussed on page 181.

HYDROPHYLLACEAE (WATER-LEAF FAMILY)

Phacelia crenulata (Desert or false heliotrope) is a viscid glandular species that blooms in March and April on dried stream beds in the desert of the west and south-west United States after a rainy winter. It has dark green rather hairy leaves and small blue to purple flowers on long stems, like a bluebell.

Every spring in Arizona this plant causes dermatitis on exposed limbs of people riding, walking or lying in the foothills or nearby desert. The eruption consists of linear vesicles and papules like a 'poison ivy' dermatitis. Only two of the 19 cases reported by Berry *et al.* (1962) were in males.

Patch tests
The dry leaf elicited positive reactions in all cases; of 10 controls, one reacted at 48 hours and two at 72 hours.

Only the viscid glandular species seem to be allergenic. Thus a patient sensitised by *P. pedicellata* reacted subsequently to *P. crenulata* but not to five other species. Nevertheless, several species are suspected of allergenicity, and were listed by Berry *et al.* (1962).

In western U.S.A. this genus should be considered as the real cause of many supposed cases of 'poison ivy' dermatitis.

Wigandia caracasana can cause dermatitis in California (Dorsey, 1962).

IRIDACEAE (IRIS FAMILY)

Iris versicolor (Iris; Blue flag), and probably other species, has rhizomes and other parts capable of causing allergic contact dermatitis (McCord, 1962).

Iris pseudacorus (Yellow flag), native to Europe, West Asia and North Africa, is quite distinct from *Iris germanica* (the 'common iris'). Its seeds are roasted for substitute coffee.

A teenager was sensitised by wearing a bracelet made of these seeds. The itchy dermatitis she developed on her wrist, under the bracelet, subsequently spread to her arms and face, causing eyelid oedema. Patch tests: seeds and leaf of the plant elicited positive reactions (Calnan, 1970).

LABIATAE (MINT FAMILY)

This is one of the families producing significant amounts of essential oils (Mitchell, 1969); the fragrant volatile oils are used in perfumes, medicines, and for culinary purposes.

Coleus blumei cultivars produced allergic contact dermatitis of the face only, in a gardener; lightly crushed leaves from 4 different cultivars each elicited positive patch tests (Saihan and Harman, 1978).

Marrubium vulgare (Hoarhound) plant juice causes dermatitis (McCord, 1962).

Mentha citrata (Mint) has caused occupational dermatitis in bar tenders (Sams, 1940).

Salvia officinalis (Sage), which contains alantolactone, has (with *Inula viscosa* and *Conyza bonariensis*) caused allergic contact dermatitis, with positive patch tests (Sertoli *et al.*, 1978).

Thyme (*Thymus*) and Rosemary (*Rosmarinus*) essences are allergenic, and many patients contact sensitive to the former, seen by Foussereau and Benezra (1970), were also allergic to thymol and its isomer carvacrol.

LAURACEAE (LAUREL FAMILY)

Well known members are the avocado pear, camphor (*Cinnamomum camphora*) and sweet bay.

1. *Cryptocarya* contains the vesicant cryptopleurine.

2. *Laurus nobilis* (Sweet bay) is an evergreen shrub of Mediterranean origin with aromatic, glossy lanceolate leaves, and dark cherry-sized berries. The berries and leaves yield both essential oils and laurel oil. These differ, for not only is some allergen (e.g. costunolide) lost during steam extraction of the essential oils, but the leaf essential oil differs chemically from that of berries.

Laurel oil is antioxidant, fungicidal, bactericidal and parasiticidal. The leaves are used to flavour and preserve food, and the oil has a place in medicines, dentistry, and the textile and cosmetic industries.

Sensitivity to laurel oil is mostly a European problem and has been recognised for over half a century. Reactions occur to ointments, felt in hats, and occasionally among grocers, cooks and housewives after contact with the leaf in foods. Among food sensitisers it is rated as common, and the sensitised patient, on ingesting it, can react with a generalised eruption and perioral dermatitis.

The incidence varies geographically, and can be common (Foussereau *et al.*, 1967) especially among Alsacians, who were sensitised, during World War II, by a German ointment containing laurel oil in high concentrations. In Strasbourg, the sensitivity still accounts for 17.8 per cent of all plant dermatitis (Asakawa *et al.*, 1974).

Indentification of the allergen is incomplete. Roots of *L. nobilis* yield laurenobiolide (Tada and Takada, 1971), but the sesquiterpene lactone in the leaf is still only a 'potential' allergen (p. 496) (Foussereau *et al.*, 1967). Laurel oil varies in its allergen content depending on its source (Foussereau *et al.*, 1975), and that from the leaf probably contains at least three sesquiterpene lactones: costunolide, desacetyl laurenobiolide and a third, unidentified, compound (Tada, 1974, quoted in Foussereau *et al.*, 1975): even so the allergen need not be a sesquiterpene lactone (Stampf *et al.*, 1978).

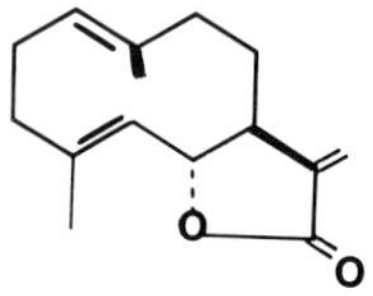

Costunolide

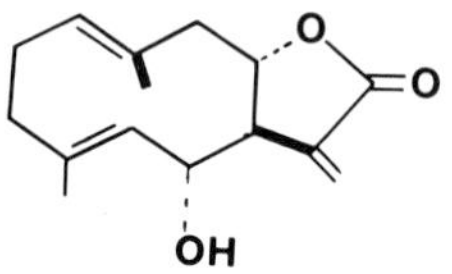

Desacetyl laurenobiolide

The clinical picture varies with the mode of contact. These are discussed elsewhere: Medicaments (p. 192); Textiles (p. 36); Foods (p. 171); and Cosmetics (p. 93).

Patch tests
Laurel oil 0.2 per cent in petrolatum, or essential oil 5 per cent in ethanol.

3. *Cinnamomum* species used for spice are:
   C. zeylanicum, in Sri Lanka, Burma, India, South America and the West Indies, yields cinnamon.
   C. loureirii (in Saigon) and *C. cassia* (in China) give cassia (Syn. Chinese, Saigon or commercial cinnamon) (Calnan, 1976).
The botanical species differ in their chemical composition, as do various parts of the plant. Thus the essential oil from *C. cassia* bark may contain 70–90 per cent cinnamic aldehyde, whereas that from *C. zeylanicum* leaf may have only 7 per cent (Fisher, 1975).
   Allergy to cinnamon oil (Fisher, 1975) is no great rarity (1.08 per cent of 1382 consecutive cases of eczema patch tested in 5 European centres). Bakers, confectioners, chemists, cooks and housewives are at risk, and if sensitised are likely to get hand eczema.

Patch testing
Cinnamon oil 0.5 per cent in petrolatum. Cross-reactions, based on cinnamates, include: balsam of Peru, balsam of Tolu, cocoa (*Theobroma cacao*), Storox, cinnamic acid and aldehyde, cinnamon oil, perfumes, flavours and sunscreens. Cinnamaldehyde is a histamine liberator and can cause contact urticaria (Nater *et al.*, 1977).

LEGUMINOSAE (PEA, LENTIL OR PULSE FAMILY)

The plants of this family range from tiny creepers to forest trees, and they provide food, ornament or dyes.

1. *Arachis hypogae* (Peanut) contains the protease arachain (see below).

2. *Mucuna pruriens* (Cowhage) produces mucunain, a highly irritant endopeptidase. Shelly and Arthur (1955) studied the species and enzyme in detail. When dry, trichomes on the pods fall off and constitute an "itch powder", which is active if the particles are adequately rubbed into the epidermis. Within 30 seconds of entry, pruritus begins, but, as the enzyme is inactivated, it lasts only 3–5 minutes. Species containing similar proteinases are shown in Table 10.8.

Table 10.8. Proteinases in plants

Species	Common name	Family	Proteinase	Activation necessary
Arachis hypogae	Peanut	Leguminosae	Arachain	—
Asclepias spp.	Milkweeds	Asclepiadaceae	Asclepain	+ (cysteine)
Carica papaya	Pawpaw	Caricaceae	Papain	+ (cysteine)
Ficus carica	Fig	Moraceae	Ficin	+ (cysteine)
Hura crepitans	Hura tree	Euphorbiaceae	Hurain	—
Mucuna pruriens	Cowhage	Leguminosae	Mucunain	—
Urtica disica	Nettle	Urticaceae	Solanain	—

LILIACEAE (LILY FAMILY)

The Liliaceae, Amaryllidaceae and Iridaceae are related (Burks, 1954). *Tulipa* and *Hyacinthus* are the Liliaceae genera of most interest dermatologically.

Tulipa is an unknown hybrid complex (Rook, 1961b) of garden tulips introduced into Holland in the mid-16th century, probably from the Caucasus (Bertwistle, 1935). In the 19th century, bulb growers produced a number of cultivars from the wild species ('botanical tulips') (Verspyck Mijnssen, 1969). The Dutch held the monopoly of the tulip industry until 1905 when some parts of England, especially around Wisbech and Spalding, started to produce tulips. Of undiminished popularity, tulips are cultivated nowadays by specialist growers in hundreds of varieties. Most cultivars are raised from seed, but new mutations ('sports') are not infrequent. The Royal Dutch Bulb Growers' Society has classified and listed the vast numbers of known tulips.

Hyacinthus is an ubiquitous house and garden plant cultivated in nurseries. All have sprung from the hardy, tall, elegant *H. orientalis*. Other species, native to the southern Mediterranean and Africa, are rarely seen outside specialist nurseries. *H. orientalis* is no longer generally grown, and its larger-flowered hybrids, so-called Dutch hyacinths, are cultivated instead. Examples are: 'L' Innocence' (white), 'City of Haarlem' (Yellow), 'General Kohler' (blue). Selective breeding from *H. orientalis* and its botanical variety *H. o. provincialis* has produced florists' varieties, some of which are sterile triploids (e.g. 'Lord Derby') (Rook, 1961b).

Botanical considerations

Tulip and hyacinth bulbs have a leathery husk (*tecta*) of dead, brown skin, formed as the outer layers die in the last weeks of growth. In tulips, this is only one layer thick and readily splits to reveal the bulb within, but in hyacinths, as in narcissi (p. 473), it is thicker and more abrasive. The tecta covers several layers of white fleshy scale leaves which are living parenchyma (Hjorth and Wilkinson, 1968).

As the bulb of the current year dies, a new daughter bulb is formed; this is peeled off by hand in the tulip bulb industry (Verspyck Mijnssen, 1969).

Tulip and hyacinth bulbs are abrasive, but only the latter contain *raphides*

(p. 473). These are formed within the root cell cytoplasm and lie in plasma strands running between expanding vacuoles. As each raphide has its own layer of plasma, the crystal sheaths are effectively united at the end of the bundle and so stay together. On opening the cytoplasmic vacuoles as the bulb is cut, the viscid mucus escapes with its embedded raphide (van der Werff, 1959).

Hyacinth varieties, like those of narcissi, differ in the raphide production and in the relative content of calcium oxalate and oxalic acid.

The allergen

Tulip allergen has been isolated an identified as α-methylene-γ-butyrolactone (tulipaline A) (Brongersma-Oosterhoff, 1967; Verspyck Mijnssen, 1968):

α-methylene-γ-butyrolactone

Patch test studies support its role as an allergen, for a dilution of 1:600 produces reactions in controls, while 1:20 000 elicits positive tests in persons contact hypersensitive to *Tulipa*, an effect nullified by cysteine.

In the plant, the lactone is bound to a glycoside as tuliposide A, which is only weakly allergenic but readily releases the free allergen on aqueous extraction. None of the other lactones in *Tulipa* spp. is a known allergen.

Most of the allergen is in the inner bulb scale epidermis, and although some is found in the outer scales, it is quickly lost in the last weeks of growth. Even during harvesting, however, some antigen remains in the outer layers of the second and other scales (Hjorth and Wilkinson, 1968). Tulipaline A is found in the rest of the plant in the following decreasing order of concentration: central tissues of scales of new bulbs; stems and leaves; flowers.

Tulipa species may differ in their allergenicity, but the point is contentious. Because *Tulipa* (and *Hyacinthus*) are hybrids from a selection of wild species, the allergen content of an individual specimen is determined quantitatively by its derivation (Rook, 1962). This explains why a florist can be sensitised to 'Keiserkroon' only (Rook, 1961b) and why a few varieties such as 'Rose Copeland' have a very bad reputation (see below). On the other hand, Klashka et al. (1964) were unable to show any difference in patch test reactions to 9 different varieties, and Verspyck Mijnssen (1969) demonstrated convincingly by gas chromatography and patch testing that only one of twelve varieties had less antigen than the others (this was 'Red Emperor' = 'Madame Lefeber', a cultivar of *T. fosterina*). Hjorth and Wilkinson (1968) interpreted these facts as being consistent with the existence of only one allergen, provided its relative concentration and distribution vary in flowers and bulbs.

Tulipaline A is also found in bulbs of *Erythronium dens canis* (Dog's tooth violet) and *E. americanum* (Cavillito and Haskell, 1946), but not in *Hyacinthus*, *Crocus* and *Narcissus* species. Tuliposide A, however, occurs in all species of *Alstroemeria* (Slob, 1973).

Hyacinthus reactions can be irritant or allergic (Rook, 1961; van der Werff, 1969), but no reference to the isolation of an allergen in this genus has been traced.

Irritants

Tulip bulbs contain no raphides, but their tecta is abrasive. Hyacinth raphides, with their surrounding cytoplasm and mucus, are potent skin irritants, both physically and chemically. The outer bulb scales and the dust surrounding hot dry bulbs can contain up to 5 per cent calcium oxalate. Hyacinth varieties differ in their ability to cause dermatitis and this applies particularly to the special varieties and subvarieties. Worst is, ironically, the pure white 'L' Innocence' (van der Werff, 1959), then 'Carnegie' and 'City of Haarlem'.

Incidence

Incidence of dermatitis from tulips and hyacinths is not known, due partly to the heterogeneity of those at risk (florists, and casual or full-time workers in the bulb industry, with differing degrees of exposure) and partly to the inconstant allergenicity and irritancy of the different plant varieties. Although dermatitis is common among Dutch bulb (especially tulip) industry workers, dermatologists see it infrequently (Hjorth and Wilkinson, 1968), possibly because patients change their job, are just seasonal workers or are stoical.

In 1935, Bertwistle reported that 85 per cent of those at risk in English bulb fields developed 'tulip fingers' whereas in Denmark, Hjorth (1969) estimated that the condition accounted for 4 per cent of plant dermatitis.

'Rose Copeland' has the worst reputation for causing dermatitis among Dutch tulip bulb handlers: 40 per cent of those sorting and skinning bulbs are affected. It is also notorious among florists (Rook, 1961b), while 'Praeludium' causes flower choppers the most trouble (van der Werff, 1959). Nevertheless, other varieties are troublesome. In patch tests, severest reactions are elicited by 'Rose Copeland' and 'Clara Butt'.

Traditional practices modify the figures. Thus, in Denmark the tulip, complete with bulb, is brought to market, but in Germany and Sweden the bulb is split with a knife to produce a longer stem, and causes dermatitis in up to 60 per cent of workers there (Hjorth and Wilkinson, 1968).

Some hyacinth varieties are particularly noxious, but all specimens contain oxalate which irritates everyone, workers and visitors alike.

Clinical features

Dermatitis from bulb handling ('Bulb fingers') is usually caused by *Tulipa* ('Tulip fingers'), much less often by *Hyacinthus* ('Hyacinth scabies') or *Allium* (p. 471).

'Tulip fingers' (Bertwistle, 1935) are due mainly to contact allergy (Rook, 1961b) but sometimes to the abrasive tecta, which can rapidly cause an increasingly severe hand dermatitis (Overton, 1926). Bulbs are usually responsible but flowers may elicit reactions and even actively sensitise (Klashka *et al.*, 1964).

The calendar of activities in the tulip bulb industry, which determines the timing of skin reactions, was described by van der Werff (1959). Flowers can produce a brisk reaction on the index finger and backs of the hands of very sensitive persons who cut or pull the flowers in the growing season. 'Tulip fingers', however, affects those who handle the bulbs whey they are being dug up, processed and stored. Much of this work is undertaken by seasonally employed women and children who tend to give it up if they develop dermatitis. Full-time employees, however, once sensitised react each time they handle bulbs, even if they have avoided contact and been trouble-free for a couple of decades.

Many years of asymptomatic recurrent seasonal work in the bulb industry antedate the onset of dermatitis, which appears on the sites of most contact during the 8 weeks of the bulb handling season. Initially, an intolerable tingling ('tulip fire'), tenderness and erythema of the finger tips, especially under the free margins of the nails, develop within 24 hours of handling bulbs (Bertwistle, 1935; Rook, 1962). After repeated exposure, desquamation appears under the nail plates distally and spreads to the finger tips and periungually to produce an irritable, painful, dry, fissuring and hyperkeratotic eczema (Hjorth and Wilkinson, 1968). The longer the nails, the worse the condition, but, early on at least, the nail plate is spared (Overton, 1926).

Deterioration takes several forms: erosion of the finger tips and intensification of the pain (Verspyck Mijnssen, 1969); exudation, granulation or abscess formation under the nail plate; onycholysis with the formation of a keratinous ridge; a shortened nail plate which becomes brittle and may split across if chipped at one corner (Bertwistle, 1935).

Other sites are often involved, especially the backs of the fingers and hands where vesicles may appear. The face and cheeks tend to become scaly, red and swollen, and the lids dry, thick and rigid. Genital involvement is not unusual, but generalisation occurs only in the severest cases. Some patients also have rhinorrhoea or asthma.

'Hyacinth itch', in the hyacinth bulb industry, is usually an irritant effect, but in the 1:60 patients who develop a papular and vesicular reaction it may be allergic (van der Werff, 1969). The latter author described the activities in the industry, which account for the timing of reactions.

In the bulb fields, exposure to raphides always elicits irritant dermatitis, which is common (Rook, 1961b). Pruritus is violent, and the affected skin becomes erythematous, swollen and sometimes studded with papules and vesicles, particularly around the follicles. Covered as well as exposed skin is affected. The sites of predilection are: flexor surfaces of the forearms; the face, especially the lids, round the nose, the lower jaw and behind the ears; sides of the neck; pressure and friction sites such as the groins, inner thighs, genitals and perianal region. Some patients have rhinorrhoea, lacrymation or bronchospasm (van der Werff, 1959).

Severity depends on the plant variety, the degree of exposure and the coexistence of contact allergy. However, despite painful fissures and secondary infection, which can be disabling, these patients contrive to remain at work.

Patch tests

The plant or bulb. It can be difficult to discriminate between the allergic and irritant reactions, particularly with hyacinths, for separation of oxalates from unidentified allergens is no easy matter (van der Werff, 1959).

Plants: The leaf is suitable for either tulip or hyacinth (p. 464)

Bulb:

(i) A thin slice, or a single inner scale (Rook, 1960);
(ii) Bulb epidermis after removal of the brown outer skin (Hjorth and Wilkinson, 1968);
(iii) Bulb extract, to eliminate seasonal variations in allergen content. An acetone extract, 1 per cent in 70 per cent ethanol, was preferred by Hjorth and Wilkinson (1968).

All possibly relevant varieties should be tested.

Cross-reactions occur between *Tulipa* and *Alstroemeria* (p. 472)

Other genera

Irritant species listed by Woods (1962) are: *Colchicum autumnale* (Meadow saffron), *Scilla* spp. (Squill) and *Veratrum album* (White hellebore).

Management

Logically, patients must avoid all contact with plants to which they are contact hypersensitive. This can be difficult in occupational dermatitis, as the patient requires an economically viable range of tulip and hyacinth varieties which are safe for him to handle. This necessitates detailed patch testing to detect safe as well as harmful plants.

MORACEAE (MULBERRY FAMILY)

The fig (*Ficus carica*), rubber plant (*Ficus elastica*) and mulberry (*Morus* spp.) are well known members of this family.

Chlorophora spp. yield the allergen chlorophorin (Mitchell, 1975a).

Ficus spp. and *Maclura pomifera* (Osage apple) latex causes dermatitis (McCord, 1962). *Ficus carica* contains the photosensitizer bergapten (Woods, 1962) (see p. 421).

MYRTACEAE (MYRTLE FAMILY)

Eugenia spp. belong to this family of aromatic trees and shrubs. *E. aromatica* (Clove tree) yields the clove of commerce from which eugenol is produced. This can, on ingestion, cause a flare-up of dermatitis in those contact hypersensitive to it. It is used in perfumes, soap, toothpaste, mouthwashes and foods, and is mentioned in the appropriate sections of this book.

ORCHIDACEAE (ORCHID FAMILY)

All members of this ubiquitous family are beautiful, and huge numbers of hybrids are available.

Cypripedium has some irritant species (Woods, 1962).

C. reginae (Lady's slipper — showy) has hairy stems and leaves, but the severe, sometimes delayed, dermatitis it causes is probably due to an acid. If the patient is hot and sweaty or if the plant is in flower the reaction is facilitated (McCord, 1962).

Vanilla planifolia pods yield the flavouring extract vanilla. The actual flavour is vanillin, a crystalline benzaldehyde formed from glycosides such as glucovanillic alcohol and glucoconiferyl alcohol in the plant. *Vanillism* refers to allergic contact dermatitis in workers handling the plant, which can sometimes be associated with bronchospasm, rhinitis and vertigo. Contact hypersensitivity to vanilla occurs in its industrial use as well as in the cultivation and trade of the substance.

This species is also associated with an urticarial, papular, pseudophytodermatitis due to the mite *Tyroglyphus farinae* which lives on the pods.

POLYGONACEAE (BUCKWHEAT OR KNOTWEED FAMILY)

Well known species are *Polygonum* and rhubarb (*Rheum rhaponticum*).

Polygonum species include common weeds as well as garden plants such as the popular Danish flower *P. cuspibatum*. Hjorth and Mitchell (1974) discussed dermatitis from *Polygonum* and listed the following as irritant:
P. aviculare (Common knot grass), *P. hydropiper* (Biting persicaria etc.), *P. persicaria* (Common persicaria) and *P. punctatum* (Poor man's pepper). *P. cuspibatum* (Japanese polygonum), however, caused a typically streaky phytodermatitis on the hands and forearms of a gardener who reacted to a patch test with the leaf.
P. nodosum (Knotgrass; spotted persicaria) is also a known sensitiser; its allergen is in the blossom, leaf and stem (Möslein, 1963).

Rheum rhaponticum leaves can cause dermatitis (McCord, 1962).

PRIMULACEAE (PRIMROSE FAMILY)

Cyclamen and *Primula* are representative of the 28 genera in this family.
Primula species all have primrose-like, occasionally bell-shaped, flowers; *P. communis* (Common primrose), *P. veris* (Cowslip) and *P. polyanthus* are well known examples. There are vast numbers of ornamental species, hybrids and selected forms, found as indoor plants, in the garden or greenhouse. Of the indoor plants, *P. obconica*, *P. malacoides* and, to some extent, *P. sinensis* are favourites in Europe, although *P.x kewensis*, *P. floribunda*, *P. denticulata* and *P. mollis* are seen occasionally.
Primula obconica has great appeal, due to its beauty, long flowering season, resilience in hostile environments and tolerance of neglect. Soon after its introduction in 1880, it was found as a greenhouse plant throughout Europe, especially

Germany, and in the U.S.A., but its popularity was tempered by a spate of reports of contact hypersensitivity to it.

Selection, hybridisation and mutation have produced the currently favourite plants which bear little resemblance to the original, wild, Chinese species whose direct descendants are termed *grandiflora*. *P.o. gigantea* is a noteworthy variety; it is the outcome of hybridising *P. obconica* and the non-allergenic *P. megaseaflora* in an endeavour to produce larger and longer-lasting flowers. It turned out to be even more allergenic than the original *grandiflora* (Maurer and Storck, 1935).

Primula obconica is a perennial species, usually grown as an annual, which reaches a height of up to 15 inches. The light green, ovate leaves are slightly hairy and the flowers, each about 1 inch across, are borne in clusters on long stalks. They can be pink, red, lilac, blue-purple or white and all are pungently scented. Representatives of the many cultivars are:

'Caerulea' (a clear purple-blue); 'Fasbender Red' (large and deep red); 'Giant White' (pure white); 'Wyaston Wonder' (rich deep crimson).

Botanical features

Primula obconica has two sorts of hair. The larger visible hairs, 1–3 mm long, are innocuous, whereas the tiny (0.05–0.3 mm) glandular variety, which can be seen only with a magnifying glass, are composed of 2–6 cells and secrete the allergen between the cell wall and cuticle. The latter is readily ruptured to release the allergen in resinuous droplets onto and around the hairs.

The long hairs are easily felt on the flower stalks and undersurface of the leaves, but the impalpable glandular hairs are distributed equally on both sides of the leaf and are densest along the margins and between the ribs. On the plant as a whole, they are found, in decreasing order of density, on the calyx, flower stalk, carpel leaf, leaf stem, inflorescent stem, and upper surface of the petal. Their number is constant, even among the varieties, so their density is greatest on the smallest young leaves.

The amount of allergen produced differs among the varieties as an individual characteristic unrelated to colour or year of growth. It is also influenced by cultural conditions. Thus warmth, nitrogenous manuring and especially sunlight increase allergen synthesis, whereas copious watering may render a highly allergenic plant wellnigh impotent within a fortnight.

Seasonal variation in the plant's allergen content is important clinically and in patch testing. Primulas are bought in the spring, produce gradually increasing amounts of allergen during summer, less in the autumn and least of all in February. Consequently, not only are sensitisation and severe reactions more frequent in summer, but patch test sensitisation and positive reactions are more likely to occur if a summer leaf or its extract is used. Indeed, a winter leaf may be responsible for false negative patch tests.

A popular characteristic of the plant is the growth of new leaves and flowers as the old ones wither. The owner keeps it tidy by removing the dead parts and in doing so is exposed to the most allergenic area — the calyx and flower stalk. It is this need to handle the plant, just when it is most allergenic, which accounts for the seasonal incidence and severity of primula dermatitis.

The allergen

The only *Primula* species found by Nestler (1904) to contain skin irritant principles were *P. obconica*, *P. sinensis* and the two *P. cortusoides* —*P. sieboldi* and *P. mollis*. The allergen, primin, was purified by Karrer (Bloch and Karrer, 1927), its biological activity confirmed by Bloch and Steiner-Wourlich (1927, 1931), and its structural formula and synthesis worked out by Schildknecht (1957, 1964):

2-Methoxy-6-*n*-pentyl-*p*-benzoquinone; primin

Primin was thought to be the only allergen in *P. obconica*, a view supported by Hjorth *et al.* (1969) finding just one peak, corresponding to primin, in gas chromatography of an ether extract of the plant. Furthermore, Fregert and Hjorth (1977) found primin in only one of 12 *Primula* species: this was *P. obconica*. Yet it was never certain that primin is the sole allergen (Cairns, 1964) or that it is almost exclusive to *P. obconica*. Hausen (1978), however, has not only shown that 16 *Primula* species contain primin but also suggested that, in the plant, primin may be present as a glycoside capable of yielding, as well as primin, an allergenic quinhydrone which could be the 'second allergen' of Cairns (1964).

Primin contains the optimal requirements for allergenicity (Hjorth *et al.*, 1969) viz. a basic formula of 2-methoxy-*p*-quinone with a 5-carbon (C_5H_{11}) side chain attached at position 6. Alteration of the side chain length or attaching it to position 5 on the ring reduces allergic potency. The side chain also seems to influence percutaneous absorption.

For patch test purposes (p. 529), primin can be synthetic or extracted from the plant. Cairns (1964) produced equally effective methanolic and ethyl acetate extracts. However, when he applied a paper chromatograph of the extract, moistened with ethylene glycol, as a patch test, there were reactions to more than one spot. (This finding was the first to cast doubts on the view that primin is the only allergen in *P. obconica*.)

The preparation of pure primin from *P. obconica*, described in detail by Agrup *et al.* (1968), is suitable for patch tests and is comparable to a standard solution of synthetic primin.

Incidence

For 60 years *Primula obconica* has caused most cases of plant dermatitis in Europe (British Medical Journal, 1965; Rook and Wilson, 1965), but latterly Hjorth (1970a) noted a declining incidence from a peak in the post-war years. Recently, Roed-Petersen and Hjorth (1976) claimed that, as florists are now reluctant to stock the plant, it may no longer cause most non-occupational dermatitis in Europe, but this awaits confirmation, and may be true only regionally.

The true incidence is unknown because cases are often unlike phytodermatitis and the diagnosis is missed, and patients rarely know what plants they own. It certainly was common and accounted for up to 8 per cent of all eczema cases seen during summer (Hjorth, 1966).

Most information comes from patch test series which record primula sensitivity rather than dermatitis. Their validity is restricted by factors such as seasonal variation. Representative, but somewhat dated series are:

Author	Incidence	Females
Bonnevie (1939)	8.8%	90%
Hjorth (1966)	3.7%	85%
Agrup et al. (1968)	5.7%	84%

This preponderance of females is probably due to greater contact with the plant. They are also affected more frequently in summer, unlike men, who show no seasonal variation. The considerable influence of season reflects the plant's allergen content and need to be handled. However, as patch tests with pure synthetic primin fail to eliminate seasonal variations, it seems that in summer the plant, or patch tests, must sensitise more people, and patch tests must pick up weak reactors more efficiently.

Geographical influences are poorly understood. Primula dermatitis is more common in Sweden than in Denmark, but in the U.S.A. it is said to be rare. This may, in part, reflect traditional attitudes to pot plants (Hjorth, 1970a).

Clinical features

Clinicians who diagnose primula dermatitis simply on suggestive clinical features and a history of exposure to the plant are likely to misdiagnose 50 per cent of the cases they see. Thus Hjorth (1966) thought that only half of his and Bonnevie's (1939) cases were typical of phytodermatitis. Several variables contribute to the difficulty: (1) Season: (2) Route of exposure; (3) Degree of hypersensitivity.

Seasonal variations are determined by the plant's allergen content and need of attention (p. 525). In spring, only trivial symptoms will occur, even in very sensitive people, but in summer episodes tend to become more severe and frequent. As winter approaches, the severity of attacks wanes. However, throughout, the degree of sensitivity modulates the intensity of reactions and mild episodes in summer generally indicate recent sensitisation. However, the author was sensitised in late winter and suffered an intense, widespread reaction.

Exposure to the plant is usually direct, and once aware of the possibility, the patient generally recognises it as the cause of the dermatitis. However, indirect contact can be devious, e.g. contaminated furniture or doorknobs, handshakes or, speculatively, resin-contaminated dust (Hjorth, 1970a).

The *degree of hypersensitivity* sets the threshold for attacks so that removing dead leaves may elicit violent reactions in some people and trivial attacks in others. Moreover, the very sensitive can react all year round, but the weakly sensitive only in summer.

History taking can be straightforward if the dermatitis is known to be caused by handling a known specimen of *P. obconica*, but it can be misleading and frustrating. Patients commonly exonerate plants they have owned for a long time and have to be persuaded that this is really a good reason for suspecting them. Most people do not know what plants they own, but many dermatologists are little better at identifying *P. obconica*. One way round this difficulty is to display in Departments of Dermatology clear colour photographs of 8 varieties of the plant. Accounts of casual contact are largely fictional (Hjorth, 1970a) and although it is hard enough to get a valid history of contact with primula in the sitting-room, it is exceptional to do so when it is in greenhouses, entrances or offices.

In a 'typical' case, allergenic resin on the fingers can be spread widely to produce a streaky dermatitis at sites of contact. Reactions can be severe, even intense, with oedema, erythema, papules, vesicles and bullae. Itch and discomfort can be extreme. The sites of predilection are the hands, upper limbs and face, sometimes with palpebral oedema, but the nostrils, ears, trunk (through dressing), genitals and buttocks can be involved too. In Rook and Wilson's (1965) series, the following distribution was recorded:

Site	No	%	Site	No	%
Cheeks and chin	16	64	Hands	9	36
Neck	14	56	Thighs and buttocks	2	8
Arms	14	56	Ankles	1	4
Lids	13	52	Ears	1	4
Fingers	12	48	Tongue	1	4

Minor reactions can take very different forms such as: only a few 'dyshidrotic' vesicles along the finger sides, possibly of just one hand; a solitary area of itchy erythema on the chin or side of the neck; recurrent attacks of erythema, swelling and pruritus of the lids.

The spectrum of a typical patterns is, however, very wide, and Hjorth (1966) provided a comprehensive list of preliminary diagnoses ranging from dyshidrotic eczema, through seborrhoeic dermatitis to erythema multiforme. He included 'poison ivy' dermatitis (p. 479), but the two conditions can be differentiated in the U.S.A., because primula dermatitis is more diffuse and has an ill-defined erythema with pruritus rather than discomfort. In clinically atypical cases, the diagnosis can be made only by patch testing.

When reactions are more typical, the differential diagnosis includes other causes of phytodermatitis. In the vast majority, primula dermatitis is due to *P. obconica*. *Primula sinensis* is rarely responsible, and although Whiting (1971) reported that he had seen two cases due to *P. malacoides*, this species is a very unlikely cause. Similar reactions can occur to *Achillea millefolium* (Yarrow) (p. 511) and to some members of the Ranunculaceae family (p. 530).

Patch tests

The major difficulty in patch testing is the avoidance of active sensitisation while ensuring that weak reactions are not missed; this has led to the argument whether or not routine patch testing with primula is justified. It was questioned by Agrup *et al.* (1969) and advocated by Hjorth (1970a) who recommended testing all female patients who have dermatitis between March and October, otherwise on the slightest suspicion.

Test material:

a. *Leaf* (Hjorth, 1967): Drawbacks are variations in allergenicity, contamination of other patches, and sensitisation of the staff. Apart from the use in summer of a piece from a large leaf of the patient's own specimen, handled carefully with forceps, the technique is essentially obsolete (Hjorth, 1970a).

b. *Ether extract of leaves and stems* (Agrup *et al.*, 1968): this is the recommended test material, applied as a closed test. It is stable and can be stored for at least 3 years in a refrigerator, its primin content is constant in all seasons, and its allergenicity can be monitored by testing known sensitive subjects or by chemical spot tests (Brachtendorf, 1956). The extract is convenient and reliable to use, curtails false negative and too strongly positive reactions, and is less likely to sensitise the operator.

c. *Synthetic primin*: is ideal but in short supply. Open tests tend to elicit stronger reactions, as the filter paper in closed tests retains some allergen. A concentration of 1:100 is always irritant, 1:1000 commonly so and although 1:10 000 does not irritate, it can actively sensitise (Agrup *et al.*, 1969). A dilution of 1:50 000 elicits reactions in all clinically sensitive patients. Fregert *et al.* (1968) recommended not more than 1 μg primin on a filter[*] under occlusion, and quoted 20 μl of a 1:10^4 solution in ethyl ether for an open test.

Active sensitisation causes most reactions that appear 1 week or more after applying the test. They are prone to occur in young women and comprise a few follicular papules which coalesce, oedema and rarely vesicles. Hjorth (1966) estimated that more than 17 per cent of reactions are of this type, and Agrup *et al.* (1969) believed that primin in routine patch tests had sensitised 10 per cent of their hand eczema patients.

If patients are tested twice, the number sensitive remains approximately the same so that, between the tests, as many are sensitised as lose their sensitivity. The ease with which primin penetrates the skin may alone explain the frequency of test sensitisation (Fregert *et al.*, 1968) and it justifies the reluctance of Agrup *et al.* (1969) to include primula in routine patch tests, especially when 16 of their 20 primula sensitive patients, and 2 of their 4 primula hand eczema patients were already aware of their allergy.

In assessing the *relevance of positive patch tests*, patients must be able to recognise *P. obconica* in all its varieties. They have little idea; they go on colour, flower size and petal shape, all of which vary, whereas it is the shape of the leaf that matters. In Hjorth's (1970a) series of 302 patients with positive primula patch tests, 100 (33 per cent) managed to trace the plant responsible; of these, 82 found it at home and the others identified it at work or in a friend's home. Clinically, another 60 were unlikely to fit any alternative diagnosis; thus, in all, 53 per cent had relevant patch tests. The residual 49 per cent were not discussed.

[*]Available commercially from Trolab, Hollister-Stier Labs as prepared test units.

Cross-reactions

Cross-reactions result from the basic quinone structure of primin which is shared with dalbergiones (p. 560). Thus primula sensitive cases can react to dalbergiones in rosewood (*Dalbergia*) and 2,3-dimethoxydalbergione in *Machaerium scleroxylon* (both Leguminosae); they possibly react to the naphthaquinone, deoxylapachol (p. 569), in teak (*Tectona*) (Verbenaceae). The reciprocal cross-reaction in primin in wood sensitive cases has not been demonstrated. These cross-reactions were discussed by Mitchell (1975b).

As *Primula obconica* was, until recently, the only known primin-containing species (Fregert and Hjorth, 1977), reactions to *P. sinensis*, *P. malacoides* and *P. variabilis* were thought to be irritant, caused possibly by saponins, flavones or glycosides. Whiting (1971), however, reported two cases of contact allergy to *P. malacoides* but did not mention the allergen. Reports of reactions to *P. siebaldi*, *P. cortusoides*, *P.x kewensis* and to several garden primulas have not indicated whether they were due to allergens other than primin. There is, in fact, no evidence that marked hypersensitivity to *P. obconica* is regularly or even frequently associated with sensitivity to other *Primula* species (Rook and Wilson, 1965). (The few reactions in their series were to species rarely found in British gardens and belonged to the *Cortusoides* section of *Primula*, some of which are known irritants.) However, Hausen (1978) used a screening (Craven) test for primin on 82 species of the Primulaceae and found the quinone and other quinoid compounds in 16 *Primula* species (and 4 other genera). Noteworthy were *P. sinensis*, *P. elatior* and *P. veris*, as they have, in the past, been suspected causes of contact dermatitis.

Prophylaxis

Nothing short of avoiding the plant with suffice. If a florist becomes hypersensitive to *P. obconica*, he will have to offer other species such as *P. sinensis* or *P. malacoides*, but his customers will scarcely agree that they are as attractive as *P. obconica*, and their shorter flowering season will disappoint.

Other genera

Cortusa matthioli regularly causes dermatitis, probably irritant (Woods, 1962).

RANUNCULACEAE (BUTTERCUP OR CROWFOOT FAMILY)

Familiar genera include *Anemone*, *Clematis* and *Delphinium*. Members of the family are notoriously irritant due mainly to the lactone protoanemonin:

Protoanemonin

When the plants are bruised, the non-irritant glycoside ranunculin they contain is broken down to protoanemonin which tightly binds sulphydryl groups and causes sub-epidermal bullae (Burbach, 1963). Ranunculin is synthesised by members of the Heleboreae and Anemoneae tribes.

Clinically, acute dermatitis occurs at sites of contact, which in children is commonly perioral from their habit of chewing stems. The vesicant effect has long been used medically, particularly in arthritis, and although its origins date back to folk medicine, the practice continues. Thus, Rudzki and Dajek (1975) recently reported the extreme irritant effect of 'buttercups' (*Ranunculus* spp.) under occlusion used for arthralgia in Poland.

Many *Anemone* species are known irritants (Woods, 1962; Mitchell, 1975b). These include *A. cylindrica*, *A. hepatica*, *A. multifida*, *A. nemorosa* (Wood anemone), *A. obtusifolia*, *A. pratensis* (Small pasque flowers), *A pulsatilla* (syn. *Pulsatilla vulgaris*) (Pasque flower) and *A. quinquefolia*. One species can be considered as representive:

Anemone patens (Prairie crocus) is a pretty spring flower that blooms from April to June on the prairies and exposed slopes of North America (Aaron and Muttitt, 1964). It can be applied topically for arthritis, when it causes severe vesiculation. Within an hour of application, there is a burning sensation, followed by extreme erythema and some swelling, then by bullae and slough formation. Crushing a leaf releases a vapour irritant to the conjunctiva. A patch test with the leaf irritates within five minutes and even if it is removed within an hour, vesiculation appears by 24 hours. The plant is reputed to be allergenic too (McCord, 1962).

Other irritant species (McCord, 1962; Woods, 1962)
These include *Clematis virginiana*, *C vitalba*, *Delphinium ajacis*, *Helleborus niger* and *Ranunculus* spp. (Buttercup; Crowfoot; Lesser celandine). *Adonia vernalis* contains *p*-dimethoxybenzoquinone, an allergen found also in some exotic woods (Foussereau *et al.*, 1975).

ROSACEAE (ROSE FAMILY)

The list of fruiting and ornamental members is incredible and includes the rose, hawthorn, plum, peach, pear, blackberry and a host of other delicacies.

Phytodermatitis, in its broadest sense, from Rosaceae species has been discussed with examples by Krauskopf (1978). The following species are noteworthy:

Agrimonia eupatoria (Common agrimony), a common, yellow-flowered, roadside weed with a pleasantly and sweetly pungent odour, especially the juice, was responsible for a couple of minor outbreaks of contact dermatitis (O'Donovan, 1942). The reaction seemed to require a hot, sweaty skin, and consisted of erythema, fine vesicles and later bullae. It began about 36–48 hours after contact. Rubbing sap from a crushed leaf onto the skin has a blistering effect which takes 3–10 days to settle. Whether light plays a part has not been studied.

Fragaria species (Strawberry) (McCord, 1962) and *Rosa odorata* (Tea Rose) (Dorsey, 1962) have been reported as causes of dermatitis; *Malus* (apple) can elicit immediate reactions in some atopic subjects.

RUBIACEAE (MADDER FAMILY)

Coffee, madder and quinine are well known products.

Contact allergy to coffee (*Coffea*) is discussed on page 183.

Rubia tinctorum root yields the dye dihydroxyanthraquinone (alazarin), a sensitizer (Calnan, 1973b).

RUTACEA (RUE FAMILY)

The genus of greatest importance dermatologically is *Citrus*, of which the following species are representative:
C. aurantiifolia (Lime), *C. aurantium* (Sour or Seville orange), *C. limona* (Lemon), *C. paradisia* (Grapefruit), *C. sinensis* (Sweet orange).
Of some importance are: *Dictamnus albus* (Gas plant) and *Ruta graveolens* (Rue).

Botanical aspects.
The structure of citrus fruit is well known. The outermost few layers of cells of the exocarp produce peel oil which in all species consists mainly (about 90 per cent) of d-limonene. The residual 10 per cent or so varies in composition among the species, especially in the aldehyde, and it includes compounds such as citronellal, geraniol and linalool (Schwartz, 1938).

All citrus fruit juices are irritant, but lemon juice is worst and has a higher citric acid content and a lower pH than orange or grapefruit juices. The flavour of orange is due to decyl aldehyde, while lemon tastes of citral. Oranges owe their colour to hesperidin and carotene.

The allergens
d-Limonene is thought to be the principal sensitizer in *Citrus* species. Minor allergens may include α-terpinene, in lemons at least (Puglisi, 1951), carotene (Hjorth, 1961; Sulzberger, 1936) and probably others, as yet unidentified.

Extraneous allergens may contaminate the fruit, and some of them are dealt with elsewhere: fertilizers and insecticides (p. 404), dyes on oranges from Florida *not* California (p. 179), and wax (which may contain the sensitiser carnuba wax) on dyed oranges.

d-Limonene   α-Terpinene

d-Limonene is both irritant and allergenic, and the former action accounts for most of the irritation and drying of the skin by peel oil.

Incidence

The incidence of contact dermatitis from *Citrus* species is unknown, but more cases are irritant than allergic in nature. In the citrus fruit industry it has been reported as common (Beerman *et al.*, 1938; Birmingham *et al.*, 1951) and much of it was due to physicochemical trauma of wet manual work. Food-handlers seem not to suffer greatly, for of 33 studied by Hjorth and Roed-Petersen (1976) none reacted to patch tests with lemon peel and flesh, and orange peel and flesh.

Consumers are known to react, especially to the juice, but how frequently is not known, partly because they are often not seen, or are cared for by their general practitioner (Jonson, 1953).

Contact hypersensitivity is mostly due to terpenes in peel oil, whereas the role of extraneous allergens (see above) is minor (Aldick, 1952).

The citrus fruit industry

By selection of varieties, oranges are now brought to maturity all year round in North America, especially in Florida and California. Comprehensive details of the industry were given by Schwartz (1938), from which it is evident that cutaneous hazards include the extraneous allergens, mechanical trauma from plant thorns, irritation and secondary infection from wet work, and handling irritant fruit or juice. In the citrus fruit canning industry (Birmingham *et al.*, 1951), some workers handle fruit for long periods in a hot, wet environment containing alkali and carbohydrate and in consequence develop irritant dermatitis, candidiasis and nail dystrophy. Most irritation, however, is due to the peel oil.

Clinical features

The *irritant effect* of peel oil can be seen as erythema, papules and vesicles, especially on the dorsa of the hands, the forearms and the lids (Schwartz, 1938).

Contact hypersensitivity is also usually to peel oil, but of Janson's (1953) 29 cases, 8 were due to the juice only, and of the rest, 19 were due to peel oil and one each to the flower and wood. Most were due to either lemon or oranges, not both. This feature was also noted by Beerman *et al.* (1938) who found cases of sensitivity to orange only or to lemon only. Yet not all sensitivities are specific, as it was found that combined sensitivity to all *Citrus* species can occur.

Patients contact hypersensitive to citrus fruit tend to have dermatitis of the hands or face. Food-handlers, for instance, generally have hand dermatitis from squeezing juice out of the fruit or preparing it for table. Handling the fruit or juice commonly elicits a pompholyx-like reaction on the palms and fingers, but involvement of only the left palm, due to holding the fruit whilst cutting it, is a recognised pattern. Consumers often present with cheilitis or perioral dermatitis (Schwartz, 1938) from drinking fruit juice or from contaminated fingers.

The symtomatology consists of smarting, irritation, erythema, swelling and vesiculation, followed by exudation and crusting. The nails are often pitted. The severity of reactions is influenced in part by the fruit and the conditions under which it was grown (e.g. climate, soil, season).

Patch tests

Peel 'as is'. If the orange is dyed, remove the wax first. Avoid rupturing the peel oil cells. A cautious technique was described by Schwartz (1938). Always test three controls with peel. Alternatives: Peel oil 1 per cent in ethanol or 25 per cent in castor oil; Fregert and Bandmann (1975) listed d-limonene 2 per cent in petrolatum, and oil of lemon or orange each 2 per cent in petrolatum (Table 10.1).

Cross-reactions based on d-limonene can be expected to Oil of Neroli, dill, bergamot, caraway oil, celery seed oil and turpentine.

Ruta graveolens leaves cause dermatitis. The plant is a well known cause of phytophotodermatitis as are several other members of the Rutaceae: *Citrus aurantiifolia*, *C. aurantium*, *C. bergamia*, *C. limon*, *C. medica* and *Dictamnus albus* (p. 420). The phototoxic principle in the latter species (5-methoxypsoralen; bergapten) has been studied in detail by Suhonen (1977) and by Möller (1978) who identified 5-methoxypsoralen and 8-methoxypsoralen.

SAXIFRAGACEAE (SAXIFRAGE FAMILY)

Currants and gooseberries are familiar products of this family.

Hydrangea caused two reported cases of allergic contact dermatitis (Apted, 1973), one in a 16-year-old girl, the other in a 59-year-old male florist. Both had erythema, vesicles and pruritus, especially on the backs and sides of the fingers. Also involved were the thenar eminences in the girl, and the backs of the hands and flexor surfaces of the wrists in the man. Patch tests with *Hydrangea* were positive in both.

Tolmiea menziesii (Pickaback plant), a native of north-west America, is a common houseplant in the U.K. It is a modest sensitiser, but as it has been much studied it has caused a considerable number of positive patch test reactions. It accounted for 7 per cent of positive patch test reactions to plants and caused 6.5 per cent of the 420 cases of plant dermatitis in Hjorth's (1969) series.

Calnan (1969) recorded the case of an elderly woman who, for several years, had had each summer a pompholyx-like eruption. This comprised pruritic vesicles on her palms and fingers, and later, pruritus and erythema of her lids and neck. Patch tests with the plant were positive; she did not react to the other plants she had at home.

SOLANACEAE (NIGHTSHADE FAMILY)

Vegetables, fruit, spice, tobacco and drugs are notable products of this family's members.

Atropa belladonna (Deadly nightshade) sap causes erythema, oedema and vesiculation (McCord, 1962).

Capsicum frutescens (Cayenne pepper), like other spices, can cause contact allergy. Flares-up at sites of previous dermatitis in the sensitised may occur if it is inhaled or ingested (e.g. eating pickles or drinking ginger ale).

Lycopersicon lycopersicum (Tomato) is a rare sensitiser of those processing the fruit (Klauder and Kimmig, 1956), and in an uncommon cause of immediate reactions in some atopic subjects.

Nicotiana tabacum (Tobacco), in several varieties, and other species such as *N. rustica*, are cultivated as an annual crop in warm countries for tobacco.

Contact dermatitis in the tobacco industry can be caused by irritants, pesticides, fertilizers, heat and humidity as well as damp tobacco leaves. Contact allergy to *N. tabacum* also occurs (Vero and Geneovese, 1941) but is reputedly rare; patch tests are usually negative.

True hypersensitivity to the plant juice is expressed as dermatitis on the palms, fingers and sometimes the face. It is stubborn as long as the patient continues his job, but clears once he is away from work.

Three cases were described by Vero and Geneovese (1941): the most exposed areas were affected, namely the fingers, especially the thumb, the hands and forearms. Patch tests with a recently fermented leaf from a batch of *N. tabacum* were positive in all three patients, but neither raw leaves nor dry tobacco elicited a reaction. The allergen is unknown: possibilities include a produce of fermentation or curing, an essential oil or glandular hairs. It is not nicotine.

Solanum tuberosum is discussed on page 183.

UMBELLIFERAE (PARSLEY FAMILY)

Familiar products of this family are carrots, parsnips, parsley and celery.

Phytophotodermatitis is the characteristic response of the skin to members of the Umbelliferae (Ch. 9) and contact is usually through food handling (Ch. 5). The photosensitisation to ultraviolet radiation, with a wavelength of 350 nm, is due to furocoumarins in the plants (p. 418), and these chemicals are found in members of other plant families especially the Rutaceae (p. 532), Moraceae (p. 563) and Leguminosae (p. 557).

The characteristic clinical picture (Rook, 1962) comprises striate or irregularly linear bullae at sites where crushed leaves or stems have contaminated the skin. It starts within 12–24 hours of contact and sun exposure, and it heals leaving pigmentation that can last for several months.

In Table 10.9 are listed the Umbelliferae species known to cause dermatitis, usually of the phytophoto variety. A few are discussed here for they may cause dermatitis unrelated to light; for the others, see Chapter 9.

Angelica archangelica (Angelica) stem, leaf and stalk are used in salads and as a cooked vegetable, the roots as a conserve; it flavours some liqueurs and gin.

Apium graveolens (Celery) has many varieties, such as white, gold and pink, the

Table 10.9. Umbelliferae Plants Known to Cause Dermatitis.

Botanical name	Common name	Botanical name	Common name
Anethum graveolens	Dill	*Foeniculum vulgare*	Fennel
Angelica archangelica	Angelica	*Heracleum mantegazzianum*	Giant hogweed
Anthriscum sylvestris	Cow parsley	*H. sphondylium*	Hogweed, Cow
Apium graveolens	Celery		parsnip
A. g. rapaceum	Celeriac	*Pastinaca sativa*	Parsnip
Carum carvi	Caraway	*Petroselinum crispum*	Parsley
Coriandrum sativum	Coriander	*Peucedanum astruthium*	Masterwort
Daucus carota sativa	Carrot	*Pimpinella anisum*	Anise

result of selective breeding within the species (Rook, 1961b). The pink is the most pungent and possibly the most potent allergenically, but in the U.S.A. 'Pascal green' may be the commonest sensitiser. The species commonly sensitises market gardeners (Rook, 1962).

Celery is associated with contact allergy, angio-oedema and urticaria (Kaupinnen *et al.*, 1978) and with parasitophytophotodermatitis. In the latter event the fungus *Sclerotinia* parasitises it, causing it to produce the psoralens which elicit photodermatitis (Birmingham *et al.*, 1961); bergapten has been isolated by Musajo *et al.* (1954).

The *contact allergen* in the essential oil may be d-limonene (p. 532), but it seems that three conditions are necessary for dermatitis to occur: the release of considerable amounts of celery oil from the plant by rupturing the cellular tissue, exposure to water, and to friction (Henry, 1938).

In a couple of reports, Henry (1933, 1938) discussed in detail the process and hazards of celery canning. Dermatitis affected about one-third of workers, all of whom were engaged in handling the plant under wet conditions. About 25 per cent of the cases started in the first month, and a good half in the second month, of the celery season.

The dermatitis consisted of erythema, papules and vesicles, but the appearance sometimes became erysipeloid, and oedema with oozing could occur. Sites of predilection were the hands, and the distal half of the forearms, usually bilaterally. In some, the face was involved, but in about half, only the forearms were affected and in around 20 per cent only the hands. The problem could be incapacitating and necessitate absence from work for a month or so.

Patch tests

An ether extract of celery is suitable (Wiswell *et al.*, 1948). There may be cross-reactions to carrot and other Umbelliferae plants and to essential oils of orange, lemon, bergamot, caraway, dill and to balsams.

Daucus carota sativa (Carrot) is the most notorious sensitiser in the vegetable processing industry (Klauder and Kimmich, 1956). The curious tendency for outbreaks to occur might conceivably be due to variations in allergenicity among batches of carrots. Usually it is contact allergy to some ingredient of carrots

(Rook, 1962) and although the oleoresin contains pinene, terpineol and cineol, the nature of the allergen is unknown (Vickers, 1941; Peck *et al.*, 1944).

Occupationally, exposure to carrot juice in wet conditions favours sensitisation which is readily acquired. However, carrot is also irritant, and although prolonged contact with raw or cooked carrot can cause allergic contact dermatitis, raw carrot, dried carrot residue, carrot juice and to some extent heated carrot, may promote irritant reactions (Peck *et al.*, 1944).

Carrot processing and the clinical pattern of carrot dermatitis have been described in detail (Vickers, 1941; Peck *et al.*, 1944; Klauder and Kimmig, 1956). The dermatitis may be limited to the hands, as in carrot scrapers, but dicers may have a more widespread eruption consisting of an acute pruritic vesicular erythema of the fingers and backs of the hands and forearms. In addition, itchy erythema with oedema on the face and neck are not unusual. The incubation period ranges from a week to a year, but commonly is two weeks, and once contact ceases the eruption clears in a fortnight. Persons contact hypersensitive to carrots can eat them with relative impunity, but lip oedema and perioral dermatitis have occurred. Certain atopic subjects are known to develop immediate contact reactions.

Patch tests
The outer surface of unpeeled carrot, or better, a slice of carrot.

Cross-reactions occur to other Umbelliferae plants e.g. *Pastinaca sativa* and *Apium graveolens* (Klauder and Kimmig, 1956).

Pastinaca sativa (Parsnip). The weed is *P. s.* var. *pratensis* and the edible variety *P.s.* var. *hortensis*. The species was reviewed by Klauder and Kimmig (1956).

The wild variety is an outstanding cause of phytophotodermatitis, especially, it is thought, when in flower. Its common names are numerous (e.g. heelroot, hookweed, bird's nest, hart's eye, madnip). If cultivated, it assumes the appearance of the edible variety, which also causes phytophotodermatitis.

A classical phytophotodermatitis (see above) results from exposure to the plant, moisture and sun. Parsnip handlers, however, can develop acute hand dermatitis if they work out-of-doors or go out in the sun during a tea-break.

Whether or not a few cases are due to true allergic contact dermatitis is a speculation based on cross-reactions to parsnip in some carrot-sensitive persons (see above).

As an occupational hazard, parsnip dermatitis is unusual as the processing season is late in the year when sunlight is at a premium.

Petroselinum crispum (Parsley) can elicit photodermatitis if the skin is wet or sweaty (Somner and Jillson, 1967): it can also cause angio-oedema and urticaria (Kaupinnen *et al.*, 1978).

URTICACEAE (NETTLE FAMILY)

Boehmeria species produce the vesicant cryptopleurine.

Laportea species leaves and stems have fine stinging hairs which inject acetyl choline, histamine, 5-hydroxytryptamine and an unknown pain-producing substance.

Urtica dioica (Nettle) induces weals by injecting histamine, acetyl choline and some other chemical. The effects are mild compared with those of its tropical counterparts which can cause severe and widely spreading pain, convulsions and even death (Woods, 1962).

(*Ulmus procera* (Elm tree) [Ulmaceae], a relative of *Urtica*, has hairy leaves that can cause dermatitis.)

ZINGIBERACEAE (GINGER FAMILY)

Many spices, including ginger, are produced by members of this family.

Elletania species, in tropical Asia, have seeds which yield cardamom, a popular flavour for baked goods and confectionery. This caused chronic dermatitis on the hands and distal arms of a baker who bare-handed manually ground the seeds and kneaded the powder into the dough (Mobacken and Fregert, 1975). Patch tests were positive to cardomom powder and to oil of cardomom; he also reacted to delta-carene, dipentene, oil of bergamot and turpentine. Whether the cardamom was the primary or a secondary allergen was undecided, but cardamon was considered to be a possible cause of occupational dermatitis in bakers and confectioners.

MISCELLANEOUS FAMILIES

Fragmentary data are available on very many species known to be harmful to the skin and to belong to plant families other than those mentioned above. The volume of information is beyond the scope of this chapter, as is evident in the treatise by Mitchell and Rook (1979). It is an encyclopaedic account, covering the literature of botanical dermatology in its entirety. The reader is referred to it for further details.

References

Aaron, T.H. and Muttitt, E.I.L. (1964) Vesicant dermatitis due to Prairie crocus (*A. patens*). *Archives of Dermatology*, **90**, 168.

Agrup, G. (1969) Hand eczema. *Acta dermato-venereologica*, **49**, Supplement 61.

Agrup, G. & Fregert, S. (1968) Patch test reactions to *Streptocarpus*. *Contact Dermatitis Newsletter*, **4**, 72.

Agrup, G., Fregert, S., Hjorth, N. & Ovrum, P. (1968) Routine patch testing with ether extract of *Primula obconica*. *British Journal of Dermatology*, **80**, 497.

Agrup, G., Fregert, S. & Rorsman, H. (1969) Sensitisation by routine patch testing with ether extract of *Primula obconica*. *British Journal of Dermatology*, **81**, 899.

Aldick, W. von (1952) Citrusarten als Ursache von Erkrankungen der Haut. *Hautarzt*, **3**, 164.

Anderson, J.W. (1923) Geranium dermatitis. *Archives of Dermatology*, **7**, 510.

Apted, J.H. (1973) Phytodermatitis from hydrangeas. *Archives of Dermatology*, **108**, 427.

Apted, J.H. (1978) Poison ivy dermatitis in Victoria. *Australasia Journal of Dermatology*, **19**, 35.

Asakawa, Y. Benezra, C., Ducomb, G. Foussereau, J., Muller, J.C. & Ourisson, G. (1974) Cross-sensitisation between *Frullania* and *Laurus nobilis*: the allergen laurel. *Archives of Dermatology*, **110**, 957.

Auerbach, R. & Baer, H. (1964) The potency of poison ivy extracts. *Journal of Allergy*, **35**, 201.

Ayres, S.Jr. & Ayres, S.III (1958) *Philodendron* as a cause of dermatitis. *Archives of Dermatology*, **78**, 330.

Baer, H., Dawson, C.R. & Kurtz, A.P. (1968) Delayed contact sensitivity to catechols IV. Stereochemical conformation of the antigen determinant. *Journal of Immunology*, **101**, 1243.

Baer, H., Srinivasan, S., Bowser, R.T. and Karmann, A. (1963) The active principles of poison ivy. *Journal of Allergy*, **34**, 221.

Baer, H., Watkins, R.C. & Bowser, T. (1966) Delayed contact sensitivity to catechols and resorcinols. The Relationship of structure and immunisation procedure to sensitising capacity. *Immunochemistry*, **3**, 479.

Baer, H., Watkins, R.C., Kurtz, A.P. Byck, J.C. & Dawson C.R. (1967) Delayed contact sensitivity to catechols III. The relationship of side chain length to sensitising potency of catechols chemically related to the active principles of poison ivy. *Journal of Immunology*, **99**, 370.

Balyeat, R.M., Rinkel, H.J. & Stemen, T.R. (1932) Contact dermatitis (venenata). Distribution and importance of *Helenium* as a cause of contact dermatitis in the United States. *American Journal of Medical Science*, **184**, 547.

Banerjee, K. (1977) A case report of sabra dermatitis. *Indian Journal of Dermatology*, **22**, 159.

Beerman, H. Fonde, G.H. Callaway, J.L. (1938) Citrus fruit dermatoses. *Archives of Dermatology*, **38**, 225.

Benezra, C. (1973) Allergènes végétaux. Méthodes chimiques d'isolement et d'identification. *Revue Francaise d'Allergologie*, **13**, 51.

Bergh, Marianne (1975) Weed dermatitis detected by oleoresins (Hollister-Stier). *Contact Dermatitis*, **1**, 61.

Berry, C.Z., Shapiro, S.I. & Dohlen, R.F. (1962) Dermatitis from *Phacelia crenulata*. *Archives of Dermatology*, **85**, 737.

Bertwistle, A.P. (1935) Tulip fingers. *British Medical Journal*, **2**, 255.

Bhutani, L.K. and Rao, D.S. (1978) Photocontact dermatitis caused by *Parthenium hysterophorus*. *Dermatologica*, **157**, 206.

Birmingham, D.J., Campbell, P.C. & Doyle, H.N. (1951) Investigation of occupational dermatoses in the citrus fruit canning industry. *Archives of Industrial Hygiene and Occupational Medicine*, **3**, 57.

Birmingham, D.J., Key, M.M. Tubick, G.E. & Perone, V.B. (1961) Phototoxic bullae among celery harvesters. *Archives of Dermatology*, **83**, 73.

Black, H. (1972) Contact dermatitis from onion weed plant. *Contact Dermatitis Newsletter*, **11**, 282.

Bleumink, E. & Nater, J.P. (1973) Contact dermatitis due to garlic. Contact reactivity between garlic, onion and tulip. *Archiv für Dermatologische Forschung*, **247**, 117.

Bleumink, E. & Nater, J.P. (1974) Contact dermatitis in a gardener caused by daffodils. *Berufsdermatosen*, **22**, 123.

Bleumink, E., Doeglas, N.M.G., Klokke, A.H. & Nater, J.P. (1972) Allergic contact dermatitis to garlic. *British Journal of Dermatology*, **87**, 6.

Bleumink, E., Mitchell, J.C. & Nater, J.P. (1973) Contact dermatitis to chrysanthemums. *Archives of Dermatology*, **108**, 220.

Bleumink, E., Mitchell, J.C., Geissman, T.A. & Towers, G.H.N. (1976) Contact hypersensitivity to sesquiterpene lactones in *Chrysanthemum* dermatitis. *Contact Dermatitis*, **2**, 81.

Bloch, B. & Karrer, P. (1927) Chemische and biologische Untersuchungen über die Primelnidiosynkrasie. *Beiblatt Vierteljahrsschrift Naturforschende Gesellschaft in Zurich*, **72**, 23.

Bloch, B. & Steiner-Wourlisch, A. (1927) Die willkuerliche Erzeugung der Primelueberempfindlichkeit beim Menschen und ihre Bedeutung für das Idosynkrasieproblem. *Archiv für Dermatologie und Syphilis, Berlin*. **152**, 283.

Bloch, B. & Steiner-Wourlich, A. (1931) Die Sensibilisierung des Meerschweinchens gegen Primeln. *Archiv für Dermatologie and Syphilis*, **162**, 349.

Bonnevie, P. (1939) *Aetiologie und Pathogenese der Ekzemkrankheiten*. Copenhagen. Nyt Nordisk Forlag.

Brachtendorf, J. (1956) Untersuchungen zum Nachweis des Primins bei *Primula obconica*. *Züchter*, **26**, 161.

British Medical Journal (1965) Editorial: Plant dermatitis, **1**, 205.

Brongersma-Oosterhoff, U.W. (1967) Structure determination of the allergic agent isolated from tulip bulbs. *Recueil des Travaux Chimiques des Pays Bas*, **86**, 705.

Brown, E.D. (1922) Experiments in the variability in susceptibility to poison ivy. *Archives of Dermatology*, **5**, 714.

Brown, A. & Brown, F.R. (1941) Mango dermatitis. *Journal of Allergy*, **12**, 310.

Brown, A., Milford, E.L. & Coca, A.F. (1931) Studies in contact dermatitis I. The nature and aetiology of pollen dermatitis. *Journal of Allergy*, **2**, 301.

Brunsting, L.A. & Anderson, C.R. (1934) Ragweed dermatitis. A report based on eighteen cases. *Journal of the American Medical Association*, **103**, 1285.

Brunsting, L.A. & Williams, D.H. (1936) Ragweed (contact) dermatitis: observations on 48 cases and report of unsuccessful attempts at desensitisation by injections of specific oils. *Journal of the American Medical Association*, **106**, 1533.

Burbach, J.P.E. (1963) Oorspronkelijke stukken: De blaartrekkende werking van boterbloemen. *Nederlandsch Tijdschrift voor Geneeskunde*, **107**, pt I, 1128.

Burks, J.W. (1954) Classic aspects of onion and garlic dermatitis in housewives. *Annals of Allergy*, **12**, 592.

Burry, J.N. (1979) Dermatitis from fleabane: Compositae dermatitis in South Australia. *Contact Dermatitis*, **5**, 51.

Burry, J.N. Kuchel, R., Reid, J.G. & Kirk, J. (1973) Australian Bush dermatitis: Compositae dermatitis in South Australia. *The Medical Journal of Australia*, **1**, 110.

Cairns, R.J. (1964) Plant dermatitis: some chemical aspects and results of patch testing with extracts of *Primula obconica*. *Transactions of the St. John's Hospital Dermatological Society*, **50**, 137.

Calnan, C.D. (1969) *Tolmiea menziesii*. *Contact Dermatitis Newsletter*, **5**, 98.

Calnan, C.D. (1970) *Iris pseudacorus* L. *Contact Dermatitis Newsletter*, **8**, 171.

Calnan, C.D. (1973a) *Dahlia* dermatitis. *Contact Dermatitis Newsletter*, **13**, 366.

Calnan, C.D. (1973b) Rose madder paint (Dihydroxyanthraquinone). *Contact Dermatitis Newsletter*, **13**, 381.

Calnan, C.D. (1975) Petty spurge (*Euphorbia peplus* L.). *Contact Dermatitis*, **1**, 128.

Calnan, C.D. (1976) Cinnamon dermatitis from an ointment. *Contact Dermatitis*, **2**, 167.

Calnan C.D. (1978a) Sensitivity to dahlia flowers. *Contact Dermatitis*, **4**, 168.

Calnan, C.D. (1978b) Dermatitis from helenium. *Contact Dermatitis*, **4**, 115.

Campolmi, P., Sertoli, A., Fabbri, P. & Panconesi, E. (1978) Alantolactone sensitivity in chrysanthemum contact dermatitis. *Contact Dermatitis*, **4**, 93.

Caron, G.A. & Calnan, C.D. (1962) Studies in contact dermatitis XIV. Resorcin. *Transactions of the St. John's Hospital Dermatological Society*, **48**, 149.

Cavillito, C.J. & Haskell, T.H. (1946) α-Methylenebutyrolactone from *Erythronium americanum*. *Journal of the American Chemical Society*, **68**, 2332.

Chicheley Plowden, C. (1972) *A Manual of Plant Names*. 3rd (corrected) edn, London, Allen and Unwin.

Clapham, A.R. Tutin, T.G. & Warburg, E.F. (1962) *Flora of the British Isles*, 2nd edn, London: Cambridge University Press.

Cohen, S.G. (1959) Seasonal ragweed dermatitis: association of immediate and delayed types of pollen sensitivity. *Archives of Dermatology*, **79**, 328.

Cohen, S.G. & Michelini, F.J. (1958) Immune responses to ragweed pollen antigens. *Journal of Allergy*, **29**, 446.

Cookson, J.S. & Lawton, A. (1953) Hop dermatitis in Herefordshire. *British Medical Journal*, **2**, 376.

Cronin, E. (1968) Sensitivity to *Humea elegans*. *Contact Dermatitis Newsletter*, **3**, 89.

Cronin, E. (1972) Sensitivity to *Tulipa* and *Alstroemeria*. *Contact Dermatitis Newsletter*, **11**, 286.

Dang, R.W.M. & Bell, D.B. (1967) anaphylactic reaction to the ingestion of mango. *Hawaii Medical Journal*, **27**, 149.

D'Arcy, W.G. (1974) Severe contact dermatitis from Poinsettia. *Archives of Dermatology*, **109**, 909.

Dawson, C.R. (1956) The chemistry of poison ivy. *Transactions of the New York Academy of Sciences*, 427.

Dawson, C.R., Wasserman, D. & Keil, H. (1946) 3-n-Pentadecylcatechol. *Journal of the American Chemical Society*, **68**, 534.

Dorsey, C.S. (1957) Contact dermatitis from Algerian ivy. *Archives of Dermatology*, **75**, 671.

Dorsey, C.S. (1958) *Philodendron* dermatitis. *California Medicine*, **88**, 329.

Dorsey, C.S. (1959) Algerian ivy dermatitis (a Californian disease). *California Medicine*, **90**, 155.

Dorsey, C.S. (1962) Plant dermatitis in California. *California Medicine*, **96**, 412.

Edelstein, A.J. (1950) Dermatitis caused by garlic. *Archives of Dermatology*, **61**, 111.

Epstein, E. (1973) *Rhus* dermatitis: a rational regimen. *Cutis*, **12**, 47.

Epstein, E. & Claiborne, E.R. (1957) Racial and environmental factors in susceptibility to *Rhus*. *Archives of Dermatology*, **75**, 197.

Epstein, S. (1960) Role of dermal sensitivity in ragweed contact dermatitis. *Archives of Dermatology*, **82**, 48.

Epstein, W.L. (1958) *Rhus* dermatitis: fact and fiction. *Kaiser foundation Medical Bulletin*, **6**, 197.

Epstein, W.L. (1959) *Rhus* dermatitis. *Pediatric Clinics of North America*, **6**, 843.

Epstein, W.L., Baer, H., Dawson, C.R. & Khurana, R.G. (1974) Poison oak hyposensitisation. Evaluation of purified urushiol. *Archives of Dermatology*, **109**, 356.

Etter, R.I. (1951) Dermatitis caused by Japanese lacquer. *U.S. Armed Forces Medical Journal*, **21**, 505.

Fasal, P. (1945) Cutaneous disease in the tropics. A clinical study based on observations in Malaya. *Archives of Dermatology*, **51**, 163.

Feinberg, S.M. (1934) Pyrethrum sensitisation: its importance and relation to pollen allergy. *Journal of the American Medical Association*, **102**, 1557.

Fernald, M.L. (1950) *Gray's Manual of Botany* 8th (centennial) edn. New York and London: van Norstrand.

Findlay, G.H. Whiting, D.A., Eggers, S.H. & Ellis, R.P. (1974) *Smodingium* (African poison ivy) dermatitis. *British Journal of Dermatology*, **90**, 535.

Fisher, A.A. (1952) Some immunologic phenomena in treatment of and patch testing for ragweed oil dermatitis. *Journal of Investigative Dermatology*, **19**, 271.

Fisher, A.A. (1975) Allergic eczematous contact dermatitis due to foods. *Cutis*, **16**, 603.

Ford, R.M. (1963) Ragweed pollinosis. *The Medical Journal of Australia*, **1**, 712.

Foussereau, J. & Benezra, C. (1970) *Les Eczémas Allergiques Professionelles*. Paris: Masson et Cie.

Foussereau, J. Benezra, C. & Ourisson, G. (1967) Contact dermatitis from laurel I. Clinical aspects; II. Chemical aspects. *Transactions of the St. John's Hospital Dermatological Society*, **53**, 141 and 147.

Fousereau, J., Muller, J.C. & Benezra, C. (1975) Contact allergy to *Frullania* and *Laurus nobilis*: cross-sensitisation and chemical structure of the allergens. *Contact Dermatitis*, **1**, 223.

Fregert, S. & Bandmann, H-J. (1975) *Patch Testing*. New York: Springer-Verlag.

Fregert, S. & Hjorth, N. (1977) The primula allergen primin. *Contact Dermatitis*, **3**, 172.

Fregert, S., Hjorth, N. & Schulz, K-H (1968) Patch testing with synthetic primin in persons sensitive to *Primula obconica*. *Archives of Dermatology*, **98**, 144.

French, S.W. (1930) A case of skin sensitivity to *Parthenium hysterophorus*. *Military Surgeon*, **66**, 673.

Frits, B., Hjorth, N., Vail, J.T. & Mitchell, J.C. (1975) Occupational contact dermatitis from *Cichorium* (chicory, endive) and *Lactuca* (lecttuce). *Contact Dermatitis*, **1**, 311.

Fromer, J.L. & Burrage, W.S. (1953) Ragweed oil dermatitis. *Journal of Allergy*, **24**, 425.

Goldman, L., Preston, R.H. & Muegel, H.R. (1956) Dermatitis venenata from English ivy (*Hedera helix*). *Archives of Dermatology*, **74**, 311.

Goldsmith, N.R. (1943) Dermatitis from *Semecarpus anacardium* (Bhilwanol or Marking Nut) spread by contaminated mail. *Journal of the American Medical Association*, **123**, 27.

Goldstein, N. (1968) The ubiquitous urushiols. Contact dermatitis from mango, poison ivy and other 'poison' plants. *Cutis*, **4**, 679.

Grater, W.C. (1975) Hypersensitivity dermatitis from American weeds other than poison ivy. *Annals of Allergy*, **35**, 159.

Greenberg, S. & Mallozzi, E.D. (1940) Experiments in poison ivy sensitivity. Effects of specific injections on the level of sensitivity to qualitative patch tests and on clinical sensitivity. *Archives of Dermatology*, **42**, 290.

Hambly, E.M. and Wilkinson, D.S. (1978) Sensitivity to variegated ivy (*Hedera canariensis*). *Contact Dermatitis*, **4**, 239.

Hand, E.A. (1944) Contact dermatitis due to capeweed (*Cryptostemma calendulacea*). *Archives of Dermatology*, **49**, 331.

Hannuksela, M & Lahti, A. (1977) Immediate reactions to fruit and vegetables. *Contact Dermatitis*, **3**, 79.

Harris, J.H. (1942) Dermatitis of the lids due to *Philodendron* (*Scindans cordatum*) plants. *Archives of Dermatology*, **45**, 1066.

Hausen, B.M. (1977) A simple method for extracting crude sesquiterpene lactones from Compositae plants for skin tests, chemical investigations and sensitising experience in guinea-pigs. *Contact Dermatitis*, **3**, 58.

Hausen, B.M. (1978) On the occurrence of the contact allergen primin and other quinoid compounds in species of the family Primulaceae. *Archives for Dermatological Research*, **261**, 311.

Hausen, B.M. (1978a) Sensitising capacity of some common weeds (Compositae). *Contact Dermatitis*, **4**, 304.

Hausen, B.M. (1978b) Identification of allergens in *Arnica montana*. *Contact Dermatitis*, **4**, 308.

Hausen, B.M. (1978c) Die *Parthenium hysterophorus* — Allergie. *Dermatosen in Beruf und Umwelt*, **26**, 115.

Hausen, B.M., Herrmann, H.D. & Willuhn, G. (1978) the sensitising capacity of Compositae plants. 1. Occupational contact dermatitis from *Arnica longifolia* Eaton. *Contact Dermatitis*, **4**, 3.

Hausen, B.M. & Schulz, K.H. (1973) Chrysanthemen-Allergie (1. Mitteilung). *Berufsdermatosen*, **21**, 199.

Hausen, B.M. & Schulz, K.H. (1975) Experimental studies on the identification of chrysanthemum allergens. *Contact Dermatitis*, **1**, 244.

Hausen, B.M. & Schulz, K.H. (1976) Chrysanthemum allergy. III Identification of the allergens. *Archives of Dermatological Research*, **255**, 111.

Hausen, B.M. & Schulz, K.H. (1977) Occupational contact dermatitis due to croton (*Codiaeun variegatum* (L-) A. Juss var. *pictum* (Lodd.) Muell. Arg.). Sensitisation by plants of the Euphorbiacea. *Contact Dermatitis*, **3**, 289.

Hausen, B.M. & Schulz, K.H. (1978) Occupational allergic contact dermatitis due to Leather-leaf fern *Arachnoides adantiformis* (Forst) Tindale. *British Journal of Dermatology*, **98**, 325.

Hausen, B.M. and Schulz, K.H. (1978a) Polyvalente Kontaktallergie bei einer Floristin. *Dermatosen in Beruf und Umwelt*, **26**, 175.

Hay, R. (1971) *The Reader's Digest Encyclopaedia of Garden Plants and Flowers*. London: The Reader's Digest.

Hay, R. & Synge, P.M. (1969) *The Dictionary of Garden Plants*. London: Michael Joseph.

Hegyi, E.A. (1967) Plant dermatitis: *Inula brittanica*. *Contact Dermatitis Newsletter*, **2**, 4.

Henry, S.A. (1933) Celery itch: dermatitis due to celery in vegetable canning. *British Journal of Dermatology*, **45**, 301.

Henry, S.A. (1938) Dermatitis due to celery in vegetable canning. *British Journal of Dermatology*, **50**, 392.

Herout, V. & Sorm, F. (1969) Chemotaxonomy of the sesquiterpenoids of the Compositae.. In *Perspectives in Phytochemistry* ed Harborne, J.B. and Swain, T. p. 138. London: Academic Press.

Hindson, C. & Oliver, R. (1975) Eczema from the *Smodingium argutum* shrub. *Contact Dermatitis*, **1**, 388.

Hjorth, N. (1961) *Eczematous Allergy to Balsams, Allied Perfumes and Flavouring Agents*. Copenhagen: Munksgaard.

Hjorth, N. (1965) European congress of allergy. *Acta dermato-venereologica*, **68**, 65.

Hjorth, N. (1966) Primula dermatitis: sources of errors in patch test sensitisation. *Transactions of the St. John's Hospital Dermatological Society*, **52**, 207.

Hjorth, N. (1967) Seasonal variations in contact dermatitis. *Acta dermato-venereologica*, **47**, 409.

Hjorth, N. (1969) Plant dermatitis. *Contact Dermatitis Newsletter*, **6**, 126.

Hjorth, N. (1970a) Primula dermatitis. *Current Problems in Dermatology*, **3**, 31.

Hjorth, N. (1970b) Active sensitisation with alantolactone. *Contact Dermatitis Newsletter*, **8**, 175.

Hjorth, N. (1974a) Sensitivity to oleoresins of wild plants (Hollister-Stier). *Contact Dermatitis Newsletter*, **15**, 449.

Hjorth, N. (1974b) Irritant reactions from patch tests with *Streptocarpus*. *Contact Dermatitis Newsletter*, **15**, 446.

Hjorth, N. (1975) Battery for testing chefs and other kitchen workers. *Contact Dermatitis*, **1**, 63.

Hjorth, N. & Fregert, S. (1972) Contact dermatitis. In *Textbook of Dermatology* (Ed. Rook, A.J., Wilkinson D.S., & Ebling F.J.) 2nd edn. Vol. 1, p. 351. Oxford: Blackwell Scientific Publications.

Hjorth, N., Fregert, S. & Schildknecht, H. (1969) Cross-sensitisation between synthetic primin and related quinones. *Acta dermato-venereologica*, **49**, 552.

Hjorth, N. & Mitchell, J.C. (1974) *Polygonum* dermatitis. *Contact Dermatitis Newsletter*, **15**, 448.

Hjorth, N. & Roed-Petersen, J. (1976) Occupational protein contact dermatitis in food handlers. *Contact Dermatitis*, **2**, 28.

Hjorth, N., Roed-Petersen, J. & Thomsen, K. (1976) Airborne contact dermatitis from Compositae oleoresins simulating photodermatitis. *British Journal of Dermatology*, **95**, 613.

Hjorth, N. & Wilkinson, D.S. (1968) Contact Dermatitis IV: Tulip fingers, Hyacinth itch and Lily rash. *British Journal of Dermatology*, **80**, 696.

Howell, J.B. (1943) Evaluation of measures for the prevention of poison ivy dermatitis. *Archives of Dermatology*, **48**, 373.

Howell, J.B. (1959) Cross-sensitisation in diverse poisonous members of the sumac family (Anacardiaceae). *Journal of Investigative Dermatology*, **32**, 21.

Howell, J.B. (1971) Sensitivity to common weeds. *Contact Dermatitis Newsletter*, **10**, 230.

Hurtado, I. de (1970) Studies on the biological activity of *Rhus striata* IV. Toxicity versus hypersensitivity of dermal reactions in guinea-pigs to *Rhus striata* ('Manzanillo') extracts. *Journal of Investigative Dermatology*, 55, 94.

Hutchinson, J. (1973) *The Families of Flowering Plants*, 3rd edn. Oxford: Oxford University Press.

Janson, P.H. (1953) Citrusfruchte and Hauterkrankungen. *Zeitschrift fur Haut- und Geschlechtskrankheiten*, 14, 144.

Johnson, R.A., Baer, H., Kirkpatrick, C.H., Dawson, C.R. & Khurana, R.G. (1972) Comparisom of the contact allergenicity of the pentadecylacatechols derived from poison ivy urushiol in human subjects. *Journal of Allergy*, 49, 27.

Jordon, J.W., Campbell, P.C. & Osborne, E.D. (1942) Ragweed dermatitis among workers in the flour and grain industries. *Archives of Dermatology*, 46, 721.

Kahn, I.S. & Grothaus, EM (1936) *Parthenium hysterophorus*: antigenic properties, respiratory and cutaneous. *Texas State Medical Journal*, 32, 284.

Kaidby, K.H. & Kligman, A.M. (1976) Assay of topical corticosteroid efficiency of suppresion of experimental *Rhus* dermatitis humans. *Archives of Dermatology*, 112, 809.

Kanof, N.M. & Rostenberg, A. (1941) Observations on the persistence of sensitivity of the eczematous type after prolonged periods of removal from contact with the allergen. *Journal of Investigative Dermatology*, 4, 175.

Kaupinnen, K., Kousa, M. & Reunala, T. (1978) Aromatic plants — a cause of severe attacks of angioneurotic oedema and urticaria. *Allergy*, 33, 341.

Keil, H., Wasserman, D. & Dawson, C.R. (1945) A quantitative study of the relation of synthetic 3-pentadecylcatechol to hypersensitiveness to *Rhus toxicodendron* (poison ivy) as shown by the patch test. *Journal of Allergy*, 16, 275.

Keil, H., Wasserman, D. & Dawson, C.R. (1946) Mango dermatitis and its relationship to poison ivy hypersentivity. *Annals of Allergy*, 4, 268.

Ketel, W.G. van (1973) Allergic contact eczema from the leaves of *Streptocarpus*. *Transactions of the St. John's Hospital Dermatological Society*, 59, 73.

Ketel, W.G. van (1975) A cauliflower allergy. *Contact Dermatitis*, 1, 324.

Ketel, W.G. van & Haan, P. (1978) Occupational eczema from garlic and onion. *Contact Dermatitis*, 4, 53.

Ketel, W.G. van. Verspyck Mijinssen, G.A.W. & Neering, H. (1975) Contact eczema from *Alstroemeria*. *Contact Dermatitis*, 1, 323.

Kingsbury, J.M. (1964) *Poisonous Plants of the United States and Canada*. p. 208. New Jersey: Prentice-Hall.

Klaschka, F. Grimm, W. & Biersdorff, H.V. (1964) Tulpen-kontaktekzem als Berufsdermatosen. *Hautarzt*, 15, 317.

Klauder, J.V. & Kimming, J.M. (1956) Sensitisation dermatitis to carrots. *Archives of Dermatology*, 74, 149.

Kligman, A.M. (1958a) Poison ivy (*Rhus*) dermatitis. *Archives of Dermatology*, 77, 149.

Kligman, A.M. (1958b) Hyposensitisation against *Rhus* dermatitis. *Archives of Dermatology*, 78, 47.

Kligman, A.M. (1958c) Cashew nut shell oil for hyposensitisation against *Rhus* dermatitis. *Archives of Dermatology*, 78, 359.

Krauskopf, J. (1978) Phytodermatitis caused by Rosaceae. *Cesklovenska Dermatologie*, 53, 252.

Krook, G. (1973) Contact dermatitis due to lettuce (*Lactuca sativa*). *Contact Dermatitis Newsletter*, 13, 346.

Krook, G. (1977) Occupational dermatitis from *Lactuca sativa* (lettuce) and *Cichorium* (endive). Simultaneous occurrence of immediate and delayed allergy as a cause of contact dermatitis. *Contact Dermatitis*, 3, 27.

Laur, W.S., Posey, R.E. and Waller, J.D. (1978) Rhus dermatitis. An unusual example of exposure to ornamental shrubs. *Cutis*, 22, 613.

Livingood, C.S., Rogers, A.M. & Fitz-Hugh, T. (1943) Dhobie mark dermatitis. *Journal of the American Medical Association*, 123, 23.

Lonkar, A. & Jog, M.K. (1972) 'Epidemic' contact dermatitis due to *Parthenium hysterophorus* (Compositae family of plants). Report of 350 cases. *Contact Dermatitis Newsletter*, 11, 291.

Lonkar, A., Mitchell, J.C. & Calnan, C.D. (1974) Contact dermatitis from *Parthenium hysterophorus*. *Transactions of the St. John's Hospital Dermatological Society*, 60, 43.

Lonkar, A., Nagasampagi, B.A. Narayanan C.R., Landge, A.B. & Sawaikar, D.D. (1976) An antigen from *Parthenium hysterophorus*. *Contact Dermatitis*, 2, 151.

Lynne-Davies, G. & Mitchell, J.C. (1974) Patch tests for irritancy — some common house plants. *Contact Dermatitis Newsletter*, 16, 501.

Mackoff, S. & Dahl, A.O. (1951) A botanical consideration of the weed oleoresin problem. *Minnesota Medicine*, 34, 1169.

Maibach, H.I. & Epstein, W.L. (1964) Plant dermatitis: fact and fancy. *Post-graduate Medicine*, 35, 571.

Maibach, H.I. & Hjorth, N. (1973) *Rhus typhina*, a possible cause of contact dermatitis. *Contact Dermatitis Newsletter*, 13, 347.

Malten, K.E. (1973) Chrysanthemum contact hypersensitivity. *Contact Dermatitis Newsletter*, 13, 357.

Martin, J.T. & Hester, K.H.C. (1941) Dermatitis caused by insecticidal pyrethrum flowers (*Chrysantheumum cinerariifolium*). *British Journal of Dermatology*, 53, 127.

Mason, H.S. & Lada, A. (1954) Allergenic principles of poison ivy VIII. Immunological properties of a hydrourushiol-albumin concentrate. *Journal of Investigative Dermatology*, 22, 457.

Maurer, E. & Storck, A. (1936) Untersuchungen zur Zuechtung einer giftreien Primel vom 'Obconica'-Typus. *Gartenbauwissenschaft*, 10, 1.

McCord, C.P. (1962) The occupational toxicity of cultivated flowers. *Industrial Medicine and Surgery*, 31, 365.

Merrill, E.D. (1944) Dermatitis caused by various representatives of the Anacardiaceae. *Journal of the American Medical Association*, 124, 222.

Milford, E.L. (1930) Studies in allergy I. The specific activity of pollen oil. *Journal of Allergy*, 1, 331.

Miller, H.E. Mabry, T.J. Turner, B.L. & Payne, W.N. (1968) Infraspecific variation of sesquiterpene lactones in *Ambrosia psilostachya* (Compositae). *American Journal of Botany*, 55, 316.

Mitchell, J.C. (1969) Allergic contact dermatitis from Compositae. *Transactions of the St. John's Hospital Dermatological Society*, 55, 174.

Mitchell, J.C. (1972) Plant dermatitis: note on inadequacy of some plant extracts. *Contact Dermatitis Newsletter*, 11, 271.

Mitchell, J.C. (1974a) Applied chemotaxonomy of plants. A biological model. *Contact Dermatitis Newsletter*, 16, 494.

Mitchell, J.C. (1974b) Contact sensitivity to *Tulipa* and *Alstroemeria*. *Contact Dermatitis Newsletter*, 16, 506.

Mitchell, J.C. (1974c) Contact dermatitis from plants of the caper family, Capparidaceae. Effects on the skin of some plants which yield *iso*thiocyanates. *British Journal of Dermatology*, 91, 13.

Mitchell, J.C. (1974d) Contact sensitivity to costus root oil—ingredient of some perfumes. *Archives of Dermatology*, 109, 572.

Mitchell, J.C. (1975a) Contact allergy from plants. In: *Recent Advances in Phytochemistry* Vol. 9, ed. Runeckles, V.C., p. 119. New York and London: Plenum Press.

Mitchell, J.C. (1975b) Biochemical basis of geographical ecology. Parts 1 and 2. *International Journal of Dermatology*, 14, 239 and 301.

Mitchell, J.C. (1975c) Vegetables, international cooperation and journal space. *Contact Dermatitis*, 1, 195.

Mitchell, J.C. & Dupuis, G. (1971) Allergic contact dermatitis from sesquiterpenoids of the Compositae family of plants. *British Journal of Dermatology*, 84, 139.

Mitchell, J.C., Dupuis, G. & Geissman, T.A. (1972a) Allergic contact dermatitis from sesquiterpenoids of plants. Additional allergenic sesquiterpene lactones and immunological specificity of Compositae, liverworts and lichens. *British Journal of Dermatology*, 87, 235.

Mitchell, J.C. Dupuis, G. & Towers, G.H.N. (1972b) Allergic contact dermatitis from pyrethrum (*Chrysanthemum* species). The roles of pyrethrosin, a sesquiterpene lactone, and of pyrethrin II. *British Journal of Dermatology*, 86, 568.

Mitchell, J.C. & Epstein, W.L. (1974) Contact hypersensitivity to a perfume material, Costus absolute. *Archives of Dermatology*, 110, 871.

Mitchell, J.C. Fritig, B., Singh, B. & Towers, G.H.N. (1970) Allergic contact dermatitis from *Frullania* and Compositae. The role of sesquiterpene lactones. *Journal of Investigative Dermatology*, 54, 233.

Mitchell, J.C., Geissman, T.A., Dupuis, ·G. & Towers, G.N.H (1971b) Allergic contact dermatitis caused by *Artemisia* and *Chrysanthemum* species. The role of sesquiterpene lactones. *Journal of Investigative Dermatology*, 56, 98.

Mitchell, J.C. & Jordan, W.P. (1974) Allergic contact dermatitis from the radish, *Raphanus sativus*. *British Journal of Dermatology*, 91, 183.

Mitchell, J.C. & Lynne-Davies, G. (1974) Contact hypersensitivity to ragweed, *Ambrosia* and to turpentine. *Contact Dermatitis Newsletter*, 16, 505.

Mitchell, J.C. & Rook, A.J. (1976) *Scindapsus* dermatitis. *Contact Dermatitis*, 2, 125.

Mitchell, J.C. & Rook, A.J. (1977) Diagnosis of contact dermatitis from plants. *International Journal of Dermatology*, 16, 257.

Mitchell, J.C. and Rook, A.J. (1979) *Botanical Dermatology: Plants and Plant Products Injurious to the Skin*. Vancouver: Greengrass.

Mitchell, J.C., Roy, A.K. & Dupuis, G. (1971a) Allergic contact dermatitis from ragweed (*Ambrosia* species). The role of sesquiterpene lactones. *Archives of Dermatology*, **104**, 73.

Mitchell, J.C. & Shibata, S. (1969) Immunologic activity of some substances derived from lichenised fungi. *Journal of Investigative Dermatology*, **52**, 517.

Mobacken, H. (1975) Allergic plant dermatitis from *Scindapsus aureus*. *Contact Dermatitis*, **1**, 60.

Mobacken, H. & Fregert, S. (1975) Allergic contact dermatitis from cardamom. *Contact Dermatitis*, **1**, 175.

Möller, H. (1978) Phototoxicity of *Dictamnus alba*. *Contact Dermatitis*, **4**, 264.

Möslein, P (1963) Pflanzen als Kontakt-Allergene. *Berufsdermatosen*, **11**, 24.

Musajo, L., Caparole, G. & Rodghiero, G. (1954) Isolamento del bergaptene dal sedano e dal prezzemolo. *Gazetta Chimica Italiana*, **84**, 870.

Nastution, D., Klokke, A.H. & Nater, J.P. (1973) A survey of occupational dermatoses in Indonesia. *Berufsdermatosen*, **21**, 215.

Nater, J.P., de Jong, M.C.J.M., Baar, A.J.M. & Bleumink, E. (1977) Contact urticarial skin responses to cinnamaldehyde. *Contact Dermatitis*, **3**, 151.

Nestler, A. (1904) *Hautreisende Primeln*. Berlin: Bornträger.

O'Donovan, W.J. (1942) Dermatitis bullosa striata pratensis. Agrimony dermatitis. *British Journal of Dermatology*, **54**, 39.

Ogden, H.D. (1957) Diagnosis and treatment of *Parthenium* dermatitis. *Journal of the Louisiana Medical Society*, **109**, 378.

Orris, L. (1958) Cashew nut dermatitis. *New York State Journal of Medicine*, **58**, 2799.

Overton, S.G. (1926) Dermatitis from handling bulbs. *Lancet*, **2**, 1003.

Palmer, W.H. (1934) 'Lily rash': an occupational dermatitis, *Lancet*, **2**, 755.

Paschoud, von J-M (1965) Kontaktekzem durch Chrysanthemen. Gekreutze Ueberempfindlichkeitstreaktion mit Arnicatinktur. *Hautarzt*, **16**, 229.

Pasricha, J.S. and Guru, B. (1979) Preparation of an appropriate antigen extract for patch tests with garlic. *Archives of Dermatology*, **115**, 230.

Passenger, R.E. (1963) A clinical evaluation of the prophylactic treatment of poison ivy dermatitis with an alum-precipitated pyridine extract of *Rhus toxicodendron*. *Journal of Allergy*, **34**, 270.

Peck, J.M. Spolyar, L.W. & Mason, H.S. (1944) Dermatitis from carrots. *Archives of Dermatology*, **49**, 266.

Polunin, I. (1951) Pineapple dermatosis. *British Journal of Dermatology*, **63**, 441.

Polunin, O. (1969) *Flowers of Europe: A Field Guide*. London: Oxford University Press.

Porter, C.L. (1967) *Taxonomy of Flowering Plants*, 2nd Edn. San Francisco: Freeman.

Powell, R.F. and Smith, E.B. (1978) Tumbleweed dermatitis. *Archives of Dermatology*, **114**, 751.

Puglisi, V. (1951) Le dermatosi da limone. *Giornale Italiano di Dermatologie e Sifilogia*, **92**, 237.

Rao, P.V. Subba, Mangola, A., Towers, G.H.N. & Rodriguez, E. (1978) Immunological activity of parthenin and its diasteriomer in persons sensitised by *Parthenium hysterophorus* L. *Contact Dermatitis*, **4**, 199.

Ratner, J.H., Spencer, S.K. & Grainge, J.M. (1974) Cashew nut dermatitis: an example of internal-external contact-type hypersensitivity. *Archives of Dermatology*, **110**, 921.

Rinkel, H.J. & Balyeat, R.M. (1932) Occupational dermatitis due to lettuce. *Journal of the American Medical Association*, **98**, 137.

Rodriguez, E., Dillon, M.O., Mabry, T.J., Mitchell, J.C. & Towers, G.H.N. (1976) Dermatologically active sesquiterpene lactones in trichomes of *Parthenium hysterophorus* L. (Compositae). *Experientia*, **32**, 236.

Rodriguez, E., Epstein, W.L. & Mitchell, J.C. (1977) The role of sesquiterpene lactones in contact hypersensitivity to some North and South American species of feverfew (*Parthenium*-Compositae). *Contact Dermatitis*, **3**, 155.

Rodriguez, E. & Mitchell, J.C. (1977) Absence of contact hypersensitivity to some perfume materials derived from Compositae species. *Contact Dermatitis*, **3**, 168.

Roed-Petersen, J. (1975) Allergic contact hypersensitivity to ivy (*Hedera helix*). *Contact Dermatitis*, **1**, 57.

Roed-Petersen, J. & Hjorth, N. (1976) Compositae sensitivity among patients with contact dermatitis. Value of Compositae oleoresins in a standard test series. *Contact Dermatitis*, **2**, 271.

Rook, A. (1960) Plant dermatitis. *British Medical Journal*, **2**, 1771.

Rook, A. (1961a) Plant dermatitis—botanical aspects. *Transactions of the St. John's Hospital Dermatological Society*, **46**, 41.

Rook, A. (1961b) Plant dermatitis. The significance of variety-specific sensitizations. *British Journal of Dermatology*, **73**, 283.

Rook, A. (1962) Plant dermatitis in general practice. *Practitioner*, **188**, 627.

Rook, A. (1965) An unrecorded irritant plant *Synadenium grantii*. *British Journal of Dermatology*, **77**, 284.

Rook, A. (1968) Contact dermatitis caused by *Streptocarpus*, a popular greenhouse plant. *Contact Dermatitis Newsletter*, **3**, 52.

Rook, A. (1970a) *Alstroemeria* causing contact dermatitis in a florist also allergic to tulips. *Contact Dermatitis Newsletter*, **7**, 166.

Rook, A. (1970b) Contact dermatitis from *Humea elegans*. *Contact Dermatitis Newsletter*, **7**, 164.

Rook, A. (1977) Personal communication.

Rook, A. & Wilson, H.T.H. (1965) Primula dermatitis. *British Medical Journal*, **1**, 220.

Rostenberg, A. & Good, C.K. (1935) *Gaillardia* dermatitis. *Journal of the American Medican Association*, **104**, 1496.

Rovito, J. (1956) Non-specific therapy in allergy; a further report. *American Practitioner and Digest of Treatment*, **7**, 1447.

Rudzki, E & Dajek, Z. (1975) Dermatitis caused by buttercups (*Ranunculus*). *Contact Dermatitis*, **1**, 322.

Rudzki, E & Grzywa, Z. (1977) Dermatitis from *Arnica montana*. *Contact Dermatitis*, **3**, 281.

Rudzki, E., Zdzislawa, G. & Brud, W.S. (1976) Sensitivity to 35 essential oils. *Contact Dermatitis*, **2**, 196.

Saihan, E.M. and Harman, R.R.M. (1978) Coleus sensitivity in a gardener. *Contact Dermatitis*, **4**, 234.

Sams, W.M. (1940) Occupational dermatitis due to mint. *Archives of Dermatology*, **41**, 503.

Satulski, E.M. (1943) Dermatitis venenata caused by the Manzanillo tree. *Archives of Dermatology*, **47**, 36.

Satulski, E.M. & Wirts, C.A. (1943) Dermatitis venenata caused by the Manzanillo tree: further observations and report of 60 cases. *Archives of Dermatology*, **47**, 797.

Schiff, B.L. (1951) Contact dermatitis caused by bamboo. *Archives of Dermatology*, **64**, 66.

Schildknecht, H. (1957) Struktur des Primelgiftstoffes. *Zeitschrift fur Naturforschung*, **22b**, 36.

Schildknecht, H. (1964) Abwehrstoffe hoeherer Pflänzen. *Angewandte Chemie*, **76**, Supp, 112, 177.

Schemedekampf, van G., Schauder, S. and Berger, H. (1978) Aktinisches Retikuloid bei einem Blumenhändler. *Dermatosen in Beruf und Umwelt*, **26**, 95.

Schmidt, H. & Ølholm-Larsen, P (1977) Allergic contact dermatitis from croton (*Codiaeum*). *Contact Dermatitis*. **3**, 100.

Schreiber, M.M., Shapiro, S.I. & Berry, C.Z. (1971) Cactus granulomas of the skin: an allergic phenomenon. *Archives of Dermatology*, **104**, 374.

Schulz, K.H., Hausen, B.M. Wallhöfer, L. & Schmidt-Loffler, P. (1975) Chrysanthemen-Allergie. Experimentelle Untersuchungen zur Identifizierung der Allergene. *Archiv für Dermatoligische Forschung*, **251**, 235.

Schwartz, L. (1938) Cutaneous hazards in the citrus fruit industry. Brief history of citrus fruit in Florida and California. *Archives of Dermatology*, **37**, 631.

Sequeira, J.H. (1936) *Pyrethrum* dermatitis. *British Journal of Dermatology*, **48**, 473.

Schaffer, B. & Burgoon, C.F. (1951) Acute glomerulonephritis following administration of *Rhus* toxin: Report of a fatal case and near-fatal case. *Journal of the American Medical Association*, **146**, 1570.

Sertoli, A., Fabbri, P., Campolmi, P. & Panconesi, E. (1978) Allergic contact dermatitis to *Salvia officinalis*, *Inula viscosa* and *Conyza bonariensis*. *Contact Dermatitis*, **4**, 314.

Shanon, J. & Sagher, F. (1956) Sabra dermatitis. An occupational dermatitis due to prickly pear handling resembling scabies, *Archives of Dermatology*, **74**, 269.

Shelly, W.B. & Arthur, R.P. (1955) Studies on cowhage (*Mucuna pruriens*) and its pruritogenic protease mucunain. *Archives of Dermatology*, **72**, 399.

Shelmire, B. (1939) Contact dermatitis from weeds: patch testing with their oleoresins. *Journal of the American Medical Association*, **113**, 1085.

Shelmire, B (1940) Contact dermatitis from vegetation. Patch testing and treatment with plant oleoresins. *Southern Medical Journal*, **33**, 337.

Shelmire, B. (1941a) Cutaneous and systemic reactions observed during oral poison ivy therapy. *Journal of Allergy*, **12**, 252.

Shelmire, B. (1941b) The poison ivy plant and its oleoresin. *Journal of Investigative Dermatology*, **4**, 337.

Shelmire, B. (1941c) Hyposensitisation to poison ivy. *Archives of Dermatology*, **44**, 983.

Shelmire, B. & Black, J.H. (1937) A method of patch testing with plant oil. *Journal of the American Medical Association*, **108**, 719.

Singh, R. and Sharma, R.C. (1978) Contact dermatitis due to *Parthenium hysterophorus*. *Indian Journal of Medical Research*, **68**, 481.

Slob, A. (1973) Tulip allergens in *Alstroemeria* and some other Liliiflorae. *Phytochemistry*, **12**, 811.

Somner, R.G. & Jillson, O.F. (1967) Phytophotodermatitis (solar dermatitis from plants) gas plant and wild parsnip. *New England Journal of Medicine*, **276**, 1484.

Sowers, W.F., Weary, P.E., Collins, O.D. & Cawley, E.P. (1965) Ginkgo tree dermatitis. *Archives of Dermatology*, 91, 452.

Stampf, J.-L., Schlewer, G. and Benezra, C. (1978a) Animal and human sensitivity to α-methylene-ℨ-butyrolactone derivatives. *Contact Dermatitis*, 4, 306.

Stampf, J.-L., Schlewer, G., Ducombs, G., Foussereau, J. & Benezra, C. (1978) Allergic contact dermatitis due to sequiterpene lactones. *British Journal of Dermatology* 99, 163.

Stanton, D.L. & Wilson, J.W. (1971) *Rhus* dermatitis. An unusual case caused by atomized spray. *Cutis*, 8, 553.

Storrs, F.J., Mitchell, J.C. & Rasmussen, J.E. (1976) Contact hypersensitivity to liverwort and the Compositae family of plants. *Cutis*, 18, 681.

Strauss, H.W. (1931) Artificial sensitisation of infants to poison ivy. *Journal of Allergy*, 2, 137.

Suhonen, R. (1977) Phytophotodermatitis. An experimental study using the chamber method. *Contact Dermatitis*, 3, 127.

Sulzberger, M.B. (1936) Discussion. *Archives of Dermatology*, 34, 1055.

Sulzberger, M.B. & Wise, F. (1930) Ragweed dermatitis with sensitisation and desensitization phenomena. *Journal of the American Medical Association*, 94, 93.

Sutton, R.L. (1919) Ragweed dermatitis. *Journal of the American Medical Association*, 73, 1433.

Tada, H. & Takeda, K. (1971) Structure of the sesquiterpene lactone laurenobiolide. *Journal of the Chemical Society and Chemical Communications*, 1391.

Tafelkeuyer, J. & Van Ketel W.G. (1976) Sensitivity to *Codiaeum variegatum*. *Contact Dermatitis*, 2, 288.

Tuft, L. & Heck, V.M. (1952) Studies in atopic dermatitis IV. Importance of seasonal inhalant allergens, especially ragweed. *Journal of Allergy*, 23, 528.

Verhagen, A.R. & Nyaga, J.M. (1974) Contact dermatitis from *Tagetes minuta*. A new sensitising plant of the Compositae family. *Archives of Dermatology*, 110, 441.

Verhagen, A.R.H.B., Koten, J.W., Chaddah, V.K. & Patel, R.I. (1968) Skin disease in Kenya. *Archives of Dermatology*, 98, 577.

Vero, F. & Geneovese, S. (1941) Occupational dermatitis in cigar makers due to contact with tobacco leaves. *Archives of Dermatology*, 43, 257.

Verspyck Mijnssen, G.A.W. (1968) De pathogenese en aetiologie van de 'tulpen vinger'. Dissertatie. Noordhoff: Leiden-Groningen.

Verspyck Mijnssen, G.A.W. (1969) Pathogenesis and causative agent of 'Tulip Fingers'. *British Journal of Dermatology*, 81, 757.

Vickers, H.R. (1941) The carrot as a cause of dermatitis. *British Journal of Dermatology*, 53, 52.

Walsh, D. (1910) Plant dermatitis. *Lancet*, 2, 811.

Werff, P.T. van der (1959) Occupational diseases among workers in bulb industries. *Acta Allergologica*, XIV, 338.

Whiting, D.A. (1971) Plant dermatitis in the South Transvaal. *South African Medical Journal*, 45, 163.

Wilkinson, D.S. (1976) Quoted in Hjorth *et al.* (1976).

Williams, O., Spears, R. & Beggs, H.W. (1960) Hypersensitivity to marshelder. Difficulties encountered in patch testing. *Journal of the Louisiana State Medical Society*, 112, 216.

Willis, J.C. (1973) *A Dictionary of the Flowering Plants and Ferns*, 8th edn. London: Cambridge University Press.

Winer, L.H. & Zeilenga, R.H. (1955) Cactus granulomas of the skin. *Archives of Dermatology*, 49, 566.

Wiswell, J.G., Irwin, J.W., Guba, E.F., Rackemann, F.M. & Neri, L.L (1948) Contact dermatitis of celery farmers. *Journal of Allergy*, 19, 396.

Woods, B. (1962) Irritant plants. *Transactions of the St. John's Hospital Dermatological Society*, 48, 75.

Woods, B. & Calnan, C.D. (1976) Toxic woods. *British Journal of Dermatology*, 94, (Suppl. 13), 47.

11.

Woods

*J.N.S. Mitchell**

GENERAL CONSIDERATIONS
  Structure and ingredients
  clinical features
  irritant and allergenic constituents
  management of dermatitis
THE PLANT FAMILIES

Apocynaceae	Meliaceae
Betulaceae	Moraceae
Bignoniaceae	Naucleaceae
Burseraceae	Pinaceae
Combretaceae	Proteaceae
Cupressaceae	Rutaceae
Ebenaceae	Salicaceae
Fagaceae	Sapotaceae
Flindersiaceae	Sterculiaceae
Hernandiaceae	Taxaceae
Lauraceae	Thymelaeaceae
Leguminosae;	Ulmaceae
Caesalpinioideae	Verbenaceae
Mimosoideae	Lichens, liverworts and mosses
Papilionoideae	

In this chapter, the first section deals in outline with wood and the dermatitis
it produces, and the second discusses briefly the commoner species of tree, and
their woods, responsible for wood dermatitis. For convenience the species have
been grouped under their respective plant families, in alphabetical order. Only
the commonest synonyms for the woods have been given. In the interests of
brevity much detail and most controversy have been omitted, and the interested
reader is referred to Hausen (1973), Woods and Calnan (1976) and above all
Mitchell and Rook (1979) for more comprehensive accounts and lists of
references.

Wood dermatitis essentially complements plant dermatitis, and much of the
general discussion in Chapter 10 is relevant here. Tree nomenclature has been
just as confusing, but that of their woods is a further muddle for a timber with
several names can share some of them with other woods. Thus it may be
extremely difficult correctly to name a timber and the species from which it
originated. Cedar wood is a good example (Calnan, 1972).

In chemical complexity, the constituents of woods equal those of other plants

*Consultant Dermatologist, Western Infirmary, Glasgow.

(p. 463), and they share the tendency for irritant and allergenic compounds to vary seasonally, regionally and between specimens. Moreover, ignorance of the chemical basis of wood dermatitis is no less profound than is the case with plants; few allergens, for instance, have been isolated, and identified, from wood.

Latterly, the confused nomenclature has been put in order, and it should now be possible to give a botanically accurate account of wood dermatitis. (The inaccuracies in past reports are irremediable.) Unfortunately, as wood dermatitis is not common, phytochemical and clinical studies are unlikely to make rapid inroads into the ignorance about basic mechanisms.

Wood is of two types, hard and soft:

Hardwood contains three cell varieties:
 (i) *Vessels*, visible on cross-sections of the wood as rings, are for conduction.
 (ii) *Fibres* impart strength to the wood.
 (iii) *Parenchymal cells*, seen as medullary rays, are for storage.

Soft ('coniferous') wood has only two cell types:
 (i) *Tracheids* serve a double purpose, being equivalent to the vessels and fibres of hardwood.
 (ii) *Parenchymal cells*.

Living cells are confined to the outer wood, the *sapwood*, where the active processes of conduction of nutriment and fluid (sap), and the storage of assimilates, take place. Sapwood may also contain latex, mucilage and resins. It is pale, lacks durability and is of little commercial value.

After a limited life, the cells die, become lignified, and form part of the inner *heartwood*, which is strong, durable and darker and redder than the sapwood. As the cells die, they release their reserve compounds, which form chemicals such as tannins and dyes, while other substances including resins, gums, pigments and minerals accumulate. These give the heartwood its strength, resistance to fungi and other parasites, hardness, and individual colour and its irritancy.

The differing constituents and uses of soft- and hardwoods determine differences in their role in wood dermatitis. Thus the outer sapwood affects fellers and local timber workers predominantly, and most of the trouble is due to lichens on the bark, and to sap, latex and resins within the wood. To some extent these vary seasonally, geographically and even between specimens. Hardwood, on the other hand, causes dermatitis when powdered and disseminated in airborne fashion, so that those working the wood are at risk. These include carpenters and joiners who saw, plane, sandpaper or polish it. A novelty is the dermatitis in undertakers through working with chipboard (p. 887) from which, in the U.K. at least, all coffins are now made (Rook, 1977). Fellers, too, are affected by sawdust created in cutting trees down. The many types of work undertaken in forestry influence the occurrence and type of dermatitis among the workers; these were discussed by Suregar (1975) in a report on the study of an Indonesian timber company.

The chemicals responsible for reactions belong to the resins, gums, fat derivatives, alkaloids, dyes, tannins etc.; the principal allergens and irritants are outlined below.

Wood is harmful to skin in several ways: local trauma; irritant dermatitis; allergic contact dermatitis; contact urticaria; pigmentary changes. (The question of photosensitivity awaits an answer.) However, additives to the wood, parasites on the bark (e.g. lichens, caterpillars) and chemicals used with the wood account for more trouble than the wood itself.

Local trauma by splinters and thorns may be slow to heal (e.g. *Octoea*, p. 557) or cause chronic sepsis (e.g. *Pseudotsuga*, p. 566).

Irritant dermatitis can be caused by bark powders on some trees (e.g. *Acacia*, p. 558) by latex (e.g. Apocynaceae, p. 553) or sap (Moraceae, p. 563). Foresters and local timber workers are affected.

The clinical picture ranges from a mild dermatitis in the finger webs and corners of the mouth to a severe, even bullous reaction mainly on exposed skin, and often with mucosal inflammation. In foresters living rough, erosions and secondary infection are common.

Some woods (e.g. *Tectona*, p. 569) are both irritant and allergenic. They can provoke a wider spectrum of reactions and give misleading patch tests.

Allergic contact dermatitis is due mainly to sensitisers in the heartwood, although the latex in sapwood (e.g. Anacardiaceae, p. 475), and parasites (*Frullania*, p. 570) on the bark can contain potent allergens.

Clinically the dermatitis has an 'airborne' distribution, and affects those working the wood. Worst affected are exposed sites, but fine particle size, dense exposure, or light or scanty clothing facilitate wider involvement, especially of the sweaty body folds and genitalia.

Characteristically, there is a dermatitis on the backs of the hands and forearms, and on the face, lids and neck. Manual spread to the genitals is the rule, and in severe cases the axillae, groins, waist, ankles and dorsa of the feet are involved.

Mild reactions consist of an itchy erythema only, but in most cases papules and vesicles, and sometimes exudation, occur. With chronicity, there appear thickening, fissuring and lichenification, and although hardening can arise, it is usual for repeated exposure to provoke more rapid and severe reactions. Occasionally there are systemic illness with late-onset erythema multiforme-like eruptions (Holst, Kirby and Magnusson, 1976). Local reactions to contact with wooden articles (e.g. musical instruments, furniture, handles, bracelets) are much less common.

Only a few of the allergens responsible have been identified, and the chemical basis of cross-reactions is, in the main, obscure.

As an example of contact urticaria, reactions to *Triplochiton* are mentioned on page 568.

Mucosal inflammation, respiratory tract irritation, asthma and systemic toxicity can be extremely severe; they can eclipse the skin effects or occur on their own.

Paranasal sinus carcinoma appears to be an occupational hazard among woodworkers.

The irritant and sensitising wood chemicals include:

1. *Phenols*, especially catechols, account for some of the most potent allergens: e.g. pentadecylcatechol in Anacardiaceae (p. 476).
2. *Quinones* include suspected and well known sensitisers. Examples of the latter are: lapachols (Bignoniaceae, p. 553; *Tectona*, p. 569); dalbergiones (*Dalbergia*, p. 560); mansonia quinone (*Mansonia*, p. 568); and thymoquinone (*Calocedras*, p. 555).
3. *Saponins* irritate mucosae and broken skin (Sapotaceae, p. 567).
4. *Stilbenes* may be antigenic, e.g. chlorophorin (p. 564) and coniferyl benzoate (in Balsam of Peru).
5. *Terpenes* (Wilkinson, 1970) number many well-known sensitisers such as sesquiterpene lactones (p. 495) in *Frullania* (p. 570) and Δ-3-carene (*Pinus*, p. 565).

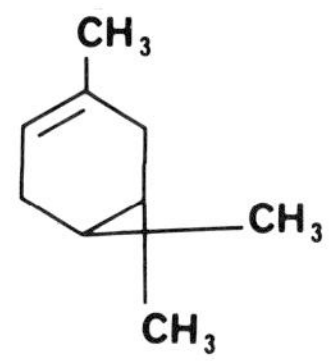

Δ-3-carene

6. *Miscellaneous allergens* include: oxyayanin (*Distemonanthus*, p. 558); β-thujaplicin (*Thuja*, p. 555); and anthothecol (*Khaya*, p. 562).

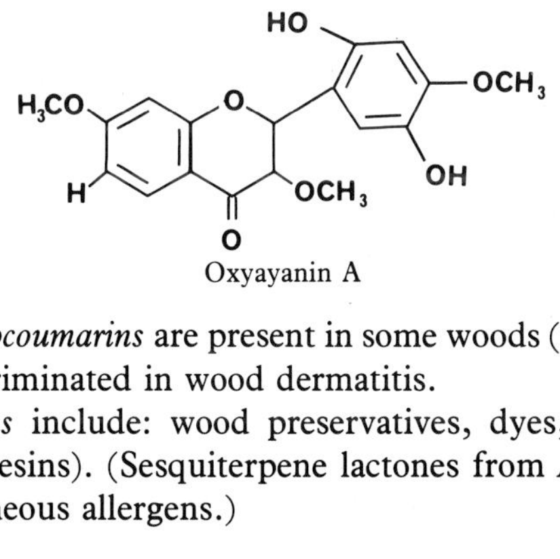

Oxyayanin A

7. *Photosensitising furocoumarins* are present in some woods (Rutaceae, p. 566), but have yet to be incriminated in wood dermatitis.
8. *Extraneous allergens* include: wood preservatives, dyes, varnishes and adhesives (e.g. epoxy resins). (Sesquiterpene lactones from *Frullania* on bark are, *sensu strictu*, extraneous allergens.)

The incidence of wood dermatitis is not known. It is uncommon, but Oleffe, Sporcq and Hublet (1975), from their study of the Belgian wood industry, thought it is probably underestimated. This seems likely for they found that 18 timbers were responsible, and Bleumink *et al.* (1973) listed 17 woods in a selection of those used in the Netherlands.

Management of wood dermatitis entails precise identification of the offending wood. If a specimen of the wood, with a note of its country of origin and its full trade name is sent to the Forest Product Research Laboratories, Institute of Forestry, or Botanical Gardens, they will willingly give invaluable help in identifying the species.

For *patch tests*, moist finely particulate sawdust should be used except for teak (p. 569) which is irritant when damp. Wood of unknown properties should also be tested on several control subjects.

Once a wood has been incriminated and identified, it may be possible to exclude it from the factory, or those sensitive to it may be able to avoid it. Sometimes, however, it is a valuable wood with no adequate substitute, and to allow its continued use, measures such as dust control, protective clothing and good washing facilities may meet with a certain amount of success. Nothing can be done about the random appearance of irritant timber as rogue specimens in a shipment of timber.

The principal genera and species of tree responsible for wood dermatitis are outlined in the following section. Table 11.1 lists the families of plants concerned, together with a representative species and its wood. The commonest causes of dermatitis are asterisked.

A brief discussion of lichens and liverworts, of major importance in woodcutter's eczema, completes the chapter.

Table 11.1. Plant families with tree species among the common causes of wood dermatitis

Family	Representative species	Wood
Apocynaceae	*Aspidosperma peroba*	[a]Peroba rosa
Betulaceae	*Alnus glutinosa*	Common alder
Bignoniaceae	*Paratecoma peroba*	[a]White peroba
	Tabebuia ipe	[a]Ipe
Burseraceae	*Acoumea klaineana*	Gaboon
Combretaceae	*Terminales superba*	Limba
Cupressaceae	*Thuja plicata*	Western red cedar
Ebenaceae	*Diospyros celebica*	[a]Macassar ebony
Fagaceae	see *Frullania* p. 570	
Flindersiaceae	*Chloroxylon swietenia*	[a]Ceylon satinwood
Hernandiaceae	*Hernandia sonora*	Toporite
Lauraceae	*Octoea barcellensis*	Louro
Leguminosae:		
Caesalpinioideae	*Distemonanthus benthamianus*	[a]Ayan
Mimosoideae	*Acacia melanoxylon*	Australian blackwood
Papilionoideae	*Brya ebenus*	[a]Cocus
	Dalbergia melanoxylon	[a]African blackwood
	D. retusa	[a]Cocobolo
Meliaceae	*Khaya anthotheca*	[a]African mahogany
	Swietena macrophylla	[a]American mahogany
Moraceae	*Chlorophora excelsa*	[a]Iroko
Naucleaceae	*Mitrogyna ciliata*	Abura
	Nauclea trillesii	Opepe
Pinaceae	*Pseudotsuga menziesii*	[a]Douglas fir
Proteaceae	*Grevillea robusta*	Grevillea
Rutaceae	*Fagara flava*	[a]W. Indian satinwood
Salicaceae	*Populus albus*	White poplar
Sapotaceae	*Tieghemella heckelii*	[a]Makoré
Sterculiaceae	*Mansonia altissima*	Mansonia
Taxaceae	*Taxus tabaca*	Yew
Thymelaeaceae	*Gonystylus bancanus*	[a]Ramin
Ulmaceae	*Ulmus procera*	English elm
Verbenaceae	*Tectona grandis*	[a]Teak

[a]Principal species responsible

The Anacardiaceae are of great importance dermatologically, but they are of no consequence as a source of timber. Even the attractive Malay wood, rengas (*Gluta renghas*; *Melanorrhoea* spp.), is scarcely exported as it is so toxic (Wilkinson, 1972). The family is discussed in detail in Chapter 10.

Apocynaceae

Several genera have species known to cause dermatitis, mainly because of their caustic sap or latex. Examples of irritant woods in commercial use are chanchito and ofurma (*Tabernaemontana* spp.) and alstonia (*Alstonia* spp.). There are others (Woods and Calnan, 1976), but their timber is little used.

Aspidosperma is the most noteworthy genus. *A. peroba* (peroba rosa) grows in Brazil and Argentina, where its wood, being fungus resistant, is highly prized. It is used in building, both indoors and out, especially for heavy duty such as floors and stairs. Its straight grain lends itself to turnery.

The sap and newly cut wood of this and some other *Aspidosperma* species cause mucosal irritation and malaise (Freise, 1937). If its sawdust contaminates damaged skin, local vesiculation and considerable systemic toxicity can result. Dermatitis and respiratory symptoms have also been reported in the trade among those processing the wood in the U.K. (Orsler, 1969). The completely dry wood, however, seems not to be toxic.

Betulaceae

Alnus glutinosa (Common alder), a species widespread in E. Europe and W. Asia, produces an easily worked wood suitable for plywood, furniture and turnery. It has caused dermatitis affecting the hands and face among those working it, with positive patch tests to the sawdust, wood (Fregert, 1974) and alder tannin (Brügel and Perutz, 1927): cross-reactions suggest that a catechol in the tannin may be an allergen.

Betula papyracea (Paper birch) produces an attractive wood, popular for veneers in furniture manufacture; it is grown expressly for this purpose in Finland.

A fine powder on the bark may cause dermatitis among workers in mills where paper birch logs are used.

Bignoniaceae

Paratecoma peroba (White peroba) has a golden brown wood, paler than other lapacho woods. It grows in Brazil and its wood, which resembles peroba rosa (see above), is hard, acid resistant, fairly strong and quite easily worked. It is used in moderate-duty construction work, and is a teak substitute.

Skin and mucosal irritation are well recognized hazards of handling white peroba in the trade. When powdered by sawing and sandpapering, it gets under the clothes onto covered skin such as groins or thighs, as well as onto exposed sites. The resultant dermatitis ranges in severity from an itchy erythema to a generalised exudative reaction (Touraine *et al.*, 1932). Sunlight may turn the skin yellow transiently. Some workers regard the splinters as poisonous.

Possible allergens in the wood are an unidentified alkaloid and several quinones including lapachol. Some cases have had positive patch tests to the sawdust and lapachonone (de Jong *et al.*, 1951).

Tabebuia spp. constitute most of the lapacho woods, so-called because of the lapachol and lapachonone they contain. The finely powdered wood irritates the skin and respiratory tract.

T. ipe (*T. avellanedae*) (Ipé) grows in northern S. America and yields a wood useful in building and for railway sleepers, furniture and turnery.

Within hours of skin contact, its fresh sawdust elicits and acute dermatitis. An initial erythema with papules leads to a fairly severe exudative reaction lasting several weeks (Freise, 1932, 1936). The dry wood, too, can cause dermatitis. Respiratory tract irritation by the dust is considerable, and systemic toxicity is common. In one case, but not in four controls, a patch test was positive (Cordero and Lynch, 1951).

T. palmeri (Amapa prieta) causes mild dermatitis.

T. serratifolia (Bethebara), a S. American species, gives a yellow-green to olive wood which is harder, more durable and weatherproof than the other species. Its uses include heavy construction work, sports equipment (e.g. fishing rods), and handles.

Making handles from the wood caused dermatitis on exposed sites, accompanied by rhinitis, in a patient described by Weitbrecht (1967). Patch testing failed to give conclusive evidence that desoxylapachol was the sensitiser.

Burseraceae

Acoumea klaineana (Gaboon: okoumé), of W. Africa, has a pale pink wood used for cigar boxes, inlays, veneers, plywood and sports boats; it is a mahogany substitute.

Working the wood is known to cause dermatitis and, more often, mucosal irritation.

Combretaceae

Terminalia superba (Limba) has a wood whose splinters are reported to cause chronicity and protracted suppuration of wounds. The sawdust is said to cause dermatitis (Hausen, 1970), contact urticaria and asthma (Oehling, 1963).

Cupressaceae

Of the half-dozen or so genera in this family with species known to cause dermatitis, the following are of some consequence:

Calocedrus decurrens (Incense cedar), from western N. America, yields wood which is used for pencils, when it can sensitise and produce dermatitis at sites of contact such as the hand or behind the ear (Calnan, 1972). This wood and virginian pencil cedar are officially recognised causes of dermatitis in the German pencil industry. In Calnan's cases, patch tests were positive to the pencil, 1 per cent thymoquinone and 1 per cent hydrothymoquinone. The latter are among several potential allergens, including thujaplicins and terpenes, in the wood, but as yet none is a proven sensitiser.

Fitzroya cupressoides (Alerce) has been little studied as a cause of wood dermatitis. A case in a woman employee at a wood factory was reported by Oleffe, Dedekin and Sporcq (1975).

Juniperus virginiana (Virginian pencil cedar) is an eastern N. American species whose wood is a recognised cause of dermatitis in the German pencil industry (see above).

Thuja occidentalis (White cedar) was reported half a century ago as a cause of hand eczema among men working the wood. It can irritate the respiratory tract in the absence of skin changes.

T. plicata (Western red cedar), indigenous to western N. America, produces a valuable commercial timber of considerable durability, and well suited to construction work. In the trade, the wood dust is a familiar cause of mucosal and skin irritation, and there are reports of its having caused asthma in Japan, the U.K. and Australia.

In one case of sensitivity to this wood, a sawyer reacted to patch tests with ɤ–thujaplicin, 7-hydroxy-4-isopropyltropolone and carvacrol, all of which are active allergens in the wood (Bleumink *et al.*, 1973). The patient also reacted to the irritant allergen thymoquinone, but so far as is known it is not present in *T. plicata*, although *Libocedrus* (*Calocedrus*) *decurrens* contains it.

T. standishii (Arbor vitae) timber, much used in Japan, has caused a considerable amount of trouble there. The fine dust from working the wood irritates the respiratory tract and can cause asthma.

Ebenaceae

Diospyros celebica (Macassar ebony), from Celebes and Molucca, has an impressively striped wood, in demand for high-class furniture and turnery for very decorative objects. It can cause a mild to severe and widespread dermatitis in those working it (Buschke and Joseph, 1927). Local reactions can occur under items such as bracelets made of it.

D. crassiflora (African ebony) is a W. African species whose wood is used for figures, handles and musical instruments.

D. ebenum (Ceylon ebony), native to India and Ceylon, is one of the few species with a black heartwood. This is popular for turnery, carpentry and, particularly, piano keys.

The allergens in these species may belong to the makassars and other naphthaquinones present in the heartwood (Hausen, 1970). In several species, the bark contains the highly vesicant quinone plumbagin.

Fagaceae

Castanea sativa (Sweet chestnut), *Fagus sylvatica* (Beech) and *Quercus robur* (Oak) are familiar trees of the countryside in temperate climates. They are associated with woodcutters' eczema (p. 569) which is caused mainly by lichens and liverworts on their bark.

Flindersiaceae

Chloroxylon swietenia (Ceylon satinwood), from India and especially Ceylon, has a silken-lustred wood, highly decorative in furniture, panelling and turnery.

Differences of opinion about the importance of the wood as a cause of dermatitis among those working it may well stem from lack of adequate identification of the 'satinwoods' incriminated; genuine satinwoods became increasingly rare.

Ceylon satinwood has caused outbreaks of dermatitis among cabinet makers (Jones, 1904). Possible allergens include chloroxylonine and the photosensitiser xanthoxin.

Flindersia spp. (e.g. Australian moah) have been held responsible for dermatitis among Australian woodworkers. One convincing case was in a cabinet maker who developed dermatitis on exposed skin through working with *F. brayleana* (Queensland maple) (McPherson, 1925): however, confirmatory patch testing was not carried out. The wide range of compounds found in the woods of these species has yet to be studied.

Hernandiaceae

Hernandia sonora (Toporite), once imported from Trinidad to the U.K. for use in joinery, is no longer used as it causes dermatitis. It contains podophyllotoxin and picropodophyllin.

Lauraceae

Several species of this family are of some dermatological importance (see also p. 517). In general, their wood is used in joinery and light construction work.

Cryptocarya pleurosperma (Poison walnut) contains the vesicant alkaloid crypto-pleurine which may have been responsible for the dermatitis elicited by handling cut bark or wood of the tree, described by Webb (1948). Starting on the hands, it spread to the face and genitals. Usage of this wood in Australia is considerable.

Laurus nobilis (Laurel; bay): see page 517.

Nectandra spp. are termed *Octoea* spp. by some botanists. Their woods can induce systemic toxicity, possibly due to their alkaloid content. The irritant bark oil of some S. Brazilian species produces intractable pyoderma in the finger webs and corners of the mouth.

Octoea rodiaei (Greenheart), from the W. Indies and northern S. America, has a wood so durable that it is eminently suited to marine use, as in waterways. Splinters cause chronicity in wounds, and its dust is a mucosal irritant.

Other S. American *Octoea spp.* yield wood called louro (e.g. *O. barcellensis*) or laurel (e.g. *O. puberula*) which can cause dermatitis, while the E. African cam-phorwood from *O. usamberensis* is known to irritate both skin and mucosae. Two definite cases of dermatitis caused by louro being worked as a veneer were seen at St John's Hospital (Woods and Calnan, 1976).

Phoebe porosa (Imbuya; Brazilian walnut) is a Brazilian species which has an eas-ily worked and polished wood that is aromatic and durable. Its unusually pretty graining secures its use as a luxury wood for furniture, panelling, parquetry, carving and the like. The sawdust not uncommonly irritates the upper respira-tory tract and, to a lesser extent, causes a vesicular dermatitis of variable severity (Schwartz, 1931).

Leguminosae: Caesalpinioideae

Species from some dozen genera of this family receive mention by Woods and Calnan (1976) as sources of dermatitis. The following are noteworthy:

Afzelia africana (Afzelia), from W. Africa, gives a dense durable wood compar-able with, and interchangeable with, iroko (p. 564). Locally, in Africa, it causes much nasal and skin irritation, but in the trade the exported wood causes more trouble in France than in the U.K. It contains catechins.

Apuleia molaris (Ferro; garapa; muiratana). Garapa, from Brazil, is valued for outdoor construction work as it resists micro-organisms. It is commoner than the Brazilian muiratana which some botanists consider is from the same species. The dark red, camphor-scented muiratana is used locally for veneers, inlays, chess boards etc. In the literature, the terminology of these and other S. American timbers has been much confused (Woods and Calnan, 1976).

The sawdust, even if the wood has been dry for years, causes systemic toxicity leading commonly to hypersensitivity. It can also elicit dermatitis of increasing severity due, possibly, to phellandrene, a saponin, and a couple of red dyes (Freise, 1936). Oxyayanin A, a known allergen, has been detected in this wood.

Cassia siamea (Tagayasan), from China and S.E. Asia, yields a general purpose wood. A yellow powder in cracks in the bark contains the irritant anthranol of chrysophenic acid. Japanese furniture workers have suffered eye inflammation, sometimes with dermatitis and violet staining of the skin, through working the wood.

Distemonanthus benthamianus (Ayan; Nigerian satinwood) wood is imported into Europe in modest amounts from W. Africa for use, *inter alia*, in house fittings and furniture.

Of twelve ayan sensitive patients seen at St John's Hospital (Woods and Calnan, 1976), eleven came from one factory shortly after this wood had been introduced as a veneer. Wood shavings and sawdust caused the dermatitis which could be quite severe and affected the arms, face, neck, lids, hands and sometimes the legs. In a case studied by Morgan and Thomson (1967), patch tests were positive to the sawdust and oxyayanins A and B. The latter may be principal allergens, with ayanin and distemonanthin minor ones. Specimens vary inversely in their content of oxyayanins and of distemonanthin, with consequent variability of allergenicity.

Melanoxylon brauna (Braúna) sawdust can produce pustules and a necrotising inflammation, especially on the legs at sites of minor skin trauma (Freise, 1932).

Peltogyne densiflora (Purpleheart) wood dust has caused asthma and urticaria in Brazilian workers engaged in polishing and working the wood. The heartwood contains the known sensitiser 4-methoxydalbergione.

(Other genera mentioned by Woods and Calnan (1976) were *Caesalpinia*, *Erythrophleum*, *Hymenaea*, *Haematoxylum*, *Koompassia* and *Zollernia*.)

Leguminosae: Mimosoideae

Several genera in this family have species known to irritate mucosae, but the following are significant causes of dermatitis:

Acacia melanoxylon (Australian blackwood) has a valuable all-purpose wood, used locally, not exported. It can cause quite a severe, even exudative, dermatitis, possibly allergic, on exposed skin of joiners and others working it (Cleland, 1925).

A. harpophylla (Brigalow) has a fine yellow bark powder which is probably the cause of 'brigalow itch' among men ringing the trees, although bag-moth shelters and coccoons may play a part (Cleland, 1925).

Other species, including *A. shirleyi* (Lancewood), can cause indolent splinter wounds. The cause of the dermatitis has not yet been found among the compounds isolated from *Acacia* spp. (Hausen, 1970).

Prosopis juliflora (Mesquite) has a general purpose wood, used only indigenously in southern U.S.A. and in Central America (Mexico). Exposure to the sawdust can cause dermatitis, with positive patch tests (Stewart, 1940). The wood contains an alkaloid but no allergen has been identified.

(Species which are irritant to mucosae belong to: *Albizia*, *Lysiloma*, *Piptadeniastrum* (*P. africanum* (Dahoma) is also a skin irritant), *Plathymenia*, *Samanea* and *Xylia*.)

Leguminosae: Papilionoideae

Many genera have species known to cause skin or mucosal irritation. A selection is presented in Table 11.2. Five are singled out for more detailed attention.

Table 11.2. More important toxic spp. of Leguminosae: Papilionoideae

Species	Wood	Irritant Skin	Irritant Mucosae	Systemic toxicity	Patch test pos.	Asthma	Troublesome splinters
Andira inermis	Angelim	√	√	√			
Bowdichia nitida	Sucupira	√			√		
Brya ebenus	Cocuswood	√					
Castanospermum australe	Black bean		√	√			
Dalbergia spp.	'Rosewood'	√	√	√	√	√	
Gossweilerodendron balsamiferum	Agba	√			√	√	
Machaerium spp.	Jacaranda	√			√		
Millettia laurentii	Wenge	√	√	√			
Pericopsis elata	Afrormosia	√	√	√	√	√	√
Pterocarpus spp.	Amboyna etc.	√	√	√		√	
Robina pseudoacacia	Robinia	Woodcutter's eczema					
Vatairea guianensis	Quassia wood	√	√				√
Vataireopsis araroba	Angelim amarello		√				√
Vouacapoua americana	Acapú	√					

Andira intermis (Angelim) grows in Trinidad, British Guyana and Brazil. The elegant striped markings in longitudinal section justify the common name, partridge wood. Once much in demand for shipbuilding, it now has a limited use in turnery and construction work.

The sawdust can cause dermatitis, urticaria and cough in those working with the wood. It contains the dalbergione-like demethylpterocarpin (see below), and biochanin A which resembles ayanin. The bark contains a poisonous alkaloid.

Brya ebenus (Cocuswood) is a West Indian species, growing especially in Jamaica and Cuba. The wood is very decorative and well suited to furniture making and for veneers, handles, pipes, jewel cases and so forth. It has been popular in flute-making. Being expensive, its market is limited.

The wood has caused dermatitis in musical instrument makers and players alike. Cocuswood flutes, for instance, have produced chronic dermatitis of the lips and chin among musicians playing them, but the subject has not been studied rigorously. The heartwood contains quinones, but no antigen has been identified.

Dalbergia spp. can be considered mostly as 'rosewood'; the following are the commoner causes of dermatitis:

D. cearensis(Kingwood; violet wood), a S. American species, produces wood used for inlays and marquetry. This was probably the wood reported by Freise (1932) as a severe irritant capable of often inducing intractable ulceration (Woods and Calnan, 1976).

D. latifolia and related spp. from Asia and Madagascar are known as Palissandre Asie. The wood of *D. latifolia* (Indian rosewood) comes from India and is used for veneers, furniture and musical instruments. It is almost interchangeable with palissandre, but is more porous.

The wood dust can cause dermatitis or urticaria with swellings in carpenters, and local reactions can occur under wearing-apparel, such as bracelets, made of the wood. It has also caused palmar eczema, spreading to the arms and lids, in a butcher whose knives had rosewood handles (Cronin and Calnan, 1975). R-4-Methoxydalbergione is one of several quinones in the heartwood.

D. melanoxylon (African blackwood). Ebony apart, this is the darkest wood in the trade. It comes from W. Africa and is used, for example, in clarinets and flutes. In the trade it is known to be irritant, and it has caused dermatitis in clarinet makers (Woods and Calnan, 1976).

Among the quinones produced by the wood are S-4'-hydroxy-4-methoxydalbergione and S-4-methoxydalbergione.

D. nigra and related spp. (Brazilian rosewood; Jacaranda; Palissander) is native to S. America, especially Brazil, and its wood finds uses in veneers, furniture, handles, necklaces, bracelets etc.

The sawdust has caused dermatitis and positive patch tests among forestry workers in Brazil (Freise, 1932), and among carpenters and cabinet makers working the wood. It also causes respiratory tract irritation and asthma. One of the quinones in the wood is R-4-methoxydalbergione.

Nowadays, as *D. nigra* is hard to come by, the even more troublesome *Machaerium scleroxylon* (see below) is used as a substitute.

D. retusa and related species (Cocobolo). The beautiful, hard, workable, resinous, golden cocuswood is of Central American origin and is in small but constant demand for items such as tableware, handles, sticks and the best flutes.

Well-known and much reported as a cause of dermatitis, cocobolo can also elicit mucosal and systemic reactions, even asthma. Most trouble is caused by fine wood dust from sawing, boring or sandpapering, while hot weather is an aggravating factor. The dermatitis affects the hands and face, then other exposed sites; sometimes it spreads widely. Reactions among those working cocobolo are not uncommon, 10–30 per cent in some firms (Record and Garrett, 1923). Local reaction can occur under articles such as handles, bracelets and musical instruments made of the wood (Levin, 1941; Leider and Schwartzfeld, 1950; Howell and Blair, 1950). Musical instruments, however, have been known to cause lid oedema and conjunctivitis of considerable severity, yet sparing the lips. In Germany, the use of cocobolo for recorders had to be discontinued as dermatitis of the mouth was so common.

Allergens in cocobolo include S-4'-hydroxy-4-methoxydalbergione and R-4-methoxydalbergione.

D. stevensonii (Honduras rosewood), from S. America, is used for handles and especially xylophones. It contains 4-methoxydalbergione (Hausen, 1970) and causes dermatitis in the trade.

The *allergens* in *Dalbergia* spp. woods are *quinones* of which R-3, 4-dimethoxydalbergione is the most potent. They have been studied by Eyton *et al.* (1965), and have been found in other genera—*Goniorrhachis, Machaerium* and *Peltogyne*. Examples are:

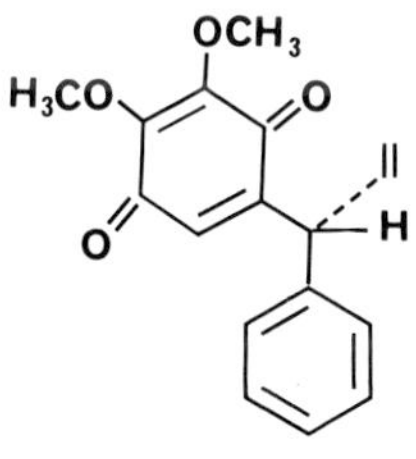

R-3,4-dimethoxydalbergione

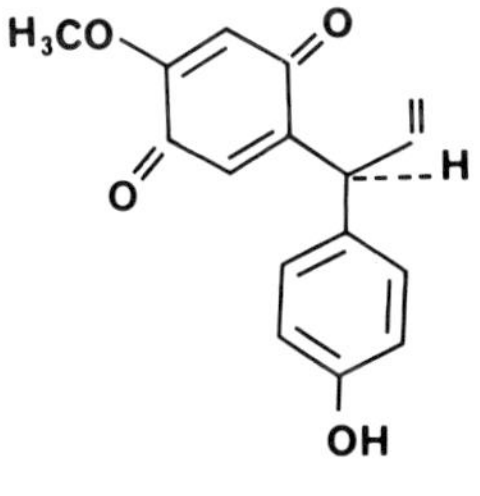

S-4'-hydroxy-4-methoxydalbergione

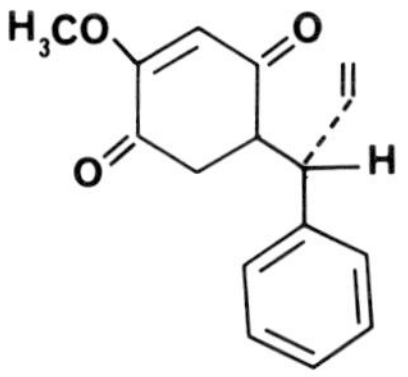

R-4-methoxydalbergione

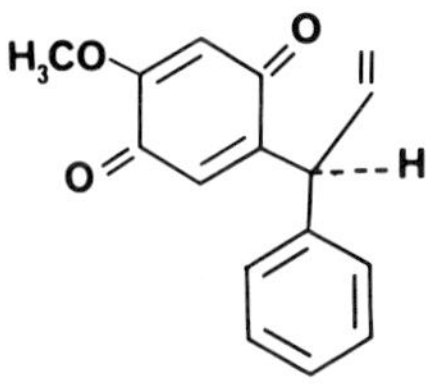

S-4-methoxydalbergione

Gossweilerodendron balsamiferum (Agba; tola branca) is a West and Central African species whose light-coloured wood is used for construction and joinery. It is known in the trade to be irritant (Orsler, 1969) but the incidence, relative to the widespread use of the wood, is probably low. Cases have been reported by Woods and Calnan (1976). The sawdust can also caused asthma.

Machaerium scleroxylon (Pao ferro) grows in Brazil, and its decorative wood is a palissandre substitute used for high-class veneers and furniture. However, it is more potently allergenic than the *Dalbergia nigra* it replaces, and it has caused a considerable amount of dermatitis in Brazil, the U.K. (Morgan *et al.*, 1968), and Germany (Hausen, 1970). In Morgan *et al.*'s (1968) series, the wood had caused dermatitis in one third of the men exposed to it in a furniture factory: patch tests with the sawdust were positive, and R-3,4-dimethoxydalbergione and its quinol were found to be the allergens. The latter are potent, and extracts in a concentration greater than 0.1 per cent can actively sensitise (Maibach, 1970).

Meliaceae

Many species yield valuable timber such as mahogany and cedar, and the following are representative of those that cause dermatitis:

Dysoxylum muelleri (Red bean), an Australian species, has a valuable red wood which is readily worked and polished. Its use is local and includes boat construction and wine casks. Notable for its potency as a systemic toxin, the sawdust can, like that of the related *D. rickii*, cause eczema.

Entandrophragma utile (Utile) from Africa and *E. cylindricum* (Sapele) are recognised irritants in the trade, and cases of allergic contact dermatitis due to them have been seen clinically (Woods and Calnan, 1976). Allowing for their extensive use, their toxicity is probably low.

Guarea spp. The Nigerian species are not only used more as timber than are the American species, but they cause more trouble and can elicit severe nasal and throat irritation. Furthermore, among the Nigerian species *G. thompsonii* is said to be more irritant to the skin and nose than is the related *G. cedrata* (Guarea).

In the trade, complaints of mucosal and skin irritation are common in England (Orsler, 1969), but infrequent in Nigeria.

Khaya spp. are known as African mahogany in the British Standard Nomenclature. They grow in tropical Africa and produce timber used in house and boat construction, furniture manufacture and veneers. Several have been incriminated in reactions to timber, but species identification is not easy.

K. anthotheca is probably the commonest sensitiser among the species (Morgan *et al.*, 1968), the principal allergen being anthothecol. The wood was responsible for a couple of outbreaks of dermatitis (associated with positive patch tests to the sawdust) in a furniture factory among those finishing the wood (Morgan and Wilkinson, 1965). In another outbreak, again with positive patch tests, the manufacturers mistakenly incriminated *K. ivorensis* (Wilkinson, 1968).

Anthothecol

Cross-reactions sometimes occur; thus positive patch tests to *K. anthotheca* sawdust occur in cases sensitive to *K. euryphylla*, but not to those sensitive to *K. ivorensis* (Wilkinson, 1971).

Whether or not *Khaya* spp. cause mucosal irritation or asthma is undecided.

Swietenia macrophylla (Honduras mahogany) and *S. mahogani* (Cuban mahogany) are both known as American mahogany. The former was first mentioned shortly after the discovery of America, and was soon used for shipbuilding in Spain. Later it became a fashionable wood in England, but the increasing demand outstripped the supply, so that it was gradually replaced by African mahogany. Very little is now exported to Europe: it is too expensive. *S. mahogani* is stronger, and was considered to be true mahogany. It, too, is scarcely exported, being too costly.

The role of *Swietenia* species' wood as causes of dermatitis seems to be a small if not an inconsequential one. Reactions are relatively mild and are sometimes associated with positive patch tests (Steiner and Schwartz, 1944).

Other species of minor importance are:

Amoora polystachya (Tasua) causes mucosal and skin irritation and toxic symptoms.

Lovoa klaineana (African walnut) produces nasal irritation, and dermatitis.

Toona sureni (Burma cedar) can cause skin irritation.

Turreanthus africanus (Avodiré) has been reported as a cause of dermatitis, with positive patch tests, in a cabinet maker (Calnan, 1970). This W. African wood is used in joinery, for plywood and as a substitute sycamore veneer in the cabinet trade.

Moraceae

Antiaris africana (Antiaris; Ako), of West and Central African origin, yields a dirty white to golden brown wood used for pit timber, containers and in construction work. It is exported in modest amounts to Europe.

The sawdust is a skin and mucosal irritant which affects the native Nigerian timber workers; the latex is highly irritant on broken or inflamed skin. *A. welwitschii* is a related species.

Chlorophora contains the most troublesome species.

C. excelsia and *C. regia* (Iroko; moule), from E. Africa, the Gold Coast and the Congo, provide a most important, durable, weatherproof wood, eminently suited to indoor and outdoor construction work, including joinery, boats (Wilkinson, 1969) and benches. Its termite-resistance is an added reason for its use as a teak substitute.

Workers sawing or planing the wood, especially in hot, humid weather, can develop dermatitis, sometimes with respiratory tract irritation. The dermatitis occurs in all degrees of severity, and outbreaks have been described in the U.K. (Davidson, 1941) and in Germany (Thinemann, 1941). The E. African wood can be troublesome if unseasoned, but tolerated when it is seasoned. Patch tests with the sawdust or an aqueous extract are positive in the sensitive.

The principal allergen is the oxystilbene, chlorophorin (Schulz, 1962):

$$HO \!-\!\! \underset{OH}{\bigodot} \!-\! CH = CH -\! \underset{OH}{\overset{OH}{\bigodot}} \!-\! CH_2\!-\!CH_2 = \underset{\underset{CH_3}{|}}{C}\!-\!CH_2\!-\!CH = C \!\!\begin{smallmatrix} CH_3 \\ \\ CH_3 \end{smallmatrix}$$

Chlorophorin

and this compound, 1 per cent in petrolatum, is satisfactory for a screening patch test.

Despite strenuous prophylactic measures, irritation by this much used wood remains a significant problem in the trade.

Ficus carica (Fig), and species, grow in Africa, India, Asia and S. America, where their elastic, porous wood is used locally for chests, frames, and occasionally furniture. The sap often irritates and may photosensitise (Behl and Captain, 1966).

Maclura pomifera (Osage orange), a N. American species, produces a solid but elastic and durable golden wood, used for veneers, turnery, carvings etc. Nowadays, its use is predominantly local. The sap is irritant and contains the chlorophorin-like tetrahdroxystilbene.

Piratinera guianensis (Snakewood; amourette) is native to northern S. America. The wood is so hard you cannot nail it. All parts of the tree, including the bark powder, are skin irritant, and working the wood results in systemic toxicity, mucosal irritation and dermatitis.

Naucleaceae

Mitragyna ciliata and *M. stipulosa* (Abura) are representative. They grow in W. Africa, and their wood is an easily worked alder substitute which is not weatherproof and is used for light construction work and turnery. The sawdust can be irritant, and reports from the trade in Nigeria, the U.K. and E. Germany indicate that it may cause dermatitis, mucosal irritation and vomiting. Woods and Calnan (1976) quoted a case of dermatitis with positive patch tests.

Nauclea trillesii (Opepe) produces W. African boxwood, a known cause of dermatitis and nasal irritation among the local Nigerian woodworkers; systemic symptoms may occur. The related *N. latifolia* may do the same.

Pinaceae

Abies alba (Silver fir) can cause dermatitis with positive patch tests to the resin in fellers.

A. balsamea (Balsam fir) has produced dermatitis and positive patch tests to the foliage in a florist.

A. grandis (Grand fir) bark and leaves have elicited positive patch tests in a lumberman with hand eczema.
    The incidence of dermatitis from 'unspecified' fir is unknown, but twelve cases were seen at the Finsen Institute, Denmark, over the period 1935–1963.

Cedrus deodora (Deodar) wood, sap and cones are skin irritants.

Larix decidua (European larch) sawdust causes contact urticaria. Larch is associated with woodcutter's eczema (p. 569).

Picea abies (European spruce) produces the most frequently used coniferous wood in W. Germany. It is used for non-weatherproof house construction — eaves, floors, etc. — and for furniture and musical instruments.
    Reports of dermatitis from working these woods are few, but it has arisen in the aircraft industry, and affected a musical instrument maker (Woods and Calnan, 1976). Sensitivity to balsam of spruce also occurs, and unexplained positive patch tests may well be even more frequent. Spruce is also a known cause of asthma.

Pinus spp., for example *P. sylvestris* (Scots pine) and *P. pinaster* (Maritime pine), are known to cause dermatitis among carpenters working them, and patch tests with sawdust and extracts of pine wood have been positive. Possible allergens are stilbenes such as pinosylvine, or balsam ingredients such as $\triangle$-3-carene or coniferyl benzoate. Pinewood foresters can develop woodcutter's eczema (p. 569).

P. radiata is grown extensively in S. Australia, though it is a N. American species. Its uses include boxes, fence posts and furniture. Those sensitive cross-react to colophony, and occult cases can be picked up among patients found to react to adhesive plaster. These have been studied by Burry (1976) who found a wide range of clinical patterns depending on the mode of exposure to the sawdust. Thus, fresh dust elicits acute reactions, but old dust, used for covering or cleaning floors or for packing, gives chronic, limited and milder responses.

Pseudotsuga menziesii (Douglas fir, Oregon pine), from N. America, gives a timber much in demand in Europe. It is a recognised cause of dermatitis, and in the trade it is prone to cause septic splinter wounds. Possible allergens are α-pinene, thunbergol and $\triangle$-3-carene.

Proteaceae

Grevillea robusta (Grevillea), an Australian species, is, however, exported mainly from East Africa. Bullous reactions can result from sawing the wood, and the sap is a recognised vesicant. Several species have vesicant phenols resembling those in Anacardiaceae plants (p. 476) (Ridley *et al.*, 1968).

Rutaceae

The species of dermatological interest either belong mainly to *Fagara* or are used as satinwood or boxwood substitutes.

Fagara flava (W. Indian satinwood; Espenille) grows in the W. Indies and Florida; it produces a golden-brown satinwood. The heartwood, when planed and polished, has an attractive, brilliant waxy surface, suitable for decorative fittings, turnery, marquetry, furniture etc.

The wood causes dermatitis in labourers in the W. Indies, and in carpenters; the latter are probably affected on a significant scale, but the relevant literature is botanically unreliable.

F. heitzii (Olon) and *F. macrophylla* (African satinwood; olonvogo), both African species, are very similar, but the latter has the harder wood. Off-white to straw-gold, the wood is homogeneous and decorative; not being waterproof, it is used for furniture, plywood and turnery.

Fine dust from dry olon is very irritant both to skin and to mucosae, and its bark is vesicant. Olonvogo and olon are known in the trade to be irritant. No allergen has so far been incriminated, but chloroxylonine is a possibility. The presence of coumarins in the wood suggests that photosensitisation might occur.

Satinwood and boxwood substitutes come from *Euxylophora paraensis* (Amarelo), *Esenbackia leiocarpa* (Guarantá), *Raputia magnifica* (Arapoca), *R. alba* (Arapoca branca) and *Balfourodendron riedelianum* (Guatambu). These are S. American species whose golden woods are solid, hard, durable and workable. All can cause dermatitis ranging from mild localised reactions on exposed sites, such as the finger webs, to severe widespread eruptions with gangrenous ulceration and systemic illness (Freise, 1936). The fresh sawdust particles are large and fail to penetrate clothing, so exposed sites are exclusively or predominantly affected.

Some of the woods contain toxic alkaloids, others the photosensitiser xanthotoxin.

Salicaceae

Populus spp. *Populus albus* (White poplar) is representative. Its bud resin can cause dermatitis, but whether sawdust also affects the skin is uncertain. However, poplar is one of the woods associated with woodcutter's eczema (p. 569), and as the liverwort allergen can soak into the wood, it can thereby elicit dermatitis indirectly.

Sapotaceae

Several species have irritant woods (Table 11.3), but only *Tieghemella heckelii* (Makore) justifies particular mention. The wood of this W. African species is light red and is much exported to Europe for furniture making, indoor and outdoor building, parquetry and stairs. It irritates mucosae and skin (Turc *et al.*, 1950), and cases of dermatitis due to it may have positive patch tests (Sandermann and Barghoorn, 1955). Its irritancy, well-known in the trade, has reduced its popularity. A saponin may be the active principle.

The related *T. africana* can cause severe respiratory tract irritation and haemoptysis.

Table 11.3. Principal irritant Sapotaceae woods.

Species	Wood	Effects
Autranella congolensis	Mukulungu	Mucosal irritation
Baillonella toxisperma	Moabi	? As Makoré q.v.
Calocarpum mammosum	Sapote	Caustic, vesicant sap
Chrysophyllum canito et spp.	Uajara	see *Manilkara*
Lucum spp.	Massaranduba	see *Manilkara*
Madhuca longifolia	Moah	Dermatitis from gummy bark juice
Manilkara bidentata	Balata rouge	Erythema, vesicles, painful skin swelling
Tieghemella heckelii	Makoré	Dermatitis and mucosal irritation

Sterculiaceae

Dermatitis has been said to be caused by several species in this family, but only two have been adequately documented.

Mansonia altissima (Mansonia), from Nigeria, has a red to violet-brown wood which is notoriously irritant. When powdered it almost invariably irritates the respiratory tract and sometimes elicits dermatitis with positive patch tests (Bourne, 1956). Skin irritation with a follicular eruption, but with negative patch tests, has also occurred.

The problem is sufficient to restrict the wood's use in veneers, parquetry and construction work. Among the quinones isolated from the heartwood, mansonia quinone has been identified as a sensitiser (Sandermann and Dietrichs, 1959).

Mansonone A

Triplochiton scleroxylon (Obeche) grows in W. Africa, and its pale wood is used on a limited scale for indoor construction and plywood as it is not weatherproof. It can cause contact urticaria and asthma (Oehling, 1963). One case of allergic contact dermatitis (due to an obeche lavatory seat), with a positive patch test, was reported by Wilkinson (1971).

Taxaceae

Taxus bacata (Yew) yields an extraordinarily valuable but increasingly scarce wood, useful in joinery, turnery and ideally for archery bows. As such it caused allergic contact dermatitis with a positive patch test in an archer.

The wood is also systemically toxic due to its alkaloids, and is a mucosal irritant due to its volatile oils.

Thymelaeaceae

Gonystylus bancanus (Ramin), from Borneo, is an oak substitute for veneers and construction work. There have been reports of skin irritation by bark fibres on logs, and a case of allergic contact dermatitis, with positive patch tests, caused by sawdust, was quoted by Woods and Calnan (1976). In the trade, the bark and sawdust are known to cause dermatitis and asthma.

Ulmaceae

Celtis brieyi (Diomia) is said to be a skin and mucosal irritant.

Ulmus procera et spp. (English elm) have an irritant hairy undersurface to their leaves.

Verbenaceae

Tectona grandis (Teak) yields one of the most outstanding and popular woods, but has one of the best known toxic timbers. It is native to the South East Asian mainland, especially Burma and Thailand. Being so stable and weatherproof and resistant to chemicals and parasites, it is one of the best woods for indoor and outdoor construction work, and is in demand for veneers in the furniture industry.

Dermatitis from working teak, often severe, is well-known (Hoffmann, 1926), contact urticaria and systemic effects less so (Schmidt, 1978). The sawdust is allergenic, but when damp it is also irritant. As this leads to false-positive patch tests, fresh native teak dust is the preferred test material (Krogh, 1962, 1964). In the furniture industry, adequate dust extraction is necessary to reduce the dermatitis problem from excessive to acceptable dimensions.

Resinous acids in the wood probably account for some of the irritation. Known sensitisers are lapachol and lapachonone, while there may be others, including tectoquinone. It is likely that desoxylapachol is the principal allergen (Schulz, 1962, 1967). The amount of this compound is variable in different specimens and its presence may be a function of the wood's quality.

Desoxylapachol

Vitex littoralis (New Zealand teak) splinters cause severe inflamation.

Lichens, liverworts and mosses

The bulk of occupational dermatitis among forestry workers, termed woodcutter's eczema, is due to contact hypersensitivity to allergens in liverworts and lichens.

Lichens comprise a fungus and an alga in symbiosis (Champion, 1971; Mitchell, 1965). The alga, usually green or blue-green, is generally unicellular or filamentous, and is active photosynthetically. It forms the lichen's medulla, but is penetrated to some extent by the fungus which constitutes a cortex. The tangle of fungus, usually ascomycetes, affords protection and provides minerals for the alga. It is the allergenic moiety.

Morphologically, lichens may be much branched and upright, but many are a single, flat, lobed leaf. The form is determined mostly by the fungus, but on bark the alga may predominate, giving a mucilaginous colony permeated by hyphae.

Lichens thrive in light and are found in woods especially when the trees are not in leaf. They are seen on the bark of deciduous or coniferous trees, even on dead wood, as orange, green, grey or yellow patches.

There are some 20 000 species in 400 or so genera, and they can be divided into three main classes. Common genera are: *Cladonia*, *Hypogymnia*, *Lecanora*, *Letharia*, *Parmelia* and *Usnea*.

Allergens produced by lichens include:

a. D-*Usnic acid*

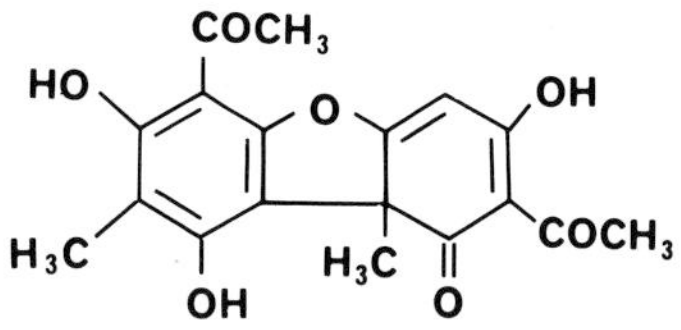

This shows stereoisomeric specificity (Mitchell and Shibata, 1969) and resembles furocoumarins (Mitchell, 1965).

b. *Depsides* e.g. atranorin, evernic acid, perlatolic acid.

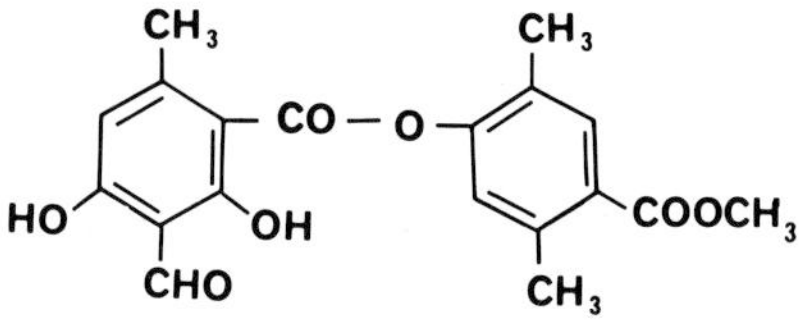

Atranorin

Some of these may photosensitise (Thune, 1977a,b).

There is no apparent correlation between hypersensitivity to these two groups of sensitisers.

Liverworts (*Hepaticae*) and mosses (*Musci*) are the two main groups of bryophytes.

Liverworts (e.g. *Frullania*) are rootless plants with stems and 'leaves', but as the latter have no veins they are not true leaves. Morphologically they are flat and lobed, or branch in a regular forking manner. They can be seen as small reddish or brown plants, compact and rope-like in appearance, growing often with mosses and lichens. They prefer moist, humid areas at low altitude, and are found in woods especially in Spring before the canopy is complete. Smooth barked trees, such as alder, oak, spruce, chestnut, beech and poplar are the preferred hosts. Sometimes the plants are invisible to the naked eye, when microscopical examination is necessary to show their presence (Foussereau *et al.*, 1975) as 1 mm leaves with turned edges. Commonly, however, they can be seen as dark patches.

Notable species include *Frullania nisquallensis* and *F. tamarisii*: a dozen were listed by Mitchell *et al.* (1970).

Allergens produced are sesquiterpene lactones (Connolly and Thornton, 1973), including L-and R-frullanolide (Foussereau *et al.*, 1975).

Frullanolide

Mosses can be tufted, cushion-like or mats, and are small. Moist areas are their preferred habitat and they tend to be abundant in wet winters in the forest. A representative species is *Isothecium spiculiferum*.

The gradual unravelling of the aetiology of *woodcutter's eczema* has been summarised by Woods and Calnan (1976). Milestones were the confirmation by Tenchio (1948) that lichens are involved, and the demonstration by LeCoulant and Lopès (1956a,b) that most cases in S.W. France are due to allergy to liverworts including *Frullania* [Jungermannales]. In their review of the subject, Le Coulant *et al.* (1966) showed the importance of liverworts among contact allergens in that part of the world. Similar conclusions were drawn by Mitchell *et al.* (1969) from their study of 'cedar poisoning' among lumbermen in British Columbia.

Overall, most cases seem to be due to sesquiterpene lactones in *Frullania*, but some are due to D-usnic acid, and to a lesser extent to depsides, in lichens. Moss allergy is rare. In a few instances, lichen allergy takes the form of contact exacerbation of atopic dermatitis (Champion, 1971). Foresters with dermatitis are as a rule allergic to *Frullania*, and only a few react to the wood or lichens alone; in fact, those who react to D-usnic acid are usually also sensitive to *Frullania* (Storrs, Mitchell and Rasmussen, 1976).

Clinically

a. *Frullania allergy* can cause a violent eczematous response (Foussereau *et al.*, 1975). It affects lumbermen, forest rangers, merchants in rough timber, truckers, sawyers and carpenters. Once the wood is debarked it is safe. The usual way that the liverwort elicits dermatitis is through close contact with the bark, but the allergen may be picked up from the undergrowth or through its volatilisation in hot weather.

The incubation period is measured in weeks to years. Exposed skin is the site of predilection — the face, neck, hands and arms; the skin under the chin may be spared, but eyelid involvement is the rule. Severe sensitivity can lead to generalised spread. There is more trouble in wet winters, and this is in direct contrast to Compositae plant allergy.

In patch testing (Mitchell *et al.*, 1970) no single allergen suffices as a screening test substance. It is best to test with small pieces (to avoid pressure reactions) of the whole plant, taking a specimen from the patient's own environment. The sample need not be bruised; in fact, reactions can be severe even if the test is applied for only 80 minutes.

Great care is needed in making the diagnosis as cross-reactions with Compositaè plants (Storrs *et al.*, 1976) and *Laurus nobilis* (Foussereau *et al.*, 1975) are common. These are complex and unique to the individual.

Once sensitive to *Frullania*, patients can stay in their employment only if they handle bark-free wood exclusively. They must also be warned about cross-reactions to Compositae plants such as chrysanthemums and 'daisy'-like weeds. The value of hyposensitisation is less than dubious.

b. *Lichen allergy* can affect foresters, and those carrying firewood or coming into contact with the allergens in wood ash, decorations and wreaths. Another presentation is an immediate-type of flare up of atopic dermatitis in children through their climbing lichen-covered apple trees; these children have positive prick tests to lichens (Rook, 1977). Indirect contact from handling contaminated clothes has been detected by Champion (1965). The problem seems to be greater in cold wet weather when usnic acid production may be greater.

Recurrent acute episodes or a chronic dermatitis can occur. Sites affected are predominantly on exposed skin — the face, neck, hands and forearms — but the genitals and the waist are often involved. Light sensitivity seems to be important, as all of Thune's (1977a) cases were light-sensitive and gave abnormal responses when tested with long wave ultraviolet light. Moreover, when he studied ten patients suffering apparently from photodermatitis he found that all were contact hypersensitive to lichens, possibly to their depsides (Thune, 1977b).

The skin reaction tends to resemble 'dermal sensitivity' i.e. an indurated dermatitis with scanty vesicle or bulla formation; however, the histological appearances are eczematous (Mitchell *et al.*, 1970).

Patients with an atopic sensitivity who come into contact with lichens may develop intense pruritus followed sometimes by long-lasting weals, especially in 'atopic sites'.

Patch tests: D-usnic acid and atranorin, each 1 per cent in petrolatum, are satisfactory (Mitchell, 1970); tests with the whole lichen are also recommended.

c. *Moss* (*Isothecium spiculiferum*) was first described as a cause of dermatitis by Robertson and Mitchell (1967). The reaction in their patient lacked vesiculation and resembled a response to lichens.

References

Behl, P.N. & Captain, R.M. (1966) *Skin-irritant and Sensitising Plants found in India*. New Delhi: Behl.

Bleumink, E., Mitchell, J.C. & Nater, J.P. (1973) Allergic contact dermatitis from cedarwood (*Thuja plicata*). *British Journal of Dermatology*, 88, 499.

Bourne, L.B. (1956) Dermatitis from Mansonia wood. *British Journal of Industrial Medicine*, 13, 55.

Brügel, S. & Perutz, A. (1927) Über Klinik und Pathogene der Erlenholz-dermatitis. *Archiv für Dermatologie und Syphilis*, 153, 661.

Burry, J.N. (1976) Contact dermatitis from radiata pine. *Contact Dermatitis*, 2, 262.

Buschke, A. & Joseph, A. (1927) Über Hautentzündung hervorgerufen durch Makassarholz. *Deutsche medizinische Wochenschrift*, 53, 1641.

Calnan, C.D. (1970) Avodiré wood sensitivity. *Contact Dermatitis Newsletter*, **8**, 190.

Calnan, C.D. (1972) Dermatitis from cedar wood pencils. *Transactions of the St John's Hospital Dermatological Society*, **58**, 43.

Champion, R.H. (1965) Wood-cutter's disease: contact sensitivity to lichens. *British Journal of Dermatology*, **77**, 285.

Champion, R.H. (1971) Atopic sensitivity to algae and lichens. *British Journal of Dermatology*, **85**, 551.

Cleland, J.B. (1925) Plants, including fungi, poisonous or otherwise injurious to man in Australia. *Medical Journal of Australia*, **2**, 443.

Connolly, J.D. & Thornton, I.M.S. (1973) Sesquiterpene lactones from the liverwort *Frullania tamarisii*. *Phytochemistry*, **12**, 631.

Cordero, A & Lynch, H. (1951) Sensibilizacion profesional al aserrin de Lapacho. *Prensa Medica Argentinia*, **38**, 838.

Cronin, E. & Calnan, C.D. (1975) Rosewood knife handle. *Contact Dermatitis*, **1**, 120.

Davidson, J.M. (1941) Toxic effects of Iroko, an African wood. *Lancet*, **1**, 38.

Eyton, W.B. Ollis, W.D., Sutherland, I.O., Gottlieb, O.R., Magalhaes, M.T. & Jackman, L.M. (1965) The Neoflavanoid group of natural products I-III. *Tetrahedron*, **31**, 2683.

Foussereau, J., Muller, J.C. & Benezra, C. (1975) Contact allergy to *Frullania* and *Laurus nobilis*: cross-sensitisation and chemical structure of the allergens. *Contact Dermatitis*, **1**, 223.

Fregert, S. (1974) Allergic contact dermatitis from alder (*Alnus glutinosa*). *Contact Dermatitis Newsletter*, **15**, 457.

Freise, F.W. (1932) Gesundheitsschädigungen durch Arbeiten mit giftigen Hölzern. Beobachtungen aus Brasilianischen Gewerbebetrieben. *Archiv für Gewerbepathologie und Gewerbehygiene*, **3**, 1.

Freise, F.W. (1936) Vergiftungen durch Brasilianische Werkhölzer, I, II. *Sammlung der Vergiftungsfällen*, **7C**, 1 and 61.

Freise, F.W. (1937) Vergiftungen durch Brasilianische Werkhölzer III. *Sammlung der Vergiftungsfällen*, **8C**, 13.

Hausen, B.M. (1970) Untersuchungen über gesundheitsschädigende Hölzer. Thesis, Hamburg.

Hausen, B.M. (1973) *Hozarten mit gesundheitsschädigenden Inhaltstoffen*. Stuttgart: DRW-verlags-Gmbh.

Hoffmann, H. (1926) Über Hautentzündungen nach teakholzarbeitung. *Zentralblatt für Gewerbehygiene*, **NF3**, 333.

Holst, R., Kirby, J. & Magnusson, B. (1976) Sensitisation to tropical woods giving erythema multiforme-like eruptions. *Contact Dermatitis*, **2**, 295.

Howell, J.B. & Blair, D.S. (1950) Eczema of the hands from wooden-handled objects. *Archives of Dermatology and Syphilology*, **62**, 400.

Jones, H.E. (1904) Acute dermatitis produced by satinwood irritation. *British Medical Journal*, **1**, 1484.

Jong, J.C. de, Lenstra, J.B. & Vermeer, J.H. (1951) Eczema due to the wood of Peroba da campos; isolation of the allergen. *Acta Dermato-venereologica*, **31**, 108.

Krogh, H.K. (1962) Contact eczema caused by true teak (*Tectona grandis*). *British Journal of Industrial Medicine*, **19**, 42.

Krogh, H.K. (1964) Contact eczema caused by true teak. *British Journal of Industrial Medicine*, **21**, 65.

Le Coulant, M.P. & Lopes, G. (1956a) A propos des dermites des bois. *Journal médicale de Bordeaux*, **133**, 245.

Le Coulant, M.P. & Lopès, G. (1956b) A propos des dermites auxsciures de bois. *Bulletin de la Societé francaise de Dermatologie et de Syphiligraphie*, **63**, 80.

Le Coulant, M.P. Texier, L., Maleville, J., Géniaux, M., Tamisier, J.-M. & Bancons, F. (1966) L'allergie au frullania: son rôle dans la'dermite du bois de chene. *Bulletin de la Societé francaise de Dermatologie et de Syphiligraphie*, **73**, 440.

Leider, M. & Schwartzfeld, H.K. (1950) Allergic eczematous contact type dermatitis caused by cocobolo wood (*Dalbergia*). *Archives of Dermatology and Syphilology*, **62**, 125.

Levin, S.J. (1941) Cocobolo wood dermatitis. *Journal of Allergy*, **12**, 498.

MacPherson, J. (1925) Dermatitis caused by Queensland Maple. *Medical Journal of Australia*, **2**, 542.

Maibach, H.I. (1970) Active sensitisation to wood extracts. *Contact Dermatitis Newsletter*, **7**, 149.

Mitchell, J.C. (1965) Allergy to lichens. *Archives of Dermatology*, **92**, 142.

Mitchell, J.C. (1970) Patch test results. *Contact Dermatitis Newsletter*, **8**, 177.

Mitchell, J.C., Fritig, B. Singh, B. & Towers, G.H.N. (1970) Allergic contact dermatitis from *Frullania* and Compositae. *Journal of Investigative Dermatology*, **54**, 233.

Mitchell, J.C. and Rook, A.J. (1979) *Botanical Dermatology: Plants and Plant Products Injurious to the Skin*. Vancouver: Greengrass.

Mitchell, J.C. Schofield, W.B., Singh, B. & Towers, G.H.N. (1969) Allergy to *Frullania*. *Archives of Dermatology*, **100**, 46.

Mitchell, J.C. & Shibata, S. (1969) Immunologic activity of some substances derived from lichen-ised fungi. *Journal of Investigative Dermatology*, **52**, 517.

Morgan, J.W.W., Orsler, R.J. & Wilkinson, D.S. (1968) Dermatitis due to the wood dusts of *Khaya anthotheca* and *Machaerium scleroxylon*. *British Journal of Industrial Medicine*, **25**, 119.

Morgan, J.W.W. & Thomson, J. (1967) Ayan dermatitis. *British Journal of Industrial Medicine*, **24**, 156.

Morgan, J.W.W. & Wilkinson, D.S. (1965) Sensitisation to *Khaya anthotheca*. *Nature*, **207**, 1101.

Oehling, A. (1963) Berufsallergie im Holzgewerbe. *Allergie und Asthma*, **9**, 312.

Oleffe, J.A. Dedekin, H. & Sporcq, J. (1975) Occupational dermatitis from alerce (*Fitzroya cupres-soides*). *Contact Dermatitis*, **1**, 319.

Oleffe, J.A., Sporcq, J. & Hublet, P. (1975) Epidemiological study of the wood industry in Belgium. *Contact Dermatitis*, **1**, 315.

Orsler, R.J. (1969) Timberlab Papers no. 11: The Effects of Irritant Timbers. Princes Risborough: Forest Products Research Laboratory.

Record S.J. & Garratt, G.A. (1923) Cocobolo. Bulletin no. 8. New Haven: *Yale University School of Forestry*.

Ridley, D.D., Ritchie, E & Taylor, W.C. (1968) Some further constituents of *Grevillea robusta* A. Cunn. *Australian Journal of Chemistry*, **21**, 2979.

Robertson, W.D. & Mitchell, J.C. (1967) Allergic contact and photodermatitis. *Canadian Medical Association Journal*, **97**, 380.

Rook, A.J. (1977) Personal communication.

Sandermann, W. & Barghoorn, A.-W. (1955) Über die Inhaltsstoffe von Makoré—und Peroba—Holz sowie ihre gesundheitsschädigende Wirkung. *Holzforschung*, **9**, 112.

Sandermann, W. & Dietrichs, H.H. (1959) Über die Inhaltsstoffe von *Mansonia altissima* und ihre gesundheitsschadigende Wirkung. *Holz als Rohund Werkstoffe*, **17**, 88.

Schmidt, H. (1978) Contact urticaria to teak with systemic effects. *Contact Dermatitis*, **4**, 176.

Schulz, K.H. (1962) Untersuchungen über die sensibilisierende Wirkung von Inhaltsstoffen Hölzer. *Berufsdermatosen*, **10**, 17.

Schulz, K.H. (1967) Berufsdermatosen—ausgewählte Kapitel. *Zeitschrift für Hautund Geschlechtskrankheiten*, **42**, 499.

Schwartz, L. (1931) Dermatitis due to contact with Brazilian walnut wood. *Public Health Reports (Washington)*, **46**, 1938.

Steiner, S.D. & Schwartz, L. (1944) Dermatitis from mahogany wood (*Swietenia macrophylla*). *Industrial Medicine*, **13**, 234.

Stewart, C. (1940) Dermatitis due to Mesquite wood. *Archives of Dermatology and Syphilology*, **42**, 937.

Storrs, T., Mitchell, J.C. & Rasmussen, J.E. (1976) Contact hypersensitivity to liverworts and the Compositae family of plants. *Cutis*, **18**, 681.

Suregar, R.S. (1975) Occupational dermatoses among foresters. *Contact Dermatitis*, **1**, 33.

Tenchio, F. (1948) Etiologie de l'eczéma des bûcherons. *Dermatologica*, **97**, 72.

Thienemann, K. (1941) Kambala-Teakholz-Dermatosen. *Archiv für Dermatologie und Syphilis*, **182**, 551.

Thune, P. (1977a) Allergy to lichens with photosensitivity. *Contact Dermatitis*, **3**, 213.

Thune, P. (1977b) Contact allergy to lichens in patients with a history of photosensitivity. *Contact Dermatitis*, **3**, 267.

Touraine, A, Hesse, J. & Golé, L. (1932) Vingt cas de dermatite par bois satiné ('Peroba grande amarella'). *Bulletin de la Societé francaise de Dermatologie et de Syphiligraphie*, **39**, 1392.

Turc, H., Brunel, R. & Tolot, F. (1950) Accidents allergiques dus aus bois de Makoré. *Archives des Maladies Professionelles*, **11**, 490.

Webb, L.J. (1948) The blistering alkaloid in 'poison walnut' (*Cryptocarya pleurosperma* Wh. and Fr.). *CSIR Forest Products Newsletter* no. **169**.

Weitbrecht, U. (1967) Allergie gegen Bethabara-Holz. *Berufsdermatosen*, **15**, 183.

Wilkinson, D.S. (1968) Khaya woods. *Contact Dermatitis Newsletters*, **3**, 44.

Wilkinson, D.S. (1969) Sensitivity to Iroko wood in a boat builder. *Contact Dermatitis Newsletter*, **6**, 142.

Wilkinson, D.S. (1970) Terpenes. *Contact Dermatitis Newsletter*, **8**, 183.

Wilkinson, D.S. (1971) Tests with different species of khaya woods. *Contact Dermatitis Newsletter*, **9**, 216.

Wilkinson, D.S. (1972) Renghas—a crosswood problem. *Contact Dermatitis Newsletter*, **11**, 262.

Woods, B. & Calnan, C.D. (1976) Toxic Woods. *British Journal of Dermatology*, **94**, (Suppl. 13).

12.

Plastics

MONOMERS WHICH SENSITISE
  Acrylic
  Epoxy
  Formaldehyde
RESIN SYSTEM WHICH CAUSES
DERMATITIS
  Polyester — unsaturated
  Allyl (Diallylglycol carbonate)
RESIN SYSTEMS WHICH RARELY
CAUSE DERMATITIS
  Polyester — saturated (Alkyd)
  Polyurethane

MONOMERS NON-ALLERGIC BUT
SENSITISING ADDITIVES
  Cellulose acetate
  Vinyl polymers
  Polyvinyl chloride
  Polyvinyl acetate
  Vinyl carbazole
  Vinyl pyridine
  Polyvinylidene chloride
OTHER POLYMERS
  Polystyrene
  Polyolefins
  Polyamides
  Fluoropolymers

MONOMERS WHICH SENSITISE

Acrylic polymers

Acrylic resins are based on a series of related compounds:

  Acrylic acid and its esters
  Methacrylic acid and its esters
  Cyanoacrylic acid and its esters
  Acrylonitrile
  Acrylamide

The monomers of these resins, and the additives used in their manufacture, are potential allergens and can sensitise workers in contact with them in industry, and the consumer handling the finished products.

ACRYLATES

$$CH_2 = CH - COOH$$

Acrylic acid

$$CH_2 = \overset{\overset{\textstyle CH_3}{|}}{C} - COOH$$

Methacrylic acid

Acrylic acid and its esters are more toxic than methacrylic acid and its derivatives, and acrylic acid is irritant and corrosive on the skin. During its manufacture, nickel bromide may be used as a catalyst and nickel carbonyl as a source of carbon monoxide.

Acrylic acid polymerises readily, but may do so with explosive force. The acrylate polymers are made as emulsions, which readily spread over surfaces and dry to form films, and, in their production, ammonium persulphate is frequently used as the catalyst. These polymers, being flexible and transparent, have a wide application as surface coatings such as leather coatings, paints, adhesives, in paper manufacture and some forms of printing. Acrylate polymers are rather soft, and to harden them methacrylates may be added.

Methyl acrylate — textile size, leather finish
Polymers of methyl acrylate, being susceptible to cold and water, are used only as a textile size and leather finish.

Ethyl and butyl acrylate — synthetic rubber
Although ethyl and butyl acrylates cross-link to produce a rubber, the product is soft and ages rapidly. However, acrylates used as copolymers form a rubber which is resistant to heat, ageing and oils, and is readily vulcanised by triethylenetetramine. Such rubbers, especially those derived from ethyl acrylate, are used for seals and gaskets in the motor industry.

Butyl, octyl and nonyl acrylates
These esters are used as leather finishes.

Causes of dermatitis

Adhesive tape Ethylhexyl acrylate

2-Ethylhexyl acrylate   N-*tert*-Butyl maleamic acid

Several adhesive tapes are composed of a plastic film and an acrylate adhesive. During predictive testing, Jordan (1975) found that seven volunteers reacted to one acrylic tape (Curad, Kendall Company, Chicago) but remained tolerant of another (Dermicel Hypoallergenic Cloth Tape, Johnson & Johnson, New Brunswick, New Jersey). All were sensitive to 2-ethylhexyl acrylate, and three to N-*tert*-butyl maleamic acid. These compounds were considered to be no more allergenic than other constituents of the adhesive, but their monomers, being less volatile, are more likely to remain after the curing process.

Patch tests: each man was tested with the four constituents of the adhesive and with methyl methacrylate:

	2-ethylhexyl acrylate (5% in olive oil)	N-tert-butyl maleamic acid (1% in petrolatum)	acrylo-nitrile (5% in olive oil)	ethyl acrylate (5% in olive oil)	methyl methacrylate (20% in olive oil)
Positive	7	3	0	0	0
Negative	0	4	7	7	7

In a further series of patch tests no evidence was found that acrylates and methacrylates cross-react. Some of the acrylates at 5 per cent in olive oil appeared to have caused active sensitisation.

Spectacle frames Butyl acrylate
A woman with dermatitis from the plastic nose pads of her spectacle frames was found on patch testing to react to butyl acrylate 1 per cent (olive oil) but not to ethyl or methyl acrylate. A spectacle manafacturer confirmed that such acrylates might be present in acrylic frames. (Hambly and Wilkinson, 1978).

Bonding agent Ammonium acrylate
Four women developed irritation of their hands, arms and eyelids while working in the trim shop of the car body section of a motor company. This was attributed to a bonding adhesive used to coat the hardboard door panels. The adhesive was a PVC emulsion containing an ethyl acrylate copolymer and ammonium acrylate as a thickening agent. After methyl cellulose had been substituted as the thickening agent and the dust in the job reduced, no further cases of dermatitis were seen. Patch test were not done (Routledge, 1971).

Diacrylates — Delayed Irritation
Butanediol diacrylate, present as a cross-linking agent in an unsaturated polyester paint used to coat doors by electron beam, caused a delayed type of irritant dermatitis in about one third of the workers exposed. Hexanediol diacrylate has the same effect. Characteristic was a latent period of 12–24 hours, circumscribed lesions and severe contamination caused bullae which ached rather than itched. Preventative measures solved the problem (Malten, den Arend and Wiggers, 1979).

MONOMETHACRYLATES

$$CH_2 = \overset{\overset{\displaystyle CH_3}{|}}{C} - COOH \qquad CH_2 = \overset{\overset{\displaystyle CH_3}{|}}{C} - COOCH_3 \qquad CH_2 = \overset{\overset{\displaystyle CH_3}{|}}{C} - COOC_2H_5$$

Methacrylic acid   Methyl methacrylate   Ethyl methacrylate

The majority of acrylic plastics are made from esters of methacrylic acid, predominantly methyl methacrylate. Varying the technique of polymerisation alters the length and molecular weight of the resin chain and the physical properties of the plastic produced.

Methyl methacrylate

Methyl methacrylate polymers are clear, colourless, rigid resins, which transmit light without heating and have good weathering properties. The monomer is stable if air and light are excluded or if an inhibitor is added. Polymerisation is initiated by heat, ultraviolet light, oxygen or peroxides: the reaction is exothermic, and during curing considerable heat may be generated. For polymerisation, heat is usually applied, but the method varies according to the type of plastic required: a polymer-monomer mixture may be used.

There are four types of polymerisation: bulk, solution, emulsion and suspension.

Bulk polymerisation, combined with casting, consists of heating the monomer, to which benzoyl peroxide has been added, to alter its consistency from a liquid to a syrup and finally to a solid. This process is used to make Perspex or Plexiglas, a methyl methacrylate transparent polymer sheet of high (10^6) molecular weight. Perspex (Plexiglas) is used for:

Glazing, particularly in aircraft
Boat windscreens
Light fittings, display signs
Bathroom fittings, furniture
Contact lenses, spectacle frames

Solution polymerisation is usually adjusted to give a polymer with a molecular weight of about 90 000.
It is used for:

Surface coatings, particularly of automobiles
Lacquers and varnishes
Printing inks

Emulsion polymerisation is used for:
Water-based paints
Surface coatings for leather, paper and textiles

Suspension polymerisation is used to make polymer-monomer doughs; the polymer has a molecular weight of about 60 000.

The polymer powder is manufactured by adding *benzoyl peroxide* as a catalyst to an aqueous suspension of methyl methacrylate monomer liquid. This mixture is stirred continuously so that, as it polymerises, it becomes first a syrup and then a suspension of solid particles which can be dried to a powder of polymethyl-methacrylate beads. Residual peroxide remains on the surface of the polymer beads and is sufficient to act as a catalyst for final polymerisation.

The monomer liquid consists of methyl methacrylate monomer to which is added 20–100 parts per million of *hydroquinone* to inhibit polymerisation during storage.

Immediately before use, the polymer powder and the monomer liquid are mixed to form a dough.

Curing (*i*) *By heat*. Heating alone polymerises the dough efficiently and leaves very little unreacted monomer in the final product.

(*ii*) *In the cold*. Cold-curing requires the addition to the monomer liquid of an accelerator, which frequently is *dimethyl*-para-*toluidine*. As cold polymerisation is rarely complete, some unreacted monomer usually remains in the final solid.

Chemicals. The chemicals mentioned above are those most commonly used, but others may be preferred in the manufacture of a particular methyl methacrylate polymer.

Resins: methyl methacrylate. Glycol dimethacrylate monomer is sometimes added to the monomer liquid, particularly in the manufacture of dentures, because it makes the final solid polymer less soluble and more resistant to saliva and organic solvents. Methacrylic acid anhydride and vinyl methacrylate may be added.

Catalyst: benzoyl peroxide.

Inhibitors: hydroquinone, methyl ether of hydroquinone, *p*-methoxyphenol, resorcinol, pyrogallol, pyridine, benzoic acid, eugenol and thymol. In the United Kingdom and Europe, 2:4-dimethyl-6-*tertiary*-butyl phenol (Topanol 'A', I.C.I.) is available.

Plasticisers: dibutyl phthalate, triphenyl phosphate, tricresyl phosphate, glycol, fatty acid alcohols.

Solvents: trichloroethylene, methylene chloride, ethylene chloride, chloroform.

Accelerators: dimethyl-*p*-toluidine, aliphatic amines, mercaptans, hydrazine compounds.

Pigments.

(Malten and Zielhuis, 1964)

Advantages of a 2-part system

 (i) Malleability: the dough can be easily moulded to desired shapes
 (ii) Speed: as part of the system is already polymerised, it requires a relatively short time for the dough to be cured to a solid.
(iii) Reduced volume of liquid in the reaction minimises shrinkage during polymerisation.
(iv) Reduced heat production: as the powder is already partly a polymer, generation of exothermic heat during completion of polymerisation is diminished. This is most important in work on human tissues.

Sensitising potential in guinea pigs

Methyl, ethyl and *n*-butyl methacrylates are strong sensitisers in guinea pigs and they mutually cross-react (Chung and Giles, 1977).

Uses

Dentures
Hearing aids
Bone cement
Artificial nails

Causes of dermatitis

Dentures and hearing aids rarely sensitise those who wear them because, being heat-cured, they usually contain only minimal amounts of free monomer. Although bone cement is cold-cured and will contain unreacted monomer it appears not to sensitise patients, probably because it is locked away in bone. Dermatitis among orthopaedic surgeons is infrequent, for although they mould the uncured dough, the duration of contact is short and the practice of wearing two pairs of gloves reduces the risk of penetration of the monomer. Artificial finger nails are cold-cured and are a definite hazard to those who have them applied.

Dentures

Most dentures are made of methyl methacrylate, but in many reports the resin is referred to loosely as 'acrylic'. Dentures when correctly heat-cured contain only traces of unreacted monomer and therefore rarely if ever sensitise those who wear them. Fisher (1954) stressed that dentures are not sensitisers because the heat cure fully polymerises the resin. He investigated four women diagnosed as being sensitive to their methacrylate dentures, although three of them had changed to rubber plates without benefit. Each was patch tested with the methyl methacrylate monomer undiluted. Only one reacted and she was thought to have been sensitised by a cold-cured relining, which may have contained free monomer, rather than by her original plate. Three patients, including the sensitised patient, continued to wear methacrylate dentures comfortably, because they were fully polymerised. Fisher emphasised that symptoms, just because they parallel the wearing of the dentures, do not indicate allergy and that testing with whole dental plates strapped to the skin is a bad technique because the pressure causes an irritant reaction which may even be bullous. Another cause of false positive patch tests was demonstrated by Salo and Hirvonen (1969). They showed that denture filings, contaminated by *Candida albicans* in saliva can cause localised infections which simulate positive responses.

However, Crissey (1965) questioned the non-sensitising character of methacrylate dentures. He reported sensitisation as a cause of denture sore mouth in four patients, but the positive patch tests were to denture filings applied to the cheeks of the patients. Another patient (Giunta and Zablotsky, 1976) reacted to a temporary dental crown and bridge made of methacrylate but she had been presensitised to methyl methacrylate monomer by an artificial nail kit. McCabe and Basker (1976), using gas chromatography, examined heat-cured dental polymers and found that with a long wet cure the content of residual monomer was 0.045 per cent whereas with a long dry cure it increased to 0.095 per cent and a self curing material contained 0.185 per cent monomer. They described a patient who developed burning discomfort in her mouth every time she wore her new dentures; despite heaving been heat-cured they were found to contain 0.233 per cent of residual monomer. The patient was not patch tested but new heat-cured dentures containing 0.023 per cent monomer were made for her and she wore them comfortably. It was likely that she had been sensitised previously because a cold-cure repair to an old denture had caused a burning sensation in her mouth.

These reports suggest that dentures do not sensitise but if a cold-cure process has sensitised the patient to methyl methacrylate then a denture with a high residual monomer content may elicit dermatitis.

Denture sore mouth. The majority of those who wear dentures learn to tolerate the discomfort, but in a few it becomes extreme and is known as denture sore mouth. The patient complains of burning, soreness and pain in the mouth which is relieved by removing the plate. On examination the mucosa under the denture may look normal or inflamed. *Candida* on the plate or palate (Davenport, 1970; Renner *et al.*, 1979) or trauma from an ill-fitting denture may be the reason, but the cause is often obscure; it is rarely considered to be due to sensitivity to the dental plate. Wakkers-Garritsen, Timmer and Nater (1975) studied this condition in detail and finding no specific cause suggested that psychological factors may be important. In complete contrast Kaaber, Thulin and Nielsen (1979) reported frequent allergy to constituents of the dental plate.

Dentists and dental technicians. Twenty years ago, sensitivity to methyl methacrylate monomer was reported among dentists and dental technicians. Such cases seem no longer to occur, probably because awareness of the risk has led to greater care in the handling of these materials.

Two dentists with dermatitis of the right hand, mainly of the first fingers, and two dental mechanics with dermatitis of both hands were described by Fisher (1954). All had positive patch tests to methyl methacrylate monomer 100 per cent; the two mechanics wore fully-polymerised acrylic dentures comfortably. A further three dentists and three dental technicians were reported by Calnan and Stevenson (1963). Each had a positive patch test to 100 per cent methyl methacrylate monomer; they warned that this concentration causes active sensitisation.

Hearing aids

Hearing aids are made in a similar way to dentures — a polymer powder and monomer liquid are mixed, shaped in a mould and heat-cured. As is the rule with heat polymerisation, the finished plastic contains either no unreacted monomer or such minute amounts that sensitisation is highly unlikely.

A patient described by Guill and Odom (1978) developed dermatitis from a new 'in the ear' hearing aid made of cold cured methyl methacrylate whereas a replacement with a heat cured aid was comfortable. Patch tests: she reacted to methyl methacrylate 10 per cent in olive oil and to pieces of a cold cured plastic but not to the heat cured one.

St John's
> In 1972 a woman (Patient 1) aged 25 years, and in 1975 a girl (Patient 2) aged 16 years were seen with eczema of the external auditory meatus, limited exactly to the sites of contact with a polymethacrylate hearing aid. Both were totally deaf. The woman had worn a hearing aid for five years and had had the eczema for two years. The girl had worn hearing aids since the age of two years for deafness following chronic otitis media; her ears had always been wet but never itchy. Both

patients wore a deaf aid in their better ear only, and both said the eczema healed when the aid was removed, but rapidly recurred after the aid was reinserted. The girl had not worn an aid in her worse ear for a year and the skin of that ear was normal.

Patch tests: In the standard series, both were sensitive to nickel, each having acquired this allergy from jewellery. Neither patient reacted to any of the patch tests relevant to their hearing aids.

	Patient 1		*Patient 2*	
Methyl methacrylate monomer	10%	—	25%	—
Methyl methacrylate polymer	10%	—	100%	—
Benzoyl peroxide	5%	—	5%	—
Hydroquinone	1%	—	1%	—
Scraping of hearing aid		—		—
Nickel sulphate	5%	+	2.5%	+

Petrolatum was the diluent used for each chemical

Conclusion: Despite the clinical picture, these two patients were not allergic to their hearing aids. Possibly the plastic acted as an irritant, and a combination of moisture, debris, friction and infection caused the dermatitis.

Bone cement

Methyl methacrylate is being used with increasing frequency in orthopaedic surgery as a bone cement for the repair of fractures and in joint replacements, particularly for knee and hip prostheses. It has occasionally caused contact dermatitis of the hands in surgeons, and collapse, cardiac arrest and even death of patients during operation, although extremely rare, is well documented.

The methacrylate cement is made by mixing a monomer liquid with a powder of polymer granules, and in the process the liquid polymerises, binding the granules into a solid aggregate. While the liquid and powder are being mixed to a pliable dough the polymerisation may generate enough heat to make the mass extremely hot; it takes 5–10 minutes to set hard. The surgeon moulds the dough in his gloved hands, and with the tips of his fingers he forces it down into the medullary cavity, which in a hip replacement is the femur, and then he inserts the tapered stem of the stainless steel head. Similarly the cement is pressed into the acetabulum prior to inserting the acetabular socket which is likely to be made of high density polyethylene.

Monomer Liquid		*Polymer Powder*	
Methyl methacrylate monomer	97.5%	Polymethyl methacrylate granules	97.5%
Hydroquinone or Ascorbic acid (stabiliser)	0.01%	Benzoyl peroxide (activator)	2.5%
Dimethyl-*p*-toluidine (catalyst)	2.0%		

(Charnely, 1970)

Orthopaedic surgeons, despite wearing rubber gloves, are at risk of being sensitised by methyl methacrylate, but it seems to occur very infrequently.

The first case reported (Pegum and Medhurst, 1971) was that of an orthopaedic surgeon in London who developed eczema on the palmar surface of the left hand and fingers, but only on the tips of the right index and little fingers. The condition was worse after operating sessions, and the sites affected corresponded with how he held the polymerising methyl methacrylate dough in his gloved hands. Patch tests: he reacted to the methyl methacrylate monomer 5 per cent in acetone, to the monomer enclosed in a piece of rubber glove and to benzoyl peroxide 10 per cent in petrolatum (? a high concentration for patch testing). An *in vitro* test confirmed that the monomer readily penetrates through a rubber glove.

During the period 1971–1973 Fisher (1973) in New York saw five orthopaedic surgeons with dermatitis of the hands from this acrylic bone cement. Three had eczema, and on patch testing reacted to methyl methacrylate monomer 10 per cent in olive oil. Two had an irritant type of dermatitis with dry and fissured finger tips, and both had negative patch tests. A striking feature was that all five complained of a burning type of paraesthesia.

Patients. It is well recognised that the insertion of bone cement may be followed by an immediate but generally transient fall in blood pressure. It can, however, cause cardiac arrest (Powell *et al.*, 1970; Kirwan, 1973) and even death.

The mechanism is uncertain. Elderly patients having immediate treatment for a fractured neck of femur with a Thompson prosthesis seem to be at greater risk than patients having the elective operation of total hip replacement by a McKee-Farrar or Charnley procedure, possibly because this second group comprises younger people better able to withstand the surgical insult (Gresham, Kuczynski and Rosborough, 1971). Death on the table was caused by massive fat emboli in five patients (Gresham *et al.*, 1971) and by widespread pulmonary marrow emboli in another (Kepes, Underwood and Becsey, 1972). The toxicity of the monomer, anaphylaxis, and the heat of polymerisation of the resin within the bone marrow have been postulated as responsible factors but they are difficult to prove. A working party set up to examine the cardiovascular toxicity of acrylic cement has published a detailed review of the literature (Working Party on Acrylic Cement in Orthopaedic Surgery, 1974).

Artificial finger nails

Methyl methacrylate has been used in the past to make artificial finger nails, and the method has again been revived. The two-part system consists of a polymer powder and a monomer liquid; the formulation is similar to that for dentures, but, as curing is in the cold, polymerisation is likely to be incomplete.

Polymer powder	Monomer Liquid	
Methyl methacrylate polymer	Methyl methacrylate monomer	97%
Benzoyl peroxide	Glycol dimethacrylate	2%
	Dimethyl-*para*-toluidine	1%

In the technique, the surface of the nail plate is first roughened then painted with a mixture of the polymer powder and monomer liquid. This layer dries and polymerises within minutes, and the newly-formed plastic nail can then be smoothed and shaped to the desired length. As the natural nail grows out it is cosmetically necessary to renew ('fill in') the resin at the base of the nail about every two weeks.

These nails look good and adhere well, but the procedure can cause an extremely painful paronychia, a nail dystrophy and an allergic contact dermatitis of the nail beds and fingers. The monomer may be absorbed through contamination of the nail folds or fingers, or possibly it penetrates through the nail plate itself.

In 1957 Fisher, Franks and Glick described four such patients. Two had applied the plastic to camouflage abnormal nails and two were demonstrators of the technique who had used it on their own normal nails. The symptoms began after two to four months in three patients, but one woman had applied it only once. In one demonstrator the paronychia, with redness and itching around her nails, were followed by a vesicular eczema of the right cheek and eyelids. In all cases the nails took weeks to months to return to normal. Patch tests: all four patients reacted strongly to the undiluted acrylic monomer.

In the U.S.A. although methyl methacrylate has been prohibited for making artificial nails it is thought to have been replaced by butyl methacrylate and ethyl methacrylate (Maibach *et al.*, 1978). A paronychial and eyelid dermatitis followed sensitisation to ethyl methacrylate nails. The patient reacted to patch tests with ethyl methacrylate, methyl methacrylate and *N*-butyl methacrylate, each 1 per cent in ethanol (Marks, Bishop and Willis, 1979).

St John's

In the latter half of 1975, women suddenly began to be referred with nail dystrophy following the application of artificial nails. One manicurist and three customers seen at St John's had had the nails applied in a manicure salon by the standard technique. The interval between the first application and the onset of symptoms varied from 2–9 months. The clinical picture in the three customers comprised onycholysis and hyperkeratosis under the distal parts of the majority of their finger nails. Brown discolouration and petechial haemorrhages were sometimes present, and one woman complained of irritable blisters around the nail folds and on the sides of her fingers. The manicurist differed in that she had an acutely painful paronychia on her right thumb and little finger but minimal changes in the rest of her nails. In each patient the nails gradually grew out normally.

Patch tests: the chemicals used for the tests were kindly supplied by the manufacturer; the diluent was petrolatum:

	Methyl methacrylate monomer 1%	Glycol dimethacrylate monomer 1%	Dimethyl-*p*-toluidine 1%
Customer 1	+	—	—
2	+	—	—
Manicurist	—	—	—

One patient refused to be tested.

The patch tests confirmed that the two customers were sensitive to the methyl methacrylate monomer, whereas the painful dystrophy in the manicurist was an irritant effect.

Hydroxyethyl methacrylate

An histology technician was sensitised to hydroxyethyl methacrylate and developed dermatitis of his hands, paresthesiae of his fingers (p. 583) and an associated nausea and diarrhoea. He reacted to patch tests with 5 per cent hydroxyethyl methacrylate in alcohol. The monomer penetrated rubber (p. 583) and vinyl plastic and the patch tests reproduced the gastrointestinal symptoms (Mathias, Caldwell and Maibach, 1979).

Lauryl methacrylate

This methacrylate ester is added to lubricating oils to improve their viscosity and to lower the temperature at which they can be poured.

DIMETHACRYLATES

$$CH_2 = \overset{\overset{\textstyle CH_3}{|}}{C} - \overset{\overset{\textstyle }{\|}}{\underset{O}{C}} - O\left(CH_2CH_2O\right)_n - \overset{\overset{\textstyle O}{\|}}{C} - \underset{CH_3}{C} = CH_2$$

Polyethylene glycol dimethacrylate
N = 4 approximately

Sealants—

Anaerobic, metal
Anaerobic sealants, based on polyethylene glycol dimethacrylate, polymerise rapidly under anaerobic conditions in the presence of metals such as copper, iron and manganese, as are found in steel and brass. In the absence of metal, curing occurs, but it is slow, whereas in air the monomer is stable as oxygen blocks polymerisation. Enclosure between a screw and its socket is ideal for polymerisation, as there are abundant metal ions and no air.

Inhibitors
Inhibitors are added to the resins in a concentration of about 0.01 per cent to prevent premature polymerisation during storage. These include 1,4-naphthoquinone, benzoquinone, hydroquinone and butylated hydroxytoluene.

Uses
Anaerobic sealants are used to lock screws firmly in position and are used particularly in car assembly. The usual technique is to insert the screw partially into its orifice, squeeze the sealant from a plastic bottle onto the thread and then drive the screw home. The polymerised resin then locks the screw. Because the work is with small parts operatives tend not to wear gloves and their hands contact the resin on contaminated bottles. Occasionally workers dip the screws into the sealant and then there is gross contamination of their fingers.

Case reports
Allergic contact dermatitis from such a sealer was first reported by Allardice (1967) in seven assembly workers in an English car factory. The men developed a dry, fissured eczema of those fingers which came into contact with the resin,

and in some it spread to the dorsa of the hands, wrists and forearms. The face was not affected. Only one man had had to stop work. Patch tests: nine men in whom this diagnosis was suspected were patch tested with the acrylic sealer 25 per cent in vaseline, and seven reacted. The identity of the acrylate in the sealer was not given. The men were warned of the risk, instructed in a no-touch technique, and the nozzle of the dispenser was lengthened and curved away from the bottle to avoid drip contamination of its surface. No new cases occurred in the following year.

From Sweden, Magnusson and Mobacken (1972) reported seven similar cases among car assembly workers. The men had used a screw sealant for a few months to two years and each had hand eczema. Patch tests: the formulation was not disclosed, so each man was tested with the sealer undiluted, and all reacted. Two men reacted when tested with methylmethacrylate 1 per cent in MEK, but not to three acrylates and N-methylol acrylamide.

A glue for screws, described as a methacryl acid ester, sensitised 34/280 workers in a car factory in Germany. After exposure varying from a few weeks to two years, they developed bullous lesions on the fingers and sometimes the hands. Patch tests with the acrylate 2 per cent and 5 per cent in acetone were positive. Undiluted, it gave irritant reactions in controls (Jansen, 1975).

St John's

From 1969 to 1976 three men and one woman were seen who had been sensitised by dimethacrylate screw sealants. The dermatitis affects principally the pulps of the fingers, causing a dry, scaly eczema which is chronic and uncomfortable rather than incapacitating. It is easily overlooked as being an allergic contact dermatitis and many months may elapse before the patient is referred for patch testing.

Patient 1. A woman, aged 43 years, used a screw sealant when assembling car parts at work, and after a month she developed a dry, scaly, fissured eczema on her fingers and palms, which spread to the inner arms and lower face. The eczema had been present for three months by the time she was seen for patch testing.

Patient 2. A 43-year-old worker in a car factory had, for two years, used a sealant to secure the screws in pressure switches; he wore gloves but the sealant soaked through them. For 18 months he had had eczema on his hands, eyes and nose, which cleared when he was on holiday.

Patient 3. A man, aged 32 years, used a screw sealant whilst assembling postage franking meters, and within two to three weeks a vesicular eczema appeared on the palms and the palmar surfaces and sides of the fingers, which at times became dry and fissured. His hands healed away from work. He was referred for investigation ten months after the onset.

Patient 4. A 56-year-old electrical engineer had had eczema of the hands for six years which had spread widely on his body; for one year the pulps of his fingers had been cracked and painful. He had used a screw sealant for five years, and was known to be sensitive to epoxy resin.

Patch tests:

Sealant monomer		Methyl methacrylate
Pt. 1. Dimethacrylate ester	5% +	25% —
Pt. 2. Tetraethylene glycol dimethacrylate	1% +	25% —
Pts. 3. Triethylene glycol dimethacrylate	5% +	10% + (Pt. 3)
and 4. Polyethylene glycol dimethacrylate	5% +	5% — (Pt. 4)

The diluent was petrolatum.

The first three patients stopped using the sealant and their eczema healed; the fourth patient avoided the sealant but improved little.

Aerobic sealants

Aerobic sealants are used in the building industry on joints of all types and also for sealing window frames. These formulations usually do not contain acrylates but may include polysulphides, phenol formaldehyde resin, *p-tert*-butyl phenol formaldehyde resin, epoxy resin or colophony compounds: those made of rubber will include an accelerator which may be a dithiocarbamate.

Acrylates. A man developed hand eczema while using a small joint sealant to secure the joints in wooden window frames. The sealant contained ethyl acrylate in polymer and monomer form and solvents. Patch tests: he reacted to ethyl acrylate, butyl acrylate and the sealant each 0.1 per cent in petrolatum: ethylhexyl acrylate (1 per cent in pet.) and methyl methacrylate (5 per cent in pet.) elicited no responses. It was not known whether the sealant contained traces of butyl acrylate or whether it cross-reacted with the ethyl acrylate (Fregert, 1978).

St John's

A man who had been a weather proofing specialist for ten years suddenly developed a hyperkeratotic, fissured eczema of the fingers and palms. He had been using a new window-frame sealant for two months. Patch tests: he reacted to the window sealant and to 1 per cent of the acrylic resin mixture it contained (Cronin, 1969). The manufacturers disclosed later that this sealant monomer was based on butyl acrylate, a methacrylate and acrylic acid.

CYANOACRYLIC ACID AND ESTERS

$$\begin{array}{c} \text{CN} \\ | \\ \text{CH}_2 = \text{C} - \text{COOH}_3 \end{array}$$

Methyl 2-cyanoacrylate

Cyanoacrylates polymerise readily in air at room temperature, they have good bonding properties, and are used as adhesives for metal, rubber, glass and plastics and also in surgery, to bind tissues and to seal wounds. Cyanoacrylates bond strongly to keratin and isobutyl cyanoacrylate which polymerises when moist has been used successfully to fix the discs and to prevent leakage from ileostomy appliances (Hale, 1970).

A typical formulation contains a cyanoacrylate, a plasticiser, a thickener which may be a methyl methacrylate polymer and a stabiliser, to inhibit polymerisation.

Irritant — humidity effect

Workers using cyanoacrylates may complain of irritation and discomfort of their faces. These symptoms are relieved by raising the humidity above 55 per cent so that the cyanoacrylate polymerises in the atmosphere before it reaches the skin (Calnan, 1979).

ACRYLONITRILE (Vinyl cyanide)

$$CH_2 = CH - CN$$

Acrylonitrile is an explosive, flammable liquid which is highly poisonous when inhaled or absorbed percutaneously, but its toxicity is not due to liberation of cyanide (Paulet, Desnos and Battig, 1966). It polymerises spontaneously in the absence of oxygen or in the presence of light or alkali. It is used for:

1. Synthetic fibres (Acrilan, Orlon, Courtelle)
   Dyeing is facilitated by the addition to the fibre of about 10 per cent of a copolymer such as methyl methacrylate or vinyl acetate.
2. Rubber
   In combination with butadiene, acrylonitrile forms nitrile rubber.
3. Acrylonitrile — butadiene — styrene copolymer
   These copolymers are tough, rigid plastics which are used for motor car parts and fittings, telephones, heels, luggage and some building panels.
4. Surface coatings

Allergic contact dermatitis

After wearing a Plexidur finger splint for five weeks a man developed vesicular eczema at the sites of contact. Patch tests: he reacted to the Plexidur splint and to acrylonitrile 0.1 per cent but not to methyl methacrylate 0.1 per cent or to benzoyl peroxide 0.1 per cent. Tests in five controls were negative to 5 per cent of each of these compounds (Balda, 1971; 1975).

Sarcoid granuloma

Acrylonitrile fibres from a carpet penetrated a woman's sole and caused a sarcoid granuloma (Cortez Pimental, 1977).

Methacrylonitrile (α-Methylacrylonitrile)

$$CH_2 = \overset{\overset{\displaystyle CH_3}{|}}{C} - CN$$

Methacrylonitrile is a poison. In animals it is absorbed through the skin, stomach and respiratory tract, and forms cyanide in the blood after intravenous injection (Pozzani, Kinkead and King, 1969). It is used as a monomer and copolymer in the manufacture of elastomers, coatings and plastics.

ACRYLAMIDE (Propenamide)

$$CH_2 = CH - CO - NH_2 \qquad (CH_3)_2NCH_2CH_2N(CH_3)_2$$

N, N, N′ N′-tetramethylethylenediamine (TMEDA)

Acrylamide readily polymerises to a hard brittle material, and can be used as a copolymer. In granulated form, the polymer is an effective flocculant for separating solids suspended in water, and as such, it is used in mining, in soil stabilisation and in the treatment of sewage and industrial waste. To a small extent it is used in dyeing, photography, plastics and the paint industry. As a copolymer it is used to increase the dry strength of paper.

Toxicity
The polymer is not toxic but the monomer is a neurotoxin and chronic poisoning causes a polyneuropathy and mid-brain damage. Six cases of poisoning in men engaged in the manufacture of flocculators were described by Garland and Patterson (1967), who thought that the monomer had been absorbed through the skin. Apart from the presenting neurological signs of numbness, paraesthesiae, weakness and ataxia, several of the men had hyperhidrosis of the hands or feet and erythema and peeling of the palms.

In vitro acrylamide has been shown to depress chemotaxis of human polymorphonuclear leucocytes (Mangan and Synder, 1978).

Immediate-type hypersensitivity to tetramethylethylenediamine
Polyacrylamide gel electrophoresis is frequently used in protein analysis. A research worker preparing such gels was sensitised by tetramethylethylenediamine added to promote polymerisation. He developed generalised pruritus, and when 5 μl was applied to his forearm, it caused intense pruritus, diffuse vasodilatation and urticaria. One control was tested and did not react (Klein, 1976).

N-Methylolacrylamide

$$CH_2 = CH - CO - NH - CH_2OH$$

Methylolacrylamide is used as a copolymer with vinyl acetate and acrylic acid. Polymers are made into coatings, varnishes, adhesives and crease-proof fabrics.

Occupational dermatitis
A man with nummular eczema had three attacks of dermatitis on his face and body while working in a plastics factory where four acrylates were being used as copolymers with polyvinyl acetate in the manufacture of paints. (Such paints may contain up to 0.3 per cent of unreacted acrylic monomer.) Patch tests: He

reacted to N-methylolacrylamide but not to ethylhexylacrylate, butylacrylate or ethyl acrylate. Each monomer was diluted to 0.1 per cent in petrolatum. Controls: 20 gave negative reactions to this concentration of N-methylolacrylamide (Fregert and Dahlquist, 1968).

LIGHT SENSITIVE ACRYLATES

Light sensitive acrylates have been developed to make
  (i) printing plates
 (ii) quick drying inks: these are used in printing and for making printed circuit boards
(iii) lacquers: for shiny coatings on gramophone record sleeves and other surfaces.

Many different acrylates are used for these purposes.

Photo-reactivity
The most photosensitive of this group of compounds are the acrylates, and on exposure to ultraviolet light, they harden in fractions of a second. Methacrylates, although photosensitive are much less so and as they require minutes to cure, they are not suitable alternatives.

Irritancy
Acrylates, diacrylates and triacrylates are all irritants but of a descending order. Methacrylates are much less toxic.

Printing plates

Technique
A metal printing plate, coated on one side with a light-sensitive acrylic monomer, is covered with a printed negative in which the lettering is white and transmits light, while the background is black and excludes it. When the plate is placed under ultraviolet light, only the exposed print polymerises and hardens; the rest remains as soft unreacted monomer which can be removed to leave the print standing in relief. The monomer can be dissolved away in alkali or sprayed with ethanol and blasted off with air. It may be necessary to file uneven edges off the plate, and this creates a dust of resin particles.

Allergic contact dermatitis and photosensitivity
At least some of the light sensitive acrylic monomers used for these plates are allergens but as manufacturers are unwilling to disclose their formulations it has required much laboratory work to identify the sensitisers. Dermatitis has occurred in those working with Dycril (Du Pont) Nyloprint (BASF) Letterflex (Grace, Ltd) and other printing plates. Persistent light sensitivity has also been reported from the Nyloprint resin.

Dycril (Du Pont) acrylic-unidentified. In Göteborg, three men were employed to file the edges of Dycril plates, and while doing so their skin was coated with the dust. Within six months of starting this work they developed dermatitis on the dorsa of the hands and fingers, on the lower arms and the face, particularly the eyelids. A fourth man handled the same acrylic plates in another printing plant and developed the same contact dermatitis. Patch tests: the four men reacted to scrap from an unexposed plate; two were tested with this material diluted to 0.1 per cent in petrolatum and they reacted; two were tested with scrap from an exposed plate and one responded. Three of the men were tested with methyl-methacrylate 1 per cent in MEK and all were negative; and one man did not react to butyl acrylate, ethyl acrylate, 2-ethylhexyl acrylate and *N*-methylol acrylamide, each 0.5 per cent and 0.1 per cent (Magnusson and Mobacken, 1972).

Nyloprint (BASF) — ?*acrylamide derivate.* Six patients using the Nyloprint technique in four printing works in Stockholm were investigated by Wahlberg (1974). Each had been splashed with a mixture of ethanol and plastic during the blasting procedure and each had developed dermatitis of the hands, forearms and face. Patch tests: the five patients patch tested reacted to scrapings from the unexposed Nyloprint plates and to the ethanol-resin mixture 100 per cent, 50 per cent and 6 per cent; two reacted to the ultraviolet-irradiated plate. Five reacted to one of the ten coded ingredients, and two to another, but their identity was not disclosed. Fifteen controls had negative tests to all ten ingredients. Two patients were tested with methyl methacrylate and neither reacted. Castelain and Piriou (1978) reported one case.

In England a 60-year-old man, after working with Nyloprint plates for five years, developed dermatitis of his hands, arms and face. Although gloves were supplied, he found it easier to remove the wet plates from the washing cabinet with his bare hands. Patch tests: the patient reacted to unexposed Nyloprint, the solvent containing the monomer and glycol amol, one of the ten coded constituents of Nyloprint supplied by BASF. It was identified as the monomer, an acrylamide derivative (Pye and Peachey, 1976). Despite careful chemical analysis Malten, van der Meer-Roosen and Seutter (1978) failed to establish precisely the significant component but on patch testing their patients had group reactions to NN' methylene bis acrylamide.

In Tasmania, a self-employed printer began using a Nyloprint photo-printing machine; he did not wear gloves whilst handling the plates or when dipping them into butyl alcohol. After one month he had an exudative dermatitis of the hands, arms, face and neck. He stopped using this new technique and the eczema healed, but three months later he was still photosensitive even to light through window glass. Patch tests: the patient reacted to the unexposed and light-exposed Nyloprint (Tilsley, 1975).

St John's

A 39-year-old maker of printing plates began Nyloprinting, and, being unaware of any hazard, he did not wear gloves. After three months he developed eczema of the sides of the thumbs and index fingers where they touched the resin when he picked up the plates. The eczema spread to his feet. Patch tests: he reacted to the unexposed and exposed Nyloprint resin.

Di- and tetraethylene glycol dimethacrylate and hydroxyethyl methacrylate. Another company made a photopolymer based on an unsaturated polyester resin with five methacrylic hardeners. A commercial laboratory tested the mixture in guinea-pigs but failed to detect its sensitising capacity. In the Netherlands, five plate makers employed by journals or newspapers used this resin system and developed an allergic contact dermatitis of their hands and arms. Four were patch tested: each reacted to 2-hydroxyethyl methacrylate 0.1 per cent in alcohol (p. 583) and two to diethylene glycol dimethacrylate 1 per cent in MEK and tetraethylene glycol dimethacrylate 1 per cent in MEK. This latter compound although a sensitiser here was a successful alternative in the plant described below (Malten and Bende, 1979).

Letterflex (Grace, Ltd) — penta-erythritol tetrakis-3-mercaptopropionate
— 3-mercaptopropionic acid (p. 641).

Irritant and allergen

Tetraethylene glycol diacrylate. An outbreak of dermatitis, in a large French newspaper plant, followed the introduction of light sensitive printing plates. The printers who handled the plates developed an irritant bullous dermatitis of the wrists, fingers, thighs and dorsa of the feet, whereas maintenance men, who cleaned the machines, had an allergic contact eczema of the fingers and forearms. Beurey, Mougeolle and Weber (1976) analysed and identified the resin as tetraethylene glycol diacrylate and they found it to be irritant to a dilution of 1 per cent in acetone. The sensitised men reacted to 0.5 per cent and 0.1 per cent concentrations; gloves failed to protect them and they had to change their jobs. After confirming that it was not irritant tetraethylene glycol dimethacrylate was substituted for the diacrylate and the dermatitis ceased.

Inks

The industrial use of photosensitive inks is growing because, compared with conventional printing inks they have distinct advantages. Their most important asset is a greatly increased speed of drying, which allows different colours to be printed in one process, they facilitate handling of the printed matter, obviate care in stacking and shorten the time required for packing. In addition these inks do not rub off.

In contrast to traditional printing inks, which are handled without harm, the new light sensitive inks require, not only a new technology but also adequate protection for those who work with them and their education to be aware of the dermatitic hazard.

Composition of light sensitive inks
Light cured inks consist of pigments dispersed in a vehicle containing compounds of the following type:

(i) multifunctional acrylic monomers (MFAs) e.g.

trimethylol propane triacrylate (TMPTA) or
pentaerythritol triacrylate (PETA)
either alone or with a monofunctional acrylic monomer
(ii) an unsaturated polymer sensitive to ultraviolet light e.g.
acrylated urethane polyester oligomer or
acrylated epoxy resin oligomer
(iii) a photoinitiator e.g.
benzophenone or
isomers of amyl dimethylaminobenzoate
(iv) diluents e.g.
alcohols or phthalates
(v) also triethanolamine, stabilisers, surfactants, fillers and polymerization
inhibitors
Curing is by mercury arc lamps.

(Emmett, Taphorn and Kominsky, 1977).

The MFAs are low viscosity liquids, whose function is to dilute the resin,
they are highly reactive and combine with the oligomers to harden the resin.

Occupational dermatitis
These inks cause occupational dermatitis which may be irritant, allergic or
phototoxic.

*Irritant—acrylic acid, diacrylate (HDODA) and triacrylates (PETA and
TMPTA).*
In 1973 after the introduction of UV cured links into a printing works in
France several workers developed acute dermatitis of the hands and arms which
in some was vesicular or bullous. Patch tests with the inks were positive. The
cause was traced to defective polymerisation of an acrylic resin in the inks with
the production of acrylic acid which acted as an irritant and caused the dermatitis (Ducombs, Derville and Texier, 1974).

Allergic
Pentaerythritol triacrylate (PETA)
Trimethylolpropane triacrylate (TMPTA)
Hexanediol diacrylate (HDODA)
Epoxy acrylate oligomer

In the U.S.A. two men while employed in making UV-cured inks developed
both a phototoxic reaction to a photoinitiator and an allergic contact dermatitis
to the resin monomers. Patch tests: both men reacted to pentaerythritol triacrylate 0.2 per cent, trimethylopropane triacrylate 1 per cent, hexanediol diacrylate
1 per cent and epoxy acrylate oligomer 1 per cent; each in petrolatum (Emmett,
Taphorn and Kominsky, 1977).
In another ink firm 26 men were exposed to ultraviolet cured ink and four
developed an allergic contact dermatitis. Patch tests: each reacted to PETA 0.2
per cent (pet.), TMPTA 0.2 per cent (pet.) and cross-reacted to dipentaery-
thritol monohydroxy pentaacrylate 0.2 per cent (pet.) to which they had not

been exposed. A fifth employee with very mild dermatitis was not sensitised (Emmett, 1977).

In a Toronto ink manufacturing plant cases of dermatitis occurred and were intensively investigated by Nethercott (1978) he established that seven men were sensitised to PETA.

In Great Britain, a printing firm introduced ultraviolet light cured inks to facilitate the rapid production of multi-coloured labels. The ink manufacturers were unaware of any dermatitic risk until the commissioning period when the two press minders developed dermatitis. Patch tests: both men reacted to their inks and, of the constituents, to the reducer pentaerythritol triacrylate (0.1 per cent in MEK). They also reacted, without having been exposed, to two alternative acrylate reducers, trimethylol propane triacrylate and tripropylene glycol triacrylate (both 0.1 per cent in MEK) (Smith, 1977).

Printed electrical circuit boards — trimethylol propane triacrylate

St John's
> In a printed circuit department a green acrylic ink was used to form a solder-resistant coating; it was flooded over the printed circuit boards and then polymerised by exposure to ultraviolet light. The foreman occasionally picked up the wet boards to inspect them prior to polymerisation and when there was ink on the edges it contaminated his hands. He suddenly developed an acute dermatitis of the hands, wrists, and face, with oedema of the eyelids. He had six attacks in eight months. Patch tests: he reacted strongly to the green ink; it was ascertained that it contained trimethylol propane triacrylate.

Phototoxic

Amyldimethylaminobenzoate. Four men (two described above) became photosensitive while preparing UV-cured inks. Symptoms of smarting and burning began within minutes of light exposure and the subsequent erythema and oedema lasted several days. By *in vitro* investigation of the ink ingredients Emmett *et al.* (1977) found that the photoinitiator used, amyl dimethylaminobenzoate, was phototoxic and tests on the patients and controls established that phototoxicity to this chemical was the cause of the reaction. Application of 10 per cent sulizobenzone prior to sun exposure blocked the effect.

Patch testing
No single monomer will screen for sensitisation to the whole group of acrylic resins; each monomer must be tested separately and to avoid active sensitisation they must be diluted. Patch tests with methyl methacrylate 100 per cent (Calnan and Stevenson, 1963) and butyl acrylate 5 per cent in petrolatum have sensitised patients in the St John's clinic. No active sensitisation was observed by Maibach *et* al. (1978) from patch testing 542 patients with 1 per cent *n*-butyl methacrylate monomer and 1 per cent ethyl methacrylate monomer.

The correct concentrations for patch testing with these compounds is at present not established, the following list is therefore only tentative.

Monomer	%	Diluent
Acrylates (methyl, ethyl, butyl)	1	Petrolatum
Methacrylates	5 and 2	Petrolatum
Dimethacrylates	5 and 1	Petrolatum
Cyanoacrylates	2	Petrolatum
Acrylonitriles	0.1	Petrolatum
Methylolacrylamides	0.1	Petrolatum
Light-sensitive monomers		
Acrylamide	0.1	Petrolatum
Tetraethylene glycol diacrylate	0.1 (and 0.5 %)	Petrolatum
Pentaerythritol triacrylate (PETA)	0.2	Petrolatum
Trimethylolpropane triacrylate (TMPTA)	0.2	Petrolatum

Epoxy resins

Epoxy resins are now used throughout the world, but because they are made of expensive materials, cost is a limiting factor in their expansion. Their total manufacture remains small compared with that of polyethylene, polystyrene and polypropylene, but their versatility and range of properties are unequalled and ensures them a growing market and a steadily increasing production.

In 1938 and 1943, Castan, a Swiss chemist working on the development of dental resins, filed patents describing the production of epoxy resin from epichlorohydrin and bisphenol A. The resin was not a success as a dental material, but in 1946 Ciba-Geigy of Basle promoted epoxy resins as adhesives. Simultaneously, in the United States, Greenlee of Devoe and Raynolds, a paint company, filed a patent in 1943 describing a similar epoxy resin, but with a higher molecular weight, suitable for use as a surface coating. By the late 1940s the commercial production of epoxy resins had begun.

Chemistry

Epoxy resins are thermosetting, cross-linked polymers which, in curing, produce almost no by-products so that shrinkage during polymerisation is minimal. Curing is an exothermic reaction. About 95 per cent of epoxy resins are made by reacting bisphenol A and epichlorohydrin to produce glycidyl ethers. These reactants are chosen because bisphenol A is relatively inexpensive and the polymers produced have a good range of properties.

Epoxy group (Epoxide, ethoxylene group)

The epoxy group is a ring structure in which the atomic bonds are so strained that they are easily broken and molecules containing these rings are highly reactive.

Glycidyl ether group

$$H_2C - CH - CH_2 - O -$$

(with epoxide O across the $H_2C - CH$)

Glycidyl ether groups are formed when epichlorohydrin reacts with an hydroxyl compound, usually bisphenol A; they are terminal on the monomer molecules.

Epichlorohydrin
1-chloro-2,3-epoxypropane; δ *-chloropropylene oxide*

$$H_2C - CH - CH_2Cl$$

(with epoxide O across the $H_2C - CH$)

In the formation of these epoxy resin monomers, epichlorohydrin and bisphenol A are mixed, heated and stirred, while sodium hydroxide is added to maintain neutrality. The reaction is exothermic and temperature control may be required. The proportioning of the reactants determines whether the resin monomer produced is a liquid of low molecular weight (400 approx.) or a solid of high molecular weight (4000 approx.). Epichlorohydrin is always present in excess to ensure that the molecules terminate in epoxy groups by which they subsequently cross-link. In a liquid resin monomer (molecular weight about 400) the proportion of epichlorohydrin is relatively high, the molar ratio being 4 epichlorohydrin : 1 bisphenol A. By increasing the bisphenol A content, the molecular weight rises and the resin becomes increasingly viscous and eventually solid. In a solid resin (molecular weight 1420) the proportions are 1.2 epichlorohydrin : 1 bisphenol A (Saunders, 1973).

Bisphenol A (4,4′-isopropylidenediphenol; 2,2-Bis(4-hydroxyphenyl) propane; diphenylolpropane)

Bisphenol A is formed from two molecules of phenol and one molecule of acetone, whence its name.

Epichlorhydrin + Bisphenol A → diglycidylether

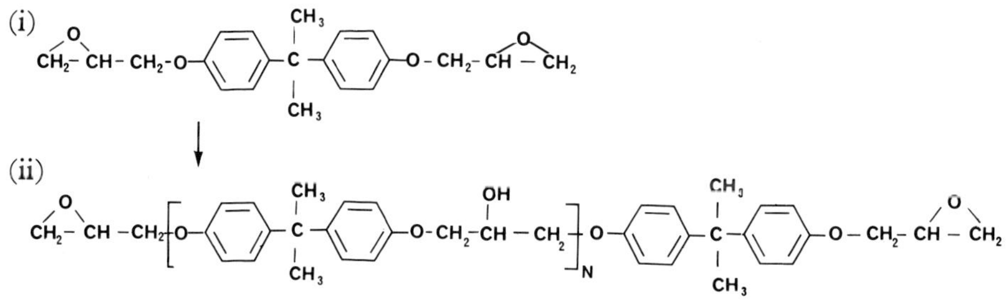

(i)

(ii)

(i) = the simplest diglycidyl ether, $n = \frac{1}{2} - 1$ molecular weight = 340, the proportion of epoxy groups is high and the reactivity of the molecules is great.

(ii) = the general formula of epoxy resin molecules based on epichlorohydrin and bisphenol A. The greater the value of n, the higher the molecular weight, and the resin changes in consistency from a thin liquid, through a viscous syrup to a solid form. When $n = 13$, the resin monomer is a solid with a molecular weight of 4000. As the molecular weight increases the molecule elongates separating the terminal epoxy groups, and the epoxy value and the epoxy reactivity fall. However, these solid epoxy compounds remain very reactive through their hydroxyl groups.

Commercial resin monomers are mixtures of epoxy molecules with n varying from 0–12.

Hardeners (cross-linking compounds)
The resin monomers are polymerised by cross-linking to become solid three-dimensional networks. Most epoxy resins are two-component systems and those which harden at room temperature are of this type. One-part epoxy resins are used, but they require heat, usually by stoving, to achieve a good result.

The curing agents are most important, as they influence the performance and properties of the cured resin, and in many systems they are incorporated into the structure as segments of the polymer network. Numerous curing or cross-linking agents are available, the choice depending upon the physical and chemical requirements of the cured resin.

Polymerisation is an exothermic reaction, heat being generated during the curing process but many curing agents require additional heat to effect complete polymerisation.

Cross-linking agents have been divided by Saunders (1973) into the three groups: tertiary amines, polyfunctional amines and acid anhydrides.

Tertiary amines act mainly as catalysts in the cross-linking of epoxy groups, and take little part in the formation of the final polymers. The following compounds are used:

Benzyldimethylamine (BDMA); 2-(Dimethylaminoethyl)phenol (DMP-10);
2,4,6-Tris(dimethylaminomethyl)phenol (DMP-30)
Triethanolamine
N-n-Butylimidazole.

These tertiary amines are used alone in some adhesives and surface coatings, but more frequently they are employed as accelerators of anhydride curing compounds.

Polyfunctional amines participate in the structure of the final polymer; they include:

Diethylenetriamine (DTA)   Triethylenetetramine (TET)
m-Phenylenediamine (MPD)   4,4′-Diaminodiphenylmethane (DDM)
                                 4,4′-Diaminodiphenylsulphone (DDS).

Amines are used for adhesives, coating and laminating operations. Aliphatic amines are economical because they harden at low concentrations and cure rapidly at room temperature, although the bond strength is greater if heat is used. Aromatic amines always require heat but the final resin has good heat and chemical resistance.

Acid anhydrides. These compounds will cure most types of epoxy resin, but they require heat:

Maleic anhydride (MA)   Dodecenylsuccinic anhydride (DDSA)
Phthalic anhydride (PA)
Hexahydrophthalic anhydride   (HPA).

Many of the epoxy resins and their catalysts and hardeners have been listed, with their structural formulae, by Malten (1973).

Adducts
Adducts are modified cross-linking agents, which have been partially reacted with the epoxy resin. Thus they still act as cross-linking agents, but may be less toxic or easier to handle technically than the original compound.

The pot life of a resin is the time the mixture remains workable after the resin and its curing agent have been mixed and before the combination begins to harden, and become unmanageable. It is particularly during this period that the resin is handled by workers when the monomer content is high and the dermatitic risk is at its greatest.

Additives
The properties of the resins can be modified and improved by the addition of various materials prior to polymerisation. These additives may be diluents, fillers and reinforcers, resin modifiers, plasticisers and pigments.

Diluents are added to the uncured resin system to reduce its viscosity, to increase its manageability and to facilitate its penetration between fibres or other materials. There are two types of diluents; reactive and non-reactive.

Reactive diluents are the more effective; they form chemical bonds with the epoxy compounds during cure and become an integral part of the final resin. In addition to reducing the viscosity of the resin, they accelerate and increase the efficiency of the curing process.

Many of the reactive diluents are low viscosity epoxy compounds. They may be the monoepoxides: allyl glycidyl ether, butyl glycidyl ether, cresyl glycidyl ether and phenyl glycidyl ether. Less frequently, they are the even more reactive diepoxides, 1,4-butanediol diglycidyl ether and butadiene diepoxide. The diepoxides have the advantage of increasing the heat resistance of the final resin.

Non-epoxy reactive diluents may be alcohols, lactams, lactones and triphenyl phosphate.

Non-reactive diluents include: dibutyl phthalate, styrene and phenolic compounds. They increase the pot life of the system by decreasing the activity of the curing agent, but the final resins have a reduced performance.

Fillers and reinforcements. Fillers are inert compounds, added to reduce the cost of the resins and to modify their physical properties. They may improve the thermal conductivity of the system, alter the hardness and handling of the resin, improve its flow, and increase fire retardation. Silica and calcium carbonate are used for these purposes.

Reinforcements are added to increase the flexural, tensile and impact strengths of the resin. Fibreglass and chopped nylon act in this way. The heat resistance of the resin is increased by asbestos or carbon black.

Resin modifiers. The combination of an epoxy resin with another type of resin gives a final polymer with the advantages of both. Thus, they can be combined with phenolic, urea, melamine, aniline formaldehyde, furfural, polyurethane, polyester, silicone, vinyl and nylon resins.

Plasticisers are used infrequently because they tend to be incompatible with the cured resin, and the same effect can be achieved by curing with long chain fatty polyamides. Dibutyl phthalate is occasionally used as a plasticiser.

Other additives. Coal tar pitches are added to paints to improve their water resistance. Bitumens reduce the cost of antiskid surfacings for roads.

Epoxidised oils

Epoxy resins react with unsaturated oils such as castor, soybean, safflower and linseed oils to form esters. These epoxidised oils are used as plasticisers and stabilisers, particularly for PVC.

Uses of epoxy resins

Epoxy resins have a range of properties which surpasses that of other plastics, and, despite their expense, their field of utilisation is increasing. Their many uses have been described in detail by Potter (1975). He listed the following attributes of epoxy resins:

1. Excellent chemical resistance
2. Excellent adhesion to many different substrates
3. Outstanding toughness

4. A high level of mechanical strength, which is retained at elevated temperatures
5. Good electrical properties
6. The ability to be cured rapidly or slowly over a wide range of temperatures
7. Low shrinkage during cure
8. The absence of volatile by-products formed during the curing reaction
9. The ability to be processed by a large number of different techniques.

Epoxy resins are used for:
1. Surface coatings
2. Electrical insulations
3. Adhesives
4. Construction industry
5. Miscellaneous applications, including polymer stabilisers and plasticisers, laminates, in sculpture, in the manufacture of jewellery and ornaments, in electron microscopy and as a home pack.

Surface coatings
The principal use of epoxy resins is as surface coatings and about half the resins produced are for this purpose. Such paints are excellent anti-corrosives, affording protection against fresh and salt water, acids, alkalis and other chemicals. They are used to coat and line steel pipes, to paint ships and marine equipment, as primers for automobiles and also as can linings. Many air-drying epoxy paints are esters produced by reacting an epoxy resin, which acts as an hydroxyl compound with a vegetable oil fatty acid. Tar, which is one of the oldest protective coverings, can be combined with epoxy resin to make paints which can withstand exposure, water, heat and chemicals.

Powder paints. Paints in powder form are becoming increasingly popular because the absence of a solvent eliminates both a risk to the operatives and pollution of the atmosphere; moreover powders can be applied as a single film of varying thickness. The surface is more likely to be completely covered, and wastage to be less. They can also be made to harden rapidly and to adhere well, and their application can be automated.

To make such powders, a solid resin ($n=11$) is partially reacted with a curing agent to form a crushable solid; this is ground to a powder and then pigments, curing agents and accelerators may be added. One way to apply these paints is by electrostatic spray. In this method, the spray and the powder are given the same electrical charge but the object to be coated is oppositely charged, so that the powder adheres to the surface by electrostatic attraction. The part is then heated to melt and polymerise the powder.

Powder paints have the disadvantages of chalking, and losing gloss on exposure.

Electrical insulation
Epoxy resins make good insulators; the total usage is small only because the parts to be covered are small. Methods of insulation are facilitated because the

resins can be cast to cover complicated and difficult shapes and small parts can be encapsulated or impregnated by the resin. Shrinkage during cure is negligible. Epoxy-glass laminates are being used increasingly for electronic circuit boards.

Epoxy resin insulation has made it possible to design small compact switchgears, and to make more efficient transformers, and they have, with advantage, replaced hot bitumen as jointing compounds for electric cables.

The addition to the resin system of small amounts of a photosensitive compound, such as a cinnamic acid resin or cinnamal ketone, reduces internal stresses in the cured resin and increases resistance to thermal shock (Breslau, 1973).

Adhesives
Epoxy resins have outstanding bonding properties, and of the total resin sold in the United States in 1969 about 12 per cent was as adhesives and bonding compounds (Lewis and Saxon, 1973). They will glue similar and dissimilar materials; thus they bond metal to metal, metal to wood and other structures, and they also bond stone, rubber, plastics, glass, china and textiles.

Most commercial adhesives are based on the diglycidyl ether of bisphenol A, but the curing agents influence the chemical structure and the physical properties of the final polymer. Aliphatic amines cure at room temperature, although the bond strength is increased by heat. Phenolic modified epoxy resins make the best high temperature adhesives, and nylon-epoxy resins provide the greatest joint strength.

As adhesives, epoxies are used in the aerospace, automobile, ship, electrical and electronics industries and also for military equipment and the small-part assembly of metals and plastics.

Construction industry
In the building industry, epoxy resins are used for floorings, repairings cracks in concrete, bonding concrete to concrete, and concrete to steel or other materials and as a jointing compound. Brick-layers use them as a laminating strip between the top rows of bricks on a wall to give them greater security.

Epoxy resins have been found to be particularly effective as a surface covering on roads and bridges, where they bond the surface and act as an efficient barrier to moisture and chemical corrosion. An increasing application is as an anti-skid road surfacing; such a coating may comprise the resin, coal tar and, to increase flexibility, pine oil.

Polymer stabiliser and plasticiser
Uncured epoxy resins have been used as stabilisers (prevent deterioration and discolouration) and plasticisers (maintain flexibility and toughness) in polyvinyl chloride plastics since the 1950s, but they are now being added to the halogenated polymers and to cellulose resins.

It is thought that epoxides protect PVC and halogenated polymers by mopping up autocatalytic hydrochloric acid formed during degradation by heat, light and oxygen (Port, 1973).

Other uses

Other uses for epoxy resins include the restoration of antiques, in sculpture, in the manufacture of jewellery, decorative plates, tiles and bowls, and as an embedding material in electron microscopy. A home pack, consisting of two tubes, one of resin and the other of a polyamide hardener, is marketed principally as a glue.

The sensitisers in epoxy resin systems

The sensitiser in an epoxy resin system may be:

(i) the epoxy monomer
(ii) a reactive diluent
(iii) the hardener
(iv) some other additive.

Allergenic component of the epoxy monomer

The epoxy group is the sensitiser in the epoxy resin molecule. This was proved experimentally by Malten, Verwilghen and Seutter (1965) using glycidyl ether epoxy resins on guinea pigs and the strong sensitising potential of the epoxy grouping was confirmed experimentally by Kligman (1966). Butylglycidyl ether at a concentration of 10 per cent for the induction and the challenge sensitised 19/24 human subjects (sensitisation grade 4), whereas epoxy resin 25 per cent for the induction and 15 per cent for the challenge sensitised 21/25 subjects (sensitisation grade 5). Zschunke (1959) demonstrated that repeated topical application of epoxy resin, triethylenetetramine and other hardeners, would induce sensitisation.

The sensitising capacity of diglycidylether-bisphenol A epoxy resins is directly related to their molecular weight (MW). This has been proved by Thorgeirsson and Fregert (1977) and Thorgeirsson, Fregert and Ramnäs (1978) using the guinea pig maximisation test. In this type of resin the lowest MW is 340 and such molecules are potent allergens, oligomers of MW 624 are less sensitising and as the MW increases to 908 and 1192 the allergenic potential disappears. Resin mixtures with an average MW of 350 were strong allergens whereas the resins with the largest molecules (MW 1850) elicited no reactions.

Epichlorohydrin is extremely irritant and has been reported as causing chemical burns in five patients (Ippen and Mathies, 1970). It is also an allergen (Fregert and Gruvberger, 1970; Epstein, 1974; Lambert *et al.*, 1978) but it is said that in the uncured resin monomer no free epichlorohydrin remains (Broughton, 1965) and guinea pigs sensitised to epoxy resins did not react to epichlorohydrin (Thorgeirsson and Fregert, 1977). However in clinical practice Calnan (1975) has found that patients sensitised by epoxy resins may react to a patch test with epichlorohydrin.

Bisphenol A was postulated as the allergen by Gaul (1957), but this was based on the results of patch testing one man sensitised by an epoxy glue at work. The problem was investigated by Fregert and Rorsman (1962) and they found that patients sensitised by epoxy resin through occupational exposure did not react to patch tests with bisphenol A, whereas those sensitised without occupational exposure did so. Most of the latter patients reacted to stilboestrol-like chemicals which were therefore considered possibly to be the primary allergens, in which case reactions to epoxy resins containing bisphenol A and to bisphenol A were cross-reactions. They had previously reported (Fregert and Rorsman, 1960) that a woman sensitised by diethylstilboestrol cross-reacted to bisphenol A. However, Krajewska and Rudzki (1976) found that of 78 subjects sensitised in industry to a Polish epoxy resin (MW 150) 13 reacted to patch tests with bisphenol A 2 per cent in water.

Epoxy reactive diluents

Low-molecular weight epoxy compounds are used as reactive diluents and many are potent sensitisers. Three glycidyl ether compounds, frequently used as reactive diluents, were selected by Fregert and Rorsman (1964) to patch test 20 patients sensitive to epoxy resin. The results were as follows:

	Positive/Tested
Phenylglycidyl ether 0.25% in acetone	14/20
Allylglycidyl ether 0.25% in acetone	3/20
n-Butyglycidyl ether 0.25% in acetone	2/20

Workers in contact with phenylglycidyl ether are frequently sensitised (Rudzki and Krajewska, 1979).

Another reactive diluent, Epoxide No. 8, purported by the manufacturer to be non-allergenic, sensitised 12/12 guinea pigs exposed in the maximisation test (Thorgeirsson, Fregert and Magnusson, 1975). In comparison, with the same method of induction, 6/12 animals were sensitised by butylglycidyl ether. Cardura® E. the glycidyl ester of the synthetic fatty acid Versatic® 911 with a molecular weight of 240–250, sensitised a man who was filling it and epoxy resin into tins from drums. Although he reacted to patch tests with both epoxy resin and Cardura E (down to 0.01 per cent in acetone) these two substances do not cross-react (Dahlquist + Fregert 1979a).

The sensitising capacity of six reactive diluents was assessed with the guinea pig maximisation by Thorgeirsson (1978a). Those of low molecular weight 175–360 sensitised (1,2-epoxydodecane, monoglycidylester of synthetic fatty acids, monoglycidylether of isomeric alcohols, diglycidylether of butanediol and diglycidylether of neopentylglycol) but aliphatic polyglycidylether with a higher MW 1700 caused no reactions. Both ethers and esters sensitised.

Hardeners

Aliphatic amines are potent allergens, and their alkalinity makes them irritants. The most sensitising have been listed by Fregert (1972) as:

ethylenediamine (EDA)	diethylenetriamine (DETA)
triethylenetetramine (TETA)	dipropylenetriamine (DPTA)
dimethylaminopropylamine	*p,p'*-diaminodiphenylmethane (DDM)

From his experience on working sites Fregert (1972) has observed that sensitisation by epoxy resins is less frequent when an amide hardener is being used instead of an amine.

Cycloaliphatic amines
Isophoronediamine (IPD) is a strong sensitiser.

Polyamide and anhydride hardeners require heat but cause much less dermatitis.

Epoxidised oils are not allergenic (Fregert and Rorsman, 1964).

The sensitising capacity of cold-curing resin hardeners was assessed with the guinea-pig maximisation test by Thorgeirsson (1978b):

Aliphatic polyamines: all sensitised (EDA, DETA, TETA, DPTA, tetraethylenepentamine TEPA, diethylaminopropylamine DEAPA and trimethylhexamethylenediamine TMDA).

Cycloaliphatic polyamines: isophoronediamine (IPD) and *N*-aminoethylpiperazine sensitised but not dimethyl-diamino-dicyclohexyl-methane.

Aromatic amine, DDM sensitised 20 per cent.

Polyaminoamides sensitised 20–67 per cent.

Adducts without aliphatic amines probably do not sensitise.

Incidence of sensitisation to epoxy resin

Epoxy resins are among the most potent sensitisers introduced into industry in the past 30 years. The incidence of dermatitis varies with the industrialisation and the local occupations of the particular community studied and the figures of sensitisation recorded also depend upon whether epoxy resin is included in a routine series for investigating all patients or whether only selected patients are tested.

The following frequencies of sensitisation, though not comparable, have been reported; the concentration of epoxy resin used for patch testing varied from 1–2 per cent.

City	Tested	Positive	%	
Lund	3057	54	1.8 (M=2.3% F=1.4%)	Fregert (1973)
Amsterdam	556	9	1.6	van Ketel (1974)
New York	340		5.6	Baer *et al.* (1973)
S. Carolina	42	2	4.7	Lepine (1976)
Auckland	214	5	2.3	Black (1972)
Adelaide	(Pts. with Contact dermatitis)			
	1000	48	4.8	Burry *et al.* (1973)

In the Lund series (Fregert, 1973), from 1966–1969, every patient was tested with epoxy resin 1 per cent in acetone, and the 1.8 per cent figure probably does reflect the true incidence of sensitivity among this community in the south of Sweden. Similarly, in Amsterdam, over an 18 month period, all patients were routinely tested with epoxy resin 1 per cent in petrolatum, and their incidence of sensitisation was 1.6 per cent. The high frequencies reported in the other centres were probably due to selection of patients.

In Warsaw due to the lack of automated production methods in some factories sensitivity to epoxy resins and triethylenetetramine is the most frequent cause of occupational dermatitis (Krawjewska and Rudzki, 1976). In Dresden also, sensitivity to epoxy resins is an important cause of occupational dermatitis (Richter, 1974).

St John's

At St John's every patient attending the Contact Clinic is routinely tested with epoxy resin 2 per cent in petrolatum. From 1971–1976 the incidence of sensitivity for all patients was 1.3–2.1 per cent (Table 12.1), for men 2–2.8 per cent and for women 0.5–1.5 per cent (Table 12.2).

Table 12.1. Incidence of epoxy resin sensitivity (St John's 1971–1976).

Year	Tested	Positive	%
1971	1558	33	2.1
1972	1606	26	1.6
1973	1546	23	1.5
1974	1433	21	1.5
1975	1858	25	1.3
1976	1982	30	1.5

Table 12.2. Incidence of epoxy resin sensitivity in men and women (St John's 1971–1976).

Year	Men			Women		
	Tested	Positive	%	Tested	Positive	%
1971	707	20	2.8	851	13	1.5
1972	738	18	2.4	868	8	0.9
1973	710	19	2.7	836	4	0.5
1974	655	13	2.0	778	8	1.0
1975	887	18	2.0	971	7	0.7
1976	937	23	2.5	1045	7	0.7

Causes of dermatitis

Fully-cured epoxy resins are harmless. The hazard occurs when there is contact with the uncured resin monomer or with hardeners, and the greatest risk is to those handling these compounds. Workers generally incriminate the hardeners as the dermatitic hazard and so treat them with circumspection whereas erroneously they regard the resins as less dangerous.

Polymerisation is exothermic (p. 596), and although the vapour pressure of these resins is low, some volatilisation probably occurs during all methods of cure, but is increased when heat is applied. Fumes from the curing resins are therefore a hazard not only to those working with them but also to others in the vicinity who may not be in direct contact.

Complete polymerisation may require two weeks at room temperature, but only one day if heat is applied. Should a newly-cured resin, or even the final resin be incompletely polymerised, dermatitis may be elicited, particularly if the product is sawn, drilled or ground with the production of dust.

Dermatitis is predominantly occupational and occurs in a variety of industries.

The resins and hardeners act both as irritants and as sensitisers. Lemon (1972) divided the resins into three grades:

(i) Solid resins are innocuous to the skin, and also when in solution but then the solvents may be mild irritants.

(ii) Liquid resins are moderate irritants and as they are sticky they have to be removed by solvents, which further irritate the skin. They may be sensitisers.

(iii) Diluted liquid grades are the most active sensitisers and they may contain reactive diluents, many of which are low-molecular weight epoxy compounds. Vapour from these liquids may also irritate the eyes and respiratory tract. The curing agents, particularly the amine hardeners, act as irritants and as sensitisers (Birmingham, 1959; Lemon, 1972; Fregert, 1972).

Allergic contact dermatitis —

Occupational

Sensitisation to epoxy resin in industry has been known for 20 years (Grandjean, 1957); the risk of dermatitis in *aircraft factories* (Calnan, 1958; Malten and Zielhuis, 1964; Bord et Castelain, 1966), *car factories* (Négri, 1959; Turner, 1964), *electrical* and *electronics industries* (Grandjean, 1957; Mehl, Fuchs and Fousseareau, 1971) is well recognised. These latter authors also reported that 18 workers had been sensitised in the manufacture of *special epoxy paints* for use on boat hulls and fuel stoves. The use of epoxy resins in *surface coatings*, their risk and its control have been described by Lemon (1972).

In 1973 Rudzki and Krajewska reported from Warsaw that, in two electrical engineering plants, 15 per cent (35/236) of the employees in contact with epoxy resin had dermatitis. Patch tests: of 26 tested, 19 reacted as follows:

epoxy resin 2 per cent in petrolatum (3), triethylenetetramine (TET) 1 per cent in water (2), phthalic anhydride (PA) 1 per cent in alcohol (1), resin and TET (6), resin and PA (1), TET and PA (1), resin, TET and PA (5).

Other sources of exposure area:

Cable jointing: A man used epoxy resin to insulate joints when connecting metal anodes on soil pipes to electric cables. He accidentally spilled the resin on his hands and developed dermatitis. He reacted to a drop of resin applied to his arm, but not to the hardener (Gaul, 1962).

For seven months a man connected telephone cables with epoxy resin and during this time he carried his contaminated tools in his right-hand trouser pocket. He stopped this work, but continued to carry the same tools in the same pocket and three months later, having been sensitised by the contaminated pocket, he developed eczema first on the fingers of the right hand, then as a patch on his right thigh and subsequently of his eyelids. Patch tests: he reacted to the lining of his pocket and to epoxy resin 1 per cent in petrolatum (Sjöberg, Tegner and Fregert, 1973).

Sealants. An electric cable jointer developed dermatitis of the hands while using a two-component putty sealant which he mixed in his palm. One part was a low molecular weight epoxy resin and the other, a hardener, was an aniline formaldehyde adduct and a phenolic mixture. Patch tests: he reacted to epoxy resin 2 per cent in petrolatum; the hardener was not available for testing (Calnan, 1969).

A gas jointer daily used pitch epoxide sealant in repair kits for mending leaks in large gas pipes. He sandblasted the joint to clean it, enclosed it with a rubber band containing nozzles, mixed the resin and activator, and poured it through the rubber nozzles on to the joint. He did not wear gloves and the uncured resin contaminated his hands. After four months, he developed severe eczema on the dorsa of his hands, which spread to his arms and face. Patch tests: he reacted to epoxy resin 1 per cent in petrolatum but not to the activator 1 per cent in petrolatum (Cronin, 1974).

Glue. A plastic film, heated with an electric current to 265°C was used to glue small metal objects to a glass plate, and in the process fumes were given off. Three men engaged in this work developed facial dermatitis, but another, who simply cut the adhesive film, was not affected. Patch tests: the three affected men reacted to the plastic film, to filter paper impregnated with the fumes and to the standard epoxy allergen. It was confirmed that the film contained epoxy resin (Fregert and Dahlquist, 1969).

Electron microscopy. A laboratory technician, sensitised by epoxy resin while making histological sections for electron microscopy, was mentioned by Mehl, Fuchs and Fousseareau (1971).

PVC containers. A woman, while filling polyvinyl chloride tubes with shampoo, developed hand dermatitis which was partly attributable to sensitization to an epoxy resin plasticiser in the PVC (Ancona-Alayon, Jimenez-Castilla and Gomez-Alvarez, 1976).

Non-occupational

Plasticers and stabilisers. Uncured epoxy resins are used as plasticisers and stabilisers in other plastics. In the course of routine patch testing 21/1502 (1.4 per cent) patients reacted to a PVC film, which at that time was part of the patch test units. After it was ascertained that the PVC film contained 3–4 per cent of an epoxy plasticiser, 13 of the patients were tested to this resin 1 per cent in acetone and all reacted. None had been exposed to epoxy resin in industry, and it was presumed that sensitisation had been by domestic plastic articles. A further three patients developed dermatitis from a PVC handbag, a PVC chamber pot and a necklace respectively (Fregert and Rorsman, 1963).

In the course of investigating a man with a spectacle frame dermatitis, Jordan and Dahl (1971) found that he had an incidental positive patch test to diglycidyl ether of bisphenol A and that he reacted to the vinyl backing of an adhesive tape. They ascertained that this uncured epoxy compound was present as a stabiliser in the tape.

Glue. Two housewives sensitised by a home pack of epoxy resin were mentioned by Fregert (1973).

Paint. Dermatitis in a kitchen worker was atrributed to her job until patch testing showed her to be unexpectedly sensitive to epoxy resin; the dermatitis was then traced to a two-component paint she had used for painting cattle fodder trays (Malten, 1977d).

Spectacle frames. A plastic material 'Optyl', made of epoxy resin, has been used in Austria to make spectacle frames, apparently without trouble (Herzberg, 1973). But Fisher (1976) has reported that Optyl spectacle frames covered with a polyurethane lacquer, which were imported from Hong Kong, caused dermatitis of the face in a woman previously sensitised by an epoxy glue. Patch tests: she reacted to scrapings from the frames but not to polyurethane resin monomers.

Pacemaker. A pacemaker with an epoxy resin coating (hardened with diethylenetriamine) caused a dermal inflammatory reaction in a man who later tolerated a replacement in a titanium capsule. Patch tests were not reproducible and the reaction remained unexplained (Andersen, 1979).

St John's

From 1971–1976, 111 men and 47 women were found to be sensitive to epoxy resin.

Among the 111 men the exposure was occupational in 81 (73 per cent), domestic glue in 12 (11 per cent) and untraced in 18 (16 per cent). The most frequent occupations were the aircraft, assembly and engineering, electrical, construction and cable industries (Table 12.3).

Table 12.3. Source of epoxy resin sensitisation in 111 men and 47 women (St John's 1971–1976).

Occupational	Men Number	%	Women Number	%
Aircraft	20			
Assembly and engineering	17		4	
Electrical	10		7	
Construction	7			
Cables	6			
Plastics factory	5			
Carpenters	3			
Cars	2			
Inks	2		1	
Paints	2			
Glue	2			
Embedding crystals	1			
General repairs	1			
Aerial manufacture	1			
Metallurgy	1			
Microscopy	1		1	
Making jewellery			4	
Sculpture			1	
		73		38
Domestic				
Glue	12		8	
Varnish			1	
		11		19
Source unknown	18	16	20	43
	111		47	

Among the 47 women the sensitisation was occupational in 18 (38 per cent), domestic glue or varnish in 9 (19 per cent) and untraced in 20 (43 per cent). The most frequent work was in the electrical and electronics industries (Table 12.3).

Clinical features

The primary sites of epoxy resin dermatitis are the face and hands, both being affected in most patients; the eczema frequently affects the arms too, and it may spread widely. Sometimes the dermatitis is confined to the hands and less often to the face.

The eruption may be acute and episodic, starting with irritation of the eyelids and progressing to an explosive attack of marked facial oedema, particularly of the eyelids, and an exudative eczema of the hands and arms. The dermatitis may then spread to the neck, retroauricular folds, scalp, skin of the thighs under pockets, and the legs. In a few cases the genitalia and perianal region are affected by contamination from the fingers (Calnan, 1958; 1975).

In those with dermatitis restricted to the hands or fingers, there may be a subacute papulovesicular eruption, or a chronic eczema with lichenification, fissuring and occasionally a psoriasiform appearance (Calnan, 1975).

In an analysis of 170 patients seen at St John's Calnan (1975) listed the sites affected in order of frequency as:

face   (86) hands (82) eyelids (75) arms   (55)
wrist   (33) neck   (25) legs   (15) genitalia (8)
scalp   (4)

Epoxy resin sensitisation should be considered in every man presenting with a sudden onset of facial eczema accentuated around the eyes.

Results of patch testing

Resin and hardener

Sensitivity to epoxy resin, whatever the source of exposure, is investigated by patch testing with a standard low molecular weight epoxy resin, and practically all those sensitised will react. It is not an absolutely reliable screen because a man who had a negative patch test to the standard epoxy resin, reacted to the one he had been using (Calnan, 1973), and two out of 31 patients with epoxy dermatitis reacted to patch tests with phenylglycidyl ether or butylglycidyl ether (1 per cent in petrolatum) but not to epoxy resin (1 per cent in petrolatum) (Behrbohm, Nehring and Nehring, 1975).

In contrast, there is no one chemical which will screen for sensitisation to the many different hardeners, and several must be used for testing. At the time of the investigation, the hardener is usually unknown and may have to be identified subsequently through the factory and manufacturer. These factors make it more difficult to establish allergy to the hardener. Of 31 patients with epoxy resin dermatitis investigated by Behrbohm, Nehring and Nehring (1975), three reacted only to hardeners, of which two were based on aromatic aminopolyamides and one contained diaminodiphenylmethane. *Meta*-phenylenediamine, used as a hardener, caused an allergic contact dermatitis of the hands in a man who had been using it at work for two years. Patch tests: he reacted to *meta*phenylenediamine, *para*phenylenediamine (PPD), benzidine and toluidine (each 2 per cent in petrolatum) and to aniline (5 per cent in petrolatum). He did not react to epoxy resin. Thin-layer chromatography confirmed that the *meta*phenylenediamine contained trace amounts of PPD. Two other men with hand eczema, working in the same factory, had positive patch tests to epoxy resin and to triethylenetriamine, but not to *meta*phenylenediamine (Rudzki and Krajewska, 1974). Three men making plastic tennis rackets were sensitised by the hardener, isophorone diamine (IPD) and the epoxy resin(Lachapelle, Tennstedt and Dumont-Fruytier, 1978). Two further patients sensitised to IPD were reported by Dahlquist and Fregert, 1979b).

Foussereau and Benezra (1970) detailed the results of patch tests with the resin and hardener in seven small series of patients by seven different investigators. The aggregate of all these results showed that over half the patients were sensitive to the resin alone, one-third were sensitive to both the resin and the hardener, and only about a tenth to the hardener alone.

	Positive	%
Resin	80	57
Hardener	13	9
Both	47	34
	140	100

(Adapted from Foussereau and Benezra, 1970)

In Warsaw Krajewska and Rudzki (1976) reported on a study of eight factories over a period of seven years, during which time 828 people were employed and 126 developed dermatitis. Ninety-nine were patch tested and approximately half (48 per cent) reacted to the resin and half (55 per cent) to triethylenetetramine and a third was sensitised to neither but some of these reacted to other hardeners or glycidyl ethers. Diethylenetriamine and ethylenediamine may cross-react (p. 245).

Anhydrides are infrequent sensitisers but dodecenyl-succinic anhydride caused an allergic contact dermatitis in an electron microscopy technician; on patch testing she reacted to this hardener 0.5 per cent in acetone but had no response to epoxy resin (Göransson, 1977).

St John's

In Calnan's (1958) series of 12 men sensitised in an aircraft factory, and 22 sporadic cases, 80 per cent were sensitive to the resin alone and two patients reacted only to the hardener.

As a routine, patients are tested with epoxy resin but testing with hardeners is selective; of the patients seen from 1971–1976, 157 were sensitive to the resin and one reacted only to a hardener, some patients were sensitised to both the resin and hardener but the total number is not known, because not all were tested with hardeners.

In summary, from the cases reported it seems that the majority of patients are sensitive to the resin, either alone or in combination with a hardener; sensitivity to the hardener alone does occur but it is less frequent.

Relevance of patch tests

In Fregert's (1973) series of 30 men sensitive to epoxy resins, the exposure was known in 23 and remained unexplained in only seven, whereas among 24 sensitised women the source was known in only four and was unknown in 20. He noted that when the resin was the only sensitiser, the allergy could usually be explained, but that if the reaction was associated with other positive patch tests, often to a balsam, its relevance was much less likely to be apparent.

The reaction to epoxy resins was found by van Ketel (1974) to be relevant in 6/9 sensitised patients, most of whom had acquired the sensitivity in the plastics industry.

St John's

Men
Of the 111 men seen from 1971–1976, the epoxy resin sensitivity was:

(i) the entire cause of the dermatitis	40	(36%)
(ii) superimposed upon an existing eczema or only partly responsible for the present contact dermatitis	34	(31%)
(iii) associated with a history of dermatitis in the past	19	(17%)
(iv) the source was untraced	18	(16%)

Women
Of the 47 women seen from 1971–1976, the epoxy resin sensitivity was

(i) the entire cause of their dermatitis	11	(23%)
(ii) superimposed upon an existing eczema, partly responsible for a present contact dermatitis, or with known domestic exposure	11	(23%)
(iii) associated with a history of dermatitis in the past	5	(11%)
(iv) the source was untraced	20	(43%)

Association with other positive patch tests

Men
Reactions to other patch test allergens occurred in about half the men presenting with epoxy resin dermatitis (19/40) and similarly in half of those with a relevant past history (11/19). Whereas, other positive patch tests were more frequent when the relevance was only partial (25/34) or when the source of exposure was unknown (15/18).

Unlike Fregert's (1973) results, reactions to balsam of Peru was infrequent in the whole group and occurred in only 13/111 patients. In 1971 and 1972 there was a significant, but unexplained, association of reactions between epoxy resin and PTBP resin 10 per cent in petrolatum (p. 618).

Women
The results were similar for the women: of those with present epoxy dermatitis, 4/11 had associated positive patch tests; of those in whom the epoxy reaction had past relevance 3/5 reacted to other allergens; of those in whom it had partial relevance 7/11 had other reactions; and among those in whom the relevance was unknown 15/20 had independent reactions. Only 3/47 reacted to balsam of Peru.

Patch testing

Resin
A low molecular weight epoxy resin monomer 2 per cent in petrolatum

Hardeners

Ethylenediamine	1 per cent in petrolatum
Diethylenetriamine	1 per cent in petrolatum
Triethylenetetramine	1 per cent in petrolatum
Dipropylenetriamine	1 per cent in petrolatum
Dimethylaminopropylamine	1 per cent in petrolatum
Boron trifluoride-ethylamine	1 per cent in petrolatum
Isophorone diamine	? 1 per cent or 0.1 per cent in olive oil
Phthalic anhydride	1 per cent in petrolatum
Hexahydrophthalic anhydride	1 per cent in petrolatum
Tri-2-ethyl hexoate of 2,4,6-tris (dimethyl-aminomethyl) phenol	1 per cent in petrolatum
2,4,6-tris (dimethylaminomethyl) phenol	1 per cent in petrolatum

Epoxy diluents:

Phenylglycidyl ether	0.25 per cent in MEK
Other glycidyl ethers	0.25 per cent in MEK

Components:

Bisphenol A	0.5 per cent and 1 per cent in petrolatum
Epichlorohydrin	1 per cent in petrolatum

Active sensitisation

Epoxy monomer. Active sensitisation was induced in 2/1690 persons tested with epoxy resin monomer (?1 per cent) by Fregert and Rorsman (1964). At St John's patch testing several thousand patients with epoxy resin monomer 2 per cent in petrolatum actively sensitised six patients—four women and two men (Calnan, 1975).

Phenylglycidyl ether, 1 per cent in acetone, sensitised 2/10 patients, without causing irritation at the patch test site (Fregert and Rorsman, 1964). Two patients were recorded by Calnan (1967) as having been sensitised by 10 per cent diglycidyl ether.

Respiratory symptoms

Epoxy resin workers have occasionally been described as developing respiratory symptoms, including rhinitis (Morris, 1959), nocturnal dyspnoea (Mehl, Fuchs and Foussereau, 1971) and asthma (Tolot *et al.*, 1961; Fawcett, Newman Taylor and Pepys, 1977). In this latter study the inhaled sensitisers were phthalic acid anhydride, trimellitic acid anhydride and triethylene tetramine.

Carcinogenicity
Some epoxy compounds are carcinogenic, but those found to be so are not used commercially, and the common commercial resin, based on epichlorohydrin and bisphenol A, apparently does not carry this risk. The work on carcinogenicity has been summarised briefly by Piper (1965).

Alopoecia. Dogs and rats were exposed to the vapour of phenyl glycidyl ether and the rats, but not the dogs developed alopecia (Lee, Terrill and Henry, 1977)

Control of the hazard
Epoxy resins are too useful in industry to be discarded because of their dermatitis risk and so the hazard has to be, and can be, greatly diminished by careful control in their handling.

Fregert (1972) has listed the following nine points for the prevention of dermatitis:

1. The workers should be informed of the risk and instructed in safety control. If possible the work should be localised in one department.
2. Instructions should be displayed in factories and reminders given regularly.
3. Warning labels and preventive measures should be present on all containers of epoxy resin.
4. Aliphatic amines should be replaced.
5. Mixing should always be done in disposable containers.
6. Protective creams should be those designed specifically for use with epoxy resins.
7. Protective clothing and gloves, preferably disposable, and aprons should be worn.
8. Cleansing should be with soap or waterless cleansers, not with solvents.
9. Good housekeeping is essential.

In his measures for the control of dermatitis, Birmingham (1959) stressed that batches of resin and hardener should be mixed under ventilation hoods which should also be used to cover sawing or grinding operations to remove the dust.

The effectiveness of a safety programme in a car factory has been described by Turner (1964), and in a plant developing and manufacturing these resins by Craigen (1975).

Demonstration of bisphenol A epoxy resins (Fregert and Trulsson, 1978)

Method A — a colour reaction. Although not specific for epoxy resin this test identifies the presence of a bisphenol A compound; it is positive with both cured and uncured epoxy resins. The sensitivity of the test is reduced by the presence of substances which darken in sulphuric acid.

About 0.1 g of material is dissolved in 2 ml of concentrated sulphuric acid by heating to 40–50°C in a water bath. If necessary the solution is diluted with acid to obtain an orange colour equivalent to 0.1 mole × 1^{-1} potassium dichromate solution. A drop of the solution is streaked across filter paper, if positive the streak turns purple within a minute and eventually becomes blue. A control test should be done simultaneously with a bisphenol A epoxy resin.

Method B—thin layer chromatography. This test identifies the presence of oligomers of low molecular weight (340, 624, and 908) in uncured epoxy resins of the bisphenol A type.

The sample, prepared as a 1 per cent solution in acetone, is compared on a chromatogram with a known standard low molecular weight epoxy solution.

Fregert and Trulsson (1978) have found these tests of practical value in demonstrating the presence of undeclared low molecular weight epoxy oligomers of the bisphenol A type.

Formaldehyde resins

Formaldehyde resins are of two types:

1. Phenol-formaldehyde polymers (Phenoplasts)
2. Amino-formaldehyde polymers (Aminoplasts: Carbamid-formaldehyde).

PHENOL FORMALDEHYDE POLYMERS

Chemistry

Phenol-formaldehyde polymers
Phenol-formaldehyde resins were the first synethetic polymers to be utilised commercially. In 1907 Baekeland patented the plastic and in 1910 he formed the General Bakelite Company in the United States.

These polymers are normally made by reacting phenol with formaldehyde, but cresols, xylenols, *p-tert*-butyl phenol, resorcinol or a mixture of phenols may be used as may furfural (furan polymers) or hexamethylenetetramine.

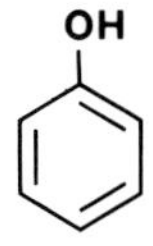

Phenol

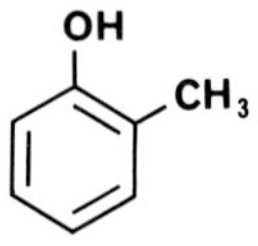

o-Cresol

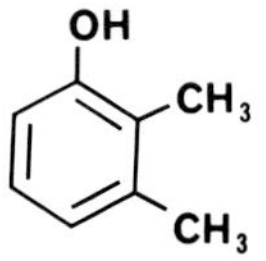

Xylenol

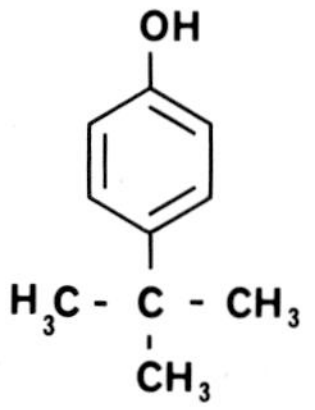

p-tert-Butylphenol

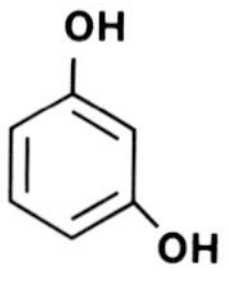

Resorcinol

Formaldehyde

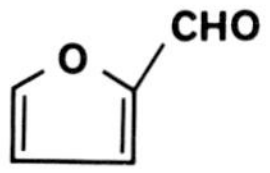

Furfural

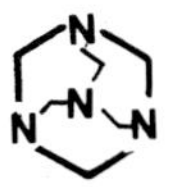

Hexamethylenetetramine

Phenol-formaldehyde resins are condensation products and are mainly utilised as network polymers. Low molecular weight resins and semi-cured resins are made and supplied commercially.

Resol resins
Resol resins are made by reacting phenol with an excess of formaldehyde in alkaline conditions; they contain reactive methylol (formaldehyde) groups and can be cross-linked by heat. The A-stage (Resol) is the initial low molecular weight resin, the B-stage (Resitol) is an intermediate partially polymerised form, and the C-stage (Resit) is the final network polymer.

Novolak resins
Novolak resins are prepared by reacting an excess of phenol with formaldehyde in acid conditions. The reaction is complete, leaving no free methylol groups in the monomers, so conversion to a final network polymer requires the addition of a chemical cross-linking agent.

Curing. Resols are cured by heat alone.

Novolaks require a cross-linking compound in addition to heat. Hexamethylenetetramine is generally used, but formaldehyde or paraformaldehyde are also effective.

Additives. Inert fillers are used to enhance the mechanical properties of the resins; wood flour is added to increase the brittle quality, cotton flock to confer toughness and asbestos for heat resistance. Pigments and dyes may also be added.

Uses
Phenol-formaldehyde resins are grey-black, hard solids which resist heat, moisture and solvents, and have good electrical resistance. They are used as:

Thermosetting moulding powders	(electrical appliances, electrical fittings, household fittings and handles)
Laminates and impregnation	
Adhesives	
Binders	(foundry sand moulds, oil-well sands)
Surface coatings	(paints, baked enamel coatings)
Brake linings and clutch facings	
Abrasive paper	(the paper is impregnated with resin, sprayed with sand and then cured)

Causes of dermatitis
The manufacture of formaldehyde resins in good working conditions carries a negligible risk of dermatitis (Harris, 1959). However, dermatitis may occur in workers using them in the course of their various occupations, and consumers are occasionally sensitised.

Phenol-formaldehyde plastics are listed by Fregert (1972) as causing both irritant and allergic dermatitis. Sensitisation has most frequently been reported as due to *p-tert*-butyl phenol formaldehyde resin, which is used as a glue.

P-TERT-BUTYL PHENOL FORMALDEHYDE (PTBP FORMALDEHYDE)

This resin is used as an adhesive because it sticks rapidly, is durable and pliable, and maintains good bond strength at raised temperatures; the flexibility of the adhesive makes it particularly useful for shoes and watch straps. It is formulated with a neoprene (synthetic rubber) base which binds the surface initially and allows the resin to cure with time.

PTBP resin is used occasionally in masonry sealants.

Leather glue — shoes — cobblers and shoe dermatitis

p-tert-Butyl phenol formaldehyde is particularly useful as a leather glue. In 1958, Malten described ten cobblers sensitised by a new adhesive used to glue the outer and inner soles of shoes. The cobbler held the outer sole in his left hand while using his right hand to brush on the glue, so that the exposed finger pulps of the left hand were often contaminated. When dermatitis supervened it affected the finger pulps particularly of the left hand, but to a lesser extent of the right hand, and, by contamination, the face, neck and, if the shoes had been held between them, the thighs. The eczema began as thickening of the skin and progressed to a painful fissured eczema. Patch tests: each man reacted to the resin 50–75 per cent in ethyl acetate and to the phenol (PTBP) 50 per cent in ethyl acetate, and two reacted to formaldehyde 1 per cent aqueous. Three patients similarly sensitised while making or repairing shoes were described by Calnan and Harman (1959). Patch tests: the three men reacted to the resin 5 per cent and the phenol 10 per cent but not to formaldehyde 2 per cent aqueous.

This shoe adhesive was subsequently reported as causing an allergic contact dermatitis of the feet (Malten and van Aerssen, 1962; de Vries, 1964; Suurmond and Verspijck Mijnssen, 1967). In van Ketel's (1974) series seven patients, of whom five had shoe dermatitis, were sensitive to this resin. Patch tests: each reacted to PTBP resin 1 per cent in petrolatum.

In 1977(c) Malten reviewed PTBP resin and its phenol as causes of occupational skin disease and shoe dermatitis.

Watch straps

When this adhesive is used to glue watch straps, it can cause an allergic dermatitis of the wearer's wrist (Foussereau, Petitjean and Barré, 1968).

Handbags

A man making handbags used this adhesive for two years and then became sensitised (Calnan and Harman, 1959).

Rubber glue — car factory

Rubber weather strips, coated with a PTBP resin adhesive, were used as seals on car doors and engines. The men wiped the rubber with a rag soaked in toluol, to make the surface tacky, before applying the strips. In three years, 50 men developed dermatitis and by patch testing 35 were found to be sensitive to the resin adhesive (Engel and Calnan, 1966). Without changing the adhesive the

outbreak was halted by discarding the toluol and by taking great care in working methods.

Domestic (do-it-yourself) glues
Adhesives for domestic odd-job enthusiasts may contain PTBP resins so that
exposure and sensitisation can occur in the home rather than at work. Such a
glue sensitised a retired man described by Moran and Martin-Pascual (1978).
He reacted to patch tests with PTBP resin and his glue but not to formaldehyde,

Incidence of sensitisation by PTBP resin

St John's
Since 1971, PTBP resin has been included in the standard series; between then
and 1976 28 men and 33 women (Table 12.4) were found to be sensitive, none of
whom reacted to epoxy resin, except for an electrician who had been exposed to
both resins.

The 32 patients seen in 1971 and 1972 with the unexplained association of reactions to PTBP resin and epoxy resin (p. 618) have been excluded.)

Table 12.4. Numbers of men and women sensitised by PTBP resin (St John's
1971–1976).

	1971	1972	1973	1974	1975	1976	Total
Men	1	1	3	8	5	10	28
Women	1	2	4	7	9	10	33

Sources of sensitisation
The various commercial PTBP resins which cause dermatitis have been
reviewed by Foussereau, Cavelier and Selig (1976). The sources of sensitisation
in their own 25 cases were: shoe manufacture (5) car industry (1) footwear (9)
watch straps (8) a belt (1) and a hat (1).

St John's
In both the 28 men and the 33 women, the source of contact was more often
domestic than occupational. The exposure was not traced in three of the men or in
nine of the women. The uses of the glue have been listed below:

Adhesives	Men	Women
Occupational		
Shoe mender or maker	3	1
Glues	6	
Can lacquer (research chemist)	1	
Non-occupational		
Woodwork	1	
Ceramics		1
Shoes	4	12
Watch strap	7	7
Glue	3	3
Unknown	3	9
	28	33

The sensitiser in PTBP-formaldehyde resin

In Malten's (1958) initial report, the ten cobblers had positive patch tests both to the phenol (PTBP) and to the resin (PTBP-formaldehyde). At that time the adhesive contained an excess of the phenol (PTBP). In his subsequent investigations (Malten and Aerssen, 1962) the findings differed, and one patient reacted only to the phenol (PTBP); the patients of Suurmond and Verspijck Mijnssen (1967) reacted only to the resin (PTBP-formaldehyde). Malten (1967) then confirmed, in guinea pigs, that the phenol (PTBP) and the resin sensitised independently. He recommended to the resin manufacturers that the adhesive be made without an excess of free PTBP, thus eliminating one allergen. Since then the resin (PTBP formaldehyde) has continued to sensitise, whereas sensitisation by the phenol (PTBP) is infrequent (Malten, 1967, 1973).

Polychloroprene glues were studied by Schubert and Agatha (1979) and they found the allergens not to be PTBP compounds but 2-hydroxy-5-tert-butyl benzyl alcohol and a four nuclear condensate derived from four PTBP molecules joined in a linear configuration by methylene bridges.

St John's

Of the 61 patients sensitive to PTBP resin, 22 were tested with the resin and with the phenol (PTBP 10 per cent in petrolatum); 10 reacted, nine to both the resin and the phenol, and one, a shoemaker, to the phenol but not to the resin.

Formaldehyde

As PTBP resin contains little or no free formaldehyde, it rarely if ever causes sensitivity to formaldehyde. In Malten's original paper, two of the ten cobblers were reported as having positive patch tests to 1 per cent formaldehyde in water, but he suggested that the source of exposure may have been antimycotic preparations in the leather rather than the resin.

St John's

Each of the 61 patients was tested with formaldehyde 2 per cent (aqueous) and none reacted.

Association of reactions to epoxy resins and to PTBP resin

In late 1971 and 1972 when PTBP resin 10 per cent in petrolatum was added to the standard series, it was found that most of the reactions occurred in patients who also reacted to epoxy resin, as follows:

	+ PTBP resin 10% + Epoxy resin 2%	+ PTBP resin 10% −Epoxy resin 2%	−PTBP resin 10% + Epoxy resin 2%
Men	22	2	1
Women	10	3	2

This association was not explained. In most patients there was no definite source of contact with PTBP resin but the use of glues at work or in the home was a possibility, and the concurrence with epoxy resin sensitivity occurred whether or not this allergy had present or past relevance or its origin was unknown. It is unlikely that these reactions to PTBP resin 10 per cent were irritant, as they did not occur in other patients. The possibility of a cross-reaction between the two resins or to an impurity was considered, but there was no evidence to support it.

In 1971 a woman was patch tested to the standard series, including epoxy resin but not PTBP resin and was negative to all of the tests; one patch test came up late but was not identified. In 1973 she returned for further investigation and was patch tested to the same standard series, to PTBP resin 10 per cent and to other selected allergens. She reacted to epoxy resin and to PTBP resin. There was no history of contact with either. It is interesting to speculate that she might have been actively sensitised by the epoxy resin patch test in 1971 which may also have sensitised her to PTBP resin.

In 1972, eight patients, who reacted to epoxy resin and PTBP resin 10 per cent, were additionally patch tested to PTBP resin 1 per cent in petrolatum from another source, and all were negative. To avoid the possibility of irritant reactions the standard allergen was changed, in 1973, to this particular PTBP resin 1 per cent in petrolatum and the curious association of positive patch tests to epoxy and PTBP resins ceased.

PHENOL FORMALDEHYDE

Phenol formaldehyde as a cause of occupational dermatitis has been reported sporadically in the literature. The sensitiser is the resin, although in an early account, formaldehyde was implicated (Bourret et al., 1958). In the experience of Hjorth and Fregert (1967) a coincidence of positive reactions to phenol formaldehyde and formaldehyde is very uncommon.

Paper

Abrasive Paper. While making abrasive paper, some workers developed dermatitis, and digestive and respiratory symptoms. The work entailed impregnating paper or textile with phenol formaldehyde resin in alcoholic solution, dusting it with abrasive particles and then drying it. Dermatitis occurred in nine of the 26 employees who did the work manually, and in seven of the 35 workers who used machines (Bompart and Smagghe, 1959).

A typewriter correction paper sensitised a secretary and caused dermatitis of her eyelids. Patch tests: she reacted to the correction paper and to a 1 per cent alcoholic solution of a modified phenol formaldehyde resin containing less than 1 per cent maleic anhydride. The formulation of the paper was not disclosed, but gas chromatography confirmed the presence of a phenol formaldehyde resin, which was assumed to be present to bind the powder to the surface of the paper. Ink, from writing on the paper, was thought to be a less likely source of the resin allergy (Jordan and Bourlas, 1975).

Filter paper and glue. A woman who operated two machines, one for making gasoline filters, the other for gluing, developed dermatitis of the eyelids, hands, arms and neck. It was confirmed that both the filter paper and the glue contained phenol-formaldehyde resin. Patch tests: she reacted to the filter paper but not to formaldehyde 5 per cent, or to phenol 1 per cent. Dilutions of phenol-formaldehyde resin in isopropyl alcohol were dabbed on her arm and she reacted to the 1 per cent solution (Gaul, 1967).

Treatment of fabric with resin
A man developed dermatitis on his face and hands while using a phenolcresol resin and melamine formaldehyde to impregnate cotton fabric and rolls of fibre, which were subsequently baked. Patch tests: he reacted to the cotton containing phenolcresol resin, the fibre containing melamine formaldehyde, and to phenolcresol resin and melamine formaldehyde resin, each 5 per cent, 2.5 per cent and 1 per cent in petrolatum. Tests with formaldehyde 2 per cent, and with the melamine formaldehyde resin used for routine patch testing were both negative (Simpson, 1972).

Glues and varnishes
Phenol formaldehyde in glues and varnishes was reported by Pardon and Bompart (1959) to be a cause of dermatitis. Of three patients in van Ketel's (1974) series, two were thought to have been sensitised by a glue.

Protective coating for cement
Eight construction workers were sensitised by phenol formaldehyde and six by formaldehyde in a resin mortar (Asplit) which they were applying to cement as a protective coating (Brunner, 1962). A similar preparation (Kramit) caused both an irritant and an allergic dermatitis in four bricklayers; three had positive patch tests to the phenol formaldehyde preparation and two to formaldehyde (Sonneck, 1964).

Airborne exposure
A clerk in a Rockwool industry was sensitised by phenol formaldehyde resin present in the atmosphere through a defective ventilation system. This particular phenol formaldehyde resin contained an excess of formaldehyde (4–5 per cent) and of phenol (3 per cent). Patch tests: he reacted to the phenolic resin used at work, the standard phenolic resin used for routine testing (both 1 per cent in petrolatum), formaldehyde, dust from his desk and ethanol in which air from the office had been dissolved (Tegner and Fregert, 1973).

Finished products
Four patients developed contact dermatitis on their hands, arms, face, neck and genitalia after sawing masonite or using grinding wheels, both of which were made of phenolic resin. It was postulated that friction generated sufficient heat to break down the resin to allergenic low molecular weight components, which were scattered as dust. Patch tests: all reacted to phenolic resin 5 per cent in ethanol but not to formaldehyde (Fregert and Tegner, 1972).

Marking pen ink
A patient reacted to the ink of a marking pen used to locate patch test sites. Patch tests: he was tested with the ingredients at the concentration used in the ink, and reacted only to a phenolic formaldehyde maleic anhydride resin. This resin was added to reduce the ink's drying time (Maibach, 1973), but it is also used in other inks as a dye fixative to prevent bleeding and to enhance dye solubility (Jordan and Bourlas, 1975).

St John's

Phenol formaldehyde resin 5 per cent in petrolatum has been included in the standard series since 1974; from 1971–1976 sensitivity to it has been diagnosed only twice. The first patient was a man who used glues in his hobby of woodwork and had had eczema of the palms and soles for four months. Patch tests: he reacted to phenol formaldehyde 10 per cent in petrolatum but not to formaldehyde. The allergy was thought to be superimposed on a constitutional eczema as the skin failed to heal despite his avoiding glues. The second patient was a housewife with hand eczema, but no source or relevance for this resin allergy was found; she reacted also to formaldehyde.

Respiratory disease

A report from the U.S.A. (Schoenberg and Mitchell, 1975) suggests that workers exposed to the fumes of phenol formaldehyde resin for more than five years may develop chronic airway obstruction.

AMINO FORMALDEHYDE POLYMERS

The only commercially successful amino polymers are urea formaldehyde and melamine formaldehyde. Thiourea formaldehyde and aniline formaldehyde are made but are of little importance.

UREA FORMALDEHYDE

Urea formaldehyde is a thermosetting resin which condenses to become a network polymer. Methylolurcas are intermediate products formed during polymerisation.

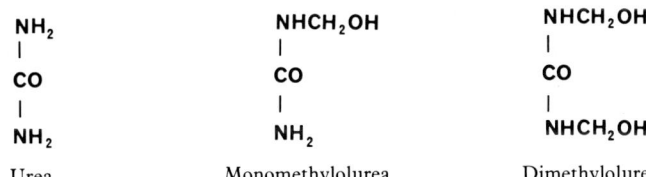

Urea   Monomethylolurea   Dimethylolurea

These resins can be modified by alcohol to make them more soluble and more reactive.

Curing

The resins are cured by heat in acid conditions.

Additives

Fillers are added to increase the mechanical strength of the resin, cellulose pulp is used if the colour is important, otherwise wood flour. Catalysts, lubricants, pigments and dyes may also be added.

Uses

The polymerised resin is a hard, insoluble material which can be made in a useful range of colours, including white. It has good electrical resistance but deteriorates and discolours with heat. It is used for:

Moulding powders (electrical fittings, bottle caps)
Wood glues
Surface coatings
Textile resins
Binder for foundry cores

Causes of dermatitis
Urea formaldehyde resins cause textile dermatitis (p. 64) and may sensitise in glues and in the manufacture of plastics. Urea formaldehyde resins break down to liberate free formaldehyde, and sensitivity to this resin and to formaldehyde are often associated. In Hjorth and Fregert's series (1967) of 67 patients sensitised by urea formaldehyde, 51 (76 per cent) reacted to formaldehyde too. Somov *et al.* (1976) used biochemical methods to investigate patients with immediate and delayed type hypersensitivity.

St John's
> A man who had been a foreman in a plastics factory for seven years suddenly developed eczema of his hands, face and neck. He wore rubber gloves at home. Patch tests: he reacted to thiurams, chemicals of the mercapto-group and repeatedly to our standard urea formaldehyde 10 per cent in petrolatum, but not to formaldehyde. As rubber chemicals were thought to be the principal allergens, he remained at work but changed to polythene gloves, and when seen subsequently he had only slight cracking of his finger pulps. Since he was able to remain at work, his contact with urea formaldehyde must have been slight, or his level of sensitivity low.

Immediate-type hypersensitivity
A woman, who developed urticaria while using a urea formaldehyde adhesive in the making of toilet rolls, was described by Jakovljevičová (1976). The urticaria was due to formaldehyde and it ceased once contact with the allergen was avoided.

MELAMINE FORMALDEHYDE
This amino resin, made from melamine and formaldehyde, forms a network polymer. Methylolmelamines are formed during polymerisation.

Melamine

Methylolmelamines can be reacted with alcohols to form methylated compounds which are used as textile resins and butylated resins which are soluble in paint solvents and are added to alkyds to enhance their properties.

Curing
Cure is effected by heat and accelerated by acidic compounds.

Additives
Fillers and colouring compounds may be added.

Uses
Melamine formaldehyde is a hard, insoluble plastic which is very similar to urea formaldehyde but has better heat and water resistance. As it also withstands staining by foods such as tea and coffee, it is used in preference to urea formaldehyde for tableware. Its uses include:
  Moulding compounds (including electrical fittings and tableware)
  Laminates
  Adhesives
  Increasing wet strength of paper
  Textile and leather treatments.

Causes of dermatitis
Melamine formaldehyde sometimes causes textile dermatitis (p. 63), otherwise it seems to be an infrequent sensitiser.

Orthopaedic plaster
Orthopaedic plaster reinforced with 10 per cent melamine formaldehyde resin caused a contact dermatitis in six patients reported by Logan and Perry (1972; 1973). Patch tests: all the patients reacted to 2.5 per cent aqueous formaldehyde but they were not tested with melamine formaldehyde.

St John's
  Apart from textile dermatitis (p. 64) cases of sensitivity have not been seen.

Patch testing

Monomers

p-tert-Butyl phenol formaldehyde	1 per cent in petrolatum
p-tert-Butyl phenol	10 per cent in petrolatum
Phenol formaldehyde	5–10 per cent in petrolatum
Urea formaldehyde	5–10 per cent in petrolatum
Melamine formaldehyde	5–10 per cent in petrolatum

These standard resins may give negative reactions when sensitivity is clinically strongly suspected; if this occurs the patient should be tested with his own resin suitably diluted.

FURAN POLYMERS

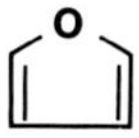

Furan

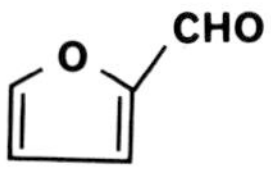

Furfural (2-furaldehyde)

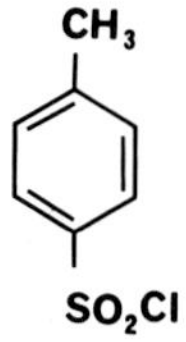

p-Toluenesulphonyl chloride (tosyl chloride)

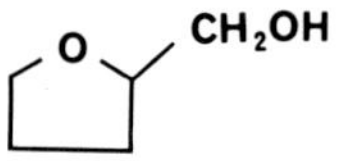

Furfuryl alcohol

Furfural and furfuryl alcohol are used to make furan resins. Furfuryl alcohol, heated in acid conditions, forms a polymer with good heat and chemical resistance. It is used in foundry sand cores, as an asphalt coating and as a corrosion resistant material in construction work. Furfural can be reacted with phenol to form a thermosetting resin.

Case report

A furan plastic, used in the construction of window frames, was polymerised by the catalytic action of p-toluenesulphonyl chloride. It caused an allergic contact dermatitis on the hands of a man after he had been handling the plastic for a year. Another man had, for 18 months, been intermittently in contact with furan resin during its use as an acid-resistant plaster in tanks of brick stone used for sulphite paper pulp. He suddenly developed dermatitis on his hands and face. Patch tests: both men reacted to p-toluenesulphonyl chloride 0.5 per cent in ethanol (Fregert, 1969).

COUMARONE-INDENE POLYMERS

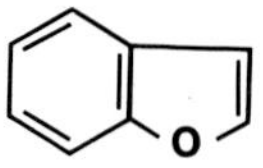

Coumarone (benzofuran)

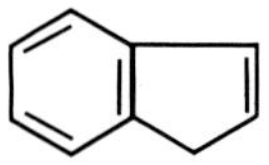

Indene

Coumarone and indene are derived from coal tar naphtha. Without separation they can be polymerised to a soft sticky material, which hardens to a solid resin. They are used in adhesives, varnishes, printing inks, waterproof materials, rubber and floor tiles.

Chemically they are inert compounds and they do not appear to cause dermatitis.

RESIN SYSTEMS WHICH CAUSE DERMATITIS

Polyester resins

1. UNSATURATED

Polyester resins are polycondensation, thermosetting compounds. They are esters and, by varying the reacting acid, alcohol or conditions of reaction, many types of polyesters can be made. The majority are unsaturated and contain sites for subsequent cross-linking. Linear unsaturated polyesters are high molecular weight syrupy compounds in which the unsaturated component is practically always the acid and not the diol. In the condensation process an anhydride is preferred to an acid because it avoids the production of water and in the presence of a catalyst and accelerator the final cross-linking can be carried out at room temperature.

Unsaturated dibasic acids or acid anhydrides

Diols

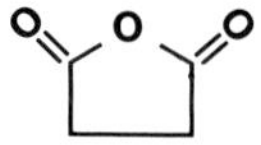

Maleic anhydride (generally used)

$$CH_3$$
$$|$$
$$HO-CH-CH_2-OH$$

Propylene glycol (preferred because its esters are compatible with styrene and it is inexpensive)

$$HC-COOH$$
$$||$$
$$HC-COOH$$

Maleic acid

$$HOCH_2-CH_2-O-CH_2-CH_2OH$$

Diethylene glycol (gives flexibility but increases water sensitivity)

$$CH-COOH$$
$$||$$
$$HOOC-CH$$

Fumaric acid (is less corrosive, gives paler products and better heat resistance than its *trans*-isomer maleic acid)

Modifiers

Modifiers are saturated dibasic acids or their anhydrides. They are added to reduce the number of unsaturated sites and by lessening the degree of cross-linking the final product is less brittle and is tougher and more flexible.

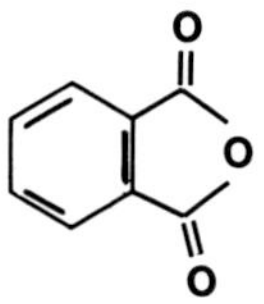

Phthalic anhydride

Phthalic anhydride polyesters are compatible with styrene, and the plastics formed are hard and rigid.

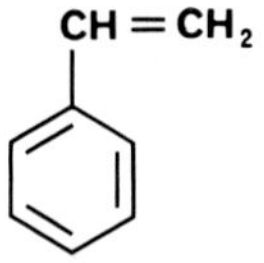

Styrene

Other modifiers are adipic and sebacic acids which give flexible products, and isophthalic acid which gives tough, heat resistant plastics.

Solvent

Styrene acts as a solvent and cross-linking agent.

Cross-linking agents

Styrene is the preferred cross-linking agent because it is compatible, easy to use and inexpensive.

Methyl methacrylate and styrene are used in the manufacture of translucent sheeting.

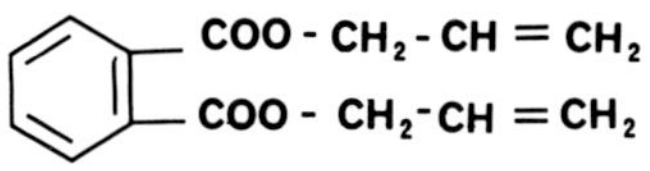

Diallyl phthalate

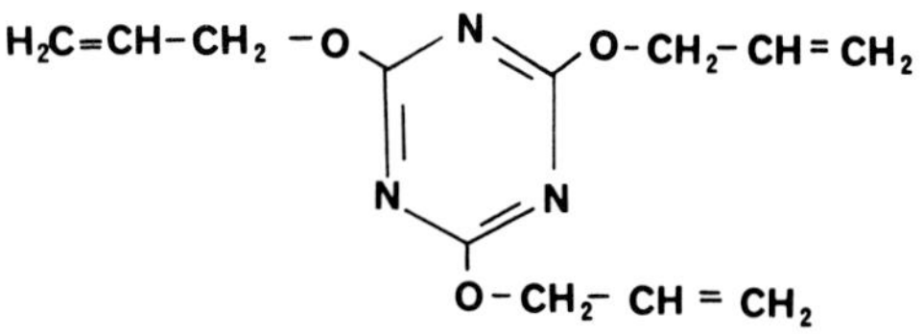

Triallyl cyanurate

Cross-linking by diallyl phthalate and triallyl cyanurate gives heat resistant products.

Catalysts and accelerators

The catalysts (initiators) are peroxides and they are always required for polymerisation regardless of whether the cure is 'hot' or 'cold'. They are supplied either undiluted or dispersed in a base such as dibutyl phthalate.

Accelerators (activators) are metal salts or tertiary amines and they are necessary only for curing in the 'cold' room temperature).

Heat curing: catalysts. In the cold, a mixture of polyester and peroxide is stable but heating decomposes the peroxides and liberates free radicals which rapidly initiate cross-linking. For heat curing benzoyl peroxide is usually used.

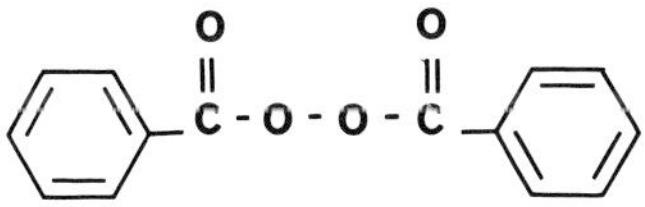

$$\text{Benzoyl peroxide}$$

Benzoyl peroxide

Cold curing: catalysts

Accelerators. For curing at room temperature a peroxy compound (catalyst) and an accelerator (activator) are necessary.

Hydroperoxides (catalysts) and metal salts (accelerators). In the 'cold' system, methyl ethyl ketone peroxide and cyclohexanone peroxide are widely used as catalysts or sources of free radicals. As commercial products neither is a single compound, both are mixtures of hydroperoxides.

These hydroperoxides are effectively decomposed by metal salts, particularly those of cobalt, but salts of iron, manganese, tin and vanadium are also used. Cobalt naphthenate is especially useful because it is freely soluble in the polyester resin, but cobalt octoate and stearate are also effective.

Peroxides (catalysts) and tertiary amines (accelerators). At room temperature, tertiary amines split peroxides, such as benzoyl peroxide, to liberate free radicals, but such resins have the disadvantage of discolouring and cracking with age. Dimethylaniline, diethylaniline and dimethyl-*p*-toluidine all react strongly with benzoyl peroxide.

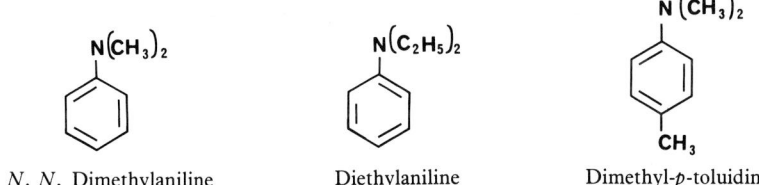

N, N, Dimethylaniline   Diethylaniline   Dimethyl-*p*-toluidine

Other additives
Polyester plastics are inflammable and may require a fire retardant; colours may also be added.

Uses
1. Reinforced plastic.
    The principal use of polyester is as a reinforced plastic in combination with fibre glass; as such it is used in the motor industry, for boat hulls, piping, roof panels and other structural applications.
2. Protective coatings, finishes and lacquers.
3. Enclosure of electrical equipment.

Technology

The manufacture of polyester resins requires considerable manual processing, and for those who work in close contact with unreacted components of the systems and who wear no protective clothing, the hazard is considerable.

For some applications the resin is used as a two component system.

1 = Resin (in styrene) + Accelerator
2 = Catalyst (peroxide).

Moulding

Fibre glass reinforced plastics are made in moulds which are either laid up by hand or with a spray machine. The glass fibre content varies from 5–90 per cent, and to enhance their adhesion to the resin, the fibres are coated with a finish of vinyl silane or methacrylate chromic chloride (Lim *et al.*, 1970).

Hand lay-up

After compounding and mixing the components of the resin system, sheets of fibre glass are immersed in the mixture and then laid by hand on to a mould until it is lined. Brushes and rollers are used to impregnate the resin and to remove any excess. Curing may be at room temperature or by heat. This technique allows for considerable skin contact.

Spray machine

The resin-glass fibre mixture can be fed into a spray gun which is then used to coat the mould. Skin contact occurs when the gun is being prepared and cleaned and also if excess resin is being rolled off the mould. Curing may be 'hot' or 'cold'.

Finishing

After curing, the mould is removed and the article is trimmed or 'flashed' to remove any excess material. This is done by cutting, sawing, grinding and sanding, and inevitably produces much polyester and fibre glass dust.

Casting

Fillers (powdered slate, chalk, glass fibre or fine mica) are added to thicken the resin system to a consistency varying from a viscous liquid to a dough. The mould is filled, if necessary, in a vacuum, and curing is by heat.

Lacquers and varnishes

A spray gun is used for coating or finishing techniques. The gun is loaded either with a freshly prepared mixture of resin and catalyst or with each component separately, the mixing taking place within the gun immediately prior to spraying.

To avoid excessive exposure during spraying, protective clothing, masks, spray booths and adequate extractor systems are essential.

Causes of dermatitis

Polyester dermatitis is an industrial disease and it extremely rarely affects the consumer. Polyester were listed by Fregert (1972) as one of the plastics commonly causing dermatitis, and in a survey of four plants making fibre glass reinforced plastics, Lim *et al.* (1970) found that dermatitis was a problem, in all four. Bourne and Milner (1963) also reported cases of dermatitis among polyester workers.

In most cases the dermatitis is irritant, not allergic.

Irritant dermatitis

Occupational

Workers are exposed to the irritant effects of fibre glass, solvents, acetone (which is used for cleansing), and the cross-linking compounds styrene and diallylphthalate.

Styrene

Styrene is a violatile liquid, with a pungent odour, which is a central nervous system poison, lethal to animals in high concentration. During manual moulding or heat curing, men may inhale sufficient vapour to cause styrene sickness, with malaise, drowsiness and anorexia. Styrene also irritates the upper respiratory tract, and this discomfort may be the main complaint of men exposed (Lim *et al.*, 1970).

Being a fat solvent, styrene can degrease and irritate the skin, and has been incriminated as causing burns (Bourne and Milner, 1963). However, Fregert (1971) stated that, even in hand lay-up procedures, polyester resin and styrene rarely cause dermatitis.

Diallyl phthalate

In a factory processing polyester resins, half the workers in a particular section developed dermatitis of the hands, arms and neck, usually within 2–4 months of starting work. There was prolonged skin contact with glass fibre and the unsaturated resin containing 60 per cent of diallyl phthalate as a cross-linking agent. In another section where styrene was used for cross-linking, there was no dermatitis. Patch tests: Styrene 50–100 per cent in acetone and diallylphthalate 0.25–1 per cent in acetone caused irritant reactions both in the workers with dermatitis and in controls (Firegert, 1971).

Peroxides —catalysts

Peroxides damage the eyes and may irritate the skin. They are supplied in solvents or plasticisers such as dimethyl phthalate (Malten and Zielhuis, 1964). Mixtures of peroxides and accelerators are explosive.

Dimethylaniline —accelerator

Dimethylaniline is absorbed through the skin, and is a poison which not only affects the central nervous system but also causes methaemoglobinaemia.

Allergic dermatitis —

Occupational

Polyester resins

There are few reports of allergic contact dermatitis. Malten and Zielhuis (1964) reported from Holland that five aircraft workers out of a group of 30 developed dermatitis within the first months of these resins being introduced. The men were unskilled in their use and no precautions were taken. They were found to be sensitive both to the resins and to other ingredients. Following this initial phase, precautions were taken and sensitisation by the resin stopped. A further three men laminating fibre glass were sensitised by additives in the system. These authors have also seen sensitisation to unsaturated polyester resins occurring in conjunction with epoxy resin dermatitis. They considered that dibutyl maleinate is a strong sensitiser.

From Germany, Wehle (1966) reported that following the introduction of polyester resins, 12 cases of sensitisation were seen in Dresden between 1962–65. Reactions were to the polyester resins and to other components of the system. In Czechoslovakia, Kadlec, Hanslian and Folprechtová (1974) reported nine cases of allergic contact dermatitis and one case of irritant dermatitis among 24 workers using two particular polyester paints, viz. B-1006 and B-1007. Three of these patients were sensitive to the polyester resin only, three to cobalt naphthenate only, and three to both. Patch tests: In the first two series, the patch test concentrations were not recorded, and in the Czechoslovakian series, the patients had been tested with the paints B-1006 and B-1007 (?undiluted) and with 2 per cent cobalt naphthenate in petrolatum.

	Malten and Zielhuis (1964)	Wehle (1966)	Kadlec et al. (1974)
Number of patients	8	12	9
Positive reactions			
Polyester resins	5	9	6
Benzoyl peroxide (paste)	3	2	
Cyclohexanone hydroperoxide	2		
Methyl ethyl ketone hydroperoxide	1		
Cobalt naphthenate	2	4	6
Dimethylaniline		1	
Dimethyl phthalate	1		
Dioctyl phthalate	1		
Adipic acid	1		
Fumaric acid	2		
Phthallic acid anhydride	1		

Diethyl ester of maleic acid

While investigating men who were working with unsaturated polyester resins, Malten and Zielhuis (1964) patch tested six volunteers with diethyl ester of maleic acid 0.5 per cent in alcohol, and in four the tests were positive at 24 hours. The reactions were considered to be allergic and they queried whether the patch tests may have actively sensitised these men.

Semi-stereate of maleic acid anhydride

A laboratory worker became sensitive to a semi-stearate of maleic acid anhydride nine days after beginning an experiment to synthesise it (Malten and Zielhuis, 1964).

Scottissue paper towels appeared to be the cause of dermatitis in a patient investigated by Klauder (1948). The patient reacted to a patch test with the paper, and when tested subsequently with resins used in paper manufacture he reacted to the diethylene glycol ester of 'abalyn' maleic anhydride. However, it was not established that this resin was in the paper.

Chromium compounds

Traces of hexavalent and trivalent chromium were detected in samples of fibre glass used to reinforce polyester resins. Its source was found to be the methacrylate chromic chloride finish (Lim *et al.*, 1970). As hexavalent chromate is a sensitiser, this finish is a potential cause of dermatitis.

Non-occupational

Cobalt

Perioral eczema in an eleven-year-old boy, who was found to be sensitive to cobalt, was attributed to the presence of cobalt in the polyester of his fountain pen and ball-point pen (Grimm, 1971).

St John's

Methyl ethyl ketone peroxide

A man, aged 53 years, had had his left leg amputated in 1942 and had worn an artificial limb with a leather socket for 20 years and a plastic socket for seven years, both without difficulty. In 1969, an exotosis was removed from the stump, and as this changed its shape, he was fitted with a new plastic socket, but within hours of wearing it he developed an acute dermatitis at the site of contact with the plastic. He resumed wearing a leather socket and his skin became normal, but on wearing the plastic socket again the dermatitis recurred. Patch tests: he reacted to methyl ethyl ketone peroxide 20 per cent, but not to the standard series, methyl, ethyl and butyl phthalates (5 per cent each), an accelerator, polyester resin rigid and polyester resin flexible (20 per cent each). Open tests: two applications of methyl ethyl ketone peroxide 20 per cent to his forearm caused itching, papules and vesicles. There was no response to the accelerator or to the rigid or the flexible polyesters.

Controls: 40 control patients were patch tested with methyl ethyl ketone peroxide 20 per cent, but none reacted.

Patch tests

	%	Diluent
Polyester monomer	? 10–20%	?
Benzoyl peroxide	1	Petrolatum
Cyclohexanone peroxide	? 5	Petrolatum
Methyl ethyl ketone peroxide	? 5	Petrolatum
Cobalt naphthenate	2	Petrolatum
Dimethylaniline	1	Petrolatum

	%	Diluent
Dimethyl phthalate	5	Petrolatum
Dioctyl phthalate	5	Petrolatum
Adipic acid	? 0.1–1	?
Fumaric acid	? 0.1–1	?
Phthallic anhydride	1	Alcohol
Maleic anhydride	1	Alcohol

Allyl resin — diallylglycol cabonate

Diallylglycol carbonate (DAGC) is a thermosetting resin and although it polymerises by polyaddition it is classified as a polyester. Heating the colourless liquid monomer with a peroxide catalyst, frequently isopropyl percarbonate, changes it to a colourless transparent solid with excellent optical properties. It is used by the optical industry for moulding into beading, tubes and transparent sheets.

Dermatitis — irritant

Those employed in filling the moulds with the monomer (DAGC) and catalyst mixture frequently develop an irritant dermatitis of the hands, sometimes of their faces, and the abdominal skin is affected if they carry contaminated trays to the ovens. The resultant erythema burns rather than itches and is aggravated by hot water. Extensive investigation by Lacroix *et al.* (1976) established that the dermatitis was due to the irritant effect of the DAGC monomer and no evidence of sensitisation was found. Patch tests with DAGC 1 per cent in olive oil gave irritant reactions in five of 22 controls. Simple protective measures greatly reduced the incidence of dermatitis.

II. SATURATED

Saturated polyesters are of several types and include alkyd resins for paints, polyester plasticisers and polyester fibres.

Alkyd resins

Alkyd resins are saturated polyesters modified by the addition of oil. The name is derived from their basic constituents, an *al*cohol and an *acid*. They are used as paints and surface coatings.

The saturated acids, anhydrides and alcohols most commonly used in their manufacture are listed below:

Saturated dibasic acids or anhydrides + polyhydric alcohols

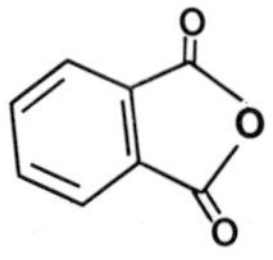

Phthalic anhydride

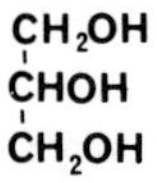

CH_2OH
$CHOH$
CH_2OH

Glycerol

Phthalic anhydride and glycerol are generally used because they are inexpensive and the resins produced are soluble, compatible and make good films.

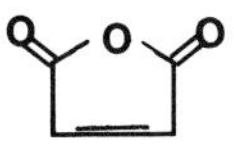

Maleic anhydride

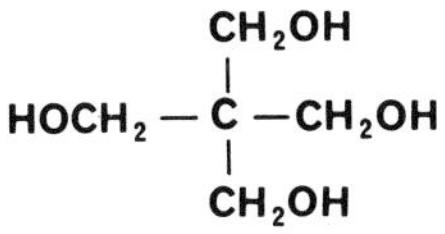

$$CH_3-CH_2-\overset{\overset{\displaystyle CH_2OH}{|}}{\underset{\underset{\displaystyle CH_2OH}{|}}{C}}-CH_2OH$$

Pentaerythritol

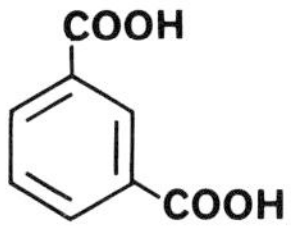

COOH

COOH

Isophthalic acid

$$CH_3-CH_2-\overset{\overset{\displaystyle CH_2OH}{|}}{\underset{\underset{\displaystyle CH_2OH}{|}}{C}}-CH_2OH$$

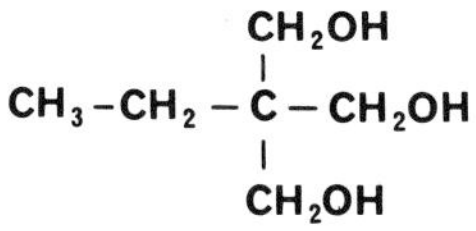

Trimethylolpropane

$$HOOC-(CH_2)_4-COOH$$

Adipic acid

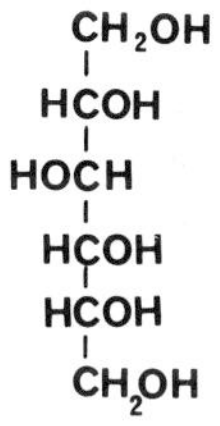

$$HOOC-(CH_2)_8-COOH$$

Sebacic acid

CH₂OH
HCOH
HOCH
HCOH
HCOH
CH₂OH

Sorbitol

MODIFYING OILS AND ACIDS

Oils

Oils are classified as drying, semi-drying and non-drying according to the length of time it takes a thin film to dry in the atmosphere. Drying oils take 2–6 days, a semi-drying oil is tacky at 7 seven days and a non-drying oil is still liquid at 20 days. Only vegetable oils are added to alkyd resins.

Drying Oils	*Semi-drying oils*	*Non-drying Oils*
Linseed	Dehydrated castor	Castor
Perilla	Safflower	Coconut
Tung	Soya bean	Cotton seed

The characteristics of alkyd resins depend largely upon the amount and type of added oil. Drying oils confer the property of drying; semi-drying oils withstand yellowing with age and so are particularly useful for white finishes.

A *short oil resin* contains less than 50 per cent oil; when a drying oil, the film is glossy, hard and suitable for signs and toys.

A *medium oil resin* contains 50–70 per cent oil; when a drying oil, the finish is glossy and durable, and is used for hardware, metal furniture, and implements.

A long oil resin contains more than 70 per cent oil; when a drying oil, the finish is glossy, durable, brushes on and dries quickly and is suitable for domestic paints.

Acids
Rosin (colophony), which contains abietic acid, and the synthetic fatty acid iso-octanoic acid and pelargonic acid may be added to the resin.

Modified alkyd resins
The inclusion of other compounds can improve the performance of alkyd resins: cellulose nitrate confers fast drying and strength, chlorinated rubber is fire-resistant and tough, and silicone resins improve heat and water resistance. Alkyd resins can also be chemically linked with other compounds: thus, phenolic resins increase their speed of drying and resistance to corrosion, while amino-resins harden and prolong the life of the resin (Saunders, 1973).

Uses
Alkyd resins are glossy, adhere well and withstand weathering, and as industrial finishes they give good protection for prolonged periods. They form the basis of most paints, varnishes and lacquers.

Causes of dermatitis
Dermatitis, whether irritant or allergic, appears to be very rare.

Irritant dermatitis

Phthalic acid anhydride (p.a.a.) or possibly contaminating impurities in it, causes irritation of the eyes, respiratory tract and gastro-intestinal tract. On moist skin, phthalic acid anhydride absorbs water to form phthalic acid which is caustic and produces burns (Malten and Zielhuis, 1964).

Maleic acid anhydride (m.a.a.) is readily hydrated to the caustic and irritant acid form (Malten and Zielhuis, 1964).

Naphthoquinone. Phthalic acid anhydride is formed by the catalytic oxidation of naphthalene, but the anhydride produced contains impurities including naph-thoquinone, which causes an indelible red-brown discolouration of wet skin (Malten and Zielhuis, 1964).

Allergic dermatitis
No report of allergic dermatitis from alkyd resins has been traced. Malten and Zielhuis (1964) suggested that naphthoquinones may act as contact sensitisers because they bind so readily to skin but they cited no other evidence.

Urticaria — phthalic anhydride. Urticaria from phthalic anhydride was described by Menschick (1955).

Rhinitis and asthma — phthalic anhydride. An industrial chemist, working in a laboratory where paints were tested, developed rhinitis and asthma which occurred only while he was at work. He suspected the dust of phthalic anhydride as the cause. Scratch tests with phthalic anhydride as crystals and as a 1/1000 solution were strongly positive in the chemist and negative in controls. A passive transfer of the patient's serum and a challenge with the 1/1000 solutions was positive (Kern, 1939). Both Baader (1955) and Menschick (1955) described asthma from phthalic anhydride as an occupational risk. Dr Menschick had asthma from it himself.

Patch testing

	%	Diluent
Phthalic acid or anhydride	1	Petrolatum
Maleic acid or anhydride	1	Petrolatum
Naphthoquinone	?	

Polyester plasticisers
Linear saturated polyesters of low molecular weight (500–8000) are viscous liquids which are used as plasticisers particularly for polyvinyl chloride. They have the advantage of being non-volatile and resistant to solvents.

Polyester fibres
Polyethylene terephthalate is a linear saturated polyester of high molecular weight (over 10 000). It is made as a fibre and is important in the manufacture of textiles, when it is often combined with wool or cotton.

Polyurethanes

Polyurethanes are polymers which contain isocyanate groups; polymerisation is by self-addition.

$$R-N=C=O \quad + \quad R'-OH \quad \longrightarrow \quad R-NH-CO-O-R'$$

An isocyanate   An alcoholic hydroxyl   A urethane

DIISOCYANATES

Diphenylmethane 4,4'-diisocyanate (MDI)

Toluene 2,4-diisocyanate (TDI; Tolylene diisocyanate)

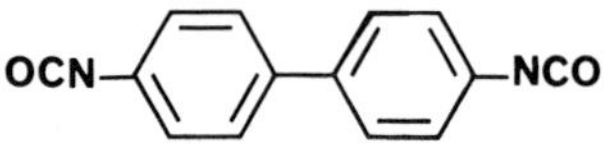

$$OCN-\hspace{-0.2cm}\langle\bigcirc\rangle\hspace{-0.2cm}-\hspace{-0.2cm}\langle\bigcirc\rangle\hspace{-0.2cm}-NCO$$

Diphenyl 4,4′-diisocyanate

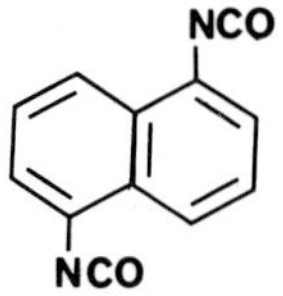

$$OCN-(CH_2)_6-NCO$$

Hexamethylene diisocyanate (HDI)

Naphthalene 1,5-diisocyanate (NDI)

The principal diisocyanates used in industry are toluene 2,4-diisocyanate, diphenylmethane diisocyanate, naphthalene 1,5-diisocyanate and hexamethylene diisocyanate. Desmodur is a trade name (Bayer AG) for these isocyanates.

Hydroxyl compounds

By varying the hydroxy compounds used in the reaction, the final polymer can vary from a soft rubbery elastomer to a rigid plastic. Polyesters and polyethers (Desmophens, Bayer AG) are most frequently used, but castor oil is employed as a hydroxy compound in the production of semi-rigid foams.

Catalysts

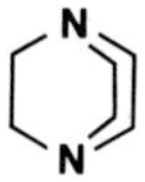

Triethylenediamine

The polymerisation reactions of isocyanates and hydroxy compounds are catalysed by tertiary amines (Desmorapid, Bayer AG), such as trie-thylenediamine, and by metal compounds, particularly the tin salts tributyltin acetate and dibutyltin diacetate. Each type of polymerisation requires its own catalyst.

Solvents

$$HCON(CH_3)_2$$

N, *N*-Dimethylformamide

$$CH_2Cl_2$$

Methylene chloride

Dimethylformamide and methylene chloride are solvents used in foam-making factories and they may be utilised to cleanse the machines of dried foam. Both are strong irritants.

Polyurethane products

Foams —flexible and rigid
During the formation of a polyurethane polymer it is possible to evolve and trap a gas so that a foam is produced. The rigidity of the foam depends upon the degree of cross-linking, which is itself controlled by the choice of reactants; a flexible foam is slightly cross-linked, and a hard foam is highly cross-linked.

Flexible foams are made in a one-stage procedure, usually with toluene diisocyanate together with a polyether in 80 per cent or with a polyester in 20 per cent. Water added to the reaction liberates carbon dioxide from the isocyanate to form a foam; the catalyst is a tin compound, a tertiary amine or both. Polyether foams have a high resilience and are used for upholstery; polyester foams have high tensile strength, they resist solvents and are suitable for textile laminates and padding.

Rigid foams are made in a similar way using a polyether, trichlorofluoromethane, which volatilises to a gas, and a tertiary amine as the catalyst. These rigid foams are good thermal and acoustic insulators and are also used in shipbuilding and motor components.

Elastomers —rubbers
These synthetic rubbers are of three types: cast, millable and thermoplastic.

Cast rubber is made by pouring the reacting compounds into a mould and curing them by heat; alteration of the technique and reactants modifies the properties of the rubber produced.

Millable elastomers are made so that they can be milled with other ingredients, and vulcanised by isocyanates, sulphur compounds and peroxides.

Thermoplastic rubbers cross-link during polymerisation and require no subsequent vulcanisation: they are elastic at normal temperatures and pliable at high temperatures.
　　These rubbers are used for printing rollers, oil seals, solid tyres, driving belts, coatings for metal buffers and bumpers, and shoe heels.

Fibres —elastomeric
Polyurethane can be made into a fibre similar to nylon, but as it is difficult to dye and feels harsh, it is of no commercial value. However, an elastomeric fibre (spandex), made by spinning, is strong, withstands ageing and is easy to dye. It has been used extensively to replace natural rubber thread in brassières, girdles, underwear and swimsuits.

Surface coatings
Surface coatings may be polymerised as a one-component system by exposure to air, moisture or heat, or as a two-component system by mixing the isocyanate

and the hydroxyl compound immediately prior to use; curing occurs after spraying or application. The hazard of the volatility of toluene diisocyanate and hexamethylene diiosocyanate is partially overcome by polymerisation to form isocyanates or by combination with polyols to give isocyanates of high molecular weight. Small amounts of the primary isocyanate are likely to remain, and the actual quantity determines the risk of the coating to the user (Lowe, 1970).

Urethane oils are one such type of coating; they form films which resist abrasion and chemical attack but require an ultraviolet light absorber to reduce their tendency to turn yellow in air. They are used as fire-resistant wood varnishes and quick-drying enamels. Other types of coating are used for insulation, wire coverings, tank linings, maintenance paints and masonry coatings.

Adhesives
There are three categories of polyurethane adhesives. (i) The isocyanate-polyol type is a two-component system which is used for bonding wood, plastics and metal. (ii) Elastomers, soluble in solvents and similar to millable elastomers, are used as adhesives particularly in the shoe industry. (iii) Polyisocyanates, especially triphenylmethane 4,4′,4′′-triisocyanate, effectively bond rubber to metal, glass, synthetic fibres and to rubber itself.

Polyurethanes, as finished products, are virtually harmless to the consumer, but during production there is a considerable occupational hazard. The risk lies in the toxicity and pulmonary complications of exposure to isocyanates (Malten and Zielhuis, 1964), not to the other components of the plastic which seem to cause little trouble. Dermatitis is rare. Accidental spillage of isocyanates is dealt with by decontaminants based on ethanol and water.

Printing plates (light-sensitive urethane)
The Letterflex printing process utilises a urethane monomer cross-linked by a polythiol, which is polymerised by exposure to ultraviolet light in the presence of an initiator, such as benzophenone. The urethane monomer is produced by reacting toluene 2,4-diisocyanate with trimethylolpropane diallylether using dibutyltin dilaurate as a catalyst, the polythiol is penta erythritol-tetrakis-3-mercapto-propionate and di*tertiary*butyl paracresol is added as an antioxidant (Malten, 1977a).

Toxicity and pulmonary complications
The systemic toxicity and pulmonry complications are caused by inhalation.

Toluene diisocyanate (TDI)
Toluene diisocyanate is a very reactive and aromatic compound, and although it is the most useful it is also the most dangerous of the industrial isocyanates. It is a volatile liquid at room temperature, and as many polymerising reactions generate heat it is readily vaporised to exceed the accepted threshold limit value (TLV) of 0.02 ppm in the atmosphere. It is used particularly in the manufacture of flexible foam.

Acute exposure. Acute massive accidental exposure to toluene diisocyanate (TDI) may cause immediate symptoms of intoxication, or the illness may be delayed for 4–8 hours. Fireman fighting a fire at a polyurethane foam factory were suddenly exposed to high concentrations of TDI when a thousand gallons leaked on to the floor of the burning building (McKerrow, Davies and Parry Jones, 1970). Their pulmonary, gastric and neurological symptoms included: cough, tightness of the chest and breathlessness; nausea and vomiting; and euphoria, ataxia and loss of consciousness, followed by a mild encephalopathy (Fullerton, 1970).

A much less severe episode occurred in a naval shipyard when steel plate backed by polyurethane foam was burned, releasing toluene diisocyanate into the atmosphere. All the men exposed developed respiratory symptoms (Bergtholdt, 1961).

Chronic exposure. Exposure to dangerous levels of TDI in industry causes irritation of the eyes and respiratory tract and may induce a crippling pulmonary sensitisation. After days or months, workers complain of tightness of the chest, breathlessness and cough, which may continue at night and simulate bronchitis; some develop severe disabling asthmatic attacks. The symptoms subside when the men are away from work and recur on their return. Nasal discomfort may precede the pulmonary symptoms. Those severely affected require systemic corticosteroids. The pulmonary symptoms usually disappear once exposure ceases (Munn, 1965), but a few men are chronically disabled. Asthma in three clerical workers was traced by Carroll, Secombe and Pepys (1976) to exposure to TDI emanating from the exhausts of a neighbouring factory and sucked into the ventilation system of the office block in which they worked. Less volatile compounds are being substituted for TDI but it may still be present as an impurity in both diphenylmethane diisocyanate (MDI) and polymethylene polyphenyl isocyanate (PAPI) (Lubach, 1978).

It is now accepted that the asthma-like syndrome is allergic in nature and those who are highly sensitised react to minute quantities of TDI in the atmosphere. As yet there is no satisfactory skin test to demonstrate the allergy, but deliberate exposure to very low levels of TDI causes a fall in FEV_1 and may reproduce the dyspnoea. Asthma from TDI has been reviewed by Lubach (1979).

Diphenylmethane diisocyanate (MDI)

Diphenylmethane diisocyanate (MDI) is much less volatile than TDI and in comparison the vapour hazard is small, but if it is applied as a spray droplets of MDI may be inhaled and cause respiratory irritation and asthma (Munn, 1965).

Hexamethylene diisocyanate (HDI)

This aliphatic isocyanate is a volatile liquid which is much less reactive than the aromatic isocyanates TDI and MDI and therefore has limited commercial value. It is toxic to the eyes and skin and can cause respiratory symptoms (Munn, 1965).

Naphthalene diisocyanate (NDI)

This isocyanate is a solid at room temperature. Munn (1965) has seen three cases of sensitisation.

Polyurethane foam. A single case report (Tolot, Bresson, Dhers and Beaupère, 1960) described the manageress of a toy factory who developed attacks of conjunctivitis, pharyngitis and then asthma, which were directly related to her being at work, where she was exposed to a fine dust of polyurethane. Other workers were not affected. She was skin tested to the various products she handled and reacted only to the polyurethane foam.

Decomposition products of burning polyurethane foam. While burning, polyurethane foam decomposes to toxic products, and experimentally rats have died after inhaling high concentrations of these products (MacFarland and Leong, 1962).

Dermatitis and other skin lesions
The isocyanates, and the hardeners occasionally cause dermatitis but the polyalcohols and polyurethane itself, rarely affect the skin. Malten and Zielhuis (1964) suggested that this is due to the care with which these irritant chemicals are handled.

ISOCYANATES

Toluene diisocyanate (TDI)

Allergic contact dermatitis. One case was described by Peschel (1970); this was a woman who had worked for many years with latex foam in a chemical factory. Two weeks after being transferred to the polyurethane foam section she developed, on one arm, an eczema which spread to her hands, arms, face and neck. She stopped work and her skin healed, and when she returned to work in another department, she remained well. Patch tests: initial tests were with mixtures of components but eight months later she was tested with toluene diisocyanate 0.5 per cent and 0.1 per cent in acetone; she reacted to the stronger solution, but not to the weaker.

Irritant contact dermatitis. Irritant dermatitis from TDI in two workers processing polyurethane has been reported by Rothe (1976).

Thrombocytopenic purpura. There is one report (Jennings and Gower, 1963) which describes the cases of two men, heavily exposed to TDI, who developed pulmonary symptoms followed by thrombocytopenia. One had a persistent, widespread purpura which eventually required splenectomy, but the other had only minimal purpura and his platelet count spontaneously returned to normal after three weeks.

Diphenylmethane diisocyanate (MDI). Isophorone Diisocyanate (IPDI)
Allergic contact dermatitis from MDI in workers processing polyurethane has been reported by Rothe (1976); isophorone diisocyanate (IPDI) and triisocyanate-triphenylmethane also caused dermatitis. The investigation suggested cross-sensitivity between MDI and diaminodiphenylmethane. There is also cross-sensitivity between isophorone diisocyanate(IPDI) and the chemically related epoxy hardener isophorone diamine(IPD) but their industrial use is entirely different (Lachapelle and Lachapelle-Ketelaer, 1979).

Diphenyl diisocyanate

Allergic contact dermatitis. Three men developed dermatitis of the hands and face after working for two weeks with a mixture containing diphenyl 4,4-diisocyanate (Desmodure VL, Bayer), castor oil and coal tar. Only one was referred for investigation. Patch tests: he reacted to diphenyl diisocyanate 1 per cent in acetone, coal tar, phenol formaldehyde resin and diaminodiphenylmethane, but not to toluene diisocyanate. The diaminodiphenylmethane sensitivity was attributed to rubber gloves, and the phenol formaldehyde resin response was tentatively explained as a cross-reaction with coal tar (Fregert, 1967).

Polymethylene polyphenyl isocyanate (PAPI)
Cases of sensitivity have been described by Rothe (1976).

Methylene bis(4-cyclohexylisocyanate)
In a small polyurethane plant seven plastic moulders were sensitised by fumes from ovens and open containers and direct skin contamination. The two patients patch tested reacted to the resin methylene bis(4-cyclohexylisocyanate) 1 per cent in pet. and to the catalyst methylenedianiline 1 per cent in olive oil. Hygienic measures stopped the outbreak (Emmett, 1976).

Trimethyl hexamethylene diisocyanate (TMDI)
A laboratory technician developed an allergic contact dermatitis from TMDI after working for one month in a paint factory. Patch tests: she reacted to TMDI 0.5 per cent in acetone. Twenty controls were negative (Hjorth, 1975).

HARDENERS

Light sensitive urethane prepolymer mixture (Penta Erythritol-tetrakis-3 mercaptopropionate) Letterflex printing plates coated with a light sensitive urethane prepolymer mixture have caused allergic contact dermatitis in printers in Holland (Malten, 1977a) and in France (Calas *et al.*, 1976, 1977). The mixture is slightly irritant and may cause a transient erythema of the skin, which is distinct from the eczema of the hands, fingers, subungual skin and sometimes arms and face that occurs in those who are sensitised. By using the guinea pig maximisation test Calas *et al.* (1977) were able to identify the allergen as the polythiol (penta erythritol-tetrakis-3 mercaptopropionate). Patch tests: Malten's (1977a) patients reacted to the unpolymerised mixture 5–10 per cent in alcohol or methyl ethyl ketone; the patients of Calas *et al.* (1977) reacted to the polythiol 0.1–1 per cent in acetone. Malten (1977b) then investigated seven more newspaper printers and found that five were sensitised to the polythiol hardener, penta erythritol-tetrakis-3 mercaptopropionate but also to 3-mercaptopropionic acid another component of the mixture (the patch test concentrations were 1 per cent in MEK).

Triethylamine. Allergic contact dermatitis. Triethylamine, used as a hardener in the manufacture of polyurethane, sensitised two men (Wodiansky, 1967). Patch tests with triethylamine 0.1 per cent were positive. Positive reactions to the hydroxyl compound (Desmophen) were attributed to contamination by amines.

POLYETHER ALCOHOL

A man developed a widespread eczema while mixing poyols and catalysts in open barrels. Patch tests with the amines and other chemicals were negative but the undiluted polyol, a polyether alcohol, Desmophen 6510, produced a strong reaction. Nine controls were negative (Verdich and Skoven, 1979).

POLYURETHANE LACQUER

Urticaria. After he had applied polyurethane lacquer to floorboards, a man developed acute asthma and urticaria and died the following day (Schürmann, 1955).

Patch testing

	%	Diluent
Toluene diisocyanate (TDI)	1.0	pet. or acetone
Methyl diisocyanate (MDI)	1.0	pet. or acetone
Isophorone diisocynate (IPDI)	1.0	pet. or acetone
Polymethylene polyphenyl isocyanate (PAPI)	3	pet. or acetone
Triphenylmethane triisocyanate	1.0	pet. or acetone
Letterflex polythiol	0.1–1.0	Acetone
(penta-erythritol-tetrakis-3 mercapto-propionate)		
Polyesters	?0.5–1.0	?Petrolatum
Polyethers	?0.5–1.0	?Petrolatum
Amine catalysts	0.5–1.0	Petrolatum

MONOMERS NON-ALLERGIC BUT SENSITISING ADDITIVES

Cellulose polymers

Regenerated cellulose

Rayon is an important textile, made by solubilising cellulose in alkali and regenerating it in acid solution. The viscose process is the principal method of production and gives viscose rayon its name.

Cellophane, which is used for packaging, is transparent sheeting of regenerated cellulose, made by the viscose process.

Cellulose nitrate

Pyroxylin is nitrocellulose.

Gun cotton is a nitrocellulose explosive.

Collodion, a protective film used for wounds, is a solution of cellulose nitrate in ether and ethanol.

Celluloid, made in 1872, was the first successful plastic, and though superseded by newer materials, it is still used as a lacquer for furniture. Essentially, it is made of cellulose nitrate plasticised with camphor, but other plasticisers, such as dibutyl phthalate or tricresyl phosphate, and also pigments may be added. It is highly inflammable.

The inflammability of cellulose nitrate limits its commercial application, but the material gives good colour effects and is used for imitation ivory knife handles and tortoiseshell spectacle frames.

Cellulose acetate

Fibre: Acetate rayon was developed in the 1920s by the British Celanese Company (UK) and is still a major textile.

Injection moulding: Moulded items are now limited to a few articles such as toothbrushes, combs and knife handles.

Film: Cellulose acetate film is used for packaging, photographic and X-ray films.

Sheet: As sheets, cellulose acetate is made into spectacle frames and display boxes.

Lacquer: Cellulose acetate is sometimes used as a lacquer to coat fabrics, glass, metal and paper.

These various types of cellulose acetate are rendered malleable by plasticisers, such as dimethylphthalate and triphenylphosphate, and colours are also often added.

Causes of dermatitis
Contact dermatitis from cellulose plastics is infrequent and cases which do occur seem to be principally, if not entirely, due to cellulose acetate. The plastic itself is non-allergenic but some of the additives used in its manufacture can sensitise. Consumers in contact with the finished products, rather than workers in the industry, are sensitised. Spectacle frames are the commonest cause of dermatitis, but it has also been reported from ball-point pens, a hearing aid, a patch test film and a steering wheel.

Spectacle frames
Most spectacle frames are made of metal or plastic; wood is occasionally used, but tortoiseshell rarely, because of its expense.

Metal. Metal frames consist of a central core plated with a silver-coloured nickel alloy or a gold film of varying carat. The nickel alloy consists of copper, zinc and nickel.

Plastic. Frames are usually made of cellulose acetate; cellulose nitrate is used infrequently, because of its inflammability. A few frames are made of perspex (polymethylmethacrylate), or of Optyl, an epoxy resin (p. 608).

During manufacture, plasticisers, ultraviolet light stabilisers, antioxidants and colourants are added to the plastic, and polishes are used for the final finish (Jordan and Dahl, 1972).

Dermatitis — clinical features

The eczema is confined to the sites where the frames touch the skin, namely the bridge and sides of the nose, the temples and behind the ears. The eyes are not in contact with the frames and are not involved and neither are the cheeks except occasionally when the lower edge of the frame touches them.

Causes of dermatitis

Nickel. Nickel is the sensitiser in silver-coloured metal spectacle frames. Very small amounts of nickel may also be present in low carat yellow gold wire used for some frames, but as the concentration is low it probably rarely gives trouble (p. 351).

Cellulose acetate — allergic

The plastic is not a sensitiser, but its additives may be. Triphenyl phosphate, resorcinol monobenzoate, *p-tert*-butyl phenol, azo dyes, ethylene glycol mono-methyl ether acetate and turpentine have all been reported as the cause of allergic contact dermatitis from spectacle frames.

1. *Plasticiser — triphenyl phosphate*. A woman, sensitive to tricresyl phosphate in polyvinyl chloride, also had dermatitis from triphenyl phosphate in her cellulose acetate spectacle frames. Patch tests: she reacted to triphenyl phosphate (1 per cent in both arachis oil and acetone), to tricresyl phosphate (5 per cent in arachis oil), her spectacle frames and PVC from various articles (Pegum, 1966).

2. *Ultraviolet light stabiliser — resorcinol monobenzoate*.

Resorcinol monobenzoate is a colourless, ultraviolet light absorber which is added to plastics to prevent deterioration by sunlight. It is no longer used in domestic articles such as spectacle frames, pens and hearing aids but is still added to outdoor plastics including signs and lighting fixtures (Jordan and Dahl, 1972).

This compound was the sensitiser in two cases of determatitis from sunglasses reported by Jordan and Dahl (1972). Patch tests: both patients reacted to resor-cinol monobenzoate 1 per cent in petrolatum but not to resorcinol. Two of three patients sensitive to resorcinol monobenzoate were patch tested to balsam of Peru and both reacted.

St John's

A woman with palmar eczema and contact dermatitis from her spectacle frames was reported by Calnan (1975). Patch tests: she reacted to resorcinol monobenzoate 1 per cent, balsam of Peru 25 per cent, and had an unexplained reaction to ethylenediamine 1 per cent, each in petrolatum. A negative patch test to her spectacle frames was considered to be a false negative reaction.

3. *Antioxidant — p-tert*-butyl phenol

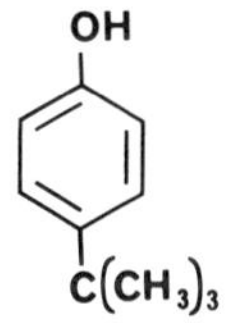

Para-tertiary-butyl phenol, in a concentration less than 0.5 per cent, is added to plastics to prevent discolouration and photo-oxidation.

A patient who was very sensitive to it developed dermatitis on the sides of the nose and temples from carbon black eye glasses, on the left breast from a ball-point pen in his shirt pocket, and on the feet from a shoe adhesive; all of these items contained this chemical. Patch tests: he reacted to *p-tert*-butyl phenol 2 per cent in petrolatum (Jordan and Dahl, 1972).

4. *Colours — azo dyes*. Solvent yellow 3 (C.I. No. 11160). Solvent red 26 (C.I. No. 26120). Pigment red 481 (C.I. No. 15865:1).

Pigments are generally added to plastics because dyes, although used, have a tendency to bleed. The pigments include carbon black, cadmium reds and yellows, chrome yellows and oranges, iron oxides, molybdate oranges, phthalocyanine blues and greens, and ultramarine blues. The dyes include azo and anthraquinone dyes, nigrosine and triphenylmethane dyes (Jordan and Dahl, 1972).

Two patients with dermatitis from mirror-black spectacle frames had been sensitised by the dyes. Patch tests: both patients reacted to the azo dye Solvent Yellow 3 (Colour Index No. 11160), and one also to an azo naphthol dye Solvent Red 26 (Colour Index No. 26120). The dyes were diluted 1 per cent in petrolatum.

St John's

Pigment Red 481 C.I. No. 15865:1 (Rubine Toner B.S. 8820; 6-Amino-4-chloro-*m*-toluenesulfonic acid)

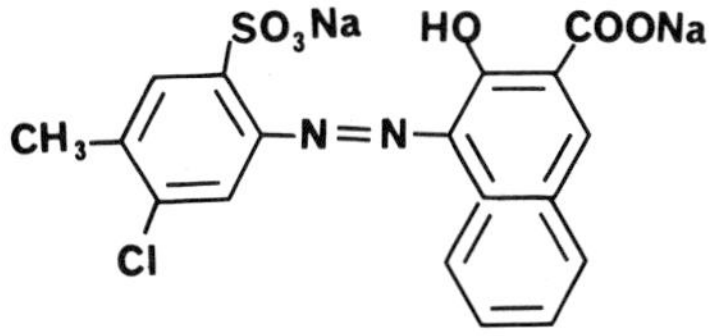

Patients suspected of having spectacle frame dermatitis are tested with a series of selected compounds, including Rubine Toner, used in the making of cellulose acetate for eye glasses. Three patients have reacted to this azo dye (50 per cent in petrolatum). One hundred controls were negative. It was not possible to confirm that this dye was present in their spectacle frames.

5. *Solvent — ethylene glycol monomethyl ether acetate*. (Methyl Cellosolve Acetate)

$$CH_3 - \overset{\overset{\displaystyle O}{\|}}{C} \underset{O - CH_2 - CH_2 - O - CH_3}{\diagdown}$$

Ethylene glycol monomethyl ether acetate (EGMEA) is a good solvent for cellulose plastics and is used to join the nosepads of spectacles to the frames. It acts as an adhesive for cellophane and may also be added to lacquers, varnish removers and wood stains.

A woman bought new eyeglasses and within a week developed acute eczema on the sides of her nose, under the nose pads. The rest of the frame was comfortable. Patch tests: she was tested to a series of chemicals including the solvents used to cement the nosepieces to the frame. She reacted to EGMEA 0.01 per cent and cross-reacted to ethyl acetate 0.1 per cent (both in MEK). Shavings from the spectacles elicited no response (Jordan and Dahl, 1971).

6. *Polish — turpentine*. A man known to be sensitive to turpentine developed an acute dermatitis from contact with his spectacle frames, and this flared when he changed to a new pair of glasses. It was ascertained that a beeswax and turpentine polish was used by the manufacturers to give eyeglass frames a glossy finish. Patch tests: he reacted strongly to his spectacle frames and to the beeswax and turpentine polish 5 per cent, but not to beeswax, other ingredients of the cellulose acetate or to the identical plastic unpolished (Jordan, 1972).

Plastic — Irritant dermatitis

Irritant dermatitis from cracked, worn and dust-laden spectacles has been described (Smith and Calnan, 1966), and some of the chemicals in the plastic are thought to cause an irritant contact dermatitis, but no compound has been specifically incriminated (Jordan and Dahl, 1972). These patients have negative patch tests, and can continue wearing their glasses. Old, roughened frames should be re-polished to smooth any abrasive surfaces.

Spectacle frame acanthoma

Mechanical trauma from the ear-piece of a spectacle frame can cause a fissured acanthoma behind the ear (Barnes, Calnan and Sarkany, 1974).

Ball-point pen

Two patients with dermatitis from ball-point pens were reported by Jordan and Dahl (1972). One, who had eczema of the lateral fingers of the right hand, had been sensitised by resorcinol monobenzoate and the other, with dermatitis of the left breast under his shirt pocket where he carried his pen, was allergic to p-*tert*-butyl phenol.

Hearing aid

A patient with retro-auricular dermatitis was found to be sensitive to resorcinol monobenzoate in a component of her hearing aid (Jordan and Dahl, 1972).

Patch test film

Plasticiser — triphenyl phosphate

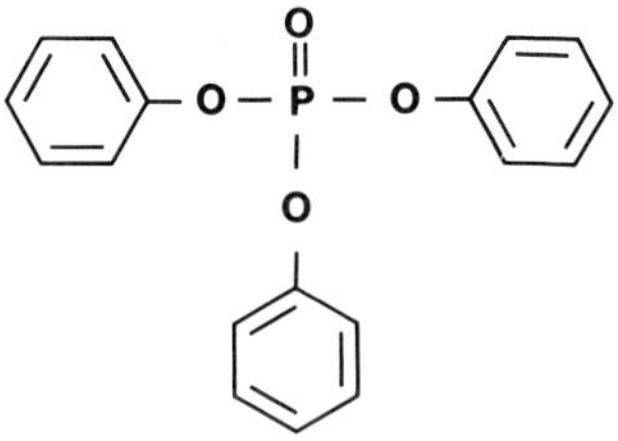

A man with hand eczema was routinely patch tested and reacted to the patch test units made with a cellulose acetate film containing, as plasticisers, 7–10 per cent triphenyl phosphate and 3–4 per cent dimethyl glycol phthalate (Hjorth, 1964). He was subsequently found to be sensitive to tricresyl phosphate in his carbon paper. Patch tests: he reacted to triphenyl phosphate 0.1–1 per cent, tricresyl phosphate 1 per cent (both in acetone) and to his carbon paper, but not to dimethyl glycol phthalate, 1 per cent in acetone.

Sellotape (p. 812)

Steering wheel

An intractable palmar eczema of a year's duration in a man aged 69 years was found to be due to sensitivity to resorcinol monobenzoate in the cellulose acetate steering wheel of his car. Patch tests: he reacted to resorcinol monobenzoate, balsam of Peru (concentrations not stated) and the plastic of the steering wheel. The wheel was encased in a protective cover and his hands remained healed.

It was ascertained (? for the U.S.A.) that cellulose acetate steering wheels made after 1971 should not contain resorcinol monobenzoate (Jordan, 1973).

Patch testing

	% in petrolatum	Diluent
Scrapings from the suspected plastic		
Plasticisers		
Tricresyl phosphate	5	Petrolatum
Triphenyl phosphate	5	Petrolatum
Dibutyl phthalate	5	Petrolatum
Diethyl phthalate	5	Petrolatum
Dimethyl phthalate	5	Petrolatum
Antioxidant		
p-*tert*-butyl phenol	10	Petrolatum

	% in petrolatum	Diluent
Light Absorbers		
Resorcinol monobenzoate	1	Petrolatum
Polish		
Turpentine peroxide	0.3	Olive oil
Solvent		
Ethylene glycol monomethyl ether acetate	0.1	MEK
Colours		
Azo dyes	1	Petrolatum
Metal spectacle frames		
Nickel	5	Petrolatum

Vinyl polymers

Vinyl polymers are used to make many of the plastics found in the home; the polymers themselves are dermatologically inert, but additives used to improve their properties may sensitise.

POLYVINYL CHLORIDE (PVC)

Polyvinyl chloride is a colourless, rigid plastic which withstands acids, alkalis and moisture, and has good insulating properties. However, on exposure to heat or ultraviolet light, it is degraded by oxidation and dehydrochlorination and loses colour and mechanical strength. It is made as film, sheet, fibre and foam, and is commercially one of the most important plastics.

Plasticisers
Plasticisers are added to facilitate processing and to increase the flexibility of the final plastic.

$$COOCH_2CH(C_2H_5)(CH_2)_3CH_3$$
$$COOCH_2CH(C_2H_5)(CH_2)_3CH_3$$

Dioctyl phthalate (DOP; Di(2-ethylhexyl)phthalate; Bis(2-ethylhexyl)phthalate)

Tricresyl phosphate (TCP; Tritolyl phosphate)

Triphenyl phosphate (TPP)

Dibutyl phthalate (*n*-butyl phthalate; phthalic acid dibutyl ester)

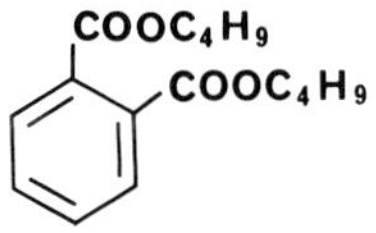

Dioctyl adipate

Dioctyl sebacate

Adipic acid polyesters

Sebacic acid polyesters

Chlorinated paraffins

Stabilisers
Stabilisers retard degradation of the polymer.
Organotin compounds

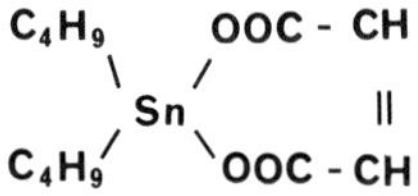

Dibutyltin maleate

$$(C_4H_9)_2 Sn \left[OOC(CH_2)_{10}CH_3 \right]_2$$

Dibutyltin dilaurate

Lead Compounds
  Basic lead carbonate
  Dibasic lead phthalate

Metal Soaps
  Barium, cadmium and zinc laurates, octoates and stearates

Epoxidised Oils
  Epoxidised linseed and soyabean soils

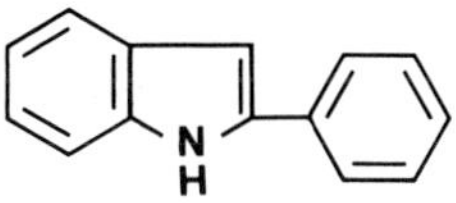

α -Phenyl indole

Ultraviolet light absorbers
These compounds slow the deterioration caused by light. Derivatives of 2-hydroxybenzophenone

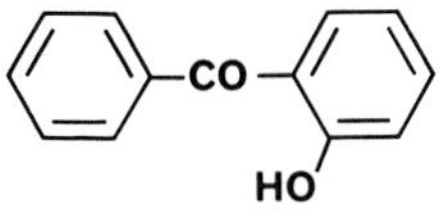

2-Hydroxybenzophenone

Hydroxyphenylbenzotriazoles

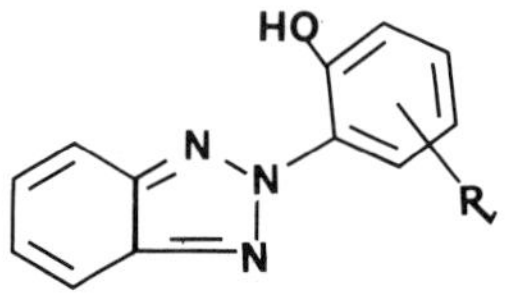

Tinuvin® P (Alkylated 2-(2-hydroxyphenyl)-2H-benzotriazole

Esters of benzoin, salicylic, terephthalic and isophthalic acids with resorcinol and phenols

Resorcinol monobenzoate

Derivatives of Cinnamic acid

$$C_6H_5CH = CHCOOH$$

Cinnamic acid

Fungicides and bactericides
The additives rather than the polymers are susceptible to attack by microorganisms.

Copper 8-quinolate + toluene sulphonamide condensates
Phenyl mercury salicylates
2,2'-Thiobis-(4,6-dichlorophenol)
8-Hydroxyquinoline

Flame retardants
Fire retardants diminish the susceptibility of the plastic to incipient and sustained burning. Chlorinated paraffins ($C_{10}-C_{30}$) and hexachlorocyclopentadiene derivatives are suitable for most plastics (Mascia, 1974).

Other additives
Lubricants, blowing agents and pigments may also be included in the formulation.

Uses
Polyvinyl chloride is used for cable and electrical insulation, plumbing and construction applications, leather cloth for clothes, shoes and upholstery, domestic containers, packaging and toys.

Causes of dermatitis
The PVC monomer does not sensitise and clinical reports of sensitisation by additives are uncommon. When it does occur it seems to be due to contact with finished articles in the home, rather than from exposure to the raw materials in industry. Additives can migrate out of the plastic, and, if skin contact is prolonged, as with PVC clothing or upholstery, then sensitisation may ensue. Positive patch test reactions to PVC, particularly in shoes, is not uncommon, but it is extremely difficult to identify the allergen.

Case reports —

Non-occupational
Two women with dermatitis on the backs of their forearms were found by Hitschmann (1950) to be allergic to their plastic tablecloths. Patch tests: both reacted strongly to their own tablecloths, but no sensitiser was identified. Kipping (1959) reported sensitivity to a vinyl thermoplastic tape used for mending tears in clothing. The patient had a positive patch test to the tape, but the sensitising component was not determined.

Tricresyl phosphate. A woman, who unexpectedly reacted to a PVC patch test tape, was found to be sensitive to the tricresyl phosphate it contained as a plasticiser. She was then tested to various PVC articles in her home and reacted to PVC upholstery, floor tiles and kitchen utensils. She discarded as many of these as she could, and her eczema improved (Pegum, 1966).

Epoxy resin. Uncured epoxy resin used as a plasticiser-stabiliser in a PVC patch test film caused reactions in some of those tested (Fregert and Rorsman, 1963) (p. 607).
   The reaction to the vinyl backing of a tape used in patch testing a patient was found to be due to the diglycidyl ether of bisphenol A, present in the vinyl as a stabiliser (Jordan and Dahl, 1971).

Occupational

Epoxy resin (p. 607)

α *-Phenyl-indole*. A man, while making PVC beer bottles, developed a rash on his arms which cleared when he was away from work. Patch tests: he reacted to alpha-phenyl-indole 1 per cent in MEK and 2 per cent in petrolatum, but not to PVC and the other ingredients of the PVC formulation (Tegner and Fregert, 1973).
   Two men who developed dermatitis while making PVC cables were found by Sonneck (1962) to have a mixture of an irritant and an allergic dermatitis.

Other plasticisers. In a study of the toxicity, irritancy and sensitising effect of plasticisers in rabbits and humans, Malette and Haam (1952) found that the following compounds, though of varying irritancy, were also moderate or slight sensitisers in man:

Moderate sensitisers	Condensation products of sebacic acid with glycols and/or glycerin
	Methylacetyl ricinoleate
	Diethylene glycol dicaprate
	? Monooctyldiphenyl phosphate
Slight sensitisers	Cyclohexyl azelate
	Dioctyl phthalate
	N,N-di-beta-(2-ethylhexyl)ethyl 2-ethylhexamide

Dioctyl phthalate. A man working with unsaturated polyester resins in an aircraft factory was found by Malten to be sensitive to dioctyl phthalate (Malten and Zielhuis, 1964).

Toxicity of PVC (vinyl chloride disease)

Workers employed in the production of PVC may develop an illness, initially called acro-osteolysis but re-named vinyl chloride disease when it became apparent that many systems are affected. There may be sclerosis of the skin, osteolysis, circulatory disturbances, thrombocytopenia, and hepatic and pulmonary damage. The symptoms include coldness and paraesthesiae of the hands and feet, Raynaud's phenomenon, fatigue, muscle and joint pain, dizziness, dyspnoea and impotence. The changes in the hands can be disabling. A scleroderma-like hardening may affect the hands, arms and face, and there may be lytic lesions in the phalanges. Many patients have thrombocytopenia. Vascular changes in the digital vessels have been shown by arteriography, and cooling causes a drop in finger blood flow and skin temperature. There may be fibrosis of the lungs with impaired perfusion, fibrosis of the liver and splenomegaly. Cryoglobulins and cryofibrinogens have been found in some patients (Veltman *et al.*, 1975; Veltman *et al.*, 1978; Walker, 1975) and circulating immune complexes have been demonstrated not only in those with the disease but also in exposed workers. It is suggested that a metabolite of vinyl chloride binds to plasma or tissue protein to form an antigen which initiates the disease (Ward *et al.*, 1976).

A monograph by Heimann, Lilis and Hawkins (1975) on the toxicity of vinyl chloride-polyvinyl chloride concludes with a comprehensive bibliography.

The extraction of vinyl chloride monomer from PVC used for packaging cosmetics and toiletries has been investigated by Tester (1976) and found to be minimal.

The *ortho* isomer of tricresyl phosphate is a dangerous neurotoxin, and has caused several outbreaks of poisoning (Susser and Stein, 1957). In the 1930s, in the U.S.A., hundreds of people were poisoned by drinking Jamaica ginger extract, which had been adulterated by the addition of 2 per cent tri*ortho*cresyl phosphate (Aring, 1942).

Both tricresyl phosphate and trixylenyl phosphate are too toxic to be used in the packaging of food (Bondy *et al.*, 1960).

Neoplasia and vinyl chloride

Angiosarcoma of the liver occurs in workers exposed to vinyl chloride gas in the manufacture of polyvinyl chloride (Heath, Falk and Creech, 1975; Thomas *et al.*, 1975) and a man with both acro-osteolysis and angiosarcoma of the liver has been reported by Legrand and Puech (1976). It seems likely that there is also an excess risk of cancer of the lungs, brain, lymphatic and haemopoietic systems (Nicholson, 1977) and a squamous cell carcinoma of the buccal mucosa in a man aged 22 years was attributed to his habit of chewing plastic containing PVC (Casterline, Casterline and Jaques, 1977). The levels of carcinoembryonic antigen(CEA) have been reported as high in these patients but the significance of the finding remains to be evaluated (Anderson *et al.*, 1978).

POLYVINYL ACETATE (PVA)

Polyvinyl acetate is dissolved by solvents, it softens in water, and deteriorates and discolours when heated. Its brittleness precludes its manufacture in bulk form, and it is used mainly as a surface coating and as an adhesive. Plasticisers, such as dibutyl phthalate, tend to migrate out of PVA, but this and other disadvantages are overcome by linking the PVA to a copolymer.

Polyvinyl acetate and polyvinyl chloride copolymer

Dibutyltin maleate

In the U.S.A., in the 1940s, a transparent flexible copolymer of PVA and PVC called 'elastiglass' was used to make garters, suspenders and wristwatch straps. Within months it had caused dermatitis. Zeisler (1940) reported that organic tin stabilisers, which in pure form are vesicants, were used to elasticise the polymer, and that they would probably be established as the cause of the dermatitis. The only confirmation found of this suggestion is Schwartz's (1945) statement that the irritants in this plastic had been identified as dibutyltin maleate and dibutyl sebacate.

A plastics factory worker with severe hand dermatitis was found by Sharvill (1971) to give a strongly positive reaction to a patch test with 1 per cent Stanclere 55, containing about 1 per cent di-*n*-butyltin bis(methyl maleate), but whether this reaction was irritant or allergic was not established.

Diacetyl (biacetyl; dimethyl glyoxal)

$$CH_3CO-COCH_3$$

An outbreak of dermatitis in workers coating fabrics with a PVC-PVA copolymer was traced to a by-product, biacetyl. This was removed and the dermatitis ceased (Schwartz, 1945). It was not stated whether or not patch tests had been done.

Patch testing

	Conc. % in petrolatum
Pieces of the suspected plastic	
Plasticisers	
Tricresyl phosphate	5
Triphenyl phosphate	5
Dibutyl phthalate	5
Diethyl phthalate	5
Dioctyl phthalate	5
Stabilisers	
Epoxy resin monomer	2
Dibutyltin maleate	? 1 and 0.1
α-phenyl-indole	2
Light absorbers	
Hydroxymethoxymethylbenzophenone	1
Hydroxyphenylbenzotriazole	1
Resorcinol monobenzoate	1
Ethoxyethyl-*p*-methoxycinnamate	1

	Conc. % in petrolatum
Antiseptics	
Phenyl mercury salicylate	1
Hydroxyquinolone	1
Colours	
Azo dyes	1
D. Yellow 3	1
D. Red. 1	1
Gentian Violet	1 (in water)
Brilliant Green	2 (in water)
Also Butylated hydroxytoluene	
Cobalt naphthenate	1
Ethylenediamine	1
Hydroquinone	1
Maleic anhydride	5
Phthalic anhydride	5
Para-tertiary-butyl phenol	10

VINYL CARBAZOLE

N-Vinyl carbazole

Polyvinyl carbazole is brittle and difficult to process, but as it has good dielectric properties, it is used as an electric insulator.

In two plants where vinyl carbazole was being used to impregnate electrical components, it caused dermatitis in many of the workers exposed. The patients were not patch tested. An effective safety programme stopped the outbreaks (Tabershaw and Skinner, 1944). The authors stated that in 1943 Dr Louis Schwartz, of the United States Public Health Service, investigated 30 cases of dermatitis in a factory making vinyl carbazole, and showed by patch testing that the monomer and polymer are strong sensitisers but not irritants.

VINYL PYRIDINE

Vinyl pyridine polymers resemble polystyrene but are harder; they are used as copolymers in the rubber industry.

4-Vinyl pyridine   Pyridine   2-Vinyl pyridine

A chemical research engineer developed hand eczema while preparing polymers with 4-vinyl pyridine. Patch tests: he reacted strongly to 4-vinyl pyridine 1 per cent in alcohol but not to 2-vinyl pyridine, pyridine or several related chemicals (Foussereau, Lantz and Grosshans, 1972).

POLYVINYLIDENE CHLORIDE

The copolymer, which consists of 85 per cent vinylidene chloride and 15 per cent vinyl chloride, is tough, durable and impermeable. As a filament, it is used for upholstery, and as a transparent film (Saran) for packaging. It is not likely to contain plasticisers as they exude from the polymer.

A case of contact dermatitis due to Saran Wrap, used as an occlusive dressing in a patient with psoriasis, was reported by Osbourn (1964). A patch test with a piece of the material caused a vesicular reaction, but the sensitiser was not identified.

OTHER POLYMERS

Polystyrene

Polystyrene, one of the major commercial plastics, is a hard, rigid, transparent, brittle material with good insulating properties. It is soluble in many solvents, is softened by boiling water, and it deteriorates in air and heat.

It is used for domestic appliances, food containers, knife handles, electrical equipment, radio and clock cabinets, toys and packaging. As a foam it is used for insulation.

Occupational dermatitis — azo dye
Solvent Yellow 14 C.I. 12055

In a plastics factory, a woman, who added dye to a thermoplast mixture, developed eczema of exposed sites. The dye was identified as Solvent Yellow 14 C.I. No. 12055 and she reacted to it on patch testing (2 per cent in petrolatum), but she was negative to the finished plastic. By making the dye in granules the dust hazard was eliminated. The patient may have been sensitised in a previous job packing? coloured oranges (Fregert and Gruvberger, 1976).

Polyolefins

The principal polyolefin polymers are polyethylene (polythene), polypropylene and polyisobutylene.

Their uses include electrical insulation, containers, squeeze bottles, domestic equipment, packaging film, refuse bags and adhesives (especially polybutylene).

These polymers are not harmful, but the aluminium alkyl compounds, used as catalysts in their production, can cause burns, and in experimental animals have caused pulmonary damage (Harris, 1959).

Polyamides

The most important polymers of this group are the linear aliphatic polyamides, which can be made into fibres and are known as nylons.

Granulomas

A woman, working in a nylon fibre bag factory, frequently injured the side of her index finger and at the site developed a sarcoidal granuloma which contained nylon particles; she also had granulomatous disease of the lungs due to inhalation of nylon dust (Cortez Pimental, 1977).

Fluoropolymers

Fluoropolymers have been developed for their ability to withstand chemical attack, extremes of temperature and weathering. They are costly and have limited application. Polytetrafluoroethylene, as Teflon, is used in non-stick cooking ware.

Polytetrafluoroethylene if heated to a high temperature gives off fumes which cause an influenza-like illness (Harris, 1959).

References

Allardice, J.T. (1967) Dermatitis due to an acrylic resin sealer. *Transactions of the St John's Hospital for Diseases of the Skin*, 53, 86.

Ancona-Alayon, A., Jimenez-Castilla, J.L. & Gomez-Alvarez, E.M. (1976) Dermatitis from epoxy resin and formaldehyde in shampoo packers. *Contact Dermatitis*, 2, 356.

Andersen, K.E. (1979) Cutaneous reaction to an epoxy-coated pacemaker. *Archives of Dermatology*, 115, 97.

Anderson, H.A., Snyder, J., Lewinson, T., Woo, C., Lilis, R. & Selikoff, I.J. (1978) Levels of CEA among vinyl chloride and polyvinyl chloride exposed workers. *Cancer*, 42, 1560.

Aring, C.D. (1942) The systemic nervous affinity of triorthocresyl phosphate. (Jamaica Ginger Palsy). *Brain*, 65, 34

Baader, E.W. (1955) Erkrankungen durch Phthalsäure und ihre Verbindungen. *Archiv für Gewerbepathologie und Gewerbehygiene*, 13, 419.

Baer, R.L., Ramsey, D.L. & Biondi, E. (1973) The most common contact allergens. *Archives of Dermatology*, 108, 74

Balda, B-R. (1971) Allergic contact dermatitis due to acrylonitrile. *Contact Dermatitis Newsletter*, 9, 219.

Balda, B-R. (1975) Akrylnitril Als Kontaktallergen. *Hautarzt*, 26, 599.

Barnes, H.M., Calnan, C.D. & Sarkany, I. (1974) Spectacle frame acanthoma (granuloma fissuratum). *Transactions of the St John's Hospital Dermatological Society*, 60, 99.

Behrbohm, P., Nehring, A. & Nehring, P. (1975) False negative tests with epoxy resin. *Contact Dermatitis*, 1, 267.

Bergtholdt, C.P.I. (1961) Recent welding practices at naval facilities. *Archives of Environmental Health*, 2, 257.

Beury, J., Mougeolle J.-M. & Weber, M. (1976) Accidents cutanés des résines acryliques dans l'imprimerie. *Annales de Dermatologie et de Syphiligraphie*, 103, 423.

Birmingham, D.J. (1959) Clinical observations on the cutaneous efects associated with curing epoxy resins. *Archives of Industrial Health*, 19, 365.

Black, H. (1972) *Contact Dermatitis Newsletter*, 12, 323.

Bompart, P.V. & Smagghe, G. (1959) Quelques remarques d'ordre pratique a propos d'une application industrielle des résines formo-phénolique. *Archives des Maladies Professionnelles de Médecine du Travail et de Sécurité Sociale*, 20, 64.

Bondy, H.F., Field, E.J., Worden, A.N. & Hughes, J.P.W. (1960) A study on the acute toxicity of the tri-aryl phosphates used as plasticisers. *British Journal of Industrial Medicine*, 17, 190.

Bord, A. & Castelain, P.-Y. (1966) Les dermatoses professionnelles dans l'industrie aéronautique. *Bulletin de Dermatologie et de Syphiligraphie*, 73, 396.

Bourne, L.B. & Milner, F.J.M. (1963) Polyester resin hazards. *British Journal Industrial Medicine*, 20, 100.

Bourret, J., Tolot, F., Pollet, M.-L. & Genevois, M. (1958) Les dermatoses professionnelles provoquées par le formal et ses dérivés industriels. *Archives des Maladies Professionnelles de Médecine du Travail et de Sécurité Sociale*, 19, 611.

Breslau, A.J. (1973) Electrical and electronic applications in epoxy resins. *Chemistry and Technology*. Ed. May, C.A. & Tanaka, Y. New York: Marcel Dekker p. 501.

Broughton, W.E. (1965) Epoxy resins in industry. The hazards and their control. *Annals of Occupational Hygiene*, 8, 131.

Brunner, L. (1962) Neuere beruflich bedingte Hauterkrankungen. *Berufsdermatosen*, 10, 61.

Burry, J.N., Kirk, J., Reid, J.G. & Turner, T. (1973) Environmental dermatitis: Patch tests in 1000 cases of allergic contact dermatitis. *Medical Journal of Australia*, 2, 681.

Calas, E., Castelain, P.-Y., Raulot-Lapointe, H., Ducos, P., Cavelier, C., Duprat, P. & Poitou, P. (1977) Allergic contact dermatitis to a photopolymerisable resin used in printing. *Contact Dermatitis*, 3, 186.

Calas, E., Castelain, P.-Y., Raulot-Lapointe, H. & Mahé, A.-M. (1976) L'allergie aux résines chez les imprimeurs. *Bulletin de la Société Franscaise de Dermatologie et de Syphiligraphie*, 83, 222.

Calnan, C.D. (1958) Studies in contact dermatitis IV. Epoxy resins. *Transactions of the St John's Hospital Dermatological Society*, 40, 12.

Calnan, C.D. (1967) Studies in contact dermatitis XX. Active sensitisation. *Transactions of the St John's Hospital Dermatological Society*, 53, 129.

Calnan, C.D. (1969) Epoxy resin putty. *Contact Dermatitis Newsletter*, 5, 89.

Calnan, C.D. (1973) False negative tests with epoxy resin. *Contact Dermatitis Newsletter*, 13, 366.

Calnan, C.D. (1975) Epoxy resin dermatitis. *Journal of the Society of Occupational Medicine*, 25, 123.

Calnan, C.D. (1975) Resorcinol monobenzoate. *Contact Dermatitis*, 1, 59.

Calnan, C.D. (1979) Cyanoacrylate dermatitis. *Contact Dermatitis*, 5, 165.

Calnan, C.D. & Harman, R.R.M. (1959) Studies in contact dermatitis X. Sensitivity to para-tertiary butylphenol. *Transactions of the St John's Hospital Dermatological Society*, 43, 27.

Calnan, C.D. & Stevenson, C.J. (1963) Studies in contact dermatitis XV.—Dental materials. *Transactions of the St John's Hospital Dermatological Society*, 49, 9.

Carroll, K.B., Secombe, C.J.P. & Pepys, J. (1976) Asthma due to non-occupational exposure to toluene (tolylene) di-isocyanate. *Clinical Allergy*, 6, 99.

Castelain, P.-Y. & Piriou, A. (1978) New case of sensitisation to Nyloprint. *Contact Dermatitis*, 4, 310.

Casterline, C.L., Casterline, P.F. & Jaques, D.A. (1977) Squamous cell carcinoma of the buccal mucosa associated with chronic oral polyvinyl chloride exposure, *Cancer*. 39, 1686.

Charnley, J. (1970) *Arrylic Cement in Orthopaedic Surgery*. Edinburgh: Churchill Livingstone.

Chung, C.W. & Giles, A.L. (1977) Sensitisation potentials of methyl, ethyl and n-butyl methacrylates and mutual cross-sensitivity in guinea pigs. *Journal of Investigative Dermatology*, 68, 187.

Cortez Pimentel, J. (1977) Sarcoid granulomas of the skin produced by acrylic and nylon fibres. *British Journal of Dermatology*, 96, 673.

Craigen, A.A. (1975) The control of dermatitis in a plastics factory. *Journal of the Society of Occupational Medicine*, 25, 127.

Crissey, J.T. (1965) Stomatitis, dermatitis, and denture materials. *Archives of Dermatology*, 92, 45.

Cronin, E. (1969) Acrylic resin in window sealant. *Contact Dermatitis Newsletter*, 5, 104.

Cronin, E. (1974) Epoxy resin dermatitis in a gas-jointer. *Contact Dermatitis Newsletter*, 15, 453.

Dahlquist, I. & Fregert, S. (1979a) Contact allergy to Cardura E, an epoxy reactive diluent of the ester type. *Contact Dermatitis*, 5, 121.

Dahlquist, I. & Fregert, S. (1979b) Contact allergy to the epoxy hardener isophoronediamine (IPD). *Contact Dermatitis*, **5**, 120.

Davenport, J.C. (1970) The oral distribution of Candida in denture stomatitis. *British Dental Journal*, **129**, 151.

Ducombs, G., Derville, E. & Texier, L. (1974) Dermites de contact dans l'imprimerie, par procede offset. *Bulletin de la Société Franscaise de Dermatologie et de Syphiligraphie*, **81**, 408.

Emmett, E.A. (1976) Allergic contact dermatitis in polyurethane plastic moulders. *Journal of Occupational Medicine*, **18**, 802.

Emmett, E.A., (1977) Contact dermatitis from polyfunctional acrylic monomers. *Contact Dermatitis*, **3**, 245.

Emmett, E.A., Taphorn B.R. & Kominsky, J.R. (1977) Phototoxicity occuring during the manufacture of ultraviolet-cured ink. *Archives of Dermatology*, **113**, 770.

Engel, H.O. & Calnan, C.D. (1966) Resin dermatitis in a car factory. *British Journal of Industrial Medicine*, **23**, 62.

Epstein, E. (1974) Allergy to epichlorhydrin masquerading as trichlorethylene allergy. *Contact Dermatitis Newsletter*, **16**, 475.

Fawcett, I.W., Newman Taylor, A.J. & Pepys, J. (1977) Asthma due to inhaled chemical agents—epoxy resin systems containing phthalic acid anhydride, trimellitic acid anhydride and triethylene tetramine. *Clinical Allergy*, **7**, 1.

Fisher, A.A. (1954) Allergic sensitisation of the skin and oral mucosa to acrylic denture materials. *Journal of the American Medical Association*, **156**, 238.

Fisher, A.A. (1973) Acrylic bone cement sensitisation and dermatitis. *Cutis*, **12**, 333.

Fisher, A.A. (1976) Epoxy resin dermatitis. *Cutis*, **17**, 1027.

Fisher, A.A., Franks, A. & Glick, H. (1957) Allergic sensitisation of the skin and nails to acrylic plastic nails. *Journal of Allergy*, **28**, 84.

Foussereau, J. & Benezra, Cl. (1970) *Les Eczemas Allergiques Professionnels*, p. 249 Paris: Masson et Cie.

Foussereau, J., Cavelier, C. & Selig, D. (1976) Occupational eczema from paratertiary-butylphenol formaldehyde resins: A review of the sensitising resins. *Contact Dermatitis*, **2**, 254.

Foussereau, J., Lantz, J.P. & Grosshans, E. (1972) Allergic eczema from vinyl-4-Pyridine. *Contact Dermatitis Newsletter*, **11**, 261.

Foussereau, M.J., Petitjean, J. & Barré, J.-G. (1968) Eczema aux bracelets—montres par allergie a des résines formol—p.t. butylphénol des colles pour cuir (Résines du type c.k.r. 1634). *Bulletin de la Société Franscaise de Dermatologie et de Syphiligraphie*, **75**, 630.

Fregert, S. (1967) Allergic contact reaction to diphenyl-4,4-diisocyanate. *Contact Dermatitis Newsletter*, **2**, 35.

Fregert, S. (1969) Allergic contact dermatitis due to p-toluenesulphonylchloride in furan plastic. *Contact Dermatitis Newsletter*, **5**, 90.

Fregert, S. (1971) Outbreak of irritant contact dermatitis from diallyl-phthalate in polyester resin. *Contact Dermatitis Newsletter*, **10**, 234.

Fregert, S. (1972) Dermatitis caused by plastics. *Proceedings of the XIV International Congress of Dermatology*. p. 212 Amsterdam: Excerpta Medica.

Fregert, S. (1973) Routine patch test reactions to epoxy resin. *Contact Dermatitis Newsletter*, **13**, 350.

Fregert, S. (1978) Allergic contact dermatitis from ethylacrylate in a window sealant. *Contact Dermatitis*, **4**, 56.

Fregert, S. & Dahlquist, I. (1968) Allergic contact dermatitis from N-methylolacrylamide. *Contact Dermatitis Newsletter*, **5**, 102.

Fregert, S. & Dahlquist, I. (1969) Allergic contact dermatitis from epoxy resins. Lack of prevential instructions. *Contact Dermatitis Newsletter*, **5**, 101.

Fregert, S. & Gruvberger, B. (1970) Sensitisation to epichlorhydrin and cross-sensitisation to propene oxide. *Contact Dermatitis Newsletter*, **8**, 172.

Fregert, S. & Gruvberger, B. (1976) Allergic dermatitis from solvent yellow 14 used in plastics. *Contact Dermatitis*, **2**, 126.

Fregert, S. & Rorsman, H. (1960) Hypersensitivity to Diethylstilbestrol. Cross-sensitisation to dienestrol, hexestrol, bisphenol-A, p-benzyl-phenol, hydroquinone monobenzylether, and p-hydroxybenzoic-benzylester. *Acta Dermato-venereologica*, **40**, 206.

Fregert, S. & Rorsman, H. (1962) Hypersensitivity to epoxy resins with reference to the role played by bisphenol A. *Journal of Investigative Dermatology*, **39**, 471.

Fregert, S. & Rorsman, H. (1963) Hypersensitivity to epoxy resins used as plasticisers and stabilisers in polyvinyl chloride (PVC) resins. *Acta Dermato-venereologica*, **43**, 10.

Fregert, S. & Rorsman, H. (1964) Allergens in epoxy resins. *Acta Allergologica*, **19**, 296.

Fregert, S. & Tegner, E. (1972) Allergic contact dermatitis due to phenolic resin in ready products. *Contact Dermatitis Newsletter*, **12**, 328.

Fregert, S. & Trulsson, L. (1978) Simple methods for demonstration of epoxy resins of bisphenol A type. *Contact Dermatitis*, 4, 69.

Fullerton, P.M. (1970) Symposium on isocyanates: discussion. *Proceedings of the Royal Society of Medicine*, 63, 382.

Garland, T.O. & Patterson, M.W.H (1967) Six cases of acrylamide poisoning. *British Medical Journal*, 4, 134.

Gaul, L.E. (1957) Sensitising structure in epoxy resin. *Journal of Investigative Dermatology*, 29, 311.

Gaul, L.E. (1962) Epoxy dermatitis from installing cathodic protection. *Archives of Dermatology*, 86, 77.

Gaul, L.E. (1967) Absence of formaldehyde sensitivity in phenol formaldehyde resin dermatitis. *Journal of Investigative Dermatology*, 48, 485.

Giunta, J. & Zablotsky, N. (1976) Allergic stomatitis caused by self-polymerising resin. *Oral Surgery, Oral Medicine, Oral Pathology*, 41, 631.

Göransson, K. (1977) Allergic contact dermatitis to an epoxy hardener: dodecenylsuccinic anhydride. *Contact Dermatitis*, 3, 277.

Grandjean, E. (1957) The danger of dermatoses due to cold-setting ethoxyline resins (epoxide resins). *British Journal of Industrial Medicine*, 14, 1.

Gresham, G.A., Kuczyński, A. & Rosborough, D. (1971) Fat embolism following replacement arthroplasty for transcervical fractures of femur. *British Medical Journal*, 2, 617.

Grimm, I. (1971) Unge wohnliche Formeiner Kontaktdermatitis durch Kobalt bei einem 11 jahrigen Kind. *Berufsdermatosen*, 19, 39.

Guill, M.A. & Odom, R.B. (1978) Hearing aid dermatitis. *Archives of Dermatology*, 114, 1050.

Hale, J.E. (1970) Isobutyl cyanoacrylate as a skin adhesive. *Postgraduate Medical Journal*, 46, 447.

Hambly, E.M. & Wilkinson, D.S. (1978) Contact dermatitis to butyl acrylate in spectacle frames. *Contact Dermatitis*, 4, 115.

Harris, D.K. (1959) Some hazards in the manufacture and use of plastics. *British Journal of Industrial Medicine*, 16, 221.

Heath, C.W., Falk, H. & Creech, J.L. (1975) Characteristics of cases of angiosarcoma of the liver among vinyl chloride workers in the United States. *Annals of the New York Academy of Sciences*, 246, 231.

Heimann, H., Lilis, R. & Hawkins, D.T. (1975) A bibliography on the toxicology of vinyl chloride and polyvinyl chloride. *Annals of the New York Academy of Sciences*, 246, 322.

Herzberg, J. (1973) Untersuchungen über einen neuen Epoxidkunststoff, 'Optyl', zur Herstellung von Brillenfassungen. *Berufsdermatosen*, 21, 1.

Hitschmann, O.B. (1950) Contact dermatitis due to table cloth cover of vinyl plastic fabric. *Archives of Dermatology*, 61, 679.

Hjorth, N. (1964) Contact dermatitis from cellulose acetate film. *Berufsdermatosen*, 12, 86.

Hjorth, N. (1975) Dermatitis from trimethyl hexamethylene diioscyanate. *Contact Dermatitis*, 1, 59.

Hjorth, N. & Fregert, S. (1967) Sensitivity to formaldehyde and formaldehyde resins. *Contact Dermatitis Newsletter*, 2, 18.

Ippen, H. & Mathies, V. (1970) Die protrahierte Verätzung (unter besonderer Berücksichtigung der Hautschaden durch Epoxide und Propansulton). *Berufsdermatosen*, 18, 144.

Jakovljeviòvá, E. (1976) Professional urticaria caused by urea-formaldehyde resin. *Č Československá dermatologie*. 51, 323.

Jansen, K. (1975) Zur Haufigkeit und Prophylaxe Allergischer Kontaktekzeme durch Acrylat-Klebstoffe. *Berufsdermatosen*, 23, 183.

Jennings, G.H. & Gower, N.D. (1963) Thrombocytopenic purpura in toluene diisocyanate workers. *Lancet*, 1, 406.

Jordan, W.P. (1972) Turpentine in eyelgasses. *Contact Dermatitis Newsletter*, 12, 309.

Jordan, W.P. (1973) Resorcinal monobenzoate, steering wheels, Peruvian balsam. *Archives of Dermatology*, 108, 278.

Jordan, W.P. (1975) Cross-sensitisation patterns in acrylate allergies. *Contact Dermatitis*, 1, 13.

Jordan, W.P. & Bourlas, M. (1975) Contact dermatitis from typewriter correction paper. *Cutis*, 15, 594.

Jordan, W.P. & Dahl, M.V. (1971) Contact dermatitis to a plastic solvent in eyeglasses. *Archives of Dermatology*, 104, 524.

Jordan, W.P. & Dahl, M.V. (1972) Contact dermatitis from cellulose ester plastics. *Archives of Dermatology*, 105, 880.

Kaaber, S., Thulin, H. & Nielsen, E (1979) Skin sensitivity to denture base materials in the burning mouth syndrome. *Contact Dermatitis*, 5, 90.

Kadlec, K., Hanslian, L. & Folprechtová, A. (1974) Výskyt kožnich onemocnéni při praci s polyesterovými laky. *Československá Dermatologie*, 49, 281.

Kepes, E.R., Underwood, P.S. & Becsey, L. (1972) Intraoperative death associated with acrylic bone cement. *Journal of the American Medical Association*, 222, 576.

Kern, R.A. (1939) Asthma and allergic rhinitis due to sensitisations to phthalic anhydride. *Journal of Allergy*, 10, 164.

Ketel, van W.G. (1974) Plastics and glues. *Contact Dermatitis Newsletter*, 16, 470.

Kipping, H.F. (1959) Dermatitis from thermoplastic tape. *Archives of Dermatology*, 80, 348.

Kirwan, W.O. (1973) Systemic phenomena and bone cement. *Irish Journal of Medical Science*, 142, 342.

Klauder, J.V. (1948) Sensitisation dermatitis from 'Scottissue' towels. *Archives of Dermatology*, 57, 415.

Klein, R.A. (1976) Occupational hazard in preparation of polyacrylamide gels. *British Medical Journal*, 2, 962.

Kligman, A.M. (1966) The identification of contact allergens by human assay. III. The maximisation test: A procedure for screening and rating contact sensitisers. *Journal of Investigative Dermatology*, 47, 393.

Krajewska, D. & Rudzki, E. (1976) Sensitivity to epoxy resins and triethylenetetramine. *Contact Dermatitis*, 2, 135.

Lachapelle, J.M. & Lachapelle-Ketelaer, M.J. (1979) Cross-sensitivity between isophorone diamine (IPD) and isophorone diisocyanate (IPDI). *Contact Dermatitis*, 5, 55.

Lachapelle, J.M., Tennstedt, D. & Dumont-Fruytier, M. (1978). Occupational allergic contact dermatitis to isophorone diamine (IPD) used as an epoxy resin hardener. *Contact Dermatitis*, 4, 109.

Lacroix, M., Burckel, H., Foussereau, J., Grosshans, E., Cavelier, C., Limasset, J.C., Ducos, P., Gradinski, D. & Duprat, P. (1976) Irritant dermatitis from diallylglycol carbonate monomer in the optical industry. *Contact Dermatitis*, 2, 183.

Lambert, D., Lacroix, M., Ducombs, G., Journet, F. & Chapuis, J.-L. (1978) L'allergie cutanée a l'épichlorhydrine. *Annales de Dermatologie et de Vénéréologie*, 105, 521.

Lee, K.P., Terrill, J.B. & Henry, N.W. (1977) Alopoecia induced by inhalation exposure to phenyl glycidyl ether. *Journal of Toxicology and Environmental Health*, 3, 859.

Legrand, J. & Puech, A.M. (1976) Chlorure de vinyle: angiosarcome hepatique associé a une acro-ostéolyse. *Archives des Maladies Professionelles de Médecine du Travail et de Sécurité Sociale*, 38, 645.

Lemon, R.C. (1972) Epoxy resins in surface coatings. *Annals of Occupational Hygiene*, 15, 131.

Lepine, E.M. (1976) Results of routine office patch testing. *Contact Dermatitis*, 2, 89.

Lewis, A.F. & Saxon, R. (1973) Epoxy-resin adhesives in epoxy resins. *Chemistry and technology*, p. 374 Ed. May, C.A. & Tanaka, Y. New York: Marcel Dekker.

Lim, J., Balzar, J.L., Wolf, C.R. & Milky, T.H. (1970) Fiber glass reinforced plastics. *Archives of Environmental Health*, 20, 540.

Logan, W.P. & Perry, H.O. (1972) Cast dermatitis due to formaldehyde sensitivity. *Archives of Dermatology*, 106, 717.

Logan, W.P. & Perry, H.O. (1973) Contact dermatitis to resin-containing casts. *Clinical Orthopaedics*, 90, 150.

Lowe, A. (1970) The chemistry of isocyanates. *Proceedings of the Royal Society of Medicine*, 63, 367.

Lubach, D. (1978) Erkrankung durch diisocyante. *Dermatosen In Beruf Und Umwelt*, 26, 184.

Lubach, D. (1979) Erkrankung durch diisocyanate. *Dermatosen In Beruf Und Umwelt*, 27, 5.

MacFarland, H.N. & Leong, K.J. (1962) Hazards from the thermodecomposition of plastics. *Archives of Environmental Health*, 4, 591.

Magnusson, B. & Mobacken, H. (1972) Allergic contact dermatitis from acrylate printing plates in a printing plant. *Berufsdermatosen*, 20, 138.

Magnusson, B. & Mobacken, H. (1972) Contact allergy to a self-hardening acrylic sealer for assembling metal parts. *Berufsdermatosen*, 20, 198.

Maibach, H.I. (1973) Marking pen dermatitis. *Contact Dermatitis Newsletter*, 14, 402 Maibach, H., Maibach, H.T., Hjorth, N., Fregert, S., Meneghini, C., Bandmann, H.-J., Malten, K., Pirilä, V., Magnusson, B., Cronin, E. Calnan, C.D., Wilkinson, D. & Marzulli, F. (1978) Butyl methacrylate monomer and ethyl methacrylate monomer-frequency of reaction. *Contact Dermatitis*, 4, 60.

Mallette, F.S. & Haam, E. von (1952) Studies on the toxicity and skin effects of compounds used in the rubber and plastics industries. II Plasticisiers. *Archives of Industrial Hygiene and Occupational Medicine*, 6, 231.

Malten, K.E. (1958) Occupational eczema due to para-tertiary butylphenol in a shoe adhesive. *Dermatologica*, 117, 103.

Malten, K.E. (1967) Contact Sensitisations caused by *p. tert.* Butylphenol and certain phenolformaldehyde-containing glues. *Dermatologica*, 135, 54.

Malten, K.E. (1973) Occupational dermatoses in the processing of plastics. *Transactions of the St John's Hospital Dermatological Society*, 59, 78.

Malten, K.E. (1977a) Contact sensitisation to Letterflex urethane photoprepolymer mixture used in printing. *Contact Dermatitis*, 3, 115.

Malten, K.E. (1977b) Letterflex photoprepolymer sensitisation in newspaper print due to penta erythritol tetrakis 3 mercaptopropionate and 3 mercaptopropionic acid *Contact Dermatitis*, 3, 257.

Malten, K.E. (1977c) Tracing back a positive reaction to epoxy resin. *Contact Dermatitis*, 3, 217.

Malten, K.E. (1977d) Les résines formaldéhyde-paratertiaire butylphénol et al paratertiaire butylphénol en médecine du travail. *Archives des maladies professionelles, de médecine du travail et de Sécurité Sociale*, 38, 427.

Malten, K.E. & Aerssen, van R.G.L. (1962) Kontaktekzeme durch Leime bei Schuhmachern und Schuhträgern. *Berufsdermatosen*, 10, 264.

Malten, K.E., den Arend, J.A.C.J. & Wiggers, R.E. (1979) Delayed irritation: hexanediol diacrylate and butanediol diacrylate. *Contact Dermatitis*, 5, 178.

Malten, K.E. & Bende, W.J.M. (1979) 2-Hydroxy-ethyl-methacrylate and di- and tetraethylene glycol dimethacrylate: contact sensitisers in a photoprepolymer printing plate procedure. *Contact Dermatitis*, 5, 214.

Malten, K.E., van der Meer-Roosen, C.H. & Seutter, E. (1978) Nyloprint-sensitive patients react to NN' methylene bis acrylamide. *Contact Dermatitis*, 4, 214.

Malten, K.E. Verwilghen, L.M.E. & Seutter, E. (1965) The sensitising capacity of a simple epoxy-resin. As demonstrated in the guinea pig nipple test 1. *The Sixth European Congress of Allergy* (Stockholm, 1965). Ed. Skog, E. p. 44. Copyright Acta Dermato-venereologica.

Malten, K.E. & Zielhuis, R.L. (1964) Industrial Toxicology and Dermatology in the Production and Processing of Plastics. pps. 79, 92, 93, 123, 125. Amsterdam: Elsevier Publishing Company.

Magnan, D. & Snyder, I.S. (1978) The effect of acrylamide on human polymorphonuclear neutrophils *in vitro*. *British Journal of Industrial Medicine*. 35, 305.

Marks, J.G., Bishop, M.E. & Willis, W.F. (1979) Allergic contact dermatitis to sculptured nails. *Archives of Dermatology*, 115, 100.

Mascia, L. (1974) *The role of additives in plastics*. p. 163. London: Edward Arnold.

Mathias, C.G., Caldwell, T.M. & Maibach, H.I. (1979) Contact dermatitis and gastrointestinal symptoms from hydroxyethylmethacrylate. *British Journal of Dermatology*, 100, 447.

McCabe, J.F. & Basker, R.M. (1976) Tissue sensitivity to acrylic resin. *British Dental Journal*, 140, 347.

McKerrow, C.B., Davies, H.J. & Parry Jones, A. (1970) Symptoms and lung function following acute and chronic exposure to tolylene diisocyanate. *Proceedings of the Royal Society of Medicine*, 63, 376.

Mehl, J., Fuchs, E. & Foussereau, J. (1971) Pathologie professionnelle des résines d'époxy. *Archives des Maladies Professionnelles de Médecine du Travail et de Sécurité Sociale (Paris)*, 32, 713.

Menschick, H. (1955) Gesundheitliche Gefahren bei der Herstellung von Phthalsäureanhydrid. *Archiv fur Gewerbe Pathologie und Gewerbehygiene*, 13, 454.

Moran, M. & Martin-Pascual, A. (1978) Contact dermatitis to para-tertiary-butylphenol formaldehyde. *Contact Dermatitis*, 4, 372.

Morris, G.E. (1959) Allergic rhinitis acquired during the processing of epoxy resins. *Annals of Allergy*, 17, 74.

Munn, A. (1965) Hazards of isocyanates. *Annals of Occupational Hygiene*, 8, 163.

Négri, R. (1959) Pathologie des matieres plastiques dans l'industrie automobile. *Archives des Maladies Professionnelles de Médecine du Travail et de Sécurité Sociale*, 20, 74.

Nethercott, J.R. (1978) Skin problems associated with multifunctional acrylic monomers in ultraviolet curing inks. *British Journal of Dermatology*, 98, 541.

Nicholson, W.J. (1977) Cancer following occupational exposure to asbestos and vinyl chloride. *Cancer*, 39, 1792.

Osbourn, R.A. (1964) Contact dermatitis caused by saran wrap. *Journal of the American Medical Association*, 188, 1159.

Pardon, N. & Bompart, P.V. (1959) Quelques formes cliniques d'intolérance aux résines phénolformal. *Archives des Maladies Professionnelles de Médecine du Travail et de Sécurité Sociale*, 20, 63.

Paulet, G., Desnos, J. & Battig, J. (1966) De la toxicité de l'acrylonitrile. *Archives des Maladies Professionnelles de Médecine du Travail et de Sécurité Sociale*, 27, 849.

Pegum, J.S. (1966) Contact dermatitis from plastics containing tri-aryl phosphates. *British Journal of Dermatology*, 78, 626.

Pégum, J.S. & Medhurst, F.A. (1971) Contact dermatitis from penetration of rubber gloves by acrylic monomer. *British Medical Journal*, 2, 141.

Peschel, H. (1970) Hautveränderungen durch Isozyanate (Desmodur). *Dermatologische Monatsschrift*, **156**, 691.

Piper, R. (1965) The hazards of painting and varnishing (1965) *British Journal of Industrial Medicine*, **22**, 247.

Port, W.S. (1973) Epoxy compounds as polymer stabilisers and plasticisers, in epoxy resins. *Chemistry and Technology* p. 635. Ed. May, C.A. & Tanaka, Y. New York: Marcel Dekker.

Potter, W.G. (1975) *Uses of Epoxy Resins*. Butterworth: London.

Powell, J.N., McGrath, P.J., Lahiri, S.K. & Hill, P. (1970) Cardiac arrest associated with bone cement. *British Medical Journal*, **3**, 326.

Pozzani, U.C., Kinkead, E.R. & King, J.M. (1969) The mammalian toxicity of methacrylonitrile. *American Industrial Hygiene Association Journal*, **29**, 202.

Pye, R.J. & Peachey, R.D.G. (1976) Contact dermatitis due to nyroprint. *Contact Dermatitis*, **2**, 146.

Renner, R.P., Lee, M., Andors, L., McNamara, T.F. & Brook, S. (1979) The role of *C. albicans* in denture stomatitis. *Oral Surgery Oral Medicine Oral Pathology*, **47**, 323.

Richter, G. von (1974) Zur Epidemiologie des Epoxidharzekzems. *Dermatologische Monatsschrift*, **160**, 785.

Rothe, A. (1976) Zur Frage arbeitsbedingter Hautschädigungen durch Polyurethanchemikalien. *Berufsdermatosen*, **24**, 7.

Routledge, R. (1971) Contact dermatitis and bronchial irritation due to ammonium acrylate in the motor industry. *Transactions of the Society of Occupational Medicine*, **21**, 59.

Rudzki, E. & Krajewska, D. (1973) Incidence of epoxy resin dermatitis. *Contact Dermatitis Newsletter*, **13**, 372.

Rudzki, E. & Kradjewska, D. (1974) Primary sensitivity to metaphenylenediamine. *Contact Dermatitis Newsletter*, **16**, 483.

Rudzki, E. & Krajewska, D. (1979) Contact Sensitivity to phenylglycidyl ether. *Dermatosen In Beruf Und Umwelt*, **27**, 42.

Salo, O.P. & Hirvonen, M.L. (1969) Yeasts as a cause of false-positive reactions in patch tests for allergy to denture materials. *British Journal of Dermatology*, **81**, 338.

Saunders, K.J. (1973) *Organic-Polymer Chemistry*, pp. 234, 375 London: Chapman and Hall.

Schoenberg, J.B. & Mitchell, C.A. (1975) Airway disease caused by phenolic (phenol-formaldehyde) resin exposure. *Archives of Environmental Health*, **30**, 574.

Schubert, H. & Agatha, G. (1979) Zur allergennatur der para-tert. butylphenolformaldehydharze. *Dermatosen In Beruf Und Umwelt*, **27**, 49.

Schürmann, D. (1955) Gesundheitsschaden durch neuartige Lacke und Schaumstoffe. *Deutsche medizinische wochenschrift*, **80**, 1661.

Schwartz, L. (1945) Dermatitis from Synthetic Resins. *Journal of Investigative Dermatology*, **6**, 239.

Sharvill, D.E. (1971) Reaction to di-n-butyl tin bis methyl maleate — 'Stanclere 55'. *Contact Dermatitis Newsletter*, **9**, 208.

Simpson, J.R. (1972) Dermatitis from phenolic and melamine formaldehyde resins. *Contact Dermatitis Newsletter*, **12**, 332.

Sjöberg, K., Tegner, E. & Fregert, S. (1973) Sensitisation to epoxy resin from contaminated pocket. *Contact Dermatitis Newsletter*, **13**, 356.

Smith, W.D.L. (1977) Allergic dermatitis due to a triacrylate in ultraviolet cured inks. *Contact Dermatitis*, **3**, 312.

Smith, E.L. & Calnan, C.D. (1966) Studies in contact dermatitis. XVII. Spectacle frames. *Transactions of the St John's Hospital Dermatological Society*, **52**, 10.

Somov, B.A., Shatskaya, N.N. Veretinskaya, A.G. & Lopukhova, K.A. (1976) Features of the pathochemical stage of allergic reaction in patients with occupational allergic dermatitis and eczema caused by formaldehyde containing polymers. *Vestnik Dermatologii I Venerologii*, No. 7, 3.

Sonneck, H.J. (1962) Berufsbedingte Hautschäden durch Polyvinyl chlorid. *Berufsdermatosen*, **10**, 38.

Sonneck, H.J. (1964) Hautschäden durch Kunstharzsäurekitte. *Berufsdermatosen*, **12**, 42.

Susser, M. & Stein, Z. (1957) An outbreak of tri-ortho-cresyl phosphate poisoning in Durban. *British Journal of Industrial Medicine*, **14**, 111.

Suurmond, D. & Verspijck Mijnssen, G.A.W. (1967) Allergic dermatitis due to shoes and a leather prothese. *Dermatologica*, **134**, 371.

Tabershaw, I.R. & Skinner, J.B. (1944) Dermatitis due to vinyl carbazole. *Journal of Industrial Hygiene and Toxicology*, **26**, 313.

Tegner, E. & Fregert, S. (1973) Exposure to phenolic resin due to badly constructed ventilation. *Contact Dermatitis Newsletter*, **13**, 354.

Tegner, E. & Fregert, S. (1973) Allergic contact dermatitis from alfa-phenyl-indol in PVC. *Contact Dermatitis Newsletter*, **13**, 356.

Tester, D.A. (1976) The extraction of vinyl chloride from PVC containers. *Journal of the Society of Cosmetic Chemists*, **49**, 459.

Thomas, L.B., Popper, H., Berk, P.D., Selikoff, I., & Falk, H. (1975) Vinyl-chloride-induced liver disease. *New England Journal of Medicine*, **292**, 17.

Thorgeirsson, A. (1978a) Sensitisation capacity of epoxy reactive diluents in the guinea pig. *Acta Dermato-venereologica*, **58**, 329.

Throgeirsson, A. (1978b) Sensitisation capacity of epoxy resin hardeners in the guinea pig. *Acta Dermato-venereologica*, **58**, 332.

Thorgeirsson, A. & Fregert, S. (1977) Allergenicity of epoxy resins in the guinea pig. *Acta Dermato-venereologica*, **57**, 253.

Thorgeirsson, A., Fregert, S. & Magnusson, B. (1975) Allergenicity of epoxy-reactive diluents in the guinea pig. *Berufsdermatosen*, **23**, 178.

Thorgeirsson, A., Fregert, S. & Ramnäs, O. (1978) Sensitisation capacity of epoxy resin oligomers in the guinea pig. *Acta Dermato-venereologica*, **58**, 17.

Tilsley, D.A. (1975) Contact and photo-dermatitis from Nyloprint. *Contact Dermatitis*, **1**, 334.

Tolot, F., Bresson, J.R., Dhers, V. & Beaupère, A. (1960) Manifestations pharyngées récidivantes d'origine allergique probable; rôle de la mousee de polyuréthane. *Archives des Maladies Professionnelles de Médecine du Travail et de Sécurité Sociale*, **22**, 147.

Tolot, F., Colin, M. & Soubrier, R. (1961) Asthma et araldite. *Archives des Maladies Professionnelles de Médecine du Travail et de Sécurité Sociale*. **22**, 163.

Turner, T. (1964) Epoxy resins in industry. *Australian Journal of Dermatology*, **7**, 225.

Veltman, G., Lange, C.-E., Jühe, S., Stein, G., & Bachner, U. (1975) Clinical manifestations and course of vinyl chloride disease. *Annals of the New York Academy of Sciences*, **246**, 6.

Veltman, G., Lange C.-E. & Stein, G. (1978) Die vinylchloridkrankheit. *Hautarzt*, **29**, 177.

Verdich, J. & Skoven, I. (1979) Allergic contact dermatitis from Desmophen®, a polyether alcohol. *Contact Dermatitis*, **5**, 120.

Vries, H.R. de (1964) Allergic dermatitis due to shoes. *Dermatologica*, **128**, 68.

Wahlberg, J.E. (1974) Contact sensitivity to nyloprint® printing plates. *Contact Dermatitis Newsletter*, **16**, 510.

Wakkers-Garritsen, B.G., Timmer, L.H. & Nater, J.P. (1975) Etiological factors in the denture sore mouth syndrome: an investigation of 24 patients. *Contact Dermatitis*, **1**, 337.

Walker, A. (1975) A preliminary report of a vascular abnormality occurring in men engaged in the manufacture of polyvinyl chloride. *British Journal of Dermatology*, **93**, (Suppl. 11) 22.

Ward, A.M., Udnoon, S., Watkins, J., Walker, A.E. & Darke, C.S. (1976) Immunological mechanisms in the pathogenesis of vinyl chloride disease. *British Medical Journal*, **1**, 936.

Wehle, U. (1966) Arbeitsbedingte Ekzeme durch Polyester. *Allergie und Asthma*, **12**, 184.

Wodniansky, P. (1967) Hautschäden bei der Erzeugung von Polyurethan-kunststoffen. *Berufsdermatosen*, **15**, 81.

Working Party on Acrylic Cement in Orthopaedic Surgery (1974) Acrylic cement and the cardiovascular system. *Lancet*, **2**, 1002.

Zeisler, E.P. (1940) Dermatitis from elasti-glass garters and wrist watch straps. *Journal of the American Medical Association*, **114**, 2540.

Zschunke, E. (1959) Über die Epoxydhartz-dermatitis. *Deutsche Gesundheitswesen*, **14**, 1810.

13.

Preservatives and antibacterials

PARABENS
PHENOLIC COMPOUNDS
  Chlorocresol
  Chloroxylenol
  Dichlorophen
  Hexachlorophane
  *Ortho*phenylphenol
MERCURY
  Metallic mercury
  Amalgam dental fillings
  Mercury compounds
    Inorganic Ammoniated mercury
           Mercuric chloride
           Mercurous chloride
           Mercury fulminate
    Organic   Phenylmercuric salts
           Mercurochrome (Merbromin)
           Merthiolate
QUATERNARY AMMONIUM COMPOUNDS
  Cetrimide
  Benzalkonium chloride
  Dequalinium chloride
  Cetalkonium chloride
  Benzethonium chloride
  Chloroallylhexaminium chloride (Dowicil 200)

BRONOPOL
CHLORHEXIDINE
CHLOROACETAMIDE
CHLOROBUTANOL
DIMETHOXANE
DOMIPHEN BROMIDE
ETHYLENEDIAMINETETRAACETATE
ETHYLENE OXIDE
IMIDAZOLIDINYL UREA COMPOUNDS
IRGASANS
  DP300 Triclosan
  CF3 Cloflucarban
LAURYL GALLATE
NORDIHYDROGUAIARETIC ACID
POTASSIUM METABISULPHITE
SORBIC ACID
TOCOPHEROLS (p. 177).

Preservatives are widely used in cosmetics, toiletries, pharmaceuticals, creams and lotions of all types. They may be added also to foods and to many substances used in industry.

Cosmetics and toiletries are easily spoiled by organisms which cause separation of emulsions, discolouration or unpleasant smells. Furthermore, Gram-negative bacilli, particularly *Pseudomonas*, can cause the decomposition of anionic detergents in shampoos. The principal bacterial contaminants belong to the genera *Pseudomonas*, *Klebsiella*, *Achromobacter* and *Alcaligenes*. These are common residents of water, and, in recent years, it has been realised that water used in manufacture is a major reservoir of contaminants.

These preparations may be infected during filling of the containers, by the user's fingers, or from the air, particularly with wide mouthed jars. Cap liners have been traced as a source of fungal growth, and powders may contain fungal spores. The bacterial and fungal contaminants of used samples of mascara, eyeliners and eye-shadows were found by Wilson *et al.* (1971) to correlate with the organisms isolated from the users' eyelid margins. Bacteria, most commonly Gram-positive micrococci, were isolated from 43 per cent of the 428 used samples, and fungi from 12 per cent.

To counter these contaminants, suitable preservatives are added to the preparations, the choice depending on safety, compatibility with the product and cost (Van Abbé *et al.*, 1970; Croshaw, 1977).

Topical pharmaceutical preparations have likewise to be preserved. Solutions for parenteral administration which cannot be autoclaved, multidose containers and vaccines also have added bactericides. Those most commonly used are the paraben esters, chlorocresol, thiomersol, phenylmercuric nitrate, phenol and chlorbutol.

Preservatives must have a low sensitising potential in the concentrations in which they are added to a product. Therefore the incidence of contact dermatitis is low in relation to the widespread presence of these chemicals in preparations handled by everyone. As might be expected, when sensitisation occurs, it is nearly always from topical medicaments used for the treatment of eczematous patients rather than from cosmetics applied to normal skin. Reactions to preservatives in cosmetics and foods do occur but are infrequent.

Esters of *p*-Hydroxybenzoic Acid (Parabens; Nipagin; Nipa esters)

Esters of *p*-hydroxybenzoic acid are effective preservatives for cosmetics, drugs and foods. They are used especially in cosmetic creams and lotions but also in many pharmaceutical preparations for topical use. They are added to some solutions for parenteral injection and to certain foods. The derivatives of greatest value are the methyl, ethyl, propyl, butyl and benzyl esters.

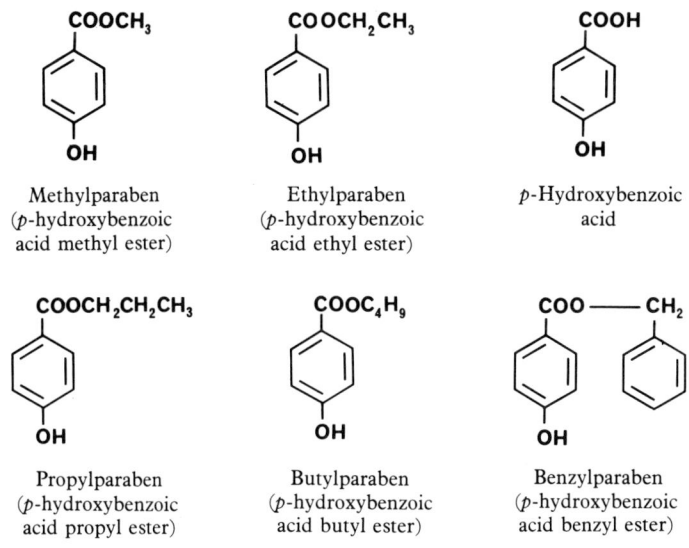

Methylparaben (*p*-hydroxybenzoic acid methyl ester)	Ethylparaben (*p*-hydroxybenzoic acid ethyl ester)	*p*-Hydroxybenzoic acid
Propylparaben (*p*-hydroxybenzoic acid propyl ester)	Butylparaben (*p*-hydroxybenzoic acid butyl ester)	Benzylparaben (*p*-hydroxybenzoic acid benzyl ester)

These esters are stable, tasteless, odourless substances of low toxicity and there is no evidence that they are harmful in foods (Marzulli and Maibach, 1974). They are neither bactericides nor fungicides but act by inhibiting the growth of organisms and they may need to be supplemented with another preservative. As each ester is effective against a different range of organisms they are used in combinations rather than singly, perhaps unnecessarily because it has been found (O'Neill *et al.*, 1979) that an adequate concentration of the most efficient ester is better than a mixture.

They are effective over a wide range of pH, but are only sparingly soluble in water. The most soluble is the methyl ester, which is effective in concentrations of 0.1 per cent to 0.3 per cent; the higher esters, being less water-soluble, are added in concentrations of 0.01 per cent to 0.025 per cent (Van Abbé *et al.*, 1970). Their activity is reduced but not abolished by oils and non-ionic emulsifiers such as the Spans and Tweens. On hydrolysis the parabens yield *p*-hydroxybenzoic acid, which has little preservative activity; the influence of temperature and pH on this reaction is important in relation to heat sterilisation. These effects have been studied by Blaug and Grant (1974).

Sensitising potential

Paraben esters are not strong sensitisers. Two reports suggest that they can be placed in the lowest grade of sensitisers. In the first, Kligman (1966) used the maximisation test to try to sensitise 25 human subjects with 25 per cent methyl paraben; the concentration of the ester for the challenge was 10 per cent. Only one person was sensitised. In the second report, Marzulli and Maibach (1973) used the Draize procedure and for induction and challenge applied mixtures of methyl and propyl parabens in concentrations up to 10 per cent of each, with and without sodium lauryl sulphate. They sensitised one of 397 subjects, a sensitisation index of only 0.3 per cent.

Incidence of sensitivity

Sensitivity to parabens varied between 0.8 per cent and 3 per cent in the following series of eczematous patients, patch tested routinely. Men and women were affected with about equal frequency (Table 13.1).

Table 13.1

	Conc.	No. Tested	M + F%	M%	F%	Report
Copenhagen	?	3629	1.13			Hjorth & Trolle-Lassen (1963)
Copenhagen	?	1835		1	1	Magnusson *et al.* (1968)
Lund		1406		1	1	
Stockholm		510		1	1	
Gothenburg		1000		2	3	
Europe	3% × 5 = 15%	4825	1.9	1.3	2.3	Fregert *et al.* (1969)
U.S.A.	5% × 1	273	0.8			Schorr (1968)
	5% × 3 = 15%	138	2			Epstein, Rees & Maibach (1968)
	3% × 5 = 15%	1200	3			N. American C.D. Group (1973)
Poland	10% mix	861	2	2	2	Rudzki & Kleniewska (1970)
New Zealand	3%	216	1.9			Black (1972)

In Australia, of 1000 patients with contact dermatitis, five were found to be sensitive to parabens (Burry *et al.*, 1973). In the U.S.A., Fisher, Pascher and Kanof (1971) patch tested 100 patients with eczema, thought to be due to topical medicaments, and found that three reacted to a mixture of methyl, ethyl and propyl parabens, 5 per cent in petrolatum.

St John's

All patients are routinely tested with a mixture of paraben esters, methyl, ethyl, propyl, butyl and benzyl, each 3 per cent, giving a total concentration of 15 per cent in petrolatum. From 1971–1976 the incidence of sensitivity varied between 0.4–1.0 per cent of the total tested, 0.5–1.4 per cent for men and 0.2–0.9 per cent for women (Table 13.2).

Table 13.2. Incidence of parabens sensitivity in the total patients and men and women (St John's 1971–1976).

	Total			Men			Women		
	Tested	+	%	Tested	+	%	Tested	+	%
1971	1558	13	0.8	707	5	0.7	851	8	0.9
1972	1606	10	0.6	738	4	0.5	868	6	0.7
1973	1546	12	0.8	710	6	0.8	836	6	0.7
1974	1433	10	0.7	655	3	0.5	778	7	0.9
1975	1858	7	0.4	887	5	0.6	971	2	0.2
1976	1982	20	1.0	937	13	1.4	1045	7	0.7

Causes of sensitivity

Contact dermatitis from paraben esters has been recognised for the past 20 years and its history falls into two phases, corresponding to their use first as medicaments and later as preservatives.

As medicaments

Initially, patients acquired the allergy from the high concentrations used therapeutically in topical medicaments. The first report came from Denmark where 5 per cent ethyl paraben was used topically as an antifungal agent (Bonnevie, 1940). Later, Hjorth and Trolle-Lassen (1963) ascribed the 1 per cent incidence of parabens sensitivity at the Finsen Institute to the use of antimycotic preparations containing these esters in a concentration of 5 per cent.

As preservatives

An antibiotic ointment containing either tetracycline or chlortetracycline was preserved with 2.4 per cent methyl paraben and 0.6 per cent propyl paraben; its use caused parabens sensitisation both in Germany (Schultheiss, 1958) and in England (Sarkany, 1960).

During the past decade, parabens sensitivity has been acquired from the low concentrations, of the order of 0.1–0.5 per cent, used as preservatives, and not by the high concentration previously described.

Cosmetics and other creams

Unless information to the contrary is obtained, it must be assumed that all cosmetic creams and lotions contain parabens, but as cosmetics are applied to normal skin, the parabens they contain rarely sensitise. Lorenzetti and Wernet

(1977) stress that they are well tried and effective preservatives and at present there is no basis for banning them from cosmetics. Very occasionally they do cause trouble as in the parabens sensitive patient described by Simpson (1978) who became intolerant of her cosmetics.

Barrier creams may contain parabens. Sensitisation to parabens in a barrier cream was reported by Husain (1975) in a telephone engineer who had noticed that the barrier cream provided at work aggravated his hand eczema. Patch tests: he was positive to the barrier cream, parabens (15 per cent) and potassium dichromate 0.5 per cent.

St John's

In the 12 years 1965–1976 seven women have been seen in whom it was thought that parabens in cosmetic creams were the source of their sensitivity to these esters and the cause of their dermatitis. During this period one man was sensitised by a sun protective cream and it caused an acute dermatitis of his face.

Women sensitised by medicaments rarely seem to get trouble from cosmetics possibly because the concentration of parabens in cosmetics is too low to elicit eczema on normal skin. This is not absolute because one woman, probably sensitised by medicaments for her stasis ulcers, noticed irritation from cosmetics as did the patient described by Simpson (1978).

Topical medicaments

Ointments, being anhydrous, do not support the growth of bacteria or moulds and therefore require no preservatives. Creams, on the other hand, must be preserved because they contain water; for this reason they contain parabens, chlorocresol or another preservative.

Medicaments, not cosmetics, are the usual source of allergy to parabens which accounts for the similar incidence in men and in women.

In the U.S.A., Schorr and Mohajerin (1966) were the first to record the condition, and their paper was followed by further case reports (Schamberg, 1967; Wuepper, 1967). In each instance the allergy had been acquired from the use of medicaments to treat an established eczema. Similar patients were seen in England (Rudner and Cronin, 1966). These preservatives are present in the occlusive bandages used to treat stasis ulcers (Visco paste P.B.7. Smith and Nephew Ltd.; Quinaband and Ichthaband, Seton Products Ltd) and have caused reactions (Verbov, 1970; Sharvill, 1971). Two of Verbov's patients had a purpuric eczema under their bandages. A surprisingly high incidence of paraben sensitivity was found in patients with stasis eczema and ulcers by Maucher (1974); of 148 patients patch tested 45 (30 per cent) were positive to parabens.

Formulations are constantly changing and lists become outdated, but in 1978, in the United Kingdom, the following topical corticosteroid preparations contained lanolin, parabens and chlorocresol:

Preparation	Chlorocresol	Lanolin or Derivative	Parabens	Manufacturer
Adcortyl creams	No	No	YES	Squibb & Sons Ltd
Adcortyl ointment	No	No	No	
Alphaderm	No	No	No	Eaton Laboratories

Preparation	Chlorocresol	Lanolin or Derivative	Parabens	Manufacturer
Betnovate cream	YES	No	No	Glaxo
Betnovate lotion	No	No	YES	Glaxo
Betnovate ointment	No	No	No	Glaxo
Cortenema	No	No	YES	Bengue & Co. Ltd
Dermovate cream	YES	No	No	Glaxo
Dermovate ointment	No	No	No	Glaxo
Efcortelan cream	YES	No	No	Glaxo
Efcortelan lotion	No	No	YES	Glaxo
Efcortelan ointment	No	No	No	Glaxo
Hydrocortistab Cream	YES	No	No	Boots Co. Ltd.
Hydrocortistab ointment	No	No	No	Boots Co. Ltd.
Hydrocortistab eye drops	No	No	No	Boots Co. Ltd.,
Hydrocortistab eye ointment	No	YES	No	Boots Co. Ltd.
Hydromycin-D ear/eye drops	No	No	No	Boots Co. Ltd.
Hydromycin-D ear/eye ointment	No	YES	No	Boots Co. Ltd.
Medrone acne lotion	No	No	YES	Upjohn Ltd.
Medrone cream	No	No	YES	
Metosyn	No	No	No	ICI Ltd.
Molivate cream	YES	No	No	Glaxo
Molivate ointment	No	No	No	Glaxo
Myciguent ointment	No	YES	No	Upjohn Ltd
Myciguent opthalmic ointment	No	YES	No	Upjohn Ltd
Neo-Cortef eye and ear ointment	No	YES	No	Upjohn Ltd
Neo-Cortef ointment	No	No	YES	Upjohn Ltd
Neo-Cortef lotion	No	No	YES	Upjohn Ltd
Neo-Medrone acne lotion	No	No	YES	Upjohn Ltd
Nerisone cream	No	No	YES	Schering Chemicals Ltd
Nerisone oily cream	No	No	No	Schering Chemicals Ltd
Nystadermal cream	No	No	YES	Squibb & Sons Ltd
Nystadermal gel	YES	No	No	Squibb & Sons Ltd
Propaderm cream	YES	No	No	Allen & Hanbury's Ltd
Propaderm lotion	YES	No	No	Allen & Hanbury's Ltd
Propaderm ointment	No	No	No	Allen & Hanbury's Ltd
Remiderm cream	No	No	YES	Squibb & Sons Ltd
Schericur ointment	No	YES	No	
Scheriproct ointment	No	No	No	
Synalar creams — except	No	No	No	
for Synalar Forte cream:	No	No	YES	ICI Ltd
Synalar combination creams	No	No	YES	ICI Ltd
Synalar ointments	No	YES	No	ICI Ltd
Terra-Cortril ointment	No	No	No	Pfizer
Terra-Cortril spray	No	No	No	Pfizer
Topilar	No	No	No	Syntex
Topilar ointment	No	YES	No	Syntex
Topisone	No	No	No	Syntex
Topisone C	No	No	No	Syntex
Triadcortyl cream	No	No	YES	Squibb & Sons Ltd
Triadcortyl ointment	No	No	No	Squibb & Sons Ltd
Ultradil cream plain	No	No	YES	Schering Chemicals Ltd
Ultradil ointment plain	No	YES	No	Schering Chemicals Ltd
Ultralanum cream plain	No	No	YES	Schering Chemicals Ltd
Ultralanum lotion	No	No	YES	Schering Chemicals Ltd
Ultralanum ointment	No	YES	No	Schering Chemicals Ltd
Ultralanum ointment plain	No	YES	No	Schering Chemicals Ltd
Ultraproct ointment	No	No	No	Schering Chemicals Ltd

This list is published through the cooperation of the various manufacturers. It is correct as of February 1978, but formulations are constantly being revised and queries regarding these compounds should be checked with the manufacturer.

St John's

Medicaments had sensitised 68 of the 72 patients seen during the six years 1971–1976. Five of the patients with stasis eczema had noticed deterioration after treatment with occlusive medicament bandages, three from an Ichthopaste bandage and two from a calamine or quinoline bandage.

Clinical features

A clinical pattern distinctive of parabens sensitivity does not exist. In most cases the allergy is acquired from topical medicaments and the resultant contact dermatitis is superimposed upon an existent eczema. As stressed by Schorr (1968) the eczema may appear to be very chronic and resistant to treatment and the underlying reason, a paraben sensitivity, remains unrecognised unless detected by routine patch testing. This aspect was emphasised by Epstein (1968) when he called parabens sensitivity a 'subtle trouble'.

St John's

Cosmetics

From 1965–1976 seven women were seen with a parabens sensitivity definitely due to their cosmetics; an eighth patient (a man) was sensitised by a sun-protective cream.

Case 1. One week before attending the hospital, a woman aged 45 years had suddenly developed itching and swelling of her face with transient irritation of her body. She had no past history of skin trouble. On patch testing, she reacted to a 15 per cent parabens mixture and to her moisturising cream, which was found to contain methyl and propyl parabens. She was reviewed periodically for six months during which time there was no recurrence.

Case 2. A woman aged 54 years gave a nine months' history of irritation and scaling of her eyes. When patch tested, she reacted to a 15 per cent parabens mixture, to her night cream and to 20 per cent neomycin. It was not confirmed that her cream contained parabens, but when she was seen one month later, her skin was clear.

Case 3. A woman, 52 years old, gave a six weeks' history of eczema spreading from her face and neck, to her arms and legs. She had had eczema as a child but this had cleared when she was aged 11 years. On patch testing, she reacted to a 15 per cent parabens mixture and to her two foundation creams, both of which contained parabens. Subsequently, the eczema cleared from her face and neck but remained on her limbs where it fluctuated in severity.

Case 4. A 21-year-old woman described the sudden onset, three weeks previously, of discomfort around her eyes and in her elbow flexures. On examination her upper eyelids were red and glazed, her face was peeling and in her antecubital fossae there was a papular eczema. She had a past history of nickel dermatitis from jewellery and clothing but she avoided contact with metal. On patch testing, her sensitivity to nickel was confirmed, but she reacted also to the 15 per cent parabens mixture. She was not tested with her cosmetics, nor was it confirmed that they contained parabens. However, she stopped using cosmetics, and her face healed. When seen two years later on account of a patchy eczema of recent onset on her body, she said her face remained clear only so long as she avoided cosmetics. She was given a list of parabens-free preparations.

Case 5. Another woman aged 43 years developed a mild eczema of her face, neck and arms, which grumbled on for three to four years, during which time she used numerous cosmetics including a body lotion. She had a past history of nickel dermatitis. On routine patch testing she reacted to nickel 2.5 per cent, to the 15 per cent parabens mixture and gave a doubtful response to a moisturising cream. It was confirmed that most of her cosmetics contained parabens; she was advised to stop using all cosmetics except a loose powder and was given an emollient cream which did not contain parabens. When she was seen four months later, her eczema had cleared completely.

Case 6. An 82-year-old lady had three months previously developed a mild eczema which began on her neck and spread to her face. Every night, for six years she had rubbed one particular emollient lotion onto her face and neck. She stopped applying this preparation and her skin healed. Patch testing: she reacted to parabens but not to the emollient lotion, despite the fact that it did contain parabens. She was given a substitute cream which was parabens free.

Case 7. A woman aged 30 years gave a nine months' history of intermittent itching, burning and swelling of her face, particularly her cheeks and for one month her neck had been affected. Patch tests: she reacted to parabens and one particular cosmetic cream, which the manufacturers revealed contained about 1 per cent methyl and propyl parabens. She stopped all cosmetics and for a time used only a pharmaceutical emollient cream without parabens. She then used in addition a cosmetic cold cream and had no relapse. She remained comfortable and six months later, having kept to these two preparations, her face was normal and this despite the fact that the cold cream she had bought herself contained 0.1 per cent methyl paraben.

Case 8. A man aged 59 years presented with an acute eczema of his face and neck which began while he was on holiday. On patch testing he reacted to parabens 15 per cent and to his sun-protective cream; it was ascertained that the cream contained parabens.

The pitfall of attributing paraben sensitivity to the use of cosmetics is illustrated by the case of another woman seen in 1973. This patient had for 18 months been experiencing episodes of eczema on her face, neck, arms and chest. She was known to be sensitive to paraben esters which were present in her cosmetics, yet she repudiated them as the cause of her eczema as she had never applied them to her body. She stopped using all cosmetics and her skin healed with topical applications; she then resumed using her cosmetics as previously. There was no recurrence of her eczema. The original diagnosis of seborrhoeic dermatitis was correct and the parabens sensitivity had been induced by medicaments. Patients, such as these, tolerate cosmetics without trouble.

Medicaments
From 1971–1976 (inclusive), 33 women and 35 men have been seen who had been

sensitised to parabens by medicaments; the majority belonged to the older age groups (Table 13.3).

Table 13.3. Ages of 68 patients sensitised to parabens by medicaments (St John's 1971–1976 (inclusive)).

Years	0–10	11–20	21–30	31–40	41–50	51–60	61–70	71–80
No. Pts.	1	3	3	7	7	32	14	1

In each patient the sensitivity was superimposed upon a constitutional eczema and all patterns were affected but 20 patients had stasis ulcers or eczema and 3 men had pruritus ani.

It was striking that on being patch tested only 16 per cent (11 patients) reacted just to parabens. The most frequently associated sensitivities were to wool alcohols 37 per cent (25 patients) and to neomycin 28 per cent (19 patients).

Systemic absorption of parabens

Parabens-sensitive patients must absorb small amounts of these esters from food and many will have been injected, inadvertently, with small quantities preserving solutions in multidose vials. This systemic exposure appears to do them no harm. However Aeling and Nuss (1974) inferred that the exacerbation of an eczema in a parabens-sensitive patient was due to a mandibular block with lidocaine (Xylocaine) containing methyl paraben 0.001 gm/ml as a preservative. This report conflicts with Fisher's (1975) experience. He investigated two parabens-sensitive patients with scratch tests and intracutaneous and subcutaneous injections of parabens without eliciting either an immediate or a systemic reaction.

Immediate-type hypersensitivity to parabens

A patient with an immediate-type reaction to local anaesthetics was mistakenly thought to be allergic to lidocaine (Xylocaine). Intracutaneous tests and Prausnitz-Küstner reactions established that she had no reaction to this anaesthetic but was sensitive to the methyl paraben used as a preservative in the multidose container. She was also sensitive to anaesthetics of the procaine group (Aldrete and Johnson, 1969). Parabens in an intravenous hydrocortisone preparation caused bronchospasm and pruritus in a ten-year-old asthmatic boy. Intradermal tests were positive and a patch test was negative but at the time he was receiving oral corticosteriods (Nagel, Fuscaldo and Fireman, 1977).

Patch testing

Patch testing with topical medicaments or cosmetics is unreliable in the diagnosis of parabens sensitivity. Four esters in graded dilutions were used separately by Hjorth and Trolle-Lassen (1963) to patch test 19 parabens-sensitive patients. They found that a 5 per cent concentration of each ester elicited a reaction to one or several of the esters in all 19 patients; 13 of the 19 reacted to 1 per cent; 11 of the 19 reacted to 0.5 per cent; and only 5 of the 19 reacted to 0.1 per cent. These results confirm that the concentration of paraben esters in topical preparations is too low to elicit positive patch test reactions in most patients. Furthermore the presence of a corticosteroid in a medicament being used for patch testing would tend to suppress an eczematous response thus increasing the possibility of a false negative patch test result.

Schorr (1968) found the methyl, ethyl, propyl and butyl esters mutually to cross-react and that testing with any one of them at 5 per cent in petrolatum established the allergy.

Routine testing. A mixture of paraben esters in petrolatum is recommended by the International Contact Dermatitis Research Group:

Methyl paraben	3 per cent	
Ethyl paraben	3 per cent	
Propyl paraben	3 per cent	Total = 15 per cent in petrolatum
Butyl paraben	3 per cent	
Benzyl paraben	3 per cent	

Alternatives

Cosmetics. This is difficult. Loose face powder does not contain parabens and compressed powder is unlikely to do so, but most other cosmetics are preserved with parabens. The range of parabens-free cosmetics is very limited although companies are now beginning to formulate such preparations. As sensitive patients are fairly infrequent and formulations are constantly changing, it is advisable to obtain current lists from manufacturers as they are required.

Emollient pharmaceutical creams such as Oily Cream B.P. which contains lanolin, or Aqueous Cream B.P. which is lanolin-free, are both preserved with chlorocresol and they can be substituted for night, cleansing and moisturising creams.

Medicaments. A list of parabens-free steroid preparations is given on page 669. Information about other medicaments and applications has to be obtained from the manufacturer.

Phenolic compounds

In 1867, Lister acclaimed the value phenol (carbolic acid) and established it as the standard disinfectant for many years. In fact, its effectiveness is limited but is increased by adding chlorine or alkyl groups to the benzene ring, thereby facilitating the dissociation of the phenolic groups.

CHLOROCRESOL (*p*-chloro-*m*-cresol)

4-Chloro-*m*-cresol (4-chloro-3-methylphenol)

Chlorocresol is an efficient bactericide which is more effective in acid than in alkaline solutions. In the U.K. it is used in pharmaceutical creams and lotions (p. 669) and particularly in the formulation of some diluted steroid creams. Aqueous solutions of drugs for parenteral use are sometimes preserved with 0.05–0.1 per cent chlorocresol. Cosmetic chemists avoid it in their formulations as it may interfere with the perfumes.

Sensitising potential

Chlorocresol has a low sensitising potential. The Draize procedure, using a concentration of 5 per cent chlorocresol for both the induction and challenge, failed to sensitise all 31 subjects tested (Marzulli and Maibach, 1973).

Incidence of sensitivity

Clinically, chlorocresol is an infrequent sensitiser. Of the 1000 patients with contact dermatitis analysed by Burry et al. (1973) in Southern Australia, 11 reacted to chlorocresol.

St John's

From 1967–1969 no cases were diagnosed; in 1970, two patients reacted to 0.1 per cent chlorocresol. Then in the latter part of 1972 chlorocresol 2 per cent in petrolatum was added to the standard patch test series and immediately cases of sensitivity were detected. The yearly incidence from 1973–1976 has varied between 0.3 and 0.6 per cent and the overall numbers of men and women sensitised were similar (Table 13.4).

Table 13.4. Incidence of chlorocresol sensitivity in the total patients and men and women (St John's 1973–1976).

	Total			Men			Women		
	Tested	+	%	Tested	+	%	Tested	+	%
1973	1546	7	0.5	710	2	0.3	836	5	0.6
1974	1433	6	0.4	655	4	0.6	778	2	0.3
1975	1858	5	0.3	887	2	0.2	971	3	0.3
1976	1982	12	0.6	937	9	1.0	1045	3	0.3
Total	6819	30	0.4	3189	17	0.5	3630	13	0.4

Causes of sensitivity

Dermatitis from chlorocresol in betamethasone creams was reported in 13 patients in Australia by Burry et al. (1975). Many were thought to have been primarily sensitised by chloroxylenol, because on patch testing although all were positive to chloroxylenol only eight were additionally positive to chlorocresol. It was suggested that in the negative reactors absorption of chlorocresol was dependent upon its incorporation into the corticosteroid cream. Another woman, who had been sensitised, possibly by betamethasone cream, was described by Parks in New Zealand (1970). Patch tests: she was strongly positive to chlorocresol 5 per cent in paraffin, while 84 controls were negative. Two patients have reacted to chlorocresol in Dermovate® (17-clobetasol propionate) cream (Oleffe, Blondeel and de Coninck, 1979).

St John's

In all the patients the sensitivity was superimposed upon an existing eczema and no pattern predominated, nor was any particular cream implicated as the source of the allergen. Of the 30 patients, 4 were sensitive to both chlorocresol and parabens.

Cross-reactions

Hjorth and Trolle-Lassen (1963) reported three patients with cross-reactions between chloroxylenol and chlorocresol.

Patch testing

Chlorocresol 2 per cent in petrolatum

Alternatives

A list of topical corticosteroid preparations with and without chlorocresol is given on page 669.

CHLOROXYLENOL (4-chloro-3,5-xylenol; *para*-chloro-*meta*-xylenol; PCMX; Dettol)

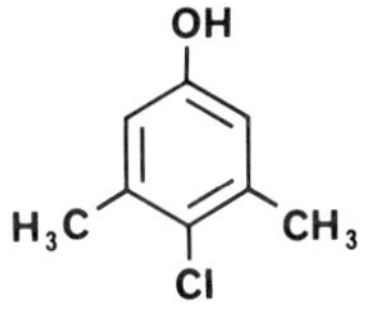

Chloroxylenol is a safe disinfectant which is active against streptococci, less so against staphylococci and almost inactive against *Pseudomonas* and *Proteus*. In a concentration of 0.5–5 per cent, it was very popular as a hospital and household disinfectant but nowadays is probably used less frequently. Occasionally, cosmetics or toiletries contain it as a preservative.

A few preparations such as chloroxylenol solution BPC and Surgical Dettol (Reckitt and Colman) contain a terpineol.

Sensitising potential

The Draize procedure using chloroxylenol in a concentration of 5 per cent for both induction and challenge failed to sensitise 208 subjects in one series; likewise in a further series none of 110 subjects was sensitised although the concentration had been increased to 20 per cent (Marzulli and Maibach, 1973).

Case reports

Reports of sensitisation are few.

In the U.S.A., carbolated vaseline (C.V.) which contains 0.2 per cent phenol and 0.5 per cent p-chloro-m-xylenol (PCMX) in a petrolatum base is a popular ethnic remedy among the Negro community. In Philadelphia, seven patients with eczema and one with intertrigo reacted acutely to this preparation. Patch tests: 4 were positive to 0.5 per cent PCMX. In the other 4 patients the reaction was diagnosed as irritation by the phenol. A further 20 patients, who had used C.V. either as a cosmetic or for mild ichthyosis, developed a dusky erythema and subsequently pigmentation which was attributed to a low-grade irritant effect of the phenol (Rubin and Pirozzi, 1973).

In Kuwait (Kanan, 1969), four nurses and two cleaners developed dermatitis of their hands from using weak Dettol solutions. Patch tests: each was positive to Dettol 0.5 per cent.

From Australia Burry *et al.* (1973) have reported another four cases.

St John's

In 1962, Calnan found chloroxylenol to be a frequent sensitiser having caused reactions in 53 of 772 patients sensitised by drugs. From 1967–1976, 26 cases of sensitivity have been seen (Table 13.5) each having reacted to 0.5 per cent or strongly to 1 per cent chloroxylenol; weak reactions to a 1 per cent concentration have been omitted as probable irritant reactions.

Table 13.5. Number of patients sensitive to chloroxylenol (St John's 1967–1976).

	1967 1968	1969 1970	1971 1972	1973 1974	1975 1976
Patients +	5	6	4	4	7

In this series there were 16 men and 10 women. Dettol was directly incriminated in five instances. One woman used it for washing bandages, another for dandruff and a third woman, who had occasionally used it undiluted in the past, added it to the water for washing floors and then developed dermatitis. A man applied neat Dettol to insect bites and his skin blistered and a second man developed dermatitis of his ear from using Dettol as a telephone disinfectant. His ear healed when this practice was stopped. A further man with pruritus ani was sensitised by suppositories, containing 0.44 per cent chloroxylenol.

Semi-cosmetic preparations containing chloroxylenol have caused dermatitis in two women. One had had eczema of her fingers for one year and was found, on patch testing, to be sensitive to a baby lotion; she was tested with its ingredients and reacted repeatedly to chloroxylenol 0.1 per cent. Her hands healed when she stopped using the lotion, but nine months later she noticed a rash under her nails. To treat this, she bathed her hands in Dettol and as a result developed an acute vesicular dermatitis of her palms and fingers. The other woman developed vesicular eczema of her palms which, after two months, became exudative. She had noticed that a proprietary skin emulsion aggravated the eruption. On patch testing she reacted to the emulsion and, on being tested to the constitutents, reacted quite strongly also to chloroxylenol 1 per cent.

Cross-reactions

Cross-reactions between chlorocresol and chloroxylenol were reported by Hjorth and Trolle-Lassen (1963).

St John's

Eleven of the chloroxylenol sensitive patients were tested with chlorocresol, 2 per cent in petrolatum and 2 were positive.

Patch testing

Chloroxylenol 0.5 per cent in petrolatum (1 per cent is a mild irritant in some patients)

DICHLOROPHEN (dichlorodihydroxydiphenylmethane; 2,2'-methylenebis(4-chlorophenol); bis(5-chloro-2-hydroxyphenyl)-methane; G4'; Panacide)

This chemical, which is soluble in fat solvents but almost insoluble in water, is a bactericide, a fungicide and an algicide. It has been used as a germicide in soaps, cosmetic and toilet preparations and industrially in water-cooling systems, storage tanks and cutting oil emulsions.

Sensitising potential

With an induction and challenge concentration of 5 per cent dichlorophen none of 208 subjects was sensitised by the Draize procedure. An increase in the induction concentration to 20 per cent resulted in the sensitisation of only one of 110 subjects (Marzulli and Maibach, 1973).

Incidence of sensitivity

St John's

> In 1972, 251 routine patients were patch tested with a mixture of sodium dichlorophen 0.4 per cent and ethylenediamine 0.04 per cent in petrolatum. They were simultaneously tested with ethylenediamine 1 per cent in petrolatum. Two of these 251 patients reacted to the dichlorophen mixture but were negative to ethylenediamine; in neither patient was the reaction found to be relevant.

Case reports

Medicaments

The first report of dichlorophen as a sensitiser was by Gaul and Underwood (1949) who described a patient whose dermatitis of the feet was greatly aggravated by a proprietary anti-fungal ointment containing this chemical. Patch testing with the ointment and corresponding powder was positive, but dichlorophen as the sensitiser was incriminated only by inference. However in another report of contact dermatitis from an anti-mycotic preparation, Bier (1958) proved by patch testing that dichlorophen was the sensitiser.

In 1970, Schorr described three patients who reacted to the 0.25 per cent dichlorophen in an Unna's boot mixture. One, a woman, was thought to have been sensitised previously by a commercial hand lotion containing 0.05 per cent dichlorophen, but the second patient was sensitised by the Unna's boot mixture; both reacted to patch tests with 0.5 per cent dichlorophen. The third patient reacted clinically to the boot but on patch testing was positive only to 5 per cent dichlorophen. None of these three patients cross-reacted to hexachlorophane.

Toothpastes

A report by Fisher and Lipton (1951) established dichlorophen ('Baxin') in a toothpaste as the cause of an allergic glossitis and cheilitis. Patch tests with the toothpaste and with dichlorophen 5 per cent in petrolatum were positive. Over a period of six months a further eight patients were seen of whom seven had been sensitised by a toothpaste and one by a tooth powder. Stomatitis, glossitis, cheilitis, perleche or circumoral dermatitis were the clinical features of these cases. Each had a positive patch test to dichlorophen 5 per cent in petrolatum; 25 controls were negative (Fisher and Tobin, 1953). Another patient developed itching, swelling and blistering of the left palm from cleaning dentures with a similar toothpaste. There was no stomatitis. Patch testing with the toothpaste was positive (Lowenthal, 1952).

Cosmetics

Contact dermatitis of the face due to dichlorophen, used as a preservative in cosmetics, was reported by Epstein (1966). One of his two patients, a 19-year-old girl had dermatitis of her face and, on being patch tested, reacted to her liquid make-up base. She was tested with its components and reacted to dichlorophen 1 per cent in petrolatum. The second patient had noticed that many cosmetics caused dermatitis; as she was found to be sensitive to dichlorophen 1 per cent, this was presumed to be a relevant allergen.

Patch testing

Dichlorophen 0.5 per cent and 1 per cent in petrolatum (1 per cent may be mildly irritant)

HEXACHLOROPHANE (2,2'-methylenebis(3,4,6-trichlorophenol); dihydroxy-hexachlorodiphenylmethane; G-11)

Hexachlorophane, a bis-phenol, was first synthesised in 1939. It is too toxic to be given systemically but it has been extensively used as a topical antiseptic. Only sparingly soluble in water, it is brought into solution by the addition of soap or a detergent and has the great advantage of retaining its potency in their presence. Active against Gram-positive bacteria, it is much less effective against Gram-negative organisms. Although its action is slow hexachlorophane attaches to skin and has a prolonged effect, which obviates the necessity for prolonged scrubbing in pre-operative disinfection. It has been used in concentrations of 0.01–2 per cent in germicidal soaps and creams, in dusting powders, deodorants and toothpastes. pHisohex (Winthrop) was 3 per cent hexachlorophane in a detergent cream; Ster-zac DC Skin Cleanser for per operative use (Hough, Hoseason & Co. Ltd.) contains hexachlorophane 3 per cent and chlorocresol 0.3 per cent.

Toxicity

Recently, the safety of hexachlorophane has been brought sharply into question. For years, 3 per cent hexachlorophane preparations were effectively used on infants' skin to combat staphylococcal sepsis. It is now known, however, that it is absorbed through intact skin (Curley *et al.*, 1971), and is neurotoxic, causing oedema and vacuolation of the cerebral white matter. In 1972, in France, due to an error in manufacture, a baby powder was made and sold containing more than 6 per cent hexachlorophane and it caused the death of at least 30 children. Suddenly babies presented with neurological signs and a striking erythema of the napkin area. Severe cases progressed to decerebrate rigidity and death but milder ones recovered, confirming that the changes are reversible (Jacquelin and Colomb, 1972; Lockhart, 1973). In California the deaths of seven premature infants were ascribed, retrospectively, to hexachlorophane (Powell *et al.*, 1973) and in 1974, Shuman, Leech and Alvord reported their evidence for a significant association between the use of hexachlorophane and a vacuolar encephalopathy. These cerebral changes are not specific; they may also be seen in the brains of infants dying without exposure to hexachlorophane (Gowdy and Ulsamer, 1976). In a study in Australia, it was found that only small premature infants are at serious risk and hyperbilirubinaemia is a contributory factor (Plueckhahn and Collins, 1976).

The washing of intact skin in guinea pigs and humans with a soap or detergent containing up to 1 per cent hexachlorophane has been assessed as harmless but the exposure time was limited (Black *et al.*, 1974).

The toxicology of hexachlorophane has been reviewed by Gump (1969), Kimbrough (1973), Lockhart (1973), Trout (1973) and in the Adverse Drug Reaction Bulletin (1974). The evidence definitely establishing hexachlorophane as a neurological toxin was summarised by Catalano (1975), criticised by McCarl (1976) and defended by Catalano (1976).

Legislation in the U.S.A. and in Great Britain now restricts the sale of products containing hexachlorophane. Only those with a concentration of 0.75 per cent or less can be bought over the counter; pHisohex has been reformulated to comply with the regulations and the 3 per cent emulsion, renamed pHiso-Med (Winthrop) can only be obtained on prescription.

Sensitising potential

This is extremely low. The maximisation test, with an induction concentration of 25 per cent, failed to sensitise all 23 subjects tested by Kligman (1966). The Draize procedure was equally ineffective in 80 subjects, the concentration for induction being 20 per cent and for challenge 1 per cent (Marzulli and Maibach, 1973). The guinea pig maximisation test was negative in all 25 animals tested (Magnusson and Kligman, 1969).

Incidence of sensitivity

Routine patch testing of eczematous patients with hexachlorophane has given few positive results. Fregert and Hjorth (1969) tested 660 patients (the concentration used was not stated) and 0.3 per cent were positive; Rantuccio and Meneghini (1970) used 5 per cent in petrolatum to test 150 patients and none reacted. In Australia, the patch test results in 1000 patients with contact dermatitis were analysed by Burry *et al.* (1973) and 6 had reacted to hexachlorophane.

St John's

Similar to experience elsewhere, the number of patients reacting to hexachlorophane has been very small. From 1967–1976 no certain cases of direct contact sensitivity to it have been seen.

It is used as 1 per cent in petrolatum in the routine photopatch testing of patients with light evoked eruptions. From 1970–1976, 2 patients have reacted but each also had positive reactions to other halogenated phenols.

Dermatitis

Allergic

Reports of sensitisation are few. In Adelaide, Burry *et al.* (1973) listed hexachlorophane as the cause of six cases of dermatitis, and in Kuwait Kanan (1969) reported three nurses who had been sensitised by using pHisohex and who all gave a positive patch test reaction to hexachlorophane 0.5 per cent. In the U.S.A. three cases have been reported. Of these, one woman had used a hexachlorophane deodorant spray then developed an axillary dermatitis which she treated with a hexachlorophane cream. She gave a positive patch test reaction to 1 per cent hexachlorophane, and when she stopped using the two preparations her dermatitis rapidly healed. A second woman described a dermatitis produced both by pHisohex (3 per cent hexachlorophane) and by a hexachlorophane first-aid cream; on patch testing she reacted to several chlorinated phenols including hexachlorophane 1 per cent (Epstein, 1966).

In 1955, Epstein used topical preparations containing 1–2 per cent hexachlorophane on several hundred patients, sometimes over large areas, and found only one sensitised patient. This patient reacted, on several occasions, to patch tests with hexachlorophane; four years previously he had noticed irritation from a soap containing hexachlorophane.

Cross-sensitivity reactions. Other reports of positive patch tests, in which details are given, seem to be cross-reactions to related halogenated chemicals.

Twenty-six men with a photocontact dermatitis due to halogenated salicylanilides were investigated by Epstein, Wuepper and Maibach (1968). They were photopatch tested with a series of chemicals; four reacted to hexachlorophane, but each patient reacted also to other members of this group of chemicals. Similarly, Wilkinson (1962) reported positive reactions to hexachlorophane in 4 of 14 patients sensitive to tetrachlorosalicylanilide. Epstein (1966) found cross-reactions between dichlorophen and hexachlorophane in two of three patients investigated, but this cross-sensitivity did not occur in the three dichlorophen-sensitive patients reported by Schorr (1970).

St John's

The cross-reactions both in men, were:

Case 1. (38 years) Bithionol, TCS, TCC, Fenticlor all with light irradiation

Case 2. (75 years) Bithionol, Fenticlor both with light irradiation.

Irritant
Hexachlorophane concentrate (Ster-zac), used in baths, has caused an irritant dermatitis of the scrotum in seven men and in two small children. This 10 per cent hexachlorophane solution contained a surface active agent, and, when the preparation was added in excess, the hexachlorophane precipitated at the bottom of the bath and caused the inflammation (Baker, Ive and Lloyd, 1969). These authors also described the case of a young man who developed acute inflammation of his scrotum and groins after applying undiluted pHisohex to his genital area. Five of these ten patients were patch tested; each gave an irritant reaction to hexachlorophane 10 per cent and each was negative to 1 per cent and 0.1 per cent.

Patch testing
Hexachlorophane 1 per cent in petrolatum

*ORTHO*PHENYLPHENOL (*o*-Phenylphenol; 2-hydroxybiphenyl)

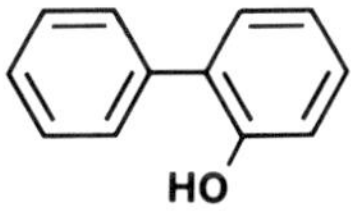

This chemical, in a concentration of about 0.25 per cent, is used in some cosmetics as a preservative; and the paper linings in the lids of cosmetic jars may be impregnated with it.

Case reports
Sensitivity has not been reported, but Kahn (1970) reported depigmentation caused by a detergent germicide containing several phenols, including 4 per cent *ortho*phenylphenol.

St John's
Two women were investigated, one in 1968 and the other in 1971, on account of episodes of facial eczema. Both reacted to the same foundation cream and, on being patch tested with its ingredients, both reacted to *ortho*phenylphenol 1 per cent. The tests on one patient were read at two days only; six controls were negative.

Patch testing
*Ortho*phenylphenol 1 per cent ? in water

Mercury

METALLIC MERCURY

Hg

As a sensitiser

Reports of sensitisation by metallic mercury are extremely rare. Gaul (1966) described a girl, who at the age of seven years while handling mercury contaminated a gold ring she was wearing and as a result developed dermatitis. Subsequently, when patch tested she reacted to mercuric chloride 0.001 per cent.

In Poland, Rudzki and Kohutnicki (1971) reported that 5 of 61 (8.2 per cent) bricklayers reacted to patch testing with 0.1 per cent mercuric chloride, and that mercury was detectable spectroscopically in samples of Polish cement. These authors pointed out that Eberhartinger *et al.* (1968) had considered the mercury sensitivity in their cement workers to be iatrogenic.

St John's

A man, aged 26 years, had eight years previously performed a series of experiments with metallic mercury, being in contact with the metal for 2–3 hours every day. After two weeks, his eyelids began to swell and an eruption appeared on his face, wrists and arms; these symptoms cleared within four days of stopping the experiments. Two years later, he was again exposed to mercury and the same eruption recurred. Since then, he had had intermittent recurrences, apparently unrelated to mercury contact. On patch testing, he reacted strongly to ammoniated mercury 2 per cent and to phenylmercuric acetate 0.06 per cent, but gave negative responses to all the other allergens.

Eliciting a contact dermatitis

A man, who had been sensitised by a mercury ointment 20 years previously, broke a clinical thermometer and stepped on the mercury. As a result, he developed a widespread dermatitis and subsequently stomatitis, enterocolitis and nephrosis; he finally died in uraemia (Frykholm and Wahlgren, 1964). Another patient, a woman, had been sensitised by a mercury medicament and later developed a generalised eruption after contact with mercury from a broken thermometer (Vickers, 1967).

In Lund, Sweden, metallic mercury 0.5 per cent in petrolatum is found to be a reliable detector of mercury sensitivity (Fregert and Hjorth, 1969).

Patch testing

Metallic mercury 0.5 per cent in petrolatum

AMALGAM DENTAL FILLINGS

An amalgam is an alloy of mercury with another metal; dental amalgam is made by combining metallic powders, usually silver 69.4 per cent, tin 26.2 per cent, copper 3.6 per cent, zinc 0.8 per cent, or sometimes gold or platinum, with equal parts of pure mercury to form a malleable mass. Tattooing of the oral mucosa by the amalgam is quite common (Weathers and Fine, 1974).

Amalgam fillings, once inserted, do not cause stomatitis. However, contamination of the facial skin and buccal mucosa during filling of the teeth can cause eczema of the face and neck which may become widespread (Case 6, Frykholm,

1957; Vickers, 1967) and a mild stomatitis was also present in the girl described by Traub and Holmes (1938). Transient erosions of the mouth and tongue, coinciding with the development of sensitisation to the mercury present in a man's tattoo, were attributed by Juhlin and Ohman (1968) to the mercury in his amalgam fillings.

Patch tests applied to the buccal mucosa are usually reported as negative. Gaul (1966) demonstrated this lack of reaction in two girls, who were sensitive to mercury, by failing to provoke a reaction to discs of amalgam placed adjacent to the buccal mucous membrane. However, he also patch tested the bite margin of an edentulous old man, and this elicited a positive response. Gaul suggested that a specific epidermal protein, not present in oral mucous membrane, may be required to conjugate with mercury to make the complete antigen. However, the difficulty may lie in maintaining apposition of the patch test to the mucosa, because in the case (No. 6) of undoubted mercury sensitivity described by Frykholm (1957), amalgams applied to the palate by means of a plate produced severe inflammation and erosions.

Systemic absorption of mercury from amalgam seems to be a rare cause of dermatitis in sensitised patients. Sidi and Casalis (1951) described such a woman who, as a child, had been sensitised by mercury applied topically; she had no stomatitis but had a chronic eczema of her face, neck and forearms. Patch tests with mercury were positive; her amalgam fillings were removed and her eczema healed.

A man with a strongly positive patch test to 5 per cent ammoniated mercury had recurrent episodes of severe dermatitis not only after amalgam fillings were inserted but also in the intervals between dental treatments. All his amalgam fillings, both new and old, were removed and he remained free of attacks (Feuerman, 1975).

St John's

A woman, aged 30 years, gave a three year history of a rash around the side of her mouth and on her neck which appeared on each of the three occasions she had been to the dentist for a filling. The retained amalgam fillings gave her no trouble. On patch testing she reacted strongly to ammoniated mercury ointment 1 per cent and less strongly to phenylmercuric nitrate 0.1 per cent.

It was suggested that further amalgam fillings were not contraindicated provided that skin contamination could be avoided during their insertion.

MERCURY COMPOUNDS

Mercurial compounds are toxic and sensitise. They are now rarely prescribed for topical treatment, although organic mercurial chemicals still have a limited role as preservatives. The various sources of mercury sensitivity in 59 patients were reported from Heidelberg by Taugner and Schütz (1966); 34 were psoriatics who had been treated with mercury precipitate; 15 had used ophthalmic preparations containing mercury; and 14 were hospital workers handling mercuric chloride and mercury oxycyanate as disinfectants, and particularly mercury sublimate for thermometers.

INORGANIC

AMMONIATED MERCURY (Mercuric chloride, ammoniated; mercury ammonium chloride)

$$Hg\,NH_2\,Cl$$

In Britain, until about 1965, ammoniated mercury ointments were commonly prescribed for psoriasis. Their efficacy is now questioned. Their undoubted absorption (Bork, Morsches and Holzmann, 1973), their potential toxicity as a cause of the nephrotic syndrome (Silverberg, McCall and Hunt, 1967) and of pink disease (Ward and Hingerty, 1967), which was reviewed by Turk and Baker (1968), makes them undesirable and they should be obsolete.

Sensitising potential
In the human maximisation test, 13 of 25 subjects were sensitised, giving ammoniated mercury a Grade 3 ranking on a 1–5 scale; the most potent sensitisers were Grade 5 on this scale (Kligman, 1966).

Incidence of sensitivity
In San Francisco, in 1968, Epstein *et al.* reported that 16 (3.5 per cent) of 462 patients, patch tested with ammoniated mercury 5 per cent, gave a positive reaction. In a study by the North American Contact Dermatitis Group (1973) 5 per cent of 1200 patients, patch tested with 1 per cent ammoniated mercury, reacted.

St John's
In 1962, Calnan reported that mercury was, at that time, the commonest sensitiser among a series of drugs tested. He attributed the high incidence, 60 (8 per cent) of 772 cases sensitive to drugs, to the use of mercury compounds in topical medicaments.
Since then, the numbers have been very small. Patients are tested with ammoniated mercury 1–2.5 per cent in simple ointment, only if indicated by the history; since 1965, the number of cases has varied from 1–3 each year (Table 13.6). The two men seen in 1975 and 1976 reacted to mercuric chloride 0.1 per cent; neither was tested with ammoniated mercury.

Table 13.6. Patients sensitive to inorganic mercury (St John's, 1965–1976).

Year	1965	1968	1969	1970	1971	1973	1975	1976
No. Pts.	1	3	1	2	2	2	1	1

The 13 patients, shown in Table 13.6, were of all ages; 9 were men of whom two had pruritus ani. Six patients had been sensitised by medicaments, 5 at some time in the past and the other, a man, in 1973 following recent treatment of his psoriasis with ammoniated mercury ointment. The source of contact differed in each of the other 7 patients as follows: metallic mercury; paint; amalgam fillings; at work as a district nurse; from a tattoo(2) and unidentified in a 16-year-old schoolgirl.

Patch testing
Ammoniated mercury 1 per cent in petrolatum

Discolouration and toxicity
Cosmetic creams containing 4 per cent ammoniated mercury caused a slate-grey pigmentation of the face and neck in two women who had applied them daily for over 50 years. The pigmentation, which was deeper round the eyes, in the nasolabial folds and in the folds of the face and neck, was due both to metallic mercury in the dermis and to an increased amount of melanin (Lamar and Bliss, 1966; Burge and Winkelmann, 1970).

Mercury is also used in skin lightening creams. The absorption and subsequent urinary excretion of mercury from such preparations have been studied in healthy young African nurses by Barr, Woodger and Rees (1973), and Barr *et al.* (1972) have reported that the 5–10 per cent amino-mercuric chloride contained in them has caused the nephrotic syndrome in young African women in Nairobi. In the German Federal Republic creams containing 5–6 per cent mercury were sold for bleaching freckles, they caused chronic mercury poisoning with signs of systemic toxicity, discolouration of the nails and loss of hair (Wustner *et al.*, 1975).

Mercuric chloride (Mercury bichloride; mercury perchloride; corrosive sublimate)

$$Hg\ Cl_2$$

Mercuric chloride solution 0.1 per cent was at one time a popular antiseptic and disinfectant. Indigo carmine is added as a safety precaution and gives solutions their distinctive pink colour.

Sensitising potential
It is a strong sensitiser. In the human maximisation test, using an induction concentration of 2 per cent and on challenge with 0.05 per cent, 23 of 25 subjects were sensitised by Kligman (1966). In the guinea pig maximisation test, 8 of 25 animals were sensitised (Magnusson and Kligman, 1969). In the Draize test, when done on the arm with an induction concentration of 2 per cent and on challenge with 0.05 per cent, two of 24 subjects were sensitised; when the same procedure was performed on the back, two of 18 subjects were sensitised. It was emphasised that, as this compound gives irritant patch test reactions, it can be difficult to differentiate an allergic from an irritant response (Marzulli and Maibach, 1973).

Incidence of sensitivity
The replacement of mercury by more effective medicaments for topical applications has reduced the incidence of sensitivity, but these chemicals are still present in the environment in an occult form. The frequency of sensitivity in a community will depend upon the extent of its exposure to mercury from all sources.

From New York, Baer, Ramsey and Biondi (1973) reported mercury to be their commonest sensitiser: of their 540 eczematous patients, 22 per cent reacted to 0.05 per cent aqueous mercuric chloride. Most reactions were weak, and few patients gave a relevant history. The sensitivities were regarded as subclinical, having been derived from mercury in a polluted environment. Epstein (1974) suggested that this incidence was artificially high due to the difficulty in distinguishing between an allergic and an irritant reaction when patch testing with mercuric chloride.

A rising incidence was reported from the Finsen Institute (Fregert and Hjorth, 1969). In the years 1962 to 1963 positive reactions were found in 2.5 per cent of 2634 patients, routinely patch tested with mercuric chloride; by 1967 the number had risen to 4.9 per cent of 1273 patients tested.

Patch testing

Mercuric chloride 0.05–0.1 per cent aqueous

Epstein (1974) thinks the irritancy of mercuric chloride precludes its use for patch testing, and suggests that ammoniated mercury should be substituted.

Mercurous chloride (Calomel)

$$Hg_2 Cl_2$$

It has been used as a diuretic, an antiseptic and in the treatment of syphilis.

Patch testing

Mercurous chloride as is (Fregert and Hjorth, 1972)

MERCURY FULMINATE (mercuric cyanate)

$$Hg(CNO)_2$$

Mercury fulminate is a grey, crystalline, highly toxic, powder which must be stored wet because it is extremely explosive when dry. It is used in the making of detonators for the military, industry and sporting pursuits.

During the last world war mercury fulminate caused many cases of contact dermatitis among workers in munitions factories. The dermatitis affected particularly the hands, face and eyelids and in some was severe (Joltrain, Hissard and Boulard, 1939; Swanston, 1943).

The powder irritates abrasions and may form ulcers, these are known as powder holes, and occur particularly on the fingers.

ORGANIC

PHENYLMERCURIC SALTS

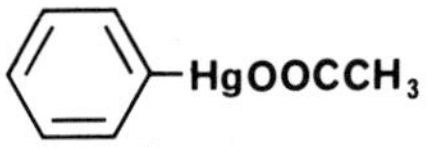

Phenylmercuric acetate (acetoxyphenylmercury)

Phenylmercuricborate ([dihydrogenborato]phenylmercury)

Phenylmercuric nitrate basic

These compounds can be used as herbicides, fungicides, antiseptics, in contraceptives and as preservatives in materials, cosmetics and pharmaceutical preparations. Phenylmercuric salts have antibacterial and antifungal properties; in concentrations of 0.002 per cent they are added to eye drops which will be given for only a limited time, and phenylmercuric nitrate is used in some solutions for parenteral injection. They are useful in concentrations of 0.001–0.004 per cent, as preservatives for some cosmetics, such as shampoos, which are only transiently in contact with the skin. In a concentration of 0.2 per cent, they are used to preserve emulsion paints and the sock part and lining of some shoes. It was reported by Sunderman, Hawthorne and Baker (1956) that during the Second World War phenylmercuric benzoate had been used by the United States Army as a preservative in camouflage cosmetics and that it did not appear to cause dermatitis.

Sensitising potential — phenylmercuric acetate
The Draize procedure was used by Marzulli and Maibach (1973) to sensitise human subjects, but the irritancy of this chemical made it difficult to interpret the challenge patch test results. The induction concentration was 0.125 per cent and graded dilutions were used for the challenge: of the 56 subjects tested, 16 reacted to a concentration of 0.1 per cent; 12 to 0.05 per cent; and only one to a 0.01 per cent challenge concentration.

Incidence of sensitivity —*phenylmercuric borate*
In Germany phenylmercuric borate, in a concentration of 0.066 per cent in an alcoholic solution, is a popular remedy for tinea pedis and is used preoperatively for preparation of the skin. It was the cause of dermatitis in 116 out of 1094 patients sensitised by a topical medicament, and many of these patients had a cross-sensitivity to other mercury compounds used as preservatives in creams and ointments (Breit and Bandmann, 1973). Its use as a thermometer disinfectant caused an acute axillary dermatitis in a cardiac surgery patient (Ippen, 1979).

St John's
In 1971, 110 patients with eczema were patch tested with phenylmercuric borate 0.025 per cent in petrolatum. One patient, a 16-year-old schoolgirl, gave a positive reaction; she also reacted strongly to ammoniated mercury ointment (inorganic mercury). Her acute, blistering eczema spread from her hands to her arms, face and thighs. A history of contact with mercury was not elicited.

Case reports

Phenylmercuric nitrate. Two patients sensitised by phenylmercuric nitrate were described by Morris (1960). One, a man, had put a weedkiller powder containing this chemical onto his lawn, and had developed an itchy, papular eruption on his legs; the other, a woman, developed dermatitis of her face from the same chemical in an ointment. Both patients reacted to patch tests with an 0.06 per cent solution of phenylmercuric nitrate.

Phenylmercuric acetate. Another woman, reported by Morris (1960), complained that her vulva itched and burned when she used a contraceptive jelly containing 0.02 per cent phenylmercuric acetate. A patch test with 0.06 per cent phenylmercuric chloride was positive.

Occupational dermatitis

Phenylmercuric benzoate. The toxicity of phenylmercuric salts has been reviewed by Ladd, Goldwater and Jacobs (1964), and they reported 12 cases of occupational dermatitis possibly due to phenylmercuric benzoate.

Phenylmercuric acetate. A man, while grinding phenylmercuric acetate, got some of the powder into his gloves and, some hours later, his hands became erythematous then bullous. Ethylmercuric phosphate had a similar effect on another worker (Goldblatt, 1945). A research chemist spilled a saturated solution of phenylmercuric acetate over his hand and, eight hours later, despite washing, it became erythematous and subsequently bullous (Sunderman *et al.*, 1956). None of these cases was patch tested, and an allergic rather than an irritant effect was not proved.

An allergic contact dermatitis from phenylmercuric acetate and phenylmercuric oleate was reported by Hartung (1965) in 8 out of 150 seamstresses handling tarpaulin treated with these chemicals. Three of these patients were patch tested with each of these chemicals in concentration of 0.025 per cent and 0.026 per cent, and all three reacted to both; they also reacted to 0.1 per cent mercuric chloride.

Patch testing

These chemicals are irritants, and phenylmercuric acetate 0.1 per cent in petrolatum has given strong, irritant reactions (Koby, 1972).

Phenylmercuric acetate 0.01 per cent aqueous
Phenylmercuric nitrate 0.01 per cent aqueous (Fregert and Hjorth, 1972).

MERCUROCHROME (Merbromin)

In Denmark mercurochrome 5 per cent in water is used extensively in surgical departments and for first-aid. On patch testing, sensitised patients usually react also to mercuric chloride (Fregert and Hjorth, 1969).

Case reports
In the report from Kuwait by Kanan (1969), four cases were listed as sensitive to mercurochrome 1 per cent. In Spain, a man whose injuries were treated with mercurochrome, developed a violent local reaction, a generalised eruption and facial and laryngeal oedema of such severity that he required treatment in an intensive care unit. Patch tests: he was strongly positive to merthiolate (0.1 per cent aqueous), mercuric chloride (0.05 per cent aqueous) and the response to Mercromina, containing 2 per cent aqueous solutions of the sodium salt of dibromohydroxy mercuric resorcinaphthalene precipitated an erythroderma and laryngeal oedema which necessitated his return to the intensive care unit (Camarasa, 1976).

MERTHIOLATE (Thiomersal; Thimerosal; sodium ethylmercurithiosalicylate)

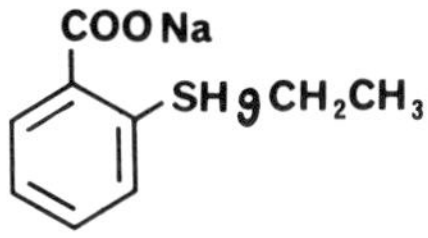

COO Na

SH 9 CH$_2$CH$_3$

Merthiolate (thiomersal; [(*o*-carboxyphenyl)thio]ethyl-mercury sodium salt)

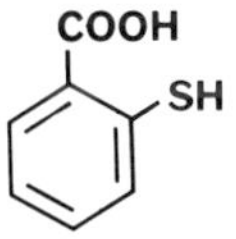

COOH

SH

Thiosalicylic acid (2-mercaptobenzoic acid)

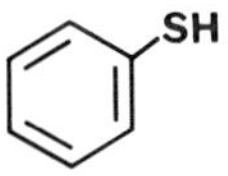

SH

Thiophenol (benzenethiol)

Merthiolate is a useful preservative, particularly for vaccines but also for antitoxins. Tincture of merthiolate, containing thiomersal 0.1 per cent in 50 per cent alcohol is still used occasionally for pre-operative skin preparation. Contact with aluminium foil must be avoided in such patients as the mercury in the merthiolate catalyses oxidation of the aluminium producing sufficient heat to burn the skin (Thelwall Jones, 1972).

There are two oddities about merthiolate. One is its sensitising component which is not necessarily mercury, and the other is the high incidence of reactions to it among healthy young men, which has been reported from Sweden.

Incidence of sensitivity

In the routine testing of eczematous patients the following incidences have been recorded:

Centre	No. Tested	Conc.	No. +ve	
Finsen Inst., Copenhagen	1880	0.1% petrolat.	25	(1.3%) (Hjorth, 1967)
Lund (Sweden)	994	0.1% petrolat.	14	(1.5%) (Fregert, 1969)
Prague	316		38	12%) (Novak and Kuicalová, 1978)
California	52	0.1% aqueous	7	(13.4%) (Epstein, Rees and Maibach, 1968)

Sensitiser

Sensitivity to merthiolate was described 30 years ago by Ellis and Robinson (1942) in four patients, none of whom reacted to other mercury compounds. This led Ellis (1947) to patch test six merthiolate-sensitive patients with a freshly prepared solution of thiosalicylic acid 0.1 per cent and five of the six were positive; three of the six also reacted to inorganic ammoniated mercury. Gaul (1958) studied a further patient and found thiophenol to be the sensitiser.

Since then, the following results have been reported:

(a) Finsen Institute (Hjorth, 1967): of 1880 patients tested, 25 reacted to merthiolate, 30 to mercuric chloride, and 8 to both

(b) Malmö, Sweden (Hansson and Möller, 1970): of 26 men tested, 18 reacted to merthiolate 0.1 per cent, 2 to mercuric chloride 0.1 per cent, and 2 to thiosalicylic acid 0.1 per cent.

These results suggest that some patients are sensitised by the mercury in merthiolate but the majority by some other component.

Case reports — parenteral injections

In the U.S.A. allergy to merthiolate seems not to be uncommon. Epstein (1963) described five patients, four of whom had given false positive reactions to intradermal tests with solutions containing merthiolate as a preservative; none of the five cross-reacted to ammoniated mercury. Ten patients were similarly detected by Reisman (1969), because each had reacted to every solution used for intradermal testing including the control solutions. Of these 10 patients, three had a past history of contact dermatitis from merthiolate, five had possibly been exposed to it, and in only two was no contact traced.

Hansson and Möller (1970, 1971), from Malmö in southern Sweden, reported that in 16 per cent of healthy young military service recruits patch tests with 0.1 per cent merthiolate in petrolatum were positive and that in 15 per cent intracutaneous tests with 0.01 per cent merthiolate in saline also were positive. These reactions to merthiolate had caused false positive responses to tuberculin as merthiolate was present as a preservative in the tuberculin solution. Contact with merthiolate in Sweden is minimal; the reactions seem to occur particularly in healthy young people, and, when eczematous subjects are tested, it is the younger rather than the older patients who are positive. These anomalies made the authors doubt initially whether such responses indicated a true delayed-type hypersensitivity but a study in twins suggested that the reactions were allergic rather than irritant (Holst and Möller, 1975). On the basis of their results they stressed that merthiolate should not be used as a preservative in solutions for the detection of delayed-type hypersensitivity but that, if it is present, a control test with merthiolate should be included in the investigation.

In the U.S.A., these misleading skin reactions are now unlikely to be seen as merthiolate is generally not used in these skin testing solutions (Maibach, 1972).

Merthiolate sensitivity is common in Prague and being without clinical relevance Novák and Kvicalova (1978) consider parenteral injections a likely source of sensitisation.

Topical applications
A man sprayed his slightly sore throat with a first-aid aerosol spray containing 0.033 per cent thiomersal and 22 per cent alcohol and within 30 hours he required adrenaline, an emergency tracheostomy, intravenous corticosteroids and antibiotics. He made a rapid recovery. Patch tests: he was strongly positive to thiomersal 0.1 per cent in petrolatum. Sensitivity to merthiolate, rather than infection, was thought to be the cause of his acute laryngeal obstruction (Maibach, 1975). Another man, who wore contact lenses, developed reddening of the conjunctivae which was traced to sensitivity to merthiolate (0.001 per cent) present in the solution in which he kept the lenses overnight. Patch tests: merthiolate 0.1 per cent in petrolatum was positive, disodium edetate 1 per cent in water (another constituent of the solution) was negative. It was emphasised that the patient had conjunctivitis without eyelid involvement (Bang Pedersen, 1976).

Patch testing.
Merthiolate 0.1 per cent in petrolatum (this concentration is slightly irritant in some patients).

Cross-reactions among mercury compounds. Cross-reactions certainly occur between the metal, the inorganic and the organic mercurials, but the incidences reported have varied. Fregert and Hjorth (1969) found a high incidence of cross-reactivity.

			Positives	Controls
mercuric chloride	(?)	0.1% aq.	28	
mercury		0.5% pet.	25/28	
These 25 were tested as follows:				
phenylmercuric acetate		0.1% pet.	13/25	0/27
ethoxyethylmercuric acetate		0.1% pet.	16/25	0/27
mercuric acetate		0.1% pet.	15/25	0/27
methoxyethylmercuric chloride		0.1% pet.	12/25	0/27
merthiolate		0.1% pet.	6/25	
ethylmercuric chloride		0.1% pet.	7/25	7/27
bisethylmercuric sulphide		0.2% pet.	6/18	1/20
methylmercuric dicyanamide		0.1% pet.	7/25	3/27

Routine patch testing

It is probably adequate to test with:

Ammoniated mercury 1 per cent in petrolatum
Phenylmercuric acetate 0.01 per cent in water or petrolatum

Quaternary ammonium compounds

Quaternary ammonium compounds are effective, water-soluble antimicrobials which are widely used in hospitals as disinfectants, sterilisers and skin cleansers. They are also formulated as antiseptic creams and as shampoos. As preservatives, they are added to pharmaceutical preparations but in cosmetics their use is restricted because of incompatability with other ingredients of the formulation, particularly with non-ionic and ionic surfactants.

Clinically they are infrequent sensitisers and as all the chemicals in this group are irritant, the interpretation of patch test results is most difficult, and it is easy to label as sensitisation an irritant response. In France, Huriez et al. (1965, 1966) have studied sensitisation by these chemicals and in Sweden Wahlberg (1962) reported two patients sensitised in the treatment of varicose ulcers and eczema. In Spain many pharmaceutical products contain quaternary ammonium compounds and they frequently cause or prolong an eczema. The difficulties of patch testing with these chemicals makes it uncertain whether their adverse effect is due to irritation or sensitisation (Garcia-Perez and Moran, 1975).

CETRIMIDE (Cetavlon; cetyltrimethylammonium bromide;
hexadecyltrimethylammonium bromide; cetrimonium bromide)

$$\left[CH_3 \left(CH_2 \right)_{15} N \left(CH_3 \right)_3 \right] Br$$

Cetrimide is frequently used in British hospitals and reports of sensitisation are extremely rare.

Case reports—Sensitisation

Four patients were described by Sharvill (1965). One reacted to a shampoo, two to pre-operative skin preparation, and the fourth was a small boy who developed a severe bullous eruption after using a 1 per cent aqueous solution to cleanse a balanitis. In two of these patients the dermatitis was severe enough to require systemic corticosteroids. Three of them were patch tested; all three reacted to 0.1 per cent cetrimide, and two reacted both to 0.01 per cent and to 0.001 per cent.

St John's

In 1962 a woman was seen with acute erythema and swelling of her upper arms due to using a cream containing 0.5 per cent cetrimide to treat axillary irritation. Patch tests: she reacted to the cream and to cetrimide 0.5 per cent, 0.1 per cent and 0.05 per cent. From 1965–1976, there have been two further patients definitely sensitised to cetrimide; both had deteriorated while using a cetrimide cream. Patch tests: the first woman reacted to the cream, to cetrimide 0.5 per cent and had a positive open test to the cream; the second woman reacted to cetrimide 0.25 per cent and 0.01 per cent.

Other patients have had positive patch test responses to various dilutions of cetrimide, but the history of relevance was indefinite, and the reactions in these patients were difficult to interpret.

Irritation

Cutaneous necrosis of an old lady's foot and leg was attributed to dressings with cetrimide powder (B.P.C.) applied daily for over two weeks. Patch tests with cetrimide 0.1 per cent and other medicaments were negative (August, 1975).

St John's

In 1974 a woman used a shampoo containing 17.5 per cent cetrimide to wash her own and her daughter's hair. That night she was awakened because her fingers, face and neck had become red, raw and acutely swollen. Her daughter was unaffected. She patch tested herself with the shampoo and produced a blister. In the clinic patch tests with cetrimide 0.25 per cent and 0.1 per cent were negative. Coded prepared samples of the shampoo were supplied by the manufacturer for patch tests; she reacted moderately to only one, which was identified as cetrimide 7 per cent!

Patch testing

Cetrimide 0.1 per cent, and 0.01 per cent in water

BENZALKONIUM CHLORIDE (Roccal; Zephiran chloride; Drapolene, a mixture of alkyldimethybenzylammonium chlorides)

This chemical is widely used in ophthalmic preparations, including contact lens solutions.

Sensitising potential

The maximisation test, with an induction concentration of 25 per cent and a challenge concentration of 10 per cent, failed to sensitise any of 24 subjects tested (Kligman, 1966).

Case reports

In 1972, Fisher and Stillman described a doctor who had been sensitised by ophthalmic solutions. They reported that this was the second case of sensitisation to be confirmed by patch testing; the first, reported by Cohen in 1952, was a woman sensitised by benzalkonium chloride in an antazoline ophthalmic solution.

Among ophthalmic patients Afzelius and Thulin (1979) report it as a significant allergen, having found sensitisation in six of 100 patients with chronic conjunctivitis.

Patch testing
Benzalkonium chloride 0.1 per cent and 0.01 per cent aqueous
Reactions to both concentrations will help to differentiate between irritant and allergic responses.
Fisher and Stillman (1972) stressed that the chemical itself should be used for patch testing, as a corticosteroid in a medicament may suppress the reaction.

DEQUALINIUM CHLORIDE (1,1'-Decamethylenebis (4-aminoquinaldinium chloride); Dequadin chloride)

This quaternary ammonium compound has been reported as a cause of necrotic ulcers on the penis (Coles and Wilkinson, 1965; Wilkinson 1970; Armijo Moreno et al., 1976), and in the vulva, perineum and body folds (Tilsey and Wilkinson, 1965).
In Helsinki, it was thought possible that patients had been sensitised as on patch testing they reacted to dequalinium chloride 0.01 per cent (Salo and Pirilä, 1968).

CETALKONIUM CHLORIDE (Benzylhexadecyldimethylammonium chloride; cetyldimethylbenzylammonium chloride; hexadecyldimethylbenzylammonium chloride)

This was the sensitiser in a roll-on deodorant (p. 108).

BENZETHONIUM CHLORIDE (Benzyldimethyl
[2-[2-(p-1,1,3,3-tetramethylbutylphenoxy) ethoxy]ethyl]ammonium chloride;
disobutylphenoxyethoxyethyl dimethyl benzyl ammonium chloride)

$$\left[\begin{array}{c} CH_3 \ CH_3 \\ | \quad | \\ CH_3CCH_2C-\langle\!\langle\bigcirc\rangle\!\rangle-OCH_2CH_2OCH_2CH_2NCH_2-\langle\!\langle\bigcirc\rangle\!\rangle \\ | \quad | \\ CH_3 \ CH_3 \end{array} \right]^+ Cl^-.H_2O$$

This compound, in a feminine hygiene spray, sensitised two patients (p. 110). Another two women were sensitised by neutral red 0.05 per cent in an alcoholic solution of benzethonium chloride which was used as a pre-operative skin disinfectant. Patch tests: both patients reacted to the whole solution, to neutral red 0.05 per cent in alcohol and to *p*-aminobenzene but were negative to benzethonium chloride 0.1 per cent (Dahlquist and Fregert, 1967).

Patch testing
Benzethonium chloride 0.1 per cent in water

CHLOROALLYLHEXAMINIUM CHLORIDE
(1-(3-chloroallyl)-3,5,7,-triaza-1-azoniaadamantane chloride; Dowicil 200).

$$\left[\begin{array}{c} CH_2CH=CHCl \\ \\ N-\!\!\!\diagup\!\!\!\diagdown-N \\ \diagdown N^+\!\!\diagup \\ N \end{array} \right] Cl^-$$

Dowicil 200, a type of quaternary ammonium compound, is a broad spectrum bactericide which is more effective against bacteria than yeasts and fungi. Highly soluble in water it has little solubility in oil. In aqueous solution it is unstable and releases formaldehyde. It is occasionally used in cosmetics and is also used in latex, paints, inks, polishes and jointing cements.

St John's
A girl was sensitised to this compound in a rouge (p. 149).

Patch testing
Dowicil 200 1 per cent in petrolatum

Bronopol (2-bromo-2-nitro-1,3-propanediol

$$HOCH_2-\overset{\overset{\displaystyle Br}{|}}{\underset{\underset{\displaystyle NO_2}{|}}{C}}-CH_2OH$$

This is a broad spectrum preservative which is very soluble in water but not in oil. Effective against Gram-negative organisms especially Pseudomonas aeruginosa (Bryce *et al.*, 1978), it is of particular importance because its activity remains in the presence of protein and is only slightly diminished by non-ionic detergents. It is unstable, being discoloured by light, and in alkaline solution it dissociates to form formaldehyde. This deterioration in the presence of light can be counteracted by adding to the formulation a light-absorber, such as benzophene. Bronopol is used in shampoos in a concentration of 0.01–0.02 per cent.

Sensitising potential

The Draize procedure, on human subjects, with an induction concentration of 5 per cent and a challenge concentration of 0.25 per cent, sensitised none of the 93 subjects tested (Maibach, 1977). This study amended a previous conclusion by Marzulli and Maibach (1973) that bronopol is a sensitiser.

Case reports

Bronopol seems to be innocuous in use, and as yet cases of sensitivity have not been reported.

St John's

Bronopol 0.25 per cent in petrolatum was used at St John's to test 149 routine patients: four reacted. In three the response was weak and easily distinguishable from a true allergic positive, and one man with a definite (++) reaction at two days did not return for the four day reading. In this group four patients had positive patch tests to 2 per cent formaldehyde and each was negative to bronopol.

These results indicate that bronopol 0.25 per cent in petrolatum is a mild irritant when used for patch testing. As the efficacy of an 0.1 per cent concentration for detecting sensitisation has not been assessed, it is suggested that both 0.25 per cent and 0.1 per cent be used for patch testing.

Patch testing

Bronopol 0.25 per cent and 0.1 per cent in petrolatum

Chlorhexidine (Hexamethylene bis-chlorphenyl biguanide; Hibitane; Nolvasan; Rotersept; Sterilon)

1,1'-hexamethylenebis[5-(*p*-chlorophenyl)biguanide]

Chlorhexidine is an effective, non-toxic germicide. It is used as chlorhexidine digluconate in creams and emulsions, and as chlorhexidine acetate and diacetate in aqueous and alcoholic solutions. Creams, ointments and dusting powders usually contain 0.1–1.0 per cent solutions. The concentration of chlorhexidine in irrigations and lotions is 0.01–0.1 per cent and in eye drops, as a preservative, it is 0.01 per cent.

Irritancy

It has been shown in rats that chlorhexidine 0.02 per cent and 0.1 per cent, applied to experimental skin wounds, impairs healing, probably by a direct toxic effect on the tissues (Mobacken and Wengström, 1974).

Case reports

Sensitisation is extremely rare.

A woman, aged 78 years, treated her stasis ulcer topically for three months with a 1 per cent chlorhexidine digluconate emulsion (Hibitane, ICI), and then developed an acute dermatitis of her left leg and thigh, the left side of her face and both eyes. She was patch tested with chlorhexidine digluconate emulsion 1 per cent and with chlorhexidine diacetate 0.5 per cent in ethanol and 0.05 per cent in water, and she reacted to each, whereas chlorhexidine diacetate 1 per cent in petrolatum elicited no reaction. Open tests with the solutions were negative; an intracutaneous test with 0.1 ml of chlorhexidine diacetate 0.005 per cent in saline was positive. On account of these results, it was suggested that chlorhexidine is not released from petrolatum and that this vehicle gives false negative reactions (Ljunggren and Möller, 1972).

The case of a man, who developed a vesicular eczema from Hibitane used as a pre-operative wound disinfectant, was described by Wahlberg and Wennersten (1971, a). Patch testing with 0.125 per cent chlorhexidine and photopatch testing with 0.0156 per cent, both gave positive reactions. The authors suggested that the lights in the operating theatre had augmented the eczematous reaction (Wahlberg and Wennertsen, 1971, b).

St John's

One case was included in the series of contact dermatitis from drugs reported by Calnan (1962). Patch tests: he was positive to Hibitane cream, Hibitane digluconate 1 per cent and Hibitane diacetate 1 per cent (Calnan, 1972).

In 1973, patch testing with 1 per cent chlorhexidine in alcohol and in petrolatum were compared in routine eczematous patients:

No. Tested	162
No. +ve to chlorhexidine 1 per cent in alcohol	22
No. +ve to chlorhexidine 1 per cent in petrolatum	1

One man reacted to chlorhexidine both in alcohol and in petrolatum; the reactions at four days were weak, but by the seventh day they were pronounced. Retesting with the same preparation failed to elicit any reaction after two and four days.

In none of the positive patients was there a relevant corresponding history. It was concluded that patch testing with chlorhexidine 1 per cent in alcohol is definitely irritant.

Patch testing

Chlorhexidine digluconate 1 per cent in emulsion
Chlorhexidine diacetate 0.5 per cent in ethanol
Chlorhexidine diacetate 0.05 per cent in water
(Ljunggren and Möller, 1972)

Chloroacetamide (Konservierungsmittel C; CA 24)

$$CICH_2C\underset{NH_2}{\overset{O}{<}}$$

2-chloroacetamide

This preservative is used as a mixture of 60–70 per cent chloroacetamide and 30–40 per cent sodium benzoate. It prevents the growth of organisms and moulds and is effective in the presence of non-ionic detergents (Smeenk and Prins, 1972). In cosmetic and pharmaceutical creams it is used in a concentration of about 0.4 per cent and it may also be used in some glues and in shoe polish.

Diallyl-chloroacetamide (Randox) is a herbicide and has once been reported as a sensitiser (p. 403).

Sensitising potential

Chloroacetamide is an active sensitiser. Marzulli and Maibach (1973), using the Draize procedure with 1.25 per cent chloroacetamide, sensitised 35 of the 205 (17 per cent) human volunteers tested.

Reports of sensitisation

Cosmetics

Allergic reactions to chloroacetamide were first described by Nater (1971), from a cosmetic cream which had been reported to the manufacturer as being irritant. He patch tested 18 controls with the cream, and two were positive. On being tested to the constituents, each reacted to 0.18 per cent chloroacetamide in water — its concentration in the cosmetic. The cream was then tested on a further 200 controls, but none reacted. Later, the source of chloroacetamide sensitivity in a woman with hand eczema was traced to her baby's body lotion, which she had started to use about the time her eczema appeared. When patch tested, she had reacted to chloroacetamide 0.18 per cent in water and to the body lotion, but not to 5 per cent sodium benzoate. The baby was not affected. A further two women were described by Klaschka (1975). One, sensitised by a skin cleanser, developed quite severe dermatitis of the face, neck, chest, hands and arms before the source and identity of the contact allergen were traced. The second woman was employed in dipping corks into an 0.5 per cent solution of chloroacetamide as a preservative. After five months she developed an incapacitating eczema. Patch tests: both were positive to chloroacetamide (one to an 0.5 per cent concentration) and the first woman reacted to her facial cleanser.

St John's

Since 1971, this sensitivity has been diagnosed in four women. The first patient, aged 26 years, had dermatitis of her eyelids and reacted to patch testing with her eye cream. When tested with the constituents, she reacted severely to chloroacetamide with sodium benzoate 1 per cent in water but not to sodium benzoate 1 per cent in water (Calnan, 1971). Since then, three women have been seen with facial contact dermatitis caused by one particular make of foundation cream. Their ages were 62, 32, and 31 years, the duration of the history varied from 1–9 months, and each complained of recurrent swelling of the eyes or face or both. All reacted on patch testing with foundation cream, and, when tested with the constituents, each reacted to a 1 per cent mixture of chloroacetamide and sodium benzoate. They were not tested to sodium benzoate on its own. One of the patients was also sensitive to perfumes. By August 1973, this preservative had been replaced and no other cosmetic made by the firm contained it.

Medicaments

In Holland, Hirudoid ointment (Luitpold-Werk, München) is a popular treatment for chronic venous insufficiency of the legs. For only a limited time, it contained chloroacetamide, yet through its use at least 17 patients were sensitised; each reacted to patch tests with chloroacetamide 0.2 per cent in water (Smeenk and Prins, 1972).

Occupational

Glue. A vinyl plastic waterproof wall paper, for use in bathrooms and kitchens, and a glassfibre fabric both required hanging with a special polyvinyl acetate glue, which contained chloroacetamide 0.1 per cent and formaldehyde 0.2 per cent as preservatives. Two house painters, both with hand eczema for several years, were sensitised by the glue. Patch tests: both men were positive to chloroacetamide 0.1 per cent and formaldehyde 2 per cent; one tested with 10 per cent of the glue was positive (Bang Pedersen and Fregert, 1976). Sensitisation in house painters by similar glues was confirmed by Wahlberg, Högberg and Skare (1978).

Nylon spin finish. Methylol chloracetamide (Grotan HD) 0.075 per cent in a spin finish caused dermatitis among workers making nylon yarn. Patch tests: they reacted to the spin finish but were not tested with its separate components (the other ingredient was a synthetic coolant). They were negative to formaldehyde (Savage, 1978).

Active sensitisation

St John's

An operating theatre sister with hand eczema was tested to many chemicals including glutaraldehyde 1 per cent in water and chloroacetamide 2 per cent in petrolatum. She reacted to the glutaraldehyde, and the chloroacetamide response was described as irritant. She returned, a month later, saying that ten days after the final visit this patch had become red and swollen. It had by then subsided to a mauve scaly area. She refused to have the patch tests repeated.

Patch testing

Chloroacetamide 0.2 per cent in water or petrolatum

Chlorobutanol (Trichlormethyl propanol; acetone chloroform; chlorbutol)

$$CH_3 - \underset{\underset{OH}{|}}{\overset{\overset{CH_3}{|}}{C}} - CCl$$

1,1,1-trichloro-2-methyl-2-propanol

Chlorobutanol has three useful properties: It has some local anaesthetic action, and is made up in clove oil as a dental analgesic. As a preservative it may be added to solutions of adrenaline or extracts of posterior pituitary. It can also act as a plasticiser for cellulose esters and ethers.

In Fisher, Pascher and Kanof's (1971) series of 100 patients suspected of having an allergic contact dermatitis from a medicament, it was used undiluted for testing and gave no positive reactions. Reports of sensitivity have not been found.

Patch testing
Undiluted (Fisher, Pascher and Kanof, 1971)

Dimethoxane (Acetoxydimethyl-dioxane;)

2,6-dimethyl-*m*-dioxan-4-ol-acetate

This chemical is active at concentrations of 0.03–0.1 per cent against a wide range of bacteria, yeasts and fungi. It is effective in cosmetics containing protein material, such as egg shampoo, and is also used in cutting oils, emulsions of resins, water-based paints and inks.

Maibach (1971) used the Draize test on 205 volunteers and sensitised 50 (25 per cent) of them with 1.25 per cent dimethoxane; this is, however, a much higher concentration than is used as a preservative.

Reports of sensitivity have not been traced.

Patch testing
Dimethoxane 0.1 per cent (Schorr, 1971) in petrolatum

Domiphen bromide (dodecyldimethyl(2-phenoxyethyl) ammonium bromide; Bradosol bromide)

This chemical is freely soluble in water and is also soluble in organic solvents. It is used in topical medicaments, is the active principle in Bradosol lozenges (Ciba) and has been present in the formulation of a plaster of Paris bandage.

Case reports
It was listed as causing dermatitis in two patients in a report by Calnan (1962).

Patch testing
Domiphen bromide 0.1 per cent in water

Ethylenediamine Tetraacetate (EDTA)

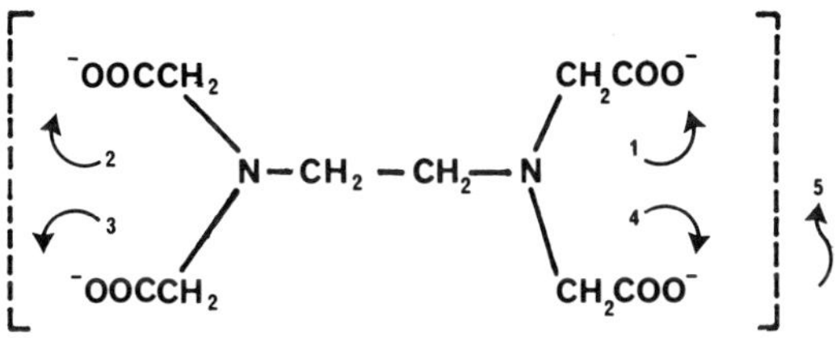

Quadruply charged anion of EDTA

Substitutions

	1.	2.	3.	4.	5.
Edetic acid	H	H	H	H	—
Monosodium edetate	Na	H	H	H	—
Disodium edetate	Na	Na	H	H	—
Trisodium edetate	Na	Na	Na	H	—
Tetrasodium edetate	Na	Na	Na	Na	—
Ferric sodium edetate	—	—	—	—	Na^+ Fe^{2+}

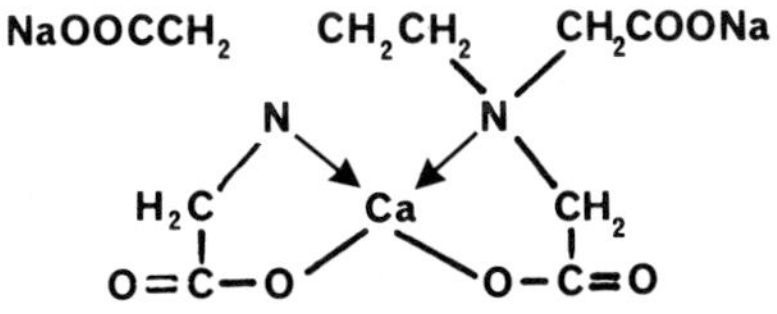

Calcium disodium edetate

This chemical is very widely used; it is added as a preservative to ophthalmic solutions, ear and nose drops, procaine solutions and solutions for contact lenses. As the calcium disodium salt (Edathamil calcium, Versene, Sequestrene) it sequesters or binds metallic ions and prevents discolouration and oxidation of pharmaceutical, cosmetic and other preparations. Systemically some of its salts are used in the treatment of hypercalcaemia and lead poisoning (Raymond and Gross, 1969). It may be added to foods, including salad oil, wine and pickled cucumbers (p. 175).

Case report

A man developed acute allergic conjunctivitis and contact dermatitis from using two ophthalmic solutions containing EDTA. The first he had bought himself, and this produced the conjunctivitis for which the second was prescribed. Another two patients reacted to EDTA on routine testing and these, but not the patient with conjunctivitis, cross-reacted to ethylenediamine (Raymond and Gross, 1969).

St John's

In 1973, 162 routine patients were tested with tetrasodium edetate (EDTA 4Na) 1 per cent in petrolatum. One patient gave a mild irritant response, and a woman with hand and arm eczema, who worked on an assembly line, gave repeatedly positive reactions. No cause was found for the sensitivity: she did not react to ethylenediamine but was sensitive to MBT, thiurams, carbamates and her rubber gloves. In 1974, a woman with eczema of her ankle which had spread to other sites had positive patch tests to ethylenediamine 1 per cent and EDTA 1 per cent both in petrolatum; it was impossible to know which was the primary allergen.

Cross-reactions. At the Finsen Institute in Copenhagen, Eriksen (1975) found that of 23 patients with a positive patch test reaction to ethylenediamine, three also reacted to EDTA. It was thought possible that EDTA was the primary sensitiser in these three patients (p. 245).

Patch testing

Ethylenediamine tetraacetate tetrasodium (EDTA 4Na) 1 per cent in petrolatum

Ethylene oxide (Oxirane, Anprolene)

$$H_2C \overset{\displaystyle O}{\diagup \diagdown} CH_2$$

Ethylene oxide is an explosive, flammable gas. Its inherent toxicity to all living cells makes it an effective steriliser for heat and moisture-sensitive articles such as plastic and pharmaceutical products. It is the simplest chemical containing an epoxy group and is highly reactive and irritant.

It is most hazardous as a vapour in industry: the threshold limit is 50 ppm, and a concentration of 5–10 per cent can be lethal within a few minutes.

The gas is absorbed by some products during sterilisation, and, unless it is completely eliminated afterwards by aeration, it causes cutaneous burns and irritation. It has been widely, and apparently safely, used in the U.K. to sterilise equipment and pharmaceutical products. The paucity of incidents probably reflects a respect for its toxicity.

Case reports

Patients

In the past few years there have been three reports from the U.S.A. of toxic reactions occurring in patients. One patient received facial burns from an anaesthetic mask which had been sterilised by ethylene oxide (La Dage, 1970). In an episode reported by Hanifin (1971) packets of nitrofurazone gauze had been sterilised with ethylene oxide, and residual gas left in the gauze caused skin irritation and burns in seven patients, five post-operatively. The toxic effect had been enhanced by semi-occlusive dressings applied over the gauze. In New York, 19 women, who had worn re-usable gowns containing residual ethylene oxide, developed a severe bullous eruption of their buttocks and lower back. The skin healed with pigmentation and scarring. The gowns contained 16–50 times the safe level of gas (Biro, Fisher and Price, 1974).

Occupational
A closed-box system, incorporating rubber gloves, was sterilised with ethylene oxide. The gloves absorbed the gas and subsequently caused an irritant dermatitis in the operators (Royce and Moore, 1955). In Belgium, four employees working in a sterile zone making vaccines developed an irritant dermatitis from overalls, gloves and masks which had been sterilised in ethylene oxide (Lamy, Lachapelle and Braekel, 1974).

Imidazolidinyl urea compounds (Germall Group)
N-*N''*-Methylenebis[*N'*-[1-(hydroxymethyl)-2,5-dioxo-4-imidazolidinyl]urea]

Germall 115 (tentative formula)

This is a new group of preservatives of which only Germall 115 (Sutton Laboratories Inc., Roselle, N.J., U.S.A.) is at present commercially available. They have particular advantages in being non-toxic, effective against both Gram-positive and Gram-negative organisms (even in the presence of protein and detergents), synergistic with other preservatives such as parabens and compatible with most cosmetic formulations (Berke and Rosen, 1970).

One case of sensitisation has been reported — a woman who developed eczema of her face two weeks after the daily use of a moisturising lotion containing 1:10000 concentration of imidazolidinyl urea (Germall 115). Patch tests: she was positive to the moisturising lotion and had a vesicular reaction to a 1 per cent solution of imidazolidinyl urea (Mandy, 1974).

Patch testing

Imidazolidinyl urea (Germall 115) 1 per cent? base? petrolatum

Irgasans

Irgasan is the Ciba-Geigy brand name for two relatively new antimicrobial agents.

TRICLOSAN (Trichloro-hydroxy-diphenyl ether; DP 300; Irgasan 3565)

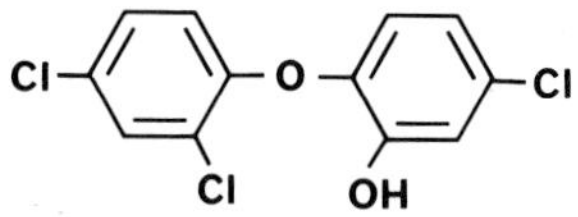

2,4,4'-Trichloro-2'-hydroxydiphenyl ether

This chemical is sparingly soluble in water; it is more soluble in dilute alkali and is readily soluble in most organic solvents.

It is being used with increasing frequency in the United States of America and in Great Britain as an antiseptic in toilet soaps (0.5–2 per cent), shampoos, bath additives and deodorants (0.1–0.2 per cent). It has also been used for impregnating some papers (Fisher, 1973). A recent antimicrobial and antimycotic cream, Logamel®, contains 3 per cent triclosan and 0.02 per cent flumethasone pivilate.

Irgasan DP300 has no action on *Pseudomonas* and was found to be a less effective skin disinfectant than hexachlorophane or chlorhexidine by Lilly and Lowburry (1974), but in their evaluation the concentrations of the antiseptics differed.

The percutaneous absorption of Triclosan was studied in rats and found to be greater from an aerosol than from a shampoo (Black and Howes, 1975).

Sensitising potential

The Draize test, with an induction concentration of 5–20 per cent and a challenge concentration of 1–5 per cent, failed to sensitise or photosensitise human subjects (Marzulli and Maibach, 1973). Similarly none of 20 humans was sensitised by Lachapelle and Tennstedt (1979) but they did sensitise one of 20 guinea-pigs.

Case reports

Despite the experimental results, clinicians are beginning to detect cases of sensitisation.

In Copenhagen, after testing 291 consecutive patients with Irgasan 2 per cent in petrolatum, none of whom reacted, two cases of sensitivity were seen. One, a 66-year-old man, developed dermatitis of his feet and right hand while using a deodorant foot powder containing 0.2 per cent Irgasan. Patch tests with the foot powder were positive, and, on testing with the ingredients, he reacted to Irgasan 2 per cent in petrolatum. His feet healed, and, when the patch tests were repeated two months later, they were still positive. A 32-year-old woman developed axillary dermatitis while using a deodorant containing 0.12 per cent Irgasan; she reacted on patch testing to the deodorant, to Irgasan 2 per cent, 1 per cent and 0.5 per cent and to several other allergens. Her axillary rash cleared, but she later developed eczema of her face. A usage test with a bar of soap containing 0.5 per cent DP300, caused mild erythema and irritation (Roed-Petersen, Auken and Hjorth, 1975). Another patient sensitised by a deodorant was reported by Hindson (1975). In Stockholm, Triclosan was added to the standard series (Wahlberg, 1976) and with concentrations of 0.5 and 1 per cent no cases of sensitisation were detected in 902 patients but with 2 per cent (petrolatum) two of 1100 patients reacted. Both were atopics and both had been sensitised by deodorants.

St John's
In 1974, a woman developed eczema of her axilla while using a deodorant containing Irgasan DP300. Patch tests: she was positive to the deodorant and to Irgasan DP300 2 per cent in petrolatum. In 1976, a woman who had had chronic eczema for ten years had a positive patch test to DP300 2 per cent in petrolatum, but neither a source nor a relevance was found for the reaction.

Patch testing
Triclosan (DP300) 1–2 per cent in petrolatum

CLOFLUCARBAN (dichloro-trifluoromethyl-carbanilide; Irgasan CF3)

3-Trifluoromethyl-4,4'-dichloro-*N*-*N*'-diphenyl urea

This bacteriostatic chemical can be used in soaps and detergents. In the U.S.A. it is present in one soap, Safeguard, and in Europe it is used in vinyl gloves and certain shampoos (Fisher, 1973). In the United Kingdom its use is practically non-existent.

There have been no reports of cases of sensitivity.

Nordihydroguaiaretic acid (NDGA 4,4'-(2,3-dimethyltetramethylene)dipyrocatechol; 2,3-bis(3,4-dihydroxybenzyl)-butane)

Nordihydroguaiaretic acid has been used as an antioxidant in foods but it is now restricted to topical products (Roed-Petersen and Hjorth, 1976).

Case reports

A total of eight cases of sensitisation have been reported by Jørgensen and Hjorth (1970) and Roed-Petersen and Hjorth (1976). A lanolin cream (Cosmea) containing 0.1 per cent NDGA was responsible in four patients: one, a pharmacist, developed an acute eczema of his face and hands, and another, a woman, became erythrodermatous after using the cream for her ichthyosis. The formulation of this particular cream has now been changed. A pharmaceutical worker while working on the production of vitamin AD tablets developed an acute dermatitis of his face with mild involvement of his hands. Patch tests: he was tested with the ingredients of the tablets and reacted to hydrogenated oil of soya bean, containing 0.15 per cent of NDGA, and to NDGA 2 per cent in petrolatum. Three patients reacted on patch testing to 2 per cent NDGA but a specific source of exposure was not traced.

A series of 435 consecutive patients was tested by Jørgensen and Hjorth (1970) to NDGA 5 per cent in petrolatum; all the tests were negative except one, which was weakly positive.

Patch testing

NDGA 2 per cent in petrolatum

Potassium metabisulphite (Potassium pyrosulfite)
$$K_2S_2O_5$$

Potassium metabisulphite prevents the oxidation of adrenaline and may therefore be added, in a concentration of 0.5 per cent, to local anaesthetic solutions containing adrenaline. Similarly, solutions of chlorpromazine for injection contain sodium sulphite 0.1 per cent and sodium metabisulphite 0.075 per cent as anti-oxidants; and potassium metabisulphite also preserves solutions of ascorbic acid. Other uses are the dyeing of textiles, in printing, photography and in disinfectants (Nater, 1968).

Case reports

A woman, while working in a pharmaceutical firm, handled potassium metabisulphite and developed hand eczema; after this had healed with treatment, she was able to resume work provided she wore gloves. Months later, within a day of receiving an injection of xylocaine with adrenaline, her hand eczema recurred. She was then extensively patch tested and found to be sensitive to potassium metabisulphite 0.5 per cent and 1.0 per cent in water. Control patch tests on ten subjects were negative (Nater, 1968).

SODIUM BISULPHITE

According to the Merck Index (1968) 'sodium bisulphite of commerce consists chiefly of sodium metabisulphite', so that the following patient may have been another case of sensitivity to sodium metabisulphite.

Case report

Epstein (1970) described the case of a woman who, while working in a cafeteria, developed hand eczema which seemed to have a definite relationship to her occupation. When patch tested, she reacted to a Veg white powder, which is an anti-oxidant, used to prevent discolouration of fruit and vegetables for salads. On patch testing with the ingredients of this powder she was strongly positive to 10 per cent and 20 per cent sodium bisulphite but was negative to 2 per cent. She was also tested with potassium metabisulphite 5 per cent and 10 per cent and reacted to both. Controls tested to 20 per cent sodium bisulphite were negative.

Patch testing

Potassium metabisulphite 1–5 per cent in petrolatum (Nater, 1968; Epstein, 1970).

Sorbic acid (2,4-hexadienoic acid; 2-propenylacrylic acid)

$$CH_3CH = CH\ CH = CH\ COOH$$

Sorbic acid is a useful preservative because, unlike parabens, it maintains its activity in the presence of non-ionic detergents. However, as it is effective only as an undissociated acid it must be used in preparations with a pH up to 6.5 but not higher; sorbates have a similar broad spectrum action but in high concentrations they may be oxidised by sunlight and discolour products. Sorbic acid is particularly useful as an antifungal agent: it inhibits the growth of moulds and yeasts and for this reason it is added to formulations in concentrations of 0.1–0.2 per cent. It not only is used in cosmetic and pharmaceutical creams but also is added to foods such as syrups, pickles, fruit juices and especially cheeses. It may be added to drying oils and to alkyd coatings to improve the gloss, and it also is used to facilitate the milling of cold rubber (Merk, 1968).

Sensitising potential

Experimentally it is a very weak sensitiser. The Draize procedure, with an induction concentration of 10 per cent, failed to sensitise all 93 human subjects tested; a concentration of 20 per cent sensitised only one of 33 subjects. Both groups were challenged with 5 per cent sorbic acid (Marzulli and Maibach, 1973).

Incidence of sensitivity

Positive reactions have been recorded in routine patch testing of eczematous patients. Prior to its use in Denmark, Hjorth and Trolle-Lassen (1962) patch tested 1489 patients with concentrations of 10 per cent and 5 per cent in soft paraffin; five patients (0.3 per cent) reacted. As they found a concentration of 10 per cent to be irritant, they recommended 5 per cent or 2 per cent for patch testing. They also noticed that sorbic acid caused an immediate reaction (within 20 minutes) and ascribed this to its acidity, as benzoic acid can evoke the same response. These authors suggested that berries and plants were the source of contact with sorbic acid.

In Germany, Klaschka and Biersdorff (1965) patch tested 736 eczematous patients with sorbic acid 2.5 per cent in eucerin; of the five patients (0.7 per cent) who reacted, three had used a medicament containing sorbic acid.

In the U.S.A. Schorr (1971) used a concentration of 2 per cent to patch test 200 eczematous patients, and found only one (0.5 per cent) positive reaction.

St John's
> In 1972, 261 consecutive patients were tested with 2.5 per cent sorbic acid in petrolatum; only one man reacted, an incidence of 0.4 per cent. The source of his sensitivity was not traced.

Case reports

Clinically, sorbic acid is a very rare sensitiser. Simpson (1971) described a woman who had been treated with Cortacreme bandages (Smith and Nephew Ltd) for gravitational eczema and had developed a disseminated eczema. On patch testing she reacted to Cortacreme bandage and to sorbic acid 10 per cent, 5 per cent, 2 per cent and 1 per cent in petrolatum; the tests with the other ingredients were negative. Sixteen controls were negative. Two patients were sensitised by the 0.2 per cent concentration of sorbic acid in Unguentum Merck® and on patch testing they reacted to Ung. Merck and to sorbic acid 5 per cent in petrolatum (Saihan and Harman, 1978; Brown, 1979).

Sorbitan monolaurate, an ingredient of Alphaderm (Eaton Laboratories), caused a bullous eruption on the legs of a woman who had been applying Alphaderm for one week. Patch tests; she reacted to Alphaderm and of its constituents she was positive to sorbitan monolaurate 5 per cent (aqueous); ten controls were negative. The patient also had a positive open test to Alphaderm (Finn and Forsyth, 1975).

Patch testing

Sorbic acid 2.5 per cent in petrolatum
Sorbitan monolaurate 5 per cent in water

References

Adverse drug reaction bulletin (1974) Hexachlorophane: risk and benefit. No. 44 February, p. 144.

Aeling, J.L. & Nuss, D.D. (1974) Systemic eczematous "contact-type" dermatitis medicamentosa caused by parabens. *Archives of Dermatology.* 110, 640.

Afzelius, H. & Thulin, H. (1979) Allergic reactions to benzalkonium chloride. *Contact Dermatitis*, 5, 60.

Aldrete, J.A. & Johnson, D.A. (1969) Allergy to local anaesthetics. *Journal of the American Medical Association.* 207, 356.

Armijo Moreno, M., Gutierrez Salmeron, M.T., Camacho Martinez, F., Naranjo Sintes, R., Armijo Lozano, R., Garcia Mellado, V. & Dulanto de F. (1976) Necrosis de pene por dequalinium. *Actas Dermo-Sifiliograficas*. **67**, 547.

August, P.J. (1975) Cutaneous necrosis due to cetrimide application. *British Medical Journal*, **1**, 70.

Baer, R.L., Ramsey, D.L. & Biondi, E. (1973) The most common contact allergens. *Archives of Dermatology*. **108**, 74.

Baker, H., Ive, F.A. & Lloyd, M.J. (1969) Primary irritant dermatitis of the scrotum due to hexachlorophene. *Archives of Dermatology*, **99**, 693.

Bang Pedersen, N. (1976) Allergy to chemical solutions for soft contact lenses. *Lancet*, **2**, 1363.

Bang Pedersen, N. & Fregert, S. (1976) Occupational allergic contact dermatitis from chloracetamide in glue. *Contact Dermatitis*, **2**, 122.

Barr, R.D., Rees, P.H., Cordy, P.E., Kungu, A., Woodger, B.A. & Cameron, H.M. (1972) Nephrotic syndrome in adult Africans in Nairobi. *British Medical Journal*, **2**, 131.

Barr, R.D., Woodger, B.A. & Rees, P.H. (1973) Levels of mercury in urine correlated with the use of skin lightening creams. *American Journal of Clinical Pathology*, **59**, 36.

Berke, P.A. & Rosen, W.E. (1970) Germall, a new family of antimicrobial preservatives for cosmetics. *American Perfumer and Cosmetics*, **85**, 55.

Bier, A.G. (1958) Allergie gegen ein Diphenylmethanderivat *Berufsdermatosen*, **6**, 40.

Biro, L., Fisher, A.A. & Price, E. (1974) Ethylene oxide burns. *Archives of Dermatology*, **110**, 924.

Black, H. (1972) Analysis of routine battery results in Auckland skin clinic. *Contact Dermatitis Newsletter*, **12**, 323.

Black, J.G. & Howes, D. (1975) Percutaneous absorption of Triclosan from toilet preparations. *Journal of the Society of Cosmetic Chemists*, **26**, 205.

Black, J.G. Sprott, W.E., Howes, D. & Rutherford, T. (1974) Percutaneous absorption of hexachlorophene. *Toxicology*, **2**, 127.

Blaug, S.M. & Grant, D.E. (1974) Kinetics of degradation of the parabens. *Journal of the Society of Cosmetic Chemists*, **25**, 495.

Bonnevie, P. (1940) Overfølsomhed for Ætylparaoxybenzoat (Mycoten). *Nordisk Medicin*, **6**, 684.

Bork, K., Morsches, B. & Holzmann, H. (1973) Zum problem der Quecksilber-Resorption aus weiber Präzipitatsalbe. *Archiv für Dermatologische forschung*, **248**, 137.

Breit, R. & Bandmann, H-J. (1973) The wide world of antimycotics. *British Journal of Dermatology*, **89**, 657.

Brown, R. (1979) Another case of sorbic acid sensitivity. *Contact Dermatitis*, **5**, 268.

Bryce, D.M., Croshaw, B., Hall, J.E., Holland, V.R. & Lessel, B. (1978) The activity and safety of the antimicrobial agent Bronopol (2-bromo-2-nitropropan-1,3-diol). *Journal of the Society of Cosmetic Chemists*, **29**, 3.

Burge, K.M. & Winkelmann, R.K. (1970) Mercury pigmentation. *Archives of Dermatology*, **102**, 51.

Burry, J.N., Kirk, J., Reid, J.G. & Turner, T. (1973) Environmental dermatitis: patch tests in 1000 cases of allergic contact dermatitits. *Medical Journal of Australia*, **2**, 681.

Burry, J.N., Kirk, J., Reid, J.G. & Turner, T. (1975) Chlorocresol sensitivity. *Contact Dermatitis*, **1**, 41.

Calnan, C.D. (1962) Contact dermatitis from drugs. *Proceedings of the Royal Society of Medicine*, **55**, 39.

Calnan, C.D. (1971) Chloroacetamide dermatitis from a cosmetic. *Contact Dermatitis Newsletter*, **9**, 215.

Calnan, C.D. (1972) Hibitane. *Contact Dermatitis Newsletter*, **11**, 281.

Camarasa, G. (1976) Contact dermatitis from mercurochrome. *Contact Dermatitis*, **2**, 120.

Catalano, P.M. (1975) Hexachlorophene — Not a Cry of 'Wolf'. *Archives of Dermatology*, **111**, 250.

Catalano, P.M. (1976) Letter. *Archives of Dermatology*, **112**, 1032.

Cohen, S.G. (1952) Antistine eyedrops. *American Journal of Ophthalmology*, **35**, 1704.

Coles, R.B. and Wilkinson, D.S. (1965) Necrosis and Dequalinium. 1. Balanitis. *Transactions St John's Hospital Dermatological Society*, **51**, 46.

Croshaw, B. (1977) Preservatives for cosmetics and toiletries. *Journal of the Society of Cosmetic Chemists*, **28**, 3.

Curley, A., Hawk, R.E., Kimbrough, R.D., Nathenson, G. & Finberg, G. (1971). Dermal absorption of hexachlorophane in infants. *Lancet*, **2**, 296.

Dahlquist, I. & Fregert, S. (1967) Allergic contact dermatitis from neutral red in quaternary ammonium salt solution. *Contact Dermatitis Newsletter*, **2**, 34.

Eberhartinger, C., Ebner, H. & Klotz, L. (1968) Beitrag zur Kenntnis der Chromat-Kontaktallergie. *Berufsdermatosen*, **16**, 147.

Ellis, F.A. (1947) The sensitising factor in merthiolate. *Journal of Allergy*, **18**, 212.

Ellis, F.A. & Robinson, H.M. (1942) Cutaneous sensitivity to merthiolate and other mercurial compounds. *Archives of Dermatology*, **46**, 425.

Epstein, E. (1966) Dichlorophene allergy. *Annals of Allergy*, **24**, 437.

Epstein, E. (1970) Sodium bisulfite. *Contact Dermatitis Newsletter*, **7**, 155.

Epstein, E. (1974) Mercury allergy and patch testing. *Archives of Dermatology*, **109**, 98.

Epstein, E., Rees, W.J. & Maibach, H.I. (1968) Recent experience with routine patch testing screening. *Archives of Dermatology*, **98**, 18.

Epstein, J.H., Wuepper, K.D. & Maibach, H.I. (1968) Photocontact dermatitis to halogenated salicylanilides and related compounds. *Archives of Dermatology*, **97**, 236.

Epstein, S. (1955) Hexachlorophene (G11) in the treatment of eczematous dermatitis. *Archives of Dermatology*, **71**, 692.

Epstein, S. (1963) Sensitivity to merthiolate: A cause of false delayed intradermal reactions. *Journal of Allergy*, **34**, 225.

Epstein, S. (1968) Paraben sensitivity: subtle trouble. *Annals of Allergy*, **26**, 185.

Eriksen, K.E. (1975) Allergy to ethylenediamine. *Archives of Dermatology*, **111**, 791.

Feuerman, E.J. (1975) Recurrent contact dermatitis caused by mercury in amalgam dental fillings. *International Journal of Dermatology*, **14**, 657.

Finn, O.A. & Forsythe, A. (1975) Contact dermatitis due to sorbitan monolaurate. *Contact Dermatitis*, **1**, 318.

Fisher, A.A. (1973) Irgasan DP 300 and Irgasan CF 3. *Contact Dermatitis Newsletter*, **14**, 416.

Fisher, A.A. (1975) Allergic paraben and benzyl alcohol hypersensitivity relationship of the "delayed" and immediate varieties. *Contact Dermatitis*, **1**, 281.

Fisher, A.A. & Lipton, M. (1951) Allergic stomatitis due to 'Baxin' in a dentifrice. *Archives of Dermatology*, **64**, 640.

Fisher, A.A., Pascher, F. & Kanof, N.B. (1971) Allergic contact dermatitis due to ingredients of vehicles. *Archives of Dermatology*, **104**, 286.

Fisher, A.A. & Stillman, M.A. (1972) Allergic contact sensitivity to benzalkonium chloride. *Archives of Dermatology*, **106**, 169.

Fisher, A.A. & Tobin, L. (1953) Sensitivity to compound G-4 ('dichlorophene') in dentifrices. *Journal of the American Medical Association*, **151**, 998.

Fregert, S. (1969) Personnal Communication to Hansson, H. and Möller, H. (1970) Patch test reactions to merthiolate in healthy young subjects. *British Journal of Dermatology*, **83**, 349.

Fregert, S. & Hjorth, N. (1969) Increasing incidence of mercury sensitivity. The possible role of organic mercury compounds. *Contact Dermatitis Newsletter*, **5**, 88.

Fregert, S. & Hjorth, N. (1972) In Textbook of Dermatology. eds. Rook, A., Wilkinson, D.S. & Ebling, F.J.G. 2nd Ed., p. 418, *Scientific Publications*, Oxford: Blackwell Scientific Publications.

Fregert, S., Hjorth, N., Magnusson, B., Bandmann, H-J., Calnan, C.D., Cronin, E., Malten, K., Meneghini, C.L., Pirilia, V. & Wilkinson, D.S. (1969). Epidemiology of contact dermatitis. *Transactions St John's Hospital Dermatological Society*, **55**, 17.

Frykholm, K.O. (1957) Mercury from dental amalgam. Its toxic and allergic effects. *Acta Odontologica Scandinavica*, **15**, Supplement 22, p. 65.

Frykholm, K.O. & Wahlgren, F. (1964) A fatal case of mercurial dermatitis with complications. *Acta Dermato-venereologica*, **44**, 362.

Garcia-Perez, A. & Moran, M. (1975) Dermatitis from quarternary ammonium compounds. *Contact Dermatitis*, **1**, 316.

Gaul, L.E. (1958) Sensitising component in thiosalicylic acid. *Journal of Investigative Dermatology*, **31**, 91.

Gaul, L.E. (1966) Immunity of the oral mucosa in epidermal sensitisation to mercury. *Archives of Dermatology*, **93**, 45.

Gaul, L.E. & Underwood, G.B. (1949) The cutaneous toxicity of dihydroxydichlorodiphenylmethane. *Journal of Indiana State Medical Association*, **42**, 22.

Goldblatt, M.W. (1945) Vesication and some vesicants. *British Journal of Industrial Medicine*, **2**, 183.

Gowdy, J.M. & Ulsamer, A.G. (1976) Hexachlorophene lesions in newborn infants. *American Journal of Diseases of Children*, **130**, 247.

Gump, W.S. (1969) Toxicological properties of hexachlorophene. *Journal of the Society of Cosmetic Chemists*, **20**, 173.

Hanifin, J.M. (1971) Ethylene oxide dermatitis. *Journal of the American Medical Association*, **217**, 213.

Hansson, H. & Möller, H. (1970) Patch test reactions to merthiolate in healthy young subjects. *British Journal of Dermatology*, **83**, 349.

Hansson, H. & Möller, H. (1971) Intracutaneous test reactions to tuberculin containing merthiolate as a preservative. *Scandinavian Journal of Infectious Diseases*, **3**, 169.

Hartung, J. (1965) Phenyl-Quecksilberacetat und Phenyl-Quecksilberoleat in textilien. *Berufsdermatosen*, **13**, 116.

Hjorth, N. (1967) Sensitivity to organic mercury compounds. *Contact Dermatitis Newsletter*, **1**, 15.

Hjorth, N. & Trolle-Lassen, C. (1962) Skin reactions to preservatives in creams with special regard to parabens esters and sorbic acid. *American Perfumer*, 77, 146.

Hjorth, N. & Trolle-Lassen, C. (1963) Skin reactions to ointment bases. *Transactions St John's Hospital Dermatological Society*, 49, 127.

Hindson, T.C. (1975) Irgasan Dp 300 in a deodorant. *Contact Dermatitis*, 1, 328.

Holst, R. & Möller, H. (1975) Merthiolate testing in twins. *Contact Dermatitis*, 1, 370.

Huriez, C., Agache, P., Martin, P., Vandamme, G. & Mennecier, J. (1965) Fréquence des sensibilisations aux ammoniums quaternaires. *Bulletin de la Société Francaise de Dermatologie et de Syphiligraphie*, 72, 106.

Huriez, C., Martin, P., Vanoverschelde, M. & Mennecier, J. (1966) L'allergie aux sels d'ammonium quaternaire. *Bulletin de la Société Francaise de Dermatologie et de Syphiligraphie*, 73, 260.

Husain, S.L. (1975) Sensitivity to parabens in Codella barrier cream. *Contact Dermatitis*, 1, 395.

Ippen, H. (1979) Akutes axillarekzem durch quecksilber-verbindungen. *Dermatosen In Beruf Und Umwelt*, 27, 54.

Jacquelin, C. & Colomb, D. (1972) Erytheme fessier et coma. Diagnostic eliologique tardif. A propos d'une trentaine de cas d'intoxication par de l'hexachlorophene surdosé dans un talc a usage infantile. *Revue d'Electroencéphalographie et de Neurophysiologie Clinique*, 2, 414.

Joltrain, M., Hissard, R. & Boulard, E. (1939) Accidents observés chez des ouvriers d'une cartoucherie. *Bulletin de L'Académie de Médecine (Paris)*, 122, 692.

Jorgensen, G. & Hjorth, N. (1970) Dermatitis from Nordihydroguaiaretic acid, and antioxidant in fats. *Contact Dermatitis Newsletter*, 7, 151.

Juhlin, L. & Öhman, S. (1968) Allergic reactions to mercury in red tattoos and in mucosa adjacent to amalgam fillings. *Acta Dermato-venereologica*, 48, 103.

Kanan, W.J. (1969) Contact Dermatitis in Kuwait. *Journal of the Kuwait Medical Association*, 3, 129.

Khan, G. (1970) Depigmentation caused by phenolic detergent germicides, *Archives of Dermatology*, 102, 177.

Kimbrough, R.D. (1973) Review of the toxicity of hexachlorophene including its neurotoxicity. *Journal of Clinical Pharmacology*, 13, 439.

Klaschka, F. (1975) Contact allergy to chloracetamide. *Contact Dermatitis*, 1, 265.

Klaschka, F. & Beirsdorff, H.U. (1965) Crux medicorum: allergie gegen nicht deklarierte Salben-konservantien. *Münchener Medizininische Wochenschrift*, 107, 185.

Kligman, A. (1966) The identification of contact allergens by human assay. III the maximisation test: a procedure for screening and rating contact sensitisers. *Journal of Investigative Dermatology*, 47, 393.

Koby, G.A. (1972) Phenylmercuric acetate as primary irritant. *Archives of Dermatology*, 106, 129.

Lachapelle, J.M. & Tennstedt, D. (1979) Low allergenicity of triclosan. Predictive testing in guinea pigs and in humans. *Dermatologica*, 158, 379.

La Dage, L.H. (1970) Facial 'irritation' from ethylene oxide sterilisation of anaesthesia mask? *Plastic and Reconstructive Surgery*, 45, 179.

Ladd, A.C., Goldwater, L.J. & Jacobs, M.B. (1964) Absorption and excretion of mercury in man. *Archives of Environmental Health*, 9, 43.

Lamar, L.M. & Bills, B.O. (1966) Localised pigmentation of the skin due to topical mercury. *Archives of Dermatology*, 93, 450.

Lamy, F., Lachapelle, J.-M. et Braekel, G. van (1974). Dermites professionnelles a l 'oxyde d'ethylene chez des des sujets travaillant en zone sterile. *Archives des Maladies Professionelles de Médicine du Travail et de Sécurité Sociale*, 35, 719.

Lilly, H.A. & Lowbury, E.J.L. (1974) Disinfection of the skin with detergent preparations of irgasan DP300 and other antiseptics. *British Medical Journal*, 4, 372.

Ljunggren, B. & Möller, H. (1972) Eczematous contact allergy to chlorhexidine. *Acta Dermato-venereologica*, 52, 308.

Lockhart, J.D. (1973) Hexachlorophene and the food and drug administration. *Journal of Clinical Pharmacology*, 13, 445.

Lorenzetti, O.J. & Wernet, T.C. (1977) Topical parabens: benefits and risks. *Dermatologica*, 154, 244.

Lowenthal, K. (1952) Eczematous contact dermatitis of the palm due to toothpaste. *New York State Journal of Medicine*, 52, 1437.

Magnusson, B., Blohm, S.-G. Fregert, S., Hjorth, N., Høvding, G., Pirilä, V. & Skog, E. (1968) Routine patch testing. IV. Supplementary series of test substances for Scandinavian countries. *Acta Dermato-venereologica*, 48, 110.

Magnusson, B. & Kligman, A. (1969) The indentification of contact allergens by animal assay. The guinea pig maximisation test. *Journal of Investigative Dermatology*, 52, 268.

Maibach, H.I. (1971) Allergic sensitisation potential (Draize test) in man of several preservatives. *Contact Dermatitis Newsletter*, **9**, 213.

Maibach, H.I. (1972) False positive intradermal skin tests and thiomersal. *Journal of the American Medical Association*, **220**, 126.

Maibach, H.I. (1975) Acute laryngeal obstruction presumed secondary to thiomersal (merthiolate) delayed hypersensitivity. *Contact Dermatitis*, **1**, 221.

Maibach, H.I. (1977) Dermal sensitisation potential of 2-bromo-2-nitropropane-1,3-diol (Bronopol®) *Contact Dermatitis*, **3**, 99.

Mandy, S.H. (1974) Contact dermatitis to substituted imidazolidinyl urea—a common preservative in cosmetics. *Archives of dermatology*, **110**, 463.

Marzulli, F.N. & Maibach, H.I. (1973) Antimicrobials: experimental contact sensitisation in man. *Journal of the Society of Cosmetic Chemists*, **24**, 399.

Marzulli, F.N. & Maibach, H.I. (1974) Status of topical parabens: skin hypersensitivity. *International Journal of Dermatology*, **13**, 397.

Maucher, O.M. (1974) Beitrag zur Kreuz-oder Kopplung sallergie auf Parahydroxybenzoesauteester. *Berufsdermatosen*, **22**, 183.

McCarl, G.W. (1976) In support of hexachlorophene. *Archives of Dermatology*, **112**, 1031.

Merck Index (1968) 8th Ed., p. 971 Ed. Stetcher, P.G. Rahway, N.J: Meick.

Mobacken, H. & Wengström, C. (1974) Interference with healing of rat skin incisions treated with chlorhexidine. *Acta Dermato-venereologica*, **54**, 29.

Morris, G.E. (1960) Dermatoses from phenylmercuric salts. *Archives of Environmental Health*, **1**, 53.

Nagel, J.E. & Fuscaldo, J.T. and Fireman, P. (1977) Paraben allergy. *Journal of the American Medical Association*, **237**, 1594.

Nater, J.P. (1968) Allergic contact dermatitis caused by potassium metabisulfite. *Dermatologica*, **136**, 477.

Nater, J.P. (1971) Allergic reactions due to chloracetamide. *Dermatologica*, **142**, 191.

North American Contact Dermatitis Group (1973) Epidemiology of contact dermatitis in North America: 1972. *Archives of Dermatology*, **108**, 537.

Novák, M. & Kvičalová, E. (1978) The problem of contact reactions to merthiolate. *Ceskoslovenská Dermatologie*, **53**, 313.

Oleffe, J.A. Blondeel, A. & de Coninck, A. (1979) Allergy to chlorocresol and propylene glycol in a steroid cream. *Contact Dermatitis*, **5**, 53.

O'Neill, J.J., Peelor, P.L., Peterson, A.F. & Strube, C.H. (1979) Selection of parabens as preservatives for cosmetics and toiletries. *Journal of the Society of Cosmetic Chemists*, **30**, 25.

Park, R.G. (1970) Chlorocresol sensitivity. *Contact Dermatitis Newsletter*, **7**, 152.

Plueckhahn, V.D. & Collins, R.B. (1976) Hexachlorophene emulsion and antiseptic skin care of newborn infants. *Medical Journal of Australia*, **1**, 811.

Powell, H., Swarner, O., Gluck, M. & Lampert, P. (1973) Hexachlorophene myelinopathy in premature infants. *Journal of Pediatrics*, **82**, 976.

Rantuccio, F. & Meneghini, C.L. (1970) Results of patch testing with cosmetic components in consecutive eczematous patients. *Contact Dermatitis Newsletter*, **7**, 156.

Raymond, J.Z. & Gross, P.R. (1969) EDTA: Preservative Dermatitis. *Archives of Dermatology*, **100**, 436.

Reisman, R.E. (1969) Delayed hypersensitivity to merthiolate preservative. *Journal of Allergy*, **43**, 245.

Roed-Petersen, J., Auken, G. & Hjorth. N. (1975) Contact sensitivity to Irgasan DP300. *Contact Dermatitis*, **1**, 293.

Roed-Petersen, J. & Hjorth, N. (1976) Contact dermatitis from antioxidants. Hidden sensitisers in topical medications and foods. *British Journal of Dermatology*, **94**, 233.

Royce, A. & Moore, W.K.S. (1955) Occupational dermatitis caused by ethylene oxide. *British Journal of Industrial Medicine*, **12**, 169.

Rubin, M.B. & Pirozzi, D.J. (1973) Contact dermatitis from carbolated vaseline. *Cutis*, **12**, 52.

Rudner, E. & Cronin, E. (1966) Contact sensitivity to para-hydroxybenzoate esters. *Dermatology Digest*, **5**, 51.

Rudzki, E. & Kleniewska, D. (1970) The epidemiology of contact dermatitis in Poland. *British Journal of Dermatology*, **83**, 543.

Rudzki, E. & Kohutnicki, Z. (1971) Sensitivity to mercury in bricklayers. *Contact Dermatitis Newsletter*, **10**, 241.

Saihan, E.M. & Harman, R.R.M. (1978) Contact sensitivity to sorbic acid in 'Unguentum Merck'. *British Journal of Dermatology*, **99**, 583.

Salo, O.P. & Pirilä, V. (1968) Sensitisation to Topical Dequaline. *Contact Dermatitis Newsletter*, **4**, 66.

Sarkany, I. (1960) Contact dermatitis from paraben. *British Journal of Dermatology*, **72**, 345.

Savage, J. (1978) Chloracetamide in nylon skin finish. *Contact Dermatitis*, **4**, 179.

Schamberg, L. (1967) Allergic contact dermatitis to methyl and propyl parabens. *Archives of Dermatology*, **95**, 626.

Schorr, W.F. (1968) Paraben allergy. A cause of intractable dermatitis. *Journal of the American Medical Association*, **204**, 859.

Schorr, W.F. (1970) Dichlorophene (G-4) allergy. *Archives of Dermatology*, **102**, 515.

Schorr, W.F. (1971) Cosmetic allergy. *Archives of Dermatology*, **104**, 459.

Schorr, W.F. & Mohajerin, A.H. (1966) Paraben sensitivity. *Archives of Dermatology*, **93**, 721.

Schultheiss, E. (1958) Uberempfindlichkeit gegenüber p-Hydroxybenzoesäuremethylester. *Berufsdermatosen*, **6**, 292.

Sharvill, D. (1965) Reaction to chlorhexidine and cetrimide, *Lancet*, **1**, 771.

Sharvill, D.E. (1971) Paraben-sensitivity. Reactivation of patch tests. *Contact Dermatitis Newsletter*, **9**, 211.

Shuman, R.M., Leech, R.W. & Alvord, E.C. (1974) Neurotoxicity of hexachlorophene in the human: 1. A clinicopathalogic study of 248 children. *Pediatrics*, **54**, 689.

Sidi, E. & Casalis, F. (1951) Les intolérances de la muqueuse buccale. *La Presse Medicale*, **59**, 730.

Silverberg, D.S., McCall, J.T. & Hunt, J.C. (1967) Nephrotic syndrome with use of ammoniated mercury. *Archives of Internal Medicine*, **120**, 581.

Simpson, J.R. (1971) Sorbic acid sensitivity from cortacream bandages. *Contact Dermatitis Newsletter*, **10**, 232.

Simpson, J.R. (1978) Dermatitis due to parabens in cosmetic creams. *Contact Dermatitis*, **4**, 311.

Smeenk, G. & Prins, F.J. (1972) Allergic contact eczema due to chloracetamide. *Dermatologica*, **144**, 108.

Sunderman, F.W., Hawthorne, M.F. & Baker, G.L. (1956) Delayed sensitivity of the skin of phenyl mercuric acetate. *Archives of Industrial Health*, **13**, 574.

Swanston, C. (1943) Effects on the skin of irritant explosives. *Proceedings of the Royal Society of Medicine*, **36**, 633.

Taugner, M. & Schütze, R. (1966) Beitrag zur Quecksilber-Allergie. *Dermatologica*, **133**, 245.

Thelwall Jones, H. (1972) Danger of skin burns from thiomersal. *British Medical Journal*, **2**, 504.

Tilsey, D.A. & Wilkinson, D.S. (1965) Necrosis and dequalinium. *Transactions St John's Hospital Dermatological Society*, **51**, 49.

Traub, E.F. & Holmes, R.H. (1938) Dermatitis and stomatitis from the mercury of amalgam fillings. *Archives of Dermatology*, **38**, 349.

Trout, m.e. (1973) Hexachlorophene in perspective. *Journal of Clinical Pharmacology*, **13**, 451.

Turk, J.L. & Baker, H. (1968) Nephrotic syndrome due to ammoniated mercury. *British Journal of Dermatology*, **80**, 623.

Van Abbé, N.J., Dixon, H. Hughes, O. & Woodroffe, R.C.S. (1970) The hygienic manufacture and preservation of toiletries and cosmetics. *Journal of the Society of Cosmetic Chemists*, **21**, 719.

Verbov, J. (1970) Parabens in paste bandages. *Contact Dermatitis Newsletter*, **8**, 170.

Vickers, C.F.H. (1967) Mercury sensitivity. *Contact Dermatitis Newsletter*, **2**, 20.

Wahlberg, J.E. (1962) Two cases of hypersensitivity to quaternary ammonium compounds. *Acta Dermato-venereologica*, **42**, 230.

Wahlberg J.E. (1976) Routine patch testing with Irgasan DP 300® *Contact Dermatitis*, **2**, 292.

Wahlberg, J.E. Hogberg, M. & Skare, L. (1978) Chloracetamide allergy in house painters. *Contact Dermatitis*, **4**, 116.

Wahlberg, J.E. & Wennersten, G. (1971(a)) Hypersensitivity and photosensitivity to chlorhexidine. *Dermatologica*, **143**, 376.

Wahlberg, J.E. & Wennersten, G. (1971(b)) Hypersensitivity and ?photosensitivity to chlorhexidine — a topical antiseptic. *Contact Dermatitis Newsletter*, **10**, 240.

Ward, O.C. & Hingerty, D. (1967) Pink disease from cutaneous absorption of mercury. *Journal of the Irish Medical Association*, **60**, 94.

Weathers, D.R. & Fine, R.M. (1974) Amalgam tattoo of oral mucosa. *Archives of Dermatology*, **110**, 727.

Wilkinson, D.S. (1962) Patch test reactions to certain halogenated salicylanilides. *British Journal of Dermatology*, **74**, 302.

Wilkinson, D.S. (1970) Durch dequalinium hervorgerufene hautnerkrosen. *Hautarzt*, **21**, 114.

Wilson, L.A., Kuehne, J.W., Hall, S.W. & Ahearn, D.G. (1971) Microbial Contamination in Ocular Cosmetics. *American Journal of Ophthalmology*, **71**, 1298.

Wuepper, K.D. (1967) Paraben contact dermatitis. *Journal of the American Medical Association*, **202**, 579.

Wüstner, H., Orfanos, C.E., Steinback, H., Käferstein, H. & Herpers, H. (1975) Nagelverfärbung und Haarausfall. *Deutsche Medizinische Wochenschrift*, **100**, 1694.

14.

Rubber

SOURCES AND STRUCTURE OF RUBBER
  Natural
  Synthetic
  Additives
SENSITISERS
INCIDENCE OF SENSITIVITY

SOURCES OF SENSITIVITY
CLINICAL FEATURES
  'Domestic' Rubber Dermatitis
  Occupational Dermatitis
  Dermatitis in the Rubber Industry
PATCH TESTING

Sources and structure

NATURAL AND SYNTHETIC

The following resumé of the sources, structure and uses of rubber has been taken from a most interesting account by Allen (1972).

Rubber and compounds with rubbery properties are linear, high polymers, which can be cross-linked to form molecular networks. Their molecular weight ranges from 100 000 to 1 000 000. It is characteristic of rubbers that, although they can be stretched without difficulty, they maintain their strength in an elongated position, and, once the tension is released, they revert quickly to their original shape. Chemically, most rubbers contain double bonds; these are reactive and allow the molecules to vulcanise by cross-linking and to polymerise by joining.

However, these double bonds also open rubber to attack and destruction by heat, light, oxygen and ozone.

The invention of the motor car and the consequent demand for rubber tyres galvanised rubber production into a most important and growing industry. In 1870, the output of wild rubber from trees in Brazil was about 7000 tons a year; now, it is estimated that the combined production of synthetic and natural rubber during the 1980s will be 15 million tons a year, of which 60–70 per cent will go into the manufacture of tyres. Before 1939, natural rubber supplied practically 100 per cent of the market, but now it provides only 35 per cent of the world's requirements. It is not that natural rubber is inferior to synthetic rubber but its production has failed to keep pace with the increased demand. Synthetic rubbers have been formulated which are as good as natural rubber, and for some purposes are better, because they can be given special properties such as resistance to oil and oxidation. In recent years, the rising cost of petroleum products has greatly increased the price of synthetic rubber and although natural rubber is still more costly its price may have greater stability and with its expanding production it is becoming a more competitive product.

Natural rubber
Wild rubber was first obtained from the tree *Hevea brasiliensis*, which is indiginous to Brazil. In 1896, seeds were collected, brought to London and replanted as seedlings in Ceylon and South East Asia. Gradually, plantations in Malaysia and Indonesia flourished and became the major producers of natural rubber; at the same time, output in South America dwindled and has remained at about 1 per cent of the world total.

Latex is tapped from the tree as a white milky fluid containing some 30 per cent rubber. It is preserved by adding ammonia or sodium sulphite, sieved to remove dirt, and coagulated, usually by the addition of formic or acetic acid which reduces the pH to less than 4. The coagulated sheets are dried and shipped in bales. Rubber in this form is not cross-linked (vulcanised) and is of little commercial use except as crepe soles for shoes. Approximately 10 per cent of the world's rubber is used as a latex concentrate in which the water content has been reduced and ammonia and sodium pentachlorophenate added as preservatives to prevent spontaneous coagulation. This liquid latex has a special use for the manufacture of gloves, contraceptives, elastic thread and adhesives. It is also added to bitumen for roads and is used to bind and back the tufted fabrics of carpets.

The monomer of natural rubber is *cis*-1,4-polyisoprene. The *trans* form, gutta percha, is a different kind of material and is used in golf ball covers.

Manufacture
An ideal rubber does not exist but, with few exceptions, natural rubber fulfills most requirements. Its advantages are ease of processing, strength, and resistance to flexing. Drawbacks are its susceptibility to environmental damage, and a lack of resistance to very high temperatures and to hot oil. In particular it is used for aircraft tyres because it retains its strength at the raised temperatures which occur in landing and take-off. It is also used for conveyor belting and many engineering components.

Synthetic rubbers
The monomers for most synthetic rubbers are made from petroleum.

Styrene/butadiene rubber
In 1933, the first important synthetic rubber was produced in Germany by combining liquid styrene and gaseous butadiene to form styrene-butadiene rubber (SBR). However, the product was not easy to process, and there was little stimulus for its development.

$$C_6H_5 — CH = CH_2 \quad + \quad CH_2 = CH — CH = CH_2$$
$$\text{styrene} \qquad\qquad\qquad \text{1,3-butadiene}$$

Up to the Second World War, only 2 per cent of all rubber was synthetic.

From 1941–1945, however, the Allies were cut off from rubber supplies, and this led to a major scheme being launched in the U.S.A. for the production of synthetic rubber. At the same time, the rubber plantations in South East Asia were severely disrupted; they have, however, made a good recovery in the post-war period. In 1950, further urgency was given to the manufacture of synthetic rubber by the Korean war; as a result, SBR was greatly improved by cold polymerisation and by the discovery that the addition of oil and oil extension greatly facilitated its processing. SBR is now the major synthetic rubber produced and comprises 40 per cent of the world's consumption.

In comparison with natural rubber, SBR is weaker and less resistant to fatigue but has the merit of ageing more slowly. Oil-extended SBR is used exclusively for the tyres of passenger vehicles because it wears well and has an excellent grip on wet roads. The great demand for car tyres in the U.S.A. explains the large American consumption of this particular type of rubber.

Polybutadiene rubber

Polybutadiene is the third most important rubber. Being difficult to process, it is unsuited to use on its own. Its value lies in its capacity to blend with SBR or natural rubber. In tyre treads, it lowers the heat build-up and improves wearing qualities, but it has the disadvantage of reducing the skid resistance.

Synthetic polyisoprene

The synthesis of isoprene meant that rubber could be produced with the same structure as the natural product which was a great achievement for the industry. Nevertheless, polyisoprene still differs from natural rubber and its main function is as a blending component with other types of rubber.

cis-1,4-Polyisoprene

Polychloroprene

This rubber is widely known as Neoprene—the Du Pont trade name. It has most of the advantages of SBR and of natural rubber and, in addition, is flame resistant and wears longer; but, despite these attributes, its high price limits its production. It is used mainly in the transport industry and for cables, sealants, coatings and adhesives.

Polychloroprene(Neoprene)

Butyl rubber

As this rubber has a low permeability for gases, it is used for the inner tubes of tyres.

Specialised synthetic rubbers
Specialised rubbers are made with particular properties, but they are expensive and their market is limited.

Silicone rubbers
These rubbers are effective in extremes of temperature, and are used in the aerospace industry. They also seem to be well tolerated by human tissues which makes them of use in surgery.

Polyurethane rubbers
Solid polyurethane has a small market; it is used, for example, for the soles and heels of shoes and for solid tyres. Polyurethane competes effectively with natural rubber when used as thread (Spandex) for underclothes or as foams, including that used in furniture upholstery. Polyurethane foams are cheaper than those made of rubber.

Polysulphide rubbers
These are known by their trade name, Thiokol; being very resistant to solvents, they are used mainly as sealant putties in the construction industry.

Chlorosulphonated polyethylene
Generally known as Hypalon (Du Pont) this rubber is used for cable coverings.

Polyacrylic rubbers
These plastic rubbers resist oil and ageing but are difficult to process; they are used in seals and gaskets for vehicles.

Fluorocarbon rubbers
These, the most costly of all the rubbers, have been used to a small extent in the aerospace programme. Viton is their Du Pont trade name.

Rubber consumption
The transport industry is the largest consumer of rubber, using about 75 per cent of the world's output. Latex probably comes second and uses less than 6 per cent; all other rubber products together amount to only 1–2 per cent of the total output (Table 14.1).

Table 14.1. Rubber consumption by various products (Allen, 1972).

	%
Tyres	60
Latex (foam and carpet backing)	5.5
Footwear	4
Rubber/metal bonded components	2.5
Belting	2
Hose and tubing	2
Wire and cable	1.5
Flooring	1
Proofed goods	1
Adhesives	1
Thread	0.5

Vulcanisation

Natural rubber latex is of limited use because it deteriorates with keeping, it is sensitive to temperature and it tends to stick to other materials. By 1833, it was realised that the addition of sulphur hardened rubber, prolonged its life and greatly improved its properties. When it was discovered that heating facilitated this combination the process was called vulcanisation, in memory of Vulcan the Roman god of fire and smiths.

The terms vulcanisation and cross-linking are synonymous; vulcanising chemicals act by forming cross-linkages (Gibbs, 1961). Sulphur remains the principal vulcanising agent but other chemicals such as nitrogen-containing compounds and organic peroxidases are also effective. Natural and synthetic rubbers have similar chemical structures and both are improved by vulcanisation.

Additives

Many hundreds of chemicals are added to rubber to improve it, to prolong its life and to give it special properties. They are constantly being changed and their number is steadily increasing. The same chemicals are used both in synthetic and in natural rubber and they belong to the following broad functional groups:

A. ACCELERATORS

These are mainly sulphur-containing compounds which speed up vulcanisation; as they vary in their rate of action, they are classified as slow, medium and fast. Which accelerator is used will depend on the type, thickness and potential use of the rubber.

1. *Thiurams*

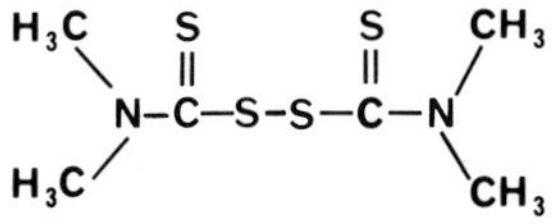

Tetramethylthiuram disulphide (TMTD; Bis(dimethylthiocarbamoyl) disulphide)

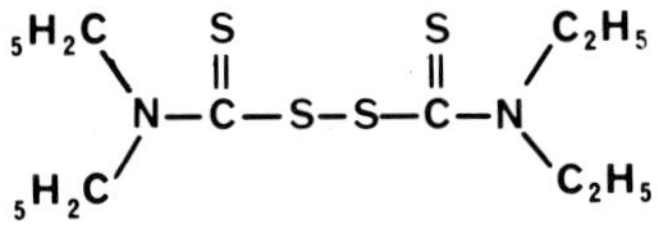

Tetraethylthiuram disulphide (TETD; Bis(diethylthiocarbamoyl) disulphide)

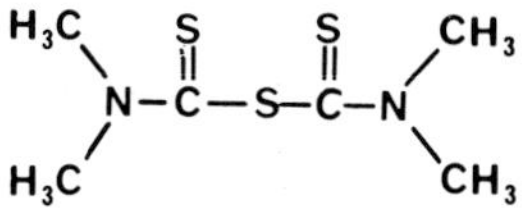

Tetramethylthiuram monosulphide (TMTM)

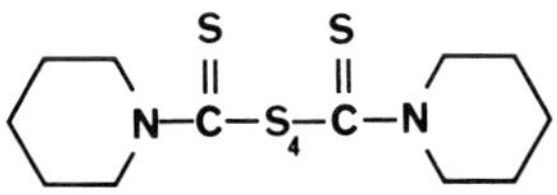

Dipentamethylenethiuram disulphide (PTD)

2. *Mercaptobenzothiazole group*

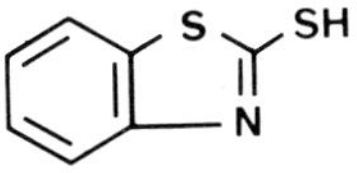

2-Mercaptobenzothiazole (MBT; 2-benzothiazolethiol)

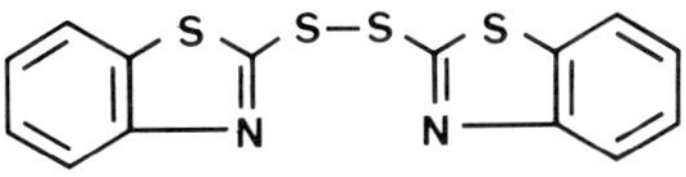

2,2′-Dibenzothiazyl disulphide (MBTS; 2,2′-Dithiobis[benzothiazole])

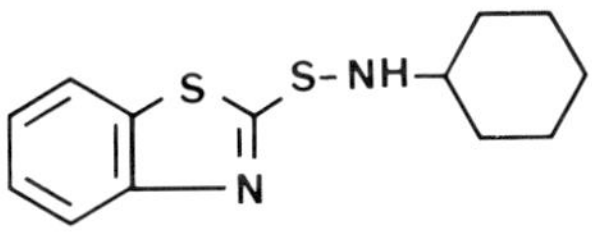

N-Cyclohexylbenzothiazyl sulphenamide (CBS)

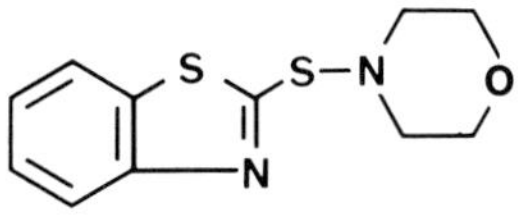

Morpholinylmercaptobenzothiazole (MMBT)

3. *Guanidines*

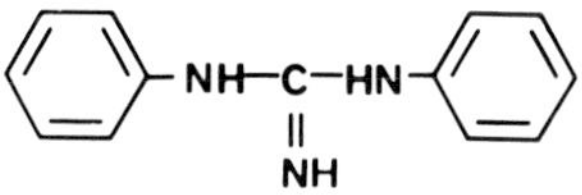

1,3-Diphenylguanidine (DPG)

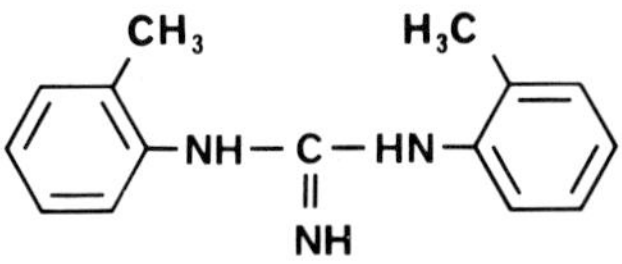

Di-*o*-tolylguanidine (DOTG)

4. *Dithiocarbamates*

Zinc diethyldithiocarbamate (ZDC; Bis(diethyldithiocarbamato)zinc)

Zinc ethylphenyldithiocarbamate (ZEP; Bis(ethylphenyldithiocarbamato)zinc)

Sodium diethyldithiocarbamate (SDC; Diethyldithiocarbamic acid sodium salt)

5. *Amines*
Hexamethylenetetramine
Triethyltrimethyltetramine

B. ANTIOXIDANTS
These chemicals prevent oxidation and ozone attack.

1. *Amines*

N-Phenylcyclohexyl-*p*-phenylenediamine (CPPD)

Diphenyl-*p*-phenylenediamine (DPPD)

Isopropylphenyl-*p*-phenylenediamine (IPPD; 4-Isopropylamino-diphenylamine)

$$H_2N - \langle\!\!\bigcirc\!\!\rangle - CH_2 - \langle\!\!\bigcirc\!\!\rangle - NH_2$$

p, p'-Diaminodiphenylmethane (DDM; 4,4'-Methylenedianiline)

Phenyl-*β*-naphthylamine (PBN)

Sym-di-*β*-Naphthyl-*p*-phenylenediamine (Nonox CI)

2. *Phenols*

$$HO - \langle\!\!\bigcirc\!\!\rangle - \langle\!\!\bigcirc\!\!\rangle - OH$$

4,4'-Dihydroxydiphenyl (DOD)

3. *Monobenzyl ether of hydroquinone (MHQ; Monobenzone; p-(Benzyloxy) phenol)*

$$HO - \langle\!\!\bigcirc\!\!\rangle - O - CH_2 - \langle\!\!\bigcirc\!\!\rangle$$

4. *Quinolines*
1,2-Dihydro-2,2,4-trimethylquinoline ('Flectol' H)

C. PEPTIZERS
Thio-*β*-naphthol (2-naphthalenethiol)

D. VULCANISING AGENTS

Sulphur

4,4'-Dithiodimorpholine ($C_4H_8ONSSNOC_4H_8$)

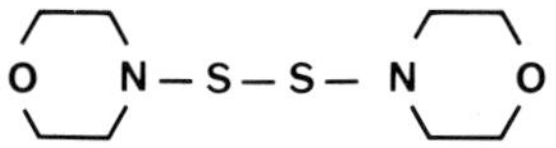

4,4'-Dithiodimorpholine (Morpholine N, N'-disulphide)

E. MISCELLANEOUS CHEMICALS

The majority of the chemicals given in the following section have been listed by Bourne, Yee and Seferian (1968).

Blowing Agents:	Sodium bicarbonate with or without stearic acid
	Dinitrosopentamethylene tetramine
	Azodicarbonamide
Dusting and dipping Agents:	Zinc Stearate
	Talc
	Soap solution
Inert fillers:	Kaolin
	Whiting
	Silica
Plasticisers:	Dibutyl phthalate
	Dioctyl phthalate
Reinforcers:	Carbon black
Retarders:	Salicylic acid
	n-Nitrosodiphenylamine

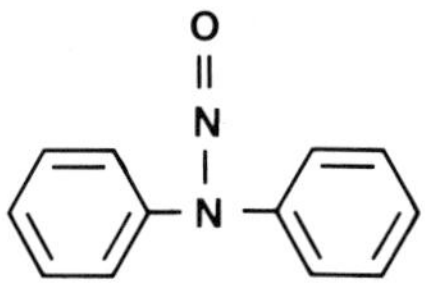

Mould lubricant:	Sodium oleyl-*para*-anisidine sulphonate
Colours:	Inorganic, mineral pigments are used, including cadium sulphides, iron oxides, chromium oxide, mercuric sulphide and nickel titanate. Organic dyes and lakes are also utilised.

Sensitisers

Rubber itself is not allergenic, it is the chemicals which are added to it during the manufacturing processes which sensitise, and, as these allergens are present in the finished product, both consumer and manufacturer are at risk of being sensitised.

In general, compounds containing sulphur act as accelerators, and the additives without sulphur have a variety of other properties. Although most of the sensitisers in rubber are either accelerators or antioxidants, the chemical properties of these compounds are of much less concern to the dermatologist than are:

(a) a knowledge of the various groups of potentially allergenic chemicals which may be present in rubber, and

(b) the cross-reaction patterns of the individual chemicals.

From a dermatological standpoint, therefore, it is better to divide rubber chemicals arbitrarily into the following sensitising groups (Hjorth, 1970):

(i) Thiurams
    Tetramethylthiuram disulphide   (TMTD)
    Tetraethylthiuram disulphide   (TETD)
    Dipentamethylenethiuram disulphide   (PTD)
    Tetramethylthiuram monosulphide   (TMTM)

(ii) Mercapto-group
    Mercaptobenzothiazole   (MBT)
    Cyclohexylbenzothiazylsulphenamide   (CBS)
    Dibenzothiazyldisulphide   (MBTS)
    Morpholinylmercaptobenzothiazole   (MMBT)

(iii) PPD group
    Phenylcyclohexyl-PPD   (CPPD)
    Isopropylphenyl-PPD (Isopropylamino-
        diphenylamine)   (IPPD)
    Diphenyl-PPD   (DPPD)
    Diaminodiphenylmethane   (DDM)

(iv) Naphtyl group
    Phenyl-β- naphthylamine   (PBN)
    sym-Di-β- naphthyl-PPD   (DBNPD)

(v) Carbamates
    Zinc diethyldithiocarbamate   (ZDC)
    Zinc dibutyldithiocarbamate   (ZBC)

(vi) Miscellaneous
    Diphenylguanidine   (DPG)
    Dioxydiphenyl   (DOD)
    Dithiodimorpholine

Most of these additives are firmly entrenched in the rubber industry — they have been used satisfactorily for many years and are unlikely to be replaced. However, the requirements of the manufacturers alter; more efficient chemicals are found and prices vary, so that any list of rubber additives needs constant revision. Kortschak (1977) has discussed sensitising chemicals and also the manufacture of rubber. Adams (1975) has suggested that mercaptobenzimidazole be substituted for mercaptobenzothiazole because it is likely to be less allergenic.

These compounds are not exclusive to the rubber industry and some of the chemicals may have other uses. For example, mercaptobenzothiazole has been used as an anti-corrosive agent (Fregert and Skog, 1962) and may also be added to antifreeze mixtures (p. 845); tetraethylthiuram disulphide is Antabuse; tetramethylthiuram disulphide and dithiocarbamates are used as pesticides (Shelley, 1964); zinc diethyldithiocarbamate is used as a preservative in zinc oxide tape (Calnan, 1978a); diaminodiphenylmethane can act as a hardener for epoxy resins; and monobezyl ether of hydroquinone is a bleaching agent.

Fregert (1971) has listed the following chemicals which may be present both in rubber and in plastics; the sensitising potential of some of these additives is unknown.

Phenyl-α-naphthylamine	Mercaptobenzimidazole
Phenyl-β-naphthylamine	2,6-Di-*tert*-butyl-4-methyl-phenol
p-Hydroxyphenyl-β-naphthyl-amine	2,6-Di(methylbenzyl)-4-methyl-phenol
Aldol-α-naphthylamine	Bis(5-methyl-3-*tert*-butyl-2-hydroxyphenyl)monosulphide
N-isopropyl-*n*-phenyl-PPD	2,5-Di-*tert*-butylhydroquinone
N,N'-diphenyl-PPD	2,5-Di-*tert*-amylhydroquinone
N,N'-di-β-naphthyl-PPD	Tri(*p*-nonylphenyl) phosphite

The plastics or synthetic fibres in which they may be found include pentaplast polyamides, polyformaldehyde, polyisobutylene, polyolefins, polyoxypropylene, polypropylene, polystryrene, polythene, polyurethane and polyvinyl chloride.

The thiurams and mercaptobenzothiazoles are present in 'domestic rubber' items such as underclothes and rubber gloves, and sensitise most frequently (p. 735), not because they are the most potent of allergens but because, in clothing, they are in contact with the skin for prolonged periods which facilitates sensitisation. Chemicals of the PPD-group occur in industrial rubbers such as tyres, hoses, belting and other heavy duty rubbers which must withstand weathering. Chemicals of the other groups are used in various types of rubber.

Latex
Sensitivity to rubber itself probably does not occur. The two reports in the literature (Keil and Bereston, 1942; Bonnevie and Marcussen, 1944) probably do not invalidate this statement.

Incidence of sensitivity

Twenty-five years ago, rubber sensitivity was considered to be a curiosity outside the rubber industry (Bonnevie and Marcussen, 1944) but this has changed radically as a result of the increasing use of rubber in the home, in clothing as well as in industry.

Several reports in the literature give the frequency of reactions to individual rubber chemicals, but the actual overall incidence of rubber-sensitive patients is rarely included. In a European study carried out in five different centres, 4000 eczematous patients were patch tested with a standard series of allergens; 5 per cent reacted to a rubber chemical. The rubber chemicals used for patch testing were tetramethylthiuram disulphide (TMTD), mercaptobenzothiazole (MBT), phenylcyclohexyl-PPD (CPPD) and diphenyl-PPD (DPPD), each 2 per cent in petrolatum (Fregert *et al.*, 1969). In Belgium (Song *et al.*, 1979) 6.8 per cent (55/810) of patients patch tested reacted to a rubber chemical and in Melbourne the incidence was 10 per cent (50/486) (Nurse, 1979).

St John's

Since 1965 every patient has been routinely tested with the following rubber chemicals:

1965–1970: TMTD and MBT, both 1–2 per cent in petrolatum, and a piece of rubber containing 15 industrial rubber chemicals.

1971: To increase the range of allergens, 5 rubber mixes were introduced (p. 766): Thiuram-mix, MBT-mix, naphthyl-mix, PPD-mix and Carba-mix; MBT 1 per cent was retained in the standard series.

During the 12 years, 1965–1976, the yearly incidence of rubber sensitivity changed little (Table 14.2), the average incidence was 6.2 per cent of all the patients tested.

Table 14.2. Incidence of rubber sensitivity (St John's 1965–1976).

Year	No. Tested	+ve	%
1965	1232	68	5.5
1966	1401	93	6.6
1967	1529	70	4.6
1968	1604	100	6.2
1969	1549	82	5.3
1970	1906	104	5.4
1971	1558	119	7.6
1972	1606	132	8.2
1973	1546	121	7.8
1974	1433	88	6.1
1975	1858	104	5.6
1976	1982	103	5.2

Sex incidence

In the European study (Fregert *et al.*, 1969) the sex incidence was equal, 5 per cent of the men and 5 per cent of the women being sensitive to rubber chemicals.

St John's

During the six years 1965 to 1970 the incidence of rubber sensitivity was greater in women (7.4 per cent) than men (3.9 per cent); but in the next six years, 1971–1976, the incidence in men rose (6.4 per cent) to equal that of women (6.9 per cent) (Table 14.3). This increase in men was due to a greater number being sensitised to chemicals in the thiuram group (p. 736) probably from rubber gloves worn at work.

Table 14.3. The incidence of rubber sensitivity in men and women (St John's 1965–1976).

| | Men | | | | Women | | | |
	Tested	+ve	%			Tested	+ve	%	
1965	618	20	3.2			614	48	7.8	
1966	731	32	4.4			670	61	9.1	
1967	809	20	2.5	} 3.9%		720	50	6.9	} 7.4%
1968	812	34	4.2			792	66	8.3	
1969	787	30	3.8			762	52	6.8	
1970	916	46	5.0			990	58	5.9	
1971	707	44	6.2			851	75	8.8	
1972	738	62	8.4			868	70	8.1	
1973	710	51	7.2	} 6.4%		836	70	8.4	} 6.9%
1974	655	37	5.6			778	51	6.6	
1975	887	51	5.7			971	52	5.4	
1976	937	52	5.5			1045	51	4.9	

INCIDENCE OF SENSITIVITY TO INDIVIDUAL CHEMICALS

Geographical variations

The results in the European series (Fregert *et al.*, 1969) showed that the incidence of sensitivity to TMTD and to MBT varies among different countries. London had the highest figures: of 800 patients tested, 29 (3.6) per cent reacted to TMTD and 38 (4.8 per cent) to MBT. The smallest numbers were in Lund (Sweden): of 800 patients tested there, only 8 (1 per cent) reacted to TMTD and 10 (1 per cent) to MBT. These dissimilarities were not explained.

The industrial PPD-derivatives showed less marked differences. Munich had the highest numbers: 17 patients reacted to CPPD and 13 to DPPD; the lowest figures were in Gothenburg where 11 patients in all reacted to these two chemicals (Table 14.4).

Incidences of sensitivity to TMTD and to MBT have also been reported from North America, Warsaw and Auckland in New Zealand. The figures are high for North America and Warsaw (Table 14.4).

Table 14.4. Incidence (%) of positive reactions to rubber chemicals in different countries.

	Tested	TMTD	MBT	CPPD	DPPD	Reference
Copenhagen	800	1.0	2.8	1.1	0.5	
Gothenburg	800	1.9	1.0	0.6	0.8	
Lund	800	1.0	1.3	1.4	1.0	
London	800	3.6	4.8	1.1	0.4	
Munich	800	2.8	1.1	2.1	1.6	Fregert *et al.* (1969)
N. America	1200	4.2	4.8	N.T.	N.T.	N. American Contact Derm. Group (1973)
Warsaw	1205	4.8	4.9	N.T.	N.T.	Rudzki and Kleniewska (1970)
Auckland	216	1.4	2.8	N.T.	N.T.	Black (1972)

TMTD = Tetramethylthiuram disulphide   MBT = Mercaptobenzothiazole
CPPD = Phenylcyclohexyl-PPD   DPPD = Diphenyl-PPD   N.T. = Not Tested

Sex differences

There are differences in the rubber chemicals to which men and women become sensitised. Women react to the 'domestic' rubber chemicals, the thiurams and MBT which are present in rubber gloves, underclothes and shoes. Although men, too, are sensitised by these groups, they may also in the course of their work become allergic to industrial rubber chemicals, which is an unusual occurrence in women who are rarely exposed to these additives. These latter chemicals include, among many others, the *para*phenylenediamine group which contains phenylcyclohexyl-PPD (CPPD), diphenyl-PPD (DPPD) and iso-propylphenyl-PPD (IPPD). The frequency of reactions to these chemicals will also depend upon the use of rubber in industry in the locality.

In each of the four series tabulated below, women were more often sensitive to TMTD and to MBT, except in the North American report in which more men than women were sensitive to MBT. Of the patients tested in Europe and Scandivania, more men than women reacted to CPPD and to DPPD (Table 14.5).

Table 14.5. Incidence (%) of sensitivity to four rubber chemicals in men and women in Europe (Fregert *et al.*, 1969); Scandinavia (Magnusson *et al.*, 1969); N. America (North American Dermatitis group, 1973) and Poland (Rudzki and Kleniewska, 1970).

	TMTD		MBT		CPPD		DPPD	
	M	F	M	F	M	F	M	F
Europe	1.6	2.3	1.7	2.3	1.8	0.9	1.2	0.6
Scandinavia	2.0	2.9	1.5	2.2	4.0	1.5	2.1	1.7
N. America	2.8	5.2	6.5	3.6	N.T.		N.T.	
Poland	4.3	5.2	4.6	5.1	N.T.		N.T.	

TMTD = Tetramethylthiuram disulphide MBT = Mercaptobenzothiazole
CPPD = Phenylcyclohexyl-PPD DPPD = Diphenyl-PPD N.T. = Not Tested

St John's

These differences between reactions to domestic and to industrial rubber chemicals, in men and women, have been consistently present in the patients investigated at St John's from 1965 to 1976 (Tables 14.6 and 14.12).

Table 14.6. Incidence of sensitivity (per cent) to thiurams and mercaptobenzothiazole (MBT) in men and women (St John's 1965–1976).

	No. Tested M + F	% Positive to a Thiuram and/or MBT		
		M + F	M	F
1965	1232	5.4	2.9	7.8
1966	1401	6.4	4.0	9.1
1967	1529	4.1	1.6	6.8
1968	1604	5.7	3.3	8.1
1969	1549	4.6	2.7	6.6
1970	1906	4.5	3.6	5.6
1971[a]	1558	6.9	5.1	8.3
1972	1606	7.0	6.2	7.7
1973	1546	7.1	5.9	8.0
1974	1433	5.4	4.6	6.2
1975	1858	5.0	4.7	5.3
1976	1982	4.8	4.8	4.8

[a]From 1971 onwards a thiuram-mix replaced TMTD in the standard patch test series.

'Domestic' rubber chemicals

Thiurams and MBT
During the twelve year period 1965–1976, the yearly incidence of patients sensitised by a thiuram, by mercaptobenzothiazole (MBT) or by both varied from 4.1 per cent to 7.1 per cent of all the patients tested. More women (4.8–9.1 per cent) than men (1.6–6.2 per cent) are sensitized (Table 14.6)

Thiurams
St John's
Women are particularly prone to acquire sensitivity to thiurams, the usual source being rubber gloves; the yearly incidence from 1965–1976 has ranged from 3.4–7.0 per cent of those tested. The incidence in men is lower, the numbers being 0.5–4.3 per cent of those tested (Table 14.7). These patients may also have reacted to chemicals of other rubber groups.

Table 14.7. Incidence of sensitivity (per cent) to thiurams in men and women (St John's 1965–1976).

| | No. Tested | | M + F | M | F |
	M	F	+%	+%	+%
1965	618	614	3.5	1.1	5.6
1966	731	670	4.5	2.2	7.0
1967	809	720	2.3	0.5	4.3
1968	812	792	3.4	2.0	4.9
1969	787	762	2.7	0.9	4.6
1970	916	990	2.5	1.4	3.4
1971[a]	707	851	5.1	3.1	6.8
1972	738	868	5.4	4.3	6.3
1973	710	836	5.4	4.1	6.6
1974	655	778	4.5	3.7	5.3
1975	887	971	4.0	3.5	4.4
1976	937	1045	3.6	2.8	4.3

[a]In 1971 the thiuram mix replaced TMTD in the standard series.

Geographical variations and testing with the thiuram mix
Many clinics now include more than one thiuram or a thiuram mix in their standard series; the mix consists of:

Tetramethylthiuram disulphide (TMTD)	0.25% in petrolatum
Tetraethylthiuram disulphide (TETD)	0.25% in petrolatum
Dipentamethylenethiuram disulphide (PTD)	0.25% in petrolatum
Tetramethylthiuram monosulphide (TMTM)	0.25% in petrolatum

The geographical variation in the incidences of sensitivity to the various thiurams is interesting.

Holland. In 1976, van Ketel reported from Amsterdam on his experience of testing with the thiuram mix. He found it to be a good detector of thiuram sensitivity and TMTD and TMTM were their most frequent allergens whereas PTD was a very uncommon sensitiser.

Poland. In Warsaw, too, the most frequent sensitiser of the three thiurams tested was TMTD and then TMTM; none of 200 patients reacted to dipentamethylenethiuram tetrasulphide (Rudzki *et al.*, 1976).

Spain. In Barcelona, TMTD was found to be the commonest sensitiser in 28 patients with an allergic contact dermatitis from rubber (Giménez Camarasa, 1968). Construction workers are also sensitised; of 100 tested with a series of chemicals, many reacted to TMTD and TMTM (Conde-Salazar Gomez and Gomez Urcuyo, 1976).

These results contrast with those of St John's, where PTD and TETD are more frequent sensitisers than TMTD and TMTM (Table 14.8). These variations between countries probably reflect the different thiurams preferred by their manufacturers for gloves and similar domestic articles.

St John's

In 1971, the thiuram mix replaced TMTD 1–2 per cent in the standard series and most of the patients who reacted to the mix were also tested with the four constituents, each being applied as 1 per cent in petrolatum. The mixture as formulated is a good detector of thiuram sensitivity, as about 95 per cent of the patients sensitive to a component reacted also to the mixture. Those recorded as not reacting to the mix usually had had weak, doubtful responses at two days which had led to testing with the components. The four thiurams do not always cross-react one with another, and the mixture is a better detector of sensitivity than is an individual chemical.

There was a remarkable similarity between the incidence and patterns of sensitivity in the men and women. In both sexes the greater number of reaction (67 per cent) was to PTD and TETD and the lesser number (57 per cent) to TMTD and TMTM (Table 14.8).

Table 14.8. Incidences of sensitivity to the constituents of the thiuram mix in men and women (St John's 1971–1976).

| | Tested | | + | | % | |
	M	F	M	F	M	F
Thiuram mix	164	296	152	282	93	95
PTD	122	221	81	147	66	67
TETD	124	223	84	152	68	68
TMTD	124	226	70	129	56	57
TMTM	125	227	73	128	58	56

(The concentration of each chemical in the mixture was 0.25 per cent; for testing separately each chemical was 1 per cent, all were diluted in petrolatum)

Mercaptobenzothiazole (MBT) and mercapto-group

During the period 1965–1969 there was an increased incidence of reactions to MBT in women (3.9–5.2 per cent) due to the occurrence at that time of a particular type of brassière dermatitis. From 1971–1976 the yearly incidence of sensitisation to MBT (or a mercapto chemical) has been similar in men (1.2–2.7 per cent) and women (1.5–2.8 per cent) (Table 14.9). These patients may also have reacted to chemicals of other rubber groups.

Table 14.9. Incidence of sensitivity to MBT and the mercapto-group in men and women (St John's 1965–1976).

	No Tested		M + F	M	F
	M	F	+%	+%	+ %
1965	618	614	3.1	2.1	4.1
1966	731	670	3.4	2.2	4.8
1967	809	720	2.4	1.1	3.9
1968	812	792	3.4	1.7	5.2
1969	787	762	3.0	1.9	4.1
1970	916	990	2.6	2.3	2.8
1971	707	851	2.5	2.3	2.7
1972	738	868	2.7	2.7	2.8
1973	710	836	2.6	2.7	2.5
1974	655	778	1.8	1.2	2.3
1975	887	971	1.7	1.9	1.6
1976	937	1045	2.1	2.7	1.6

In 1971, MBT 1 per cent was continued in the routine series but a mercapto-mix was added, consisting of:

Mercaptobenzothiazole	(MBT)	0.25% in petrolatum
Cyclohexylbenzothiazyl sulphenamide	(CBS)	0.25% in petrolatum
Dibenzothiazyl disulphide	(MBTS)	0.25% in petrolatum
Morpholinylmercaptobenzothiazole	(MMBT)	0.25% in petrolatum

The mercapto-mix is an extremely useful addition to the standard series but to avoid active sensitisation the concentration of its components has necessarily to be kept low and false negative reactions to its 0.25 per cent concentration of MBT occurred in about 30 per cent (64/216) of the patients.

Date	Total + Mercapto Chemical	Total + MBT	MBT + Mix +	MBT + Mix ?	MBT + Mix –
1971–76	224	216	152	23	41

Similar experience has been reported from other clinics (Mitchell *et al.*, 1976).

The concentration of MBT in the mix has been increased to 0.5 per cent but false negative reactions still occur. Retaining mercaptobenzothiazole 1 per cent in the standard series compensates for this short-coming of the mercapto-mix.

False negative reactions to MBT 1 per cent occurred in 10 of the 216 (5 per cent) patients; each had a positive reaction when again tested with MBT 1 per cent as part of the mercapto-mix. In 3 of these patients the mercapto-mix was positive, in 5 it was doubtful and in 2 it was negative.

MBT – to + Mix +	MBT – to + Mix ?	MBT – to + Mix –
3	5	2

The results of testing with the separate constituents of the mercapto-mix have been tabulated (Table 14.10). In both men and women the greatest number of reactions was to MBT and in both sexes there was a decreasing incidence to MMBT, CBS and MBTS.

Table 14.10 Positive reactions in105 men and 119 women to constituents of the Mercapto-Mix (St Johns 1971–1976).

	Tested		+		%	
	M	F	M	F	M	F
MBT 1%	105	119	101	115	96	97
Mercapto-Mix	105	119	81	77	77	65
MMBT 1%	77	72	64	57	83	79
CBS 1%	78	71	61	45	78	63
MBTS 1%	78	70	50	33	64	47

MMBT	= Morpholinylmercaptobenzothiazole
CBS	= Cyclohexylbenzothiazylsulphenamide
MBTS	= Dibenzolthiazyl disulphide
Diluent	= Petrolatum

Carbamates and diphenylguanidine

Dithiocarbamates are frequently present in domestic type rubber such as that used for gloves, clothing and contraceptive sheaths. Six patients who reacted to the elastic of their bleached underclothes but not to unbleached rubber were investigated by Jordan and Bourlas (1975). They found that the accelerator in the rubber, zinc dibenzyldithiocarbamate, was affected by the hypochlorite bleach and produced compounds, one of which, N,N-dibenzylcarbamyl chloride, was a strong allergen.

Diphenylguanidine (DPG) is used in heavier industrial rubbers. Although DPG is an infrequent allergen in the U.K., it may be a common sensitiser in other countries, as in Spain (Gimenez Camarasa 1968) and Venezuela (Soto, 1974).

St John's

Since 1971, a carba-mix, containing 2 dithiocarbamates and diphenylguanidine, has been used for testing:

Zinc diethyldithiocarbamate	(ZDC)	1 per cent petrolatum
Zinc dibutyldithiocarbamate	(ZBC)	1 per cent petrolatum
Diphenylguanidine	(DPG)	1 per cent petrolatum

Sensitivity to the carba-mix alone was infrequent and occurred in only 31 patients; it was more frequent in men (27) than women (4). However simultaneous reactions to the carba-mix and thiuram-mix were not infrequent and were seen in 154 patients, among whom there were more women (102) than men (52). This association of reactions is explained by the similarity between the chemical formulae of the two groups (pp. 718, 720).

Table 14.11 Reactions in Men and Women to the Carba-mix and Thiuram-mix (St John's 1971–1976).

Date	Tested		Carba-Mix only + No. Patients		Carba-Mix + Thiuram-mix + No. Patients	
	M	F	M	F	M	F
1971–76	4634	5349	27	4	52	102

When the patient reacts only to the carba-mix then the diphenylguanidine

(DPG) is the most likely sensitiser. As DPG is an industrial rubber chemical, it sensitises more men than women (Table 14.12).

Table 14.12. Sensitisation to components of the carba-mix in patients who reacted only to this group of rubber chemicals.

	Carba-mix		ZDC		ZBC		DPG	
	M	**F**	**M**	**F**	**M**	**F**	**M**	**F**
Tested	27	4	18	2	9	1	17	2
+	22	3	2	0	1	0	14	2

ZDC = Zinc diethyldithiocarbamate   ZBC = Zinc dibutyldithiocarbamate
DPG = Diphenylguanidine

Industrial rubber chemicals
Industrial rubber chemicals belong principally to the PPD-group, the naphthyl-group, the mercapto-group, and also include diphenylguanidine.

In contrast to domestic rubber, only a few patients are seen each year, who have been sensitised by industrial rubber chemicals. During the decade 1967–1976, the average was 11 patients a year. As the exposure is mainly industrial, more men than women are sensitised; from 1967–1976, the diagnosis was made in 82 men as compared with 25 women (Table 14.13).

Table 14.13. Annual numbers of men and women sensitised by Industrial Rubber Chemicals (St John's 1967–1976).

Year	1967	1968	1969	1970	1971	1972	1973	1974	1975	1976
No. Men	7	7	9	11	5	13	10	6	6	8
No. Women	3	2	2	2	1	6	3	4	1	1

PPD-group
Most of the patients who reacted to industrial rubber compounds had been sensi-tised by chemicals of the PPD-group; a few reacted, in addition, to chemicals of other groups.

Since 1971, all patients have been tested with a PPD-mix consisting of:

Phenylcyclohexyl-PPD	(CPPD)	0.25% in petrolatum
Diphenyl-PPD	(DPPD)	0.25% in petrolatum
Isopropylphenyl-PPD	(IPPD)	0.1% in petrolatum

From 1971–1976, the overall incidence of reactions to this group of chemicals was as follows:

Tested		+		%	
M	**F**	**M**	**F**	**M**	**F**
4634	5349	39	14	0.8	0.3

The majority of the 53 patients who had a positive response to the PPD-mix were tested with its separate constituents; CPPD and DPPD were each 1 per cent in petrolatum but IPPD was 0.1 per cent to avoid active sensitisation by this potent allergen. The strongest sensitiser in the group was IPPD to which 45 of 48 patients reacted; less potent was CPPD to which 38 of 45 patients reacted and least sensitising was DPPD to which 17 of 43 patients responded. PPD is a poor detec-tor of sensitisation to this group of chemicals, only a third (17 of 53) of the patients reacted (Table 14.14).

Table 14.14. Reactions to the PPD-mix, IPPD, CPPD, DPPD and PPD in patients sensitised by a PPD rubber chemical.

	Tested		+		%	
	M	F	M	F	M	F
PPD-mix	39	14	39	13	100	93
IPPD	35	13	34	11	97	85
CPPD	33	12	28	10	85	83
PPD	31	12	14	3	45	25
PPD	39	14	13	4	33	29

Naphthyl-group

Reactions to this group of chemicals are uncommon. Since 1971 patients have been tested with a naphthyl-mix consisting of:

Phenyl-β-naphthylamine	(PBN)	0.5% in petrolatum
Di-β-naphthyl-p-phenylenediamine	(DBNPD)	0.5% in petrolatum

From 1971–1976 the number of patients who reacted to this mix was as follows:

Tested		+		%	
M	F	M	F	M	F
4634	5349	15	6	0.3	0.1

About half the patients were tested with two separate constituents of the mix, each at a concentration of 1 per cent in petrolatum. DBNPD was tested in 9 patients and each reacted, PBN was tested in 11 patients and 7 were positive (Table 14.15).

Table 14.15. Reactions to the naphthyl-mix, DBNPD and PBN in patients sensitised by this group of chemicals.

	Tested		+	
	M	F	M	F
Naphthyl-mix	15	6	15	6
DBNPD	6	3	6	3
PBN	8	3	6	1

Mercapto-group

Patients are routinely tested with the mercapto-mix (p. 730) but as nearly all the sensitised patients reacted to MBT, it is impossible to separate accurately those patients primarily sensitised by MBT from those sensitised by other members of the group.

Diphenylguanidine (p. 732).

SOURCES OF SENSITIVITY

Rubber dermatitis can be divided into two arbitary groups:
Domestic
Industrial

This division is specious in that rubber gloves, classified as domestic rubber, may be worn at work rather than in the home, particularly by men; the same applies to rubber boots and finger stalls. Nevertheless, this separation is convenient because the sensitising chemicals in light domestic rubber differ from those in heavy-duty industrial rubber.

Domestic rubber

This group includes rubber gloves, brassières, suspenders, roll-ons and girdles, shoes, contraceptives and fingerstalls.

The sensitising chemicals are the thiurams, carbamates and mercaptobenzothiazole. Sensitisation to carbamates has not been dealt with separately because reactions to these chemicals are so frequently associated with sensitisation to the thiurams and the sources of exposure are similar.

St John's

Women

During the 12-year period 1965–1976, the numbers of women sensitised by rubber gloves has gradually increased and concurrently sensitisation by brassières, girdles and suspenders has greatly diminished. The incidence of reactions to shoes and fingerstalls has changed little.

The major sources of sensitisation to the thiuram chemicals and mercaptobenzothiazole (MBT) have been tabulated as:

thiurams 'only'   = + a thiuram – MBT
                     (with or without a reaction to other rubber groups)
MBT 'only'   = + MBT – a thiuram
                     (with or without a reaction to other rubber groups)

Some women had dermatitis from several rubber contacts

Thiurams

Sensitisation 'only' to thiurams is likely to be due to rubber gloves; it is unlikely to be due to shoes. Occasionally the cause is rubber or elastic in underclothes or a rubber fingerette. Individual patients have complained of dermatitis from a rubber apron, pillow, sponge, balloons and powder puff.

MBT

Patients who react 'only' to MBT have probably been sensitised by gloves or shoes. Nowadays rubber or elastic in underclothes is a less frequent cause. A few patients had dermatitis from a rubber fingerette, elastic stockings, bathing caps, a gas-mask, rubber bands, antifreeze and rubber handles on a hockey stick and domestic tools.

Thiurams and MBT

Similarly allergy to both thiuram and MBT relates equally to gloves and shoes, other sources have been rubber bands, rubber handlebars, an insecticide and a rubber sponge.

Thiurams 'only'

	Tested	+	%	Gloves Present	PH	Bras. Susp. etc. Present	PH	Shoes Present	PH	Fingerette Present	PH
1965–67	2004	73	3.6	34(48%)		24(33%)		9			
1968–70	2544	70	2.6	40(57%)		13(19%)	4	4		2	
1971–73	2555	131	5.1	113(86%)		2(1.5%)	5	2	1	1	
1974–76	2794	99	3.5	78(79%)	12	1(1%)	4	3			

MBT 'only'

	Tested	+	%	Gloves Present	PH	Bras. Susp. etc. Present	PH	Shoes Present	PH	Fingerette Present	PH
1965–67	2004	42	2.1	4(9.5%)		28(66%)		3		3	
1968–70	2544	58	2.3	18(31%)		22(38%)		14			
1971–73	2555	34	1.3	15(44%)		4(12%)	2	12		6	
1974–76	2794	21	0.8	4(19%)	1	3(14%)		9	1	2	

Thiurams + MBT

	Tested	+	%	Gloves Present	PH	Bras. Susp. etc. Present	PH	Shoes Present	PH	Fingerette Present	PH
1965–67	2004	43	2.1	3(7%)		32(74%)		14		1	
1968–70	2544	42	1.7	14(33%)		17(40%)	5	18	1	4	1
1971–73	2555	33	1.2	15(45%)		4(12%)	3	15		1	
1974–76	2794	30	1.1	15(50%)	6	1(3%)	6	15	1	1	

Men

The incidence of rubber glove dermatitis has increased in men from 8 cases (0.4 per cent) in the triennium 1965–1967 to 53 (2.1 per cent) cases during the years 1974–1976. The numbers with dermatitis from shoes and boots remained similar each year; men still occasionally present with dermatitis from a rubber contraceptive sheath or from a finger stall. The numbers of patients with dermatitis have been tabulated as for the women.

Thiurams

Sensitisation 'only' to a thiuram is usually from rubber gloves. A few patients have dermatitis from shoes, contraceptives and fingerettes. In this series other sources of exposure were insecticides, trouser waist band, antiperspirant shields, wet suit, elastic bands, balloons, cushion foam, carpets, a mask, rubber pipes and a hearing aid.

MBT

Shoes and boots are the principal source of sensitisation to MBT, gloves seem relatively infrequent and fingerettes are occasionally to blame. Other causes of dermatitis have been masks, elastic bands, printing blankets, hot water bottles, bicycle and golf club handles, domestic rubber handles, flexes and tubing, antifreeze, elastic and rubber in a trouser waist band.

Thiurams and MBT

Allergy to thiurams and MBT is likely to be from footwear, rather than gloves.

These patients also had dermatitis from contraceptives, fingerettes, masks, rubber bands, elastic, antifreeze and balloons.

Thiurams 'only'

	Tested	+	%	Gloves		Shoes-boots		Contraceptives		Fingerette	
				Present	PH	Present	PH	Present	PH	Present	PH
1965–67	2158	22	1.0	3(14%)		4		2	2		
1968–70	2515	30	1.2	15(50%)		4		1			
1971–73	2155	69	3.2	34(49%)	1	1		3	3	1	
1974–76	2479	67	2.7	48(72%)	3	5	1	3	8		

MBT 'only'

	Tested	+	%	Gloves		Shoes-boots		Contraceptives		Fingerette	
				Present	PH	Present	PH	Present	PH	Present	PH
1965–67	2158	34	1.6	5		15(44%)				1	
1968–70	2515	44	1.7	7		19(43%)				4	
1971–73	2155	39	1.8	5		22(56%)					
1974–76	2479	36	1.5	2		24(66%)	1				

Thiurams + MBT

	Tested	+	%	Gloves		Shoes-Boots		Contraceptives		Fingerettes	
				Present	PH	Present	PH	Present	PH	Present	PH
1965–67	2158	4	0.2			2				1	
1968–70	2515	7	0.3			3					
1971–73	2155	15	0.7			9		2			
1974–76	2479	14	0.6	3		8			2		

Industrial rubber

Industrial heavy-duty rubbers contain many chemicals, some of which are potent sensitisers; because of the type of occupational exposure, cases of dermatitis occur principally in men. This type of rubber is used for tyres, belting, hoses, seals, cables and agricultural equipment, and in rubber used in the engineering construction industries.

PPD group

These chemicals are added to rubber to prevent it cracking on exposure to air and light, but their tendency to accumulate on the surface of the rubber enhances their sensitising potential (Schønning and Hjorth, 1969).

Isopropylaminodiphenylamine (Phenylisopropyl-PPD) (IPPD; Nonox ZA)

This is the most potent sensitiser in the PPD group and its dangers in this respect are well recognised. It is an anti-oxidant and anti-ozonant, which is added to rubber in a concentration of about 2 per cent to prevent weathering — that is, cracking and deterioration of the rubber on exposure to air, heat and light. It is present in tyres, cables, industrial belting and hoses. Its hazard to tyrebuilders, who were at particular risk, has been reduced by automation, but cases sensitised by tyres still occur, especially in workers in the transport industry. Those handling other industrial heavy-duty rubbers also may develop dermatitis. Eight patients who became allergic to IPPD were described by Bieber and Foussereau (1968): four men had been sensitised by tyres, a miner and another man by their boots, a builder by his gloves and boots and a painter by gloves. In France, Hervé-Bazin·*et al.* (1977) and Foussereau and Cavelier (1977) have described 42 cases sensitised by tyres; 17 were employed in the manufacture of tyres, 5 were tyre dealers and 20 worked in transport or in its servicing. A woman employed in fixing metal caps on car braking tubes was acutely sensitised by the 1 per cent IPPD in the rubber tubing (Raith, 1976). A policeman was sensitised by his black rubber truncheon and he developed a dry fissured eczema of the right palm (Menezes Brandão, 1978).

Phenylcyclohexyl-PPD (CPPD)
This chemical is another antioxidant which has been added to tyre rubber (Hjorth and Fregert, 1968) but its efficacy is limited and so its use has declined.

Diphenyl-PPD (DPPD)
This antioxidant sometimes sensitises; it, too, is used in tyre rubber to increase its resistance to heat and cracking. Two men were sensitised by this chemical which was present in rubber packing used to join cement tubes (Fregert, 1969). In a series of 24 patients with contact dermatitis from rubber bank note counters, 3 reacted to DPPD 1 per cent in yellow vaseline (Eriksson and Ostlund, 1968).

N-dimethyl — 1.3 butyl-N'-phenyl-paraphenylenediamine (*DMPPD*)
This compound, though claimed to be non-sensitising, elicits positive patch test reactions in patients sensitised to IPPD (Hervé-Bazin *et al.*, 1977).

St John's

Men
From 1965–1976, a total of 66 men were found to be allergic to these chemicals. Over half were sensitised by rubber used in the transport industry, principally tyres. The following sources of exposure were incriminated; in the case of the squash ball, it was ascertained from the manufacturers that it did contain IPPD.

a. Industrial:
Tyres, vehicles, aircraft	38
Rubber boots and shoes	6
Rubber factory	4
Milking machine (cowmen)	2
Boiler gaskets and flanges	1
Black rubber construction pipe	1
Laboratory tubing	1
Face mask	1
Earphones	1

b. Non-industrial:
Squash ball	1
Cushion	1
Bootee	1
Shoe soles, walking stick handles	1

In 7 men, a likely source of contact was not discovered; their occupations were pipe-layer, electronics engineer, maintenance engineer, in a paint shop, in an oil refinery and two were clerks.

Women

During this same period 13 women were sensitised by these chemicals. The reactions were relevant in 3, one of whom worked in a rubber factory, one in a cable factory and the other as a car polisher. The source was doubtful in a physiotherapist, but she may have handled rubbers containing those allergens. Another woman was possibly sensitised in a previous job making Wellington boots, although she had had no dermatitis at the time. In the remaining 8 there was no apparent source of contact.

Alfonzo (1979) reviewed 51 patients seen at St John's and his results were similar.

Diaminodiphenylmethane

This additive is used in tyres and other heavy duty rubbers. It is also used as an epoxy hardener, a corrosion inhibitor and chemical intermediate. It contaminated flour and caused 84 cases of jaundice in Epping (Kopelman et al., 1966).

St John's

In 1968, DDM 1 per cent in petrolatum was used in the routine testing of 834 patients; of the 23 who had positive tests, 20 reacted also to PPD. In only one patient was the reaction found to be significant; he was a 30-year-old motor engineer with a three month history of eczema of his fingers, the backs of his hands and his arms. When patch tested he reacted to DDM and to PPD. It was subsequently ascertained from the manufacturers that DDM was present in the tyres he was handling. DDM has a limited use in industry and as it is thought not to be an important allergen it is not used for routine patch testing.

N-dimethyl-1,3-butyl-N'-phenylparaphenylenediamine (DMPPD)

DMPPD, introduced as a non-sensitising antiozonant, has been found by Hervé-Bazin et al. (1977) to cross-react with IPPD. They found DMPPD to be a pure product and they were able to detect its presence in one brand of tyres.

NAPHTHYL CHEMICALS

These chemicals are widely used; phenyl-β-naphthylamine in tyres and general rubber goods, and di-β-naphthyl-PPD in latex products. They may contain trace amounts of the carcinogen β-naphthylamine and, though the level is not considered a hazard, its presence has led one rubber company in England to abandon their use.

Phenyl-β-naphthylamine

This accelerator was reported by Bieber and Foussereau (1968) to be the sensitiser in four men who had come into contact with it by handling tyres, another man by wearing rubber boots and one woman by using an elastic band.

St John's

Men

Between 1967 and 1976 a total of 24 men reacted to the naphthyl group; the pattern of their reactions to the rubber groups was as follows:

naphthyl group only	5
naphthyl group + PPD group ± other groups	17
naphthyl group + thiurams	1
naphthyl group + thiurams + carbamates + MBT	1

Sensitisation to the naphthyl group alone was not associated with any particular source of contact. Of the 5 patients, one was an aircraft fitter, one an aircraft engineer, one had dermatitis from a mask and another from earphones; the fifth man was a maintenance engineer with no apparent relevance for the sensitivity.

In this whole group of 24 men the sources of rubber contact in 18 cases were:

Aircraft	4	(Fitter (2) Engineer (2))
Tyres	3	(Garage attendant. Car washer. Lorry driver)
Earphones	2	(Telephone technician. Merchant Navy Radio Operator.)
Rubber boots	4	
Mask	1	(Glass decorator)
Cables	1	(Post Office engineer)
Gaskets and flanges	1	(Boiler maintainance)
Laboratory tubing	1	(Chemist)
Rubber factory	1	

In 6 men, neither a source of nor a relevance for the sensitivity could be found. Their occupations were maintenance engineer, carpenter, pipe layer, train driver, in an oil refinery and in a paint shop.

Women

In this same period 5 women were found to be sensitised. Three had foot eczema, shoes being a possible source of the allergen. The fourth was a housewife with mainly hand eczema and the fifth had stasis ulcers, but in neither was there an obvious contact with rubber which might have contained these chemicals.

MERCAPTO CHEMICALS

Chemicals of this group are widely used in the rubber industry. Cyclohexylbenzothiazyl sulphenamide (CBS) is a common accelerator, and morpholinylmercaptobenzothiazole (MMBT) is being used with increasing frequency. Post Office workers sensitised by CBS in rubber bank note counters have been described by Eriksson and Ostlund (1968) (p. 764).

St John's

As practically all the patients sensitised to a mercapto chemical cross-reacted with MBT it is impossible to know with certainty which mercapto compound was the primary allergens.

Diphenylguanidine

This accelerator is used in medium weight industrial rubber including articles such as mats and face masks. Rubber coated hose pipes (ascertained to contain diphenyl guanidine) sensitised and caused dermatitis of the wrists and face in a project engineer who was handling the hoses, while installing new machinery (Calnan, 1978b). Diphenylguanidine (DPG) caused allergic rhinitis in a tyre worker, application of DPG, 1 per cent in pet. produced an urticarial weal (Camarasa and Alomar, 1978).

OTHER CHEMICALS

Diethylthiourea

This accelerator was present in foam rubber weather strips, which caused an outbreak of dermatitis in 15 car assembly workers. The hands, the arms and sometimes the face were affected. The sensitised men came into contact with the rubber when it was already in place as seals round the doors and bonnet. The men who fitted the strips were not affected (White and Vickers, 1970). This difference may be explained by the way these men came into contact with the seals; those who applied them handled them only with their palms, whereas the assembly men touched the rubber with all parts of their hands and arms, sites where percutaneous absorption takes place more readily than through palmar skin. Ethyl butyl thiourea in a rubber adhesive has caused shoe dermatitis (p. 70).

Dioxydiphenyl

This additive has been a sensitiser in surgical rubber gloves (p. 744) in a rubber sheet (p. 753) and in one of the 28 patients reported by Giménez Camarasa (1968) but the source of contact in this patient was not recorded.

Dithiodimorpholine

4,4'-Dithiomorpholine was one of several rubber compounds which caused dermatitis in a Danish rubber factory. Subsequently dithiomorpholine 1 per cent in petrolatum was used in the investigation of patients with contact dermatitis and of 110 patients tested 6 gave positive reactions (Heydenreich and Ølholm-Larsen, 1976).

Clinical features

Rubber sensitivity may be the direct cause of a dermatitis or it may be superimposed upon an already existing eczema. As rubber sensitivity often has no distinctive clinical pattern, cases will be missed unless patients are patch tested routinely with rubber chemicals. A positive reaction to a rubber chemical is significant, and it usually is relevant to the existing eczema. In the European series (Fregert *et al.*, 1969), the rubber chemicals were high on the list of allergens found to be relevant to the patient's eczema (Table 14.16).

The source of rubber contact can nearly always be identified and eliminated, thereby either curing or greatly alleviating the patient's eczema. It is a mistake to rely on clinical acumen alone in diagnosing rubber dermatitis.

Table 14.16. Relevance of sensitivities to rubber chemicals (Fregert *et al.*, 1969)

	Male %	Female %
TMTD	73	91
Diphenyl-PPD	84	65
MBT	66	76
Phenylcyclohexyl-PPD	81	48

Chronic melanodermatitis of the face occurred in a Japanese ferry boat captain from contact and sensitisation to the rubber covering on the aperture of a radarscope (Hamada and Horiguchi, 1978).

'DOMESTIC' DERMATITIS

Gloves
Sensitivity to rubber gloves occurs predominantly in housewives who wear them to protect their hands during housework. In Wilson's series (1960), the sequence of events was remembered by 30 patients. Seventeen of them had had no eczema before starting to wear gloves, whereas the other 13 had begun to wear them on account of hand eczema which they had attributed to detergents.

St John's
> Most of our patients wear gloves to protect their hands which have already become eczematous and the sensitivity is therefore superimposed upon an existing eczema. In 1972–1973, 94 women were seen with rubber glove dermatitis, 38 wore gloves after the onset of the eczema, 12 before and in 44 this information was not recorded.

Clinical features
Any patient who has eczema on the dorsal surfaces of the fingers and hands and who wears rubber gloves may be sensitive to rubber. Features suggestive of the diagnosis are:

1. A sharply delineated *band of* eczema on the mid forearm corresponding to the upper border of the glove.
2. An eczema which is diffuse or patchy on the dorsa of the hands and on the flexor or extensor surfaces of the lower arms, and thus corresponds to glove area and does not extend beyond it.
3. A history of sensitivity to other rubber articles such as shoes, brassières or suspenders.

St John's
> The classical distribution of a rubber glove dermatitis was seen in very few patients. The majority had a non-specific pattern of hand eczema, and in some the wrists or lower arms were also affected. In most patients, the diagnosis could not have been made with certainty without routine patch testing; the diagnosis was made if a patient with hand eczema had worn rubber gloves and reacted to a thiuram or to MBT. In the series reported by Cronin (1972) 25 women had rubber glove dermatitis but in only 3 was the sensitivity thought to be the entire cause of their hand eczema and in none had the diagnosis been made prior to patch testing. The value of making this diagnosis was emphasised in a follow-up of 20 women

and 4 men with rubber glove dermatitis diagnosed in 1971. Fourteen had started to wear gloves after the onset of the eczema, and 5 before; this information was not recorded in 5 patients. All were requested to return to the clinic: fourteen did so and the other 10 replied to a questionnaire. By changing to plastic gloves or discarding gloves 7 patients' hands had healed completely; 16 had improved, some considerably; and only one man said that he had noticed no benefit from avoiding rubber.

Results of patch testing

At the present time, the chemicals in ordinary household rubber gloves in Britain are:

Accelerators		**Antioxidants**
Dipentamethylenethiuram disulphide	(PTD)	2-*p*-Methylcyclohexyl-4,6-dimethylphenol
Zinc Mercaptobenzothiazole	(MBT)	Methylene bis-methyl-cyclohexyl-*p*-cresol
Zinc diethyldithiocarbamate	(ZDC)	
Zinc dimethylpentamethylene-dithiocarbamate.		

Wilson (1960, 1969) studied, over a ten-year period, patients with this sensitivity and found that PTD was consistently the commonest sensitiser. The first group of 42 patients, all with rubber glove dermatitis, comprised 38 females and 4 males; 71 per cent reacted to PTD, 48 per cent to TMTD, 36 per cent to MBT and 5 per cent to ZDC. In the second series, there were 43 patients with glove dermatitis of whom 79 per cent were sensitive to PTD, 45 per cent to TMTD, 30 per cent to MBT and 15 per cent to ZDC (Table 14.17). In both series patch tests were done using the chemicals in a concentration of 1 per cent petrolatum; in the second series not every patient was tested to each of the four chemicals.

Table 14.17 Percentage of patients with rubber glove dermatitis positive to four rubber chemicals (Wilson, 1960; 1969).

Year	No. Tested	% Positive			
		PTD	TMTD	MBT	ZDC
1960	42	71	48	36	5
1969	43	79	45	30	15

PTD	= 1 per cent dipentamethylenethiuram disulphide
TMTD	= 1 per cent tetramethylthiuram disulphide
MBT	= 1 per cent mercaptobenzothiazole
ZDC	= 1 per cent zinc diethyldithiocarbamate

St John's

Women

From 1971–1976 a total of 257 women with rubber glove dermatitis were patch tested: 205 (80 per cent) reacted to a thiuram and were negative to MBT, 18 (7 per cent reacted to MBT and not to the thiurams and 34 (13 per cent) reacted to both (Table 14.18).

Table 14.18. Incidence of reactions to thiurams and mercaptobenzothiazole in 143 women with rubber glove dermatitis (St John's 1971–1976).

	Women with rubber glove derm.	Thiuram + MBT –	MBT + Thiuram –	Thiuram + MBT+
1971	46	36	5	5
1972	44	36	2	6
1973	53	43	6	4
1974	35	27	2	6
1975	37	30	3	4
1976	42	33	0	9
Total	257	205(80%)	18(7%)	34(13%)

Constituents of the thiuram-mix

Testing with the thiuram-mix and its constituents confirms Wilson's (1960, 1969) finding that PTD is the commonest sensitiser in British rubber gloves. These results also show that to detect thiuram sensitivity by patch testing it is essential to use several chemicals of the group, or a mixture of them (Table 14.19).

Table 14.19. Results of patch testing with the thiuram-mix and its constituents in women with rubber glove dermatitis (St John's 1971–1976).

Thiuram-mix		PTD		TMTD		TETD		TMTM	
Tested	+	Tested	+	Tested	+	Tested	+	Tested	+
239	227(95%)	180	130(72%)	180	106(59%)	181	107(59%)	181	101(56%)

Methylcyclohexyldimethylphenol

One patient seen had been sensitised by this antioxidant in rubber gloves. On preliminary testing, she twice reacted to her own gloves but not to TMTD 2 per cent or to MBT 2 per cent. When subsequently tested with each constituent chemical of the glove, she reacted only to 1 per cent methylcyclohexyldimethylphenol. Her eczema improved greatly after she stopped wearing rubber gloves.

Gloves

Patients who bring their gloves to the clinic are tested with them, but they may give false negative reactions and testing with them is not relied upon to make the diagnosis.

Men

Although most of the men had acquired their rubber glove dermatitis from gloves worn at work, their patch test results were essentially the same as those of the women.

In all, 99 men with this dermatitis were seen in the six years 1971–1976: 82 (83 per cent) reacted to a thiuram and were negative to MBT, 8 (8 per cent) reacted to MBT and were negative to a thiuram, and 9 (9 per cent) reacted to both a thiuram and MBT (Table 14.20).

Thiuram-mix

Reactions to the thiuram mix were positive in 87 of 91 men (96 per cent) and testing with the separate constituents showed that, as with women, PTD was the commonest sensitiser (Table 14.21).

Table 14.20. Incidence of reactions to thiurams and mercaptobenzothiazole in 99 men with rubber glove dermatitis (St John's 1971–1976).

	Men with rubber glove derm.	Thiuram + MBT −	MBT + Thiuram −	Thiuram + MBT +
1971	11	9	2	1
1972	15	10	1	3
1973	17	13	2	2
1974	19	19	0	0
1975	19	14	3	2
1976	18	17	0	1
Total	99	82(83%)	8(8%)	9(9%)

Table 14.21. Results of patch tests with the thiuram-mix and its constituents in men with rubber glove dermatitis (St John's 1971–1976).

Thiuram-mix		PTD		TETD		TMTM			
Tested 91	+ 87(96%)	Tested 68	+ 53(78%)	Tested 70	+ 46(66%)	Tested 73	+ 39(53%)	Tested 73	+ 38(52%)

Alternatives

Plastic gloves are available, similar in weight and strength to ordinary domestic rubber gloves, and are suitable for home use.

Similar or heavy plastic gloves can be used by men in industry.

Surgical rubber gloves

Surgeons and nurses may become sensitive to their gloves. In The Hague, four surgeons and one theatre sister developed dermatitis from a particular type of rubber glove. They were patch tested with the constituents and all reacted to dioxydiphenyl 1 per cent in ung. cetyl (Polano, 1958). Five surgeons with hand eczema were investigated by Lintum and Nater (1973) in the Netherlands; each reacted to their rubber gloves and to thiuram chemicals, and one was also sensitive to carbamates. In 1975 Nater again found thiurams to be the principal cause of an occupational rubber dermatitis among 12 members of an operating theatre staff.

The formulation of surgical gloves varies according to the manufacturer. In Great Britain one widely used standard make of glove contains the following chemicals:

Zinc diethyldithiocarbamate (Accelerator)
Polymerised 2,2,4-trimethyl-1,2-dihydroquinoline (Antioxidant)

Cases of dermatitis are few but continue to crop up. Sometimes, but not always, positive patch tests are obtained with one of the standard rubber chemicals; in patients with negative tests, it is possible that the dermatitis is due to a mild irritant remaining in the rubber after manufacture.

Surgical glove powder

An inflammatory response was evoked in guinea pigs by starch glove powder in

Freund's adjuvant. It was thought to be a combination of an irritant and a delayed hypersensitivity reaction (Grant, Davies and Verrier Jones, 1975).

Alternatives

1. *Puritee gloves*: These are made of natural rubber and combined sulphur, they contain the antioxidant

    2,2′-methylene-bis (4-methyl-6-*tert*-butylphenol)

    They are manufactured by Searle Medical Products, P.O. Box 88, Lane End Road, High Wycombe, Bucks, England HP12 3TD.

2. *Elastyren gloves*: are made of a styrene-butadiene polymer and contain less than 0.5 per cent of the antioxidant:

    zinc dithiocarbamate

    They are manufactured by Danpren A/S, 272 Vigerslevvej, DK 2500 Valby, Denmark.

3. *U.S.A.* Fisher (1975) has given details of the American suppliers of 'hypo-allergenic' gloves.

Brassières

Elastic is present in nearly all brassières to a greater or lesser extent, and in deep brassières there may be wide elastic panels. In many patients a localised pattern of eczema on the chest and upper trunk is strongly suggestive of dermatitis from elastic in a brassière, but in others the diagnosis is not so obvious. In them, a patch of eczema on the sternum may be called seborrhoeic dermatitis, and an itchy plaque on the back be passed off as just 'eczema', without considering a contact dermatitis from elastic in the front of a brassière or from the elastic band at the back. In brassières, the allergen nearly always is a thiuram or mercaptobenzothiazole.

About 1966, there was a flurry of cases of brassière dermatitis in Britain due to one particular make called 'Playtex'. This garment had deep elastic panels made of polyurethane Spandex yarn, and the women who became sensitised had plaques of eczema imprinted on their chest wall directly under the elastic in their brassière. The clinical picture was striking, and cases closely resembled one another. The sensitiser was mercaptobenzothiazole in the polyurethane Spandex yard (Allenby, et al., 1966). Such cases are no longer seen but, at the time, similar patients were reported from America (Joseph and Maibach, 1967; Tannenbaum, 1967).

Spandex is a generic term for polyurethane fibres and does not imply the presence or absence of any particular chemical. These fibres are manufactured by various companies and have different trade names: Lycra, for example, is made by Du Pont. Spandex is better than rubber for certain uses as it is stronger, lighter and whiter; also it takes dyes easily and is resistant to oils and perspiration. Such advantages have made it particularly suitable for underclothes and swimsuits (Couzens and Yarsley, 1968). It is likely that different chemicals are used by different companies in the manufacture of polyurethane yarn, and that some, being sensitisers, have been reported in the literature as being the cause of Spandex dermatitis.

Three women with dermatitis from Spandex brassières were reported from Holland (van Dijk, 1968). On patch testing, 2 reacted to 2 per cent mercaptobenzothiazole and all 3 reacted to 2 per cent zinc diethyldithiocarbamate and to 2 per cent phenylisopropyl-PPD; however, it may be that this latter chemical, in a concentration of 2 per cent, is an irritant.

Sensitivity to Lycra has not been reported from Britain but has from the U.S.A. Porter and Sommer (1967) described 5 women with brassière dermatitis, who were sensitive both to Lycra thread in their brassières and to 1 per cent mercaptobenzothiazole. Similarly, the 9 patients reported by Carr (1967) had developed dermatitis from Lycra in their brassières, and one also reacted to it in her girdle. Patch tests with the Lycra thread were positive, but those with mercaptobenzothiazole were negative. Owing to the lack of information from the manufacturer it was not possible to trace the sensitising chemical. The composition of Lycra obviously is variable because other American authors (Snider, 1966; Dickey, 1967) have recommended it as an elastomer that does not cause dermatitis.

Brassière cups padded with rubber foam may cause dermatitis over the breasts. A patient with this condition was investigated by Verbov (1969). When patch tested, she reacted to mercaptobenzothiazole and to the rubber foam filling from the cups of two brassières made by different firms. Verbov was told by one firm that their rubber foam contained 2 per cent mercaptobenzothiazole as an accelerator. They suggested that a terylene fibre padding would be a suitable alternative for his patient.

Being a potent sensitiser, isopropylaminodiphenylamine (IPPD) must rarely be used in elastic for underclothes, yet patients have been seen in Bulgaria with contact dermatitis caused by it from this source (Batschvarov and Minkov, 1968). These 23 patients developed an eczematous and purpuric eruption under the elastic of their underclothes, and in nine women there was a purpuric secondary spread. The patients were patch tested with IPPD 1 per cent in acetone: all tests were positive and many gave intense reactions.

St John's

A few patients are seen each year with dermatitis from the elastic in their brassières. From 1965–1970, the number increased as a result of the outbreak of 'Playtex' dermatitis which boosted the figures from the usual 2–3 per annum to 8–15 each year over this particular period. The 'Playtex' brassière was modified, and by 1971 cases had stopped appearing (Table 14.22).

Patch testing

'Playtex' brassière. All but one of the 42 patients with dermatitis from 'Playtex' brassières reacted to mercaptobenzothiazole. The exception reacted strongly to TMTD and produced a doubtful response to MBT. She was wearing a 'Playtex' brassière when seen in the clinic, but she was not tested with its elastic thread.

Table 14.22. Number of women with brassière dermatitis, those due to Playtex brassières and those with present and past dermatitis (St John's 1965–1975).

	Women with Bra dermatitis	Present dermatitis	Playtex	Past dermatitis	Playtex
1965	10	10	7	0	
1966	15	15	8	0	
1967	14	11	8	3	
1968	14	12	9	2	
1969	8	5	3	3	
1970	8	7	4	1	
1971	4	2	0	2	
1972	3	2	0	1	
1973	2	1	0	1	
1974	5	3	0		2
1975	3	1	0	1	1
1976	0	0	0	0	

Other types of brassière. In all, 44 women reacted to other types of brassière; no particular pattern of sensitisation was seen, and equal numbers reacted to a thiuram (14) to MBT (16) or to both (14).

Alternatives

Brassières which do not contain elastic are the safest alternative but they may be difficult to find. So far, in Britain, brassières made with Lycra and labelled as such also seem to be suitable. Terylene fibre may be used instead of foam rubber as padding for brassières, but unless this information happens to be given on the label of the garment it would be safer for the doctor or patient to write to the manufacturer to find out the composition of the padding.

Suspenders

Suspender dermatitis has become a clinical rarity since the introduction of tights or panty hose. Stockings, however, are still worn by some older women, and they can be sensitised by the rubber buttons on the suspenders. These usually cause four well defined patches of eczema on the fronts and backs of the thighs corresponding to the position of the four suspenders. Sometimes a band of eczema continues up the thighs towards the groins and is due to contact with the elastic that joins the suspender to the corset. The sensitising chemical is likely to be either a thiuram or mercaptobenzothiazole.

St John's

The number of women with suspender dermatitis seen each year gradually decreased from 15 in 1965 to 0–2 after 1972 (Table 14.23).

Patch testing

Over half (53 per cent) of the 105 women with suspender dermatitis reacted to both a thiuram and MBT; fewer (38 per cent) reacted to a thiuram and were negative to MBT, and only 9 per cent reacted to MBT and not to a thiuram (Table 14.24). The 90 patients seen between 1965 and 1970 were tested with only one thiuram, TMTD 2 per cent in petrolatum.

Table 14.23. Numbers of women seen Each Year with a present or past history of suspender dermatitis (St John's 1965–1976).

	Women with suspender dermatitis	Present dermatitis	Past dermatitis
1965	15	13	2
1966	23	18	5
1967	15	13	2
1968	14	12	2
1969	15	5	10
1970	8	5	3
1971	5	1	4
1972	2	0	2
1973	0	0	0
1974	6	2	4
1975	2	0	2
1976	0	0	0

Table 14.24. Reactions to thiurams and MBT in 105 Women with suspender dermatitis (St John's 1965–1976).

	Thiuram and MBT	Thiuram + MBT –	MBT + thiuram –
Numbers	56 (53%)	40 (38%)	9 (9%)

Girdles

Dermatitis from roll-ons, girdles or corsets appears under those parts of the garment which are made of elastic. Of 7 patients with girdle dermatitis in Wilson's series (1969), 4 reacted to MBT, 2 to PTD and the other to thiurams and to MBT.

St John's

Patients with this contact dermatitis are rarely seen these days, perhaps because women now replace these garments more frequently, and the elastic no longer becomes old and frayed with exposure of the rubber threads. Only 11 cases were diagnosed between 1965 and 1976; 8 presented with the dermatitis and in 3 it had occurred in the past (Table 14.25).

Table 14.25. Numbers of women with girdle dermatitis (St John's 1965–1976).

	Women with girdle dermatitis	Present dermatitis	Past dermatitis
1965–67	7	6	1
1968–70	1	1	0
1971–73	0	0	0
1974–76	3	1	2

Patch testing

There was no particular pattern of chemicals to which these 11 women had been sensitised. Four were sensitised to a thiuram, 4 to MBT and 3 to both (Table 14.26).

Table 14.26. Patch test reactions to thiuram and MBT in 11 Women with girdle dermatitis (St John's 1965–1976).

Thiuram	MBT	Both
4	4	3

Alternatives

In Britain, garments with the elastic part made of Lycra (polyurethane) only, and labelled as such, seem to be suitable for these patients. As yet (1977), no patient has been seen at St John's who has reacted to Lycra. Alternatively, garments which do not contain elastic can be worn, but these can be difficult to find.

Contraceptives

In Wilson's (1969) series of patients sensitised to rubber, 9 reacted to condoms; each was sensitive to PTD 1 per cent, 4 to TMTD 1 per cent, 1 to MBT 1 per cent and 1 (or 6 tested) to ZDC 1 per cent. Over a ten-year period at St John's, 43 patients were seen with contraceptive dermatitis; their clinical features and the results of patch testing were reviewed by Hindson (1966). Of this group, 33 men and 2 women were diagnosed as having dermatitis due to rubber condoms. The presenting feature in the women was pruritus vulvae and in the men it was recurrent episodes of itching, frequently with oedema of the penis after intercourse. Of the 40 men with all types of contraceptive dermatitis, 3 had balanitis only, 4 had eczema of the shaft of the penis only, 21 had dermatitis of the penis, scrotum, groins and suprapubic region, the other 12 had involvement of all these sites with a secondary spread to the eyes, sides of the neck, axillae and antecubital fossae. In typical cases of dermatitis due to condoms, the diagnosis is easy because there is a clear relationship to intercourse and the irritation of the penis is often accompanied by marked oedema.

In England, the standard types of condoms contain the following chemicals:

Accelerators
Zinc mercaptobenzothiazole
Dipentamethylenethiuram
disulphide
Zinc diethyldithiocarbamate

Antioxidant
Polytrimethylhydroquinolone

Patch testing

The 43 patients in Hindson's series were not tested with dipentamethylenethiuram disulphide because it was not in routine use at that time. However, tetramethylthiuram disulphide 1 per cent was used and 28 of 38 tested reacted; in addition 6 of 38 reacted to mercaptobenzothiazole 1 per cent; 6 of 19 were sensitive to zinc dithiocarbamate 1 per cent; and when tested with their condoms, 34 of 43 reacted. Hindson stressed that a condom of the same type as that used by the patient must be used for patch testing, otherwise false negative reactions occur. But even when the correct type of condom is applied, the test is occasionally negative; this he thought was due either to a lipid film on the rubber or to insufficient allergen leaching out of the rubber.

The dermatitis is not frequent, 1–2 men are seen each year (p. 736) with eczema from this cause and occasionally women, who are sensitive to thiurams, notice vulval irritation from contraceptive sheaths.

Patch testing series

Hindson (1966) suggested that the following chemicals should be used for patch testing a patient thought to have contraceptive dermatitis:

1. Rubber condom (as is)
2. Chemical contraceptive used (as is)
3. Zinc mercaptobenzothiazole (1 per cent petrolatum)
4. Dipentamethylenethiuram disulphide (1 per cent in petrolatum)
5. Zinc dithiocarbamate (1 per cent in petrolatum)
6. Zinc lupetimide (2 per cent in petrolatum)
7. Quinine hydrochloride (1 per cent in water)
8. Phenyl mercuric acetate (0.01 per cent in petrolatum)
9. Hexyl resorcinol (1 per cent in petrolatum)
10. Oxyquinoline sulphate (1 per cent in petrolatum)
11. Phenoxypolyethoxy ethanol (0.5 per cent in petrolatum)

Alternatives

Sheaths, made with zinc dibutyl dithiocarbamate, or zinc lupetimide, are said to be suitable. In rare cases sheaths made from raw rubber or animal gut are used.

Elastic stockings

Sensitivity to dyes and rubber chemicals explained the itching felt by a patient every time he wore elastic stockings. In Malten's (1977) experience this is not unusual and he advocates undyed elastic stockings with rubber additives declared on the label.

St John's

Three or possibly four women have been seen at St John's with a contact dermatitis from elastic stockings. The first attended in 1965: she was aged 47 years and had a past history of dermatitis from the rubber of her suspenders. Following operative treatment for her varicose veins, she began to wear elastic stockings, but had to stop because of severe irritation of her feet. The second woman, seen in 1969, was 53 years old; the skin of her legs was dry and she had had varicose veins for many years. Wearing elastic stockings produced irritation of her legs, and later exudative eczema appeared; subsequently she developed a generalised eruption for which she had to be given a course of systemic corticosteroids. A third, more doubtful case was seen in 1972. This was a 70-year-old woman who, a month after starting to wear elastic stockings, developed redness of the skin around her ankles; this spread to her legs despite discarding the stockings. The skin later improved with topical therapy. The fourth patient, aged 58 years, was seen in 1974; she had previously been sensitised by rubber gloves and subsequently developed eczema of her legs from wearing elastic stockings.

Patch testing

Each patient was sensitive to MBT and 2 reacted also to thiurams. The elastic thread of the stocking may give a false negative reaction. Only 2 of the 4 reacted to the elastic threads although in the case of Patient 4 it was confirmed from the manufacturers that the rubber did contain MBT.

Patients	MBT	Thiuram	Elastic thread
1	+		
2	+	–	+
3	+	–	–
4	+	+	–

Alternatives
Elastic stockings made of Lycra (polyurethane) are obtainable, although they are not suitable for patients with severe varicose veins.

Elastic in men's socks
A man with bilateral lower leg eczema, which simulated stasis eczema, was found to have a contact dermatitis to the Lycra thread in the elastic of his socks. He had previously been sensitised by MBT in rubber gloves (Fregert, 1973).

Dress and coat shields
Rubber dress shields are seldom worn nowadays, but they are still sold and are an occasional cause of axillary dermatitis. Two cases due to dioxydiphenyl in the rubber have been described (Shultz and Hermmann, 1960).

St John's
One patient, seen in 1968, was a man with a two-year history of an intermittent axillary rash; in the previous weeks, the eczema had spread to involve his soles, heels and palms. On patch testing he reacted to tetramethylthiuram disulphide 2 per cent, to dipentamethylenethiuram disulphide 1 per cent and to the outer soles of a shoe and slipper.

He was not tested with the heel stiffeners. The axillary rash was traced to rubber shields which had been sewn into his coats because his axillae sweated excessively.

Alternative
Probably none is necessary, but, if desirable, a detachable, washable fabric shield could be made.

Rubber apron

St John's
A woman, aged 58 years, was seen in 1965 with eczema on her neck where the neckband of a rubber apron came into contact with the skin. She had a six-year history of patchy eczema on her body, which was not due to rubber contact. Patch tests showed her to be sensitive to TMTD, but she was not tested with her apron.

Scuba diver face mask
In San Francisco, scuba diver face masks containing *N*-isopropyl-*N*-phenyl-PPD (IPPD) caused a mini-epidemic of facial dermatitis among the divers. Patch

tests: those tested reacted to shavings from the rubber and IPPD 0.5 per cent. These patients were able to wear other masks without trouble (Maibach, 1975).

Bathing cap

St John's

Two women have had dermatitis from bathing caps. In the first it had occurred when she was a child, the second attended with dermatitis from brassieres and shoes and she had noticed that her rubber bathing cap was causing irritation. Both were sensitive to MBT.

Disulfiram implants

Two alcoholic patients were sensitised by repeated subcutaneous implants of disulfiram (tetraethylthiuram disulphide, TETD). Both men developed eczema at the implantation sites and in the first patient the eruption became generalised and he required systemic steroids. The pellets were removed. Patch tests: both patients reacted to TETD and TMTD 2 per cent in petrolatum. Oral provocation with a 400 mg tablet of disulfiram elicited a reaction in the first patient but not in the second (Lachapelle, 1975).

Haemodialysis unit

In one particular haemodialysis unit in Miami, pruritic skin rashes became a problem among their patients. Twenty-one patients were patch-tested; sensitivity to various thiurams was found in eight, of whom 4 had dematitis. It was hypothesised that the thiurams were eluted from the haemodialysis apparatus, and sensitised the patients who were then at risk of developing dermatitis (Penneys, Edwards and Katsikas, 1976).

Tourniquet

A tourniquet applied to a patient's arm prior to giving an intravenous injection elicited a contact dermatitis. The sensitiser was identified as thio-β-naphthol, a peptizing agent added to rubber to facilitate its flow during moulding. The patient reacted to 0.1 per cent thio-β-naphthol in xylene, acetone or ethanol (Schamberg and Flesch, 1953).

Hearing aid pad

St John's

In 1968, a man, aged 37 years, was seen with eczema behind his ear under the pad of his hearing aid. He reacted to TMTD and weakly to the rubber of the hearing aid.

Rubber pillows

St John's

In 1967, a 56-year-old woman, with a past history of rubber dermatitis, presented with eczema under her suspenders and also on her face and neck. She slept on a rubber pillow. When patch tested, she reacted to TMTD 1 per cent, MBT 1 per cent and a piece of the pillow. After discarding the pillow, the eczema healed.

A girl, aged 17 years, was seen in 1970 with a history of repeated episodes of facial eczema since childhood. Patch tests showed she was sensitive to TMTD 1 per cent; it was then found that she not only used a rubber sponge, but also slept on a rubber pillow; these items were incriminated by implication, but the diagnosis was not proved by patch testing.

Hot water bottle

St John's

Three patients have been seen, a woman and two men all with dermatitis from their rubber hot water bottles. The woman, aged 49 years, lay in bed with her arm against a hot water bottle and developed a rash at the site of contact; during the previous year she had noticed that a rubber finger-stall, rubber gloves, a brassière and the elastic of a hair net had all caused irritation. One man, aged 34 years, had eczema of his palms and soles. The other, aged 81 years, had eczema of the dorsa of his hands; in his case, positive patch tests to MBT were the clue to the diagnosis and it was eventually discovered, with some difficulty, that he lay in bed with his hands under a hot water bottle.

Patch testing

Patients	MBT	Hot water bottle
1	+	+
2	+	+
3	+	+

Rubber sheet

St John's

A 53-year-old man who had urinary incontinence, always slept on a rubber sheet; he presented with a 7 months' history of an itchy, scaling, weeping eczema on the outer thighs, calves and upper arms. The condition was severe and required admission to hospital. On patch testing, he reacted to the rubber sheet and to dioxydiphenyl 1 per cent in petrolatum.

Sponge rubber cushion

St John's

A man, aged 50 years, had a 2 months' history of a rash which began on his buttocks and spread to his groins, abdomen and legs. When first seen, the eczema was widespread and weeping. After preliminary patch testing, it was discovered that he sat on a sponge rubber cushion at work. He reacted when tested with the rubber cushion, and with dimethylpentyl-PPD, methylheptyl-PPD and MBT, each 1 per cent in petrolatum. The test with PPD was negative. After he discarded the cushion, his eczema healed rapidly.

Rubber on household equipment

Rubber is present in the home in flexes, electrical plugs, vacuum cleaners and to a variable extent on other electrical equipment; it is also found in cushions, mats, rubber sleeves on handles, rubber draw sheets and on some gadgets. This type of rubber is likely to have a composition similar to that of industrial rubbers and may contain not only mercaptobenzothiazole and thiurams but also other mercaptochemicals, diphenylguanidine and possibly compounds of the PPD group. Sensitivity to the PPD rubber derivatives does sometimes occur in women (p. 732) and the source may be household equipment. In Prague phenyl-isopropyl-*para*phenylenediamine (IPPD) in the rubber sleeves on the flexes of electric irons caused dermatitis in 36 housewives and 9 others using irons at work. The eczema was purpuric, it affected principally the medial side of the hand and wrist and 5 patients developed widespread purpura. Patch tests with IPPD were positive in all the patients (Jirásek and Kalenský, 1975).

St John's

Rubber utensils in the home, and handles on bicycles and sports equipment such as hockey sticks and golf clubs are sometimes incriminated as causing or contributing to a hand eczema, but it is difficult to prove. Two typical examples are described.

A man aged 47 years, who worked as a cleaner, developed hand eczema, and when patch tested was found to be sensitive to MBT, CBS, MBTS and MMBT. The only recognisable sources of contact were rubber-handled polishers and the cables of similar utensils. A trainee chef, aged 16 years, developed palmar eczema; he too was shown to be sensitive to MBT, CBS, MBTS and MMBT, and it was thought that he may have been sensitised by rubber-handled cooking utensils and rubber grips on his bicycle. Neither patient was tested with the rubber he handled.

Rubber cosmetic sponges and eyelash curlers

About 20 years ago, rubber sponges were used by women to apply their cosmetics and were an occasional cause of dermatitis. Twenty-six women with contact dermatitis from their sponges were described by Furman, Fisher and Leider (1950), but the sensitising chemicals were not identified. Rubber in eyelash curlers caused eyelid dermatitis in 7 women; five were patch tested with the ingredients and each reacted to phenyl-β-naphthylamine 1 per cent in 90 per cent alcohol (Curtis, 1945). This type of sponge and eyelash curler is practically never used now and these cases are rarely seen.

Balloons

Occasionally, patients are seen who develop dermatitis of the lips and adjacent parts of the face from blowing up balloons. The eczema can be very acute, as happened to two patients described by Gaul (1957); in them, the oedema was severe enough to close their eyes and to evert their nostrils and lips. The sensitiser was monobenzyl ether of hydroquinone. Patients may either recognise the cause and effect relationship themselves, or present with recurrent episodes of eczema of the lower half of the face.

St John's

Three patients have been seen; two were men, the other was a woman. Both men gave a 5-year history of episodic swelling of the face after blowing up balloons, and both had noticed the association. One described cracking of his lips, but the other insisted that his lips were unaffected. The woman gave a 6-year history of repeated attacks of swelling of her face, neck and eyelids, each attack beginning on the right side of her neck. Although her lips and mouth were affected, this appeared as part of the generalised facial eczema and was not a prominent feature. The diagnosis was only made after patch-testing, and even then it was made by the patient herself.

Each patient was sensitive to a thiuram (1 per cent); none was tested with balloons.

Patient 1 :	Male	TMTD + (only thiuram tested)
Patient 2 :	Male	TETD +, PTD +, TMTD —
Patient 3 :	Female	TMTD +, TETD +, PTD +, TMTM +

Toys

A semi-solid rubber called Flubber was used to make children's toys in the U.S.A. where it caused dermatitis, mainly on the face, in 40 per cent of the children who played with them. Results of patch testing with constituents of the Flubber were inconsistent and were not suggestive of an allergic contact dermatitis. The condition was thought to be an irritant effect, principally of the follicles, caused by an oil used in the manufacture of the Flubber (Sauer, 1965).

Squash ball

St John's

A carpenter, aged 26 years, complained of itching, redness and cracking of the centre of his left palm for 4 months. When he was off work for two weeks with tonsillitis, his palm healed. His hobby was playing squash, but it was only after he had reacted to the PPD rubber mix in the standard patch test series that the importance of his squash ball was realised.

Patch tests

He reacted to the PPD-mix, isopropylphenyl-PPD (IPPD) 0.1 per cent in petrolatum and the rubber of the squash ball; he was negative to p-phenylenediamine, phenylcyclohexyl-PPD and diphenyl-PPD.

Holding the squash ball in his left hand for one hour on each of two successive days reproduced this dermatitis exactly. The manufacturers of the squash ball confirmed that it contained isopropylphenyl-PPD (Cronin, 1973).

OCCUPATIONAL DERMATITIS

Transport industry

TYRES

Chemicals in tyres

In the motor industry synthetic rubber is used predominantly for the treads of tyres for cars and vehicles. Natural rubber is used for the sidewalls of these tyres and also for the complete tyres on aircraft. The physical properties of natural rubber make it better suited for these special situations; in particular it generates less heat build-up during the continuous flexing which occurs in the sidewall of a tyre, or during the strains of take-off and landing on aircraft tyres.

The same chemicals are used in both types of tyres; although the exact formulations vary with different manufacturers, the following list is representative:

Accelerators

Tetramethylthiuram disulphide
Dipentamethylenethiuram tetrasulphide
Zinc diethyldithiocarbamate
Zinc dimethyldithiocarbamate
Zinc dibutyldithiocarbamate
2-Mercaptobenzothiazole
Zinc mercaptobenzothiazole
Dibenzothiazyl disulphide
Cyclohexylbenzothiazylsulphenamide
Morpholinylmercaptobenzothiazole
Dicyclohexylbenzothiazylsulphenamide
Ethylene thiourea

Antioxidants and Antiozonants

Isopropylphenyl-*p*-phenylenediamine
   (Nonox ZA:ICI. 4010 NA:Bayer)
Dicylohexyl-*p*-phenylenediamine
   (UOP 26:Universal Oil Products).
N,N'-bis (1-ethyl-3-methylpentyl)-*p*-phenylenediamine
   (Santoflex 17:Monsanto. UOP88).
N,N'-bis(1,4-dimethylpentyl)-*p*-phenylenediamine
   (Santoflex 77:Monsanto. Antioxidant 4030:Bayer. UOP788).
N-1,3-Dimethylbutyl-*N'*-phenyl-*p*-phenylenediamine
   (Santoflex 13:Monsanto. Nonox ZC:ICI).
N,N'-di-β-naphthyl-*p*-phenylenediamine
   (Santowhite CI:Monsanto. Antioxidant DNP : Bayer. Nonox CI:ICI).
Diphenylamine-acetone condensation products
   (BLE 25: Rubber Regenerating. Nonox BL, BLN:ICI).
Phenyl-β-naphthylamine
   (Nonox D, DN:ICI. Neozone D:Du Pont. Antioxidant PBN : Bayer).
Phenyl-α-naphthylamine
   (Nonox AN:ICI. Antioxidant PAN : Bayer. Neozone A : Du Pont).
Polymerised trimethyldihydroquinoline
   (Flectol flakes: Monsanto).
2,2'-methylene-bis (4-ethyl-6-*tert*.-butylphenol)
   (Antioxidant 425: Anchor).

Retarders

N-nitroso diphenylamine (Vulkatard A:ICI).
N-'cyclohexylthiophthalimide (Santogard PVI:Monsanto).
Phthalic anhydride (Retarder PD : Anchor).

Other compounding ingredients

Stearic acid
Resorcinol
Hexamethylenetetramine
Zinc oxide
Titanium dioxide

Peptisers

Pentachlorothiophenol   (Renacit VII: Bayer).
Di-(*o*-benzamidophenyl) disulphide   (Pepton 22:Anchor).

Process Oils

These fall into the following types: paraffinic, naphthenic, aromatic pine tar, reclaim oils.
Resins, which are both petroleum based and synthetic.
Carbon blacks.
Sulphur.

Dermatitis

Four men, who handled finished tyres at work and became sensitised by the isopropylphenyl-PPD (IPPD) contained in the rubber, were reported by Bieber and Foussereau (1968). Subsequently Hervé-Bazin *et al*. (1977) investigated 42 men sensitised to IPPD through handling tyres in their various occupations and 15 of these men were tested with *N*-dimethyl-1,3-butyl-*N'*-phenyl-*para*phenylenediamine (DMPPD) and all reacted. Another man developed hand eczema every time he washed his Volkswagen car; he was found by Jordan (1971) to have a contact dermatitis from this same chemical (IPPD), present in the car tyres. When patch tested, he reacted to 0.1 per cent IPPD in petrolatum and produced a bullous response to a shaving from the tyre. Jordan stated that IPPD is not used by the larger tyre manufacturers in the U.S.A.

A man, who had previously been sensitised by diphenyl-PPD and cyclohexyl-PPD in black rubber gloves, developed eczema on the palmar aspects of his hands the day after a long car drive. During the journey, he had felt the tyres on several occasions to check their temperature. The antioxidants and antiozonants, which accumulate on the tyre surface, were thought to have contaminated his hands and caused the relapse (Fregert, 1973).

St John's

Between 1966 and 1976, 20 men and 1 woman have been seen with rubber sensitivity acquired by handling finished tyres. The occupations of the men were:

Tyre fitter	2
Tyre remoulder (past history)	1
Motor industry: assembly, mechanic	2
Garage: motor mechanic, tyre mender	4
Drivers delivering and unloading tyres	2
Transport contractor	1
Engineers: motor, aircraft	2

Labourers: moving and washing cars, changing tyres	2
Car park attendant	1
Wooden case maker, handling tyres occasionally	1
Servicing own cars	2

The woman was a car polisher

The duration of employment was variable. Of the two drivers, one had been doing the job for 21 years, whereas the other had done it for only nine months; and one of the garage men, after working on the petrol pumps for 15 years, had his job changed to mending tyres, and within two months he had developed hand eczema.

Most were past middle age; the ages of the 2 tyre fitters were 16 and 18 years, 3 men were aged 30 to 39, 4 were between 42 and 49, and 11 were between 50 and 60 years of age.

The lengths of many of the histories were relatively short being measured in weeks or months rather than years, and although some of the older patients had had hand eczema for several years, its onset seemed to coincide with their handling of tyres. One man, with palmar eczema for a year because of it, changed his job from an aircraft engineer to chemical work. His hands failed to improve and only after patch tests had revealed his sensitivity to IPPD was it discovered that he owned three cars which he serviced himself, handling all the various rubbers in them, including the tyres.

Pattern of eczema

The eczema has an unusual pattern for a contact dermatitis, because it characteristically affects the palms and the flexor surfaces of the wrists; consequently, it is easily mistaken for a constitutional hand eczema. The skin becomes red, dry, scaly and cracked; the thenar eminences may bear the brunt, or there may be a confluent sheet of eczema covering the palm. It is unusual for the fingers and dorsa of the hands to be the principal sites involved.

In several patients, it was only after patch testing had revealed sensitivity to the PPD chemicals that a history of handling tyres was sought and obtained.

One of the men affected was a truck driver for a tyre company; while loading and unloading the tyres, he carried them suspended from his arms. After 3 months, he developed a mauve-brown lichenoid dermatitis of the flexor surfaces of his wrists and lower forearms. The histology showed changes both of lichen planus and of dermatitis. He was patched tested and reacted to IPPD 0.25 per cent in petrolatum, but not to colour developers with which he had never been in contact (Calnan, 1971).

Patch testing

These patients are sensitised by PPD chemicals, characteristically by IPPD. In this group only 7 of the 21 patients tested reacted to PPD, showing it to be a completely unreliable detector of this allergy.

IPPD (0.1–0.5 per cent in petrolatum)	19/19 positive
CPPD (0.25 per cent–1.0 per cent in petrolatum)	14/18 positive
PPD (0.5 per cent–1.0 per cent in petrolatum)	7/21 positive

Pulmonary disease

Workers with prolonged and intense exposure to tyre-curing fumes have been found in the U.S.A. to have an increased incidence of chronic bronchitis (Fine and Peters, 1976).

Transport drivers

Van and lorry drivers may be sensitised by rubber parts of their vehicles and develop hand eczema.

St John's

Four such drivers have been seen; 3 reacted to phenylcyclohexyl-PPD (CPPD) and one to mercaptobenzothiazole, cyclohexylbenzothiazyl sulphenamide and morpholinyl mercaptobenzothiazole.

Motor bicycle rubber

St John's

A man, aged 55 years, worked as a truck driver in a motor bicycle factory for 25 years without any trouble. Two years after being transferred to the assembly line he developed eczema of his palms, the dorsa of his fingers and the flexor surfaces of his arms. He was found to be sensitive to IPPD, CPPD and rubber foam from the battery carrier and foot rest of the motor cycles.

Aircraft

Aircraft workers come into considerable contact with rubber as seals, linings, tubing and tyres, and, as a result, some are sensitised by rubber chemicals particularly those of the PPD-group.

St John's

From 1965–1976, 9 aircraft workers were seen who had been sensitised by rubber. Their jobs were fitter (4), inspector (1), mechanic (1), and engineer (1), aircraft loader (1) and storeman (1).

The hands and arms principally were affected, but in 4 men the eczema had spread to the face, neck or thighs, and one man had generalised eczema which had begun on his hands. The distribution on the hands was not characteristic, the dorsa, the palms or the fingers being involved. Striking bands of eczema were seen on the forearms of a man who had worked with an arm through a ring of tubing lined with rubber.

Patch testing

The predominant sensitisers among the 9 men were chemicals of the PPD-group.
PPD Group: All 8 men tested with the separate PPD chemicals reacted and 4 men were sensitive to this group only. The results were as follows:

Isopropylphenyl-PPD	(IPPD),	6/8 positive
Cyclohexyl-PPD	(CPPD),	5/7 positive
Diphenyl-PPD	(DPPD),	2/7 positive
p-Phenylenediamine	(PPD),	1/8 positive

Napthyl
Group: Two men were additionally sensitised to this group, both to phenyl-β-naphthylamine and to di-β-naphthyl-PPD.

Mercapto-
group: Three men were sensitive, two to mercaptobenzothiazole and the other to morpholinyl mercaptobenzothiazole.

Dairy farmers

Dairy farmers can be sensitised by isopropylphenyl-PPD (IPPD) in the rubber hoses, tubing and caps of milking machines. This antioxidant is said to be irreplaceable in the rubber (Black, 1972), which has to withstand detergents, disinfectants and weathering. IPPD in a concentration of 1.5 per cent is one of the chemicals allowed in dairy rubber by German regulations which are adhered to also by manufacturers of dairy rubber for the European Common Market (Lintum and Nater, 1974; Nater, 1975).

In New Zealand, Black (1972) reported that 5 consecutive dairy farmers with dermatitis of their palms were allergic to IPPD. Some were also tested with and reacted to the rubber from rings on the steering wheels of their tractors.

In Holland, dairy workers with hand eczema were investigated by Lintum and Nater (1973, 1974), who found that 44 per cent (14/32) were sensitive to rubber chemicals as compared with 12 per cent (9/70) of patients with leg ulcers and 11 per cent (7/60) of a control group with hand eczema. In the later (1974) study they tested 6 dairy men, aged from 33 to 64 years, with a series of individual rubber chemicals; all reacted to IPPD (isopropylaminodiphenylamine) 0.1 per cent in petrolatum, CPPD (phenylcyclohexyl-PPD) 0.25 per cent in petrolatum and rubber from their milking machines. Two also responded to other rubber chemicals but only one of the six was sensitive to PPD.

St John's

Three dairy men have been investigated and each was sensitive to IPPD.

Patient 1. For 30 years this 53-year-old man had been a milker, and for the past 12 years he had had recurrent hand eczema. On two occasions the eczema had been generalised, requiring hospital admission. He wore rubber gloves constantly at work.

Patient 2. This 51-year-old man had used milking machines for six years and soon afterwards developed a fluctuating eczema of the sides of his fingers, his hands and his arms.

Patient 3. A 52-year-old man, who had been milking cows for 20 years, had had hand eczema for 12 years which in the previous year had spread to his arms, forehead and neck. He wore rubber gloves to protect his hands.

Patch Tests:

	IPPD 0.1%	DPPD 1%	CPPD 1%	PPD 0.5% or 1%	Thiurams	Rubber from machines
Patient 1	+	+	−	−	+	+
Patient 2	+	+	+	−	+	+
Patient 3	+	+	−	−	+	+

(Patients 1 and 3 were sensitised to thiurams by rubber gloves)

Earphones

St John's

Two patients have been seen with dermatitis from rubber earphones, and both had been sensitised by phenyl-β-naphthylamine.

Patient 1. A telephone engineer, aged 40 years, had had eczema on his left pinna and adjacent scalp for ten months. The right ear was slightly affected.

Patch tests: He reacted to phenyl-β-naphthylamine 1 per cent and rubber from his earphones.

Patient 2. A 64-year-old merchant navy radio operator developed irritation of his ears and cheeks after new rubber covers had been put on his earphones. He stopped using them and the condition cleared.

Patch tests: He reacted to phenyl-β-naphthylamine 1 per cent and diaryl-PPD 1 per cent. It was impossible to test him with the earphone covers because they had been left on his ship in Germany.

Rubber packing for cement tubes

Two men developed hand eczema while making cement tubes and connecting them with rubber packing. Neither wore rubber gloves. Patch tests showed them to be sensitive to the rubber packing and, in the routine series, to diphenyl-PPD; they did not react to either chromium or cobalt. Both continued working with cement tubes, but once they avoided rubber, their hands healed (Fregert, 1969).

St John's

Two pipe layers were investigated:

Patient 1. A man, aged 63 years, was seen with a dry lichenified eczema which had affected the dorsa of his hands for one month. He used rubber for sealing the pipe joints.

Patch tests: He reacted to morpholinyl MBT and his own rubber. He was negative to MBT.

Patient 2. This 67-year-old pipe layer had had eczema on his hands, arms and ankles for 3 months.

Patch tests: He reacted to diphenyl-PPD, phenyl-β-naphthylamine and potassium dichromate.

Lycra conveyor belt

A male, leather factory employee worked at a conveyor belt made of Lycra (polyurethane and nylon). Friction caused dust particles to disperse from its surface and these produced dermatitis of his hands, axillae and face, which was directly related to his being at work. A patch test with MBT was positive (Fregert, 1972).

Face masks

Rubber face masks can cause either an allergic or an irritant contact dermatitis or both; these can be differentiated only by patch testing. Scuba divers face masks have caused dermatitis (p. 751)

Allergic contact dermatitis

St John's

From 1966–1976, 12 men and 1 woman were seen who had had an allergic contact dermatitis from rubber face masks. The dermatitis had occurred in the past in 6 of these patients, 5 of whom were men who had worn oxygen masks while serving in the Royal Air Force. The sixth was a woman, aged 44 years when seen, who remembered having had a rash from her gas mask when she was about 10 years old.

Seven men presented with this dermatitis; their occupations were:

Royal Air Force	3
Paint sprayers (aircraft companies)	2
Boiler attendant	1
Glass decorator	1

The diagnosis is obvious when the pattern of dermatitis on the face traces out the areas of contact with the mask, but the eczema can be less defined, as in one man in whom only the sides of the face were affected. The history is sometimes misleading in that the patient may blame the fumes from which the mask is supposed to protect him rather than the mask itself.

Patch testing

The results of patch testing these 13 patients were:

MBT and related chemicals	11/13 positive
Phenyl-β-naphthylamine	1/13 positive (glass decorator, Swedish mask)
PPD group (IPPD, CPPD, DPPD)	1/13 positive (paint sprayer)
Rubber from mask	3/3 positive

Three of the patients sensitised by the mercapto-group reacted also to thiurams and two were also sensitive to diphenylguanidine.

Irritant contact dermatitis

Face masks occasionally cause an irritant dermatitis. The mechanism may be friction and chafing on a sweating skin or sometimes the toxic material, which the mask is meant to exclude, accumulates under the mask and inflames the skin. The oxygen masks worn by aircrew for pressure breathing in combat aircraft at high altitude cause dermatitis because these masks are so tightly clamped on to the men's faces.

When patch tested, these patients do not react to any of the rubber chemicals, and if tests with the rubber of the mask also are negative, the diagnosis is confirmed. Sometimes, testing with the rubber of the mask elicits a misleading false positive reaction because it is contaminated with toxic material. In such patients the diagnosis is established only if there are negative patch tests with the constituents of the rubber obtained from the manufacturers and also with rubber from an identical but unworn mask.

Rubber bands

In 1969, among a group of 30 Post Office sorters using wide rubber bands, 4 men and 2 women developed eczema of the fingers for the first time. Some, but not all, had positive patch tests to cyclohexylbenzothiazyl sulphenamide (CBS) and other chemicals of the mercapto-group, the reactions to mercaptobenzothiazole being weak; one patient reacted to tetramethylthiuram disulphide. Friction and trauma were considered to have caused the eczema in some of the patients. It was later ascertained that the rubber bands contained a mixture of benzothiazyl disulphide, hexamethylenetetramine and diphenylguanidine. To explain this unusual outbreak, it was queried whether these patients might have handled a particular batch of incorrectly-formulated rubber bands (Kirton and Wilkinson, 1972).

Phenyl-β-naphthylamine was the sensitiser in a case of rubber band dermatitis reported by Bieber and Foussereau (1968).

St John's

From 1965–1976, 11 men and 3 women have been seen with occupational dermatitis from rubber bands. Four of the men worked in the Post Office, where rubber bands have replaced string in the packaging of mail; 3 were bank clerks putting rubber bands round bundles of Treasury notes; and 2 were computer operators who used elastic bands to secure rolls of computer tape. The occupations of the other 5 patients were a florist, a surveyor, a clerk, a secretary and a storekeeper.

Patchy dermatitis of the fingers is the most characteristic pattern, but several of these patients had a nondescript hand eczema, affecting the palmar and dorsal surfaces.

In 6 patients, rubber bands were thought to be the entire cause of their hand eczema, and in another man, rubber bands and a finger-stall had caused his dermatitis.

Patch testing

Eleven of the patients reacted to MBT. Five of these were tested with other chemicals of the mercapto-group and reacted to them, but these patch-test results do not clarify which mercapto chemical was the primary sensitiser. Three patients responded only to thiurams.

Patch tests:

	MBT	CBS	MBTS	MMBT	Thiuram	Rubber band
Tested	14	5	5	5	14	9
+	11	3	2	2	6	7

All the chemicals were diluted 1% in petrolatum.

MBT   (Mercaptobenzothiazole)
CBS   (cyclohexylbenzothiazyl sulphenamide)
MBTS (dibenzothiazyl disulphide)
MMBT (morpholinyl mercaptobenzothiazole).

Rubber bank-note counters

Twenty-four Post Office workers, who developed hand eczema from rubber bank note counters, were investigated by Eriksson and Ostlund (1968). Of this group 17 had been sensitised by cyclohexylbenzothiazyl sulphenamide in the counters; patch tests with this chemical, 5 per cent in yellow vaseline, were positive in all. The patients were also tested with MBT 1 per cent in vaseline, and 15 of them reacted.

Finger-stalls

Clinically, it is easy to miss a contact dermatitis due to rubber finger-stalls (fingerettes) and to misdiagnose the condition as simply 'hand eczema'. When the dermatitis exactly corresponds to the area of rubber contact, the diagnosis is straightforward and can be made by both patient and doctor. In other patients the cause may not be so obvious: the dermatitis begins with redness and irritation of the tip and pulp of one finger, but, failing to implicate the finger-stall, the patient moves it to another finger. This process may be repeated until several fingers of both hands are affected and the eczema has spread along the fingers. The patient does not mention that a finger-stall is being worn and the clinician does not enquire into this possibility. In the absence of routine patch testing the diagnosis tends to be overlooked in such patients. Sensitivity to MBT in a patient with eczema which began on the fingertips will suggest the diagnosis.

Isopropylphenyl-PPD (IPPD). An outbreak of fingertip dermatitis (sparing the pulps) in 51(2.5 per cent) Danish Post Office workers was caused by IPPD 0.1 per cent in their red rubber finger-stalls. The presence of IPPD in the rubber was confirmed, not by the manufacturers, but by gas chromatography (Roed-Petersen et al., 1977).

St John's

From 1965–1976, 26 women and 8 men were seen with dermatitis from finger-stalls. The clinical features were:

Eczema confined to one or more fingertips	14
Hand eczema beginning under a finger-stall	4
Hand eczema worse on the pulps	2
Eczema of the fingers	1
Hand eczema, sequence of events uncertain	5
Hand eczema, ?finger-stall irrelevant	1
Past history	7

One woman had hand eczema and though she wore a finger-stall, it did not appear to aggravate her eczema. She was sensitised to thiurams only, and the finger-stall was probably irrelevant.

In 16 patients, a finger-stall was the only source of rubber to which they were sensitive. All of the remaining 10 patients, in whom the finger-stall dermatitis was of present and certain relevance, had dermatitis from other sources of contact with rubber such as gloves, shoes and rubber bands.

Patch testing
Mercaptobenzothiazole was the predominant sensitiser; 30 of the 34 patients reacted to it:

+ MBT	+ MBT + Thiuram	+ Thiuram
20	10	4

Eighteen were tested with their finger-stall; 9 had a positive response and in 9 the reaction was either doubtful or negative.

Dermatitis in the rubber industry

With increasing automation in the rubber industry, the incidence of dermatitis among workers has decreased, but some contact with solvents and sensitising chemicals continues and cases of dermatitis still occur. There are few recent reports in the literature.

When first used, the sensitising potential of isopropylphenyl-PPD (IPPD) was not realised and it was only after the occurrence of cases of dermatitis that the hazard was appreciated (Munn, 1967). The incidence of sensitisation has been reduced by automation in tyre building and by limiting the amount of IPPD used to 2 per cent or less of the total rubber mix (Munn, 1970, personal communication). A man who developed eczema of the dorsa of his hands and of his forearms, and who was sensitised by this chemical in a rubber factory, was investigated by Wilkinson (1968). He reacted to 0.1 per cent IPPD in MEK.

Over a five year period, Herrmann and Schulz (1960) investigated 29 patients with occupational dermatitis due to rubber; of these, 16 worked in the rubber industry. The commonest sensitisers were mercaptobenzothiazole and tetramethylthiuram disulphide. Dithiodimorpholine has caused dermatitis in a Danish rubber factory (p. 740).

An unusual cause of chronic contact dermatitis in a rubber factory worker was reported by Sharvill (1971), who identified the allergen as dioctyl phthalate used as a plasticiser. The patient reacted so strongly to 2 per cent dioctyl phthalate in soft paraffin that 1 per cent was recommended as a more suitable concentration for patch testing.

St John's
From 1965–1976, 6 male and 2 female employees in rubber factories were seen and found to have been be sensitised by rubber chemicals.

The occupations of the men were tyre builder (2), tyre inspector (1), storeman in a tyre firm (1) packer in a tyre firm (1) and the sixth man made rubber parts for cars. Both women worked for rubber companies. One stuck rubber sheets to metal, and the other operated a machine cutting cylinders of rubber into rings, which she then tied into bundles.

All the patients had hand eczema; in five it had spread to their shins and the storeman's neck was also affected.

Patch tests: The positive reactions in these 8 patients were:

IPPD and CPPD	5
IPPD, CPPD and di-β-naphthyl PPD	1
IPPD, CPPD, DPPD, MBT, CBS and MMBT	1
MBT, CBS and MMBT	1

Own rubber: 4 were tested and each reacted

Carcinogenicity

The evidence in two Russian reports that exposure to chloroprene is associated with skin and lung cancer has been reviewed by Lloyd, Decoufle and Moore (1975). They also discussed the toxicity of chloroprene. In the U.S.A. an epidemiologic study of the rubber industry showed an excess of deaths from cancer of the stomach, colon and prostate and neoplasms of the lymphatic and haemopoietic systems. An association was found between lymphatic leukaemia and solvent exposure, lung cancer and work in the curing room, and bladder and stomach carcinomas with exposure to raw ingredients and precured rubber (McMichael, Andjelkovic and Tyroler, 1976). In a British survey of the rubber and cable-making industries (Fox and Collier, 1976), there was a statistically significant increase in lung cancer in the tyre sector, and an excess of deaths from bladder cancer throughout the industries required further investigation.

Patch testing

To detect cases of rubber sensitivity, it is essential to include rubber chemicals in a standard patch test series, for if patients are tested only when there is a clinical suspicion of the allergy, many cases will be missed. The following 5 mixes can be used for routine testing, and, if a positive reaction occurs to one of them, its constituents can then be tested separately. The naphthyl-mix is no longer used because of the sparcity of reactions. To avoid patch test sensitisation, the concentration of each chemical in the mixture is less than when these constitutents are used separately.

1. *Thiurams*

Mixture =		%	*Diluent*
Tetramethylthiuram disulphide	(TMTD)	0.25	pet.
Tetraethylthiuram disulphide	(TETD)	0.25	pet.
Dipentamethylenethiuram disulphide	(PTD)	0.25	pet.
Tetramethylthiuram monosulphide	(TMTM)	0.25	pet.

Separately, each is tested 1 per cent in petrolatum.
None of these chemicals on its own can be used instead of the mixture because it will fail to detect all cases of sensitivity.

2. *Mercapto chemicals*

		%	*Diluent*
Mercaptobenzothiazole	(MBT)	1.0	pet.
Mixture =			
Mercaptobenzothiazole	(MBT)	0.5	pet.
Cyclohexylbenzothiazyl sulphenamide	(CBS)	0.5	pet.
Dibenzothiazyl disulphide	(MBTS)	0.5	pet.
Morpholinyl mercaptobenzothiazole	(MMBT) (MOR)	0.5	pet.

Separately, each is tested 1 per cent in petrolatum.
The concentration of MBT in the mix has been raised from 0.25 per cent to

0.5 per cent but false negative reactions to this increased concentration still occur, and therefore all patients should be routinely tested with MBT 1 per cent as well as the mercapto-mix.

Cross-reactions. The pattern of cross-reactions among the mercapto-group was studied by Fregert (1969). He found that the combination of a benzene and a thiazole ring and a thiol group in the 2-position were necessary for cross-sensitivity.

3. *Naphthyl chemicals*

Mixture =		%	Diluent
Phenyl-β-naphthylamine	(PBN)	0.5	pet.
Di-β-naphthyl-p-phenylenediamine	(DBNPD)	0.5	pet.

Separately each is 1 per cent in petrolatum.

4. *PPD chemicals*

Mixture =		%	Diluent
Phenylcyclohexyl-p-phenylenediamine	(CPPD)	0.25	pet.
Phenylisopropyl-p-phenylenediamine (Isopropylaminodiphenylamine)	(IPPD)	0.1	pet.
Diphenyl-p-phenylenediamine	(DPPD)	0.25	pet.

Separately CPPD and DPPD are 1 per cent in petrolatum.
IPPD   is 0.1 per cent in petrolatum.

Cross-reactions. Only about half of those sensitive to this group of chemicals cross-react with PPD.

Patch test sensitisation. IPPD is a potent allergen and if used in too high a concentration for patch testing it causes active sensitisation. This has been reported by Schønning and Hjorth (1969) who used 2 per cent and sensitised 12 of 440 patients tested.

5. *Carbamates and diphenyl guanidine*

Mixture =		%	Diluent
Diphenylguanidine	(DPG)	1	pet.
Bis (diethyldithiocarbamate) zinc	(ZDC)	1	pet.
Bis (dibutyldithiocarbamate) zinc	(ZBC)	1	pet.

Separately each is tested 1 per cent in petrolatum.

6. *Other chemicals.*

	%	Diluent
Dioxydiphenyl	1	pet.
Dithiodimorpholine	1	pet.

7. Rubber

Thin shavings of the suspected rubbers; if thick pieces of rubber are applied, false positives, due to pressure, will occur.

Irritant patch tests

Doubtful reactions to all these rubber mixes occasionally occur but particularly with the Carba-mix. Testing with the separate constituents of the mixture will clarify whether the weak response was an irritant or an allergic reaction.

References

Adams, R.M. (1975) Possible substitution for mercaptobenzothiazole in rubber. *Contact Dermatitis*, 1, 246.

Alfonzo, C. (1979) Allergic contact dermatitis to isopropylaminodiphenylamine (IPPD) *Contact Dermatitis*, 5, 145.

Allen, P.W. (1972) *Natural Rubber and the Synthetics*. London, Crosby Lockwood.

Allenby, C.F., Crow, K.D., Kirton, V., Munro-Ashman, D. (1966) Contact dermatitis from spandex yarn. *British Medical Journal*, i, 674.

Batschvarov, B. & Minkov, D.M. (1968) Dermatitis and purpura from rubber in clothing. *Transactions St John's Hospital Dermatological Society*, 54, 178.

Bieber, Ph. & Foussereau, J. (1968) Rôle de deux amines aromatiques dans l'allergie au caoutchouc; PBN et 4010 NA, amines anti-oxydantes dans l'industrie du pneu. *Bulletin Société Français de Dermatologie et de Syphilographie*, 75, 63.

Black, H. (1972) *Contact Dermatitis Newsletter*, 12, 323.

Bonnevie, P. & Marcussen, P.V. (1944–45) Rubber products as a widespread cause of eczema; Report of 80 cases. *Acta Dermato-venereologica*, 25, 163.

Bourne, H.G., Yee, H.T. & Seferian, S. (1968) *Archives of Environmental Health*, 16, 700.

Calnan, C.D. (1971) Lichenoid dermatitis from isopropylaminodiphenylamine. *Contact Dermatitis Newsletter*, 10, 237.

Calnan, C.D. (1978a) Diethyldithiocarbamate in adhesive tape *Contact Dermatitis*, 4, 61.

Calnan, C.D. (1978b) Diphenyl guanidine in rubber hoses. *Contact Dermatitis*, 4, 241.

Camarasa, J.M.G. & Alomar, A. (1978) Allergic rhinitis from diphenyl guanidine. *Contact Dermatitis*, 4, 242.

Carr, R.D. (1967) Spandex dermatitis. *Archives of Dermatology*, 96, 642.

Conde-Salazar Gomez, L & Gomex Urcuyo, J.F. (1976) Sensibilidad a los componentes de la goma en obreros de la construcción. *Actas Dermo-Sifiliograficas*, 67, 297.

Couzens, E.G. & Yarsley, V.E. (1968) *Plastics in the Modern World*. Harmondsworth: Penguin Books.

Cronin, E. (1972) Clinical prediction of patch test results. *Transactions St John's Hospital Dermatological Society*, 58, 153.

Cronin, E. (1973) Squash ball dermatitis. *Contact Dermatitis Newsletter*, 13, 365.

Curtis, G.H. (1945) Contact dermatitis of eyelids caused by an anti-oxidant in rubber fillers of eyelash curlers. *Archives of Dermatology*, 52, 262.

Dickey, R.F. (1967) Allergic contact-type dermatitis due to Spandex in brassiere. *Archives of Dermatology*, 95, 89.

Dijk, E. van (1968) Contact dermatitis due to Spandex. *Acta Dermato-venereologica*, 48, 589.

Eriksson, G. & Ostlund, E. (1968) Rubber bank note counters as the cause of eczema among employees at the Swedish Post Giro Office. *Acta Dermato-venereologica*, 48, 212.

Fine, L.J. & Peters, J.M. (1976) Respiratory morbidity in rubber workers. *Archives of Environmental Health*, 31, 5.

Fisher, A.A. (1975) 'Hypoallergenic' surgical gloves for special situations. *Cutis*, 15, 797.

Fox, A.J. & Collier, P.F. (1976) A survey of occupational cancer in the rubber and cablemaking industries: analysis of deaths occurring in 1972–74. *British Journal of Industrial Medicine*, 33, 249.

Foussereau, J. & Cavalier, C. (1977) La N-isopropyl-N'-phénylparaphénylenediamine a-t-elle sa place dans la batterie standard d'allergènes? Importance de cet allergène dans l'intolerances au caoutchouc. *Dermatologica*, 155, 164.

Fregert, S. (1969) Cross-sensitivity pattern of 2-mercaptobenzothiazole (MBT). *Acta Dermato-venereologica*, **49**, 45.

Fregert, S. (1969) 'Cement dermatitis' caused by rubber packing. *Contact Dermatitis Newsletter*, **6**, 123.

Fregert, S. (1971) Chemicals used in both rubber and plastic. *Contact Dermatitis Newsletter*, **9**, 204.

Fregert, S. (1972) Dermatitis due to conveyor Belt of Lycra. *Contact Dermatitis Newsletter*, **12**, 325.

Fregert, S. (1973) Relapse of hand dermatitis after short contacts with tyres. *Contact Dermatitis Newsletter*, **13**, 351.

Fregert, S. (1973) Lower leg dermatitis from Lycra in socks. *Contact Dermatitis Newsletter*, **13**, 352.

Fregert, S., Hjorth, N., Magnusson, B., Bandmann, H.J., Calnan, C.D., Cronin, E., Malten, K. Meneghini, C.L., Pirilä, V., Wilkinson, D.S. (1969). *Epidemiology of contact dermatitis. Transactions St John's Hospital Dermatological Society*, **55**, 17.

Fregert, S., & Skog, E. (1962) Allergic contact dermatitis from mercaptobenzothiazole in cutting oil. *Acta Dermato-Venereologica*, **42**, 235.

Furman, D., Fisher, A.A. & Leider, M. (1950) Allergic eczematous contact-type dermatitis caused by rubber sponges used for the application of cosmetics. *Journal of Investigative Dermatology*, **15**, 223.

Gaul, L.E. (1957) Results of patch testing with rubber antioxidants and accelerators. *Journal of Investigative Dermatology*, **29**, 105.

Gibbs, F.W. (1961) *Organic Chemistry Today*. Harmondsworth: Penguin Books.

Giménez Camarasa, J.M. (1968) Dermatitis por la goma. *Medicina Cutanea*, **3**, 281.

Grant, J.B.F., Davies, J.D. & Verrier Jones J. (1975) Starch dermatitis: evidence of immunogenicity of surgical glove powder in the guinea pig. *British Journal of Experimental Pathology*, **56**, 396.

Hamada, T. & Horiguchi, S. (1978) Chronic melanodermatitis due to the rubber peephole of a ship radarscope. *Contact Dermatitis*, **4**, 245.

Herrmann, W.P. von & Schulz, K.H. (1960) Hilfsstoffe der Gummiindustrie als Ekzemnoxen. *Dermatologica*, **120**, 127.

Hervé-Bazin, B., Gradiski, D., Duprat, P., Marignac, B., Foussereau, J., Cavelier, C. & Bieber, P. (1977) Occupational eczema from N-Isopropyl-N'-phenylparaphenylenediamine (IPPD) and N-dimethyl-1,3 butyl-N'-phenylparaphenylenediamine (DMPPD) in tyres. *Contact Dermatitis*, **3**, 1.

Heydenreich, G. & Ølholm-Larsen, P. (1976) 4,4'-dithiodimorpholine, a new rubber sensitiser. *Contact Dermatitis*, **2**, 292.

Hindson, T.C. (1966) Studies in contact dermatitis. xvi Contraceptives. *Transactions St John's Hospital Dermatological Society*, **52**, 1.

Hjorth, N. (1970) Personal Communication.

Hjorth, N. & Fregert, S. (1968) *Textbook of Dermatology*. Ed. Rook A., Wilkinson, D.S. & Ebling, F.J.G. p. 1896. Scientific Publications. Oxford and Edinburgh: Blackwell

Jirásek, L. & Kalenský, J. (1975) Kontakní alergický ekzém způsobený gumovými součástmi zěhličky. *Ceskoslovenská Dermatologie*, **50**, 174.

Jordan, W.P. (1971) Contact dermatitis from N-Isopropyl-N-Phenylparaphenylenediamine. *Archives of Dermatology*, **103**, 85.

Jordan, W.P. & Bourlas, M.C. (1975) Allergic contact dermatitis to underwear elastic. *Archives of Dermatology*, **111**, 593.

Joseph, H.L. & Maibach, H.I. (1967) Contact Dermatitis from Spandex brassieres. *Journal of the American Medical Association*, **201**, 880.

Keil, H. & Bereston, E.S. (1942) Dermatitis due to a transparent adhesive tape. *Archives of Dermatology*, **45**, 1052.

Ketel, W.G. von (1976) Thiuram-mix. *Contact Dermatitis*, **2**, 232.

Kirton, V. & Wilkinson, D.S. (1972) Rubber band dermatitis in Post Office sorters. *Contact Dermatitis Newsletter*, **11**, 257.

Kopelman, H., Robertson, M.H. Sanders, P.G. & Ash, I. (1966) The epping jaundice. *British Medical Journal*, **1**, 514.

Kortschak, E (1977) Rubber chemicals. *Australasian Journal of Dermatology*, **18**, 127.

Lachapelle, J.M. (1975) Allergic 'contact' dermatitis from disulfiram implants. *Contact Dermatitis*, **1**, 218.

Lintum, J.C.A. Te & Nater, J.P. (1973) Sensitisation to rubber chemicals in different professions. *Contact Dermatitis Newsletter*, **14**, 396.

Lintum, J.C.A. Te & Nater, J.P. (1973) Contact dermatitis caused by rubber chemicals in dairy workers. *Berufsdermatosen*, **21**, 16.

Lintum, J.C.A. Te & Nater, J.P. (1974) Allergic contact dermatitis caused by rubber chemicals in dairy workers. *Dermatologica*, **148**, 42.

Lloyd, J.W., Decoufle, P. & Moore, R.M. (1975) Background information on chloroprene. *Journal of Occupational Medicine*, **17**, 263.

Magnusson, B., Blohm, S.G. Fregert, S., Hjorth, N., Høvding, G., Pirilä, V., & Skog, E. (1968) Routine Patch Testing IV. *Acta Dermato-venereologica*, **48**, 110.

Maibach, H.I. (1975) Scuba diver facial dermatitis: allergic contact dermatitis to N-isopropyl-N-phenylparaphenylenediamine. *Contact dermatitis*, **1**, 330.

Malten, K.E. (1977) Sensitisers in leg bandages. *Contact Dermatitis*, **3**, 217.

McMichael, A.J., Andjelkovic, D.A. & Tyroler, H.A. (1976) Cancer mortality among rubber workers: an epidemiologic study. *Annals New York Academy of Sciences*, **271**, 125.

Menezes Brandão, F. (1978) Occupational contact dermatitis from rubber antioxidants. *Contact Dermatitis*, **4**, 246.

Mitchell, J.C., Clendenning, W.E., Cronin, E., Fregert, S., Kanof, N.B. & Maibach, H.I. (1976) Patch testing with mercaptobenzothiazole and mercapto-mix. *Contact Dermatitis*, **2**, 123.

Munn, A. (1967) Health hazards in the chemical industry. *Transactions of the Society of Occupational Medicine*, **17**, 8.

Munn, A. (1970) Personal communication.

Nater, J.P. (1975) Überempfindlichkeit gegen Gummi. *Berufodermatosen*, **23**, 161.

North Americar Contact Dermatitis Group (1973) Epidemiology of Contact Dermatitis in North America: 1972. *Archives of Dermatology*, **108**. 537.

Nurse, D.S. (1979) Rubber sensitivity. *Australasian Journal of Dermatology*, **20**, 31.

Penneys, N.S., Edwards, L.S. & Katsikas, J.L. (1976) Allergic contact sensitivity to thiuram compounds in a hemodialysis unit. *Archives of Dermatology*, **112**, 811.

Polano, M.K. (1958) Ekzem durch Gumminhandschuhe. *Dermatologica*, **116**, 105.

Porter, P.S. & Sommer, R.G. (1967) Contact dermatitis due to Spandex. *Archives of Dermatology*, **95**, 43.

Raith, L. (1976) Contact dermatitis from 4-isopropyl-amino-diphenylamine. *Contact Dermatitis*, **2**, 362.

Roed-Petersen, J., Hjorth, N., Jordan, W.P. & Bourlas, M. (1977) Postsorters' rubber fingerstall dermatitis. *Contact Dermatitis*, **3**, 143.

Rudzki, E. & Kleniewska, D. (1970) The epidemiology of contact dermatitis in Poland. *British Journal of Dermatology*, **83**, 543.

Rudzki, E., Ostaszewski, K., Grzya, A. & Kozlowska, A. (1976) Sensitivity to some rubber additives. *Contact Dermatitis*, **2**, 24.

Sauer, G.C. (1965) Flubber dermatitis. *Archives of Dermatology*, **91**, 465.

Schamberg, I.L. & Flesch, P. (1953) Contact dermatitis from rubber caused by allergic sensitivity to thio-beta-naphthol. *Journal of Investigative Dermatology*, **21**, 59.

Schønning, L. & Hjorth, N. (1969) Cross-sensitisation between hair dyes and rubber chemicals. *Berufsdermatosen*, **17**, *100*.

Sharvill, D.E. (1971) Reaction to dioctyl phthalate in a rubber worker. *Contact Dermatitis Newsletter*, **9**, 208.

Shelley, W.B. (1964) Golf-course dermatitis due to thiuram fungicide. *Journal of the American Medical Association*, **188**, 415.

Shultz, K.H. & Herrmann, W.P., (1960) 4,4'-Dioxydiphenyl als ursache von schweibblattekzemen. *Dermatologische Wochenschrift*, **141**, 124.

Snider, B.L. (1966) Synthetics cause new reaction. *Medical World News*, **7**, 98.

Song, M., Degreef, H., de Maubeuge, J., Dooms-Goossens, A. & Oleffe, J. (1979) Contact sensitivity to rubber additives in Belgium. *Dermatologica*, **158**, 163.

Soto, J.M. (1974) Sensibilidad por contacto en dermatitis eczematosas. *Dermatologia Venezolana*, **13**, 29.

Tanenbaum, M.H. (1967) Spandex dermatitis. *Journal of the American Medical Association*, **200**, 899.

Verbov, J. (1969) Rubber in brassiere cups. *Contact Dermatitis Newsletter*, **5**, 98.

White, W.G. & Vickers, H.R. (1970) Diethyl thiourea as a cause of dermatitis in a car factory. *British Journal of Industrial Medicine*, **27**, 167.

Wilkinson, D.S. (1968) Sensitivity to N-Isopropyl-N-phenyl-p-phenylenediamine. *Contact Dermatitis Newsletter*, **3**, 42.

Wilkinson, D.S. Bandmann, H.J., Calnan, C.D. Cronin, E., Fregert, S., Hjorth, N., Magnusson, B., Maibach, H.I., Malten, K.E., Meneghini, C.H. & Pirilä, V. (1970). The role of contact allergy in hand eczema. *Transactions St John's Hospital Dermatological Society*, **56**, 19.

Wilson, H.T.H. (1960) Rubber glove dermatitis. *British Medical Journal*, **2**, 21.

Wilson, H.T.H. (1969) Rubber dermatitis. An investigation of 106 cases of contact dermatitis caused by rubber. *British Journal of Dermatology*, **81**, 175.

15.

Other allergens

LANOLIN
COLOPHONY
FORMALDEHYDE
  Compounds which release formaldehyde
  Paraformaldehyde
  Hexamethylenetetramine
  Bronopol   (p. 695)
  Chloroallylhexaminium chloride;
  Dowicil 200 (p. 695)
GLUTARALDEHYDE
OIL OF TURPENTINE
ALCOHOLS
  Ethyl alcohol
  Isopropyl alcohol
  Benzyl alcohol
  Cetyl alcohol
  Stearyl alcohol
  Oleyl alcohol
GLYCOLS
  Ethylene glycol
  Propylene glycol
  Hexylene glycol
  Polyethylene glycol
  Glyceryl monostearate

SURFACTANTS—SOAPS AND
SYNTHETIC DETERGENTS
COMPOSITION OF SURFACTANTS
Soaps
  The soap compound Irritant
  Additives   Allergic
                  Germicides
                  Perfume
                  Lanolin
                  Colophony
Synthetic detergents
  The detergent compound
    Irritant
    Allergic
      Lauryl ether sulphate
      Sodium lauryl sulphate
    Tego
  Additives
    Irritant
      Enzymes—dermatitis
    Allergic
      Enzymes—pulmonary
      Fluorescent whitening agents (p. 81)
      Perfumes
MATCHES
TATTOOS

Lanolin

Lanolin is derived from the sebum of sheep. A crude grease is recovered from the wool, cleansed with detergent to rid it of dirt and extraneous matter and then further refined to give anhydrous lanolin (adeps lanae) or wool wax. Chemically, wool fat is more like a fat than a wax, and more than 99 per cent of it consists of a complex mixture of esters which by hydrolysis can be separated into alcohols and acids:

Wool Fat B.P.	free fatty acids	0.3%	
	ash	0.02%	
	water	0.08%	
			Hydrocarbons 1%
	esters etc.	99.6%	Free fatty alcohol 3%
			Esters 95.6%

Hydrolysis of wool fat esters

Alcohols (52%)			Acids (48%)			
21%	29%	27%	28%	7%	22%	29%
n-Aliphatic	Sterols	Triterpenoid	hydroxy	normal	iso	ante-iso
C_{18}–C_{28}	Cholesterol	Lanosterol				
	Cholestanol	Dihydrolanosterol				
	Cyclic diols	Agnosterol				
	Cyclic triols	Dihydroagnosterol				
		Others				

The 3 per cent free fatty alcohol in the original esters is scattered through these alcohols

The percentages are approximate

Other chemicals in wool fat

Antioxidants: The manufacturers add an antioxidant, which usually is butylated hydroxytoluene but occasionally is butylated hydroxyanisole; the concentration used in anhydrous lanolin is 200 parts per million and in wool alcohols is 500 parts per million.

Detergents: Residues may remain from the initial washing of the wool.

Uses and properties of lanolin and its derivatives
Lanolin and its derivatives are widely used in cosmetic and in many pharmaceutical bases. Lanolin is present also in diverse products such as paints, some adhesive plasters, polishes, textiles and occasionally soaps. Lanolin fatty acids are added to lubricants for their water-repellant properties.

The cosmetic and pharmaceutical industries use lanolin and its derivatives for their texture and for their emollient, emulsifying and stabilising properties.

Lanolin is occlusive and has excellent emollient properties; it is added to creams and lotions to impart a smooth and soft texture to the skin. However, lanolin itself is tacky, yellow and has a faint but definite odour, and so to overcome these disadvantages derivatives have been prepared.

Wool alcohols
On extraction from the lanolin, wool alcohols form a brown solid. They are excellent emulsifiers, forming water-in-oil emulsions; they retain the emollient property of lanolin but are not so sticky and have less colour and smell.

Ung. Aquosum B.P.: is an emulsion containing 3 per cent wool alcohols.

Eucerin: Unna used wool fat as an emulsifier in dermatological preparations, but in 1907 he found that a specific wool fat alcohol fraction called eucerit was more effective. This is obtained by the saponification of wool fat: it contains cholesterol and related sterols; lanosterol and related C_{30} sterols; aliphatic C_{15} and C_{30} alcohols; and butylated hydroxytoluene (Ional) as an antioxidant (de Beukelaar, 1963). Eucerin (eucerinum anhydricum) is 6 per cent eucerit in a petrolatum-paraffin base.

Aquaphor (Hartolan; eucerinum cum aqua) is a water-in-oil cream of eucerin and water.

Superlan is a purified derivative of Aquaphor (Hartolan). It is paler because 15 per cent of the dark material is removed during purification.

Acetylation
Acetylation esterifies lanolin (Modulan, American Cholesterol Products Inc.), removing the free alcohols. The product no longer emulsifies, but it stabilises emulsions, and, although it is more hydrophobic than lanolin, it is still emollient and feels soft and waxy. Acetylated wool alcohols (Acetulan, American Cholesterol Products Inc.) have similar properties and spread well on the skin.

Hydrogenation
Hydrogenation of lanolin increases the alcohol content by converting the esterified fatty acids to alcohols. It is added to a base because it feels soft and spreads well, but its use is extremely limited.

Ethoxylation
Ethoxylation increases water solubility.
Lanolin, its compostion and derivatives have been reviewed by Schlossman and McCarthy (1979).

The sensitiser
The allergens in lanolin remain unknown. Attempts to identify them are bedevilled by the enormous amount of chemical work required to isolate even partially pure compounds and by the variability in response of patients to these fractions.

It is generally agreed that the sensitisers are present in the lanolin alcohol fraction.

Aliphatic alcohols
In 1950, Sulzberger and Lazar established in 4 lanolin-sensitive patients that the lanolin alcohols and not the lanolin fatty acids contained the sensitiser. Nineteen lanolin-sensitive patients were then studied (Sulzberger, Warshaw and Hermann, 1953), and each was found to react to one or more test substances containing lanolin alcohols; three patients reacted to lanolin fatty acids, and two to lanosterol, but these reactions were attributed to contamination of the samples by lanolin alcohols. The greatest reaction was to the aliphatic alcohol fraction, and in 8 out of 10 patients this response was blocked by acetylation. Two patients reacted to cetyl alcohol.

Fractionation by thin layer chromatography was found by Peter, Schröpl and

Franzwa (1969) not to be sufficiently precise to identify the allergen. They confirmed that the aliphatic alcohols elicited positive patch tests and that the alcohols with between 12 and 26 carbon atoms varied in their potency.

Free fatty alcohols
In the original esters of lanolin there are approximately 3 per cent free fatty alcohols and these are scattered through all the lanolin alcohols. There is now evidence from patch testing patients that the allergens are present in these natural free fatty alcohols rather than in the total alcohols as previously supposed. It has also been found that the presence of residual detergent in the samples of lanolin used for patch testing increases the incidence of positive results. Lanolin without either free fatty alcohols or detergent elicited very few positive patch test reactions (Clark, Cronin and Wilkinson, 1977).

Derivative of lanosterol
One patient was intensively investigated by Everall and Truter in 1954. They confirmed that the allergen was an alcohol but that it was neither in the aliphatic fraction nor pure cholesterol. They identified it as a yellow glassy solid with an optical rotation of +25.0° and a maximum wavelength absorption of 250 nm. Acetylation inactivated it. Further study showed that 7,11-dioxolanosterol was weakly reactive: this substance is always present as an impurity being an autooxidation derivative of lanosterol (Truter, 1956, 1963).

Hydrogenated lanolin
Two patients, sensitised by the hydrogenated lanolin in a steroid ointment base, were reported by Vollum (1969). In both patients, patch tests with hydrogenated lanolin were positive, and those with lanolin were negative; in one patient, patch testing with wool alcohols was negative. Similarly in Japan, patients sensitised by this same corticosteroid ointment base reacted on patch testing with hydrogenated lanolin but only about half of them were positive to anhydrous lanolin (Sugai and Higashi, 1975). In Belgium relatively feis(4/30) lanolin sensitive patients reacted to their hydrogenated lanolin (Oleffe, Blondeel and Boschmans, 1978).

Incidence of sensitivity
Lanolin and its derivatives are ubiquitous substances and to the majority they are a benefit and not a hazard; nevertheless, a few people, particularly those with eczema, become sensitised.

Many centres have reported finding sensitivity to lanolin or wool alcohols during the routine investigation of eczematous patients. These figures have been criticised, particularly by cosmetic chemists, not only because the subjects tested are a selected population but because of the diversity of test substances used in different series. Until the allergens in lanolin are known, such variation is inevitable but does not invalidate the results.

The incidence of lanolin sensitivity is not strictly comparable in different clinics because the selection of patients so greatly influences the results. For example, if many patients with hypostatic eczema are tested, the incidence is likely to

Country,City	Year	Test substs.	Ecz. Pts. No. Tested	% +ve			Reference
				M & F	M	F	
Europe	1969	Wool alc 30%	4825	2.6	2.0	3.1	Fregert et al. (1969)
Scandinavia	1968	Lanolin	5558	1.5	1.2	1.8	Magnusson et al. (1968)
Belgium	1976	Wool alc. 30%	1376	5.5			Oleffe et al. (1978)
Copenhagen	1961	Eucerin	1878	1.8			Hjorth & Trolle-Lassen (1963)
Copenhagen	1962	Wool alc.	1664	1.6			
Copenhagen	1968	Lanolin	1835	3.3	2.0	4.0	Magnusson et al. (1968)
Copenhagen	1969	Wool alc. 30%	800				Fregert et al. (1969)
Gothenburg	1968	Lanolin	1000		2.0	1.0	Magnusson et al. (1968)
Gothenburg	1969	Wool alc. 30%	800	2.6			Fregert et al. (1969)
Lund	1968	Lanolin	1406		1.0	3.0	Magnusson et al. (1968)
Lund	1968	Wool alc. 30%	800	1.4			Fregert et al. (1969)
Stockholm	1969	Lanolin	510		1.0	1.0	Magnusson et al. (1968)
Helsinki	1968	Lanolin	500		0	0	Magnusson et al. (1968)
Nijmegen	1969	Wool alc. 30%	378	1.0			Fregert et al. (1969)
Munich	1960–66	Eucerin	9185	2.1			Bandmann & Bandmann (1968)
Munich	1969	Wool alc. 30%	800	3.8			Fregert et al. (1969)
Warsaw	1970	Eucerin + 5% alc. sal.	791	5.9	3.3	8.1	Rudzki & Kleniewska (1970)
		Lanolin + 5% alc. sal.	791	2.5	1.4	3.5	
North America	1972	Wool alc. 30%		3.0			N. Am. Contact Derm. Gr. (1973)
New York	1953	Anhydrous Lanolin	1048	1.1			Sulzberger et al. (1953)
San Francisco	1968	Lanolin	202	2.0			Epstein, Rees, Maibach (1968)
Auckland	1972	Lanolin	218	2.3			Black (1972)

be high. Nevertheless, the reported incidence of sensitivity to wool alcohols 30 per cent in petrolatum is of interest: for subjects in Europe it was 2.6 per cent (Fregert *et al.*, 1969) and in North America 3.0 per cent (North American Contant Dermatitis Group, 1973), and although 3.8 per cent reacted in Munich, only 1 per cent did so in Nijmegen (Fregert *et al.*, 1969).

Selected series of patients

		Test substance	No. tested	+%	Reference
Oslo	In-Patients	Lanolin and/or Eucerin	270	7.4	Wereide (1965)
Oslo	Stasis eczema	Lanolin + 5% Ac. Sal.			
		Eucerin + 5% Ac. Sal.	230	7.0(?)	Thune (1969)
Adelaide	Pts. with contact derm.	Wool alc. 30%	1000	1.8	Burry *et al.* (1973)

St John's

From 1953–1965 inclusive, patients were patch tested with lanolin or with wool alcohols only if indicated by the history; during this time, 41 patients were diagnosed (Table 15.1). The patients have been reported previously (Cronin, 1966).

Table 15.1. Numbers of patients diagnosed as sensitive to lanolin or wool alcohols (St John's 1953–1965).

Year	1953	1954	1955	1956	1957	1958	1959
Pts. attending clinic	1039	887	885	1009	1014	926	1099
No. +	3	0	1	1	2	0	1

	1960	1961	1962	1963	1964	1965	Total
Pts. attending clinic	1338	1461	1309	1116	1215	1232	14 530
No. +	0	5	1	10	5	12	41

In 1966, a standard patch test series was introduced for use in all patients; wool alcohols 30 per cent in soft paraffin was included as one of the allergens. Immediately, the number of patients detected as being sensitive to wool alcohols rose, and from 1968 to 1976 the incidence has ranged from approximately 2–4 per cent of all patients tested (Table 15.2).

Table 15.2. Incidence of sensitivity to wool alcohols (St John's 1966–1976).

Year	1966	1967	1968	1969	1970	1971	1972	1973	1974	1975	1976	Total
No. Tested	1401	1529	1604	1549	1906	1558	1606	1546	1433	1858	1982	17972
No. +	26	19	40	31	50	63	53	50	29	43	59	463
%	1.9	1.2	2.5	2.0	2.6	4.0	3.3	3.2	2.0	2.3	3.0	2.3

Sex incidence

In the eleven years, 1966–1976, the incidence of lanolin sensitivity has been similar in men and women; an average of 2.5 per cent of the men and 2.6 per cent of the women were found each year to be sensitive to wool alcohols. The increased number of men sensitised from 1971–1973 is unexplained (Table 15.3).

Table 15.3. Incidence of sensitivity to wool alcohols in men and women (St John's 1966–1976).

	M			**F**		
	Tested	+	%	Tested	+	%
1966	731	10	1.4	670	16	2.4
1967	809	10	1.2	720	9	1.3
1968	812	23	2.8	792	17	2.1
1969	787	14	1.8	762	17	2.2
1970	916	23	2.5	990	27	2.7
1971	707	39	5.5	851	24	2.8
1972	738	26	3.5	868	27	3.1
1973	710	30	4.2	836	20	2.4
1974	655	11	1.7	778	18	2.3
1975	887	14	1.6	971	29	3.0
1976	937	19	2.0	1045	40	3.8
Total	8689	219	2.5	9283	244	2.6

Causes of sensitivity

Medicaments
These are the major source of sensitisation.

Cosmetics
Facial cosmetics rarely sensitise. Hand creams, emollients and protective creams are sometimes used on damaged skin, giving them a greater potential to induce sensitivity.

Soaps
The few soaps which contain lanolin seem to cause little, if any, trouble.

Protective metal coatings
In industry metals are coated with greasy films to protect them from rust and corrosion. Some of these coatings contain 15–30 per cent lanolin, which may cause or contribute to the persistence of an eczema, as in the patient described by Calnan (1979a).

Relevance
Lanolin is a significant allergen: in the European study on contact dermatitis (Fregert et al., 1969), it was considered relevant in 80 per cent of the patients found to be sensitised.

Entire cause of a contact dermatitis
In a facial cosmetic, lanolin, or a derivative, can be the sole cause of an allergic contact dermatitis. In a very few patients seen at St. John's, lanolin, in an emollient hand cream or in an ointment used for the treatment of psoriasis, has been completely responsible for an allergic contact dermatitis.

Aggravating factors
In the great majority of patients this allergy is an unsuspected aggravating factor

engrafted upon an existing eczema. Without routine patch testing of eczematous patients it remains unrecognised. Emollients and topical medicaments are the usual sources; many of the latter contain a corticosteroid which suppresses acute exacerbations, and the patient and clinician may, in consequence, remain unaware that sensitisation has occurred. In an analysis of pre-patch test diagnoses, wool alcohol sensitivity was suspected in only 7 of 44 patients (16 per cent) (Cronin, 1972).

Clinical features

At the Finsen Institute, Hjorth and Trolle-Lassen (1963) analysed the clinical findings in 50 consecutive patients sensitised by lanolin. Thirty-five were women, and 40 of the patients were over 50 years of age; thirty-two had leg eczema with spread to other sites in 23, 8 had hand eczema, 5 had eczema of the head, 2 of the thigh, 1 of the trunk and in 2 the site was not stated. They explained the frequency in elderly women by emphasising that patients with chronic leg eczema, particularly those with stasis eczema, are prone to lanolin sensitivity because they use so many topical medicaments.

In Munich, 43 patients sensitive only to Eucerin were studied: thirty-four were women, 34 were more than 50 years old, and 31 had stasis dermatitis with or without leg ulcers (Bandman and Bandman, 1968). In New York, Fisher, Pascher and Kandf (1971), using a 'vehicle tray', patch tested 100 patients suspected of having a contact dermatitis due to a medicament; six reacted to lanolin ('as is'), but there were only three positive patch tests to suspected medicaments.

St John's

Forty lanolin-sensitive patients seen from 1953–1965 inclusive have previously been reported. The eczema was hypostatic in 14, involved the face in 13, the hands in 9, the lower leg in 2 and the arm in 1; in one case the distribution was widespread (Cronin, 1966).

From 1966–1976, a total of 463 patients reacted to wool alcohols on patch testing. In contrast to other series, there was no significant preponderance of women: there were 219 men and 244 women (Table 15.3).

Age

Of these 219 men and 244 women, the majority (320) (approximately 70 per cent) were over 40 years old (Table 15.4).

Table 15.4. Ages of 219 men and 244 women sensitive to wool alcohols (St John's 1966–1976).

Ages yrs.	0–10	11–20	21–30	31–40	41–50	51–60	61–70	71–80	81–90
Men	1	4	29	25	62	51	34	12	1
Women	0	14	35	35	47	56	42	14	1

Patterns of eczema

To clarify whether individual patterns of eczema are prone to develop sensitivity to wool alcohols, these patients have been divided into five clinical groups. Many patients had more than one site involved; allocation to a group was determined by the principal site of the eczema. If there was no obvious source of lanolin contact in an existing eczema but there was a past history of varicose ulcers or eczema, the patient was included in the stasis eczema group. The patients with cosmetic facial eczema are described on page 98.

Clinical group	Men	Women
1. Stasis eczema	48	71
2. Cosmetic facial eczema	1	26
3. Hand eczema ± other sites	73	59
4. Leg eczema	17	6
5. Other patterns of eczema	80	82
	219	244

Patients sensitised by medicaments rarely complain of cosmetic dermatitis, although they occasionally remember being irritated by a lanolin emollient cream. This apparent anomaly can be explained by the facts that, in cosmetics, the concentration of lanolin or a derivative is low and that absorption through the intact facial skin is minimal.

Stasis eczema and ulcers
Patients with varicose or stasis eczema and ulcers are undoubtedly prone to 'lanolin' sensitivity (Breit and Bandman, 1973) and, in these patients, secondary eruptions are often precipitated by such sensitisation (Hjorth and Trolle-Lassen, 1963).

In 1965, Reichenberger patch tested 150 patients with leg ulcers and 50 (33 per cent) of them reacted to Eucerin. A series of 230 patients with stasis eczema were patch tested by Thune (1969) with anhydrous lanolin containing 5 per cent salicylic acid and also with anhydrous Eucerin containing 5 per cent salicylic acid. Although 43 reacted, he concluded, on the basis of provocation tests in which Eucerin was applied to eczematous skin, that only 16 (7 per cent) were sensitised to wool fat. In Munich, Breit (1972) patch tested 326 cases of eczema and ulcers of the lower leg, caused mainly by venous insufficiency, and found that 13.2 per cent had positive reactions to wool alcohols 30 per cent.

St John's
Patients with varicose ulcers were studied by Perera (1970), who found that of the 37 patch tested, 13 were sensitive to lanolin (wool alcohols 30 per cent in petrolatum being used for patch testing). The commonest associated sensitivity was neomycin.

Number each year.
There is no varicose ulcer clinic at St John's, and therefore relatively few of these patients are seen compared with other centres: of 1000 consecutive patients investigated in the contact dermatitis clinic in 1971–72, only 11 women and 9 men (2 per cent) had been referred on account of hypostatic dermatitis or stasis ulcers. Despite this low attendance in this present series of 463 wool alcohol-sensitive

patients, 119 (25 per cent) had this diagnosis of whom 48 were men and 71 were women (Table 15.5).

Table 15.5. Numbers of men and women with statis eczema or ulcers sensitised to wool alcohols (St John's 1966–1976).

Year	1966	1967	1968	1969	1970	1971	1972	1973	1974	1975	1976	Total
Nos. of Men	3	1	5	3	4	9	8	6	3	2	4	48
Nos. of Women	0	4	6	6	12	5	6	5	7	6	14	71

Age
Most of the patients had passed middle age but 10 per cent (11 of 119) were less than 40 years old (Table 15.6).

Table 15.6. Ages of patients with stasis eczema or ulcers sensitised to wool alcohols (St John's 1966–1976).

Age (years)	21–30	31–40	41–50	51–60	61–70	71–80	81–90
Nos. of Men	1	4	12	16	12	2	1
Nos. of Women	1	5	13	22	22	8	0

Secondary spread
A secondary spread of the eczema to distant sites had occurred in 15 of 48 men (31 per cent) and in 37 of 71 women (52 per cent).

Patch testing
Each patient was routinely patch tested with wool alcohols 30 per cent in petrolatum, and 109 of the 119 patients (92 per cent) were positive. The ten that were negative reacted to other preparations containing wool alcohols; these included hydrogenated lanolin and Ung. Aquosum BP which contains 3 per cent wool alcohols.

Associated sensitivities
All 119 patients were also patch tested with neomycin 20 per cent in petrolatum and with Vioform 5 per cent in petrolatum.

Sixty-three (53 per cent) were found to be sensitive to neomycin and 15 (13 per cent) to Vioform.

Hand eczema
In her study of hand eczema in Sweden, Agrup (1969) used lanolin with 5 per cent salicylic acid for patch testing; she found positive reactions in 2 of 210 males (1 per cent) and in 16 of 378 (4 per cent) females. In 9 of these 18 patients, the lanolin sensitivity was contributing to their hand eczema. In one man, it caused an occupational dermatitis as he used a lanolin-containing hand cream at work. Five patients, who reacted repeatedly to patch tests with 30 per cent wool alcohols in petrolatum, were reported by Epstein (1972). One, an atopic woman, had had persistent hand eczema for one year and had been using two hand lotions containing lanolin. She improved greatly by avoiding lanolin. In contrast, a patient with hand eczema, described by Jordan (1974), failed to improve by avoiding lanolin hand cream.

St John's

Number each year
Since 1966, all patients attending the contact clinic have been tested routinely with wool alcohols 30 per cent in petrolatum and this has led to the detection of sensitivity in patients presenting primarily with hand eczema. Each year 2–16 men and in 3–10 women have been found to be sensitised. From 1966–1976 the total of these patients was 132; each had hand eczema, either alone or in association with involvement of other sites. There were 73 men and 59 women (Table 15.7).

Table 15.7. Numbers of men and women with hand eczema sensitive to wool alcohols (St John's 1966–1976).

	1966	1967	1968	1969	1970	1971	1972	1973	1974	1975	1976	Total
Men	4	2	5	5	7	16	11	11	2	4	6	73
Women	7	3	3	4	5	3	9	8	4	3	10	59

In 1970–1971 approximately half the patients attending the Contact Clinic had hand eczema (Cronin, 1972). On the assumption that this proportion is similar each year, a very approximate estimate of the incidence of wool alcohol sensitivity among patients with hand eczema is 2 per cent for men and 1 per cent for women (Table 15.8).

Table 15.8. Approximate incidence (%) of wool alcohols sensitivity in men and women with hand eczema (St John's 1966–1976).

	Patch tested 1966–1976	Hand eczema Approx. No.	+ Wool Alc.	% approx.
Men	8689	4345	73	2
Women	9283	4642	59	1

Ages
In women with hand eczema, this sensitivity occurs in all decades from the age of 20 years, whereas in men it occurs after 40 years (Table 15.9). This reflects the earlier onset of hand eczema in women than in men.

Table 15.9. Ages of men and women with hand eczema sensitive to wool alcohols (St John's 1966–1976).

	0–10	11–20	21–30	31–40	41–50	51–60	61–70	71–80
Men	0	3	10	6	23	18	10	3
Women	1	4	12	13	7	12	8	2

Length of History
Approximately half the men and one-third of the women had had their hand eczema for longer than three years when the sensitivity was detected (Table 15.10).

Table 15.10. Length of history in men and women with hand eczema sensitive to wool alcohols (St John's 1966–1976).

	< 1 mth	> 1–6 mths	> 6–12 mths	> 1–3 yrs	> 3 yrs	No Inf
Men	3	13	10	14	32	1
Women	0	12	10	15	20	2

Hand and other sites affected
Sensitivity was almost as frequent in those with eczema confined to the hands as in those with other sites also affected. In these 132 patients the distribution was:

    hands only   : 53
    hands and elsewhere : 79

Occupation
The allergy was not associated with any particular type of work.

Patch Testing
Patch tests with wool alcohols 30 per cent in petrolatum were positive in 125 of 132 patients (95 per cent); the seven negative patients reacted to hydrogenated lanolin, or another preparation of wool alcohols.

Leg eczema

St John's
Among this series of 463 wool alcohol-sensitive patients, only 23 patients, 17 men and 6 women, had mainly leg eczema. This is probably due to such patients rarely being referred to this clinic for patch testing.

Nineteen were over 40 years old; in 13, the duration of the eczema was less than a year, in five it was 1–3 years and in five it was even longer. Twenty-one had positive patch tests with wool alcohols 30 per cent, and two negative patients reacted to hydrogenated lanolin.

Other patterns of eczema

St John's
Very diverse patterns of eczema occurred in about one-third (162/463) of the patients, comprising 80 men and 82 women. No particular distribution was especially susceptible. The eczema was very widespread in 18, was recorded as atopic in 15, as discoid in 7 and as seborrhoeic in 11 patients. Nine men and four women had pruritus ani. One patient was a Burmese student who developed generalised pruritus from asteatosis; he had been sensitised to wool alcohols, probably through the use of emollients.

Patch testing
Until the allergens in lanolin are identified, the compounds used for patch testing will remain imperfect.

Wool alcohols 30 per cent in vaseline and olive oil was first proposed by Hjorth and Trolle-Lassen (1963), and this has been confirmed as the most reliable patch test material; it can, however, give weak irritant responses (Cronin, 1966; Epstein, 1972). It will not detect all cases of sensitivity as confirmed by Mortensen (1979).

Lanolin
Lanolin as such is completely unreliable, as is shown in the following table of reported series of patch test results:

'Lanolin' sensitive		Positive patch tests		References
Pts	Tested	Lanolin	Wool alcohols	
	40	10 (Lanolin)	37 (Eucerin)	Hjorth & Trolle-Lassen (1968)
	30	2 (Adeps Lanae)	30 (Eucerin)	Reichenberger (1965)
	24	2 (Adeps Lanae)	24 (Eucerin)	Bandmann & Bandmann (1968)
	5	?1 (Lanolin)	5 (Wool Alcohols 30%)	Epstein (1972)

Lanolin with salicylic acid gives irritant reactions (Cronin, 1966; Thune, 1969).

St John's

The likelihood of diagnosing sensitivity to wool alcohols is enhanced by broadening the range of allergens used; this is done by applying several test compounds. Since 1966, every patient has been tested with wool alcohols* 30 per cent in petrolatum; moreover, from 1970 onwards, hydrogenated lanolin and Ung. Aquosum B.P. (which contains 3 per cent wool alcohols) have been applied, too, when the allergy is suspected, and they have also been used as the principal confirmatory test substances.

Patch testing with medicaments cannot be relied upon. Their content of lanolin or a derivative is often too low to elicit a reaction on normal skin, and many contain a corticosteroid which will tend to suppress a response. This suppression does not always occur. Five patients experienced exacerbation of their dermatitis when they used a betamethasone valerate ointment which contained hydrogenated lanolin. All had positive patch tests to the ointment and to hydrogenated lanolin, and four of them reacted also to wool alcohols. In 1972, lanolin was omitted from this particular formulation.

The results of patch tests done from 1966–1976 are tabulated below:

Years	Wool Alcohols 30%		Hydrogenated lanolin		Ung. aquosum B.P.	
	Tested	+	Tested	+	Tested	+
1966–1969	116	114(98%)				
1970–1976	347	307(88%)	219	165(75%)	168	113(67%)

In this series 226 patients were tested both with wool alcohols 30 per cent in petrolatum (W.A.) and with hydrogenated lanolin (Hydrg. lan.); the results endorse wool alcohols 30 per cent as the more reliable patch test compound, but it does not detect all cases of sensitivity.

Tested	+ WA +Hydrg. lan.	+ WA – Hydrg. lan.	– WA + Hydrg. lan.	– WA – Hydrg. lan.
226	144(64%)	52(23%)	26(11%)	4(2%)

Ocassionally wool alcohols 30 per cent in petrolatum causes weak irritant reactions which show as a mild erythema at two days but have practically gone by four days. These doubtful responses are evaluated by repeating the test and by testing with other wool alcohol or lanolin preparations.

* The wool alcohols are obtained from Westbrook Lanolin Co. of England, and they conform to the quality for wool alcohols in the British Pharmacopoeia.

Routine patch testing
1. Wool alcohols 30 per cent in petrolatum
2. One or two additional wool alcohols or lanolin preparations (e.g. Hydrogenated lanolin, Eucerin, Aquaphor, Ung. Aquosum B.P.)
3. Relevant ointments or cosmetics.

Alternatives
A list of corticosteroid preparations with and without lanolin is given on page 669.

Colophony

Colophony (rosin) is derived mainly from *Pinus palustris* and *Pinus caribaea* and is extracted in three ways: (i) Gum rosin is obtained by tapping living trees and distilling the oleoresin to yield turpentine oil and the rosin residue; (ii) Wood rosin is a distillate from pine tree stumps; (iii) Tall oil rosin is a by-product of pulping pine wood.

Crude colophony is a soft, sticky, amber-coloured material which, in air, is rapidly oxidised. Purification removes the colour until it becomes water white (Grade W-W). Esterification increases its stability as does hydrogenation to hydroabietic acid and tetrahydroabietic acid.

Rosin consists of 90 per cent resin acids and 10 per cent neutral matter. The major component of the acid fraction is abietic acid but also present are dehydroabietic, neoabietic, pimaric and isopimaric acids. The various abietic acids have a common structure but they differ in their double bonds.

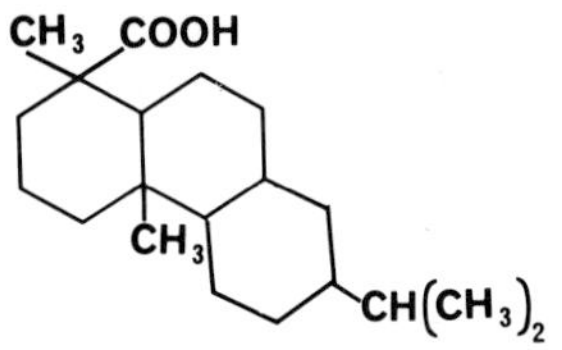

Abietic acid

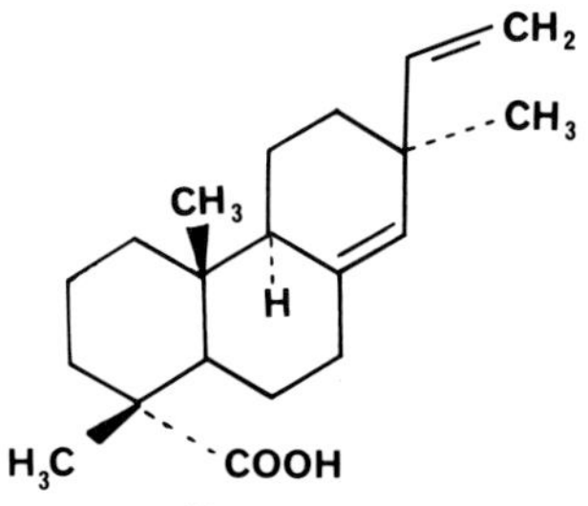

Pimaric acid

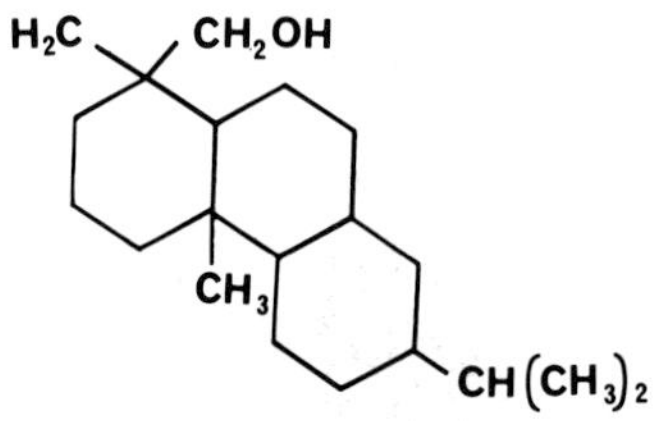

Hydroabietyl alcohol

The sensitisers
Colophony contains several allergens. Foussereau *et al.* (1971) investigated one colophony-sensitive patient, and the abietic acids with a double bond elicited reactions but pimaric acids and completely hydrogenated colophony did not.

Abietic acid 5 per cent in petrolatum was added to the standard series by Wahlberg (1978) and of 15 patients who reacted to colophony 20 per cent in petrolatum, nine reacted to abietic acid.

Esterification of colophony reduces its allergenicity. At St John's patients were tested with colophony and a maleic ester of colophony (each 20 per cent in pet.): 29 reacted to colophony and were negative to the ester, four reacted to both and two patients gave equivocal reactions to the ester and were negative to colophony.

Patients sensitised to hydroabietyl alcohol (Abitol) may react to colophony (p. 111).

Uses

Colphony is used in many different products:

Adhesive tapes, insulating tapes (now less often), jointing tapes, flypaper.

Glues, mastics and sealants.

Surface coatings and varnishes.

Paper size (rosin is added to paper to increase its water resistance and to prevent feathering or spreading of ink).

Printing inks (sometimes); also as a finishing film to protect the print.

Solders

As a tacky substance to prevent slipping: in industry on machine belts, by musicians on bows for stringed instruments, by sports players on racquet handles, and a colophony finish may be applied to leather tennis racquet and golf club grips.

Cutting oils and soap water

Colophony is in the tall oil fatty acids added to some soluble cutting oils and potassium soap waters and it sensitises (Fregert, 1979) (p. 848).

Soaps (transparent soaps may contain colophony)

Cosmetics, eyeshadows and mascara occasionally.

Shoe polishes sometimes and floor polishes occasionally

Medicaments: a few proprietary preparations contain colophony and it is used in dentistry.

Linoleum

Chewing gum

Causes of sensitisation

Adhesive tapes — *Colophony based*

Irritant reactions. The older types of sticking plasters adhere well but they frequently cause irritant plaster reactions.

Allergic reactions — Colophony. Most of these older tapes contain colophony and they are the most frequent source of colophony sensitisation. They can cause a severe dermatitis if inadvertently applied to a sensitised person.

Hydroabietyl alcohol (abitol) was found to be the sensitiser in a patch test tape which caused a severe dermatitis in one patient. She reacted to hydroabietyl alcohol 20 per cent (pet.) but not to colophony in the standard series or to the colophony esters also present in the tape (Cronin and Calnan, 1978). Abitol in mascara has caused dermatitis (p. 111).

Lanolin or a derivative is present in some of the adhesive films and is occasionally the cause of an allergic plaster reaction.

Zinc diethyldithiocarbamate may be a constituent of the adhesive mass and is a rare cause of a plaster dermatitis. Cases have been reported (Cronin, 1972; Calnan, 1978).

–Resin based
Newer tapes do not contain colophony and their adhesive films are resin-based; they rarely irritate the skin and sensitisation is most uncommon. One acrylic tape has caused an allergic dermatitis (p. 576).

In the U.S.A. Scotch tape caused an acute reaction in a patient known to be sensitive to sticking plaster. Patch testing identified the allergen in both tapes as diamyl hydroquinone (Murphy, Reif and January, 1958). In Great Britain, Sellotape, which is made of a cellophane backing with an adhesive film, adversely affected a patient and on patch testing she reacted to polyethylene glycol (10 per cent in acetone) which was present as a plasticiser in the cellulose backing (p. 812).

Salicylic Acid plaster. Two patients developed an allergic contact dermatitis while applying 40 per cent salicylic acid plaster to their plantar warts. Patch testing identified the allergen as dehydroabietic acid (Rasmussen and Fisher, 1976).

Insulating tape
An electrical engineer with dermatitis of the hands for five years was found to be sensitive to colophony. His source of contact was traced to insulating tape wrapped round the handles of his tools to prevent electric shocks. He discarded the tape and his hands healed (Calnan, 1972).

Industrial non-slip applications
An engineer, while honing crankshafts, applied powdered rosin to the machine's leather driving belt to prevent it slipping, and was thereby sensitised and developed dermatitis (Wilkinson and Calnan, 1975). A dredgerman used colophony to service the clutch of his machine and was sensitised (Breit, 1968).

Protective coating on print
A colophony coating may be used to protect a printed surface and such a film on a tube of lozenges caused dermatitis of a girl's hand after she had held the tube for 90 minutes. A similar finish on beer labels caused an occupational dermatitis of the hands and face in a woman factory worker (Fregert, 1968).

Dentistry
Following gingivectomy a paste containing colophony (42 per cent) and eugenol (7 per cent) is applied to the raw gum margin, and after several operations patients may react to this periodontal dressing with inflammation of the mucosa varying from redness to blister formation and some have developed urticaria. Koch, Magnusson and Nyquist (1971) confirmed by patch testing that patients, none of whom had had previous plaster reactions, had been sensitised to colophony and eugenol by this dental dressing.

Cosmetics
Colophony, or one of its derivatives, is occasionally present in a cosmetic and it has caused dermatitis in mascara (p. 111), eye shadow (p. 113) and rouge (p. 149).

Soaps (p. 815).

Clothing
In Australia, a man who was sensitive to colophony developed a dermatitis of his neck from shirt collars cleaned with a pre-wash preparation containing trichloroethane and colophony (Kirk, 1976).

Polythene patch test units
A patient described by Foussereau *et al.* (1971) reacted to polythene in the patch test unit, and was sensitive to colophony and abietic acids. Similar reactions have occurred with the Al-test (p. 3).

Solder

Dermatitis. Colophony is used in many soldering fluxes, as in 'Multicore' solder, which consists of a tin lead alloy, an amine hydrochloric activator and a central core of colophony. It is widely used in the U.K. for soldering steel wires. This solder occasionally causes dermatitis in industry and rarely from its use in the home.

Asthma. Occupational asthma occurs from this and other colophony solders and from hot-melt colophony adhesives (Fawcett, Newman Taylor and Pepys, 1976; Burge, Green and Pepys, 1977; Burge *et al.*, 1978).

Patch testing
Colophony	20 per cent
Abietic acid	10 and 20 per cent
Hydroabietic acid	?10 and 20 per cent
Hydroabietyl alcohol (abitol)	10 and 20 per cent
Pimaric acid	10 and 20 per cent
	each in petrolatum

Formaldehyde HCHO; oxymethylene; methanal

HCOH

Formaldehyde is a pungent-smelling gas which readily polymerises. Formalin is a 37–50 per cent solution of formaldehyde gas in water to which 15 per cent methyl alcohol is often added to prevent polymerisation.

Sources of contact

Formaldehyde resins, including those for crease-resistant textiles: urea formaldehyde is particularly likely to break down and release formaldehyde.

Nitrogenous fertilisers: formaldehyde forms insoluble urea formaldehyde which is slowly released to the plants; it is sometimes combined with inedible fish oils.

Disinfectant, and as an insecticide on flypapers.

Preservative: as a bactericide formaldehyde is slow but effective. It is used as a preservative in detergents (particularly lauryl ether sulphate), medicaments, cosmetics and it may be present in household products such as furniture creams and domestic cleansers.

Deodorising solutions, because it absorbs gases.

Tanning agent for pale washable leather, because it preserves the colour and it makes the skin water-resistant.

Fur trade: it may be used in the preparation of furs.

Dyeing and improving fastness of textile dyes.

Anti-rust agent: it protects metals and inhibits corrosion in oil wells.

Photography: it reduces silver salts and hardens the gelatin coating on films; in colour processing it is added to the stabliser bath as it prevents the diffusion of colour.

Paper manufacture: formaldehyde increases the wet strength and water resistance of paper and it is used to make parchment.

Medicaments: formaldehyde is used to treat warts.

Pathology: in histology formaldehyde fixes tissues.

Embalming: it has the same purpose.

Rubber industry: formaldehyde is added to latex as a preservative; it is an antioxidant and is used in the production of synthetic rubbers.

Sensitising potential

In the Draize procedure Marzulli and Maibach (1973), using induction concentrations of 10 per cent and 5 per cent aqueous formaldehyde solutions and challenging with a 1 per cent solution, sensitised nearly 8 per cent of the 154 subjects exposed. Even a 0.01 per cent concentration elicited a reaction in one of five subsequently tested with further dilutions. Formaldehyde preparations were applied topically with the following results: 5 of 10 reacted to a skin lotion containing 0.5 per cent formaldehyde; 4 of 10 reacted to a creme rinse containing 0.4 per cent formaldehyde and 2 of 10 to a bubble bath oil containing 0.6 per cent formaldehyde. In the maximisation test Kligman (1966) exposed 25 subjects to 5 per cent formalin and when challenged with a 1 per cent concentration

18 (72 per cent) reacted, giving formaldehyde a high rating as a sensitiser which is not in accord with clinical experience.

Incidence of sensitisation

The following incidences of formaldehyde sensitisation have been recorded in the routine investigation of eczematous patients.

	No. tested	Formaldehyde positive	Author
Europe	4825	3.5%	Fregert *et al.* (1969)
Poland	1205	6.3%	Rudzki *et al.* (1970)
N. America	1000	4.0%	N. American Contact Derm. Group (1973)
New Zealand	216	3.2%	Black (1972)

St John's

Each patient who attends the Contact Clinic is routinely tested with formaldehyde 2 per cent in water. From 1971–1975 the incidence has varied from 0.7–1.4 per cent of the patients tested (Table 15.11). Men and women are sensitised with equal frequency: 0.6–1.5 per cent of the men and 0.6–1.4 per cent of the women (Tables 15.12 and 15.13).

Table 15.11. The incidence of formaldehyde sensitivity (St John's 1971–1975).

Year	1971	1972	1973	1974	1975
Total tested	1558	1606	1546	1433	1858
+	15	12	21	11	25
%	1	0.7	1.4	0.8	1.3

Table 15.12. The incidence of formaldehyde sensitivity in men (St John's 1971–1975).

Year	1971	1972	1973	1974	1975
Males tested	707	738	710	655	887
+	4	6	11	6	11
%	0.6	0.8	1.5	0.9	1.2

Table 15.13. The incidence of formaldehyde sensitivity in women (St John's 1971–1975).

Year	1971	1972	1973	1974	1975
Females tested	851	868	836	778	971
+	11	6	10	5	14
%	1.3	0.7	1.2	0.6	1.4

Causes of allergic contact dermatitis

Formaldehyde allergy may be associated with dermatitis from urea formaldehyde resins but formaldehyde sensitivity also occurs without this association and the source of contact may then be difficult to trace. In a European study (Fregert *et al.*, 1969), patch test reactions to formaldehyde 2 per cent in water were considered relevant in less than half of the patients sensitised. Exposure to formaldehyde occurs occasionally at home but more commonly at work.

Non-occupational dermatitis

Cosmetics. Contact dermatitis from formaldehyde in cosmetics is rare. Shampoos, nail hardeners, deodorants and cosmetics, contaminated unintentionally, are possible sources of exposure. In Sweden and Japan formaldehyde is forbidden in cosmetics (Fisher, 1976).

Shampoos. Lauryl ether sulphate, which contains formaldehyde as a preservative, is the basis of many shampoos but the concentration of formaldehyde in the final shampoo formulation is small (about 0.08 per cent or less) unless it has been added specifically as a preservative. Hairdressers may occasionally get dermatitis from this source of contact with formaldehyde (p. 138) but the ordinary user rarely, Bork, Heise and Rosinun (1979) have described one case.

Nail hardeners have been formulated with 6–7 per cent formaldehyde but they caused nail dystrophy and had to be withdrawn.

Deodorants or antiperspirants rarely contain formaldehyde.

Contaminated cosmetics and other preparations. In Sweden, despite their ban on formaldehyde in cosmetics, formaldehyde has been found in cosmetics contained in polythene tubes. The melamine or urea formaldehyde coating on the outer surface of the tubes was confirmed as the source by storing emulsions, free of formaldehyde, in such tubes for two months and then finding that half the emulsions contained formaldehyde, probably in the water phase. The presence of an emulsifier seemed to increase the incidence of contamination (Tegner and Fregert, 1973). Other preparations, such as liquid soaps and cleaning products, have been found to be similarly contaminated from formaldehyde resins on the containers (Fregert, 1977).

Medicaments. Solutions of formaldehyde are used in the treatment of viral warts and an unexpected sensitivity to formaldehyde can sometimes be traced to this exposure.

Hidden Sources of formaldehyde in the home. Formaldehyde in an air cleaner can contaminate gelatin and make it impossible to melt and formaldehyde vapour from varnish on kitchen cupboards containing flour may affect the gluten, and dough made from such flour fails to rise (Thomsen, 1973).

Occupational dermatitis

Offset printing is a system of rollers in which the image from a plate is transferred to a rubber blanket and then to paper or other surface. In the process a watery solution which may contain formaldehyde as a preservative is used to wet the printing plate.

A clerk whose duties involved the use of two offset printing machines developed dermatitis of her hands. Patch tests: she reacted to the autoprime from one of the machines and on being tested with its constituents she responded only to formaldehyde 2 per cent (Simpson, 1969).

St John's
   Between 1968 and 1975, three similar patients were seen, two women and one man. Each had hand eczema.

Paper for weekly journals, cheap pamphlets and advertisements is coated with kaolin, which can be fixed by a urea or melamine formaldehyde resin mixed with starch or casein containing formaldehyde as a preservative or hardening agent. An alternative method of kaolin-fixation is with styrene-butadeine resin which contains no formaldehyde. Kaolin coating is not used for newspapers, better quality books, or glossy magazines. Urea formaldehyde resin is used to make wrapping-paper waterproof.

A woman who worked in a printing office handling weekly journals developed eczema of her face and uncovered arms. Patch tests: she reacted only to formaldehyde. Several samples of the papers were shown to contain formaldehyde (Fregert, 1974).

A maintenance man employed by a daily newspaper suddenly developed an acute eczema on the sides and dorsa of his fingers. Patch tests: he reacted to formaldehyde 2 per cent in water and at two days was positive to blank newsprint but there was no subsequent reading of this latter test. He was negative to all other tests applied. The free formaldehyde content of the newsprint was found to be 0.02 per cent (in the hospital paper towels it was 0.03 per cent) (Black, 1971).

A patient whose formaldehyde allergy plagued her existence was described in detail by Fisher (1976). She reacted to many papers including the paper sheet on Dr Fisher's examination couch and the glossy paper of the first edition of his textbook 'Contact dermatitis'.

A steel foundry worker who made moulds from sand and 'sulfidablaugen', a syrupy mixture made of paper waste, developed widespread dermatitis while doing this particular job. Patch tests: he was positive to formaldehyde. It was ascertained that the 'sulfidablaugen' contained 0.3 per cent formaldenyde (Fabry, 1968).

Renal dialysis units. Formaldehyde solutions (4 per cent and 2 per cent approx.) are used for sterilisation in some renal dialysis units and for home kidney machines. In one such unit (Sneddon, 1968) six out of 13 staff members developed dermatitis of the eyelids, face and hands. Patch tests: four were sensitive to formaldehyde. The dermatitis ceased when formaldehyde was replaced by Portex (alloylamino sulphonic acid with iodine and a surfactant, Alan Glasby Ltd.). In another centre (Abdel-Aziz and Hodgson, 1974) a man who used formaldehyde to sterilise his wife's kidney machine presented with extensive eczema of his hands and arms and patch testing confirmed his sensitivity to formaldehyde. Three cases of formaldehyde dermatitis occurred in the hospital's dialysis unit. For home dialysis an iodophor sterilising solution was substituted for formaldehyde.

St John's

> In 1975 a nurse was seen with an 18 months' history of hand eczema which began while she was working on a renal unit; it cleared when she left that department but subsequently recurred. She wore rubber gloves both at work and at home. Patch tests: she reacted to formaldehyde 2 per cent in water and to thiuram chemicals.

Pathology laboratories. Technicians and others working in pathology and histology laboratories are exposed to formaldehyde as a tissue fixative and sensitisation sometimes occurs.

St John's

> A 58-year-old mortician was investigated because for the 13 years he had worked in a post-mortem room he had had chronic hand eczema, nail dystrophy and some irritation of the face. He wore protective clothing. Patch tests: he was positive to formaldehyde 2 per cent in water, potassium dichromate 0.5 per cent and balsam of Peru 25 per cent, both in petrolatum. His formaldehyde sensitivity was thought to be the main cause of his hand eczema; his dichromate sensitivity had been acquired from occasional cementing at home. A definite source for the balsam of Peru sensitivity was not found. He gave up his pathology work and the skin of his hands became almost normal and his nails began to improve.

Embalming

St John's

> A man who had been an embalmer for 30 years was referred with a chronic lichenified eczema of the hands which sometimes spread to his wrists and arms; it had begun three to four years after starting this work. Patch tests: he reacted to formaldehyde and also to cobalt and balsam of Peru. It was ascertained that the embalming fluid contained a high percentage of formaldehyde; there was no obvious relevance for the other reactions.

Deodorant solution

St John's

> A man who had owned a fish shop for a year was seen with a six weeks' history of hand eczema. He began wearing rubber gloves after the onset. Patch tests: he was positive to formaldehyde 2 per cent in water, thiuram-mix and pentamethylenethiuram disulphide 1 per cent in petrolatum. His formaldehyde sensitivity was traced to a 'miracle' deodorant advertised for fish and meat premises; it contained 40 per cent formaldehyde. His rubber glove sensitivity was superimposed on this initial contact allergy.

Brewery. In some breweries formaldehyde solutions are used as disinfectants for cleansing and storing equipment. A brewer who doused his hands with a 40 per cent formaldehyde solution developed acute eczema of the hands which spread to his arms. Patch tests: he was positive only to formaldehyde 1 per cent in petrolatum. He moved to another brewery where formaldehyde was not used and his skin remained clear (Bandmann, Breit and Mutzeck, 1974).

Mushroom farming. Solutions of formaldehyde are used as a disinfectant in mushroom farming to spray the buildings and clean the boxes. Wilkinson (1970) described a young man who developed hand eczema initially and then an increasing watering and irritation of his eyes when exposed to formaldehyde vapour. Patch tests: he was strongly positive to formaldehyde 2 per cent (aqueous). With adequate protection he was able to remain at work.

Gum arabic, used in adhesives, is preserved with formaldehyde (2 per cent approximately). This source of contact sensitised a lithoprinter and he developed hand eczema. Patch tests: he reacted to the gum arabic, formaldehyde 2 per cent (aqueous) and cobalt. He was negative to 10 per cent and 1 per cent dilutions of gum arabic (Cooke and Wilkinson, 1973).

Oil tanning. A man developed dermatitis of his hands and face after 10 months of using cod-liver oil to tan chamois leather. Patch tests: he reacted to formaldehyde but was negative to the oil. Analysis of the tanning agent confirmed the presence of formaldehyde, probably formed in the oil through (?atmospheric) oxidation (Fregert, 1968).

Rubber manufacture. Trimene base is a dark brown viscous liquid formed by reacting ethyl chloride, formaldehyde and ammonia. It is used as an accelerator in the manufacture of rubber. Contact dermatitis from formaldehyde-ethylamine in Trimene base has been reported by Weiler (1970). Patch tests were positive to formaldehyde-ethylamine 10 per cent but negative to 1 per cent and 0.1 per cent.

Plastics factory. Four women, operating a machine which cut and sealed polythene bags at a high temperature, were exposed to acrolein and formaldehyde fumes which irritated their mucuous membranes and caused dermatitis of exposed skin (Høvding, 1969).

St John's

From 1971–1975, a total of 84 patients (38 men and 46 women) have been seen who reacted to the patch test with 2 per cent aqueous formaldehyde. The sources of sensitisation have been listed below. In about half the men and half the women no relevance for the reaction was found; it is highly likely that many of these responses were irritant, and had the tests been repeated after an interval they would have been negative. (Table 15.12).

Occupational asthma

Formaldehyde is used to sterilise artificial kidney machines and has caused asthma and productive coughs among the staff of a haemodialysis unit and in a young girl similarly exposed to formaldehyde vapour. As with other types of chemically-induced asthma, the response to an inhalation was delayed two to three hours; it sometimes lasted days or weeks and the duration of the response reflected the degree of exposure (Hendrick and Lane, 1977).

Table 15.12 Sources of sensitisation to formaldehyde (St John's 1971–1975).

	Men	Women
Non-occupational		
Clothing resin dermatitis	7	17
Wart cures	2	3
Cosmetics (Dowicil)		1
Occupational		
Pathology	1 (Autopsies)	1 (Histology)
Renal Unit		1
Embalming	1	
Hairdressing	1	1
Duplicating machine	1	1
?Oil ??Grotan	1	
Photography	1	
Deodorising solution	1	
No relevance	22	21
Total	38	46

Patch testing

Formaldehyde is an irritant and too high concentrations used for patch testing give misleading irritant responses; 5 per cent and 4 per cent (Epstein and Maibach, 1966) and 3 per cent (Eberhartinger and Ebner, 1964) have been so reported.

Formaldehyde 2 per cent in water

(with 0.5 per cent–0.6 per cent methyl alcohol to prevent polymerisation)

Occasionally this concentration is a mild irritant causing slight erythema and scaling at two days which has usually gone or greatly diminished by four days.

COMPOUNDS WHICH RELEASE FORMALDEHYDE

PARAFORMALDEHYDE   paraform

$$HO(CH_2O)_nH \qquad n = 8 - 100$$

Formaldehyde has a tendency to polymerise forming paraformaldehyde which is a white solid with a slight smell of formaldehyde. It is used as a bactericide and fungicide and may be present in shoes for this purpose; it is also used as a hardener of gelatin and in the making of resins and adhesives.

A series of 1714 patients were routinely patch tested with paraformaldehyde 5 per cent in petrolatum and formaldehyde 2 per cent in water. Twenty-seven were positive to both chemicals and 13 (0.7 per cent) reacted to paraformaldehyde alone. The causes of these reactions to paraformaldehyde were not discussed (Breit, 1969).

Patch testing
Paraformaldehyde 5 per cent in petrolatum

HEXAMETHYLENETETRAMINE   methenamine, aminoform, hexamine.

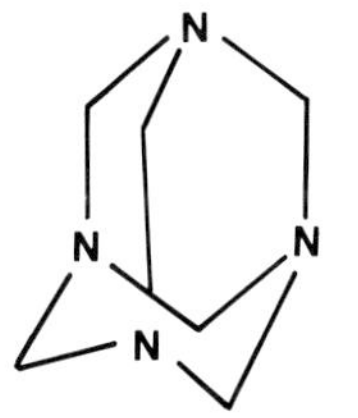

Hexamethylenetetramine, an odourless powder or crystals, liberates formaldehyde. It is used as a urinary antiseptic and occasionally added to dusting powders. In industry it is used in the manufacture of formaldehyde resins, rubber and the explosive cyclonite.

BRONOPOL (p. 695).

CHLOROALLYLHEXAMINIUM CHLORIDE (DOWICIL 200) (p. 695)

Other formaldehyde releasers are:

Methylal=dimethoxymethane=formal;
MDM hydantoin=dantoin MDMH=monomethyloldimethyl hydantoin = 1-hydroxymethyl-5,5-dimethylhydantoin;
Polynoxyline=oxymethylene urea=poly
methylenedi(hydroxy methyl) urea;
Dimethylol urea;
Preventol D1 (Bayer) 1-(3-chloroallyl)-3,5,7-triaza-1-azonia-adamantan-chloride benzylhemiformal;
Preventol D2 (Bayer) benzylhemiformal
Preventol D3 (Bayer) chlormethylacylaminomethanol;
Bakzid (Bacillolfabrik Dr. Bode and Co) cyclical amino-acetal;
Bakzid P cyclical aminoacetal + organic amine salts;
Parmetol K 50 (Schülke & Mayr;) N-methylolchloracetamide+o-formal of benzyl alcohol;
Grtoan BK (p. 846) Germall 115 (p. 703);
KM103 (Gerbstaoff Chemie Fr. Margold) substituted triazine;
Biocide DS 5249=Proxel T (ICI) 1,2-bezoisothiazoline-3-one + formaldehyde releaser   (Dahlquist and Fregert, 1978).

GLUTARALDEHYDE pentanedial

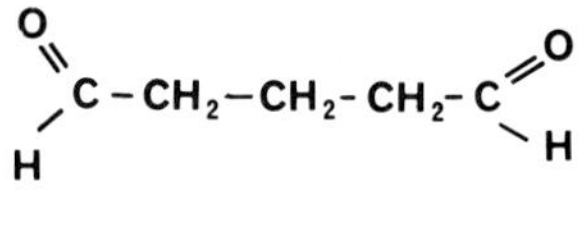

Glutaraldehyde is a moderately irritant dialdehyde which readily polymerises; it is available as 99 per cent, 50 per cent and 25 per cent solutions. It is used as a sterlising solution, tissue fixative, embalming fluid, and for tanning clothing and shoe leather because it enhances the resistance of the hide to sweat. Glutaraldehyde increases the water resistance of wallpaper and hardens photographic gelatin; it is used as an intermediate in the manufacture of resins and dyes, and is prescribed for plantar hyperhidrosis, onychomycosis and warts.

Sensitising potential
Glutaraldehyde is a weak allergen. A liquid fabric softener containing 550 p.p.m. of glutaraldehyde was used to launder cotton T-shirts and they provoked no reaction in 14 glutaraldehyde-sensitive subjects who wore them for two weeks (Weaver and Maibach, 1977). In another usage test, six glutaraldehyde-sensitive subjects applied 25 per cent aqueous glutaraldehyde to their soles twice daily for a week without ill-effect, whereas a 2.5 per cent concentration applied to the antecubital fossae caused a severe dermatitis within two days. It is likely that penetration on the sole is poor because glutaraldehyde binds to keratin (Maibach and Prystowsky, 1977).

Allergic contact dermatitis

Cold sterilising solution. Sensitisation to glutaraldehyde has occurred mainly through its use as a cold sterilising solution in hospitals and dental clinics. Contact dermatitis has been reported in operating theatre staff (Sanderson and Cronin, 1968; Skog, 1968; Harman and O'Grady, 1972), in an assistant in a renal dialysis unit (Neering and van Ketel, 1974), in an inhalation therapy aide (Gordon, 1974) and in dental assistants (Jordan, Dahl and Albert, 1972; Lyon, 1971).

Topical medicament. A man used a glutaraldehyde solution for the hyperhidrosis of his feet and was sensitised, and another man who used a 10 per cent solution to treat a chronic fungus infection of his finger nails developed after six weeks dermatitis of the nail folds (Jordan, Dahl and Albert, 1972).
Clinically the severity of the dermatitis has varied from a mild patchy eczema affecting the dorsa of the hands and fingers to a severe eczematous eruption at the sites of contact.

Leather. Although not sensitised by leather, the five patients described by Jordan, Dahl and Albert (1972) had positive patch tests to chrome and glutaraldehyde tanned glove leather. They were negative to chromate.

Cross-reactions to formaldehyde
Cross-reactions between glutaraldehyde and formaldehyde do not occur. In the case reports referred to above, patch tests with formaldehyde were negative in all the patients except the renal dialysis assistant (Neering and van Ketel, 1974) who was in contact with formaldehyde and glutaraldehyde and on patch testing reacted to both. This point was particularly studied by Maibach (1975) and he

found that 20 patients with positive patch test reactions to 1 per cent aqueous glutaraldehyde were all negative to 2 per cent aqueous formaldehyde.

Patch testing
Glutaraldehyde 1 per cent in water

Oil of turpentine

Turpentine
Turpentine is an oleoresin (oil and rosin) obtained as a yellow, sticky gum from pine trees. It is soluble in organic solvents but not in water.

Oil of turpentine
Oil of turpentine, often loosely called turpentine, is the volatile oily fraction distilled from turpentine and there is one part of this fraction to five parts of the non-volatile residue known as rosin or colophony. In warm climates oil of turpentine is obtained in the summer months by wounding the pine trees, harvesting the exuding tree gum and then by steam or vacuum distillation separating it into its two component parts. The oil of turpentine extracted in this way is known as gum turpentine or balsam oil. In cold climate it is a by-product of the sulphate extraction process in which pine wood is used to make cellulose fibre and then paper pulp. This oil of turpentine is known as sulphate oil or sulphate turpentine.

Terpenes
Plants contain in addition to carbohydrates, proteins and glycerides, essential oils most of which are terpenes and essential oils which are not terpenes such as oils wintergreen, aniseed and mustard. True terpenes (e.g. limonene, pinene and camphene) are unsaturated hydrocarbons with the molecular formula $C_{10}H_{16}$. Most are liquids with a pleasing smell and they are used as flavours and perfumes. Their botanical function is uncertain; they may attract or repel insects or be waste metabolites.

Terpene alcohols, aldehydes and ketones are also widespread and important.

Geraniol $(C_{10}H_{18}O)$ is a straight chain alcohol which occurs in many Indian grasses and as a glucoside in *Pelargonium odorantissimum*.

Citral $(C_{13}H_{21}O)$ is the aldehyde of lemon grass oil.

Citronellol is an alcohol found in rose oil and geranium oil; it is also present in the glandular secretion of the alligator.

Linalool $(C_{10}H_{18}O)$ has many botanical sources.

Differences in structure classify terpenes as acyclic, monocyclic or dicyclic.

Acyclic
Mycerene is found in oil of bay and oil of hops.

Monocyclic

(+) *Limonene* is found in the oils of lemon, neroli, dill, bergamot, orange peel and caraway.

(–) *Limonene* is found in spearmint and pine needles.

Cineole is found in the oils of wormseed, cajeput, eucalyptus and rosemary.

(++) *Phellandrene* is found in the oils of elemi, ginger grass, cinnamon and bitter fennel.

(–) *Phellandrene* is found in the oils of eucalyptus, pimento, Canada balsam and Japanese peppermint.

(+) *Phellandrene* is found in water fennel and lemon.

Carvone is found in the oils of dill and caraway.

(–) *Methone and* (–) *menthol* are found in peppermint oils.

Dicyclic

α *Pinene* is a principal ingredient of oil of turpentine obtained from coniferous trees.

(+) *Camphor* is obtained from camphor laurel.

Camphene occurs in many plants, the (–) form is obtained particularily from the oil of *Abies sibrica*.

Borneol is found in many oils.

(Wilkinson, 1970).

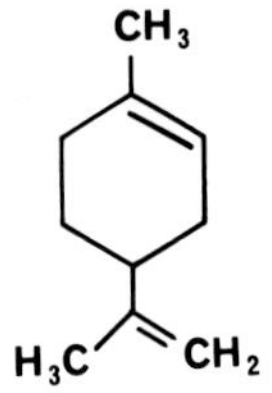

CH₃

H₃C—CH₂

dl-form inactive limonene; Dipentene

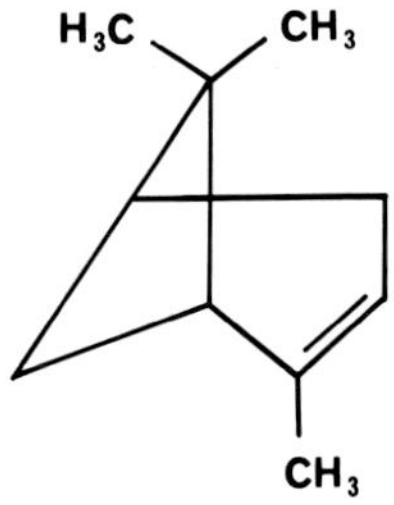

H₃C   CH₃

CH₃

2-Pinene; Pinene; α -pinene

Myrcene

$\triangle^3$-Carene; 3-carene

White spirit
White spirit (turps substitute; mineral turpentine, petroleum spirits, petroleum thinner) is a petroleum product, consisting of a mixture of hydrocarbons with a narrow range of boiling points. It has replaced oil of turpentine as a thinner in paints and varnishes. White spirit and other thinners and solvents such as toluene and methyl ethyl ketone may contain dipentene or α-pinene.

Composition of oil of turpentine
Oil of turpentine consists of a variable mixture of:

α-pinene	(2-pinene)
β-pinene	(nopinene)
$\triangle^3$-carene	(3-carene)
d- and *l*-limonene	(dipentene)

The composition of the oil varies with the botanical species and the geographical source. All turpentines contain high proportions of α-pinene but the amount of $\triangle^3$-carene differs: it is high, 30–40 per cent, in the sulphate oils of Sweden, Finland and Russia but low or negligible in the balsam oils of southern Europe, in the south of France and the U.S.A. A high content of $\triangle^3$-carene is undesirable not only because of its sensitising properties but also commercially because there is as yet no industrial outlet for it.

The composition of various botanical oils of turpentine was given by Brus, Bentejac and Prevot (1968) as follows:

		α-pinene %	β-pinene %	$\triangle^3$-carene %	Camphene %	Mycrène %
Pin maritime	Landes	71.1	26.2	0	0.7	0.7
Pin maritime	Portugal	78.5	17.0	0	1.0	1.0
Pin d'Alep	Greece	96.6	2.2	0	1.2	0
Pin Sylvestre	Russia	63.7	3.1	24.9	0.9	1.1
Pinus longifolia	India	27.3	6.0	60.8	0.3	2.2
Oil of turpentine	China	90.5	5.3	0	1.5	1.0
Oil of turpentine	Mexico	90.0	4.5	2.2	1.7	traces
Oil of turpentine	America	65.3	29.5	0	1.4	0.5
Sulphate oil (paper mills)	France	73.3	21.7	0.8	0.8	0.9
Sulphate oil (paper mills)	Sweden	57.1	6.4	32.1	1.3	traces

Sources of oil of turpentine
Nowadays the major commercial sources of oil of turpentine are Portugal, Spain, Mexico, China and India. For industrial reasons the amounts of gum turpentine produced by France and the U.S.A. have greatly diminished.

Irritancy of the terpenes of oil of turpentine
Fresh unoxidised samples of α-pinene, β-pinene, $\triangle^3$-carene and limonene were tested for irritancy on 28 control patients using the adhesive chamber method (Pirilä, Siltanen and Pirilä, 1964). At concentrations of 70–80 per cent they were each definitely and equally irritant, at 50 per cent weak reactions occurred in some patients and at 20–30 per cent no responses occurred. Oxidation of the four terpenes with the formation of hydroperoxides increased their irritancy. Thus inadvertent or deliberate oxidation of turpentine increases its irritancy and may lead to incorrect interpretation of patch test results (Kirton, 1972).

Allergens in oil of turpentine
Oil of turpentine is not a standard product; its composition and, in parallel, its sensitising potential, varies with its geographic source. The differences in the various oils of turpentine explains why in the Northern Scandinavian countries, Russia and Germany, oil of turpentine has been a significant allergen whereas American oil of turpentine is much less allergenic and sensitisation in the United States is rare. In Finland much work has been done by Pirilä and his colleagues to identify the sensitisers in turpentine and the subject is well reviewed by Pirilä (1970). Unfortunately animals are poor models for the study of turpentine allergy and the major part of the work has had to be done on man. The terpenes themselves are not thought to be sensitisers, but their auto-oxidation products, the hydroperoxides, are allergens, particularly those of $\triangle^3$-carene, which is particularly readily oxidised.

Hydroperoxides of $\triangle^3$-carene (Finnish and Swedish oils of turpentine)
In 1939 Hellerström showed that in painters the greater dermatitic effect of Swedish turpentine, as compared with the French product, was due to the presence of $\triangle^3$-carene in the oil of turpentine made in Sweden and its absence from that made in France. The allergen, an oxidation product in the turpentine, was identified as a hydroperoxide of $\triangle^3$-carene by Hellerström, Thyresson, Blohm and Widmark (1955) and confirmed by Pirilä and Siltanen (1958). In his monograph Rokstad (1946) described patch testing at the Finsen Institute with $\triangle^3$-carene and other fractions of oil of turpentine.

This hydroperoxide of $\triangle^3$-carene is the principal sensitiser in Swedish and Finnish oils of turpentine.

$\triangle^4$-carene (2-carene)
It has been shown that 2-carene also sensitises, possibly through hydroperoxides common to both 2-carene and 3-carene (Pirilä and Pirilä, 1964).

α-pinene (2-pinene) and Limonene
In general, reactions to α-pinene are due to $\triangle^3$-carene, present as an impurity.

However, four patients reacting specifically to α-pinene and one to limonene have been described by Pirilä *et al.* (1969).

Epoxides (German oil of turpentine)
In Berlin 12 patients sensitised to oil of turpentine were found to react to the epoxides: 2,3-epoxipinane, 2,10-epoxipinane, 3,4-epoxipinane and 1,2-epoxi-*p*-menthene, confirming the presence of sensitisers (?in balsam oils) which differ from those in the sulphate oils of Finland and Sweden (Grimm and Gries, 1968).

French oil of turpentine
The reduced allergenicity of French turpentine was demonstrated by Klashka (1975) in West Germany. He tested 18 turpentine-sensitive subjects to turpentines from different countries and found that all 18 reacted to the Finnish turpentine, 17 to the German one, 16 to the American and only 7 to the French turpentine. Sensitisation in France was reviewed by Carbillet(1973).

Sensitising potential
Experimentally turpentine is quite a potent allergen. In the human maximisation test Kligman (1966) sensitised 18 of 25 subjects (Grade 4) using an induction concentration of 50 per cent turpentine and a challenge concentration of 20 per cent. In the guinea pig, 16 of 25 animals were sensitised to turpentine (Grade 3) (Magnusson and Kligman, 1969).

However, the sensitising properties of oils of turpentine will vary with their botanical source.

Incidence of Sensitivity
In the 1950s oil of turpentine was a frequent cause of allergic occupational dermatitis but its gradual withdrawal from general use in many countries led to a sharp decline in the incidence of sensitisation. This occurred in Belgium, where by the 1970s the numbers of cases of turpentine allergy had decreased considerably and by then sensitisation was no longer a problem (Oleffe, 1973). The general rarity of sensitisation (Cronin, 1979) is explained by its replacement by the petroleum product white spirit, its deliberate exclusion from industrial products and the absence of Δ^3-carene from the balsam oils used currently. As it is such an infrequent allergen the International Contact Dermatitis Group no longer include it in their standard patch test series.

Oil of turpentine is irritant, and too strong patch test concentrations may give misleadingly high incidences of sensitisation. In the European series (Fregert *et al.*, 1969) 4825 patients were patch tested with 5 per cent turpentine and 5.2 per cent of the men and 6.4 per cent of the women reacted. However, the reaction was considered relevant in less than half (41 per cent), suggesting that a proportion of these positive responses may have been toxic effects.

St John's
The numbers of patients with positive patch test reactions to oil of turpentine from 1971–1975 are listed below. To avoid the possibility of toxic effects, in 1972 the

patch test concentration of turpentine peroxides was changed from 1 per cent to 0.3 per cent. Immediately the number of positive patch test reactions dropped and the present level 0.7 per cent for the total patients (1.0 per cent for the men and 0.4 per cent for the women) is thought to be a more genuine incidence of sensitisation. Men always have been more frequently sensitised than women (Table 15.13).

Table 15.13. Incidence of patch test reactions to turpentine peroxides (St John's 1971–1975).

	Total			Men			Women		
	Tested	+	%	Tested	+	%	Tested	+	%
1971	1558	49	3.1	707	28	4.0	851	21	2.5
1972	1606	29	1.8	738	15	2.0	868	14	1.6
1973	1546	12	0.8	710	7	1.0	836	5	0.6
1974	1433	10	0.7	655	7	1.1	778	3	0.4
1975	1858	11	0.6	887	9	1.0	971	2	0.2

Sources of contact

Countries differ greatly in the amount and the allergenic properties of the oil of turpentine they produce, the quantity they need to import and the products in which is used. In many countries the replacement of oil of turpentine, which is expensive, by white spirit, which is cheap and effective, has greatly reduced the level of exposure. In East Germany oil of turpentine has been severely restricted in paints, solvents and polishes for shoes and furniture with the specific purpose of reducing occupational dermatitis (Behrbohm, 1966).

In Great Britain in 1976 oil of turpentine and its fractions were imported and used as follows; the quantities stated are approximate:

Oil of turpentine

700 tons/year (with a low Δ^3-carene content)

Pottery industry:

For colours

Polishes:

Furniture and floor polishes are generally made with petroleum solvents; a few may contain oil of turpentine or pine oil. In the U.K. shoe polishes may contain a small quantity of pine oil but are unlikely to be made with oil of turpentine or a terpene; an exception is black shoe polishes, some of which contain a small amount of oil of turpentine. In other countries polishes may be formulated differently.

Paints:

Artists' oil paints contain oil of turpentine and artists use it for cleaning their brushes and palettes. Household paints are generally based on white spirit but a few specialised paints may contain oil of turpentine or α-pinene.

Solvents and thinners for paints,
varnishes and lacquers:

Although predominantly petroleum solvents they may sometimes contain some oil of turpentine or a terpene.

Liniments:

Turpentine liniment B.P. contains 65 per cent oil of turpentine, and white liniment BPC contains 25 per cent; it may also be present in cold remedies, balsams and rubefacients.

α-pinene

2000–2500 tons/year

Synthetic perfumes and fragrances: It is used as a basic raw material.

Synthetic camphor:

α-pinene is the starting material but the final camphor contains none or practically none.

Engine oil additive

Disinfectants:

Chloroxylenol is often formulated with a terpene.

β-pinene

1500 tons/year

Synthetic perfumes
Terpene resins

Reports of sensitisation

Paints

Paints were a former source of oil of turpentine sensitivity but with the substitution of white spirit in industry turpentine allergy has become infrequent, as reported from Belgium by Oleffe (1973) and other countries by Cronin (1979). The hazard does still exist because in a report on causes of allergic occupational dermatitis in Poland turpentine is listed as having caused dermatitis in three house painters (Rudzki, 1976).

An 'epidemic' of turpentine allergy occurred in Limoges among decorators of porcelain when imported oil of turpentine replaced their own innocuous French product. The sensitiser was identified as Δ^3-carene (Benezra, Foussereau and Maleville, 1970).

Paint thinner

A paint mixer in a car factory was sensitised by dipentene, which comprised 40 per cent of a paint thinner (Calnan, 1979b).

Polishes

Shoe. A soldier used his socks to give the final sheen to his boots and developed dermatitis under his socks. The cause was traced to contamination of his socks by α-pinene in the boot polish. Patch tests: he reacted to α-pinene 20 per cent in petrolatum (Hindson, 1969).

Floor

In Belgium, waxes still contain turpentine (Oleffe, 1973) and in Poland dermatitis of the soles of a woman who was sensitive to turpentine was attributed to her walking barefoot on her frequently polished floors. Her feet healed when she desisted, but the presence of turpentine in the polish was not confirmed and she did not develop hand eczema from handling the polish (Rudzki, 1976). A second woman, sensitised by turpentine in floor polish, was included in Rudzki's (1976) list of patients with occupational dermatitis.

Spectacle frame manufacture

A man known to be sensitive to turpentine developed spectacle frame dermatitis. It was traced to a turpentine-beeswax mixture used in the final polishing. Patch tests: he was positive to the turpentine-beeswax polish and a piece of buffed plastic; he was negative to beeswax and unbuffed plastic (Jordan, 1972).

Industrial soaps

In Belgium, special soaps used by mechanics contain turpentine, and cleansers of all types accounted for more than half the cases of sensitisation among a group of 30 patients (Oleffe, 1973).

St John's

From 1971–1975 a total of 66 men and 45 women had a positive patch test reaction to turpentine peroxides. Among the men, 27 had a known source of exposure or they were employed in occupations where contact with turpentine was likely; in 39 no source of contact was elicited. Of the 45 women the exposure was definitely known or supposed in 9 but not in 36.

The source of exposure in these 27 men and 9 women are listed below:

	Men	Women
Printers	6	1
Painters	5	
Shoe repairers (?polishes)	3	
sales	1	
Artists or sculpturers	2	1
Violin maker	1	
Home decorating	7	3
Medicaments	1	1
Sewing leather bags (?polish)		1
Patient aware of sensitivity		
but source not stated	1	2
Total	27	9

Reactions to balsam of Peru and colophony

Among these patients associated reactions to balsam of Peru (25 per cent in petrolatum) and colophony (20 per cent in petrolatum) were not frequent:

+ Turps peroxides	+ B. Peru	+ colophony
111	13 (12%)	16 (14%)

Patch testing
Turpentine peroxides 0.3 per cent in olive oil
α-pinene   15 per cent in olive oil
dipentene   10 per cent in MEK

Alcohols and glycols

Alcohols are a class of organic compounds in which a hydroxyl (–OH) group is common to each member; they are mono-, di- or trihydric according to the number of hydroxyl groups they contain. Alcohols are colourless liquids with a wide range of boiling points. The lower alcohols methyl to butyl (C_1–C_4) are volatile liquids, from C_5–C_{11} they are oily liquids and above C_{12} they are solid.

Alcohols are used as general solvents and as solvents and thinners in paints, lacquers and varnishes; they are added to antifreeze and de-icing mixtures and brake fluids; in pharmaceuticals they are used as antiseptics; in cosmetics as preservatives and solvents; and in foods and beverages they are a considerable asset.

Glycols are dihydric alcohols with properties and uses similar to alcohols.

ETHYL ALCOHOL Alcohol; ethanol. C_2H_5OH

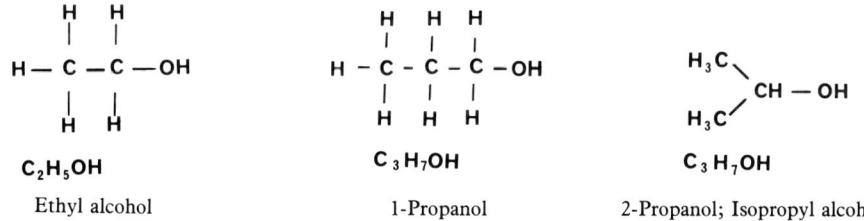

Ethyl alcohol	1-Propanol	2-Propanol; Isopropyl alcohol
C_2H_5OH	C_3H_7OH	C_3H_7OH

Ethyl alcohol is used as a solvent, chemical intermediate, preservative, for its antibacterial and antifungal properties, a cleansing solution and in surface coatings, cosmetics, pharmaceuticals and beverages.

Contact dermatitis
Sensitivity to ethyl alcohol has been described in eight women. In three the exposure was occupational: one, a medical student, developed hand eczema after washing with spirit (Haxthausen, 1944), and two were pathology technicians, one of whom splashed herself with spirit and the sites because eczematous (Martin-Scott, 1960) and the other had an acute bullous hand eczema after contact with alcohol (Fregert et al., 1969). Drinking alcohol caused a flare of the hand eczema in Haxthausen's (1944) patient and it was the presenting symptom in the patient described by Drevets and Seebohm (1961). Two women experienced burning and discomfort of the mouth after drinking alcohol (Fregert et al., 1969). Other patients were detected by reacting to allergens diluted in ethanol (Fregert et al., 1963; 1969) or through a post-operative eruption (Ketel and Tan-Lim, 1975).

Positive patch tests to ethanol confirmed the sensitivity in all these patients. Chromatographically pure undiluted ethanol was used for patch testing by Fregert *et al.* (1963 and 1969) and purified alcohols by Ketel and Tan-Lim (1975) and they gave positive reactions. Vodka, beer and red wine also elicited positive patch tests. The alcohol groups to which these patients were sensitised were investigated in detail and reported in both papers. It was found that patients had positive patch test reactions to the primary alcohols methanol, ethanol, propanol and butanol, but reactions to secondary alcohols were less frequent, and tertiary alcohols gave negative tests. Aldehydes were rarely positive. The doctor described by Haxthausen (1944) was re-investigated by Fregert *et al.* (1969) and was found to be still sensitive to primary alcohols.

Urticaria

A woman whose urticaria was attributed to all sorts of alcoholic drinks from beer to Finnish vodka was reported by Karvonen and Hannuksela (1970). Oral challenges with alcohol and 4 per cent acetic acid were positive; avoiding them stopped the urticaria.

Patch tests

Purified alcohol	100 per cent
Unpurified alcohol	1 per cent and 10 per cent in water

ISOPROPYL ALCOHOL 2-propanol;isopropanol;dimethylcarbinol. C_3H_7OH

$$\begin{array}{c} H_3C \\ \diagdown \\ \diagup \quad CH - OH \\ H_3C \end{array}$$

Isopropyl alcohol is used in the manufacture of acetone, glycerol and isopropyl acetate. It is used as a solvent and in the formulation of perfumes, pharmaceuticals, lacquers and preservatives.

Many of the small pre-packed medical swabs used for cleansing the skin prior to injections contain 70% isopropyl alcohol as the cleansing agent. A woman who developed eczema at the site of an injection and a haemorrhagic bullous eczema of the pulps of the fingers with which she held such a swab was described by Wasilewski (1968). Patch tests: the patient reacted to isopropyl alcohol diluted to 5 per cent, and was negative to the primary alcohols methyl, ethyl, butyl and amyl alcohols 95–99 per cent.

A similar patient, who developed eczema at the site where such a swab was used, was described by Kurwa (1970). Patch tests: the swab itself gave a strongly positive persistent reaction; isopropyl alcohol 20 per cent (aqueous) was positive but 5 per cent (petrolatum) was negative at 5 days. There were also negative reactions to ethyl alcohol 70 per cent (aqueous) and benzyl alcohol 5 per cent (petrolatum). Propylene glycol, another constituent of the swab, was negative (10 per cent aqueous).

Patch tests

Isopropyl alcohol	?10% in water

BENZYL ALCOHOL α-hydroxytoluene, phenylmethanol, phenylcarbinol, C_7H_7OH

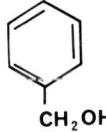

Benzyl alcohol is used as a solvent and in perfumes, flavours, photography, dyestuffs, plastics, inks and pharmaceuticals. As a preservative it is added to allergen extracts and solutions for injections.

Two patients with contact dermatitis, one from a perfume and the other from an after-shave lotion, were found by Fisher (1975) to be sensitised by benzyl alcohol. Both had positive patch tests to benzyl alcohol 1 per cent in petrolatum. Neither had evidence of immediate-type hypersensitivity. Another patient in contact with flavours for drinks reacted on patch testing to benzyl alcohol 0.5 per cent in olive oil; he had previously been sensitised to balsam of Peru (Schultheiss, 1957).

Patch tests
Benzyl alcohol 1 per cent in petrolatum
Patch test reactions need careful interpretation as they may be irritant.

CETYL ALCOHOL alcohol C–16; 1-hexadecanol; $C_{16}H_{33}OH$

$$CH_3(CH_2)_{14} CH_2 OH$$

Cetyl alcohol is a white, waxy solid used widely in cosmetics as an emulsifier and emollient and also in pharmaceuticals. It acts as a foam stabiliser in detergents, is used as a chemical intermediate and may be sprayed on water reservoirs and plants to retard evaporation. It is insoluble in water.

A woman who treated an eczema of her arm with various medicaments developed a widespread dermatitis and on subsequent patch testing reacted to one proprietary medicament. When patch tested with the constituents she was positive to cetyl alcohol 5 per cent and stearyl alcohol 3 per cent, both in petrolatum (Gaul, 1969).

In an investigation of lanolin sensitive patients Sulzberger, Warshaw and Herrmann (1953) patch tested 18 to cetyl alcohol 5 per cent or 1 per cent in olive oil and two were positive.

The possibility that positive patch test reactions to 40 per cent and 20 per cent cetyl alcohol in petrolatum were due to irritant chemical impurities was suggested by Dr K. Burdick and confirmed in a patient investigated by Epstein (1974).

Patch tests
Cetyl alcohol 5 per cent and 1 per cent in petrolatum

STEARYL ALCOHOL 1-octadecanol; octadecyl alcohol; $C_{18}H_{37}OH$

$$CH_3(CH_2)_{16}CH_2OH$$

This solid alcohol, made as whiteflakes or granules, is used in cosmetic and pharmaceutical creams, as a lubricant and antifoam agent and in textile oils and finishes.

An impurity in stearyl alcohol rather than the alcohol itself was thought by Shore and Shelley (1974a) to have sensitised a woman who applied fluocinonide cream containing stearyl alcohol under occlusion. Patch tests: she reacted to commercial stearyl alcohol (containing 6 per cent impurities) 100 per cent and 30 per cent in petrolatum, but when tested with purified stearyl alcohol (1 per cent impurities) she was positive to 100 per cent and negative to 30 per cent in petrolatum. Reactions to propylene glycol 10 per cent in water were interpreted as irritant. On subsequent testing (Shore and Shelley, 1974c) she was negative to 30 per cent oleyl alcohol and 30 per cent panthenol, both 99 per cent pure and both diluted in petrolatum. A suggestion that the positive patch tests had been irritant rather than allergic reactions (Epstein 1974) was not accepted by the authors (Shore and Shelley, 1974b). A very similar case reported by Black (1975) was that of a woman who applied Metosyn (fluocinoide) cream under occulsion and developed a contact dermatitis. Patch tests: she was positive to the cream, and of its constituents she reacted to stearyl alcohol 30 per cent in liquid paraffin. The manufacturers stated that the stearyl alcohol in this base was 93–95 per cent pure.

Five patients sensitised to stearyl alcohol in Topsym ointment were reported by Pevny and Uhlich (1975). Patch tests: each was positive to stearyl alcohol 20 per cent in petrolatum. Sensitisation to stearyl alcohol in medicament bases has also been reported by Gaul (1969) in a patient who reacted on patch testing to 3 per cent stearyl alcohol in petrolatum. Another woman with varicose ulcers and dermatitis was patch tested by Bandmann and Vogel (1970) and was positive to 100 per cent stearyl alcohol and 100 per cent panthenol (the alcohol of pantothenic acid, vitamin B5).

Patch tests
Stearyl alcohol?30 per cent and 10 per cent in petrolatum
Purified Stearyl alcohol ?100 per cent

OLEYL ALCOHOL Octadecenol; Ocenol; $C_{18}H_{35}OH$

$$CH_3(CH_2)_7 CH = CH(CH_2)_7 CH_2OH$$

Oleyl alcohol is an oily liquid used in the manufacture of surfactants, lubricants, papers, printing inks, textiles and sometimes in cosmetics, but rarely in medicaments.

Three women with lipstick cheilitis due to oleyl alcohol in the base were described by Calnan and Sarkany (1960). Patch tests: each reacted to oleyl alcohol 100 per cent and the purer samples appeared to be more allergenic. One patient was also tested with oleyl alcohol 5 per cent in liquid paraffin and was positive. In a letter Fisher (1974) mentions that oleyl alcohol in a dermatological base sensitised quite a few patients and he has found that stearyl and oleyl alcohol sensitisations cause cross-reactions, one with the other.

Patch tests
Oleyl alcohol 100 per cent and 10 per cent in petrolatum

ETHYLENE GLYCOL 1,2-ethanediol

$$HOCH_2 CH_2 OH$$

Ethylene glycol, the simplest glycol, is a colourless, syrupy liquid which is soluble in water and organic solvents. It is hygroscopic. It lowers the freezing point of water and is used in coolant and antifreeze solutions and also as a solvent and in lacquers, inks, stains, resins and adhesives. Ethylene glycol is toxic if ingested.

A case of primary sensitisation to ethylene glycol was reported by Hindson and Ratcliffe (1975) in a woman who was employed cutting glass contact lenses. The lenses, while being shaped with a diamond, were sprayed with a 25 per cent aqueous solution of ethylene glycol to prevent splintering. The woman became wet with the solution above her rubber gloves and it soaked through the front of her clothes. After three months she developed an acute eczema of the arms, chest and abdomen. Patch tests: 5 per cent ethylene glycol in water was positive; ten controls were negative. A steroid base containing 50 per cent fatty alcohol propylene glycol gave a positive patch test and applied to the patient's axilla it caused eczema in two days, suggesting that she had a cross-sensitivity to propylene glycol.

A similar patient reported by Dawson (1976) was a boy aged 17 years who operated a machine which burnished spectacle glass lenses while bathing them with a solution of 33 per cent propylene glycol in water. After 14 months he developed eczema of the hands, wrists, forearms and dorsa of the feet. Patch tests: ethylene glycol 3 per cent in ethanol was strongly positive, but ethylene glycol 1 per cent and 5 per cent in water were negative. Nine controls were tested with ethylene glycol 3 per cent in ethanol and one gave a faint, transient reaction. Dawson suggested that ethanol is a more reliable diluent than water for patch tests.

Patch tests
Ethylene glycol 5 per cent and 1 per cent in water and ethanol

PROPYLENE GLYCOL 1,2-propanediol

$$CH_3CHOH CH_2 OH$$

Propylene glycol is a viscous, colourless, odourless and tasteless hygroscopic liquid which is miscible with water, alcohols and many solvents. It is used as an organic solvent in industry, as a hygroscopic agent, a coolant, a plasticiser and in brake fluids, de-icing compounds and in the synthesis of polyester resins. It also inhibits the growth of moulds and fungi. It has been suggested that propylene glycol acts as a carrier for the cutaneous blanching factor in white soft paraffin (Woodford and Barry, 1974). Propylene glycol has almost replaced glycerin and now is widely used in cosmetics and pharmaceutical bases, and recently topical steroid preparations have been formulated containing about 60 per cent propylene glycol. It is present in some intravenous, intramuscular and oral pharmaceutical preparations, and the food industry uses it as a solvent for colours and flavours, to prevent fermentation and the growth of moulds, and as a humectant and softening compound. Dermatologically it is used to remove scales from skin, which it does by partly denaturing the epidermal proteins and making them more soluble. It also hydrates the stratum corneum by an osmotic effect (Goldsmith, 1978).

Sensitising potential
Propylene glycol has a low sensitising potential. Marzulli and Maibach (1973) failed to sensitise 204 subjects with the Draize procedure using propylene glycol 12 per cent in a cream base for induction and challenge.

Allergic contact dermatitis
Propylene glycol is an irritant when applied under occlusion, as in patch testing, and the difficulty of distinguishing irritant from allergic responses has confused the interpretation of many results. Published reports establish that propylene glycol does very occasionally sensitise but the majority of patch test reactions are irritant.

In 1952 Warshaw and Herrman patch tested patients with undiluted propylene glycol and found that 16 per cent (138/866) reacted; of these, 23 were tested with 10 per cent propylene glycol in water and and 5 were positive. Fifteen women who had positive patch tests to propylene glycol did a usage test with a lipstick containing propylene glycol and only one developed cheilitis, although when patch tested with the lipstick she was negative. They found that the incidence of reactors fell in hot humid weather and rose in dry cold weather. Their conclusion was that the patch test reactions in their patients were more likely to have been irritant than allergic responses.

Patch test reactions to propylene glycol have also been studied by Hannuksela, Pirilä and Salo (1975). They patch tested 1556 cases to glycols and 12.5 per cent were positive to undiluted propylene glycol; on the clinical appearance they interpreted 70 per cent of the reactions as irritant and 30 per cent as allergic. Steroid bases containing 50 per cent and 70 per cent propylene glycol also gave positive patch tests. They confirmed the seasonal variation, there being 17.8 per cent positives in winter compared with 9.2 per cent at other times. They patch tested 42 patients who had reached to undiluted propylene glycol with propylene glycol diluted in water — with the 10 per cent solution 12/42 were positive, with 3.2 per cent 9/42 were positive. They also had two patients who reacted to 2 per cent. An exposure test in 15 patients thought to have an allergic patch test reaction was negative in 11 and positive in 4 of the subjects. They concluded that the majority of patch test reactions to propylene glycol were irritant but that the four patients who reacted to the exposure test were sensitised. In this series 4.9 per cent of the patients reacted to ethylene glycol and 0.3 per cent to polyethylene glycol 400; both glycols were tested undiluted.

Patch test reactions to 38 per cent propylene glycol in water were reported by Huriez, Martin and Vanoverschelde (1966) in 33 leg ulcer patients and five others who had been treated with medicaments containing propylene glycol. However, the significance of these results is doubtful as the concentration of propylene glycol used for patch testing was irritant.

Patients suspected of having become allergic to medicament bases were patch tested with propylene glycol 10 per cent in water by Fisher, Pascher and Kanof (1971). Of 100 tested, two gave eczematous patch test reactions which were thought likely, but not certainly, to be evidence of sensitisation. Positive patch tests to 10 per cent propylene glycol in water were taken as evidence of sensitisation by Pevny and Uhlich (1975) in five of the eight patients who had reacted to Topsym ointment.

Sensitisation to propantheline bromide in a particular deodorant with a 90 per cent propylene glycol base has been reported by Hannuksela (1975) and Ågren-Jonsson and Magnusson (1976). On patch testing to the constituents of the deodorant, two of Hannuksela's (1975) patients also reacted to 2 per cent propylene glycol and another patient (Ågren-Jonsson and Magnusson, 1976) reacted only to propylene glycol (10 per cent, 1 per cent and 0.1 per cent in water). The dilutions to which this patient reacted strongly confirmed her sensitisation to propylene glycol. It was thought that the irritant effect of propylene glycol in the occlusive conditions of the axilla predisposed to sensitisation to the active ingredients.

Ingestion of propylene glycol
Thirty-eight patients considered to have allergic patch test responses to propylene glycol (2 per cent, 10 per cent, 32 per cent or 100 per cent) were challenged orally with propylene glycol 2, 5 or 15 ml in 250 ml of water. Fifteen of the 38 patients developed an exanthem which appeared within 3–16 hours and faded within 1–2 days except in one patient whose reaction was so severe that she required systemic steroids; 20 controls had no reaction (Hannuksela and Förström, 1978). A patient of Fisher's (1978a) with facial dermatitis from propylene glycol in cosmetics developed recurrences which were unexplained until it was found that she was eating propylene glycol in her salad dressing.

Patch tests
Propylene glycol 20 per cent in water.

HEXYLENE GLYCOL 2-methyl-2,4-pentanediol

$$\text{CH}_3 \text{ CH CH}_2 \overset{\overset{\displaystyle \text{CH}_3}{|}}{\underset{\underset{\displaystyle \text{OH}}{|}}{\text{C}}} \text{CH}_3$$
$$\phantom{\text{CH}_3 \text{ CH}}\underset{\text{OH}}{|}$$

Hexylene glycol is used in hydraulic brake fluids, inhibitors of ice formation in carburettors and as an emulsifying agent.

In South Africa an increased incidence of coma and death in a children's burns unit was traced to the use of a proprietary mesh dressing containing 80 per cent hexylene glycol (Procter, 1966).

POLYETHYLENE GLYCOL Carbowaxes (trade name)

$$H\left(O\ CH_2\ CH_2\right)_n OH \qquad n \geqslant 4$$

Polyethylene glycols are condensation polymers of ethylene glycol. As their molecular weight rises from 200 to 6000 they change from viscous liquids to waxy solids. Their numerical designation indicates their approximate molecular weight. These glycols are soluble in water and are also good solvents. They are used as lubricants, plasticisers and bases for medicaments and cosmetics.

Sensitising potential of polyethylene glycol 300

A soap was screened for sensitisation by the Draize test on 200 volunteers (Maibach, 1975). One subject was sensitised and when patch tested with the ingredients of the soap he reacted to polyethylene glycol 300 three per cent in petrolatum. He was also positive to polyethylene glycol 600, 1000, 4000 and 6000, each 3 per cent and 1 per cent in petrolatum. However, an open test with 3 per cent polyethylene glycol 300 in petrolatum, continued for one week, was negative.

Contact dermatitis

Contact dermatitis from the polyethylene glycols is rarely reported.

Two patients who appeared to react to Furacin soluble dressing, and one to other ointments, were investigated by Strauss (1950). Patch tests: both patients reacted to nitrofurazone solution 0.2 per cent and of the ingredients of the base they were positive to polyethylene glycol 400 and carbowaxes ES 1500 and 4000 in dilutions down to 5 per cent (?in water); further reductions in the concentration to 1 per cent, 0.5 per cent and 0.1 per cent gave some positive reactions. Propylene glycol 12 per cent was negative in both patients. These carbowaxes at 30–40 per cent, the highest concentration used for patch testing, were negative in 25 controls. In 1969 Braun reported 40 patients also sensitised by Furacin soluble dressing. Patch tests: positive reactions occurred to Furacin soluble dressing in 40; furacin 0.2 per cent in 37; polyethylene glycol 300 in 12; polyethylene glycol 400 in 5; polyethylene glycol 1500 in 1 and polyethylene glycol 600 in 1 patient. Each glycol was tested at 10 per cent in water. Fisher (1978b) described one patient sensitised by Furacin soluble dressing and another by Furacin solution. Patch tests: both reacted to polyethylene glycol 300 and 400 (as is) and neither reacted to polyethylene glycol 1000 and 4000.

Sellotape made of cellophane (cellulose with approximately 20 per cent polyethylene glycol) and an adhesive caused a reaction in a woman reported by Smith and Meara (1966). Patch tests: she was positive to the plain and adhesive sides of Sellotape, cellophane film and polyethylene glycol 10 per cent in acetone and also to wool alcohols and Elastoplast. The molecular weight of the polyethylene glycol was not stated.

Immediate-type hypersensitivity

Two patients with an immediate reaction to medicaments were reported by Fisher (1978b). One was sensitised by polyethylene glycol 400 and the other by 300 and when rubbed on to normal skin each patient reacted with an urticarial weal.

Patch testing

Polyethylene glycol 300 or 400 undiluted (Fisher, 1978)

GLYCERYL MONOSTEARATE Monostearin; glycerol monostearate

$$\left(C_{17} H_{35} \right) COOCH_2 CHOH CH_2 OH$$

Glyceryl monostearate is a white waxy solid or flakes; the commercial product may also contain glyceryl monopalmitate. Soluble in hot organic solvents, it is used in foods, cosmetics and pharmaceuticals.

One case of sensitisation has been reported by Schwartzberg (1961): this was a woman who developed dermatitis from a cream deodorant. Patch tests: she reacted to the deodorant, and of the constituents was positive only to glyceryl monostearate (?undiluted). Two controls were negative. A series of 1206 patients was tested with synthetic emulsifiers and none reacted to glyceryl monostearate (Hannuksela, Kousa and Pirilä, 1976).

Surfactants, soaps and synthetic detergents

Composition of surfactants

Surfactants, sometimes referred to as tensides or syndets, reduce the surface tension of water and by concentrating at oil water interfaces they emulsify fat and facilitate cleaning. The oldest surfactants are soaps, but in the last 30 years synthetic detergents have been widely developed for use in the home and in industry. Surfactant molecules consist of long, fat-soluble but water-repellent carbon chains (of 10–20 carbon atoms) linked to polar groups with a strong attraction for water.

Soaps and synthetic detergents facilitate the cleansing action of water by:

(i) lowering the surface tension of water and allowing it to penetrate a fabric
(ii) emulsifying oil droplets by surrounding and separating them
(iii) wetting and suspending particles of dirt.

The soil is loosened by mechanical agitation and the suspended dirt, together with the suds, can be rinsed away. The efficiency of these cleansers is influenced by the temperature and hardness of the water, washing time and the mechanical action.

Various additives may be incoporated into soaps and synthetic detergents:
Builders: enhance cleansing by suspending the soil and preventing its redeposition; they may also soften the water, maintain the pH and prevent oxidation of metal. They include sodium sulphate, carbonate or phosphate, sodium tripolyphosphate and sodium carboxymethyl cellulose.

Preservatives: sodium silicate acts as a preservative in soaps. In detergents , it improves the firmness of the granules and prevents corrosion of aluminium. During manufacture formalin is added to lauryl ether sulphate as a preservative and industrial users of this detergent may be unaware of its presence.

Bleach: sodium perborate

Abrasives: increase mechanical removal of dirt

Germicides

Dyes and pigments

Perfumes.

Synthetic detergents may contain:

Proteolytic enzymes

Brighteners or fluorescent compounds

Suds stabilisers: substitute amines

Suds controllers: surface active agents.

Other additives may be used in washing and laundering:

Water softeners: reduce the hardness of water by sequestering calcium and magnesium ions; sodium hexametaphosphate and zeolites (hydrated silicates) are effective softeners.

Fabric softeners: these compounds coat and lubricate textile fibres. They facilitate the movement of the fibres one against the other and by reducing static electricity they prevent the clinging of textiles. The handling and feel of fabrics, particularly of woollens, are improved. Sulphonated oils, used in the past, have been superceded by long chain quaternary ammonium compounds, which now form the basis of all these softeners. One fabric softener, Bounce (Proctor and Gamble), consists of dialkyldimethylammonium methyl sulphate and a fatty acid ester of a polyhydric alcohol; after a series of skin tests and clinical wear tests it was reported to be neither irritating nor sensitising (Weaver, 1976).

A perfume and a preservative are usually included in the formulation.

The chemistry and action of soaps and detergents were reviewed in a symposium on skin cleansing (1965). Factors influencing the irritancy of surfactants have been studied in guinea pigs and rats by Prottey and Ferguson (1975).

SOAPS

Soaps are made from animal or vegetable fat and alkali.

Fatty acid + sodium or potassium hydroxide → a water-soluble soap

Toilet soaps are usually made from palmitic, stearic or oleic acids. The sodium soaps, being hard, are suitable for bars, flakes and powders, whereas the potassium soaps are more soluble and are used for liquid soaps.

The heavy metals aluminium, calcium, magnesium and zinc form soaps but they are insoluble in water. These metallic soaps are used in lubricating greases, polishes, paints and printing inks. In hard water the soluble sodium and potassium soaps precipitate as insoluble calcium and magnesium salts so that soap is wasted and a nasty scum is formed. This undesirable side-effect instigated the development of synthetic detergents, which do not have this reaction.

Dermatitis

The soap compound — irritant
Soaps vary in their irritant effect on the skin. Bettley (1963) demonstrated by closed patch tests and penetration through excised skin that potassium laurate was more irritant than potassium octonate or potassium palmitate. Soaps de-fat the skin to some extent and they tend to make the surface alkaline, but assessment of any damage from normal use is extremely difficult. Suskind (1957) found no deleterious effect from immersing patients' eczematous hands in a solution of a soap or of a detergent. Howeve, the excessive use of soap, detergents or other cleansers by housewives or workers in industry is harmful.

Additives — allergic
Soaps of themselves are not sensitisers, but during their formulation compounds may be added which are allergens; these include germicides, perfume, lanolin and colophony.

Germicides are sometimes added to soaps and the chlorinated phenols, acting as photosensitisers, have been particularly harmful (p. 434).

Perfumes. In Copenhagen 78 (4 per cent) of 1943 consecutive patients reacted on patch testing to the perfumes of two toilet soaps and two detergents. Benzyl salicylate was a sensitiser in two of the perfumes. Allergy to these perfumes was thought to be a factor in the chronicity of the patients' eczema rather than its primary cause (Rothenborg and Hjorth, 1968) (p. 160).

Lanolin. Soaps are made superfatted by leaving unsaponified fat in the soap or by adding lanolin or mineral oil. In fact few soaps contain lanolin and those that do are probably little or no hazard. Soaps containing lanolin or a derivative will not necessarily be so labelled but even so will probably be described as having special moisturising or emollient properties.

Colophony is occasionally added to soaps, and in Great Britain a popular brand of transparent soap contains colophony. A man with eczema of the face, neck and hands due to colophony in a soap was reported by Cooke and Kurwa (1975).

SYNTHETIC DETERGENTS

The discovery that the water-solubility of soap is increased by replacing its carboxyl group by a sulphate or sulphonate group initiated the production of synthetic detergents. The efficient washing action of these compounds in hard and soft water has led to their replacing soap in laundry preparations and many other washing products such as shampoos and dishwashing liquids. Synthetic detergents are classified as:

Anionic: sulphates, e.g. sodium lauryl sulphate, lauryl ether sulphate, sodium lauroyl isothionate.
sulphonates, e.g. sodium dodecylbenzene sulphonate.
Cationic: quaternary ammonium compounds.
Nonionic: ethoxylates.
Amphoteric

Harm arising from the use and manufacture of detergents may be due to the detergent compound.

Additives
enzymes
fluorescent whitening agents (p. 81)
perfumes.

Dermatitis

The detergent compound

Irritant

Excessive exposure
Excessive exposure of the skin to detergents is undoubtedly irritant and both this effect and their absorption can be readily demonstrated in the laboratory under experimental conditions (Prottey and Ferguson, 1975; Howes, 1975). Bathing in a solution of triethanolamine-lauryl sulphate for five successive days caused a reduction in surface free fatty acids and an increase in triglycerides (Gloor, Döring and Kümpel, 1976).

Occupational dermatitis. The effect of prolonged exposure to detergents is clinically exemplified by the hand eczema of junior hairdressers doing many shampoos each day. Their hands may progress from the effects of chapping and dryness to frank and often severe eczema. Once they stop work the skin recovers.

Housewives' dermatitis. In Spain domestic cleaning cloths impregnated with a high concentration of detergent caused a dry fissured eczema of the pulps of the fingers in 52 patients seen by Piñol Aguadé, Grimalt Sancho and Romaguera Sagrera (1972). Patch tests with the detergents gave irritant responses. A change to brushes with handles healed the dermatitis.

Repeated minor exposure
More problematic is the harm done to hands by repeated minor exposures to dilute concentrations of detergents by housewives at home and workers in industry. Bettley, who has done much work on the effects of detergents on the skin has reviewed the evidence for and against the irritancy of detergents (Bettley, 1972).

Industrial hand cleansers

Industrial hand cleansers are often incriminated or at least suspected of causing industrial dermatitis. By their very purpose, which is to remove heavy industrial grease and dirt, it is inevitable that at the same time they will de-fat the skin. However, apart from detergents and soaps they often contain about 20 per cent of hydrocarbon solvents and it is likely that these rather than the surfactants in the formulation, have the greater drying and damaging effect on the skin.

Allergic

Only in the most exceptional circumstances have the detergent compounds lauryl ether sulphate and sodium lauryl sulphate acted as sensitisers.

Lauryl ether sulphate Dodecyl ether sulphate; LES

$$C_{12}H_{25}\text{-O-}(C_2H_4O)^N\text{-SO}_3^- \quad N = 3\text{-}9$$

lauryl ether sulphate $\qquad$ Cation $=$ Na, K or NH_4

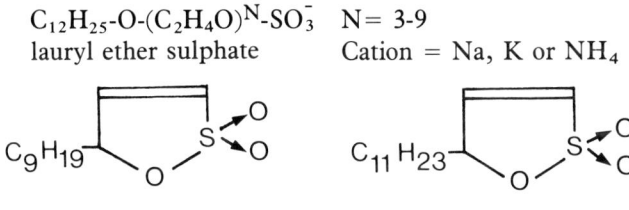

1-dodecene-1,3-sultone $\qquad\qquad$ 1-tetradecene-1-3-sultone

Alkyl ether sulphates (alkyl ethoxy sulphates) are anionic surfactants which have been widely used for years. Compounds with alkyl chains of 12 carbon atoms, called lauryl groups [hence lauryl ether sulphate (LES)] are often used for dishwashing liquids, which contain about 20 per cent LES, and for shampoos and bath foams. Normally LES is completely innocuous; however certain batches manufactured have, through a technical aberration, contained impurities which are potent contact sensitisers. The allergenic Swedish batch LES 13-2035 was shown to sensitise guinea pigs (Magnusson and Gilje, 1973; Walker *et al.*, 1973) and the allergens in this material have now been identified by Connor *et al.* (1975) as:

 unsaturated sultones
 2-chloro-sultones

(1-dodecene-1,3-sultone and 1-tetradecene-1,3-sultone, and tentatively identified were 2-chloro-1,3-dodecanesultone and 2-chloro-1,3-tetradecanesultone). Certain sultones have been shown by Ritz, Connor and Sauter (1975) to be as potent sensitisers, in the guinea pig, as dinitrochlorobenzene (DNCB).

Three outbreaks of contact dermatitis have occurred from allergenic batches of LES, the first in Norway (1966), the second in Sweden (1968) and the third in Denmark (1971).

The most extraordinary episode was that in Norway (Magnusson and Gilje, 1973) where of 200 000–500 000 people exposed, 500–1000 women were affected, the majority being housewives. About two weeks after the first exposure, a severe vesicular dermatitis affected their hands which sometimes spread to the arms and face. Oedema and irritation were striking features and some patients were febrile and ill.

Patch tests:

8/24 were positive to Swedish LES (13-2035) 0.02 per cent
6/24 were positive to Norwegian LES   0.003 per cent
controls were negative.

Higher concentrations of LES gave a greater incidence of reactions in the patients but these concentrations were also irritant as a few of the controls reacted. One patient developed general symptoms within 30 minutes of the patch test being applied, indicating an immediate-type hypersensitivity. It was followed by a flare-up of her dermatitis.

One worker in the Swedish factory making LES 13-2035 developed dermatitis. His sensitisation was confirmed by a positive patch test to 1 per cent LES 13-2035 in water (Magnusson and Gilje, 1973). The Norwegian outbreak has been reviewed by Lindup and Nowell (1978).

In 1971 six out of 12 cleaners in a Danish boarding school developed dermatitis from LES in a liquid detergent cleanser. Patch tests: 5/6 were positive to 5 per cent of the detergent in water (containing 1 per cent LES). Twenty Danish dermatologists then included the allergenic LES in their standard series, and they found that a few patients were positive; some of these gave relevant histories of having reacted acutely to a shampoo or a detergent. It was thought that clinical cases of this sensitivity were undoubtedly missed (Sylvest, Hjorth and Magnusson, 1975).

Patch testing
Lauryl ether sulphate 1 per cent and 0.2 per cent in water or petrolatum

Sodium lauryl sulphate Dodecyl sodium sulphate. SLS

$$NaC_{12}H_{25}SO_4$$

Sodium lauryl sulphate is a surfactant. It is used particularly as a wetting agent in the textile industry and is also added to cosmetics and toiletries, including toothpaste.

During the period 1953–1954 in Sweden there was an outbreak of dermatitis from a particular detergent containing 6 per cent lauryl sulphate. Nilzen (1958) saw 210 cases. Some had eczema of the hands and arms and others a textile dermatitis, particularly of the breasts and buttocks, from underclothes washed in the detergent.

Patch tests: patients were tested and were positive to the detergent 5 per cent (containing 0.3 per cent lauryl sulphate).

In 1958, Nilzen re-tested six affected patients who were then clear and they still reacted to the original detergent and to lauryl sulphate (?concentration). The composition of the detergent was changed and the dermatitis ceased.

A patient of Foussereau, Petitjean and Lantz (1974) with a leg ulcer reacted on patch testing to 5 per cent sodium lauryl sulphate. There was no corresponding history of eczema other than stasis eczema. Prater, Göring and Schubert (1978) used the lymphocyte transformation test to confirm sensitisation in ten patients.

Patch testing
Sodium lauryl sulphate, ?0.5 per cent in water or petrolatum

Tego
Dodicin: There are several Tego preparations designated by name or number; they differ in the chain length of the alkyl radical.
Tego 103 S for hand disinfection

$$CH_3(CH_2)_{11} \, NH(CH_2)_2 \, NH(CH_2)_2 \, NHCH_2 \, COOH$$
dodecyldi(aminoethyl)glycine

Tego 103 G (Tego MHG) for surface disinfection, particularly hospitals and baths. The active components are

$$C_{12}H_{25}\text{-}NHC_2H_4NHC_2H_4\text{-}NHCH_2COOH$$
dodecyldiethylenediaminoglycine

$$C_{12}H_{25}\text{-}NHCH_2CH_2CH_2 \text{-}NHCH_2COOH$$
dodecylaminopropyglycine

Tego compounds are high molecular weight amino acids which combine the detergent action of an anionic compound with the bactericidal properties of a cationic compound. They remain active in the presence of protein but are inactivated by soaps and synthetic detergents (Frisby, 1959). Tegos are used as antiseptics in hospitals, animal laboratories and as general germicidal cleaning agents. Tego 103 G is used particularly for surface disinfection in hospitals and baths.

The first case of sensitisation was reported by Bowers (1968) in an operating theatre nurse who developed dermatitis of exposed sites every time she worked in theatre. Fregert and Dahlquist (1969) then described a woman who was sensitised by a 1 per cent aqueous solution of Tego she was using to disinfect hospital beds.

St John's

Case 1
In 1969 a woman aged 24 years who had worked as an animal technician for six months presented with a four month history of eczema affecting her fingers, neck, around her eyes and behind her knees. She used Tego for cleaning the animals' cages. She was advised to avoid all contact with Tego and when seen six weeks later her skin was normal.

Case 2

A telephone disinfectant containing Tego sensitised a woman telephone cleaner (Calnan, 1974). She developed dermatitis of her hands which spread to her face and neck.

Patch tests: *Tego*

	Concentration			Diluent
	1%	0.1%	0.01%	
Bowers (1968)	+++	+	—	?
Fregert and Dahlquist (1969)	+	—	NT	?
St John's Case 1	++	NT	?	Water
Case 2 (Calnan, 1974)	+	NT	NT	Water

Tego, as identified in these three case reports = dodecylaminoethylglycine hydrochloride.
NT = Not Tested.

Calnan's (1974) patient also reacted to the telephone germicide 1 per cent in water. Twenty controls tested to 1 per cent Tego were negative (Fregert and Dahlquist, 1969).

Patch testing
Tego 1 per cent in water.

ADDITIVES

Enzymes, fluorescent whitening agents (p. 81) and perfumes are possible causes of dermatitis in synthetic detergents.

Enzymes

Hypochlorite bleaches are the oldest method of fading stains, but they harm fabrics and they discolour dyes. Proteolytic enzymes were introduced to remove protein and soil, to improve laundering and to eliminate the necessity for bleaches. The first successful enzyme detergent was marketed in Holland in 1963 and was sold as a pre-soak product for the immersion of clothes prior to washing. Gradually enzymes were developed which were capable of withstanding high temperatures and they could then be added to the detergents used for laundering. Since 1967 enzyme detergents have been sold in Europe and the United States, but adverse publicity has considerably affected their sale particularly in the United States where they are now almost confined to a few soaking products. In the U.K. about a third of the detergents contain enzymes.

There are two types of proteolytic enzyme, subtilisin A and subtilisin B; both are alkaline proteases obtained from fermentation of certain strains of *Bacillus subtilis*. Alcalase is made in Denmark (Novo Industri A/S Copenhagen), Maxatase in Holland (Gist-Brocades): both are derived from particular strains of *Bacillus subtilis* and chemically and biologically they are considered to be identical. These enzymes hydrolyse denatured protein and to some extent native protein, and thus in a washing product they facilitate the cleansing of soiled clothes. The crude commercial material contains only 5–15 per cent of proteolytic enzymes and about 0.08–1.0 per cent of this crude product is added to a laundry detergent and 1.2–5.0 per cent to a pre-soak formulation (Griffith *et al.*, 1969). Protease activity is measured by Anson units, the reference standard being Alcalase with an enzyme activity of 1.5 Anson units (A.U.) per gram on an appropriate protein substrate.

During manufacture the enzyme powder is fixed on to granules of sodium tripolyphosphate, which are then sprayed to make them dust-free. In this encapsulated form the enzyme is added to the detergent. Thus in the final detergent powder the enzyme concentration is low and the dust hazard is reduced to a minimum.

The effect of subtilisin on human stratum corneum was studied by Loomans and Hannon (1970) using the electron microscope. They found that the enzyme digested the cytoplasm of the outermost cells of the stratum corneum and the effect was enhanced by cellular damage but not by a surfactant.

OCCUPATIONAL DISEASE

Skin disease – irritant
Handled in a concentrated form, proteolytic enzymes irritate the skin but they do not sensitise.

Detergent factories. Dermatitis is not a problem in detergent workers provided that contamination of the skin by the enzyme is prevented. At the onset of production in one factory, rashes occurred on the hands particularly on the finger tips from handling drums of Alcalase (Newhouse *et al.*, 1970). Irritant lesions around and under the nails have been caused by the concentrated enzyme and one worker developed haemorrhagic ulcers under the nails (Gothe *et al.*, 1972). Chafing by collars and cuffs may cause irritation (Flindt, 1969; Gothe *et al.*, 1972) and men working in dusty atmospheres have complained of erythema around the edges of their face masks (Newhouse *et al.*, 1970).

Preventative measures have eliminated this skin hazard.

Enzyme factories. Workers making Alcalase are at greater risk but in two Danish factories prophylactic measures reduced the incidence of skin disease from 43 per cent to 21 percent in two years. These employees complained of itching and burning principally of the hands, forearms and face and to a lesser extent of the axillae and groins. Erosions and pustules occurred on the pulps of the fingers. Sweating was important because enzymes are only active in solution. Powdering the skin to keep it dry was an effective safeguard.

Affected workers were patch tested. Initially 18 workers and 12 controls were tested to Alcalase 0.5 per cent, 0.1 per cent and 0.01 per cent in water. Four controls and two workers gave irritant responses to 0.5 per cent; none reacted to 0.05 per cent. Subsequently 61 workers were tested to 0.01 per cent and all were negative (Zachariae, 1973).

In a Budapest research laboratory four workers engaged in the experimental production of proteolytic enzymes developed hyperaemia of the palms and fingers. The skin of their finger tips was thinned and fissured and was tender on pressure (Valer, 1975a).

Pulmonary disease — predominantly allergic
Workers exposed to these enzymes in detergent factories develop a Type I (immediate-type) hypersensitivity with rhinitis, asthma and peripheral lung involvement. These respiratory diseases were first reported by Flindt (1969) and three patients were intensively investigated by Pepys *et al.* (1969). In one factory practically all the workers were prick tested: 57/271 (21 per cent) were positive and of these 42 (74 per cent) had acute pulmonary symptoms. Of the 214 negative reactors 75 (35 per cent) had some chest symptoms. Sensitisation was most prevalent in workers compounding the enzyme complex and in those mixing it with detergent. High titres of IgG antibodies to the protease were present in the sera of those with symptoms and positive skin tests. Atopics were particularly prone to sensitisation (Newhouse *et al.*, 1970). In an American factory 66/238 (27 per cent) were affected; five had rhinitis, 35 had asthma and 26 had both (Slavin and Lewis, 1971). The correlation between symptoms and positive skin tests has been found to be good; serological reactions and passive transfer reactions have also been studied (How and Cambridge, 1971). In Sweden enzyme specific IgE antibodies have been correlated with positive prick tests (Göthe *et al.*, 1972).

Inhalation of dust is the greatest danger to these workers. Dust control, automation, enclosure of operations and improved ventilation has effectively reduced the incidence of disease. Protective clothing, respirators and masks are also essential.

A medical sub-committee has recommended safeguards for workers in the U.K. These include pre-employment screening to exclude atopics and those with chest disease, and, for those employed, a six-monthly review including prick tests (Soaps and Detergent Industry Association, 1971).

HOUSEWIVES

Skin disease — irritant
Evidence that dermatitis is caused by the domestic use of enzyme-containing detergents is meagre. Their effects have been reported from four different aspects:

(i) outbreaks of dermatitis
(ii) effects of domestic exposure and usage tests
(iii) patch tests
(iv) two committee reports.

(i) *Outbreaks of dermatitis*. In England in 1970 three outbreaks of hand dermatitis were attributed to the use of enzyme detergents. Jensen (1970) described 13 adults who developed burning and irritation of the hands within hours to a week of using the product. A secondary spread to light-exposed areas occurred in 10 patients. Chronicity and a failure to respond to treatment were features of the eczema. Patch tests suggested an irritant rather than an allergic mechanism. Another paper reported that at least 12/238 (5 per cent) home helps had developed dermatitis from enzyme detergents (Ducksbury and Dave, 1970). Six had used the detergent only once and within two hours to two days developed an acute blistering dermatitis of the hands. In six the exposure was greater but the dermatitis was less severe. Patch tests with 0.1 per cent detergent in water were negative. One woman relapsed when she used a similar detergent again. Eczema was thought to have been aggravated or precipitated by enzyme detergents in 30 patients seen over six months in a general practice (Bamji and Bamji, 1970).

Similar patients were seen in Cologne; of 42 patch tested with an enzyme detergent 33 were positive (Steigleder, 1970). In Zurich, Wuthrich *et al.* (1971) thought the combination of enzyme and detergent was particularly irritant in eczematous subjects. Two patients with hand eczema were patch tested to protease — one was negative to 10 per cent and the other was positive to 20 per cent.

(ii) *Effects of domestic exposure and usage tests.* The effects of detergents with and without enzymes was assessed by usage tests in 4000 housewives by Mason Bolam *et al.* (1971). They detected no differences in their effects on the skin of the hands, nor was there an adverse reaction in 130 women with already damaged hands. A similar conclusion was reached by Schneider *et al.* (1972). They observed 537 subjects using detergents, with and without enzymes, over a nine-week period, and 72 subjects after immersion tests for five days. They found no evidence that the presence of the enzymes affected tolerance of detergents. However, Wüthrich, Schwarz and Eichenberger-de Beer (1971) were of the opposite opinion and thought that domestic contact with these proteases did cause eczema.

(iii) *Patch tests.* The irritant potential of Tenzyme prilled (Grindstedvoerket, Denmark) and Maxatase (Gist-Brocades, Netherlands) was studied by Valer (1975a) using 0.25–5 per cent aqueous solutions of the enzymes for patch testing. They had no effect on normal or slightly damaged skin but once their penetration was increased by applying them in dimethyl sulfoxide (DMSO), or by stripping the skin, they caused irritation. In his investigations he found no evidence that the enzymes were contact sensitisers (Valer, 1975b). Patch tests applied to skin which was normal, slightly irritated, chemically damaged or stripped, and the enzymes applied in DMSO, all failed to sensitise any of the subjects.

In contrast Gottmann-Lückerath and Steigleder (1972) patch tested 542 patients with 0.15 per cent aqueous solution of Alcalase and Maxatase, and 38 (7 per cent) were positive to one or both enzymes. They also found that one enzyme detergent gave 14 per cent positive patch tests compared with another which gave only 6 per cent of those tested 5 per cent reacted to a detergent without enzymes. Each was tested as 0.5 per cent in acqueous solution.

(iv) *Two committee reports.* A committee in the United States undertook a detailed study on behalf of the National Academy of Sciences (1971) to determine if there was evidence that the use of enzymes in detergents was harmful. As regards domestic use they found no evidence that the average enzyme detergent caused more irritation of the skin than a similar product without enzymes.

To assess whether a problem of dermatitis from enzyme detergents existed in Great Britain and to estimate its extent, dermatologists were asked to send the details of such cases, seen over six months, to an advisory group of dermatologists. In all, 41 cases were reported: in none was it established that the enzyme in the detergent was solely reponsible. It was concluded that although some cases of dermatitis could be attributed to enzyme detergents, the incidence was small in relation to their use (C.M.O. Notes, 1972).

St John's

The incidence of cases in which dermatitis from enzyme detergents was suspected has not been recorded. A purpuric eruption in one man was attributed to his clothes having been washed with an enzyme detergent (Calnan, 1967).

Pulmonary disease — allergic

Encapsulation of the enzyme greatly reduced the dust hazard and its low concentration in the detergent probably explains the sparcity of cases of sensitisation among housewives.

In the early days the enzyme was added to the detergent in powder form and the mixture was dusty. It was in this initial period that Belin *et al.* (1970) from Sweden described pulmonary symptoms in one housewife, secretion from the eyes and nose in another, and irritation in the eyes of a third woman. Prick tests to the enzyme were positive and circulating IgE antibodies to the enzyme were demonstrated in each patient. In the report of the National Academy of Sciences (1971) on Enzyme-Containing Laundering Compounds and Consumer Health there were another five cases of pulmonary sensitisation personally reported to the committee. Four had responded to bronchial challenge and their serum gave positive passive transfer tests. Another eight cases of respiratory allergy among consumers have been reported by Rosemeyer and Wüthrick (1974).

Perfumes

Nearly 2000 eczematous patients in Copenhagen were screened by patch testing for sensitivity to two detergent and two soap perfumes. They were applied as 2.5–5 per cent dilutions in petrolatum and 78 (4 per cent) reacted to one or more of the tests. Benzyl salicylate was the main sensitiser in one of the detergent perfumes (Rothenborg and Hjorth, 1968).

Fluorescent whitening agents (p. 81)

Matches

Contact dermatitis occurs from phosphorus sesquisulphide and very occasionally from potassium dichromate in match heads and many years ago it was described from phosphorus sesquisulphide in the striking surface of match boxes.

PHOSPHORUS SEQUISULPHIDE ($P_4 S_3$)
(Tetraphosphorus trisulphide)

Match boxes

Fifty years ago cases were described in America, Denmark and Germany of dermatitis from phosphorus sesquisulphide in the striking surfaces of match boxes containing safety matches. These case reports were reviewed by Klaber (1938) who explained that the condition did not occur in Britain because phosphorus sesquisulphide was not used in match boxes. Ive (1967) in his review of the literature included Esteves̀ (1943) report from Portugal of an epidemic of match box dermatitis due to phosphorus sesquisulphide.

In the United States Foerster (1923) reported a further patient with dermatitis from a match box but also described 6 patients who had acquired the dermatitis from the heads of strike anywhere matches. He observed that the clinical picture was the same whatever the source of the allergen. An Italian patient with contact dermatitis of the thighs from an unknown allergen in a match box developed, at the eczematous sites, hypopigmentation which was still present 3 months later although the eczema had healed (Meneghini and Angelini, 1975).

In Spain two men sensitised by the striking surfaces of match boxes developed thick indurated plaques, first on the thighs then on the face and other sites, which fluctuated in severity and were initially diagnosed clinically and histologically as mycosis fungoides. Another two men had patches confined to the thighs. Patch tests: the four men were positive to the striking surface of a match box. The allergen was not identified, but they were not tested with match heads or with phosphorus sesquisulphide (Gómez Orbaneja et al., 1976).

Strike anywhere match heads

Strike anywhere matches ignite readily if struck on an abrasive surface, and although safety matches are also lit by frictional heat, the temperature necessary is higher. British standards require: (i) that safety matches cannot be struck on grade 00 glass paper, and (ii) that the ignition temperature for safety matches must exceed 170°C and for strike anywhere match heads it must exceed 140°C.

Although one popular brand of strike anywhere matches (Swan Vestas) sold in the U.K. and Ireland is red-headed it is erroneous to use the terms red-headed and strike anywhere synonymously as other manufacturers use different colours for these matches and safety match heads may be red. Strike anywhere matches are sold only in boxes, whereas book matches are always safety matches because of the danger of ignition by friction.

This type of match is popular in the north of England, in Scotland and in both Northern and Southern Ireland. They are also sold in the U.S.A. and Canada but only to a limited extent as safety matches, book matches and cigarette lighters are preferred. They are made in Sweden for export but they are not marketed in the Scandanavian countries or other countries of Western Europe. Although advertised as the pipe-smoker's match they are also used by non-pipe-smokers.

The igniting chemical, present in the match head, is phosphorus sesquisulphide. The composition of a typical match head is as follows:

Phosphorus sesquisulphide 10 per cent
Potassium chlorate
Powdered glass
Zinc oxide
Animal glue
Eosin or Rhodamine dye (Ive, 1967).

The striking surface on the box contains:

Sand
Urea formaldehyde resin.

Allergic contact dermatitis

Contact dermatitis from phosphorus sesquisulphide in strike anywhere match heads was reported from the United States by Foerster (1923). He described 6 patients; they were not patch tested but each one recovered on avoiding contact with these matches. In Canada, Burgess and Forsey (1951) reported a man and a woman with facial eczema both of whom had positive patch tests to match heads and in Britain, Klaber (1938) recorded the sequence of events which led him to recognise his own sensitivity.

St John's

In 1967, Ive described 7 patients (5 men and 2 women) all but one of whom had been investigated at St John's. One of the men with eczema of the eyes and face did not use strike anywhere matches himself but had been sensitised at work by a neighbouring clerk who used them frequently to light his pipe. This man refused to change his matches so that patient changed his job and his eczema cleared. Patch tests: 6 patients were tested with phosphorus sesquisulphide 1 per cent in petrolatum and each was positive; one patient, not tested with this chemical, reacted to the match head.

Contact dermatitis to phosphorus sesquisulphide continues and is important, because, it is nearly always the entire cause of the presenting dermatitis. This allergen is not included in our routine series so that clinical recognition, prior to patch testing, is essential for the appropriate tests to be applied. Once the clinical picture is familiar it is an easy spot diagnosis. In this clinic it is practically always caused by one popular brand of red-headed strike anywhere matches (Swan Vestas).

From 1968–1976, 3–10 men and 0–3 women have been seen each year with this contact dermatitis (Table 15.15).

Table 15.15. Numbers of patients with contact dermatitis from phosphorus sesquisulphide seen at St John's (1967–1976).

	1967	1968	1969	1970	1971	1972	1973	1974	1975	1976
Men	1	7	3	5	4	4	5	3	7	10
Women	0	1	0	0	1	2	1	1	3	2

Clinical features

This dermatitis occurs predominantly in men and it is distinguished by the following features:

(i) it is acute and episodic
(ii) it affects the eyes and face, particularly the left side
(iii) it affects the thighs
(iv) it may involve the hands.

This tendency for the dermatitis to be on the left side is also apparent in the case reports in the literature. It is probably explained by the majority of patients being right handed and lighting their pipe or cigarette on the left side of their mouth so that the left side of the face has the greatest exposure to the match head fumes.

The ages of the 60 patients seen at St John's from 1967 to 1976 varied from 22–75 years. Men were predominantly affected, there being 49 men and 11 women. The length of history was generally 2–3 months but in some it was as short as one month or as long as 6 years.

The dermatitis affected the face, thighs and hands, and the pattern was the same in men and women, except that in women the thighs were not involved.

Face

The usual history was that of a well man who suddenly developed an acute oedematous eczema of the face. In a quarter of the patients (16 of 54), who had their face, ears or neck affected, the eruption began or remained worse on the left side. The face was involved in most patients (52 of 60), the eyelids being particularly vulnerable. Redness, swelling, irritation and scaling of the eyelids were often the presenting symptoms. In 6 patients the left eye was the only one involved and in one patient the right eye. In association with dermatitis of the face, the pinnae and the neck may be eczematous.

The history of this facial eczema was often episodic, definite attacks being recorded in 26 of the 60 patients.

One woman's facial eczema appeared to be due to the use of strike anywhere matches by her colleagues at work. She avoided these smokers and her face cleared.

Thighs

Large patches of eczema occurred on the fronts of the thighs in half the men (26 of 49). In 5 men one or both thighs were the only sites affected and in one patient the eczema was followed by post inflammatory depigmentation of the thigh.

Hands

Although patients did not present with hand eczema as their principal symptom, the hands were involved in one third (21 of 60). The web spaces, the sides of the fingers and the palms were affected. The palms become involved by contact with the contaminated striking surface of the match box while holding the box to light a match.

Other sites
One patient was seen with a patch of eczema on his left breast which corresponded with the pocket of his shirt in which he carried his box of matches. Another patient in addition to the conventional sites had widespread involvement of his abdomen.

In the 28 patients in whom the information was recorded, 18 smoked cigarettes, 8 were pipe smokers and 2 smoked cigars.

Patch testing
Each of the 60 patients was tested with phosphorus sesquisulphide 1 per cent in petrolatum and each was positive. Forty-three were tested with the crushed strike anywhere red match head and all reacted.

A true allergic response to phosphorus sesquisulphide is nearly always raised, red and oedematous; it may blister and can be severe enough to cause a spread of eczema well beyond the patch test site. To avoid these severe reactions, when this diagnosis is strongly suspected, a weaker dilution (0.1 per cent) should be used initially and only if negative should the stronger concentration be applied.

Phosphorus sesquisulphide is an unstable substance and after a time in petrolatum it breaks down to release small amounts of phosphorus acid which is then oxidised to phosphoric acid. This makes the chemical test substance a mild irritant and patients to whom it is applied often give a slight erythema which is a toxic effect and does not indicate sensitisation. This irritant effect does not apply to the match head because any phosphoric acid produced from its phosphorus sesquisulphide is neutralised by the zinc oxide it contains and the pH of the match head is thus maintained constant.

Active sensitisation
Sensitisation by patch testing with phosphorus sesquisulphide 1 per cent in petrolatum occurred in one of the patients reported by Ive (1967). In 1973, another patient who had no contact with matches was possibly sensitised. She reacted weakly to phosphorus sesquisulphide 1 per cent in petrolatum at 4 days and had a definite reaction at 10 days, but the patch tests were not repeated and so sensitisation was not confirmed.

Recommended for patch testing
Phosphorus sesquisulphide 1 per cent in petrolatum
Phosphorus sesquisulphide 0.1 per cent in petrolatum
Crushed strike anywhere match head

Otitis externa
It is not unusual for patients to use match heads for cleaning or scratching their ears, and otitis externa caused by a contact dermatitis from a strike anywhere match head was reported in one man by McKelvie and McKelvie (1966).

St. John's
    In Ive's (1967) series one man and one woman had dermatitis of their ears. A

further 3 patients were seen in 1976; 2 presented with facial eczema and described previous otitis externa from strike anywhere matches. The third man had an existing eczema of the ears which was attributed to cleaning his ears with matches; he had eczema elsewhere which was not considered to be related to his matches.

POTASSIUM DICHROMATE

Safety matches
Safety matches are so named because they can only be ignited by being struck on the abrasive surface of a match box.

The composition of these matches is as follows:

Match Head:
Potassium chlorate	40–60 per cent
Hide glue	10–12 per cent
Starch	1– 3 per cent
Zinc oxide	½ per cent
Sulphur	3– 6 per cent
Infusorial earth	3– 8 per cent
Ground glass, silica and flint	20–30 per cent
Potassium dichromate	¼–½ per cent
Dye	¼–½ per cent

Striking Surface
Glue	15–20 per cent
Red phosphorus	40–60 per cent
Abrasive	20–40 per cent

(Siedlecki, 1966).

Potassium dichromate is only present in a ¼–½ per cent concentration in a safety match head and this small quantity does not seem to elicit the explosive dermatitis caused by phosphorus sesquisulphide.

Otitis externa
In 1962 Fregert reported that 9 of 62 patients with otitis externa used the head ends of safety matches for cleaning their ears and of these 7 were positive to 0.5 per cent potassium dichromate. Six were followed up; 2 had healed, 3 had only minimal irritation and one who had not recovered was exposed to cement. A further case, reported by McKelvie and McKelvie (1966), was a surveyor who worked in contact with cement.

Hand eczema
The burnt heads of safety matches are very friable and if returned to a pocket the head is easily crushed and chromate contamination of the pocket occurs. Fregert (1961) found this contact to be one cause of the chronicity of hand eczema in chromate sensitive patients.

Tattoos

The practice of decorative tattooing has been examined in detail by Scutt and Gotch (1974). They list the following colours as now being used in tattoos:

Colour	Common (probably harmless)	Rare (potentially sensitising)
Black	Carbon (charcoal suspended in ammoniacal solution containing phenol) e.g. black waterproof ink	Logwood (containing chrome)
Red	Scarlet lake (organic pigment) Carmine (dried insect bodies) Cochinilla	Cinnabar, Vermillion (mercuric sulphide) Cadmium red (selenide)
Brown	Venetian Red (hydrate of ferric oxide)	Cadmium salts
Yellow	Yellow ochre (hydrate of ferric oxide)	Cadmium sulphide Chrome zinc and lemon yellow (chrome salts)
Green	Chlorinated copper phthalocyanine	Viridian, emerald green (Chromium sesquioxide)
Blue	Copper phthalocyanine	Cobalt aluminate
White	Titanium white (titanium oxide) Zinc white (zinc oxide)	Flake white (lead carbonate)

(Scutt and Gotch, 1974)

In general tattoos are inert and the reason for removal is usually cosmetic, not medical. Only rarely do these pigments excite an inflammatory response and sometimes the reaction occurs in a tattoo that has been dormant for several years. Suddenly the area becomes swollen red and uncomfortable with itching and scaling of the skin and occasionally superficial erosions and crust formation. One or several of the colours may be inflamed. In some cases the reaction is due to the development of sensitivity to one of the pigments and patch tests with the appropriate allergens are positive. In others the reaction is a foreign body type of granuloma with sarcoidal features, and as this response is less likely to be associated with sensitisation, patch tests in these patients are more often negative. Tattoos sometimes become inflamed for no obvious reason and settle spontaneously without treatment (Scutt, 1972).

Allergic reactions

Red

Cinnabar (mercuric sulphide) may be used to produce the red colours in tattoos and is the pigment most frequently reported as causing dermatitis.

A man who developed dermatitis from mercury in kerosene was tattooed a few months later and had an immediate reaction to the red mercury pigment and a flare and spread of his previous eczema. Patch tests: he reacted to 0.5 per cent mercury metal in petrolatum (Fregert, 1975). Another man who had a localised and then a generalised eczema from sensitisation to mercury in a tattoo was reported by Biro and Klein (1967). Patch tests: he reacted strongly to 5 per cent ammoniated mercury cream. A young man tattooed himself with cinnabar and fourteen months later developed reactions at the sites and also ulceration of the buccal mucosae from amalgam fillings. Patch tests: he reacted to amalgam, mercuric chloride 0.025 per cent in water, and 50 per cent cinnabar in petrolatum but he was negative to pure cinnabar (Juhlin and Öhman, 1969). Two other patients, one with an allergic reaction and the other with a sarcoidal granuloma to mercury in red tattoos, were investigated by Sulzberger and Tolmach (1959). The electron microscope appearances of mercuric sulphide, present in the skin for ten years, were studied by Silberberg and Leider (1970).

A granulomatous reaction with the features of lichen planus was described by Taaffe, Knight and Marks (1978) in four men, only one of whom was sensitive to mercury. Three of the men and possibly the fourth had been tattooed by the same man. No mercury was found in the pigment he supplied for analysis. Four more cases have been described, each with a red mercury tattoo, only one of whom was sensitive to mercury and his positive patch tests did not become lichenoid (Clarke and Black, 1979; Winkelmann and Harris, 1979).

Green

Several green colours are used by tattooists including the trivalent chromic oxide (CR_2O_3; chrome green; Casalis green) chromic hydrate ($CR_2O(OH)_4$) and hydrated chromium sesquioxide (Guignet's green). Allergy to these green stains is rare.

Three cases, two of whom had cement eczema, were reported by Björnberg (1969); another two men with cement dermatitis and inflammation of their green tattoos were investigated by Cairns and Calnan (1962), and this combination also occurred in a patient of Lowenthal's (1960). In each of these patients the cement dermatitis preceded the tattoo reaction and each had a positive patch test to dichromate. Cairns and Calnan (1962) suggested that oxidation of the trivalent chromium occurs in the tissues to produce the sensitising hexavalent form.

Blue

Light blue tattoo markings are produced by cobalt blue (azure blue, cobaltous aluminate, $CoOAl_2O_3$) or indigo (Björnberg, 1961).

A man whose tattoo healed except for the blue sites was investigated seven months later and found to have developed a tuberculous granuloma in these inflamed areas and cobalt was demonstrated in the altered skin. Patch tests: he reacted to cobalt chloride 2 per cent in water (Björnberg, 1961). A further three patients had granulomatous reactions to their light blue tattoos and each had an associated uveitis. Patch tests: two of the three reacted to cobalt chloride 2 per cent in petrolatum (Rorsman et al, 1969). Another patient with hand eczema who developed nodules in the light blue part of his tattoo, was found on patch testing to react to potassium dichromate 0.5 per cent and cobalt chloride 2 per cent, both in water. However although chromium could be demonstrated in the tattoo no cobalt could be found (Tazelaar, 1970).

Yellow

Yellow tattoos are produced by cadmium sulfide, ochre or curcurma yellow.

Cadmium sulphide has marked photoconducting properties and tattoos with this pigment swell when exposed to wavelengths of 380 to 450 nm. Yellow is used in the Swedish flag and this is a popular design among Swedish sailors. In Sweden of 24 men with yellow tattoos 18 noticed swelling of this colour in sunlight and 4 had observed a similar change in the red areas (Björnberg, 1963). This author demonstrated the reaction in his own skin; a photopatch test was negative and he considered the effect to be phototoxic. Nguyen and Allen (1979) tried to reproduce this effect, noticed by a sailor in his yellow tattoo, but experimental exposure of this tattoo to longwave ultraviolet light was unsuccessful.

Purple

Manganese is used for a purple colour.

Swelling and itching in a purple tattoo was attributed to manganese by Nguyen and Allen (1979); the patient was not patch tested.

References

Abdel-Aziz, A.H.M. & Hodgson, C. (1974) Formalin dermatitis in a renal dialysis unit. *Contact Dermatitis Newsletter*, **15**, 441.

Ågren-Jonsson, S. and Magnusson, B. (1976) Sensitisation to propantheline bromide, trichlorocarbanilide and propylene glycol in an antiperspirant. *Contact Dermatitis*, **2**, 79.

Agrup, G. (1969) Hand eczema and other hand dermatoses in South Sweden. *Acta Dermatovenereologica*, **49**, Supplementum 61, 54.

Bamji, E. and Bamji, N. (1970) Severe dermatitis and 'biological' detergents. *British Medical Journal*, **1**, 629.

Bandmann, H.-J. & Bandmann, M. (1968) Eucerin. *Contact Dermatitis Newsletter*, **4**, 78.

Bandmann, H.-J., Breit, R. & Mutzeck, E. (1974) Allergic contact dermatitis from formaldehyde in a brewer. *Contact Dermatitis Newsletter*, **15**, 452.

Bandmann, H.-J. and Vogel, P. (1970) Stearyl alcohol and Panthenol sensitivity. *Contact Dermatitis Newsletter*, **8**, 187.

Behrbohm, P. (1966) Arbeitshygienische Massnahmen zur Verhütung des Terpentinölekzems. *Allergie und Asthma*, **12**, 175.

Belin, L. Falsen, E., Hoborn, J. & André, J. (1970) Enzyme sensitisation in consumers of enzyme-containing washing powders. *Lancet*, **2**, 1153.

Benezra, C., Foussereau, J. & Maleville, J. (1970) L'identification chimique des allergénes végétaux et son intéret dans la prevention de nombreux eczémas allergiques professionels. *Archives de Maladies Professionnelles de Médecine du Travail et de Securité Sociale*, **31**, 539.

Bettley, F.R. (1963) The irritant effect of soap in relation to epidermal permeability. *British Journal of Dermatology*, **75**, 113.

Bettley, F.R. (1972) The irritant effect of detergents. *Transactions of the St John's Hospital Dermatological Society*, **58**, 65.

Beukelaar, de, L. (1968) Allergic reactions to wool fat alcohols. *Dermatologica*, **136**, 434.

Biro, L. & Klein, W.P. (1967) Unusual complications of mercurial (cinnabar) tattoo. *Archives of Dermatology*, **96**, 165.

Björnberg, A. (1959) Allergic reactions to chrome in green tattoo markings. *Acta Dermatovenereologica*, **39**, 23.

Björnberg, A. (1961) Allergic reaction to cobalt in light blue tattoo markings. *Acta Dermatovenereologica*, **41**, 259.

Björnberg, A. (1963) Reactions to light in yellow tattoos from cadmium sulfide. *Archives of Dermatology*, **88**, 267.

Black, H. (1971) Contact dermatitis from formaldehyde in newsprint. *Contact Dermatitis Newsletter*, **10**, 242.

Black, H. (1972) *Contact Dermatitis Newsletter*, **12**, 323.

Black, H. (1975) Contact dermatitis from stearyl alcohol in Metosyn (flucinonide) cream. *Contact Dermatitis*, **1**, 125.

Bork, K., Heise, D. & Rosinus, A. (1979) Formaldehyde in harshampoos. Dermatosen In *Beruf Und Umwelt*, **27**, 10.

Bowers, R.E. (1968) Tego (dodecylic aminoethyl glycine hydrochloride). *Contact Dermatitis Newsletter*, **4**, 76.

Braun, W. (1969) Kontaktallergen gegen Polyaethylenglykole. *Zeitschrift für Haut und Geschlechts-Krankheiten*, **44**, 385.

Breit, R. (1968) Kolophonium-Kontaktallergie bei einem Baggerführer. *Berufsdermatosen*, **16**, 161.

Breit, R. (1969) Formaldehyde and paraformaldehyde. *Contact Dermatitis Newsletter*, 5, 94.

Breit, R. (1972) Medikamentöse Kontaktallergie beim Ekzem und Geschwür des Unterschenkels. *Münchener medizinische Wochenschrift*, **114**, 22.

Breit, R. & Bandmann, H.-J. (1973) Contact dermatitis XXII. Dermatitis from lanolin. *British Journal of Dermatology*, **88**, 414.

Brus, G., Bentejac, R. & Prevot, F. (1968) Analyse par chromatographie en phase gazeuse des produits Résineux. *Annales des falsification et de l'expertise chimique*, **61**, 233.

Burge, P.S., Green, M. & Pepys, J. (1977) Occupational asthma due to sensitivity to colophony (pine resin). *American Review of Respiratory Diseases*, **115**, no. 4, part 2, 203.

Burge, P.S., Harries, M.G., O'Brien, I.M. & Pepys, J. (1978) Respiratory disease in workers exposed to solder flux fumes containing colophony (pine resin). *Clinical Allergy*, **8**, 1.

Burgess, J.F. & Forsey, R.B. (1951) Contact dermatitis of the face due to matches. *Archives of Dermatology*, **64**, 636.

Burry, J.N., Kirk, J. Reid, J.G. & Turner, T. (1973) Environmental dermatitis: Patch test in 1000 cases of allergic contact dermatitis. *Medical Journal of Australia*, **2**, 681.

Cairns, R.J. & Calnan, C.D. (1962) Green tattoo reactions associated with cement dermatitis. *British Journal of Dermatology*, **74**, 288.

Calnan, C.D. (1967) Detergents with proteolytic enzymes. *Contact Dermatitis Newsletter*, **1**, 9.

Calnan, C.D. (1972) Colophony dermatitis from insulated tools. *Contact Dermatitis Newsletter*, **11**, 281.

Calnan, C.D. (1974) Tego dermatitis (telephone cleaner). *Contact Dermatitis Newsletter*, **15**, 439.

Calnan, C.D. (1978) Diethyldithiocarbamate in adhesive tape. *Contact Dermatitis*, **4**, 61.

Calnan, C.D. (1979a) Lanolin in protective metal coatings. *Contact Dermatitis*, **5**, 267.

Calnan, C.D. (1979b) Allergy to dipentene in paint thinner. *Contact Dermatitis*, **5**, 123.

Calnan, C.D. & Sarkany, I. (1960) Studies in contact dermatitis: XII. Sensitivity to oleyl alcohol. *Transactions of the St. John's Hospital Dermatological Society*, **44**, 47.

Carbillet, F. (1973) Les allergie a l'essence de térébenthine et a la colophane. These, Université Louis Pasteur, Faculté de Médecine de Strasbourg, No. 71.

Clark, E.W., Cronin, E. & Wilkinson, D.S. (1977) Lanolin with reduced sensitising potential. *Contact Dermatitis*, **3**, 69.

Clarke, J. & Black, M.M. (1979) Lichenoid tattoo reactions. *British Journal of Dermatology*, **100**, 451.

C.M.O. Notes (1972) Enzyme detergents. *Health Trends*, **4**, 21.

Connor, D.S., Ritz, H.L., Ampulski, R.S., Kowollik, H.G., Lim, P., Thomas, D.W. & Parkhurst, R. (1975) Identification of certain sultones as the sensitisers in an alkyl ethoxy sulfate. *Fette-seifen-anstrichmittel*, **77**, 25.

Cooke, M.A. & Kurwa, A.R. (1975) Colophony sensitivity. *Contact Dermatitis*, **1**, 192.

Cooke, M.A. & Wilkinson, J.F. (1973) Formalin sensitivity in gum arabic. *Contact Dermatitis Newsletter*, **13**, 379.

Cronin, E. (1966) Lanolin dermatitis. *British Journal of Dermatology*, **78**, 167.

Cronin, E. (1972) Sensitivity to zinc diethyldithiocarbamate. *Contact Dermatitis Newsletter*, **11**, 286.

Cronin, E. (1972) Clinical prediction of patch test results. *Transactions of the St. John's Hospital Dermatological Society*, **58**, 153.

Cronin, E. (1979) Oil of turpentine — a disappearing allergen. *Contact Dermatitis*, **5**, 308.

Cronin, E. & Calnan, C.D. (1978) Allergy to hydroabietic alcohol in adhesive tape. *Contact Dermatitis*, **4**, 57.

Dahlquist, I. & Fregert, S. (1978) Formaldehyde releasers. *Contact Dermatitis*, **4**, 173.

Dawson, T.A.J. (1976) Ethylene glycol sensitivity. *Contact Dermatitis*, **2**, 233.

Drevets, C.C. & Seebohm, P.M. (1961) Dermatitis from alcohol. *Journal of Allergy*, **32**, 277.

Ducksbury, C.F.J. & Dave, V.K. (1970) Contact dermatitis in home helps following the use of enzyme detergents. *British Medical Journal*, **1**, 537.

Eberhartinger, C. & Ebner, H. (1964) Beitrag zur Kenntnis der Formalin — Kontakt — Allergie. *Berufsdermatosen*, **12**, 301.

Epstein, E. (1972) The detection of lanolin allergy. *Achives of Dermatology*, **106**, 678.

Epstein, E. (1974) Patch test reactions (letter). *Archives of Dermatology*, **110**, 299.

Epstein, E. & Maibach, H.I. (1966) Formaldehyde allergy. *Archives of Dermatology*, **94**, 186.

Epstein, E., Rees, W.J. & Maibach, H.I. (1968) Recent experiences with routine patch test screening. *Archives of Dermatology*, **98**, 18.

Esteves, J. (1943) Amatus Lusitanus. 2, 608. quoted by Ive, F. A. (1967) *Transactions of the St John's Hospital Dermatological Society*, **53**, 135.

Everall, J. & Truter, E.V. (1954) Cutaneous hypersensitivity to lanolin: investigation of one case. *Journal of Investigative Dermatology*, **22**, 493.

Fabry, H. (1968) Formaldehyde sensitivity. *Contact Dermatitis Newsletter*, **3**, 51.

Fawcett, I.W., Newman Taylor, H.J. & Pepys, J. (1976) Asthma due to inhaled chemical agents — fumes from multicore soldering fluz and colophony resin. *Clinical Allergy*, **6**, 577.

Fisher, A.A. (1974) Contact dermatitis from strearyl alcohol and propylene glycol. *Archives of Dermatology*, **110**, 636.

Fisher, A.A. (1975) Allergic paraben and benzl alcohol hypersensitivity relationship of the 'delayed' and immediate varieties. *Contact Dermatitis*, **1**, 281.

Fisher, A.A. (1976) Formaldehyde: some recent experiences. *Cutis*, **17**, 665.

Fisher, A.A. (1978a) Propylene glycol dermatitis. *Cutis*, **21**, 166.

Fisher, A.A. (1978b) Immediate and delayed allergic contact reactions to polyethylene glycol. *Contact Dermatitis*, **4**, 135.

Fisher, A.A., Pascher, F. & Kanof, N.B. (1971) Allergic contact dermatitis due to ingredients of vehicles. *Archives of Dermatology*, **104**, 286.

Flindt, M.L.H. (1969) Pulmonary disease due to inhalation of derivatives of bascillus subtilis containing proteolytic enzyme. *Lancet*, **1**, 1177.

Foerster, O.H. (1923) Match and match box dermatitis. *Journal of the American Medical Association*, **81**, 1186.

Foussereau, J., Lantz, J.P., Escarde, J.-P., Grosshans, E. & Basset, A. (1971) L'allergie a la colophane des rondelles en polyéthylene des patch-tests. *Bulletin de la Société Francaise de Dermatologie et de Syphiligraphie*, **78**, 604.

Foussereau, J., Petitjean, J. and Lantz, J.P. (1974) Allergy to sodium lauryl sulphate. *Contact Dermatitis Newsletter*, **15**, 433.

Fregert, S. (1961) Eczema and matches. *Acta Dermato-venereologica*, **41**, 433.

Fregert, S. (1962) Otitis externa due to chromate of matches. *Acta Dermato-venereologica*, **42**, 473.

Fregert, S. (1968) Allergic contact dermatitis from formaldehyde formed at oil tannage. *Contact Dermatitis Newsletter*, **3**, 45.

Fregert, S. (1968) Contact dermatitis from colophony used as a print proteoline coating. *Contact Dermatitis Newsletter*, **4**, 58.

Fregert, S. (1974) Allergic contact dermatitis from formaldehyde in paper. *Contact Dermatitis Newsletter*, **15**, 459.

Fregert, S. (1975) Sensitisation to mercury in kerosene and exacerbation from red tattoo. *Contact Dermatitis*, **1**, 255.

Fregert, S. (1977) Contamination of chemico-technical preparations with formaldehyde from packages. *Contact Dermatitis*, **3**, 109.

Fregert, S. (1979) Colophony in cutting oil and in soap water used as cutting fluid. *Contact Dermatitis*, **5**, 52.

Fregert, S. & Dahlquist, I. (1969) Allergic contact dermatitis from Tego (dodecyclic aminoethyl glycine hydrochloride). *Contact Dermatitis Newsletter*, **5**, 103.

Fregert, S., Groth, O., Hjorth, N., Magnusson, B., Rorsman, H. & Övrum, P. (1969) Alcohol dermatitis. *Acta Dermato venereologica*, **49**, 493.

Fregert, S., Håkanson, R., Rorsman, H., Tryding, N. & Övrum, P. (1963) Dermatitis from alcohols. *Journal of Allergy*, **34**, 404.

Fregert, S., Hjorth, N., Magnusson, B., Bandmann, H.-J., Calnan, C.D., Cronin, E., Malten, K., Meneghini, C.L., Pirillä, V. & Wilkinson, D.S. (1969) Epidemiology of contact dermatitis. *Transactions of the St John's Hospital Dermatological Society*, **55**, 17.

Frisby, B.R. (1959) 'Tego' compounds in hospital practice. *Lancet*, **2**, 57.

Gaul, L.E. (1969) Dermatitis from cetyl and stearyl alcohols. *Archives of Dermatology*, **99**, 593.

Gloor, M., Döring, W.J. & Kümpel, D. (1976) Uber den einfluss synthetischer Tenside auf die zusammensetzung der Hautoberfüchenlipide. *Fette-Seifen-Anstrichmittel*, **78**, 40.

Goldsmith, L.A. (1978) Propylene glycol. *International Journal of Dermatology*, **17**, 703.

Gómez Orbaneja, J., Iglesias Diez, L., Sánchez Lozano, J.L. & Conde Salazar, L. (1976) Lymphatoid contact dermatitis. *Contact Dermatitis*, **2**, 139.

Gordon, H.H. (1974) Glutaraldehyde contact dermatitis *Contact Dermatitis Newsletter*, **15**, 442.

Gothe, C.-J., Nilzén, A., Holmgren, A., Szamosi, A., Werner, M. & Wide, L. (1972) Medical problems on the detergent industry caused by proteolytic enzymes from bacillus subtilis. *Acta Allergologica*, **27**, 63.

Gottmann-Lückerath, I. & Steigleder, G.K. (1972) Uberempfindlichkeit gegen Enzym-haltige Waschmittelenzyme. *Archiv für Dermatologische Forschung*, **245**, 63.

Griffith, J.R., Weaver, J.E., Whitehouse, H.S., Poole, R.L., Newman, E.A. & Nixon, G.A. (1969) Safety evaluation of enzyme detergents. Oral and cutaneous toxicity, irritancy and skin sensitisation studies. *Toxicology*, **7**, 581.

Grimm, W. & Gries, H. (1968) Untersuchungen über die Terpentinol-Allergie. *Berufsdermatosen*, **16**, 190.

Hannuksela, M. (1975) Allergy to propantheline in an antiperspirant (Ercoril lotion). *Contact Dermatitis*, **1**, 244.

Hannuksela, M. & Förström, L. (1978) Reactions to peroral propylene glycol. *Contact Dermatitis*, **4**, 41.

Hannuksela, M., Kousa, M. & Pirillä, V. (1976) Contact sensitivity to emulsifiers. *Contact Dermatitis*, **2**, 201.

Hannuksela, M., Pirilä, V. & Salo, O.P. (1975) Skin reactions to propylene glycol. *Contact Dermatitis*, **1**, 112.

Harman, R.R.M. & O'Grady, K.J. (1972) Contact dermatitis due to sensitivity to Cidex (activated glutaraldehyde). *Contact Dermatitis Newsletter*, **11**, 279.

Haxthausen, H. (1944–'45) Allergic eczema caused by ethyl alcohol. Elicited both by epicutaneous and by internal application. *Acta Dermato-venereologica*, **25**, 527.

Hellerström, S. (1939) Hypersensitivity tests in professional eczema, their applicability and sources of error (Discussion). *Acta Dermato-venereologica*, **20**, 657.

Hellerström, S., Thyresson, N., Blohm, S.-G., & Widmark, G. (1955) On the nature of the eczematogenic component of oxidised Δ^3-carene. *Journal of Investigative Dermatology*, **24**, 217.

Hendrick, D.J. & Lane, D.J. (1977) Occupational formalin asthma. *British Journal of Industrial Medicine*, **34**, 11.

Hindson, T.C. (1969) Contact allergy to α-pinene in boot polish. *Contact Dermatitis Newsletter*, **6**, 116.

Hindson, C. & Ratcliffe, G. (1975) Ethylene glycol in glass lens cutting. *Contact Dermatitis*, **1**, 386.

Hjorth, N. & Troile-Lassen, C. (1963) Skin reactions to ointment bases. *Transactions of the St John's Hospital Dermatological Society*, **49**, 127.

Hovding, G. (1969) Occupational dermatitis from pyrolysis products of polythene. *Acta Dermato-venereologica*, **49**, 147.

How, M.J. & Cambridge, G.W. (1971) Prick tests and serological tests in the diagnosis of allergic reactivity to enzymes used in washing products. *British Journal of Industrial Medicine*, **28**, 303.

Howes, D. (1975) The percutaneous absorption of some anionic surfactants. *Journal of the Society of Cosmetic Chemists*, **26**, 47.

Huriez, Cl., Martin, P. & Vanoverschelde, M. (1966) L'allergie au propyleneglycol. *Bulletin de la Société Francaise de Dermatologie et de Syphiligraphie*, **73**, 263.

Ive, F.A. (1967) Studies in contact dermatitis. XXI Matches. *Transactions of the St. John's Hospital Dermatological Society*, **53**, 135.

Jensen, N.E. (1970) Severe dermatitis and 'biological' detergents. *British Medical Journal*, **1**, 299.

Jordan, W.P. (1972) Tuperntine in eyeglasses. *Contact Dermatitis Newsletter*, **12**, 309.

Jordan, W.P. (1974) Allergic contact dermatitis in hand eczema. *Archives of Dermatology*, **110**, 567.

Jordan, W.P., DAHL, M.V. & Albert, H.L. (1972) Contact dermatitis from glutaraldehyde. *Archieve of Dermatology*, **105**, 94.

Juhlin, L. & Öhman, S. (1968) Allergic reactions to mercury in red tattoos and in mucosa adjacent to amalgam fillings. *Acta Dermato-venereologica*, **48**, 103.

Karvonen, J. & Hannuksela, M. (1976) Urticaria from alcoholic beverages. *Acta Allergologica*, **31**, 167.

Ketel, van, W.G. & Tan-Lim, K.N. (1975) Contact dermatitis from ethanol. *Contact Dermatitis*, **1**, 7.

Kirk, J. (1976) Colophony collar dermatitis. *Contact Dermatitis*, **2**, 294.

Kirton, V. (1972) Reactions to ageing turpentine. *Contact Dermatitis Newsletter*, **11**, 302.

Klaber, R. (1938) Match and match box dermatitis. *British Journal of Dermatology*, **50**, 451.

Klashka, F. (1975) Allergy to turpentine: Examination of systemic trigger action. *Contact Dermatitis*, **1**, 319.

Kligman, A.M. (1966) The identification of contact allergens by human assay. III. The maximisation test: A procedure for screening and rating contact sensitisers. *Journal of Investigative Dermatology*, **47**, 393.

Koch, G., Magnusson, B. & Nyquist, G. (1971) Contact allergy to medicaments and materials used in dentistry. *Odontologisk Revy*, **22**, 275.

Kurwa, A.R. (1970) Contact dermatitis from isopropyl alcohol. *Contact Dermatitis Newsletter*, **8**, 168.

Lindup, W.E. & Nowell, P.T. (1978) Role of sultone contaminants in an outbreak of allergic contact dermatitis caused by alkyl ethoxysulphates: a review. *Food and Cosmetics Toxicology*, **16**, 59.

Loomans, M.E. & Hannon, D.P. (1970) An electron microscopic study of the effects of subtilisin and detergents on human stratum corneum. *Journal of Investigative Dermatology*, **55**, 101.

Lowenthal, L.J.A. (1960) Reactions in green tattoos. *Archives of Dermatology*, **82**, 237.

Lyon, T.C. (1971) Allergic contact dermatitis due to Cidex. *Oral Surgery*, **32**, 895.

Magnusson, B., Blohm, S.—G., Fregert, S., Hjorth, N., Høvding, G., Pirilä, V. & Skog, E. (1968) Routine patch testing IV. *Acta Dermato-venereologica*, **48**, 110.

Magnusson, B & Gilje, O. (1973) Allergic contact dermatitis from a dish-washing liquid containing lauryl ether sulphate. *Acta Dermato-venereologica*, **53**, 136.

Magnusson, B. & Kligman, A.M. (1969) The identification of contact allergens by animal assay. The guinea pig maximisation test. *Journal of Investigative Dermatology*, **52**, 268.

Maibach, H. (1975) Polyethylene glycol: allergic contact dermatitis potential. *Contact Dermatitis*, **1**, 247.

Maibach, H. (1975) Glutaraldehyde: cross reaction to formaldehyde. *Contact Dermatitis*, **1**, 326.

Maibach, H.I. & Prystowsky, S.D. (1977) Glutaraldehyde (Pentanedial) Allergic contact dermatitis. *Archives of Dermatology*, **113**, 170.

Martin-Scott, I. (1960) Contact dermatitis from alcohol. *British Journal of Dermatology*, **72**, 372.

Marzulli, F.N. & Maibach, H.I. (1973) Antimicrobials: experimental contact sensitisation in man. *Journal of the Society of Cosmetic Chemists*, **24**, 399.

Mason Bolam, R., Hepworth, R. & Bowerman, L.T. (1971) In-use evaluation of safety to skin of enzyme-containing washing products. *British Medical Journal*, **2**, 499.

McKelvie, M. & McKelvie, p. (1966) Some aetiological factors in otitis externa. *British Journal of Dermatology*, **78**, 227.

Meneghini, C.L. & Angelini, G. (1975) Hypopigmentation following acute contact dermatitis from a match box. *Contact Dermatitis*, **1**, 55.

Mortensen, T. (1979) Allergy to lanolin. *Contact Dermatitis*, **5**, 137.

Murphy, J.C., Reif, A.E. & January, H.L. (1958) Cutaneous hypersensitivity to adhesive and scotch tapes. *Journal of Investigative Dermatology*, **31**, 45.

National Academy Of Sciences (1971) *Enzyme-Containing Laundering Compounds and Consumer Health*. p. 15, 23. Washington D.C.

Neering, H. & Ketel, Van, W.G. (1974) Glutaraldehyde and formaldehyde allergy. *Contact Dermatitis Newsletter*, **16**, 518.

Newhouse, M.L., Tagg, B., Pocock, S.J. & McEwan, A.C. (1970) An epidermological study of workers producing enzyme washing powders. *Lancet*, **1**, 689.

Nguyen, L Q. & Allen, H.B. (1979) Reactions to manganese and cadmium in tattoos. *Cutis*, **23**, 71.

Nilzén, Å. (1958) Some aspects of synthetic detergents and skin reactions. *Acta Dermato-Venereologica*, **38**, 104.

North American Contact Dermatitis Group (1973) Epidemiology of contact dermatitis in North America: 1972: *Archives of Dermatology*, **108**, 537.

Oleffe, J. (1973) Epidemiologic, social and economical aspects of occupational dermatoses in Belgium. *Archives Belges de Dermatologie*, **29**, 93.

Oleffe, J.A., Blondeel, A. & Boschmans, S. (1978) Patch testing with lanolin. *Contact Dermatitis*, **4**, 233.

Pepys, J., Hargreave, F.E., Longbottom, J.L. & Faux, J. (1969) Allergic Reactions of the lungs to enzymes of bacillus subtilis. *Lancet*, **1**, 1181.

Perera, P. (1970) An investigation of varicose ulcers. *Transactions of the St John's Hospital Dermatological Society*, **56**, 175.

Peter, G., Schröpl, F. & Franzwa, H. (1969) Experimentelle Untersuchungen Über die allergene Wirkung von Wollwachsalkoholen. *Hautarzt*, **20**, 450.

Pevny, I & Uhlich, M. (1975) Allergie gegen Bestandteile medizinischer und kosmetischer externa. *Hautarzt*, **26**, 252.

Pinol Aguadé, J., Grimalt Sancho, F. & Romaguera Sagrera, C. (1972) Sobre el mecanismo de establecimiento de las pulpitis secas y fisurarias de las manos de las amas de casa. *Medicina Cutanea*, **VI**, 379.

Pirila, V. (1970) Eczema due to oil of turpentine. *Therapeutische Umschau/Revue thérapeutique*, **27**, 509.

Pirilä, V., Kilpio, O., Olkkonen, A., Pirila, L. & Siltanen, E. (1969) On the chemical nature of the eczematogens in oil of turpentine. *Dermatologica*, **139**, 183.

Pirilä, V. & Pirilä, L. (1964) Terpentinallergie. *Berufsdermatosen*, **12**, 163.

Pirilä, V. & Siltanen, E. (1958) On the chemical nature of the eczematogenic agent in oil of turpentine, III. *Dermatologica*. **117**, 1.

Pirilä, V., Siltanen, E. & Pirilä, L. (1964) On the chemical nature of the eczematogenic agent in oil of turpentine. *Dermatologica*, **128**, 16.

Prater, E., Göring, H.D. & Schubert, H. (1978) Sodium lauryl sulphate — a contact allergen. *Contact Dermatitis*, **4**, 242.

Proctor, D.S.C. (1966) Coma in burns — The cause traced to dressings. *South African Medical Journal*, **40ii**, 1116.

Prottley, C. & Ferguson, T. (1975) Factors which determine the skin irritation potential of soaps and detergents. *Journal of the Society of Cosmetic Chemists*, **26**, 29.

Rasmussen, J.E. & Fisher, A.A. (1976) Allergic contact dermatitis to a salicylic acid plaster. *Contact Dermatitis*, **2**, 237.

Reichenberger, M. (1965) Zur epicutanen sensibilisierung bei Ulcus cruris-Kranken. *Archiv für Klinische und Experimentelle Dermatologie*, **223**, 56.

Ritz, H.L., Connor, D.S. & Sauter, E.D. (1975) Contact sensitisation of Guinea pigs with unsaturated and halogenated sultones. *Contact Dermatitis*, **1**, 349.

Rokstad, I. (1946) Skin reactions caused by fractions of oil of turpentine and hexanitrodiphenylamine. *Acta Dermato-venereologica*, **26**, Suppl. 15.

Rorsman, H., Brehmer-Andersson, E., Dahlquist, I., Ehinger, B., Jacobsson, S., Linell, F. & Rorsman, G. (1969) Tattoo granuloma and uveitis. *Lancet*, **2**, 27.

Rosemeyer, G. & Wüthrich, B. (1974) Inhalationsallergien auf WashmittelProtease. *Berfusdermatosen*, **22**, 107.

Rothenborg, H.W. & Hjorth, N. (1968) Allergy to perfumes from toilet soaps and detergents in patients with dermatitis. *Archives of Dermatology*, **97**, 417.

Rudzki, E. (1976a) Occupational contact dermatitis in 100 consecutive patients. *Berufsdermatosen*, **24**, 100.

Rudzki, E. (1976b) Foot dermatitis due to Turpentine. *Contact Dermatitis*, **2**, 127.

Rudzki, E. & Kleniewska, D. (1970) The epidemiology of contact dermatitis in Poland. *British Journal of Dermatology*, **83**, 543.

Sanderson, K.V. & Cronin, E. (1968) Glutaraldehyde and contact dermatitis. *British Medical Journal*, **3**, 802.

Schlossman, M.L. & McCarthy, J.P. (1979) Lanolin and derivatives chemistry: relationship to allergic contact dermatitis. *Contact Dermatitis*, **5**, 65.

Schneider, W., Tronnier, H., Schneider, H.J. & Schmitt, G.J. (1972) Ergebnisse einer Vergleichsstudie enzymhaltiger und enzymfreier Waschmittel. *Berufsdermatosen*, **20**, 63.

Schultheiss, E. (1957) Überempfindlichkeit gegenüber Jonon und Benzylalkohol. *Dermatologische Wochenschrift*, **135**, 629.

Schwartzberg, S. (1961) Allergic eczematous contact dermatitis caused by sensitisation to glyceryl monostearate. *Annals of Allergy*, **19**, 402.

Scutt, R.W.B. (1972) The medical hazards of tattooing. *British Journal of Hospital Medicine*, **8**, 195.

Scutt, R. & Gotch, C. (1974) *Skin Deep. The Mystery of Tattooing.* p. 135 London: Peter Davies.

Shore, R.N. & Shelley, W.B. (1974a) Contact dermatitis from stearyl alcohol and propylene glycol in fluocinonide cream. *Archives of Dermatology*, **109**, 397.

Shore, R.N. & Shelley, W.B. (1974b) Patch test Reactions (reply). *Archives of Dermatology*, **110**, 300.

Shore, R.N. & Shelley, W.B. (1974c) Contact dermatitis from stearyl alcohol and propylene glycol. *Archives of Dermatology*, **110**, 636.

Siedlecki, J.T. (1966) Toxicology of matches. *Journal of the American Medical Association*, **197**, 160.

Silberberg, I. & Leider, M. (1970) Studies of a red tatto. *Archives of Dermatology*, **101**, 299.

Simpson, J. (1969) Formalin sensitivity — offset printing machine. *Contact Dermatitis Newsletter*, **6**, 133

Skog, E. (1968) Sensitivity to glutaraldehyde. *Contact Dermatitis Newsletter*, **4**, 79.

Slavin, R.G. & Lewis, C.R. (1971) Sensitivity to enzyme additives in laundry detergent workers. *The Journal of Allergy and Clinical Immunology*, **48**, 262.

Smith, E.L. & Mcara, R.II. (1966) Allergic dermatitis from Sellotape. *British Medical Journal*, **2**, 239.

Sneddon, I.B. (1968) Formalin dermatitis in a renal dialysis unit. *Contact Dermatitis Newsletter*, **3**, 47.

Soap and detergent industry association (1971) Recommended operating procedures for U.K. factories handling enzyme materials. *The Annals of Occupational Hygiene*, **14**, 71.

Steigleder, G.K. (1970) Hautveranderungun durch biologisch aktive Washmittel. *Deutsche Medizinische Wochenschrift*, **95**, 1372.

Strauss, M.J. (1950) Sensitisation to polyethylene glycols (carbowaxes®). *Archives of Dermatology*, **61**, 420.

Sugai, T. & Higashi, J. (1975) Hypersensitivity to hydrogenated lanolin. *Contact Dermatitis*, **1**, 146.

Sulzberger, M.B. & Lazar, M.P. (1950) A study of the allergenic constituents of Lanolin (wool fat). *Journal of Investigative Dermatology*, **15**, 453.

Sulzberger, M.B. & Tolmach, J.A. (1959) Allergische Aufflammungs-Reaktionen in roten tätowierungen. *Hautarzt*, **10**, 110.

Sulzberger, M.B., Warshaw, T. & Herrmann, F. (1953) Studies of skin-hypersensitivity to lanolin. *Journal of Investigative Dermatology*, **20**, 33.

Suskind, R.R. (1957) Cutaneous effects of soaps and synthetic detergents. *Journal of the American Medical Association*, **163**, 943.

Sylvest, B., Hjorth, N. & Magnusson, B. (1975) Lauryl ether sulphate dermatitis in Denmark. *Contact Dermatitis*, **1**, 359.

Symposium on skin cleansing (1965) *Transactions of the St. John's Hospital Dermatological Society*, **51**, 133–252.

Taaffe, A., Knight, A.G. & Marks, R. (1978) Lichenoid tattoo hypersensitivity. *British Medical Journal*, **1**, 616.

Tazelaar, D.J. (1970) Hypersensitivity to chromium in a light-blue tattoo. *Dermatologica*, **141**, 282.

Tegner, E. & Fregert, S. (1973) Contamination of cosmetics with formaldehyde from tubes. *Contact Dermatitis Newsletter*, **13**, 353.

Thomsen, H.F. (1973) Hidden sources of formaldehyde. *Contact Dermatitis Newsletter*, **13**, 380.

Thune, P. (1969) Allergy to wool fat. *Acta Dermato-venereologica*, **49**, 282.

Truter, E.V. (1956) Wool wax. p. 326. London: Cleaver-Hume Press.

Truter, E.V. (1963) Personal Communication.

Valér, M. (1975a) Skin irritancy and sensitivity to laundry detergents containing proteolytic enzymes. Part I. *Berufsdermatosen*, **23**, 16.

Valér, M. (1975b) Skin irritancy and sensitivity to laundry detergents containing proteolytic enzymes. Part II. Berufsdermatosen, **23**, 96.

Vollum, D.I. (1969) Sensitivity to hydrogenated lanolin. *Archives of Dermatology*, **100**, 774.

Wahlberg, J.E. (1978) Abietic acid and colophony. *Contact Dermatitis*, **4**, 55.

Walker, A.P., Ashforth, G.K. Davies, R.E., Newman, E.A. & Ritz, H.L. (1973) Some characteristics of the sensitiser in alkyl ethoxy sulphate. *Acta Dermato-venereologica*, **53**, 141.

Warshaw, T.G. & Herrmann, F. (1952) Studies of skin reactions to propylene glycol. *Journal of Investigative Dermatology*, **19**, 423.

Wasilewski, C. (1968) Allergic contact dermatitis from isopropyl alcohol. *Archives of Dermatology*, **98**, 502.

Weaver, J.E. (1976) Dermatologic testing of household laundry products: a novel fabric softener. *International Journal of Dermatology*, **15**, 297.

Weaver, J.E. & Maibach, H.I. (1977) Dose response relationships in allergic contact dermatitis: Glutaraldehyde-containing liquid fabric softener. *Contact Dermatitis*, **3**, 65.

Weiler, K.-J. (1970) Berufliche Hautschäden durch Formaldehydaethylamin. *Berufsdermatosen*, **18**, 239.

Wereide, K. (1965) Contact allergy to wool fat ('Lanolin'). *Acta Dermato-venereologica*, **45**, 15.

Wilkinson, D.S. (1970) Formalin sensitivity in mushroom farming. *Contact Dermatitis Newsletter*, **7**, 162.

Wilkinson, D.S. (1970) Terpenes. *Contact Dermatitis Newsletter*, **8**, 183.

Wilkinson, D.S. & Calnan, C.D. (1975) Rosin used for belt-drive machine. *Contact Dermatitis*, **1**, 64.

Winkelmann, R.K. & Harris, R.B. (1979) Lichenoid delayed hypersensitivity reactions in tattoos. *Journal of Cutaneous Pathology*, **6**, 59.

Woodford, R. & Barry, B.W. (1974) Placebo response to white soft paraffin/propylene glycol. *British Journal of Dermatology*, **90**, 233.

Wüthrich, B., Schwarz, K. & Eichenberger-de-beer, H. (1971) Hautschaden durch Proteasenhaltige Waschmittel. *Schweizerische Medizinische Wochenschrift*, **101**, 43.

Wüthrich, B., Schwarz, K. Eichenberger-De-Beer, H. (1971) Zur Pathogenese von Hautschaden durch biologisch aktive, proteasenhaltige waschmittel. *Dermatologica*, **142**, 265.

Zachariae, H., Thomsen, K. & Gowertz Rasmussen, G. (1973) Occupational enzyme dermatitis. *Acta Dermato-venereologica*, **53**, 145.

16.

Miscellaneous occupational

OILS
PAPERS
  Paper
  Carbon paper
  No carbon required
  Computer paper
  Typewriter correction paper
COPYING
  Dyeline — diazo
  Thermofax
  Photocopying
  Electrostatic — xerographic
PRINTING AND DUPLICATING
  Letterpress
  Lithography
    Offset

Silkscreen
Photogravure
Light-sensitive acrylates (p. 590)
INKS
  Printing
  Writing
PHOTOGRAPHY
  Black and white
  X-ray developing
  Colour
FLUXES
CHEMICAL DEPIGMENTATION
BARRIER CREAMS

Oils

Oils can be classified according to their type and function.

1. *Mineral oils* are formed by the decomposition of animal and vegetable matter under the earth's crust over the course of millions of years. Their composition varies geographically; some oils are aliphatic or wax-based, others are aromatic or asphalt based, and others are mixed. Crude oil is separated by distillation into fractions:

1. gaseous hydrocarbons
2. petrol
3. naphthas: including solvents such as white spirit
4. kerosene: paraffin oil
5. fuels: gas, diesel and furnace oils
6. lubricants: engine, machine and cutting oils
7. paraffin waxes
8. residues consisting of asphalt and bitumen.

2. *Vegetable oils* are derived from nuts and seeds; industrially they are grouped according to their drying properties and many vegetable oils are edible:

1. Drying: linseed, tung

2. Semi drying: safflower, soybean
3. Non drying: castor, cotton seed, coconut
4. Edible: olive, corn, peanut.

3. *Animal oils* may be solid fats like tallow and lard, or liquid fats such as fish oils. They are used industrially and for cooking.

4. *Essential oils* are derived from plants and are used for perfumery and for flavouring.

Only mineral oils and their derivatives are considered in this section.

Cutting fluids
Cutting fluids have 2 main functions: to cool and to lubricate the cutting action of metal on metal. In addition they flush away unwanted metal debris and they help to prevent rusting. These cutting fluids are based mainly, but not entirely, on mineral oil; some of the water-miscible fluids do not contain oils. Cutting fluids are divided into 2 main types:

1. cutting oils
2. water miscible fluids.

1. *Cutting oils* (neat, insoluble oils)
Insoluble cutting oils are based on mineral oil and are used mainly for their lubricating action, but mineral oil alone has a limited effect and its properties can be greatly enhanced by additives. Animal or vegetable oils improve the wetting of the metal sufaces and reduce friction. Sulphur, because it has an affinity for metal, lowers the surface tension and is used as an extreme pressure (E.P.) additive, as are chlorine and phosphorous. Corrosion inhibitors, such as zinc dithiophosphate, react with non-ferrous metals to form protective films which adhere strongly to the metal surfaces. These cutting oils are often recycled after centrifugation and heating.

There are various types of insoluble cutting oils:

i. Straight mineral oils have limited lubricating properties. They are used for light work on single spindle automatics and for some capstan and turret lathe work.
ii. Mineral and fatty oil mixtures. The addition of lard oil or rape-seed oil (colza oil) increases the lubricating film properties of the oil and makes it suitable for lathes, milling and general purposes.
iii. Sulphurised oils. The addition of free or combined sulphur greatly improves the performance of the oil, but has the disadvantage of staining metal. These oils are widely used in lathe work, gear-cutting, thread grinding and screwing.
iv. Sulphur or chlorine additives give oils of good performance with extreme pressure properties. They are suitable for lathes and automatic screwing, tapping and gear cutting machines.

Additives. Cutting oils usually contain few or no other additives but sometimes phenols may be present as antioxidants, bactericides to protect against rancidity, and other compounds to prevent rust (see soluble oils).

2. Water miscible fluids

The action of water miscible fluids is to cool and lubricate the metal surfaces during metal machining, tool grinding and similar engineering processes. The water content lowers the temperature, and the oil lubricates and diminishes corrosion of the metal surfaces. The use of these coolant fluids is growing in industry and they now claim about two-thirds of the cutting fluid market (Key, Ritter and Arndt, 1966).

There are 3 main types of soluble cutting fluids:

(i) *Soluble oil.* 'Soup' (USA) 'Suds' (U.K.). Soluble oils are oil in water colloidal suspensions stabilised by the addition of emulsifying agents. When the proportion of emulsifier is 15–25 per cent the appearance is milky, but when it is 35–40 per cent the micro-suspension is so fine that the fluid is clear. Opaque milky fluids are those most commonly used. Soluble oils are widely used being effective coolants, relatively inexpensive and adaptable; but they are unstable if incorrectly mixed or infrequently changed, and their composition is subject to the whim of the operators. Loss of water or oil, increase in alkalinity or content of bactericide, phenol or cresylic compounds are all changes which may occur and be unnoticed.

Additives. Basically, soluble oils are colloidal suspensions of spindle oil and petroleum sulphonate soaps but they are usually formulated with many additives:

1. Coupling agents to stabilise the emulsion: phenols, cresylic acid or alcohols.
2. Germicides.
3. Antioxidants: phenols and amines including diamines, triamines, phenyl-α-naphthylamine, phenyl-β-naphthylamine and tetramethyldiaminodiphenylmethane.
4. Anti-rust agents: metal salts of dithiophosphates and dithiocarbamates; sulphurised and phosphosulphurised terpenes.
5. Corrosion inhibitors: soluble sodium mercaptobenzothiazole protects copper; very occasionally chromates are included in the formulation.
6. Extreme pressure additives are used in heavy duty soluble oils to increase their lubricating effect.
7. Anti-foaming compounds: silicones.
8. Dyes: sometimes added e.g. fluorescein.
9. Water conditioners: polyphosphates, borax or sodium carbonate may be added to the water prior to making the emulsion.

(ii) *Synthetic (chemical) coolants* are true aqueous solutions and do not contain petroleum oils; many are based on polyglycols or polyglycol derivatives and they may contain sodium nitrite and triethanolamine as corrosion inhibitors. Fluorescein is often added giving the fluid a yellow fluorescent colour. Other additives include hygroscopic compounds, wetting agents, biocides and metal passivators.

These synthetic coolants were introduced for special engineering requirements and not for oncogenic reasons. They are used especially by the motor industry when cooling rather than lubrication is important.

(iii) *Semi-synthetic oils*. These fluids contain 15–40 per cent of mineral oils. They require emulsifiers and have additives similar to those in soluble oils.

Fuel oils

Fuel oils are petroleum products which are burned in furnaces for heat or used in engines for power. They are generally obtained by distillation. The various fractions differ in their properties and are examplified by gasoline (petrol), diesel oil and kerosene.

In the U.K. heating oils are duty-free and to distinguish them from the taxable transport fuels, diesel and petrol, which contain no markers, customs regulations require that gas oil (which is diesel oil) contains the two chemical markers, furfuraldehyde and quinizarin (1,4-dihydroxyanthraquinone) and the red dye C.I. Solvent Red 24. Kerosene contains furfuraldehyde and quinizarin but not the red dye. The French marker is diphenylamine.

Lubricating oils

Lubricating oils are selected stable fractions of refined mineral oil, which reduce friction between moving parts, usually metals. Their uses range from precision instruments to the heaviest equipment.

Different grades of oil vary in their viscosity and colour:
    thin spindle oil — pale brown
    medium engine oil — red, medium viscosity
    cylinder oils — green-black, heavy viscosity.

The properties of the oils are improved by additives:
    antioxidants: sulphur and phosphorus compounds, sulphides, phosphites, metal salts of dithiophosphoric acid, terpenes, phenols and amines (phenyl-α-naphthylamine)
    detergents.
    anti-rust agents: petroleum sulphonates, wool grease, amines, hydroxyl compounds, diolyl malate
    foam suppressors: silicones, 3 per cent *ortho*cresyl phosphate has been used in lubricating oils for jet aircraft
(Hodgson, 1961).

Greases

Greases are mixtures of mineral oils and soaps; in colour they vary from transparent to black, and in consistency from liquids to solids. They may contain inert fillers such as barytes, chalk, molybdenum disulphide or graphite, and lithium compounds are added for water resistance. Stable greases are neutral, but others may occasionally contain 0.2 per cent alkali or 5 per cent organic acids (Hodgson, 1961). Amines (phenyl-α-naphthylamine, phenyl-β-naphthylamine) are added to some greases.

SKIN HAZARDS

Mineral oils can cause the following skin changes:

1. Dermatitis: irritant and allergic from oil additives
2. Folliculitis: acneiform eruption
3. Oil melanosis and photosensitivity
4. Malignancy.

Dermatitis — irritant

Cutting fluids
Oils are one of the commonest causes of occupational dermatitis and the incidence will vary with the degree of exposure. Some workers have their hands and arms constantly immersed in cutting oils, and sprays of oil may soak their clothing. In Birmingham in the U.K. 33 per cent of all cases of occupational dermatitis were attributed to oil (Kipling, 1963) and in 1972 crude oil products accounted for 17.3 per cent of notified occupational skin diseases in Ceskoslovakia and for 14.8 per cent in the U.S.S.R. (Šak, Hegyi and Miglierini, 1975). The incidence varies in different plants, but Gellin (1970) estimated that 1 per cent of all workers exposed to oils develop skin disorders which are a major cause of loss of time from work. In one tappet assembly plant where the workers did not wear gloves an insoluble mineral seal oil caused dermatitis in the extraordinarily high figure of 60 per cent of the workers (Gellin, Possick and Davis, 1970).

It is the soluble cutting oils (fluids) and much less frequently the insoluble oils which cause irritant contact dermatitis (Key, Ritter and Arndt, 1966). In Birmingham of 190 cases of occupational eczema from all causes, 44 were due to soluble oils and 8 to insoluble oils (Kipling, 1963). The occurrence of dermatitis over a 5-year period in a medium engineering factory employing approximately 2000 manual workers and 2000 non-manual workers was reported by Wilson (1961). Eczematous conditions occurred in 121 manual workers of whom 45 had a contact dermatitis; this was irritant in 42 (paraffin — 7, soluble oils — 18, cleansers — 5) and allergic in 3 (epoxy resin sensitisation). Eczematous conditions were seen in 65 non-manual workers, of whom only 6 had a contact dermatitis which in 3 was allergic (suspenders — 2, aminoazotoluene in red biro ink — 1).

The cause of oil dermatitis is basically unknown. A single cause is very unlikely; different factors are likely to contribute to different outbreaks, but even with the most detailed investigation an exact aetiology may not be uncovered. The fault must lie in the oil (cutting fluid), the working conditions or in the susceptibility of the worker. Ippen (1978, 1979) has studied the factors which contribute to the development of skin lesions in metal workers.

A cresylic acid disinfectant added to the sumps was stated by Hodgson (1969) to be the cause of an epidemic of dermatitis among automatic lathe operators. In other outbreaks the cause is less defined. Repeated wetting and drying is thought to damage the skin (Key, Ritter and Arndt, 1966), and perhaps this makes it vulnerable to abrasions from swarf, to damage from the alkaline oil with its content of minor irritants, and to harm from solvents and cleansers.

The composition of used oil varies with the cleanliness of the plant and the supervision of the operatives. Additives, particularly bactericides added in excess, evaporation of water and contamination of the oil (fluid) by debris will all change it from its prescribed formulation. Bactericides are added to preserve the emulsion not to protect the workers; however, despite bacterial contamination of these fluids, pyogenic infection is not thought to be a cause of dermatitis (Kipling, 1963; Ritter and Arndt, 1966) although viral warts have been spread through a common oil supply (Kipling, 1963).

Predisposing factors in the workers were found by Hodgson (1969) to include dryness of the skin, poor peripheral circulation and ageing. However, this vulnerability of older workers was not confirmed by Johnson and Wilson (1971). From his experience Hodgson (1969) thought it was impossible to forecast at pre-employment examination which man was likely to develop dermatitis.

Two patterns of irritant dermatitis were described by Hodgson (1961): (i) acute and (ii) dryness and redness of the hands and arms followed by a discoid pattern of eczema.

Clinically patients are often seen with a history of increasing dryness of the hands, followed by painful cracking of the skin over the dorsal surfaces of the joints or on the pulps of the fingers and these changes may be succeeded by frank eczema of the hands spreading to the wrists and arms. Some find work impossibe, others struggle on. Many give a definite history that the dermatitis heals or improves away from work, or at the weekends, and recurs on their return.

The prognosis of 81 patients who developed skin disease while working with oil, mostly (73) as machine operators, was investigated with questionnaires by Johnson and Wilson (1971). They found that of the 52 cases with oil dermatitis 60 per cent were clear and 23 per cent were better and that the outlook was not influenced by age. The majority (46) had changed their jobs and if this was done early, within a year of the onset of the oil dermatitis, their prognosis was improved. Six with mild dermatitis stayed in the same job and 5 had cleared; this was attributed to increased protection or a change in the oil.

The control of oil dermatitis may be summarised as: improve the environment, clean the man and monitor the oil. Extremely important is the maintenance of a clean working area with adequate protective guards on the machines. Cleanliness of working clothes, the use of protective clothing, washing facilities, bland cleansers to replace solvents, and the working technique of the men all require supervision. In conjunction with these measures the oil should be repeatedly checked to ensure that its correct formulation is maintained.

Fuel oils

Fuel oils, including petrol (gasoline), diesel oil and kerosene, are fat solvents and may irritate the skin by their degreasing action. The oils themselves are not allergens but occasionally an additive may sensitise (p. 846)

Kerosene in camping equipment contaminated a boy's clothing and caused an acute eruption similar to that of toxic epidermal necrolysis but without the systemic illness (Barnes and Wilkinson, 1973).

Koilonychia

Koilonychia is not uncommon in motor mechanics, possibly due to contact with motor oils. The amino acid analysis of the keratin of these nails was normal (Dawber, 1974).

Dermatitis — allergic

Although oils, particularly soluble oils and synthetic fluids, seem to contain many additives which are potential sensitisers, reports of allergic contact dermatitis are in fact very few.

In the following summary the sensitising additives have been grouped according to their function and not according to the type of oil in which they occurred.

4-tertiary-Butyl catechol (TBC). Antioxidant — insoluble mineral seal oil

In a tappet assembly plant with a 60 per cent incidence of dermatitis 3 workers were sensitised to 4-*tertiary*-butyl catechol, an antioxidant in the mineral seal oil. The catechol also caused depigmentation in these and one other worker. Patch tests: the 3 patients reacted to TBC 0.1 per cent in acetone; in one patient the positive reaction became depigmented (Gellin, Possick and Davis, 1970).

Phenolic calcium salt. Antioxidant — lubricating oil

Two motor mechanics developed dermatitis from one particular car lubricating oil. Patch tests: both reacted to the oil and one coded component (50 per cent in mineral oil). This was identified as an anti-oxidant, the calcium salt of a high molecular weight phenol; 4 per cent was present in the commercial oil. Patch tests with this phenol in 100 control patients actively sensitised at least one woman (Hjorth and Brodthagen, 1956).

2-Mercaptobenzothiazole. Corrosion inhibitor — soluble oil

The water soluble sodium salt of mercaptobenzothiazole (MBT) was added to a soluble cutting oil to lower the pH and thus prevent corrosion of copper and tin. The concentrated oil contained 1 per cent MBT, but after dilution for use the aqueous emulsion contained only 0.05–0.01 per cent. In 3 factories, 25 men had considerable exposure to this soluble oil and 12 developed dermatitis of the hands and in some the arms. Patch tests: 7 reacted to MBT but only one of these reacted to the cutting oil (2 per cent dilution) containing 0.02 per cent MBT. The undiluted oil was irritant and could not be used for patch testing. The 5 patients with negative patch tests were diagnosed as having an irritant oil dermatitis. The irritancy of the oil was thought to have facilitated sensitisation to the MBT. The oil was changed and the patient's dermatitis healed (Fregert and Skog, 1962).

Sodium mercaptobenzothiazole. Antifreeze mixtures

Sodium mercaptobenzothiazole which is soluble is added to some antifreeze formulations to inhibit corrosion of copper in the radiator; very occasionally it sensitises those in frequent contact with these mixtures. Four patients with dermatitis from antifreeze mixtures have been seen at St John's. Two were employed in filling containers with antifreeze mixtures one of which contained 0.2 per cent and the other 0.83 per cent sodium mercaptobenzothiazole (Calnan, 1974). The third patient was a driver who had noticed that antifreeze irritated his hands, and the fourth patient was a motor mechanic and it was thought that antifreeze mixtures were contributing to his hand eczema. All four patients were sensitive to MBT.

Grotan BK (hexahydro-1,3,5-tris (2-hydroxyethyl) triazine). Bactericide —
soluble oils
Bacterial contamination shortens the life of a coolant fluid by breaking the emulsion; this reduces its efficiency and is altogether economically undesirable. As it is impossible to prevent contamination, the bacterial population is controlled by bactericides, usually phenols or formaldehyde liberators; salicylamides are used less frequently because of their dermatological risk (Keczkes and Brown, 1976).

Grotan BK is a triazine bacteriocide and a formaldehyde liberator and has been widely used in soluble oils for over a decade the recommended usage concentration is 0.15 per cent. Its dermatological hazard is in dispute. Borelli and Düngemann (1964) reported it as a fairly common sensitiser in metal workers but Schneider *et al.* (1965) found no evidence of this in their examinations of workers in 10 factories. A more recent report by Keczkes and Brown (1976) attributed the cause of a soluble oil dermatitis in 4 men to sensitisation to Grotan BK on the basis of positive patch test reactions to Grotan BK 0.2 per cent in water. However, when re-patch tested about 1 year later only one of these men reacted to Grotan BK 0.2 per cent, one responded to 1 per cent and 2 were negative to all concentrations from 0.1–5 per cent. These results indicate that only one or perhaps two of these men were sensitised by Grotan BK. Like formaldehyde, Grotan is an irritant and is likely to give irritant patch reactions which are misleading.

This sparcity of reports suggests that Grotan BK may occasionally sensitise but that the incidence is small. In guinea pigs its sensitising potential is low, but poor percutaneous absorption was a significant factor in the failure of animals to react to a topical challenge test (Poitou and Marignac, 1978).

The problem of sensitivity to Grotan BK has been reviewed by Rycroft (1979); for patch testing he recommends Grotan BK 1 per cent in water.

Chromates and nickel
Chromate and nickel dermatitis from cutting fluids is probably rare but cases are occasionally reported.

The presence of nickel and chromate in cutting fluids being currently used was sought but not found by Samitz and Katz (1975). In two plants, in neither of which did the men have dermatitis, spot tests for nickel and chromates were negative on the machinery, working areas and on ashed samples of new and used cutting oil and wipe rags. However by soaking metal turnings and chips in saline or sweat they found that 9.7 μg and 6.3 μg of nickel but no chromium could be leached out of one of the stainless steels. In another study Einarsson *et al.* (1975) did detect metals by atomic absorption analysis in used cutting oils. After 14 days use in a tool-grinding machine, a tungsten carbide alloy containing 10 per cent cobalt released into the oil emulsion 217 μg Co/g, 0.13 μg Cr/g and 0.61 μg Ni/g. A steel alloy with 1 per cent chromium was used in two machines, and in centrifuged oil samples there were 0.10 μg–0.15 μg/g of chromium and nickel and in uncentrifuged samples 0.87 μg Cr/g and 0.72 μg Ni/g. The clinical significance of these findings was to be investigated.

Chromate dermatitis in a man making ventilation pipes from zinc-galvanised iron was attributed to chromate contamination of the machine oil by the chromate coating on the sheet metal. The used oil contained 215 μg Cr_6/ml (Fregert and Gruvberger, 1976).

A series of 134 patients with dermatitis attributed to oil was investigated by Anderson (1960). He found that 6 men employed to grease ships and 2 men repairing coachwork on buses reacted to dichromate. Spectrographic and spot tests of the oils for chromate were negative and as each of the men was working with anti-rust paints these seemed the most likely source of their sensitisation.

A soluble oil formulated with 0.8 per cent potassium dichromate, giving an in use concentration of 0.01 per cent, sensitised an engineer working on grinding machines (Calnan, 1978).

Dyes — azo and anthraquinone

Orange G (benzeneazo-β-naphthol 6,8-disulphonic acid). Anti-rust oil. A fascinating account of how a scattered outbreak of dermatitis in a new tractor plant was traced to a dyed oil was told by Prout (1973). The eczema affected 25 of 370 (7 per cent) of the men and usually occurred on the arms or wrists but in some was confined to the hands. The common factor was identified as a travelling conveyor arm from which engines were suspended in their journey through the factory. At one stage the engines were sprayed with an anti-rust oil and it incidentally coated the conveyor arm. About 3 months before the dermatitis began an orange dye had been added to the oil to facilitate seeing it on the metal. The dye was Orange G (benzeneazo-β-naphthol 6,8-disulphonic acid).

Patch tests: 12 of the affected men agreed to be patch tested and 10 reacted to one or more of the tests with the dye (0.5 per cent), oil and dye, or oil and dye 50 per cent in olive oil; 6 controls were negative. Total withdrawal of the dye cured the dermatitis.

Oil red (azobenzeneazo-2-naphthol, methyl derivatives) ⎱ Gasoline dyes
Oil yellow (*p*-dimethylaminoazobenzene). ⎰

Three men with a contact dermatitis from gasoline dyes were described by Lamb and Lain (1951). One patient worked for an oil company and mixed the powdered dyes, another, a farmer, spilled a bronze coloured gasoline on his hands while filling the tanks of his tractor, and the third was a dentist who used a coloured gasoline in his mower.

Patch tests:

> Du Pont Oil Red (methyl derivatives of azobenzeneazo-2-naphthol (powder)) — 2 were positive, 1 weakly.
> Du Pont Oil Yellow (*p*-dimethylaminoazobenzene (powder)) — 1 was positive.

It was uncertain whether these dyes were primary sensitisers or whether the men had been previously sensitised by cross-reacting allergens.

A petrol station employee with long standing eczema reacted on patch testing to one particular coloured octane. It was inferred that the sensitiser was the *anthraquinone dye 1,4-dialkylaminoanthraquinone* but it was not used for patch testing (Garcia-Perez and Aparicio, 1975).

Ethylenediamine (p. 244).

Colophony

A turner with hand eczema became worse when he tried using a potassium soap water instead of cutting oil. Patch testing showed him to be sensitive to colophony. It was then ascertained that the cutting oil was emulsified with 10 per cent soap made of triethanolamine and tall oil fatty acids containing 25 per cent colophony. The potassium soap too was made of tall oil fatty acids containing 20 per cent colophony, mainly abietic acid and its isomers (Fregert, 1979).

Methyloctylbenzenesulphonate. Antistatic lubricant

During the development stages of the compound methyltriethylammonium-octylbenzenesulphonate for addition to an antistatic lubricant, an intermediate chemical, an ester, methyloctylbenzenesulphonate, was found to be a potent sensitiser. Ten persons handled the ester and all developed dermatitis, particularly of the arms from spilling the liquid, and there was an associated swelling of the eyelids.

Patch tests: 9 patients were tested with the ester 0.1 per cent in acetone and 8 reacted. For full scale production the process was enclosed and the cases of dermatitis ceased (Cruikshank and Howard-Swaffield, 1953).

Patch testing

Cutting fluids diluted as for use at work are usually not irritant and can be applied as such for patch testing. Occasionally they cause a slight toxic soap-like reaction and a few are stronger irritants. However, there is also a danger of false negative reactions to allergens present in low concentration, and dilution to avoid irritancy increases this error. Cognisant of these defects the general rule for patch testing with cutting fluids has been to apply them undiluted to avoid the error of missing an allergen, knowing that at this concentration they may be slightly irritant.

Cutting fluids

Insoluble cutting oils	Undiluted
Soluble cutting oils	Undiluted
Synthetic coolants	Undiluted (more likely to be irritant)
Additives	1–2 per cent or less (check individual chemicals)

Fuel oils
   Diesel oil   5 per cent in methyl ethyl ketone
   Kerosene   5 per cent in methyl ethyl ketone
   Petrol   5 per cent in methyl ethyl ketone
Lubricating oils   Undiluted
Greases   Undiluted

Oil folliculitis and oil acne

Oil folliculitis is an irritant effect of petroleum oils.

Oil acne is caused principally by insoluble cutting oils particularly those containing heavier distillate fractions and greases composed of heavy lubricating oils such as colliery black greases. The primary lesions are comedones causing mechanical blockage of the follicular openings. These may be associated with perifollicular papules and pustules caused by the irritant effect of the oil or by leakage of sebum from obstructed follicles into the tissues. The sites affected are the dorsa of the hands and fingers, the arms, thighs, face, neck and waist. The condition occurs where there is heavy oil exposure, poor personal cleanliness and dirty oil soaked clothes which constantly chafe the skin. Dark skinned hirsute workers are particularly susceptible but anyone may be affected. The acne is often chronic and may persist for months even though oil exposure has ceased (Hodgson, 1961). With increased personal hygiene and improved working conditions the incidence of oil acne has greatly decreased.

Oil folliculitis and oil acne are clinically and aetiologically distinct from chloracne.

Oil melanosis and photosensitivity

Sunbathing may occasionally produce marked melanosis of sites heavily exposed to cutting oils. Such a case with reticulate pigmentation of the arms and forehead was shown at a clinical meeting by Rook (1950). He suggested that the photodynamic chemicals originated in paraffin and heavy lubricating oils in the machines and these contaminated the cutting oil during work. A similar patient with facial pigmentation and exposure to cutting oils was shown at a later meeting by Warin (1959) but he did not describe the patient's brown discolouration as reticulate.

Cutaneous carcinomas

The importance of mineral oil as a cause of cutaneous carcinomas became evident in the early 1900s with recognition of the association between carcinoma of the scrotum and the oil soaked job of mule spinning in the cotton industry. This is now of historical interest but has been replaced by the realisation of this same hazard from mineral oil in the engineering industry. In Great Britain, in Birmingham, where many cases have occurred, it was established in the 1950's that there is a significant connection between occupational exposure to cutting oils and cancer of the scrotum, hands and arms (Cruikshank and Squires, 1950; Cruikshank and Gourevitch, 1952). Since then, in Birmingham, Dr Kipling has been a mainspring in the study of oil carcinomata, and Waterhouse (1971) at the Regional Cancer Registry has recorded the incidence of cases over the years.

There is a strong possibility that oils which are carcinogenic to the skin also affect internal organs because it has been shown that patients with carcinomas of the scrotum have an increased incidence of malignancies of the respiratory and gastrointestinal tracts (Holmes, Kipling and Waterhouse, 1970) due to exposure to oil mist. In France, the almost epidemic number of cases of scrotal and other cutaneous carcinomas among workers in small engineering factories in the Savoy Alps, has been intensively studied by Thony et al. (1975). Small numbers of cases are seen elsewhere in France (Desoille et al., 1973). These cases in England and France contrast strongly with the absence of cases in the Netherlands over the past 20 years and the small numbers reported from Germany, Scandanavia, America and Australia (Kipling, 1974). However cases are still reported, such as the 39-year-old lathe workers in Germany who first had oil acne and then 10 years later was seen with multiple carcinomas of the scrotum (Hundeiker and Glossman, 1975).

Tool setters and operators setting machines appear to be at particular risk of developing scrotal carcinomata, perhaps because of their exposure to insoluble cutting oils and the oil contamination of their groins while bending over the machinery (Kipling, 1968).

The characteristic skin lesions are keratoses and squamous cell carcinomata and they affect particularly the scrotum, but also the hands and arms and rarely the face and neck. The keratoses are hard, raised rough lesions, which sometimes resemble warts. Areas of skin which become hard and discoloured are described as shagreen or shark skin. It is less easy to relate keratoacanthomata and basal cell carcinomas to oil exposure.

The carcinogens in mineral oils have been shown experimentally to be polycyclic aromatic hydrocarbons; solvent refined oils are less hazardous.

PAPERS

Paper

Paper is made by chemically processing cellulose fibres, derived mainly from the softwoods of spruce, pine, hemlock and other conifers. During manufacture the stiffness, strength and smootheness of the paper is increased by the addition of a sizing compound which is usually colophony (rosin), although alkaline sizing materials may be used in preference. A glossy surface is achieved by coating the paper with a finish such as china clay which is bonded to the surface with latex or a synthetic resin. Size press gelatines may also be used as a gloss finish particularly for photographic paper. It contains 3 per cent aluminium chromium sulphate. This was thought to have been the source of chromate exposure in a wood pulp machine operator who developed hand eczema and was found to be sensitive to dichromate (Connor, 1972).

Finally, colophony may be applied as a protective coating for print on containers or on labels. A girl who developed acute palmar eczema from clutching a plastic tube with a colophony print protective finish was reported by Fregert (1968).

Wet strength papers are made by the incorporation of a formaldehyde resin; melamine formaldehyde has a high degree of wet strength, but urea formaldehyde is cheaper.

Paper pulp industry

Some of the chemicals used in the processing of paper pulp contain traces of chromium and cobalt and were the source of contact in two patients investigated by Fregert, Gruvberger and Heijer (1972). A case of occupational dermatitis in the paper trade was attributed to chromium compounds by Pirilä and Kilpiö (1954). Slimicides used in the paper pulp industry have been listed by Fregert (1976) and include mercaptobenzothiazole, dithiocarbamate, piperazine and ethylenediamine compounds. Solvents or wetting agents may be necessary; among these are ethylenediamine, iso-propanol and ethylene glycol. Preservatives used in the industry include formaldehyde, halogenated carbanilides, quinolines and sodium pentachlorophenolate.

1,2-Benzisothiazoline-3-one (with ethylene diamine is Proxel CRL)

Proxels (ICI) are a group of preservatives formulated to prevent the growth of microorganisms in the aqueous phases of paints, adhesives, glues, polishes, starches, engineering fluids and for slime control in paper mills. The recommended concentration is 0.01 per cent. Proxels are irritants and sensitisers and skin contact should be avoided.

Two men, while making polyacrylate emulsions for paints and floor waxes, handled undiluted Proxel CRL which is an aqueous solution of 1,2-benzisothiazolin-3-one and ethylene diamine. After two to three years both men developed hand eczema, which in one man affected the palms, wrists and arms. Patch tests: both patients reacted to Proxel CRL (0.1 per cent in water) and to 1,2-benzisothiazolin-3-one (0.1 per cent in ethanol); one man was also sensitised to ethylene diamine (the second component of Proxel CRL) and the other man to formaldehyde, which he also added to the emulsion (Bang Pedersen, 1976).

The related compound, 3-ethylaminobenzisothiazol hydrochloride (Ectimar) is used as a veterinary fungicide and sensitised a kennel owner; he reacted to a patch test with 1 per cent in petrolatum (Dahlquist, 1977).

St John's

A man, aged 24 years, while working in a paper mill mixed the paper ingredients, and when adding Proxel (1,2-benzisothiazolone) as a preservative he wore gloves, but his hands were contaminated when he removed them. He described three attacks of hand eczema, with occasional blisters on the dorsa of the feet, which were directly related to his being at work. Patch tests: he reacted to Proxel 1 per cent and 1,2-benzisothiazolone 0.1 per cent, both in MEK. He was changed to another part of the plant and remained well.

Men making the emulsion for NCR paper have also been sensitised (p. 853)

Patch testing

1,2-benzisothiazolin-3-one	0.1 per cent in MEK
Proxel	0.1 per cent in MEK

Carbon paper

Typescript is reproduced by three varieties of carbon:

1. typewriter ribbon
2. simple carbon paper
3. specialised carbon paper.

The constituents of the dye coating on carbon are:

(i) waxes — carnuba, candelilla, oricony, montan, paraffin wax and beeswax
(ii) oils — mineral and castor oils, stearic and oleic acids
(iii) pigments and dyes — carbon black, methyl and crystal violet, miliori blue, Victoria blue and nigrosine.

In Britain ordinary carbon paper does not contain dyes, the colour is carbon; some carbon papers may be made with oil of violet and others with methyl violet.

Case reports of sensitisation

Contact dermatitis from carbon paper is rare. Three cases of sensitisation have been reported, one from tricresylphosphate, one from nigrosine and one from methyl violet.

Tricresylphosphate. A particular carbon paper with an unusual coating, containing 30 per cent tricresyl phosphate, was formulated to be non-staining and effective with various types of pen. A salesman who handled the carbon paper many times a day developed eczema of the hands and was found on patch testing to be sensitised to the carbon paper and to the tricresylphosphate in the coating (Hjorth, 1964).

Nigrosine base. Solvent black 7, C.I. No 50415B

Nigrosine base is a mixture of compounds. It is widely used in crayons, shoe polishes, typewriter ribbons, carbon papers, inks and leather finishes and occasionally in plastics and lacquers.

A man with a previous history of seborrhoeic eczema suddenly developed a vesicular eczema affecting principally the palmar surfaces of the fingers and hands with lesser involvement of the dorsal surfaces, which he associated with handling computer documents. Patch testing revealed that he was sensitive to the special computer carbon paper and when tested with its ingredients he reacted to nigrosine base 1 per cent in petrolatum. The concentration of the nigrosine base in the carbon paper was 0.5 per cent. He avoided this carbon and his skin healed (Calnan and Connor, 1972).

Methyl violet 2 BN base; 4,4′,4′′-pentamethyltriaminotriphenylhydroxy methane

The dye, which is of the Rosaniline type, is not a pure compound.

The chief engineer of a company manufacturing carbon paper developed eczema of the face, neck, ears, arms and hands. His suspicion that one of two dyes was implicated was confirmed when on patch testing he reacted to methyl

$$\text{NH(CH}_3)_2$$

H₃CHN — ⬡ — C — OH

$$\text{NH(CH}_3)_2$$

violet 2BN, but was negative to methyl violet 10 BN. He was patch tested again six years later with the same result. Despite retiring he continued to have dermatitis (Calnan, 1974).

'No carbon required' (NCR) paper

A specialised paper, devised so that copies could be made without the necessity of using carbon, was introduced by the National Cash Register Company as NCR paper (No Carbon Required). The emulsion used to impregnate the paper contained gelatine, gum arabic and the two dyes, crystal violet lactone and benzoyl leucomethylene blue which were originally dissolved in chlorinated diphenyl, but this has now been replaced. Sensitisation by the paper has not been reported but women handling the original paper complained of headaches, irritation of the eyelids and hands, swelling of the nose and dryness and burning of the mouth, and even asthma. Patch testing with the paper was negative and the symptoms disappeared with improved ventilation in one outbreak, and with a change to a new quality paper in another (Calnan and Connor, 1972; Magnusson, 1974; Calnan, 1979).

St John's

Two men doing the same job in a factory making the emulsion for NCR paper were referred with hand eczema which had been present for four years in Patient A and on the palms of Patient B for 10 years. In both men the feet and other areas had been involved intermittently. The firm supplied details of the manufacturing process including the use, for 18 months, of two Proxel (ICI) compounds as preservatives for the gelatin. Both of these contained 1,2-benzisothiazolin-3-one, and one also contained ethylenediamine.

Patch test results in the two patients and in controls were as follows:

	Patients A and B	Controls
1,2-Benzisothiazolin-3-one:	1%(MEK) A and B tested, both were positive.	21 tested, 2 +
	0.1%(MEK) A tested and was positive	30 tested, 1 +
Proxel:	1%(MEK) A tested and was positive	33 tested, 2 +
	0.1%(MEK) B tested and was positive	50 tested, 0 +
Ethylenediamine:	1%(pet) A and B tested, only A was positive.	

Patient A was additionally sensitised to potassium dichromate and glutaraldehyde.

Subsequently two further men employed in the same work at this plant attended with hand eczema. Patch tests: both reacted to benzisothiazolone 0.1 per cent and one to ethylenediamine.

Conclusion. In the first two men their hand eczema pre-dated their contact with benzisothiazoline or ethylenediamine and this sensitisation was thought to be an aggravating factor in their dermatitis rather than its complete cause.

Sensitisation to benzisothiazolone has also been seen in a paper mill worker (p. 851) and has been reported as a sensitiser in plastic emulsions by Bang Pederson (1976) (p. 851).

Computer paper

The composition of computer paper is likely to be similar to that of ordinary paper. It may contain colophony. 'Long-life' computer tape, which is used repeatedly but only for certain applications, such as machine tools, may contain epoxy resin. Rubber bands are used to secure the computer coils and may be overlooked as a possible cause of hand eczema in computer workers.

Typewriter correction paper

A secretary with dermatitis of the upper eyelids was investigated by Jordan and Bourlas (1975). Patch tests: she reacted to two types of typewriter correcting paper and to a modified phenol formaldehyde resin containing less than 1 per cent maleic anhydride, Arochem 455 (1 per cent in alcohol). Although the formulation of the paper was not disclosed, the resin was identified by gas chromatography. It was thought to be present as a binder for the powdery coating on the paper. Patch tests should therefore be done with the powdered side of the paper. This same resin has caused dermatitis in a marking pen ink (p. 860)

COPYING

Copying is an office procedure suitable for a limited number of reproductions. There are four technical methods: the dyeline or diazo process, photocopying, the heat process, and the electrostatic or xerographic procedure (Harman and Sarkany, 1960).

Thiourea is likely to be present in photocopy paper; it has been reported to be a photosensitiser (p. 441).

Dyeline or diazo method

Original manuscripts, which must be translucent, are placed in contact with light-sensitive paper and by means of a fluorescent light the image is transferred as a negative to the copy, which is then developed by ammonia or other chemical to give a blue (blueprint), brown or black copy. This technique is widely used in drawing offices because it is simple and cheap.

The sensitised paper is coated with a diazonium compound, *p*-diethylaminobenzene diazonium chloride, which is allergenic until exposed to light, but once irradiated it is harmless. Nickel salts are present in some of these papers, as can be shown by a positive reaction to dimethylglyoxime.

Allergic dermatitis

The contact dermatitis affects the fingers and hands primarily but may spread to the face and trunk. Sensitisation from Amonax paper has been described by Harman and Sarkany (1960) and from Ozalid and Radex papers by Verspijck Mijnssen (1963). Five similar cases were reported by Gianotti and Meneghini (1963) and two by Foussereau and Benezra (1970). In 1963 Gertler and Laubstein made a detailed study of the methods and procedures for making blueprints and described the eczema and asthma which affects these workers.

Irritant dermatitis

An irritant dermatitis of the hands may occur from contact with the ammonia used in this process.

Patch tests

Unexposed sensitised paper

p-Diethylaminobenzene diazonium chloride 0.5 per cent in petrolatum or other diazonium salt 0.5 per cent in petrolatum

Phloroglucinol	1 per cent in petrolatum
Resorcinol	2 per cent in petrolatum
Potassium hydroquinone sulphonate	1 per cent in petrolatum

Heat process (Thermofax)

In the 1950s this method of copying was popular but 4-*tertiary*-butyl catechol in the Thermofax paper caused allergic contact dermatitis. Two cases were described by Harman and Sarkany (1960) and they listed the other cases described about that time. They stated that this catechol had been replaced by another chemical. In France, two clerical workers were sensitised by the antioxidant methyl gallate in Thermofax paper. Patch tests: both reacted to the paper and methyl gallate powder (?undiluted) Degos, Lépine and Akhoundzadeh, 1968).

Patch tests

Copy paper

4-*tertiary*-Butyl catechol 0.5 per cent in petrolatum

Methyl gallate   1–2 per cent in petrolatum

Photocopying

Verifax is a photocopying method, and two men who were sensitised while employed making the powder for the sensitised emulsion were described by Harman and Sarkany (1960). Both developed severe and widespread eczema and both were sensitised by 4-phenyl catechol.

Patch tests

Copy paper

4-phenyl catechol 0.5 per cent in petrolatum

Electrostatic or xerographic process

This Rank-Xerox method does not seem to sensitise.

PRINTING AND DUPLICATING

The three methods of printing differ in that the image is raised in letterpress, it is flat in lithography, and it is depressed in photogravure.

Letterpress

Letterpress is the oldest form of printing; it is based on transferring an image from a raised type to paper pressed against it. Cylinders have replaced the flat typed surfaces and composing the type, originally done manually by a compositor, is now done mechanically from a key-board on to a galley which delivers a proof for correction. For high speed newspaper production web (sheet or web of paper)-fed rotary presses are used with curved printing plates usually cast in metal and duplicated by stereotyping. Photographs or drawings are reproduced in metal by photoengraving.

Irritants
Solvents

Sensitisers
Dichromate, used for cleaning the plates, is the principal sensitiser.

Lithography

Lithography is the technique of printing on a flat surface utilising the principle that an oily impression will accept a greasy ink, while the background can be protected by a watery solution.

Lithographic plates

Deep etch lithographic plates are made in the following way: A sheet of anodised aluminium is washed with water or 2 per cent sulphuric acid, rinsed, and then coated with a layer of gum arabic containing dichromate. Once dry, the plate is placed in an exposure frame, covered with a positive, and exposed to ultraviolet light for sufficient time to harden the exposed background coating, leaving the covered printed areas soft. After exposure the plate is processed with solutions containing high concentrations of inorganic salts and lactic acid — first a developer and then an etching liquid which also contains dichromate and a borofluoride salt. These clean and etch the printed areas. The etch is removed by repeated washing with isopropyl alcohol, and an image lacquer is applied which bonds to the exposed plate. A greasy ink is next applied and is held by this lacquer. Finally the background of hardened dichromate-gum arabic is soaked and washed off in water or dilute acid to reveal the clear background metal.

Irritants
Acids, alkalis, solvents, white spirit, toluene, alcohols and detergents.

Sensitisers
Principally dichromate; a remote possibility is formaldehyde in the gum arabic. The inks may contain cobalt, chromate or mercury pigments and phenol for-

maldehyde or occasionally epoxy resins. Acrylic resins are sometimes added and if polymerisation is defective acrylic acid is released and has caused irritant dermatitis (p. 593) (Ducombs, Derville and Texier, 1974).

Offset (litho) printing

Offset printing is based on the principles of lithography but a series of rollers are utilised for the printing process. It is used for printing on paper and on other surfaces and it is becoming an increasingly popular method of printing. Small offset machines are used in many offices and large web-fed offset machines are replacing the old letterpress machines for printing newspapers. The term web-fed pertains to the method of feeding the paper into the machine.

Regardless of the size of the machines the principles of the method are the same. A flexible metal plate is printed with type which accepts an oil-based ink, while the rest of the plate is made oil repellant with gum arabic and an aqueous solution containing glycerine and 1–2 per cent phosphoric acid. The printed plate is attached to a rotating cylinder, it is coloured by ink rollers and moistened by the watery solution. The image in ink is reversed on to a rubber blanket cylinder which in turn transfers the print — the correct way up — to paper on the impression cylinder.

Irritants

It is a wet job.

The blanket wash and blanket restorer, which are used frequently to keep the rubber blanket clean and free of ink smudges, are fat solvents, usually white spirit or methyl ethyl ketone with a small amount of dye. These solvents may cause an irritant dermatitis of the hands.

Sensitisers

Aqueous solutions. Formaldehyde added as a preservative in the solutions has caused allergic dermatitis (Simpson, 1969); phenol may be added for the same purpose. Occasionally nickel salts are included in the formulation to increase the water repellent effect (p. 361).

The gum arabic is preserved with formaldehyde.

Working materials. Sensitisation to cobalt and chromium in three offset printers from the same factory was explained when these metals were detected by atomic absorption spectrophotometry of working materials from the plant (Malten, 1975; Spriut and Malten, 1975).

Inks have a similar composition to paints except that paints are thicker. Cobalt, mercury or chromate pigments may occasionally sensitise.

Paper may contain a small amount of colophony.

Silk screen printing

Silk screen printing is a simple technique which has the advantage of being able to print on flat, round or shaped surfaces. A silk or nylon screen is tightly secured in a frame and a stencil placed over it so that ink can be rolled over the stencil to print on a surface pressed to the undersurface of the silk. In other methods the design is outlined on the silk itself by making the silken background impervious to ink.

Irritants
White spirit, the screenwash of petroleum solvents and detergents.

Sensitisers
Potassium dichromate; cobalt pigments and oil of turpentine or one of its derivatives in inks.

Photogravure

This method of printing is based on etching the design on to the surface of a copper cylinder or plate so that the depressions can be filled with ink and the image transferred to paper pressed against the metal. A photographic process imprints the design on the plate using gelatin containing dichromate which can be hardened by exposure to light. Soft unexposed gelatin can be washed away and the design etched into the plate.

Irritants
Acids, alkalis and solvents used in etching.

Sensitisers
Dichromate and possibly oil of turpentine.

Light sensitive acrylates (p. 590)

INKS

Inks are of two types: printing and marking pen inks, and writing inks. Both are rare sensitisers.

Printing inks

Printing inks are viscous to semi-solid suspensions; they are used in letterpress for newspapers, in lithography and in many other occupational printing techniques. They may contain:

1. Drying oils: such as heat bodied linseed oil.
2. Pigments: include carbon black for newsprint, and yellow colours may be lead chrome or barium chromate.
3. Varnish: may contain esterified rosin, glycerol or pentaerythritol.
4. Resins: phenol formaldehyde and alkyd resins are used in many printing

inks; epoxy and acrylic resins occasionally. Resins are added to achieve quick setting, gloss, durability and rub resistance.
5. Solvents: petroleum distillates of the kerosene type.
6. Driers: cobalt, manganese and lead soaps are added to catalyse drying.
7. Waxes: are present occasionally.

Occupational dermatitis — allergic

p-Aminoazbenzene (aniline yellow). A postal worker developed eczema of the pulp of his right thumb and the tip of his nose. Patch tests clarified the cause: he reacted to stamp ink and *p*-aminobenzene (1 per cent in petrolatum), one of its constituents; he was also positive to *p*-phenylenediamine (5 per cent in petrolatum) (Braun, 1975).

Light sensitive acrylates. (p. 592)

Epoxy resin

St John's

> *Silk screen printing.* Two silk screen printers were sensitised by epoxy resin in their white inks; both were printing on glass or plastic bottles. The first patient, a man aged 28 years with a previous history of hand eczema, complained that after three years as a silk screen printer his hands became worse, the skin of his fingers split and he developed an intermittent facial rash. The second patient, a woman aged 60 years, had worked for the same firm for eight years when she developed eczema of the dorsa of her hands which spread up her arms. She admitted getting paint and thinners on her hands and though supplied with gloves she did not wear them. Patch tests: both patients reacted to epoxy resin 2 per cent in petrolatum. The man was tested with his white ink and was positive; he was also sensitive to potassium dichromate, but not to the other chemicals he handled.

> *Printing ink manufacture.* A man aged 55 years who had worked in an ink manufacturers for six years blending inks suddenly developed eczema of his inner arms and face which fluctuated in severity. Despite wearing rubber gloves and protective clothing, he described considerable contamination by the materials he handled. Prior to the onset of his dermatitis epoxy resin had been added as a stabiliser to a particular range of inks destined mainly for export to West Africa. Patch tests: he was positive to epoxy resin 2 per cent in petrolatum and his own epoxy ink; he was negative to all his other inks.

> *Phenol formaldehyde.* An apprentice printer aged 20 years who was employed as a letterpress machine minder developed eczema of his hands and arms. Patch tests: he was positive to phenol formaldehyde (10 per cent in petrolatum) but was negative to his inks and the standard series of allergens. It was confirmed from the ink suppliers that phenol formaldehyde was used in the formulation of their inks.

Fast-drying marking pen. A fast drying marking pen used to demarcate patch test sites sensitised one subject. He reacted to the ink marks and to an open test with the ink. Patch tests: when tested with the constituents he was strongly positive to the resin Arochem 455, 6 per cent in ethanol. It was identified as a modified phenolic formaldehyed maleic anhyrdride resin (Maibach, 1975). This same resin was the sensitiser in typewriter correction paper (p. 854).

The blue component, 1,4-bis(isopropylamino)anthraquinone, Colour Index Solvent Blue 36, of the black ink in a felt-tip marker pen sensitised two adults (Miller, Goldberg and Wilkerson, 1978).

Antabuse — alcohol reaction. N-Butyraldoxime (butanol oxime) is an antioxidant and has been added to inks as an anti-skimming compound. It is a volatile chemical and in a printing plant it was found that if men inhaled it and then drank alcohol the acetaldehyde level of their blood rose and they developed the unpleasant symptoms of an antabuse-like reaction (Lewis and Schwartz, 1956).

Writing inks
Inks for fountain pens are coloured aqueous solutions; those for ball-point pens are oily with a paste-like consistency.

These inks may contain:

Colours: water or oil soluble dyes; drawing inks are dispersions of carbon black in a colloid.

Preservative: may be parabens in watery inks.

Washable inks: contain glycerol.

Other additives: tannic or gallic acid.

Dermatitis — allergic

Aminoazotoluene is a yellow, oil-soluble, aniline dye which has been used in red and green semi-solid inks for ball point pens. Three women who developed eczema of the arms, hands or face where the ink had touched their skin were described by Meara and Martin-Scott (1953). Patch tests: each patient was positive to the red and green inks and to aminoazotoluene 0.01 per cent in petrolatum; blue and black inks were negative.

Similar cases have been seen in Norway and France. Björnstad's (1957) patient had positive patch tests to aminoazotoluol, *para*-phenylenediamine and *para*-aminophenol, and Castelain's (1967) patient reacted to a patch test with 0.01 per cent aminoazotoluene.

Patch testing
Inks	undiluted (very occasionally inks are irritant)
p-aminobenzene	1 per cent in petrolatum
p-aminoazotoluene	1 per cent in petrolatum

For printing or occupational inks:
phenol formaldehyde	10 per cent in petrolatum
epoxy resin	2 per cent in petrolatum
?other resins	

Light sensitive inks (p. 595).

PHOTOGRAPHY

Some of the chemicals used in photography are sensitisers; those for black and white developing rarely cause allergic dermatitis, but those for colour developing do cause trouble if exposure is not prevented during their handling.

Black and white processing

Potential allergenis are present in several of the solutions but metol in the developing formulation is the most likely to sensitise; however metol-free developers are obtainable. Lichen planus has now been described from a black and white developer (p. 862).

Developers and replenishers

Hydroquinone (1,4-benzenediol)   Resorcinol (1,3-benzenediol)   Pyrocatechol (1,2-benzenediol)

Pyrogallol (1,2,3-benzenetriol)   Phloroglucinol (1,3,5-benzenetriol)

Metol (*p*-methylaminophenol suphate)

Amidol (2,4-diaminophenol dihydrochloride)

Phenidone (1-phenyl-3-pyrazolidinone)

TSS
(4-amino-*N*, *N*-diethylaniline sulphate *N*, *N*-diethyl-*p*-phenylenediamine sulphate)

Developers and replenishers are alkaline aqueous solutions of similar composition, except that the replenisher is more concentrated and has a higher pH.

Many of these chemicals are phenols; some are primary amines. They include hydroquinone, resorcinol, pyrocatechol, pyrogallol, phloroglucinol, metol (*p*-methylaminophenol sulphate), phenidone (1-phenyl-3-pyrazolidinone), amidol (2,4-diaminophenol dihyrdochloride).

Fixers are aqueous solutions of sodium thiosulphate with acetic acid, sodium hydroxide, and boric acid, none of which sensitises.

Sodium metabisulphite may be present and it is a weak sensitiser (p. 706).

Bleaches are used for reversal processing and may contain potassium ferricyanide, sodium bromide, disodium phosphate anhydride and phosphate glass. Potassium dichormate may be included in some older formulations.

Photographic dish cleaners and stain removers. These are often dilute solutions of sulphuric acid and contain potassium dichromate.

Other chemicals. Other sensitising chemicals used in photography include: formaldehyde, glutaraldehyde, ethylenediamine salicylaldoxime and triazine compounds.

Salicylaldoxime (2-hydroxybenzaldehyde oxime)

Report of dermatitis
Dermatitis in photographic factories in Sophia was investigated by Popchristov, Balevska and Michajlov (1957). They found the main causes to be an acetone adhesive and a colour film developer; less important were acids, solvents and black and white developer. In London, a man working for a photographic company developed a contact dermatitis of his hands which was directly related to his work. The sensitiser was eventually traced after a visit to the factory. Patch tests: he reacted to salicylaldoxime 0.1 per cent (30 controls were negative); he was also sensitive to mercury (Calnan, 1967). A laboratory worker developed an acute hand aczema after one month's contact with a triazine film hardener. Patch tests: she reacted intensely to the triazine hardener 0.5 per cent in water (Baker, 1971).

Lichen Planus (TSS; 4-amino-*N,N*-diethylaniline sulphate). The same chemicals as those used in colour developing are now being used in processing high-speed black and white film. One such developer containing TSS and metol caused hand eczema in two newspaper photographers. The first patient stopped using the developer and his hands healed; the second man continued to use it and after one year the eruption changed from eczema to lichen planus. Patch tests: both men reacted to TSS (0.5 per cent aqueous) but only the first patient reacted to metol (1 per cent petrolatum) and CD2 (1 per cent in petrolatum). Both were negative to CD3 (1 per cent in petrolatum) (Roed-Petersen and Menné, 1976).

Patch testing

	%
Ammonium persulphate	2.5
Amidol	2.0
Pyrocatechol	2.0
Ethylenediaminetetra-acetate	1.0
EDTA sodium salt)	
Hydroquinone	1.0
Metol	1.0
Phenidone	1.0
Pyrogallol	1.0
TSS; 4-amino-*N,N*-diethylaniline sulphate	1.0
Sodium metabisulphite	1–5
Potassium dichromate	0.5
Salicylaldoxime	0.1 each in petrolatum
Formaldehyde	2.0 aqueous
Glutaraldehyde	1.0 aqueous
Triazine compound	0.1–0.5 aqueous

X-ray developers
The developing of X-ray plates can be a wet job and this of itself may cause dermatitis of the hands in radiographers.

The developing solutions contain the same sensitisers as are used in black and white developing (p. 861).

Colour developing
The proclivity of colour developers to produce a contact dermatitis, which closely resembles lichen planus, was first recognised by Graciansky *et al.* (1958) in France and by Buckley (1958) in the United States. The initial spate of cases ceased when colour processing was automated and now only sporadic cases occur in small firms, or among amateur photographers.

Colour developers include:

Kodak

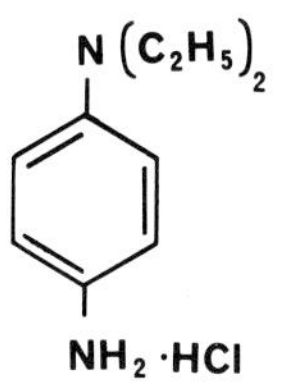

CDI (4-*N*, *N*-diethylphenylenediamine monohydrochloride)

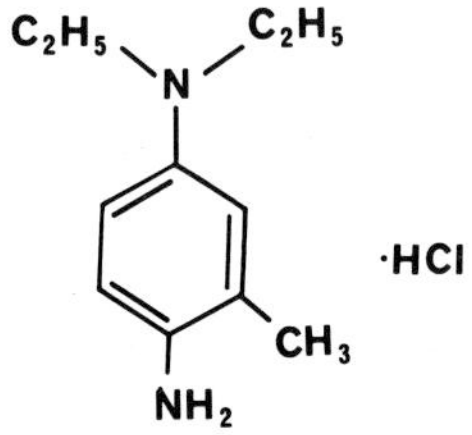

$$C_2H_5 \diagdown N \diagup C_2H_5$$

·HCl

$$CH_3$$

$$NH_2$$

CD2 (4-N, N-diethyl-2-methylphenylenediamine monohydrochloride)

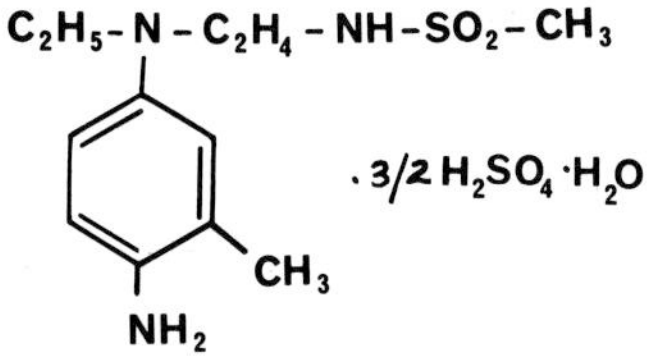

$$C_2H_5-N-C_2H_4-NH-SO_2-CH_3$$

· 3/2 H$_2$SO$_4$ ·H$_2$O

$$CH_3$$

$$NH_2$$

CD3 (4-(N-ethyl-N-2-methanesulphonylaminoethyl)-2-methyl-phenylenediamine sesquisulphate monohydrate)

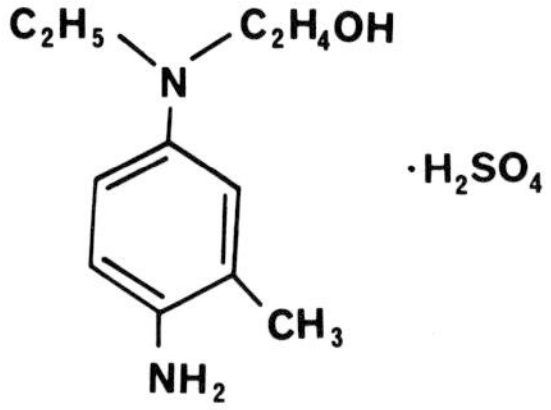

$$C_2H_5 \diagdown N \diagup C_2H_4OH$$

·H$_2$SO$_4$

$$CH_3$$

$$NH_2$$

CD4 (4-(N-ethyl-N-2-hydroxyethyl-2-methylphenylenediamine sulphate)

CD6: 4-amino-N-ethyl(2-methoxyethyl)-m-toluidine di-p-toluene sulphonate

Agfa
TSS: 4-amino-N-diethylaniline sulphate

Ilford
MI 210: N-ethyl-N-(5 hydroxy-amyl)-p-phenylenediamine hydrogen sulphate

Reports of dermatitis
Sensitisation from these chemicals has been most frequently reported with CD2 (Mandel, 1960; Knusden, 1964; Fry, 1965; Miranda *et al.*, 1978), occasionally from CD3 (Fry, 1965) and one case each from Agfa TSS (Knusden, 1964) and MI 210 (Fry, 1965).

In the early days, before the use of preventive measures, sensitisation from colour developers was frequent. An incidence of 25 per cent in one plant was quoted by Buckley (1958), and Knusden (1964) stated that 50 per cent in those exposed were affected.

Colour developers cause both an eczematous contact dermatitis and a lichen planus-like eruption. In some patients the changes are not clear cut and there are clinical features of both conditions.

The lichen planus-like eruption begins around the nail folds and on the sides of the fingers and then spreads to the hands, arms, face, neck, genitalia and other covered parts of the body. Wickham's striae occur in the lesions (Canizares, 1959; Graciansky and Boulle, 1966) and the mouth, although not usually involved (Buckley, 1958; Canizares, 1959; Fry, 1965), can be affected (Knudsen, 1964; Graciansky and Boulle, 1966; Miranda *et al.*, 1978). Healing is with hyperpigmentation as in idiopathic lichen planus. The histology shows features of lichen planus.

Three technicians employed in the French television service developed an intensely itchy, fissured dermatitis of the dorsa of their fingers and vesicles on the fronts of the wrists. They were accustomed to immerse their hands in various solutions including one called chromogène, containing CDI (*N,N*-diethyl*para*-phenylenediamine chlorhydrate). Patch tests: they gave eczematous reactions to the CD1 diluted to 5 per cent and 2 per cent in lanolin-petrolatum (Textier, Delaunay and Ducombs, 1976).

Patch tests with the colour developers are not always positive in either the eczematous or the lichenoid eruptions; when a reaction does occur it is eczematous.

The prognosis for healing is generally good once contact with the colour developers ceases and the eruption clears within weeks to a few months. However, Canizares (1959) found it to persist for 6–12 months.

Patch testing
Colour developers each 1 per cent in petrolatum

Fluxes

A solder is a metal alloy with a relatively low melting point, used to join together metals of higher melting points. It is important that the metal surfaces to be fused are clean and wettable. A flux is used for this purpose.

A flux is applied to the metals to be soldered; it cleans their surfaces by removing oxide films and when heated it facilitates the flow of the solder. Fluxes are reducing agents: some are amines, they inhibit oxidation by atmospheric oxygen and thus prevent tarnishing of the metal surfaces.

Some fluxes such as zinc chloride are strong irritants, others like ammonium chloride have a low toxicity. Hydrazine and aminoethylethanolamine are strong sensitisers but colophony, widely used as a flux, seems, in this capacity, to sensitise only occasionally.

COLOPHONY (p. 784)

HYDRAZINE

$$H_2 N NH_2$$

Hydrazine is a colourless, fuming hygroscopic liquid with a sweet ammoniacal smell. It is miscible with water, is a strong reducing agent and is highly reactive. In combination with acids it forms hydrazine hydrobromide and hydrazine hydrochloride, both of which are used as solders. In the anhydrous form it is more caustic and more explosive than when hydrated. The vapour is highly irritant to the eyes, mucous membranes, nasopharynx and respiratory tract, and if absorbed hydrazine is a systemic poison.

Hydrazine has many uses, one of which is as a flux, particularly for soldering brass and copper and sometimes aluminium and other metals. In fluxes it is present in a concentration of 10–20 per cent. Hydrazine derivatives are also used as chicken feed additives and as precursors of photographic chemicals.

Sensitising potential
Hydrazine was found by Kligman (1966) to be a potent allergen, using 5 per cent for induction and 0.5 per cent for challenge in the maximisation test he sensitised all those exposed.

Occupational dermatitis
Hydrazine monohydrochloride and stanno-chloride in aqueous solution were introduced as a new flux into a tin factory in Copenhagen and caused dermatitis of the hands and arms in 12 of 34 women workers. (Frost and Hjorth, 1959). Patch tests: hydrazine sulphate 1 per cent in water gave positive reactions in 6 of 12 affected; 30 controls were negative. Another outbreak of dermatitis from a flux containing 10–20 per cent hydrazine monohydrobromide was reported from an electric plant in Virginia by Wheeler, Penn and Cawley (1965). About half of those soldering developing mild to severe dermatitis of the fingers, hands, arms, face and eyelids. Vesicular eczema of the palmar sides of the fingers and hands simulated a constitutional eczema. Contaminated articles or walking through the soldering department caused relapses in those highly sensitised. Patch tests: hydrazine flux 0.1 per cent was positive in four patients tested.

Cross-sensitivity to hydrazine was investigated in one patient by Frost and Hjorth (1959). She reacted to aqueous dilutions of apresoline (1-hydrazinophthalazine hydrochloride) 2.5 per cent, phenylhydrazine 0.2 per cent and isonicotinic acid hydrazine 10 per cent.

A factory worker was sensitised to hydrazine while making one of its derivatives, aminoguanidine hydrochloride, a chicken feed additive (Suzuki and Ohkido, 1979).

Patch tests
Hydrazine sulphate or hydrobromide 1–2 per cent in water or petrolatum.

Testing with the same hydrazine concentration by diluting the whole flux can give false negative results (Crow, 1969).

AMINOETHYLETHANOLAMINE N-(2-Hydroxyethyl)ethylenediamine. AEE.

$$NH_2CH_2CH_2NHCH_2CH_2OH$$

Aminoethylethanolamine (AEE), a hygroscopic liquid, is used in textile finishing and in the manufacture of resins, rubbers and insecticides. It is also used as a flux.

Occupational dermatitis

In the 1950s and 1960s the scarcity and expense of copper led to the use of aluminium as an alternative metal for the conducting cores in power cables. An initial difficulty in soldering aluminium was overcome when an efficient soldering flux (Kynal) was developed, based on fluoroborate and about 55 per cent AEE. Unfortunately the amine was found to be a strong sensitiser by Crow, Harman and Holden (1968) who investigated in detail dermatitis in cable jointers employed by the Electricity Supply Industry in England. The clinical picture in these cable jointers was variable: some had finger tip and nail fold lesions with distortion of the nail plates, others had eczema of the hands, arms face and eyelids. The fingers tip lesions simulated those of chronic paronychia. Patch tests: 23 patients were patch tested and all were positive to AEE 5 per cent in water and it was notable that this preparation elicited stronger reactions than the flux itself containing 55 per cent AEE. A series of 200 control patients were patch tested with 1 per cent 5 per cent aqueous solutions of AEE, monoethanolamine, diethanolamine and triethanolamine and all were negative; it was also considered safe to use undiluted Kynal for patch testing.

Patch testing

Aminoethylethanolamine 5 per cent and 1 per cent in water or petrolatum.

CHEMICAL DEPIGMENTATION

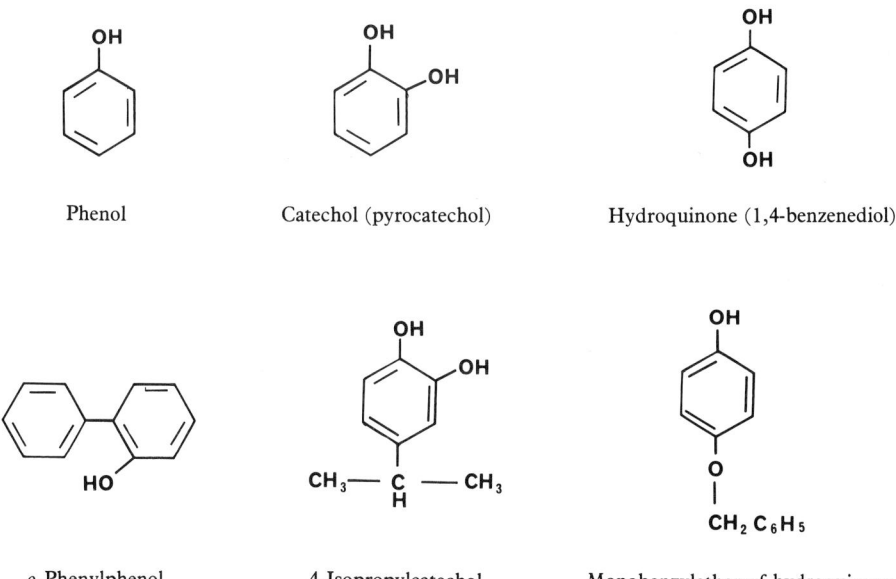

Phenol   Catechol (pyrocatechol)   Hydroquinone (1,4-benzenediol)

o-Phenylphenol   4-Isopropylcatechol   Monobenzylether of hydroquinone

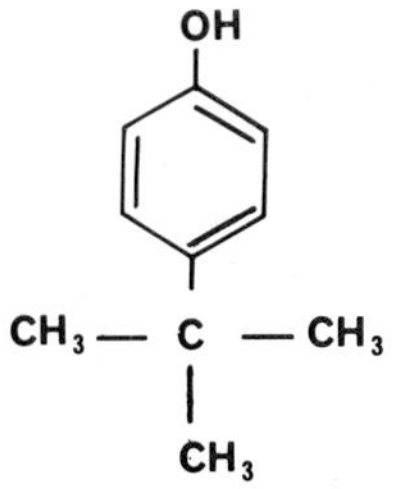

PTB phenol (*p-tert*-butylphenol)

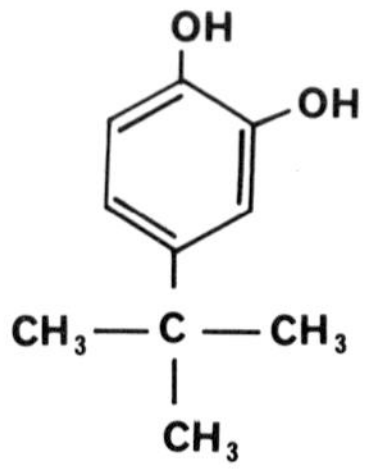

PTB catechol

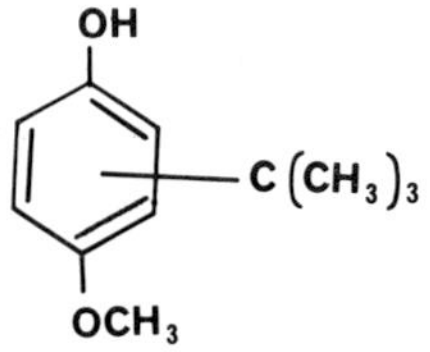

Butylated hydroxyanisole (BHA)

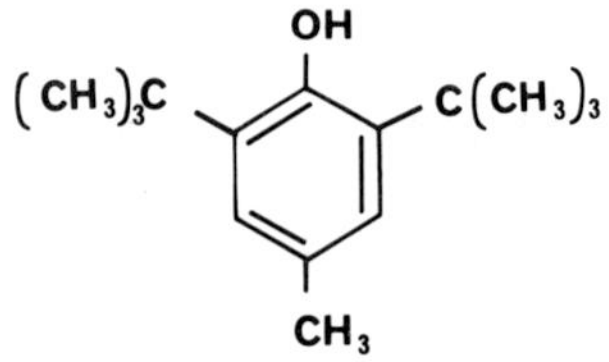

Butylated hydroxytoluene (BHT)

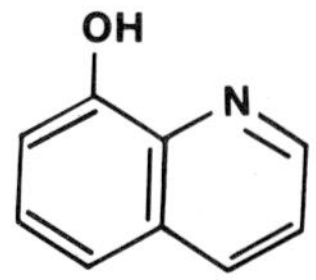

8-Hydroxyquinoline

Phenolic compounds depigment the skin by damaging or destroying the melanocytes. This toxic effect was first described from monobenzyl ether of hydroquinone in rubber but more recently phenolics in adhesives and disinfectants have also been incriminated. Clinically the appearance may be indistinguishable from idiopathic vitiligo and therefore the correct aetiology is easily overlooked.

The mechanism of the depigmentation has been studied in laboratory animals by Riley (1969), Zaumseil and Wohlrab (1976) and Wohlrab and Zaumseil (1976) Gellin *et al.* (1979). Bleehan *et al.* (1968) found that the bleaching potency of the chemicals is greatest when the substituting alkyl is in the *para* (4) position as in 4-*iso*propylcatechol. Within the melanosomes these phenolic compounds act as a substrate for tyrosinase and form semiquinone free radicals which diffuse into the cytoplasm and, by initiating lipid peroxidation, cause cell damage (Riley, 1971).

Monobenzyl ether of hydroquinone (MHQ)
Occupational leucoderma was first described by Oliver, Schwartz and Warren (1939, 1940) among tannery workers who wore rubber gloves containing mono-

benzyl ether of hydroquinone (MHQ, agerite alba). In most of the men only the hands and arms were depigmented, but covered areas were also affected in several cases. It was noted that the hairs remained coloured and that the skin repigmented in many of the men once they discarded the gloves. In those affected, patch tests with MHQ elicited reactions and the sites depigmented within a few days. Similar reported cases were due to rubber dust and debris (Zakon and Goldberg, 1951). Therapeutically, MHQ has been used to bleach the skin, but it is an irritant and a sensitiser and the depigmentation it causes is often mottled and unsightly; in addition positive patch test reactions become white (Spencer, 1962).

Hydroquinone
The topical application of hydroquinone was shown to depigment the skin by Denton, Lerner and Fitzpatrick (1952). In clinical practice its efficacy as a bleaching agent is moderate and transient, and it may cause disfiguring, confetti-like depigmentation. In a cream base 2 per cent hydroquinone was reported to be as effective as 5 per cent and caused less inflammation; sensitisation was uncommon, whereas irritation was frequent particularly with the higher concentrations (Arndt and Fitzpatrick, 1965; Spencer, 1965).

Hydroquinone damages melanocytes by interfering with the formation and melanisation of the melanosomes, destroying the membranous organelles and finally causing necrosis of the cell (Jimbow et al., 1974).

In South Africa the bleaching effect of creams containing 6–8 per cent hydroquinone has been followed by darkening of the skin due to ochronosis and the formation of pigmented colloid milia (Findlay, Morrison and Simson, 1975).

p-tert-Butyl Phenol (PTBP)

Manufacturing process
In the 1960s, it was first observed that workers engaged in the production of p-tert-butyl phenol (PTBP) developed depigmentation of the skin. Cases were reported initially in the USSR, then in Japan and subsequently in Holland. Malten et al. (1971) described their clinical findings and the experimental work done at that time. This depigmentation, which was non-inflammatory, occurred both on exposed skin and in a strikingly symmetrical distribution on covered areas such as the shoulders and buttocks, indicating absorption not only through the skin but also by inhalation or possibly by ingestion. Transient and rather indefinite systemic symptoms were described by some of the patients. Once contact ceased there was a tendency for spontaneous but slow repigmentation, the prognosis being better in those with short histories and limited leucoderma. In a British plant, of 198 men exposed, 47 (24 per cent) had obvious leucoderma, and in a further 7 (4 per cent) it was detectable by Wood's light. Clinically it was indistinguishable from vitiligo and its occurrence related to the duration and intensity of exposure. Twenty men were patch tested with 2 per cent PTBP and all were negative. Over the course of a year there was partial return of pigment in half (16/35) the men. Workers handling octyl or nonyl

phenols in another factory were unaffected (James, Mayes and Stevenson, 1977).

Adhesives

Occupational leucoderma occurred in an automobile factory among men using a PTBP resin adhesive to secure trim linings (Calnan and Cooke, 1973, 1974). One operative was patch tested with the adhesive; he had a positive reaction and one month later the site was depigmented. Concentrations of free phenol, as high as 10 per cent, were demonstrated in the resin by careful chemical analysis. A shoemaker, described by Wozniak and Hamm (1977), developed an allergic contact dermatitis of his hands, arms and face from PTBP and two years later the skin of his hands, feet and scrotum became depigmented.

Consumer. A chemist repaired his leather watch strap with a neoprene adhesive and developed leucoderma of his wrist (Calnan and Cooke, 1974); a similar patient was reported by Malten (1975).

Disinfectants (PTBP and *p-tert*-amyl phenol)
Phenolic disinfectants have depigmented the skin of hospital workers (Kahn, 1970). The compounds implicated were PTBP and *p-tert*-amylphenol, and they also sensitised some of those exposed. Experimentally, occlusion was required to reproduce the leucoderma and repigmentation was more rapid in the controls than in the patients. This same PTBP germicide (0-Syl) has caused leucoderma in other hospitals; in one man inflammation preceded the loss of pigment which progressed despite cessation of contact (Odom and Stein, 1973), whereas in other cases the onset was insidious and the pigment returned (Bentley Philips, 1974).

Lubricating oil (*tert*-Butylcatechol)
In a tappet assembly plant, 75 workers were in contact with a mineral oil containing 0.005 per cent *tert*-butylcatechol (TBC) present as a rust inhibitor and anti-oxidant. Four developed leucoderma and, in three of these, covered areas were affected; three had had a preceding dermatitis which had also affected many of the employees (60 per cent) in that section. Of the four patients with leucoderma, three had a positive patch test to TBC 0.1 per cent in acetone, and one developed, at the test site, depigmentation which was still present 20 months later. In control subjects the oil elicited irritation of the skin but not depigmentation (Gellin, Possick and Davis, 1970).

Orthophenylphenol and p-phenylphenol
In a chemical factory, workers manufacturing *o*-phenylphenol and *p*-phenylphenol developed leucoderma; and it was found that the hair of black mice was bleached by feeding them with these compounds (Ito, Nishitani and Hara, 1968).

p-Cresol
The topical application of *p*-cresol to black mice in the anagen phase of the hair cycle caused permanent depigmentation of the hairs (Shelley, 1974).

Systemic effect — PTBP
Systemic disease from absorption of PTBP was first reported from West Germany by Rodermund, *et al.* (1975) and Rodermund (1976). They described three cases all with abnormal liver function tests, abnormal liver biopsies and goitres with some impairment of thyroid function; splenomegaly was detectable in two. In a British study (James, Mayes and Stevenson, 1977) liver damage was confirmed but other disease was not detected. Of their 54 men with leucoderma, six had extensive depigmentation and increased aspartate aminotransferases. Three of these, although not jaundiced, had a raised serum bilirubin, and in all six of them a liver biopsy showed moderate to severe focal fatty change. The liver disease was not progressive because within six months of ceasing contact with PTBP the liver function tests returned to normal. Goldmann and Theiss (1976) found patients with occupational leucoderma to be indistinguishable from those with idiopathic vitiligo as regards the triad of vitiligo, and hepatic and thyroid abnormalities.

Butylated Hydroxytoluene (BHT)
Butylated Hydroxyanisole (BHA)
Two Negro children developed depigmentation at sites treated with betamethasone 17-valerate under polythene occlusion. The steroid was not considered responsible and the leucoderma was attributed to butylated hydroxytoluene (BHT), present in the polytheme film as an anti-oxidant (Vollum, 1971). Experimentally, Maibach, Gellin and Ring (1975) applied BHT repeatedly to dark-skinned subjects but failed to produce depigmentation.

Another antioxidant, butylated hydroxyanisole (BHA), was included by Riley (1971) in a list of phenolic compounds shown, *in vivo*, to have, depigmenting effect.

8-Hydroxyquinoline
The application of 8-hydroxyquinoline to mouse skin at a critical stage in the hair cycle causes depigmentation of the hair; 8-hydroxyquinaldine has a similar effect (Searle, 1972). The development of leucoderma of the face, and other areas, in a girl with acne was attributed by Calnan (1973) to her use of a cream containing hydroxyquinoline sulphate 0.5 per cent. A patch test with the cream was negative.

Steroids
The depigmenting action of corticosteroids has been studied experimentally in animals (Arnold, Anthonioz and Marchand, 1975) and described as a result of their therapeutic use in man (Marchand, Arnold and Ndiaye, 1976).

Carbamate (p. 398)

Barrier creams

Barrier creams became popular after the Second World War, but the idea of a protective cream had been in existence for fifty years.

White (1923) suggested that a greasy application should be rubbed well into the pores, creases and cracks before work in order to protect the skin. Further belief in the possibility of protection by ointments was expressed by Schwartz (1942) who thought that although they should be low on the list of preventive measures they ought to be used in industry as they might be the only available means of protection. He divided protective ointments into six types according to their function: (i) to facilitate washing; (ii) to form an 'invisible glove' to prevent irritants touching the skin; (iii) to fill the pores with a harmless fat, blocking the entrance of irritants; (iv) to incorporate a bland chemical which would detoxify irritants; (v) to coat the skin with protective inert powders; and finally (vi) to guard against the photosensitising action of tars, oils and excessive sunlight.

In 1946 Sadler and Marriott tried in the laboratory to justify their statement that 'the ability of barrier creams to prevent deleterious substances reaching the skin of operatives has been amply proved in practice and it can be asserted that the so-called 'invisible glove' produced when these preparations are properly applied has done much to limit the incidence of dermatitis'. They immersed films of barrier cream in industrial liquids, dropped substances onto them until they disintegrated, and then shook the creams and liquids to see if dispersion occurred. To improve on these methods they coated paper with barrier creams and timed penetration through the paper. Their results were not conclusive and they decided that 'the final arbiter of quality must rest on the clinical testing of the cream'. Porter (1959) used a similar method of coating paper with cream and testing it for penetration through the layer, but he employed a machine which bent the paper continuously in order to try to simulate conditions of use. He tested 11 creams but found they did not 'give the degree of protection claimed by the makers'.

Cruickshank (1948) in a more realistic approach tested 26 barrier creams by applying them to the forearm, followed by a layer of machine oil. After washing them off, he examined the underlying skin for the presence of oil. He found that the degree of protection paralleled the thickness of the layer of cream, but that even a layer 120 μ thick, left on for as long as one hour, did not protect the skin from oil. This thickness of cream would be impracticable in working conditions where the recommended film depth is 30μ. He thought, however, that greasy creams were useful as they facilitated cleansing. He emphasised that these experiments took no account of the friction and perspiration which occurred under working conditions.

In the 1950s Morris and Maloof (1953) and Morris (1954) investigated the efficacy of barrier creams and also found them wanting. Morris tested 24 creams for their ability to protect the skin from oil and found that only two prevented contamination when the oil was applied for 30 minutes. However, five of the creams could not be washed off, even with a strong industrial cleanser. He also tested two silicone creams (containing 20–50 per cent silicone) by applying them to areas of skin prior to patch testing with chemicals to which the patient was known to be sensitive. They failed to prevent the development of reactions. They were also used on three patients with treated dermatitis, for several days before they returned to work in accordance with the manufacturer's instructions. They did not protect any of them from an immediate relapse on return to work. In contrast, Suskind (1954 and 1955) gave a favourable opinion of silicone barrier creams if used in the correct concentration, namely 30–50 per cent. He found that a cream containing 52.5 per cent silicone in a bentonite base gave considerable protection in an aircraft engine plant. It was useful 'against light petroleum oils and irritants such as rust preventives dissolved in such media and against insoluble cutting oils, soluble coolants, aqueous solutions of sulphuric acid and metallic dusts'.

More recently, Wahlberg (1971) used an isotope technique in guinea pigs to study the effect of four barrier creams on the topical absorption of sodium chromate. He found that the barrier effect was slight until a film 1 mm in thickness was applied; paradoxically, increasing the film thickness diminished the protection given by some creams. Perhaps by acting as vehicles they facilitated absorption. The efficiency of barrier creams in protecting against the percutaneous absorption of solvents, such as toluene, can be assessed by measuring the excretion of the solvent in the breath. This method has been found simple and effective by Guillemin et al. (1974).

The claim that barrier creams facilitate skin cleansing after work (Cruickshank, 1948) has been investigated (Crow, 1969) by assessing the ease with which a mixture of soot and oil could be removed from the arms of workmen who had previously applied a barrier cream. A marginal benefit in favour of the presence of a barrier cream was obviated by using a more efficient cleanser.

In the past decade there has been considerable scepticism about the value of barrier creams. The reports of Engel and Calnan (1963, 1966) showed that, when used in a car factory, they were ineffective in preventing two outbreaks of allergic contact dermatitis — one due to chromate in a primer paint and the other to a resin in an adhesive. In both outbreaks approximately 70 per cent of the men had used a barrier cream and were not protected. Bettley (1960) in a review of the subject strongly criticised the claims made for barrier creams as being completely unsupported by experimental evidence. He further indicted them as being possible mild irritants due to the high soap concentration in some of them, which may cause a chapping-like effect and enhance the penetration of chemicals handled. He concluded that whether these creams diminish or increase the risk of dermatitis is unknown and he deplored the support they have received from the medical profession.

Patch testing
Barrier cream — As Is (may be a mild irritant).

The irritancy of barrier creams, when used for patch testing, particularly those which are oil-resistant, was demonstrated by Kuske, Klayman, and Schwartz (1956) and Tas (1957).

References

Anderson, F.E. (1960) Cement and oil dermatitis. The part played by chrome sensitivity. *British Journal of Dermatology*, **72**, 108.

Arndt, K.A. & Fitzpatrick, T.B. (1965) Topical use of hydroquinone as a depigmenting agent. *Journal of the American Medical Association*, **194**, 965.

Arnold, J., Anthonioz, P. & Marchand, J.P. (1975) Depigmenting action of corticosteroids. *Dermatologica*, **151**, 274.

Baker, H. (1971) Contact dermatitis — triazine film hardener. *Transactions of the St John's Hospital Dermatological Society*, **57**, 243.

Bang Pedersen, N. (1976) Occupational allergy from 1,2-benzisothiazolin-3-one and other preservatives in plastic emulsions. *Contact Dermatitis*, **2**, 340.

Barnes, R.L. & Wilkinson, D.S. (1973) Epidermal necrolysis from clothing impregnated with paraffin. *British Medical Journal*, **4**, 466.

Bentley-Phillips, B. (1974) Depigmentation caused by a phenolic detergent — germicide. *Archives of Dermatology*, **110**, 296.

Bettley, F.R. (1960) Some dermatological hazards of today. *British Medical Journal*, **2**, 1467.

Bjornstad, R. (1957) Acute eczema due to dry ink. *Acta Dermato-Venereologica*, **37**, 408.

Bleehan, S.S., Pathak, M.A., Hori, Y. & Fitzpatrick, T.B. (1968) Depigmentation of skin with 4-isopropylcatechol, mercaptoamines and other compounds. *Journal of Investigative Dermatology*, **50**, 103.

Borelli, S. & Dungemann, H. (1964) Aktuelle Kontaktekzem-Ursachen in der Metollindustrie. *Berufsdermatosen*, **12**, 1.

Braun, W.P.H. (1975) Contact dermatitis from a stamp-ink of the German Post Office. *Contact Dermatitis*, **1**, 189.

Buckley, W.R. (1958) Lichenoid eruptions following contact dermatitis. *Archives of Dermatology*, **78**, 454.

Calnan, C.D. (1967) Salicylaldoxime. *Contact Dermatitis Newsletter*, **1**, 17.

Calnan, C.D. (1973) Leucoderma with Quinoderm. *Contact Dermatitis Newsletter*, **13**, 378.

Calnan, C.D. (1974a) Methyl violet in carbon paper. *Contact Dermatitis Newsletter*, **15**, 426.

Calnan, C.D. (1974b) Antifreeze dermatitis. *Contact Dermatitis Newsletter*, **15**, 440.

Calnan, C.D. (1978) Chromate dermatitis from soluble oil. *Contact Dermatitis*, **4**, 378.

Calnan, C.D. (1979) Carbon and carbonless copy paper. *Acta Dermato-venereologica*, **59**, Suppl. 85, p. 27.

Calnan, C.D. & Connor, B.L. (1972) Carbon paper dermatitis due to nigrosine. *Berufsdermatosen*, **20**, 248.

Calnan, C.D. & Cooke, M.A. (1973) Leucodermie par adhesifs au Néoprene. *Archives des Maladies Professionnelles de Medecine du Travail et de Sécurité Sociale*, **34**, 236.

Calnan, C.D. & Cooke, M.A. (1974) Leucoderma in industry. *Journal of the Society of Occupational Medicine*, **24**, 59.

Canizares, O. (1959) Lichen planus-like eruption caused by colour developer. *Archives of Dermatology*, **80**, 81.

Castelain, P.-Y. (1967) Eczema des mains a episodes multiples par sensibilisation a l'aminoazotoluene. *Bulletin de la Société Francaise de Dermatologie et de Syphiligraphie*, **74**, 561.

Connor, B. (1972) Chromate dermatitis and paper manufacture. *Contact Dermatitis Newsletter*, **11**, 265.

Crow, K.D. (1969) Anomalous tests with hydrazine in flux. *Contact Dermatitis Newsletter*, **6**, 121.

Crow, K.D. (1969) Barrier creams. *Practitioner*, **202**, 127.

Crow, K.D., Harman, R.R.M. & Holden, H. (1968) Amine flux sensitisation dermatitis in electricity cable jointers. *British Journal of Dermatology*, **80**, 701.

Cruikshank, C.N.D. (1948) The evaluation of skin cleansers and protective creams for workmen exposed to mineral oil. *British Journal of Industrial Medicine*, **5**, 204.

Cruikshank, C.N.D. & Gourevitch, A. (1952) Skin cancer of the hand and forearm. *British Journal of Industrial Medicine*, **9**, 74.

Crukshank, C.N.D. & Howard-Swaffield, H. (1953) Methyloctylbenzenesulphonate; a new industrial sensitising agent. *British Journal of Industrial Medicine*, **10**, 121.

Cruikshank, C.N.D. & Squire, J.R. (1950) Skin cancer in the engineering industry from the use of mineral oil. *British Journal of Industrial Medicine*, **7**, 1.

Dahlquist, I. (1977) Contact allergy to 3-ethylamino-1,2-benzisothiazol-hydrochloride, a veterinary fungicide. *Contact Dermatitis*, **3**, 277.

Dawber, R. (1974) Occupational koilonychia. *British Journal of Dermatology*, **91**, Supplement 10, 11.

Degos, R., Lépine, J. & Akhoundzadeh, H. (1968) Sensibilisation cutanée due a la manipulation de papier "reprographie". *Bulletin de la Société Francaise de Dermatologie et de Syphiligraphie*, **75**, 595.

Denton, C.R., Lerner, A.B. & Fitzpatrick, T.B. (1952) Inhibition of melanin formation by chemical agents. *Journal of Investigative Dermatology*, **18**, 119.

Desoille, H., Philbert, M., Ripault, G., Cavigneaux, A. & Rossignoli, H. (1973) Action cancérogene des huiles minérales utilisées en métallurgie. *Archives de Maladies Professionelles de Médecine du Travail et de Sécurité Sociale*, **34**, 669.

Einarsson, O., Kylin, B., Lindstedt, G. & Wahlberg, J.E. (1975) Chromium, cobalt and nickel in used cutting fluids. *Contact Dermatitis*, **1**, 182.

Engel, H.O. & Calnan, C.D. (1963) Chromate dermatitis from paint. *British Journal of Industrial Medicine*, **20**, 192.

Engel, H.O. & Calnan, C.D. (1966) Resin dermatitis in a car factory. *British Journal of Industrial Medicine*, **23**, 62.

Findlay, G.H., Morrison, J.G.L. & Simson, I.W. (1975) Exogenous ochronosis and pigmented colloid milium from hydroquinone bleaching creams. *British Journal of Dermatology*, **93**, 613.

Foussereau, J. & Benezra, Cl. (1970) *Les Eczémas Allergiques Professionnels*, p. 419 Paris: Masson et Cie.

Fregert, S. (1968) Contact dermatitis from colophony used as a print protective coating. *Contact Dermatitis Newsletter*, **4**, 58.

Fregert, S. (1976) Registration of chemicals in industries. Slimicides in the paper-pulp industry. *Contact Dermatitis*, **2**, 358.

Fregert, S. (1979) Colophony in cutting oil and in soap water used as cutting fluid. *Contact Dermatitis*, **5**, 52.

Fregert, S. & Gruvberger, B. (1976) Chromate dermatitis from oil emulsion contaminated from zinc-galvanised iron plate. *Contact Dermatitis*, **2**, 120.

Fregert, S., Gruvberger, B. & Heijer, A. (1972) Sensitisation to chromium and cobalt in processing of sulphate pulp. *Acta Dermato-Venereologica*, **52**, 221.

Fregert, S. & Skog, E. (1962) Allergic contact dermatitis from mercaptobenzothiazole in cutting oil. *Acta Dermato-Venereologica*, **42**, 235.

Frost, J. & Hjorth, N. (1959) Contact dermatitis from hydrazine hydrochloride in soldering flux. Cross-sensitisation to apresoline and isoniazid. *Acta Dermato-Venereologica*, **39**, 82.

Fry, L. (1965) Skin disease from colour developers. *British Journal of Dermatology*, **77**, 456.

Garcia-Perez, A. & Aparicio, M. (1975) Dermatitis from a dye in petrol. *Contact Dermatitis*, **1**, 265.

Gellin, G.A. (1970) Cutting fluids and skin disorders. *Industrial Medicine and Surgery*, **39**, 38.

Gellin, G.A., Possick, P.A. & Davis, I.H. (1970) Occupational depigmentation due to 4-tertiarybutyl catechol (TBC). *Journal of Occupational Medicine*, **12**, 386.

Gellin, G.A., Maibach, H.I., Misiaszek, M.H. & Ring, M. (1979) Detection of environmental depigmenting substances. *Contact Dermatitis*, **5**, 201.

Gertler, H. & Laubstein, H. (1963) Uber berufsbedingte Erkrangkungen bei Lichtpausern. *Berufsdermatosen*, **11**, 125.

Gianotti, F. & Meneghini, C.D. (1966) Observations concernant certaines dermatites eczémateuses par contact chez les travailleurs affectes a la fabrication des papiers sensible. *Dermatologica*, **132**, 106.

Goldmann, P.J. & Thiess, A.M. (1976) Berufsbedingte Vitiligo durch paratertiar-Butylphenol eine Trias von Vitiligo. *Hautarzt*, **27**, 155.

Graciansky, P. de & Boulle, S. (1966) Skin disease from colour developers. *British Journal of Dermatology*, **78**, 297.

Graciansky, P. de, Boulle, S., Quercy, P. & Cardot, J.-L. (1958) Éruptions lichénoides et lichen plans vrais chez les ouvriers du development des films en couleurs. *Bulletin de la Société Francasie de Dermatologie et de Syphiligraphie*, **65**, 498.

Guillemin, M., Murset, J.C. Lob, M. & Riquez, J. (1974) Simple method to determine the efficiency of a cream used for skin protection against solvents. *British Journal of Industrial Medicine*, **31**, 310.

Harman, R.R.M. & Sarkany, I. (1960) Studies in contact dermatitis. XI. copy paper dermatitis. *Transactions of the St John's Hospital Dermatological Society*, **44**, 37.

Hjorth, N. (1964) Contact dermatitis from cellulose acetate film. *Berufsdermatosen*, **12**, 86.

Hjorth, N. & Brodthagen, H. (1956) Contact dermatitis from lubricating oil additives. *Acta Dermato-Venereologica*, **36**, 146.

Hodgson, G. (1961) Petroleum oils and lubricants. *Transactions of the St John's Hospital Dermatological Society*, **47**, 123.

Hodgson, G. (1969) Cutaneous hazards of lubricants. *Transactions of the Society of Occupational Medicine*, **19**, 9.

Holmes, J.G., Kipling, M.D. & Waterhouse, J.A.H. (1970) Subsequent malignancies in men with scrotal epithelioma. *Lancet*, 2, 214.

Hundeiker, M. & Glossman, V. (1975) Olkeratosen und Skrotalkarzinom, eine vermeidbare Berufskrankheit des Metalldrehers. *Berufsdermatosen*, 23, 174.

Ippen, H. (1978) Hautschaden in der metallverarbeitenden Industrie. *Dermatosen In Beruf und Umwett*, 26, 25.

Ippen, H. (1979) Allergische hautschaden bei der metallbearbeitung. *Dermatosen In Beruf Und Umwelt*, 27, 71.

Ito, K., Nishitañi, K. & Hara, I. (1968) A study of cases of leucomelanodermatosis due to phenylphenol compounds. *Bulletin of the Pharmaceutical Research Institute*, 76, 6.

James, O., Mayes, R.W. & Stevenson, C.J. (1977) Occupational vitiligo induced by *p-tert*-butylphenol. A systemic disease? *Lancet*, 2, 1217.

Jimbow, K., Obata, H., Pathak, M.A. & Fitzpatrick, T.B. (1974) Mechanism of depigmentation by hydroquinone. *Journal of Investigative Dermatology*, 62, 436.

Johnson, M.L. & Wilson, H.T.H. (1971) Oil dermatitis: an enquiry into its prognosis. *British Journal of Industrial Medicine*, 28, 122.

Jordan, W.P. & Bourlas, M. (1975) Contact dermatitis from typewriter correction paper. *Cutis*, 15, 594.

Kahn, G. (1970) Depigmentation caused by phenolic detergent germicides. *Archives of Dermatology*, 102, 177.

Keczkes, K. & Brown, P.M. (1976) Hexahydro, 1, 3, 5, tris (2-hydroxyethyl) triazine, a new bacteriocidal agent as a cause of allergic contact dermatitis. *Contact Dermatitis*, 2, 92.

Key, M.M., Ritter, E.J. & Arndt, K.A. (1966) Cutting and grinding fluids and their effects on the skin. *American Industrial Hygiene Association Journal*, 27, 423.

Kipling, M.D. (1963) Oil and the skin. *Transactions of the Association of Industrial Medical Officers*, 13, 22.

Kipling, M.D. (1968) *Oil and the Skin*. Annual Report, H.M. Chief Inspector of Factories 1967. p. 105 London: H.M. S.O.

Kipling,M.D. (1974) Oil and cancer. *Annals of the Royal College of Surgeons*, 55, 71.

Kligman, A.M. (1966) The identification of contact allergens by human assay. *Journal of Investigative Dermatology*, 47, 393.

Knudsen, E.A. (1964) Lichen planus-like eruption caused by color developer. *Archives of Dermatology*, 89, 357.

Kuske, von H., Klayman, M., & Schwartz, K. (1956) Zur Prufung von Gewerbeschutzsalben. *Dermatologica*, 112, 316.

Lamb, J.H. & Lain, E.S. (1951) Occurrence of contact dermatitis from oil soluble gasoline dyes. *Journal of Investigative Dermatology*, 17, 141.

Lewis, W. & Schwartz, L. (1956) An occupational agent (N-Butyraldoxime) causing reaction to alcohol. *Medical Annals of the District of Columbia*, 25, 485.

Maibach, H. (1965) Marking pen dermatitis: allergic contact dermatitis due to a fast drying resin (Arochem 455). *Contact Dermatitis*, 1, 268.

Maibach, H.I., Gellin, G. & Ring, M. (1975) Is the antioxidant butylated hydroxytoluene a depigmenting agent in man? *Contact Dermatitis*, 1, 295.

Magnusson, B. (1974) Irritation of the skin and mucous membranes by NCR paper. *Contact Dermatitis Newsletter*, 15, 450.

Malten, K.E. (1975a) Cobalt and chromium in offset printing. *Contact Dermatitis*, 1, 120.

Malten, K.E. (1975b) Paratertiary butylphenol depigmentation in a 'consumer'. *Contact Dermatitis*, 1, 181.

Malten, K.E., Seutter, E., Hara, I. & Nakajima, T. (1971) Occupational vitiligo due to paratertiary butylphenol and homologues. *Transactions of the St John's Hospital Dermatological Society*, 57, 115.

Mandel, E.H. (1960) Lichen planus-like eruptions caused by a color-film developer. *Archives of Dermatology*, 81, 516.

Marchand, J.-P., Arnold, J. & Ndiaÿe, B. (1976) Dépigmentation de la peau du noir africain provoquée par les corticoides. *Bulletin de la Société Francaise de Dermatologie et de Syphiligraphic*, 83, 17.

Meara, R.H. & Martin-Scott, I. (1953) Contact dermatitis due to aminoazotoluene. *British Medical Journal*, 1, 1142.

Miller, M.M. Goldberg, H.S. & Wilkerson, W.G. (1978) Allergic contact dermatitis to 1,4-bis(isopropylamino)anthraquinone. *Archives of Dermatology*, 114, 1793.

Miranda, A., Garcia Muñoz, M., Quiñones, P.A. & Perez-Oliva, N. (1978) Liquen plano por revelador CD-2. *Actas Dermo-Sifiliograficas*, 69, 127.

Morris, G.E. (1954) Silicone protective creams. *Archives of Industrial Hygiene and Occupational Medicine*, **9**, 194.

Morris, G.E. & Maloof, C.C. (1953) Some causes of cutting-oil dermatitis Part II. A study of protective creams. *Industrial Medicine and Surgery*, **22**, 327.

Odom, R.B. & Stein, K.M. (1973) Depigmentation caused by a phenolic detergent-germicide. *Archives of Dermatology*, **108**, 848.

Oliver, E.A., Schwartz, L. & Warren, L.H. (1939) Occupational leukoderma. *Journal of the American Medical Association*, **113**, 927.

Oliver, E.A., Schwartz, L. & Warren, L.H. (1940) Occupational leukoderma. *Archives of Dermatology*, **42**, 993.

Pirila, V. & Kilpio, O. (1954) On occupational dermatoses in Finland. *Acta Dermato-Venereologica*, **34**, 395.

Poitu, P. & Marignac, B. (1978) Sensitising effect of Grotan BK in the guinea pig. *Contact Dermatitis*, **4**, 166.

Popchristov, P., Balevska, N. & Michajlov, P. (1957) Berufsdermatitiden und allgemeine Schädigungen bei Arbeitern in filmerzeugenden Laboratorien. *Berufsdermatosen*, **5**, 70.

Porter, R. (1959) Occupational dermatitis. Its prevention with special reference to barrier substances. *British Journal of Dermatology*, **71**, 22.

Prout, J. (1973) Allergic dermatitis due to aniline dye additive. *Proceedings of the Royal Society of Medicine*, **66**, 261.

Riley, P.A. (1969) Hydroxyanisole depigmentation: *in vivo* studies. *Journal of Pathology*, **97**, 185:

Riley, P.A. (1971) Aquired hypomelanosis. *British Journal of Dermatology*, **84**, 290.

Rodermund, O.-E. (1976) Occupational vitiligo caused by paratertiary butylphenol. *Archives of Dermatology*, **112**, 554.

Rodermund, O.-E., Jorgens, H., Müller, R. & Marsteller, H.-J. (1975) Systemische Veranderungen bei berufsbedingter Vitiligo. *Hautarzt*, **26**, 312.

Roed-Peterson, J. & Menne, T. (1976) Allergic contact dermatitis and lichen planus from black and white photographic developing. *Cutis*, **18**, 699.

Rook, A. (1951) Occupational melanosis. *British Journal of Dermatology*, **63**, 159.

Rycroft, R. (1978) Is Grotan BK a contact sensitiser? *British Journal of Dermatology*, **99**, 346.

Salder, C.G.A. & Marriott, R.H. (1946) The evaluation of barrier creams. *British Medical Journal*, **2**, 769

Sak, M., Hegyi, E. & Miglierini, K. (1975) Dermatropic effect of some derivatives of crude oil. 1. Investigation of the dermatotropic effect of mineral oil extracts containing paraffin and paraffin-free extracts. *Ceskoslovenská Dermatologie*, **50**, 183.

Samitz, M.H. & Katz, S.A. (1975) Skin hazards from nickel and chromium salts in association with cutting oil operations. *Contact Dermatitis*, **1**, 158.

Schenider, W., Huber, M., Kwoczek, J.J., Popp, W., Schmitz, R. & Tronnier, H. (1965) Weitere Untersuchungen zur Frage der Hautverträglichkeit hochverdunnter Kuhlmittel. *Berufsdermatosen*, **13**, 65.

Schwartz, L. (1942) Protective ointments and industrial cleansers. *Medical Clinics of North America*, **26**, 1195.

Searle, C.E. (1972) The selective depigmenting action of 8-hydroxyquinoline on hair growth in the mouse. *British Journal of Dermatology*, **86**, 472.

Shelley, W.B. (1974) p-Cresol: cause of ink-induced hair depigmentation in mice. *British Journal of Dermatology*, **90**, 169.

Simpson, J.R. (1969) Formalin sensitivity — offset printing machine. *Contact Dermatitis Newsletter*, **6**, 133.

Spencer, M.C. (1962) Leukoderma following monobenzyl ether or hydroquinone bleaching. *Archives of Dermatology*, **86**, 615.

Spencer, M.C. (1965) Topical use of hydroquinone for depigmentation. *Journal of the American Medical Association*, **194**, 962.

Spruit, D. & Malten, K.E. (1975) Occupational cobalt and chromium dermatitis in an offset printing factory. *Dermatologica*, **151**, 34.

Suskind, R.R. (1954) Industrial and laboratory evaluation of a silicone protective cream. *Archives of Industrial Hygiene and Occupational Medicine*, **9**, 101.

Suskind, R.R. (1955) The present status of silicone protective creams. *Industrial Medicine and Surgery*, **24**, 413.

Suzuki, Y. & Ohkido, M. (1979) Contact dermatitis from hydrazine derivatives. *Contact Dermatitis*, **5**, 113.

Tas, J. (1957) Primary irritant activity of barrier creams. *Journal of Investigative Dermatology*, **29**, 223.

Textier, L., Delaunay, M.M. & Ducombs, G. (1976) N.N.Diethyl-paraphenylenediamine chlorohydrate. *Contact Dermatitis*, **2**, 236.

Thony, C., Thony, J., Lafontaine, M., Limasset, J.C., Boulanger, M. & Gosgnach, C. (1975) Concentrations en hydrocarbures polycycliques aromatiques cancérogénes de quelques huiles minérales. *Archives des Maladies Professionnelles de Médecine du Travail et de Sécurité Sociale*, **36**, 37.

Verspijck Mijnssen, G.A.W. (1964) Preliminary report on a case of contact dermatitis due to ozalid and radex copy papers. *Dermatologica*, **128**, 93.

Vollum, D.I. (1971) Hypomelanosis from an antioxidant in polyethylene film. *Archives of Dermatology*, **104**, 70.

Wahlberg, J.E. (1971) Absorption—inhibiting effect of barrier creams. *Berufsdermatosen*, **19**, 197.

Warin, R.P. (1959) Melanosis of face from 'Cutting' oil. *Proceedings of the Royal Society of Medicine*, **52**, 847.

Waterhouse, J.A.H. (1971) Occupational oils and cancer. *Annals of Occupational Hygiene*, **14**, 161.

Wheeler, C.E., Penn, S.R. & Cawley, E.P. (1965) Dermatitis from Hydrazine hydrobromide solder flux. *Archives of Dermatology*, **91**, 235.

White, P.R. (1923) *Occupational Affections of the Skin*. 2nd ed. p. 124. New York: Paul B. Hoeber.

Wilson, H.T.H. (1961) Dermatoses in a medium engineering factory. *Transactions of the St. John's Hospital Dermatological Society*, **47**, 135.

Wohlrab W. & Zaumseil, R.-P., (1976) Über die experimentelle Depigmentierung der Haut. 2. Mitteilung: Epidermale Reaktion bei externer Applikation depgimentierender Substanzen. *Derpatologische Monastsschrift*, **162**, 980.

Wozniak, K.-D. und Hamm, G. (1977) Allergisches kontaktekzem und vitiligoartige depigmentierungen durch parateritiares butylphenol. *Berufsdermatosen*, **25**, 215.

Zakon, S.J. & Goldberg, A.L. (1951) Occupational leucoderma from rubber dust and debris. *Archives of Dermatology*, **64**, 441.

Zaumseil, R.-P. & Wohlrab, W. (1976) Uber die experimentelle Depigmentierung der Haut. 1. Mitteilung: Experimentelle und klinische Erfahrungen. *Dermatologische Monatsschrift*, **162**, 974.

17.
Irritants and sensitisers in various occupations
Allergens for selected patients
Miscellaneous compounds

Irritants and sensitisers in various occupations

In 1960, a department of occupational dermatology was established in Lund in southern Sweden by Fregert. In 1975 he reviewed 1496 cases of contact dermatitis seen in the decade 1960–1969. The dermatitis was of an allergic type in approximately 75 per cent of the men and 50 per cent of the women and an irritant dermatitis was proved in 17 per cent of the men and 12 per cent of the women. The most frequent allergens in men were chromium, rubber and resins, and in women nickel, rubber and chromium. Half the men were employed in metal, concrete or building industries, and half the women in hospital or cleaning work (Fregert, 1975).

Low risk occupations
The following list of occupations was compiled by Fregert and Calnan (1969) as suitable for atopics or those with hand dermatitis:

air stewardess	prison warden
bus driver	receptionist
cinema operator or usher	security guard
computer assistant	switchboard operator
electronics technician	taxi driver
glass blower of instruments	teacher
map drawer	time checker in industry
oto-audiology assistant	typist
optician	typewriter repairer
policeman	TV technician
porter in office, hospital	warden
postman	

Possible occupations, but requiring consideration of the working environment:

assembler

carpenter (not cabinet maker)

crane operator

electrician (not in industry
  or car service)

fork lift truck driver
  (industry)

machine fitter

operator of half-automatic
  machine

packer (not glue)

salesman

shop assistant (not meat, fish,
  delicatessen, vegetables, flowers,
  and not with nickel allergy)

sorter in wood industry
  (not exotic woods)

spare parts distributor

storeman

teacher in occupations

truck driver (road)

wrapping industry

Unsuitable for nickel-sensitive subjects:

bus and train conductor or guard

clerical and related work

dressmaker

night watchman

telephone operator

The following list of irritants and allergens encountered in various occupations has been taken largely from Fregert (1974a):

Agricultural workers

Irritants: Artificial fertilisers, disinfectants and cleansers for milking machines, petrol and diesel oil.

Sensitisers: Rubber (clothing and milking equipment), oats, barley, animal feed (antibiotics, preservatives, additives and cobalt), veterinary medicaments, cement, plants, pesticides, wood preservatives.

Artists and sculptors

Irritants: Solvents, clay, plaster.

Sensitisers: Turpentine, pigments (cobalt, nickel and chromium), azo, dyes, colophony, epoxy resin.

Automobile and aircraft mechanics

Irritants: Solvents, cutting oils, paints, hand cleansers.

Sensitisers: Chromate (primers, passivators, anticorrosives, welding fumes, oils), nickel, cobalt, rubber, epoxy and dimethacrylate resins, dipentene in thinners.

Bakers and confectioners

Irritants: Flour, detergents.

Sensitisers: Flavours and spices (cinnamon, eugenol, vanilla, cardamon), orange, lemon, essential oils, dyes. Ammonium persulphate and benzoyl peroxide (improvers in flour).

Bartenders

Irritants: Detergents, citrus fruit, wet work.

Sensitisers: Orange, lemon, lime, flavours, *ortho*-phenyl-phenol (in some detergents).

Bookbinders
Irritants: Solvents, glues.
Sensitisers: Glues, resins, leathers.

Butchers
Irritants: Detergents, meat, offal.
Sensitisers: Meat (contact urticaria), teak (knife handles), nickel, sawdust.

Cabinet makers, French polishers, carpenters
Irritants: Detergents, solvents, thinners for cleaning metal (as a cause of koilonychia (Ancona-Alayón, 1975), wood preservatives.
Sensitisers: Stains (including dichromate), glues (urea, phenol, PTBP-formaldehyde resins), woods, turpentine, varnishes, colophony.

Cable-jointers
Irritants: Solvents.
Sensitisers: Epoxy resin, fluxes (aminoethylethanolamine).

Cleaners
Irritants: Detergents, solvents, wet work.
Sensitisers: Rubber gloves, chromates (bleaches in some countries).

Coal-miners
Irritants: Dust (coal, stone), cement, wet conditions.
Sensitisers: Rubber boots and masks.

Construction workers
Irritants: Cement.
Sensitisers: Chromate, cobalt, gloves (rubber, leather), resins (epoxy and formaldehyde), woods.

Cooks and Catering
Irritants: Detergents, food juices, wet work.
Sensitisers: Foods (contact urticaria), onion, garlic, spices, flavours, rubber gloves, sodium metabisulphite, lauryl and octyl gallate, formaldehyde (deodorising solution, fishmongers).

Dentists and dental technicians
Irritants: Detergents, hand cleansers, wet work.
Sensitisers: Local anaesthetics (amethocaine, procaine), methacrylates, eugenol, (eugenol and colophony gingivectomy dressing), mercury, disinfectants, rubber, dental impression material (Impregum and Scutan: the sensitisers are the catalysts methyldichlorobenzene sulphonate and methyl-*p*-toluolsulfonate (Cronin,

1973; Nally and Storrs, 1973; Groeningen and Nater, 1975; Kulenkamp, Hausen and Schulz 1977; Ketel, 1977a).

Dry cleaners
Irritants: Solvents.
Sensitisers: Rubber gloves.

Electricians
Irritants: Soldering fluxes.
Sensitisers: Fluxes (colophony, hydrazine), insulating tape (colophony), resins (epoxy and formaldehyde), rubber.

Electroplaters
Irritants: Acids, alkalis.
Sensitisers: Nickel, chromium, other metals, rubber gloves.

Embalmers and morticians
Sensitisers: Formaldehyde.

Floor-layers
Irritants: Solvents.
Sensitisers: Cement, resins (epoxy and formaldehyde), woods, varnish, linoleum (colophony).

Florists
Irritants: Manure, fertilisers, pesticides, wet work.
Sensitisers: Plants, pesticides, rubber gloves.

Foundry workers
Irritants: Cleansers.
Sensitisers: Phenol and urea formaldehyde (resin coated sand), colophony, (nitrogen-free sand), gloves (rubber, chromium).

Funeral directors
Sensitisers: Floral tributes.

Garage workers
Irritants: Petrol, diesel fuel, cleansers, solvents.
Sensitisers: Rubber gloves, chromate, epoxy resin, antifreeze (MBT).

Gardeners
Irritants: Artificial fertilisers.
Sensitisers: Pesticides, rubber gloves and boots.

Hairdressers
Irritants: Shampoos, perming and bleaching solutions, wet work.
Sensitisers: Dyes   (p-phenylenediamine, p-toluylenediamine, o-nitro-

para-phenylenediamine, *p*-aminiphenol), persulphates, rubber gloves, perfumes, formaldehyde (shampoos), resorcinol, pyrogallol, nickel.

Hospital workers

Irritants: Detergents, disinfectants, foods, wet work.

Sensitisers: Rubber gloves, disinfectants, flower, foods, polishes, hand creams (perfumes) (Dahlquist and Fregert, 1970).

Housework

Irritants: Detergents, cleaners, foods, disinfectants, wet work.

Sensitisers: Rubber gloves, foods (onions, garlic, citrus fruit; contact urticaria) spices, flavours, hand creams, nickel, chromate (bleaches), flowers, polishes.

Jewellers (jewellers' rouge is red iron oxide 87 per cent and fat 13 per cent)

Irritants: Detergents, solvents.

Sensitisers: Epoxy resin, metals, sawdust (used for drying jewellery).

Metal workers

Irritants: Cutting and drilling oils, solvents, hand cleansers.

Sensitisers: Chromates, additives in cutting oils (antibacterials and antioxidants).

Nurses

Irritants: Disinfectants, detergents, wet work.

Sensitisers: Rubber gloves, formaldehyde, glutaraldehyde, Dettol, disinfectants, medicaments (including antibiotics, chlorpromazine), flowers.

Office workers

Irritants: Photocopying (ammonia).

Sensitisers: Rubber (finger stalls), nickel (clips, photocopying solutions), copy papers, carbon papers, correction paper and ? fluids.

Painters

Irritants: Solvents, thinners, wallpaper adhesives, hand cleansers.

Sensitisers: Turpentine, dipentene, cobalt (driers, colours), chromate (colours), wallpaper adhesives (formaldehyde, chloroacetamide and fungicides), paints (preservatives, e.g. mercurials).

Photograph developers (*X-ray technicians*)

Irritants: Wet work, solvents.

Sensitisers: Rubber gloves, *p*-aminophenol (Metol), colour developers, hydroquinone, phenindone, sodium metabisulphite, EDTA, glutaraldehyde, pyrogallol, amidol, ethylenediaine, resorcinol, triazine, salicylaldoxime.

Plastics industry
Irritants: Solvents, acids, styrene, oxidising agents.
Sensitisers: Monomers, hardeners, additives.

Plating industry
Irritants: Acids, alkalis, solvents.
Sensitisers: Nickel, chromate, cobalt, mercury.

Plumbers
Irritants: Wet work, cleaners.
Sensitisers: Chromate (cement), rubber (gloves, packing).

Printers
Irritants: Solvents.
Sensitisers: Chromate, UV-cured inks, colophony (paper), turpentine, rubber gloves, rubber blanket in offset printing, formaldehyde (gum arabic).

Radio and television workers
Irritants: Fluxes.
Sensitisers: Resins (epoxy), fluxes (colophony and hydrazine), chromate.

Rubber workers
Irritants: Solvents, talc, zinc stearate.
Sensitisers: Rubber chemicals, dyes, colophony.

Secretaries
Irritants: Bosses.
Sensitisers: Carbon paper, photocopy paper (azo compound, thiourea — photosensitiser), correcting paper, rubber (fingerstall and rubber bands).

Shoemakers and cobblers
Irritants: Solvents.
Sensitisers: Glues (PTBP resin, colophony), leather, rubber, turpentine.

Tannery workers
Irritants: Acids, alkalis, reducing and oxidising agents, wet work.
Sensitisers: Tanning agents (chromium, vegetable tans, glutaraldehyde, formaldehyde), rubber (gloves and boots), fungicides, dyes.

Textile workers
Irritants: Fibres, bleaching agents, solvents.
Sensitisers: Formaldehyde resins, dyes, chromate (mordant), nickel.

Veterinarians (and slaughterhouse workers)
Irritants: Disinfectants, wet work, entrails and animal secretions.

Sensitisers: Rubber gloves, medicaments used to treat animals and which
                contaminate their fur.
                medicaments:
                    tuberculin (Hjorth and Schønning, 1968)
                    Penethamate, benzylpenicillin (Hjorth, 1967)
                    Spiramycin, Tylosin, Penethamate (Hjorth and Weismann,
                    1973)
                    Neomycin in a calf drench (Simpson, 1974)
                    Mercaptobenzothiazole in a medication (Adams, 1974)
                    Benzisothiazolone fungicide (Dahlquist, 1977)
                Contact urticaria from animal tissues. Cow hair and dander
                (Prahl and Roed — Petersen, 1979)
                In bacon factories, workers eviscerating or cleaning the guts
                develop an eczema of the fingers, known as 'gut or fat' eczema;
                it's cause is unknown (Hjorth, 1978)

Woodworkers
Sensitisers: Woods, lichens, glues, varnishes, colophony, turpentine, balsams

Selected allergens for particular patients

The following additions to the standard series of allergens have been found useful in the investigation of particular patients.

Eyelid eczema
Santolite resin (nail varnish), extra lanolins, hair dyes, all cosmetics, phosphorus
sesquisulphide (strike anywhere matches), medicaments, phenylmercuric nitrate,
and possibly the following preservatives: triclosan (Irgasan DP 300), imidazolidinyl urea (Germal 115) Bronopol and Dowicil 200.

Contact lens solutions
Benzalkonium chloride, EDTA, phenylmercuric nitrate, chlorhexidine, merthiolate.

Leg ulcers
Extra lanolins, Dettol, Cetavlon, benzocaine, tetracycline, demethylchlortetracycline, chlortetracycline, gentamicin sulphate, gramicidin, soframycin, streptomycin, bacitracin, fucidin, polymyxin, chloramphenicol, nystatin, extra perfumes.

Shoe dermatitis
Shoes (appropriate pieces from inner and outer parts, including heel stiffeners
of bedroom slippers), PTBP resin glue, D. Red 1, D. Yellow 3, D. Orange 3
and D. Blue 3 (for stocking or sock dermatitis), specially-tanned leathers if
available.

Textile dermatitis
Clothing dyes, clothing resins, pieces of material from suspected garments, deodorants (?deodorant dermatitis).

Ileostomies and colostomies
Inflammation of the skin around an ileostomy or colostomy is not uncommon and is generally an irritant effect. Psoriatics may develop psoriasis around the stoma. Occasionally the skin is secondarily infected with candida or bacteria. Patch testing should include all parts of the appliance (including the plastic or rubber bag), colophony and adhesive tapes and medicaments, including balsam of Peru (Fussell, 1976; Stevenson, 1975; Martin-Scott, 1976). An ostomy deodorant (DOR) sensitised two patients, both of whom reacted to a patch test with DOR (1 per cent in acetone), and in one the allergen was identified as a perfume component consisting mainly of citronella oil (Davies, Hodgson and Evans, 1978).

Amputation stumps
The dermatological problems occurring in amputation stumps in patients attending a prosthetic clinic were reviewed by DesGroseillers *et al.* (1978). Of 50 patients seen in one year, 17 were affected. The commonest lesions were due to a badly fitting prosthesis or to poor hygiene causing callus formation or breakdown of the skin with or without ulceration (12 patients). An allergic contact dermatitis was diagnosed in two patients; the source was leather in one but in the second the allergen was not specified. One patient had eczeme craquelé, one a non-specific dermatitis and another a virus wart. Other skin changes which may occur are maceration, folliculitis, fungal infections, intertrigo of stump folds, epidermoid cysts and chronic oedema which may lead to verrucous hyperplasia. The oedema, ulceration and hyperplastic changes are discussed by Levy (1977) and he reported a patient who died within months of developing a squamous cell carcinoma in a stump with ulceration and verrucose hyperplasia of long standing. Van Ketel (1977b) described sensitisation in seven patients with amputations: from Hexomedine (an antibacterial) (2), chromate (2), *paratertiary*butylphenol and *paratertiary*butylphenonl formaldehyde (1), the chamois leather of the prosthesis (1) and *para*phenylenediamine (1) Patch tests: Pieces from all parts and all layers of the socket and relevant medicaments and antibacterial compounds. Despite careful investigation it may be difficult to identify an allergen, particularly in limbs made of polyester (p. 631).

Miscellaneous compounds

The following compounds have been reported as causing dermatitis:

Amidotrizoate. A radiopaque substance used in angiography and renography. Allergic contact dermatitis. P.T. concentration 10–50 per cent aqueous (Rothe, Yousifand and Zschunke, 1977).

Ammonyx® LO. A surface active agent used in dishwashing products, shampoos, electroplating baths, paints and fuel additives. As an ingredient of the antiseptic Hibiscrub, it caused allergic contact dermatitis. P.T. concentration 1 per cent aqueous (Muston, Boss and Summerly, 1977).

Arecoline. Apurgative and teniacide given to dogs for tape worm infection. A hydatid control officer developed allergic contact dermatitis. P.T. arecoline hydrobromide 2 per cent in pet. (Wishart, 1979).

Benzamine lactate. Used in ointments as a local anaesthetic. Allergic contact dermatitis. P.T. concentration 1 per cent petrolatum (Calnan, 1975).

Borax (Sodium borate). Toxic alopecia due to occupational absorption of borax from a hand washing powder, containing nearly 80 per cent crystalline borax, was reported by Tan (1970).

1-Bromo-2,4-dinitrobenzene. Allergic contact dermatitis in a schoolboy (Thompson, 1975).

Brome-ethyl-dibromo-benzene. As an intermediate product of dibromo-styrene it sensitised laboratory workers. A concentration of 5 per cent actively sensitised controls (Bettley, 1969).

Dicyclohexyl-carbodiimide. A chemical intermediate, is used in the preparation of Angiotensin® and Acidoquost®. Irritant and sensitiser. P.T. concentration 0.1 per cent aqueous, but only patch test if necessary (Zschunke and Folesky, 1975). A laboratory worker using it to couple a bile acid to albumin was sensitised. P.T. 0.1 per cent in pet. (White and MacDonald, 1979).

Chipboard. Consists of wood chips (principally Spruce, Pine and Fir, with some Larch, Poplar and Sycamore), a resin binder (usually urea formaldehyde catalysed by ammonium chloride, very occasionally melamine formaldehyde is used instead) and wax emulsion.

α-Chlorobenzaldehyde phenylhydrazone. It is a strong sensitiser and has caused allergic dermatitis in students (Philp, 1972).

2-Chloroethanol (Ethylene chlorohydrin). Is a highly toxic solvent which is absorbed through the skin (Wahlberg and Boman, 1978). Industrially it is used as a solvent for polymers and lacquers, and in the manufacture of insecticides and for treating sweet potatoes before planting.

Chlormethylbenzol. A chemistry student developed a bullous eczema (Ippen and Liebeskind, 1978).

Chlorphenoxamine. An antihistamine, present in Systral® Salbe. Allergic contact dermatitis. P.T. concentration 1.5 per cent pet. or aq. (van Ketel, 1976b).

Chloroacetophenone (Mace). A lachrimator, is used in tear gas. Allergic contact dermatitis. P.T. concentration 0.009 per cent. Open test with Mace (Penneys, Israel and Indgin, 1969; Frazier, 1976).

Cigarettes. Menthol cigarettes caused an allergic contact dermatitis of the lips, perioral area and hands. P.T. menthol 1 per cent pet. (Camarasa and Alomar 1978)

Citraconic anhydride. Contact urticaria and dermatitis in guinea pigs. (Hunziker and Brun, 1978).

Cockroaches (Periplaneta americana). Contact urticaria, dermatitis and asthma (Zschunke, 1978).

Croton. Croton oil, derived from *Codiaeum tiglium*, is a strong irritant. Aqueous but not ether extracts of the sap cause allergic contact dermatitis (Schmidt and Ølholm-Larsen, 1977).

2,6-Dichlorobenzaldoxim. A chemical laboratory worker was sensitised. P.T. concentration 1 per cent in alcohol (Nater, 1969). Salicylaldoxime was the sensitiser in a photographic solution (p. 862).

Dichloropropiophenone. Allergic contact dermatitis in chemical plant workers. P.T. concentration 0.01 per cent in oil (Holzegel, 1976).

Dimethyl sulphoxide (DMSO). Topical toxicity (Malten and den Arend, 1978).

Dinitrofluorobenzene (DNFB) DNFB is used in the laboratory to split proteins and polypeptides. Sensitisation in two biochemistry students has been reported. One had used Sanger reagent (5 per cent DNFB) and on patch testing reacted to DNFB and DNCB (dinitrochlorobenzene) (Garcia-Perez, 1978). The other student split neat DNFB on her skin and she developed immediate erythema and one week later a severe bullous dermatitis. She refused to be patch tested (Ridley, 1969).

Dioxane. A toxic solvent. A man who frequently dipped his hand into it to degrease small metal parts was sensitised. P.T. concentration 0.5 per cent aq. (Fregert, 1974b).

Diphenylamine. Stabiliser (0.1 per cent) in amyl cinnamic aldehyde and hexyl cinnamic aldehyde. Sensitisation not reported. P.T. concentration 1 per cent pet. (Calnan, 1978).

Diphenylcyclopropenone. The preparation of this aromatic compound is a frequent experiment for chemistry students. One student developed a severe bullous allergic contact dermatitis. P.T. concentration 0.1 per cent in acetone (Whittaker, 1972).

Dogger bank itch. Dermatitis in trawler men. (Newhouse, 1966; Audebert and Lamoureux, 1978). Reactions to marine organisms (Manowitz and Rosenthal, 1979).

ECG electrode jelly and paste Allergic contact dermatitis has been reported from parachlormetaxylenol (Storrs, 1975), gum tragacanth (Coskey, 1977), parabens, tartrazine (FD & C Yellow no. 5) and pine oil (Fisher, 1977).

Ethyl chloride. Caused reactions in patients allergic to propellants. P.T. undiluted (van Ketel, 1976a).

Ethoxy methylene ethyl malonate. Used as an intermediate in the formation of oxychlorquinoline for the production of Nivaquine. Allergic contact dermatitis. P.T. concentration 1 per cent, 0.1 per cent and 0.01 per cent (Droin *et al.*, 1977).

Fuchsin — silver nitrate. Used as an alcoholic solution for marking patch test sites. If concentrated by evaporation it becomes irritant and causes skin necrosis (Björnberg, 1977).

Hexamidine. (Hexomidine® is the di-isothionate salt). A topical bacteriocide; sensitisation is not uncommon and the eczema is persistent. P.T. concentration 0.15 per cent in water (van Ketel, 1975; Robin, 1978).

Hydroxylamine sulphate. Salts of hydroxylamine are used as bactericides and fungicides, for the synthesis of dyes, rubber and pharmaceuticals and in photography. Allergic contact dermatitis. P.T. concentration 1 per cent and 0.1 per cent aq. (Pellerat and Chabeau, 1976).

Hydroxypolyethoxydodecane (Thesit). Is an antipruritic and local anaesthetic. A woman with anogenital pruritus was sensitised by Anacal Rectal Ointment (Luitpold-Werk, Munich) containing 5 per cent hydroxypolyethoxydodecane. Patch tests: she reacted to the ointment and of its constituents to hydroxypolyethoxydodecane 5 per cent; 15 controls were negative (Calnan, 1978). It was added to a routine patch test series by Hartung and Rudolph (1970) and of 2551 patients tested 38 were positive.

Sodium hypochlorite. Used as a swimming pool disinfectant, it has caused onycholysis (Coskey, 1974). It is also added to some dishwashing powders, scouring powders and bleaching agents. Allergic contact dermatitis has been described by Osmundsen (1978); the patient reacted severely to sodium hypochlorite 0.5 per cent (aq.) and to chloramine 0.5 per cent (aq.) and to hexachlorophene 1 per cent (pet.).

Iruxol® (*collagenase mixture*) An enzyme mixture, collagenase A, from *Clostridium histolyticum*, consisting of many polypeptidases. It has sensitised in an ointment for leg ulcers. P.T. concentration: collagenase A 1.2 mg/g pet. (Braun, 1975).

Musicians 'Fiddlers neck' occurs in violin and viola players, it is lichenification and sometimes inflammatory papules below the angle of the left mandible (Peachey and Matthews, 1978). Allergic contact dermatitis to a violin rest made of palisander wood (Hausen and Mau, 1979). Flautist's chin is acneiform lesions due to pressure and moisture (Dahl, 1978; Gardiner, 1978). Clarinettist's cheilitis occurs from pressure on the centre of the lower lip (Hindson, 1978).

Psychic possession. Two outbreaks of skin disorders labelled as industrial but proven to be psychological. A gem of an article, highly recommended (Maguire, 1978).

Solvent Yellow 33 (C.I. no. 47000). Used to colour smoke in detonators; it has caused occupational allergic contact dermatitis (Noster and Hausen, 1978).

Squaric-acid-diethylester. Squaric acid and its derivatives are not as yet used commercially; squaric-acid-diethylester is a strong sensitiser and caused dermatitis in a chemistry student. P.T. concentration 0.01 per cent alcohol (Noster *et al.*, 1976).

Stannous chloride. Irritant; sensitisation in one man has been reported; the P.T. concentration was not stated (Ogier and Duverneuil, 1977).

Sulphur. Allergic contact dermatitis has been reported in two patients. (Schneider, 1978).

Tetrachlorodibenzodioxin (TCDD; often abbreviated to dioxin). Highly toxic chemical formed as a contaminant during the synthesis of trichlorophenol; amongst other effects it causes porphyria and even trivial exposure causes chloracne (May, 1973; Oliver, 1975).

Tetraphosphoric trisulphide. Allergic contact dermatitis (D'Angelo, 1975).

p-Toluene sulphochloride. Sensitised a chemistry student. P.T. concentration 1 per cent acetone (Nater, 1968).

Toluic acids. p-Toluic acid and o-toluic acid were found experimentally to be potent sensitisers in man (Emmett and Suskind, 1973).

p-Toluoyl chloride phenylhydrazone (TCHP) A drug for animal use only was being developed as an anti-helminthic. It is a strong irritant and a powerful allergen. Two veterinary research pharmacists were sensitised. P.T. concentration 0.01 per cent in MEK (Abell and Cronin, 1973).

Trichloroethylene (Trichloroethene, Trilene, Trethylene, Tri-Clene). is toxic to the central nervous system, probably through the action of its metabolite trichloroethanol. Due to lack of appreciation of the hazard, poisoning is usually industrial rather than from an anaesthetic. Massive inhalation causes unconsciousness, hepatitis, renal damage and cardiac arrhythmias. Chronic exposure results in malaise, mental confusion simulating drunkenness, cranial nerve neuropathy, hepatitis and cardiac arrhythmias. Its solvent action causes dryness and cracking of the skin through direct contact and from its retention in clothing (Bauer and Rabens, 1977). Four patients with a generalised exfoliative dermatitis or scarlatiniform eruption have been described, (Bauer and Rabens, 1974).

Epichlorhydrin, present as a stabiliser in trichloroethylene, caused an allergic contact dermatitis in two metal platers using the solvent as a degreasing agent. Patch tests: both reacted to epichlorhydrin 0.01 per cent in isopropyl alcohol (Epstein, 1974).

References

Abell, E. & Cronin, E. (1973) Contact Dermatitis to *p*-Toluoyl chloride phenylhydrazone. Transactions of the St John's Hospital Dermatological Society, **59**, 118.

Adams, R.M. (1974) Mercaptobenzothiazole in veterinary medications. *Contact Dermatitis Newsletter*, **16**, 514.

Ancona-alayón, A. (1975) Occupational koilonychia from organic solvents. *Contact Dermatitis*, **1**, 367.

Audebert, C. & Lamoureux, P. (1978) Eczéma professionnel du marin pêcheur par contact de Bryozoaires en baie de Seine. *Annales de Dermatologie et de Syphiligraphie*, **105**, 187.

Bettley, F.R. (1969) Bromo-ethyl-dibromo-benzene. *Contact Dermatitis Newsletter*, **5**, 91.

Bauer, M. & Rabens, S.F. (1974) Cutaneous manifestations of trichloroethylene toxicity. *Archives of Dermatology*, **110**, 886.

Bauer, M. & Rabens, S.F. (1977) Trichloroethylene Toxicity. *International Journal of Dermatology*, **16**, 113.

Bjornberg, A. (1977) Toxic reactions to a patch test skin marker containing fuchsin-silver nitrate. *Contact Dermatitis*, **3**, 101.

Braun, W.P.H. (1975) Contact allergy to collagenase mixture (Iruxol). *Contact Dermatitis*, **1**, 241.

Calnan, C.D. (1975) Sensitivity to benzamine lactate. *Contact Dermatitis*, **1**, 56.

Calnan, C.D. (1978) Oxypolyethoxydodecane in an ointment *Contact Dermatitis*, **4**, 168.

Calnan, C.D. (1978) Diphenylamine. *Contact Dermatitis*, **4**, 301.

Camarasa, G. & Alomar, A. (1978) Menthol dermatitis from cigarettes. *Contact Dermatitis*, **4**, 169.

Coskey, R.J. (1974) Onycholysis from sodium hypochlorite. *Archives of Dermatology*, **109**, 96.

Coskey, R.J. (1977) Contact Dermatitis Caused by ECG Electrode Jelly *Archives of Dermatology*, **113**, 839.

Cronin, E. (1973) Impregum (Dental impression material). *Contact Dermatitis Newsletter*, **13**, 362.

Dahl, M.G.C. (1978) Flautist's chin: a companion to fiddler's neck, *British Medical Journal*, **2**, 1023.

Dahlquist, I. (1977) Contact allergy to 3-ethylamino-1, 2-benzisothiazol hydrochloride, a veterinary fungicide. *Contact Dermatitis*, **3**, 277.

Dahlquist, M.D. & Fregert, S. (1970) Occupational dermatoses in hospital personnel. *Berfusdermatosen*, **18**, 261.

D'Angelo, I. (1975) Quadri eczematosi diffusi da trisolfuro tetrafosforico. *Giornale Italiano di Dermatologia*, **110**, 496.

Davies, M.G., Hodgson, G.A. & Evans, E. (1978) Contact dermatitis from an ostomy deodorant. *Contact Dermatitis*, **4**, 11.

Desgroseilliers, J–P., Desjardins, J–P., Germain, J–P., & Krol, A.L. (1978) Dermatologic problems in amputees. *Canadian Medical Association Journal*, **118**, 535.

Droin, M., Duverneuil, G., Pellerat, Melinat & Chabaud, (1977) Dermites a l'eéthoxy méthylene malonate d'ethyle. *Archives des Maladies Professionnelles de Médecine du Travail et de Sécurité Sociale*, **38**, 836.

Emmett, E.A. & Suskind, R.R. (1973) Allergic contact sensitisation to the toluic acids. *Journal of Investigative Dermatology*, **61**, 282.

Epstein, E. (1974) Allergy to Epichlorohydrin masquerading as Trichlorethylene Allergy. *Contact Dermatitis Newsletter*, **16**, 475.

Fisher, A.A. (1977) Dermatologic Hazards Of Electrocardiography *Cutis*, **20**, 686.

Frazier, C.A. (1976) Contact allergy to Mace. *Journal of the American Medical Association*, **236**, 2526.

Fregert, S. (1974A), *Manual of Contact Dermatitis*. p. 69. Copenhagen; Munksgaard.

Fregert, S. (1974 b) Allergic contact dermatitis from dioxane in a solvent for cleaning metal parts. *Contact Dermatitis Newsletter*, 15, 1974.

Fregert, S. (1975) Occupational dermatitis in a 10-year material, *Contact Dermatitis*, 1, 96.

Fregert, S. & Calnan, C.D. (1969) Low risk occupations. *Contact Dermatitis Newsletter*, 6, 111.

Fussell, K. (1976) Common problems of ileostomies and colostomies. *Practitioner*, 216, 655.

Garcia-Perez, A. (1978) Occupational dermatitis from DNFB with cross sensitivity to DNCB. *Contact Dermatitis*, 4, 125.

Gardiner, L.D. (1978) Flautist's chin. *British Medical Journal*, 2, 1295.

Groeningen, G. van, & Nater, J.P. (1975) Reactions to dental impression materials *Contact Dermatitis*, 1, 373.

Hartung, J. & Rudolph, P.O. (1970) Epidermale Allergie gegen Hdroxypolyaethoxydodekan. *Zeitschrift für Haut- und Geschlechtskrankeiten*, 45, 547

Hausen, B.M. & Mau, H.H. (1979) Contact allergy by a violin chinrest made of palisander. *Dermatosen In Beruf Und Umwelt*, 27, 18.

Hindson, T.C. (1978) Clarinettist's cheilitis. *British Medical Journal*, 2, 1295.

Hjorth, N. (1967) Occupational dermatitis among veterinary surgeons caused by Penethamate (Benzyl Penicillin-β-diethylaminoethylester). *Berufsdermatosen*, 15, 163.

Hjorth, N. (1978) Gut eczema in slaughterhouse workers. *Contact dermatitis*, 4 49.

Hjorth, N. & Schonning, L. (1968) Occupational dermatitis from tuberculin among veterinary surgeons. *Contact Dermatitis Newsletter*, 4, 64.

Hjorth, N. & Weismann, K. (1973) Occupational dermatitis among veterinary surgeons caused by Spiramycin, Tylosin and Penethamate. *Acta Dermato-venereologica*, 53, 229.

Holzegel, K. (1976) Kontaktallergische Ekzeme durch Dichloropropiophenon. *Berufsdermatosen*, 24, 152.

Hunziker, N. & Brun, R. (1978) Contact urticaria and dermatitis to citraconic anhydride in guinea pigs. *Contact Dermatitis*, 4, 236.

Ippen, H. & Liebeskind, H. (1978) Kontaktekzem durch 1,4-bis-chlormethylbenzol. *Dermatosen In Beruf Und Umwelt*, 26, 97.

Ketel, W.G. van (1975) Allergic contact eczema by Hexomedine®. *Contact Dermatitis*, 1, 332.

Ketel, W.G. van (1976a) Allergic contact dermatitis from propellants in deodorant sprays in combination with allergy to ethyl chloride. *Contact Dermatitis*, 2, 115.

Ketel ,W.G. van (1976b) Sensitivity to chlorphenoxamine H Cl. *Contact Dermatitis*, 2, 121.

Ketel, W.G. van (1977a) Reactions to dental impression materials. *Contact Dermatitis*, 3, 55.

Ketel W.G. van (1977b) Allergic contact dermatitis of amputation stumps. *Contact Dermatitis*, 3, 50.

Kulenkamp, D., Hausen, B.M. & Schulz, K-H. (1977) Kontaktallergie durch neuartige, zahnarztlich verwendete Abdruckmaterialen. *Hautarzt*, 28, 353.

Levy, S.W. (1977) Disabling Skin Reactions Associated With Stump Edema. *International Journal of Dermatology*, 16, 122.

Maguire, A. (1978) Psychic possession among industrial workers. *Lancet*, 1, 376.

Malten, K.E. & Arend, J. den (1978) Topical toxicity of various concentrations of DMSO recorded with impedance measurements and water vapour loss measurements. *Contact Dermatitis*, 4, 80.

Manowitz, N.R. & Rosenthal, R.R. (1979) Cutaneous-systemic reactions to toxins and venoms of common marine organisms. *Cutis*, 23, 450.

Martin-Scott, I. (1967) Skin problems of ileostomies. *Practitioner*, 199, 657

May, G. (1973) Chloracne from the accidental production of tetrachlorodibenzodioxin. *British Journal of Industrial Medicine*, 30, 276.

Muston, H.L., Boss, J.M. & Summely, R. (1977) Dermatitis from Ammonyx® LO, a constituent of a surgical scrub. *Contact Dermatitis*, 3, 347.

Nally, F.F. & Storrs, J. (1973) Hypersensitivity to a dental impression material. *British Dental Journal*, 134, 244.

Nater, J.P. (1968) Allergic contact dermatitis due to paratoluene sulphochloride. *Contact Dermatitis Newsletter*, 4, 65.

Nater, J.P. (1969) 2.6-dichlorobenzaldoxim. *Contact Dermatitis Newsletter*, 5, 97.

Newhouse, M.L. (1966) Dogger bank itch: survey of trawler-men. *British Medical Journal*, 1, 1142.

Noster, U. & Hausen, B.M. (1978) Berufsbedingtes Kontaktekzem durch gelben Chinophthalonfarbstoff (Solvent Yellow 33; C.I. 47000.) *Hautarzt*, 29, 153.

Noster, U., Hausen, B.M., Krische, B. & Schulz, K.H. (1976) Squaric-acid-diethylester—a strong sensitiser. *Contact Dermatitis*, 2, 99.

Ogier, M. & Duverneuil, G. (1977) Dermite allergique au chlorure stanneux. *Archives des Maladies Professionnelles de Médicine du Travail et de Sécurité Sociale*, 38, 835.

Oliver, R.M. (1975) Toxic effects of 2,3,7,8, tetrachlorodibenzo, 1,4 dioxin in laboratory workers. *British Journal of Industrial Medicine*, **32**, 49.

Osmundsen, P.E. (1978) Contact dermatitis due to sodium hypochlorite. *Contact Dermatitis*, **4**, 177.

Peachey, R.D.G. & Matthews, C.N.A. (1978) 'Fiddler's neck'. *British Journal of Dermatology*, **98**, 669.

Pellerat, M. & Chabeau, G. (1976) Hydroxylamine et dermatoses professionnelles. *Bulletin de la Société Francaise de Dermatologie et de Syphiligraphie*, **83**, 238.

Penneys, N.S., Israel, R.M. & Indgin, S.M. (1969) Contact dermatitis due to 1-chloroacetophenone and chemical Mace. *New England Journal of Medicine*, **281**, 413.

Philp, J. McL. (1972) α-Chlorobenzaldehyde Phenylhydrazone. *Contact Dermatitis Newsletter*, **12**, 334.

Prahl, P. & Roed-Petersen, J. (1979) Type 1 allergy from cows in veterinary surgeons. *Contact Dermatitis*, **5**, 33.

Ridley, C.M. (1969) Accidental sensitisation to dinitrofluorobenzene (DNFB). *Contact Dermatitis Newsletter*, **6**, 118.

Robin, J. (1978) Contact dermatitis to hexamidine. *Contact Dermatitis*, **4**, 375.

Rothe, A., Yousif, S.H. & Zschunke, E. (1977) Allergic contact eczema from sodium amidotrizoate — a radiopaque substance in angiography and renography. *Contact Dermatitis*, **3**, 284.

Schmidt, H. & Olholm-Larsen, P. (1977) Allergic contact dermatitis from croton (*Codiaeum*). *Contact Dermatitis*, **3**, 100.

Schneider, H.G. (1978) Schwefelallergie. Hautarzt, **29**, 340.

Simpson, J. (1974) Dermatitis from neomycin in a calf drench. *Contact Dermatitis Newsletter*, **15**, 447.

Stevenson, C.J. (1975) Skin problems with surgical stomata. *Contact Dermatitis*, **1**, 243.

Storrs, F.J. (1975) Para-chlor-meta-xylenol allergic contact dermatitis in seven individuals. *Contact Dermatitis*, **1**, 211.

Tan, G.T. (1970) Occupational Toxic Alopecia Due To Borax. *Acta Dermato-venereologica*, **50**, 55.

Thompson, D.M. (1975) Accidental sensitization to 1-bromo-2,4 dinitrobenzene. *Proceedings of the Royal Society of Medicine*, **68**, 647.

Wahlberg, J.E. & Boman, A. (1978) 2-Chloroethanol — Percutaneous Toxicity of a Solvent. *Dermatologica*, **156**, 299.

White, I.R. & MacDonald, D.M. (1979) Dicyclohexyl carbodiimide sensitivity. *Contact Dermatitis*, **5**, 275.

Whittaker, M. (1972) Severe Dermatitis caused by Diphenylcyclopropenone. *Contact Dermatitis Newsletter*, **11**, 264.

Wishart, J. (1979) Contact dermatitis to arecoline. *Contact Dermatitis*, **5**, 61.

Zschunke, E. (1978) Contact urticaria, contact dermatitis, and asthma from cockroaches. *Archives of Dermatology*, **114**, 1715.

Zschunke, E. (1978) Contact urticaria, contact dermatitis and asthma from cockroaches. *Contact Dermatitis*, **4**, 313.

Zschunke, E. & Folesky, H. (1975) Some effects of dicyclohexyl-carbodiimide on human Skin. *Contact Dermatitis*, **1**, 188.

Index

Abies, 565
Abitol, 111, 786
Abura wood, 565
Acacia harpophylla, 559
    melanoxylon, 558
    shirleyi, 559
Acanthoma due to spectacle frames, 646
Acetic acid, 174
Acetone chloroform, 700
Acetoxydimethyl-dioxane, 700
Achromycin, systemic, phototoxicity, 425, 427
Acne due to oil, 849
Acoumea klaineana, 554
Acrex, 394
Acriflavine, 202
Acriflex cream, 203
Acrylamide, 589
Acrylates, 59, 575
    light-sensitive, 590
Acrylic monomer, 25
    polymers, 575–95
    resins, patch tests, 594
Acrylonitrile, 588
ACTH, 246
Adhesive tapes, 576, 785
Adhesives causing leucoderma, 870
    in shoes, 69, 73
Adonia vernalis, 531
Adrenaline, 256
Afrormosia wood, 559
After-shave lotions, 141
Afzelia wood, 557
Agba wood, 561
Agricultural workers, occupational irritants and
                sensitisers, 880
Agrimonia eupatoria, 531
Aircraft mechanics, occupational irritants and
                sensitisers, 880
    workers, rubber sensitivity, 759
Ako wood, 563
Alantolactone, 496
Alcalase, 820, 821
Alcohols, 805–9
Alder wood, 555
Aldrin, 408
Alerce wood, 555
Algae, 22
Alizarin, 38

Alkyd resins, 632, 634
Alkylamines, 234
Allergen, base, 6
    concentration, effect on patch test result, 5
    replacement in contact dermatitis, 31
    storage, 6
    supply, 7
    systemic absorption, 17
Allergens causing sensitisation, 16
    contact, reactions to systemic absorption, 26
    in elderly patients, 21
    in standard (battery) series, 9
    reactions in patch testing, 10
Alliaceae, 471
    allergens, 471
    dermatitis, clinical features, 471
    patch tests, 472
Allium, 471
Allyl resin, 631
Alnus glutinosa, 553
Alstonia wood, 553
Alstroemeria, 472, 473, 520
Al-test unit, 2
Aluminium salts in antiperspirants, 107
Amalgam dental fillings, 682
Amantidine, systemic, photosensitivity to, 447
Amaranth, 179
Amarelo wood, 566
Amaryllidaceae, 473
    dermatitis, clinical features, 474
Amboyna wood, 559
Ambrosia, 468, 494
    allergenic sesquiterpene lactones in, 497
    allergens, 498
    dermatitis, clinical features, 501
    differential diagnosis, 503
Ambrosin, 497
Ambrosiol, 497
Amethocaine, 194
Amide herbicides, 403
Amidotrizoate, 886
Amino formaldehyde polymers, 621
Aminoacridine, 203
p-Aminoazobenzene, 859
Aminoazotoluene, 860
p-Aminobenzoic acid, 28
    esters, 193
    photosensitivity to, 453

Aminoethylethanolamine, 866
Aminophylline, 241, 244
Aminopyrine, 26
Aminothiazole, 25
Ammonia, 25
Ammonium acrylate bonding agent, 577
    persulphate, 126, 137, 181
    quaternary compounds, 692
    thioglycollate, 129, 137
Ammonyx LO, 887
Amoora polystacha, 563
Amourette wood, 564
Ampicillin, 217
Amputation stumps, allergens, 886
Amyldimethylaminobenzoate, photosensitivity
        to, 452, 594
Amylocaine, 195, 198
Anacardiaceae, 475
    allergens, 476
    dermatitis, clinical features, 479
        cross-reactions, 483
        patch testing, 482
        prophylaxis, 483
        treatment, 484
Anacardium occidentale, 476, 477, 481, 483
Anaesthetics, local, 192, 193
Ananus comosus, 490
Andira intermis, 559
Anemone, 530
Anethole, 180
Anethum graveolens, 536
Angelica archangelica, 421, 535, 536
Angelim wood, 559
Aniline yellow, 859
Animal feeds, additives, 184
Animals, reactions to, 25
Anprolene, 702
Antabuse, 28
Antazoline, 235
Anthemis cotula, 507
Anthothecol, 562
Anthranol, 558
Anthraquinone dyes, 38
Anthriscum sylvestris, 536
Anthriscus, photyphotodermatitis due to, 420
Antiaris wood, 563
Antibacterials, 173, 202–27, 664–713
Antibiotics, 27, 202–27
    as food preservatives, 174
Anticandidal compounds, 227
Antidepressants, 253
Antifreeze mixtures, 845
Antihistamines, 233
    cross-reaction to ethylenediamine, 245
Antimicrobial food additives, 173
Antimitotic compounds, 237
Antimony, 81, 279
Antioxidants, 174
Antiperspirants, 107
Anti-rust oil, 847
Antistin, 235
Antu, 411
Apigenin, 116

Apium graveolens, 535, 536
Apocynaceae woods, 553
Apomorphine, 251
Apple packers, 185
Apron, rubber, 751
Apuleia molaris, 557
Aquamox, systemic, photosensitivity to, 446
Arabis albida, 513
Araceae, 487
Arachis, 518
Arachnoides adiantiformis, 489
Araliaceae, 488
Arapoca wood, 566
Arecoline, 887
Argimony, phytophotodermatitis due to, 421
Argyrol, 373
Arnica, 507
Arochem, 455, 860
Arsenic, 280
    carcinogenicity, 280
    trioxide, 281
Arsenicals, inorganic, 280
    organic, 28, 282
Arsphenamine, 28, 283
Arteglasin A, 498
Arthropods, 25
Artists, occupational irritants and sensitisers,
        880
Arum family, 487
Ashes, chromate in, 307
Aspidiaceae, 489
Aspidosperma, 553
Aspirin, 25
Asteroideae, 492
Astringents, cosmetic, 106
Atarax, 260
Atranorin, 570
Atropa belladonna, 534
Aureomycin, 224
    systemic, phototoxicity, 425, 426
Australian Bush dermatitis, 511
Automobile mechanics, occupational irritants
        and sensitisers, 880
Avodiré wood, 563
Ayan wood, 558
Azidoamphenicol, 206
Azo dyes, 28, 37, 179
    in lipsticks, 141, 143
Azulene, 147
Azure blue, 831

Bacitracin, 25, 27, 203
    cross-reaction to neomycin, 214
Bacterial contaminants, 664; *see also*
            Antibacterials.
Bakers, occupational irritants and sensitisers,
        880
BAL, 255
Balata rouge wood, 567
Balloons, rubber, 754
Ball-point pens, 646
Balsam of Peru, 26, 28, 162
    sensitisation in children, 20

Balsam of Tolu, 162
Bamboo, 515
Bank-note counter, rubber, 764
Barban, 398
Barrier creams, 668, 872
Bartenders, occupational irritants and
sensitisers, 880
Bathing caps, 752
BCNU, 240
BCSA, photosensitivity to, 435
Bed-linen, dermatitis due to, 67
Bee-keepers, dermatitis in, 101
Beeswax, 101, 111
Begoniaceae, 489
Belladonna, 534
Benadryl, 235, 236
photo-allergy to, 439
Benomyl, 397
Benzalkonium chloride, 21, 693
Benzamine lactate, 887
Benzene hexachloride, 407
Benzethonium chloride, 110, 694
Benzisothiazoline, 851
Benzocaine, 21, 195
Benzoic acid derivatives, 193
Benzoin tincture, 251
Benzophenones, 25, 252
Benzoyl peroxide, 181
Benzyl alcohol, 807
salicylate, 160
o-Benzyl-p-chlorophenol, 393
Bergamot, phytophotodermatitis due to, 420
Berloque dermatitis, 421
Beryllium, 283
Beryllium granuloma, 284
respiratory effects, 285
Betamethasone 17-valerate, 248
Betnovate rectal ointment, 256
Betula papyracea, 553
Betulaceae woods, 553
Bignoniaceae woods, 553
Bindweed, phytophotodermatitis due to, 421
Biomycin, 224
systemic, phototoxicity, 425, 426
Biostat, systemic, phototoxicity, 427
Bipyridylium herbicides, 403
Birch wood, 553
Bismarck brown, 37, 38
Bisphenol A epoxy resins, 596, 602, 607, 613
Bithionol photosensitivity, 423, 433, 436, 442,
443
Black dermographism, 335
Blackwood, 560
Australian, 558
Bleaches, chromates in, 309
Blush-on, 148
Boehmeria, 537
Boiler lining, chromate in, 307
Bokomake, 86
Bone cement, methyl methacrylate, 582
Bookbinders, occupational irritants and
sensitisers, 881
Boots, sensitisers in, 69, 884

Boraginaceae, 489
Borax, 887
Bowen's disease, 423
BPPS, 410
Bradosol bromide, 700
Brassica, 512
Brassicol, 400
Brassières containing elastic, 745
Brauna wood, 558
Brewery, formaldehyde disinfectant in, 792
Brilliant green, 240
Brilliant Lake Red R, 144
Bromochlorosalicylanilide, photosensitivity to,
433, 435
5-Bromo-4'-chlorosalicylanilide, photosensitivity
to, 433, 435
1-Bromo-2,4-dinitrobenzene, 887
Bromo-ethyl-dibromo-benzene, 887
Bromofluorescein, 142
9-Bromofluorine, 29
Bronopol, 695
Brya ebenus, 560
Buckwheat, 524
Buclizine, 260
Buclosamide, photosensitivity to, 433, 437, 442,
443
Bufexamac, 252
Burseraceae wood, 554
Busulphan, 239
Butanediol diacrylate, 577
Butchers, occupational irritants and sensitisers,
881
Buttercup, 530
Butyl acrylates, 576, 577
4-tert-Butyl catechol, 845, 855
n-Butyl methacrylate, sensitising potential in
guinea pigs, 579
p-tert-Butyl phenol, depigmentation due to, 869
dermatitis, 645
systemic disease due to, 871
p-tert-Butyl phenol formaldehyde, 69
sensitisation to, 21, 616
incidence, 617
sensitiser, 618
N-Butyl-4-chlorosalicylamide, photosensitivity
to, 433, 437
Butylated hydroxyanisole, 175
hydroxytoluene, 175

CA24, 698
Cabinet makers, occupational irritants and
sensitisers, 881
Cable-jointers, occupational irritants and
sensitisers, 881
Cactaceae, 490
Cactus, 25
Cadmium, 286
sulphide, 832
Caesalpinioideae woods, 557
Calf's liver, 26
Calocedrus decurrens, 555
Calomel, 686

Camphorwood, 557
Camyna, 267
Cananga oil, 161
Canestan, 227
Cannabidaceae, 491
Cape primrose, 514
Capers, 492
Capparidaceae, 492
Caprolactam, 86
Capsicum frutescens, 535
Captan, 399
Caraway, 536
    seed oil, 180
Carbamates, 410
    sensitisers in rubber, 720, 723
        patch testing, 767
Carbamide perhydrate, 129
Carbamol, 48
Carbon paper, 852
Carbowaxes, 812
Carbutamide, systemic, photosensitivity to, 447
Carcinoma, cutaneous, due to mineral oil, 849
Cardamom, 180, 538
Carenes, 800
Carmine, 144
Carpenters, occupational irritants and
        sensitisers, 881
Carrot, 25, 536
    phytophotosensitivity to, 421
Carum carvi, 536
Carvone, 180
Casalis green, 831
Cashew, 475
Cassia siamea, 558
Castellani's paint, 264
Castor bean pomace, 25
Cat saliva, 25
Catechols, allergenic, in wood, 551
Catering, occupational irritants and sensitisers,
        881
Cattle food, cobalt sensitivity due to, 324
Cedar wood, 555, 563
Cedrus deodora, 565
Celeriac, 536
Celery, 420, 535, 536
Cellulose acetate, allergy to, 644
    polymers, 642–8
        causes of dermatitis, 643
Celtis brieyi, 568
Cement, 24, 296–304
    chromate content, 296
    dermatitis, as occupational disease, 300
        clinical features, 301
        incidence, 300
    eczema, 302
        prognosis, 303
    irritants and sensitisers, 298
    phenol formaldehyde resin coating, 620
    tubes, rubber packing, 761
Cephalosporins, 26
Cetalkonium chloride, 108, 694
Cetavlon, 692
Cetrimide, 133, 692

Cetyl alcohol, 25, 807
Chamomile, 116
Chancito wood, 553
Chebulagic acid, 76
Chebulinic acid, 76
Cheilitis due to lipstick, 142
    due to nail varnish, 154
Chelators, 175
Chenopodiaceae, 492
Chicory, 182
China clay, cobalt pigments in, 322
Chipboard, 887
Chlorambucil, 237
Chloramphenicol, 204
Chloranil, 395
Chlorbutol, 700
Chlordantoin, 232
Chlordiazepoxide, systemic, photosensitivity to,
        447
Chlorfenicone, 207
Chlorhexidine, 110, 696
Chlormethylbenzol, 887
Chloroacetamide, 698
    in cosmetic creams, 98, 115, 698
Chloroacetophenone, 888
Chloroallylhexaminium chloride, 695, 795
α-Chlorobenzaldehyde phenylhydrazone, 887
p-Chlorobenzenesulphonylglycolic acid nitrile,
        29, 253
Chlorobutanol, 700
Chlorocresol, 673
p-Chloro-o-cresol, 392
2-Chloroethanol, 887
4-Chloro-2-hydroxytoluene, 392
Chloromycetin, 204
Chloronitrobenzenes, 400
Chlorophene, 393
Chlorophenoxamine, 887
Chloro-2-phenylphenol, photosensitivity to, 433,
        437
Chlorophora, 523, 564
Chlorothiazide, systemic, photosensitivity to,
        445
Chloroxylenol, 97, 675
    in cosmetic creams, 97
Chloroxylon swietenia, 556
Chlorphenesin, 227
Chlorpromazine, 25
    photo-allergy to, 438, 442, 443
    systemic, phototoxicity, 425, 428, 442,
        443
Chlorpropamide, systemic, photosensitivity to,
        446
Chlortetracycline, 224
    systemic, phototoxicity, 425, 426
Chromar, 254
Chromate, 41
    and nickel, combined allergy to, 366
    in cutting fluids, 846
    oral ingestion, 311
    patterns of dermatitis, 295
    photosensitising properties, 311
    sensitivity, age distribution, 295

anti-chrome barrier cream, 312
  causes, 293
  in cement workers with normal skin, 303
  incidence, 290
    in patients with cement dermatitis, 302
  patch testing, 312
  prognosis, 311
sources, 296–311
Chrome tanning compounds, 70
  ulcers, 295
Chromic oxide, 831
Chromium, 76, 287–313, 857
  combined with cobalt, 316
  compounds in polyester resins, 631
Chromonar, 253
Chrysanthemum, 495
  allergens, 498
  dermatitis, clinical features, 504, 508
    patch tests, 506
    treatment, 506
Cichorium, 182, 508
Cinchocaine, 194, 198
Cinnabar, 830
Cinnamate, photosensitivity to, 454
Cinnamic aldehyde, 26, 160, 180
Cinnamon, 180
Citraconic anhydride, 888
Citronella oil, 159
Citrus, 532
  photodermatitis due to, 420
Citrus red 2, 179
Cleaners, occupational irritants and sensitisers, 881
Clematis, 530
Clindamycin, 207
Clioquinol, 220
Cloflucarban, 705
Clothing, 36–92
  causing sensitivity, 39
  dyes, 38
  fire retardants in, 80
  sensitivity, incidence, 59
    patch testing, 41
Clotrimazole, 227
Coal tar, phototoxicity, 418
Coal-miners, occupational irritants and sensitisers, 881
Cobalt, 25, 184, 313–26, 857
  absorption, 314
  and nickel, combined allergy to, 366
  blue, 831
  -chrome alloy, 320
  combined with nickel and chromium, 316
  hard metal dust dermatitis, 324
  in cement, 317
  in polyester resin, 631
  industrial properties, 314
  sensitising properties, 314
  sensitivity, incidence, 315
    occupational causes, 322
  sources of exposure, 319
  toxicity, 314

Cobblers, occupational irritants and sensitisers, 884
Coccine, 179
Cockroaches, 888
Cocuswood, 560
Cod liver oil, 25
Codiaeum variegatum, 513
Coffee beans, 183
Coins, 350, 372
Colchicum autumnale, 523
Cold, 25
Coleus blumei, 517
Collagenase mixture, 889
Colophony, 70, 110, 111, 113, 149, 784, 848
  sensitivity, causes, 785
    due to cosmetics, 787
    in periodontal dressing, 787
    patch testing, 787
Colostomy, allergens, 886
Colour additives in foods, 178
  photography, developers, 863
Combretaceae woods, 554
Compositae, 492
  allergens, 495
  cross-reactions, 499
  dermatitis, 500
    differential diagnosis, 503
    patch tests, 505
    treatment, 506
Computer paper, 854
Condoms, 749
Confectioners, occupational irritants and sensitisers, 880
Construction workers, occupational irritants and sensitisers, 881
Contact lens solution, allergenic, 885
Contraceptives, intra-uterine, copper dermatitis due to, 327
  oral, phototoxicity, 425, 429
  rubber, 749
Conyza bonariensis, 517
Cooks, occupational irritants and sensitisers, 881
Coolants, synthetic, 841
  patch tests, 848
Copper, 326, 327
Copying procedures, 854
Coriander, 536
Coriandrum sativum, 536
Coronopilin, 497
Corrosion preventives in water system, chromate in, 306
Corrosive sublimate, 685
Corsets, 748
Corticosteroids, 246, 668
  depigmentation due to, 871
Corticotrophin, 246
Cortusa matthioli, 530
Cosmetic creams, patch testing
    positive — ingredients negative, 103
  types, 94
  sponge, rubber, 794
Cosmetics, 25, 93–170

containing formaldehyde, 790
containing lanolin, 777
containing parabens, 670
dermatitis, pigmented, 94
intolerance, 104
stinging compounds, 104
Costus root oil, 161, 510
Coumarin, 254
whitening agents, 81, 84
Coumarone-indene polymers, 624
Creams, cosmetic, *see* Cosmetic creams.
p-Cresol, depigmentation due to, 871
Cresylic acid, 843
Crinium, 474
Crotamiton, 254
Croton oil, 21, 888
Crotonaldehyde, 21
Crowfoot, 530
Cruciferae, 511
Cryptocarya pleurosperma, 517, 557
Cryptopleurine, 517, 557
Cryptostemma calendulaceae, 509
Cumambrin A, 498
Cumanin, 497
Cupressaceae woods, 555
Curad adhesive tape, 576
Cutting oils, 840
patch testing, 848
skin hazards, 843
Cyanoacrylic acid and esters, 587
Cyclamate, sodium, systemic, photosensitivity to, 448
Cyclodienes, 408
Cycloheximide, cross-reaction to neomycin, 214
Cyclohexylbenzothiazyl sulphenamide, sensitiser in rubber, 719, 730, 739, 763
Cyclohexyl-PPD, sensitiser in rubber, 757, 759
Cyclomethycaine, 198
Cynareae, 510
Cypripedium, 524

D and C Orange, 146
D and C Red, 144, 145, 149
D and C Yellow, 145, 146, 149
Dairy farmers, rubber sensitivity, 760
DBS, photosensitivity to, 435
Dahlia, 509
Daisy family, 492, 495
Daktarin, 229
Dalbergia, 560
Damsin, 497
Danders, animal 25
Daucus carota sativa, 536
Dazomet, 410
DDT, 406
Deadly nightshade, 534
Declomycin, systemic, phototoxicity, 426
Delphinium, 530
Demethylchlortetracycline, systemic, phototoxicity, 425, 426
Dentists and dental technicians, occupational irritants and sensitisers, 581, 881

sensitivity to amethocaine, 195
Dentures, cobalt dermatitis due to, 320
gold, 332
methyl methacrylate, 580
Deodar wood, 565
Deodorants, 106
formaldehyde, 792
granuloma due to zirconium, 375
Deoxybenzone, photosensitivity to, 453
Depigmentation, chemical, 867–71
Depilatories, 130
Depsides, 570
Dequadin chloride, 694
Dequalinium chloride, 694
Dermatitis, allergic, and atopic eczema, 22
allergic contact, in children, 20
associated with immediate type hypersensitivity, 26
bullosa striata pratensis, 419
contact, pigmented, 49
irritant, and atopic eczema, 22
seasonal variations, 24
lichenoid, due to stocking dyes, 50
Dermicel adhesive tape, 576
Dermographism, black, 335
Desoxylapachol, 569
Detergents, 81, 82, 815–24
additives, 820
chromates in, 309
nickel in, 352
Dettol, 675
Developers, photographic, 861, 863
Diabinese, systemic, photosensitivity to, 446
Diacetyl, 179, 653
Diacrylates, 577
Diallyl phthalate, 629
Diallylglycol carbonate resin dermatitis, 631
p,p'-Diaminodiphenylmethane, 603
sensitiser in rubber, 720, 738
Diamyl hydroquinone, 786
Diazo copying, 854
Diazonium compound, 854
Dibenzothiazyl disulphide, sensitiser in rubber, 719, 730, 763
Dibenzthione, 228
5,4'-Dibromosalicylanilide, photosensitivity to, 433, 435
Dibromsalan, photosensitivity to, 433, 435
Di-*tert*-butyl hydroquinone, 98, 113
N-Dibutyl phthalate, 108
Dibutyltin maleate, 653
Dichlone, 395
2,6-Dichlorobenzaldoxin, 888
Dichlorodiphenyltrichloroethane, 406
Dichlorophen, 96, 677
Dichlorphene, 393
Dichloropropiophenone, 888
Dichromate, 24, 76, 856, 858
Dicyclohexyl-carbodiimide, 887
Dieldrin, 408
Diethyl ester of maleic acid sensitisation, 630
Diethyl pyrocarbonate, 174

Diethylenetriamine, 603
  cross-reaction to ethylenediamine, 245
Diethylstilboestrol, 266
Diethylthiourea, sensitiser in rubber, 740
Diethyltoluamide, 25, 26
Difolatan, 400
Diiodohydroxypropane, 258
Diisocyanates, 635
Di-isopropanolamine, 114, 149
Dill, 420, 536
Dimercaprol, 255
Dimethacrylates, 585
Dimethoxane, 700
Dimethyl sulphoxide, 25, 888
Dimethylaminopropylamine, 603
Dimethylaniline, toxic effects, 629
N-Dimethyl-1,3-butyl-N'-phenylparaphenyl-
    enediamine, sensitiser in rubber, 737,
    738, 757
Dimethyloldihydroxyethylene urea, 56, 57
Di-β-naphthyl-p-phenylenediamine, sensitiser in
    rubber, 721, 733
Dinitolmide, 184
p-Dinitrobenzene, cross-reaction to
    chloramphenicol, 205
Dinitrochlorobenzene, 30, 401
  cross-reaction to chloramphenicol, 205
4,6-Dinitro-o-cresol, 393
Dinitrofluorobenzene, 888
Dinobuton, 394
Dinocap, 395
Diomia wood, 568
Diospyros, 555, 556
Dioxane, 888
Dioxydiphenyl, sensitiser in rubber, 719, 723,
    740
  patch testing, 767
Dipentamethylenethiuram disulphide, sensitiser
    in rubber, 719, 729
Diphenhydramine, 235, 439
Diphenyl diisocyanate, 641
Diphenylamine, 888
Diphenylcyclopropenone, 888
Diphenylguanidine sensitisers in rubber, 719,
    723, 731, 732, 740
  patch testing, 767
Diphenylmethane diisocyanate, 637, 640
Diphenyl-PPD, sensitiser in rubber, 720, 726,
    727, 732, 737, 757, 759, 760
Dipropylenetriamine, 603
Diquat, 404
Disinfectants, depigmentation due to, 870
Disperse blue 35, 423
  dyes, 41
Distemonanthus benthamianus, 558
Disulfiram implants, 752
Dithianone, 395
Dithiocarbamates, 396
Dithiodimorpholine, sensitiser in rubber, 722,
    723, 740
  patch testing, 767
Diuril, systemic, photosensitivity to, 445
DNCB, 30, 205, 401

Dodecyl gallate, 177
  mercaptan, 69, 70
Dog saliva, 25
Dogger Bank itch, 889
Domiphen bromide, 700
Dowicil 200, 149, 695, 795
Doxycycline, systemic, photosensitivity to, 425,
    427
Drapolene, 693
Dress shields, rubber, 751
Droxaryl, 252
Drugs, photoallergenic, 414, 437–9
  systemic, photoallergic, 414, 444–50
    photoallergic and phototoxic, 449
    phototoxic, 414, 424–31
    phototoxicity tests, 431
Dry cleaning, 76
  occupational irritants and sensitisers, 77, 882
Duhring chamber test unit, 4
Dycril printing plates, 591
Dyeline copying, 854
Dyes, 36–55, 240
  carcinogenicity following photodye therapy,
    423
  disperse group, 41, 43
  in shoe leather, 71, 74
  phototoxic, 422
Dysoxyllum muelleri, 562

Earphones, rubber, 761
Earrings, 347, 355
Ebenaceae woods, 555
Ebony, 555, 556
ECG electrode jelly and paste, 889
Eczema, association with lanolin, 779–82
  atopic, and allergic dermatitis, 22
    and irritant dermatitis, 22
  due to cement chromate, 302
  facial, due to cosmetics, 96
  'hybrids', 171
  of hand, in nickel sensitivity, 357
  photosensitive, 416
EDTA, 701
Eggs, 26
Elderly, contact dermatitis, 21
Electricians, occupational irritants and
    sensitisers, 882
Electroplaters, occupational irritants and
    sensitisers, 882
Electroplating, chrome ulceration due to, 308
  nickel, 346, 361
Elletania, 538
Elm tree, 538
  wood, 568
Embalmers, occupational sensitisers, 882
Embalming fluid, 792
Emulsifiers in cosmetic cream, 101
Encephabol, systemic, photosensitivity to, 448
Endesmanolide, 496
Endive, 183, 508
Entandrophragma, 562
Entero-Vioform, 220
Enzyme additives in detergents, 820

Eosin, 142
Ephedrine, 256
Epichlorhydrin, 596, 602, 891
Epinephrine, 256
Epiphytodermatitis, 467
Epontol, 201
Epoxide, 595
  in oil of turpentine, 801
Epoxy acrylate oligomer photosensitive ink, 593
  resins, 595
    as plasticisers, 607
    as stabilisers, 607
    carcinogenicity, 613
    chemistry, 595–604
    dermatitis, causes, 605
      clinical features, 609
    hardeners, sensitising, 603
    hazards, control, 613
    monomers, allergenic component, 602
      sensitisation to, 612
    patch tests, 609, 612
    reactive diluents, sensitising, 603
    sensitisation to, incidence, 604, 608
      respiratory symptoms, 612
    uses, 599
Ercotina Derm, 262
Eremophilanolide, 496
Erythema multiforme, 29
Erythromycin, 207
Erythronium, 520
Escalol, photosensitivity to, 452
Espenille wood, 566
Ethanediol, 809
Ethanol, 805
Ethanolamines, 234
Ethinyloestradiol, phototoxicity, 429
Ethoxy methylene ethyl malonate, 889
Ethoxyquin, 185
Ethyl acetate, 179
  acrylate, 576
  alcohol, 805
  butyl thiourea, 70
  chloride, 889
  methacrylate, sensitising potential in guinea
    pigs, 579
Ethylene chlorohydrin, 887
  glycol, 809
    monomethyl ether acetate, toxic effects, 646
  oxide, 174, 702
Ethylenediamine, 27, 234, 241, 603
  dihydroiodide, 186
  sensitisation to, 21
  tetraacetate, 701
  tetra-acetic acid, cross-reaction to
    ethylenediamine, 244
2-Ethylhexyl acrylate, 576
Eugenia, 523
Euphorbiaceae, 512
Eurax, 255, 256
Evernic acid, 570
Eye cosmetics, 110
  creams, 115
  shadows, 112

Eyelash curlers, 754
Eyelid eczema, allergens, 885
Eyeliners, 115

Fabric softeners, 78
Fabrics, chromates in, 310
  treated with phenol formaldehyde resin, 620
Face masks, rubber, 761
Fagaceae woods, 556
Fagara, 566
Falicain, 200
Feet, hyperhidrosis, 74
Feminine hygiene sprays, 109
Fennel, 536
Fentichlor, photosensitivity to, 140, 420, 433,
    436, 442, 443
Ferro wood, 557
Fibre glass, 78, 79
Ficus carica, 564
'Fiddler's neck', 890
Fig, 523
  phytophotodermatitis due to, 421
  wood, 564
Filter paper, 619
Finger nails, methyl methacrylate, 583
Finger-stall, rubber, 764
Finn chamber test unit, 3
Fir wood, 565, 566
Fire Red 2513, 144
Fire retardants, 80
Fishing nets, 86
Fitzroya cupressoides, 555
Flame retardants, 80
Flavouring agents, 179
Flindersiaceae woods, 556
Flogocid, 252
Floor waxes, turpentine in, 804
Floor-layers, occupational irritants and
    sensitisers, 882
Florists, occupational irritants and sensitisers,
    882
Flour, 25, 181
Fluorescent whitening agents, 81
Fluoropolymers, 656
5-Fluorouracil, 238
Fluxes, 787, 865
Focal flare, 16
Foeniculum vulgare, 536
Food, 171–91
  additives, 173, 184
  colouring agents, 178
  flavouring agents, 28, 179
  laboratory, chromate dermatitis in, 309
  nickel content, 359
Formaldehyde, 22, 24, 25, 48, 788–97, 857
  causes of allergic contact dermatitis, 789
  clothing dermatitis, 60, 61,
    diagnostic criteria, 64
    management, 66
    prophylaxis, 66
  cyanoguanidine compounds, 135
  in hair shampoos, 134, 138
  in nail varnish, 155, 156

in textiles, 55, 63
  detection, 65
occupational asthma due to, 793
  dermatitis due to, 66
releasers, 97, 794
resins, 614–21
  dermatitis, causes, 615
sensitisation, incidence, 789
sensitising potential, 788
sensitivity, patch testing, 63, 794
sources of contact, 788
Foundry workers, occupational irritants and
    sensitisers, 882
Fragaria, 531
Framycetin, 207
  cross-reaction to neomycin, 213
French polishers, occupational irritants and
    sensitisers, 881
Freon 11 and 12 propellants, 108
Frullania, 570, 571
Frullanolide, 571
Frusemide, systemic, phototoxicity and
    photosensivity to, 425, 429, 446
Fuchsin-silver nitrate, 889
Fucidin, 208
Fuel oils, 842, 844
  patch tests, 849
Fumigants, 85
Funeral directors, 882
Fungicides, 392–403
Fungiplex, 228
Fungistats, 227
Fur, 26
  workers, asthma in, 47
Furacin, 186, 215
Furan polymers, 624
Furazolidone, 186
Furocoumarins, 467
  photosensitising, in wood, 551
  phototoxicity, 418
  systemic, phototoxicity, 431
Fusidate, 208

Gaboon wood, 554
Gaillardia, 509
Galanthus, 473
Galvanised sheets, chromate in, 304
Gammexane, 407
Garage workers, occupational irritants and
    sensitisers, 882
Garapa wood, 557
Gardeners, occupational irritants and sensitisers,
    882
Garment sensitivity, 39, 60
Gas plant, phytophotodermatitis due to, 420
Gasoline dyes, 847
Genetris pessary, 207
Gentamicin, 208
  cross-reaction to neomycin, 214
Gentian violet, 240
Geraniaceae, 514
Germall group, 703
Gesneriaceae, 514

Ginger, 538
Ginkgoaceae, 515
Girdles, 748
Giv-Tan, photosensitivity to, 454
Gloxinia, 515
Glue, chromate in, 309
  epoxy, 607
  formaldehyde, 616
  with phenol formaldehyde, 620
  see also Adhesives.
Gluta renghas, 477
Glutaraldehyde, 795
Glyceryl monostearate, 813
Glyceryl *p*-aminobenzoate, photosensitivity to,
    452
Glycidyl ether epoxy resins, 596
Glycols, 809–13
Gold, 328
  industrial dermatitis from, 333
  orbital implant, 332
  patch testing, 334
  salts, 333
  sensitising potential, 330
  sensitivity, causes and clinical features, 330
    incidence, 330
Gonystylus bancanus, 568
Goosefoot, phytophotodermatitis due tó, 421
Gossweilerodendron balsamiferum, 561
Grains, 182
Gramineae, 515
Grasses, 515
Greases, 842
  patch tests, 849
Greenheart wood, 557
Grevillea wood, 566
Griseofulvin, systemic, phytotoxicity, 430
Grofas, photo-allergy to, 440
Grotan BK, 846
Guaianolide, 496
Guanidine sensitisers in rubber, 719, 731
Guanine in nail lacquer, 156
Guaranta wood, 566
Guarea wood, 562
Guatambu wood, 566
Gum arabic, 793

Haemanthus, 474
Haemodialysis apparatus, sensitivity to, 752,
    791, 793
Hair bleaches, 25, 126
  creams for men, 139
  depilatories, 130
  dyes, 26, 115–26
    carcinogenicity, 125
    metallic, 117
    sensitivity, clinical features, 122
      incidence, 121
      patch testing, 123
    synthetic organic, 117
    vegetable, 116
  green, 126
  net dermatitis, 54
  permanent waving, 129

preparations, 115–40
repigmentation, 126
restorers, 132
setting lotions, 130
sinuses, interdigital, 139
sprays, 25, 130
straighteners, 130
tonics, 132
Hairdressers, occupational irritants and
    sensitisers, 134–9, 882
  patch testing, 139
Haloprogin, 228
Halotax, 228
Halquinol, 187
Hand eczema, association with lanolin, 780
    due to match heads, 829
    in hairdressers, 135
Hat bands, 76
Hearing aids, 581, 647
  rubber pads, 752
Heartwood, 549
Heat, 25
Hedera, 488
Heel stiffeners, 72
Helenium, 494
Heliantheae, allergenic sesquiterpene lactones,
    497
Helleborus, 531
Hemp family, 491
Henna, 116
Heracleum, phytophotodermatitis due to, 420
  mantegazzianum, 536
  sphondylium, 536
Herbicides, 403
Hernandiaceae woods, 556
Herpes simplex inoculation in patch test, 17
Hexachlorocyclohexane, 407
Hexachlorophane, 106, 678
  dermatitis, 680
  photosensitivity to, 432, 433, 436, 442, 443
  sensitivity, incidence, 679
  toxicity, 679
Hexamethylene bis-chlorophenyl biguanide, 696
  diisocyanate, 639
Hexamethylenetetramine, 795
Hexamidine, 889
Hexamine, 795
Hexanediol diacrylate photosensitive ink, 593
Hexylene glycol, 811
Hibitane, 696
Hippeastrum, 473, 474
Hippomane mancinella, 513
Hirudoid ointment, 699
Histamine, 233
Hogweed, 420, 536
Homomenthyl salicylate, photosensitivity to,
    454
Hop pickers' dermatitis, 491
Hordeum vulgare, 515
Horse serum, 25
Hospital workers, occupational irritants and
    sensitisers, 883
Hot water bottle, rubber, 753

Housework, occupational irritants and
    sensitisers, 883
Humea elegans, 509
Humidity indicator, cobalt salt in, 323
Humulus, 491
Hutchinson's summer prurigo, 416
Hyacinth itch, 522
Hyacinthin, 161
Hyacinthus, 519
Hydrangea, 534
Hydrazine, 865
Hydroa vacciniforme, 416
Hydroabietyl alcohol, 786
Hydrochlorothiazide, systemic, photosensitivity
    to, 445
Hydrocortisone, 246
Hydro-Diuril, systemic, photosensitivity to, 445
Hydrogen peroxide, 126
Hydromox, systemic, photosensitivity to, 446
Hydroperoxide of Δ^3-carene, 800
Hydrophyllaceae, 516
Hydroquinone, 187, 786
  depigmentation due to, 868, 869
Hydrosaluric, systemic, photosensitivity to, 445
Hydroxyanisole, butylated, depigmentation due
    to, 871
4-Hydroxybenzoic acid, 179
p-Hydroxybenzoic acid esters, 665
Hydroxyethyl methacrylate, 585
Hydroxylamine sulphate, 889
p-Hydroxyphenylbutazone, 259
Hydroxypolyethoxydodecane, 889
Hydroxyquinolines, 218
8-Hydroxyquinoline, depigmentation due to,
    871
Hydroxytoluene, butylated, depigmentation due
    to, 871

Ice red TR, 48
Ichthammol, 257
Ichthyol, 257
Idoxuridine, 209
Ileostomy, allergens, 886
Ilotycin, 207
Imbuya wood, 557
Imidazolidinyl urea compounds in cosmetic
    creams, 97, 703
Imperacin, systemic, phototoxicity, 427
Indigo, 831
Ineral, 135
Inks, acrylic, photosensitive, 592
  printing, 857, 858
  with phenol formaldehyde resin, 620
  writing, 860
Insect repellant, 26
Insecticides, 404
Insulating tape, 786
Intensain, 254
Inula, 509, 517
Iodine, 257
Ipé wood, 554
Irgasan BS200, photosensitivity to, 432, 434
Irgasan DP300, 108, 109

Irgasans, 704
Iridaceae, 516
Iris, 516
Iroko wood, 564
Iron, 336
Irritants causing dermatitis in elderly, 21
Iruxol, 889
Isabelin, 497
Isoamyl-*p*-N,N-dimethylaminobenzoate,
        photosensitivity to, 452
Isocyanates, 640
Isonicotinic acid hydrazide, 210
Isophoronediamine, 604
Isopropyl alcohol, 806
    myristate, 110
Isopropylaminodiphenylamine, 75, 87
Isopropylphenyl-PPD, sensitiser in rubber, 720,
        732, 736, 757, 759, 764
Isothecium spiculiferum, 572
Iva microcephala, 509
Ivy family, 488

Jacaranda wood, 559, 560
'Jackman's blue' rue, photodermatitis due to,
        420
Jadit, photosensitivity to, 433, 437, 442, 443
Jasmin oil, 161
Jecovital, 254
Jewellers, occupational irritants and sensitisers,
        883
Jewellery, gold, 331
    nickel, 347, 351, 355
    silver, 372
Juniper oil, 180
Juniperus virginiana, 555

Kanamycin, cross-reaction to neomycin, 214
Keloid due to patch test, 16
Kerosene, 842, 844
Khaya, 562
Kidney machines, formaldehyde sterilisation,
        791, 793
Kingwood, 560
Koilonychia, 845
Konservierungsmittel C, 698
Kurasan, 185

Labiatae, 516
Lactones, sesquiterpene, allergenic, in
        Compositae, 495, 496
Lactuca sativa, 510
Lactucoideae, 492
Lakes (pigments), 141, 143, 144
Lancewood, 559
Lanette N, 102
Langerhans cells, role in allergic contact
        dermatitis, 31
Lanolin, 98, 105, 113, 771–84, 786
    allergens, 773
    in lipstick, 147
    sensitivity, 777
        clinical features, 778
        incidence, 774

patch testing, 782
    with stasis eczema and ulcers, 779
Lapacho woods, 534
Lapachol, 569
Laportea, 538
Larch wood, 565
Largactil, systemic, phototoxicity, 428
Larix decidua, 565
Latex, 715, 724
    allergens, 550
Lauraceae, 517
    woods, 557
Laurel oil, 76
Laurus, 517
Lauryl ether sulphate, 817
    gallate, 175, 176, 177
    methacrylate, 585
Lawsone, 116
Laxagen, systemic, photosensitivity to, 448
Lead, 337
    in Asian eye cosmetics, 114
Leather dyes, 71, 74
    sensitisation in children, 21
    tans, 70, 73
Ledermycin, systemic, phototoxicity, 425, 426
Leg ulcers, allergens, 885
Leguminosae, 518
    phytophotodermatitis due to, 419
    woods, 557–9
Lemon, 532
    flavouring, 179
    oil of, 160
    phytophotodermatitis due to, 420
Lemongrass oil, 160
Lentil, 518
Letterflex printing plates, 638, 641
Lettuce, 183, 510
Leucoderma, occupational, 868
Librium, systemic, photosensitivity to, 447
Lichen planus associated with copper
        sensitivity, 327
    due to photographic developer, 862, 865
Lichens, 22, 569
    allergens, 570
    allergy, 572
Light, 25
    persistent reactor, 416
Lignocaine, 199
Liliaceae, 519
Lilliflorae, 472
Limba wood, 554
Limes, 532
    phytophotodermatitis due to, 420
d-Limonene, 532, 536
Lindane, 25, 407
Lipstick, 141–9
    intolerance, 148
    patch tests, 148
    sensitivity to, incidence, 142
Lithographic plates, 856
Liverworts, 570
    allergens, 571
Locan, 195

Lorexane, 407
Louro wood, 557
Lovage, 180
Lovoa klaineana, 563
Lubricating oils, 842
    cobalt compounds in, 324
    leucoderma due to, 849
    patch tests, 849
Lycopersicon lycopersicum, 535
Lycra, 745, 746, 761

Machaerium scleroxylon, 562
Maclura pomifera, 523, 564
Madder, 532
Mafenide, 223
Magnetic tapes, chromium sensitisation due to,
    324
Mahogany, 562, 563
Makoré wood, 567
Malathion, 409
Maleic acid, 630, 631
Malus, 531
Mancozeb, 397
Maneb, 396
Manganese, 832
Mangifera indica, 476, 477, 481, 483
Mansonia wood, 568
Maple wood, 556
Marfanil, 223
Marigold, Mexican, 510
Marine plants, 25
Marrubium vulgare, 517
Mascara, 110
Massaranduba wood, 567
Masterwort, 536
    phytophotodermatitis due to, 421
Mastisol, 267
Matches, 824– 9
Mechlorethamine hydrochloride, 25
Meclofenoxate, 258
Medicaments, 192– 278
    containing dichlorophen, 677
    containing parabens, 668, 671, 673
Melamine formaldehyde, 55, 57, 63, 622
Melanosis due to oil and photosensitivity, 849
Melanoxylon densiflora, 558
Meleril, systemic, photosensitivity to, 444
Mediaceae woods, 562
Mellaril, systemic, photosensitivity to, 444
Mentha citrata, 517
Menthol cigarettes, 888
Mepyramine, 236
Merbromin, 688
Mercapto chemicals, sensitisers in rubber, 719,
    739
    patch testing, 766
Mercaptobenzothiazole, 69, 70, 71, 75, 402
    sensitisers in rubber, 719, 723, 726, 727, 729,
    734, 735, 763
2-Mercaptobenzothiazole, 845
Mercuric chloride, 24, 685
    cyanate, 686
    sulphide, 830

Mercurochrome, 688
Mercurous chloride, 686
Mercury, 681– 92
    amalgam dental fillings, 682
    ammoniated, 684
    compounds, 683
        cross-reactions, 691
        fungicidal, 401
    fulminate, 686
    metallic, 681
Merfen sensitivity in children, 21
Merthiolate, 21, 689
Mesquite wood, 559
Mesulphen, 228
Metal workers, occupational irritants and
        sensitisers, 883
Metals, 279– 390
Metaoxedrine ointment, 256
Methacrylonitrile, 588
Methanal, 788
Methoxydalbergione, 561
5-Methoxypsoralen, photoactivity, 418
8-Methoxypsoralen, phototoxicity, 418, 423, 448
Methyl acrylate, 576
        ethyl ketone peroxide dermatitis, 631
        heptine carbamate, 161
    methacrylate, 578
        causes of dermatitis, 580
        sensitising potential in guinea pigs, 579
        uses, 579, 580
    salicylate, 265
    violet, 852
Methylanisate, 161
Methylcyclohexyldimethylphenol, sensitiser in
        rubber, 743
2,2'-Methylenebis(3,4,6-trichlorophenol),
        photosensitivity to, 433, 436
Methyloctylbenzenesulphonate, 848
Methylol chloroacetamide, 86
Methylolacrylamide, 589
Mexenone, photosensitivity to, 453
Miconazole nitrate, 229
Micturin, 231
Milk testers, chromium dermatitis in, 308
Millet, 515
Momosoideae woods, 558
Mineral oil in cosmetic creams, 102
    occupational use, 839
        carcinogenicity, 849
Miranols in cosmetic creams, 97
Mitragyna, 565
Moabi wood, 567
Moah wood, 556, 567
Monoamylamine, 25, 26, 232
Monomers non-allergic but sensitising additives,
        642– 55
    sensitising, 575– 624
Monomethacrylates, 577
Monomethylol dicyandiamide, 135
Monosodium glutamate, 180
Monostearin, 813
Moquizone, photosensitivity to, 440
Moraceae, 523

phytophotodermatitis due to, 419
woods, 563
Mordants, 36, 41
Morpholinylmercaptobenzothiazole, sensitiser in rubber, 719, 730, 737, 763
Mosses, 571
Moth proofing, 85
Motor bicycle rubber, 759
Moule wood, 564
Mouth, cancer in textile workers, 86
Mucuna pruriens, 518
Mucunain, 518
Muiratana wood, 557
Mukulunga wood, 567
Mulberry, 523
Multergan, 438
Multifungin, photosensitivity to, 433, 435
Mushroom farming, formaldehyde disinfection in, 793
Musicians, allergic contact dermatitis, 890
Mussel itch, 172
Mustard, oil of, 180
Mycil, 227
Mycolog cream, 21, 162, 233, 242
Myleran, 239
Mylone, 410
Myrabolam, 76
Myrtaceae, 523

Nadisan, systemic, photosensitivity to, 447
Nail base coats, 157
covers, synthetic, 157
hardeners, 158
polish, 25
preparations, 150–58
varnish, 150
dermatitis, distribution, 153
patch testing, 154
Nails, discolouration, non-allergic, 156
photo-onycholysis due to drugs, 425, 428
Naled, 409
Nalidixic acid, systemic, phototoxicity, 425, 430
Naphthalene diisocyanate, 639
Naphthyl sensitisers in rubber, 721, 723, 738
patch testing, 767
Narcissus, 473
Naucleaceae woods, 565
NDGA, 176, 705
Nectandra, 557
Neomycin, 21, 22, 27, 210
cross-reactions, 213
Nettle, 25, 537
Neutral red, contact allergy, 422
phototoxicity, 422
Nickel, 23, 24, 28, 338–67
absorption and localisation in skin and nails, 340
alloys, 349
and chromate, combined allergy to, 366
and cobalt, combined allergy to, 366
combined with cobalt, 316, 317
dermatitis, treatment, 365
domestic sources of contact, 346

electroplating, 346, 361
in cutting fluids, 847
in detergents, 352
in footwear, 72
industrial uses, 339
occupational dermatitis, 360
oral ingestion, 359
pustular patch test reactions, 23
sensitisation in children, 21
sensitising potential, 340
-sensitive subjects, occupations unsuitable for, 880
sensitivity, associated patterns of eczema, 357
causes, 345
clinical features, 353
clinical patterns, 355
in hairdressers, 136, 137, 138
incidence, 341–5
patch testing, 362
secondary spread, 356
systemic reactions, 349
Nicotiana tabacum, 535
Nigrosine base, 852
Nipa esters, 665
Nipagin, 665
Nitrates, 174
Nitrites, 174
p-Nitrobenzene-azo-β-naphthol, 143
p-Nitrobenzoic acid, cross-reaction to chloramphenicol, 205
Nitrofen, 394
Nitrofurazone, 186, 215
Nitrogen mustard, 26, 238
Nitroglycerin, 258
Nitrophenols, 393
'No carbon required' paper, 853
Nolvasan, 696
Nordihydroguaiaretic acid, 176, 705
Novolak resins, 615
Nurses, occupational irritants and sensitisers, 883
Nylon factories, occupational dermatitis in, 86
stocking dermatitis, 49–54
taffeta, 58
Nyloprint plates, 590
Nystaform-HC ointment, 220, 233, 268
Nystatin, 232, 233

Obeche wood, 568
Occupational irritants and sensitisers, 879–85
Octadecanol, 808
Octoea, 557
Octyl gallate, 175, 177
Oestrogen, systemic, phototoxicity, 429
Oestrogenic cream, 25
Office workers, occupational irritants and sensitisers, 883
Offset printing, 361, 857
Ofurma wood, 553
Oil acne, 849
folliculitis, 849
red oil dye, 847

yellow oil dye, 847
Oils, chromate in, 306
  occupational use, 839–50
    patch testing, 848
    skin hazards, 843, 845
  see also Lubricating oils; Mineral oil.
Okoumé wood, 554
Oleoresins, 464
Oleyl alcohol, 147, 808
Olonvogo wood, 566
Omite, 410
Opuntia, 490
Optyl, 608
Orange, phytophotodermatitis due to, 420
  skin dyes, 179
  wood, 158, 564
Orange G oil dye, 847
Orchidaceae, 523
Organocyanates, 405
Organophosphorus insecticides, 408
Organo-tin compounds, fungicidal, 401
Orinase, systemic, photosensitivity to, 447
Orthodichlorobenzene, 76
Orthopaedic appliances, 28
  plaster with melamine formaldehyde, 623
  surgeons, sensitisation to methyl methacrylate,
    582
Orthophenylphenol, 681
  leucoderma due to, 870
Ortho-toluene-azo-beta-naphthylamine, 179
Osage wood, 564
Otitis externa due to match heads, 828, 829
  due to nail varnish, 153
Oxirane, 702
Oxyayanins, 558
Oxymethylene, 788
Oxyphenbutazone, 260
Oxytetracycline, 22, 224
  systemic, phototoxicity, 425, 427

PABA, photosensitivity to, 450
Pacemaker, epoxy resin coated, 608
Padimate A, photosensitivity to, 452
Paint, chromate in, 305
  drier, cobalt, 323
  primers, chromate in, 305
  thinner, turpentine in, 803
  turpentine in, 803
Painters, occupational irritants and sensitisers,
    883
Palladium, 367, 368
Pancratum, 474
Pantocaine, 194
Pao ferro wood, 562
Paper industry, chromium dermatitis in, 308
Papers, abrasive, 850–54,
  abrasive, 619
  formaldehyde fixative in, 791
  'no carbon required', 853
  pulp, 851
  with phenol formaldehyde resin, 619
Papilionoideae woods, 559
Para-aminobenzoic acid, photosensitivity to, 450

Parabens, 665
  esters as food additives, 173
    in corticosteroid preparations, 668
    in cosmetic creams, 96, 105, 679
    in medicaments, 668, 672, 673
  patch testing, 672
  sensitising potential, 666
  sensitivity, causes, 667
    clinical features, 670
    index, 666
  systemic absorption, 672
Paraformaldehyde, 794
Paranasal sinus carcinoma in woodworkers,
    550
Paraquat, 404
Parasitophytophotodermatitis, 467
Paratecoma peroba, 553
Parathion, 408
Parsley, 535, 536
Parsnip, 536
  phytophotodermatitis due to, 420
Parthenin, 497
Parthenium hysterophorus, 467, 468, 494
  allergens, 499
  dermatitis due to, 500
    clinical features, 503
    patch testing, 505
    treatment, 506
Pastinaca sativa, 536, 537
Patch testing, allergen concentration, effect on
    result,
  allergic reactions, 10
  amount of test material, 6
  complications, 14
  deterioration of test substances, 7
  effect of prednisone on reactions, 14
  false negative reaction, 13
  false positive reaction, 12
  focal flare, 16
  interpretation, 11
  irritant reactions, 10
  open, 17
  reactions, histology, 29
  reading time, 7
  recording of results, 8
  relevance of reactions, 11
  scars and keloids due to, 16
  sensitisation, active, 15
  site of application, 4
    marking, 4
  standard series (battery), 9
  technique, 1–19
  unit, 2
  usage test, 17
  vehicles, 6
Patent blue violet, 241
PCMX, 97, 675
PCNB, 400
Pea, 518
Peanut, 518
Pecilocin, 230
Pelargonium, 514
Peltogyne densiflora, 558

Penicillin, 25, 216
Pentachloronitrobenzene, 400
Pentachlorophenol, 392
Pentaerythritol triacrylate photosensitive ink, 593
Pentanedial, 795
Pentazocine, 202
Perchloroethylene, 76, 77
Perfumes, 25, 109, 110, 141, 158–64
  dermatitis, clinical features, 163
    patch testing, 163
  detergent, 824
  in cosmetics, 100, 105
  in lipstick, 147
  in medicaments, 162
Pericopsis elata, 559
Perlatolic acid, 50
Permanent Orange, 146
Permaton Red, 144
Peroba rose wood, 553
  wood, 553
Peroxides, irritant effects, 629
Peru balsam, 20, 26, 28, 162
Pesticides, 391–413
Petrol, 842, 844
  dyes in, 847
Petrolatum as base for allergens, 6
Petroselinum crispum, 536, 537
Peucedanum astruthium, 536
Phacelia crenulata, 516
Phaltan, 399
Pharynx, cancer in textile workers, 86
Phenergan, 237, 437, 444
Pheniramine, 236
Phenol formaldehyde polymers, 614
  chemistry, 615, 619, 859
  uses, 615
  resin, airborne exposure, 620
Phenolic calcium salt, 845
  compounds, 673–81
    depigmentation due to, 868, 879
Phenols, allergenic, in wood, 550
  fungicidal 392
  halogenated, cross-reactions, 437
    photosensitivity to, 432–7
  in cosmetic creams, 96
Phenothiazines, 27, 235
  derivatives, photoallergenic, 437
  systemic, photosensitivity to, 444
Phenoxybenzamine, 261
4-Phenyl catechol, 855
α -Phenyl indole dermatitis, 651
Phenyl mercuric nitrate, 401
Phenylacetaldehyde, 161
Phenylbutazone, 259
Phenylcyclohexyl-PPD, sensitiser in rubber, 720, 726, 727, 732, 736, 737
p-Phenylenediamine, 22, 438, 859
  hair dyes, 118–20, 124, 137
  patch testing, 42
Phenylephrine hydrochloride, 256
Phenylmercuric acetate, 687, 688
  benzoate, 688

borate, 687
  sensitivity in children, 21
propionate, 25
salts, 686
Phenyl-β-naphthylamine, sensitiser in rubber, 721, 733, 738
o-Phenylphenol, 97
  leucoderma due to, 870
Phoebe porosa, 557
Phosphonium compounds, 80
Phosphorus fire retardants, 80
  sesquisulphide in match boxes, 825
Phosphothioate, 402
Photo-allergens, topical, 432–4
Photo-allergy due to drugs, 414, 437–9
  photopatch testing, 441, 443
Photocopying, 855
Photodermatitis due to plants, 419
Photodermatoses, 416
Photograph developers, occupational irritants and sensitisers, 883
Photography, 861–5
Photogravure printing, 858
Photo-oncolysis, systemic, drugs causing, 425, 428
Photopatch tests, 8
Photosensitisers, 414–60
  photoallergic, 414, 432–48
    photopatch testing, 441, 443
  phototoxic, 414, 417–32
    systemic, 414, 424–32
    topical, 417–24
    topical, phototesting, 424
Photosensitivity, tests for, 417
Phototoxicity due to systemic drugs, 424–31
Phthalic acid or anhydride, 634, 635
Phytodermatitis, 461–547; *see* Plant dermatitis,
Phytomenadione, 250
Phytophotodermatitis, 419, 470
Picea abies, 565
Picropodophyllin, 556
Pigmentation due to whiteners, 82
Pigments, 36
  alteration in patch test patients, 16
  used in tattooing, 830
Pillow, rubber, 752
Pimpinella anisum, 536
Pinaceae woods, 565
Pine wood, 565, 566
Pineapple, 490
Pinus, 565
Piperazines, 234, 260
  cross-reaction to ethylenediamine, 235
Piratinera guianensis, 564
Pitch, phototoxicity, 417
Plants, 461–547
  allergens, 463
  dermatitis, allergic contact, 466, 469
    classification, 466
    clinical features, 468
    cross reactions, 464
    incidence, 467
    irritant, 466, 469

patch testing, 464
 sex and age preference, 468
 treatment, 470
identification, 462
nomenclature, 462
selection for testing, 462
Plaster reaction, 14
Plastics, 575–663
 cobalt pigment in, 322
 industry, occupational irritants and
  sensitisers, 884
Platinum, 367
 hyposensitisation, 370
 salts, 25, 368
  histamine-releasing agents, 371
 sensitivity, clinical features, 369
'Playtex' brassière, 745
Plondrel, 402
Plumbers, occupational irritants and sensitisers,
 884
Podophyllotoxin, 556
Poison ivy, 375, 467, 468, 475, 477
 cross-reactions, 478
 sensitisation in children, 20
Polishes, turpentine in, 803
Polyacetylenic compounds, phototoxicity, 421
Polyamides, 656
 aliphatic, 25
Polyester, cobalt in, 323
 cotton resin, 56
 fibres, 635
 plasticisers, 635
 resins, 625–35
  chemistry, 625
  dermatitis, 629, 630
  technology, 628
Polyether alcohol, 642
Polyethylene alcohol, 26
 glycol, 812
Polygonaceae, 524
Polymers, acrylic, 575–95
Polymethylene polyphenyl isocyanate, 641
Polymyxin B, 217
 cross-reaction with bacitracin, 204
Polyolefins, 655
Polystyrene, 655
Polyurethane, 635
 foams, 637, 640
 hardeners, 641
 in shoes, 71
 lacquer, 642
 products, 637
 toxicity and pulmonary complications, 638
Polyvinyl acetate, 653
 chloride, 648–55
  in shoes, 71
  toxicity, 652
  uses, 650
Polyvinylidene chloride, 655
Ponceau Red 6 R, 179
Poplar wood, 567
Populus, 567
Porphyrins, systemic, phototoxicity, 431

Potassium chromate, 48
 dichromate, 22
  in match heads, 829
 metabisulphite, 174, 706
 persulphate, 181
 pyrosulphite, 706
Potato, 25, 26, 183
Pottery, cobalt pigments in, 322
PPD chemicals, patch testing, 767
 sensitisers in rubber, 720, 723, 726, 727, 732,
  736
Practolol, 261
Prednisone, 247
 effect on patch test reactions, 14
Preservatives, 664–713
 in textiles, 85
Prilocaine, 200
Primin, 526
Primrose, *see* Primulaceae.
Primula, 24, 29
 obconica, 467
Primulaceae, 524
 allergen, 526
 botanical features, 525
 dermatitis, clinical features, 527
  cross-reactions, 530
  incidence, 526
  patch tests, 528
  prophylaxis, 530
Printers, occupational irritants and sensitisers,
 884
Printing, 856
 industry, chromium dermatitis, 308
 ink, cobalt in, 322
 offset, formaldehyde dermatitis due to, 790
 plates, with light-sensitive acrylates, 590
Pristinamycin, 226
Proban, 80
Procaine, 196
Proctosedyl, 199
Proflavine, 203
Promethazine hydrochloride, 235, 237, 437, 444
 photo-allergy due to, 437, 442, 443
 systemic, photosensitivity to, 444
Prontosil album, systemic, photosensitivity to,
 450
Propanediol, 809
Propanidid, 201
Propantheline bromide, 262, 811
Propenamide, 589
Propionates, 174
Propipocaine, 200
Propolis, 101
Propranolol, 261
Propyl gallate, 147, 175, 176
Propylene glycol, 174, 809
 oxide, 174
Prosopis juliflora, 559
Prostheses, cobalt, toxicity, 320
 nickel alloy, 349, 351
Proteaceae wood, 566
Protein, 171
 in food, 26

Protoanemonin, 530
Proxels, 851
Proxymetacaine, 197
Pseudoguaianolide, 496
Pseudophytodermatitis, 467
Pseudophytophotodermatitis, 467
Pseudotsuga menziesii, 576
Psoralen, photoactivity, 418
Psychic possession in industrial workers, 890
PTBP, *see p-tert*-Butyl phenol.
Pterocarpus, 559
Pulse family, 518
Purpleheart wood, 558
Purpura due to rubber antioxidant, 87
    due to textiles, 87
Pyrazoline, 83
Pyrethrin II, 499
Pyrethrosin, 499
Pyrethrum, 405
    allergens, 499
Pyrithioxin, systemic, photosensitivity to, 448
Pyritinol, systemic, photosensitivity to, 448
Pyrocarbonic acid diethyl ester, 174
Pyrovatex, 80
Pyrrolnitrin, 231

Quebracho extract powder, 76
Quinazoline Yellow, 145, 146
Quindoxin, 187, 440
Quinethazone, systemic, photosensitivity to, 446
Quinidine, 263
    systemic, photosensitivity to, 449
Quinine, 263
    photosensitivity to, 439, 442, 443
Quinolines, 217
Quinones, 395
    allergenic, in wood, 551
Quinoxalone, photo-allergy to, 440

Radio workers, occupational irritants and
        sensitisers, 884
Radiodermatitis from radioactive rings, 336
Radiographic film developers, 863
Radish, 512
Ragweed, 494, 500
Ramin wood, 568
Randox, 403
Ranunculaceae, 530
Raphanus sativus, 512
Rayon, 58
Red bean wood, 562
Renal dialysis units, formaldehyde sterilisation,
        791, 793
Rengas, 553
Resin systems causing dermatitis, 625–42
Resins in textiles, 55
    polyterpene, 59
Resol resins, 615
Resorcinol, 264
    monobenzoate dermatitis, 644, 647
Reticuloid, actinic, 416
Retinoic acid, 248
Rheum rhaponticum, 524

Rhodamine B, 145
Rhubarb, 524
Rhus, 25
    oleoresins, 23
    succedanea, 477
    typhinia, 477
Rice, 515
Ricin, 514
Rings, gold, 331
    platinum, 368
    radioactive, 336
Roccal, 693
Rockwood, 80
Rodannitrobenzene, 405
Rodenticides, 411
Rosaceae, 531
Rosaniline dyes, 240
Rosemary, 517
Rosewood, 560
Rosin, *see* Colophony.
Rotersept, 696
Rouge, 148
Rubber, 714–70
    additives, 718
    bands, 763
    composition, 717
    gloves, 734, 741, 742
        surgical, 744
    in boots and shoes, 69, 74, 75
    in household equipment, 753
    industry, occupational dermatitis, 755, 765,
        884
    manufacture, accelerators, 756
        antioxidants, 720, 756
        antiozonants, 756
        formaldehyde, 793
        peptisers, 721, 757
        retarders, 756
        sensitisers, 722
    natural, 715
    purpura, 87
    sensitivity, clinical features, 740–66
        domestic articles, 734
        'domestic' dermatitis, 741–55
        incidence, 724
        industrial rubbers, 736
        occupational dermatitis, 755–66
        patch testing, 758, 766
        sources, 733–40
        to individual chemicals, incidence, 726
    sheet, 753
    sources, 714
    structure, 714
    synthetic, 715
    workers, occupational irritants and sensitisers,
        884
Rubiaceae, 532
Rue, phytophotodermatitis due to, 420
Rust preventives as source of chromate
        dermatitis, 304
Rusters, 337
Ruta graveolens, 534
Rutaceae, 532

allergens, 533
dermatitis, 533
photodermatitis, 419
Rutaceae woods, 566

S7, photosensitivity to, 433, 436
Sage, 517
St John's wort, phytophotodermatitis due to, 421
Salicaceae woods, 567
Salicylaldoxime, 862
Salicylic acid, 265
  plasters, 786
Salsola kali, 492
Saluric, systemic, photosensitivity to, 445
Salvia officinalis, 517
Sand, foundry, chromate in, 307
Santophen, 392, 393
Santoquin, 185
Sapele wood, 562
Saponins, irritant, in wood, 551
Sapotaceae woods, 567
Sapwood, 549
Satinwood, 566
  Ceylon, 556
  Nigerian, 558
Saussurea lappa, 510
Saxifrage, 534
Scar due to patch test, 16
Scilla, 523
Scotch tape, 786
Scotchgard stain repellant, 78
Scrotum, cancer, due to mineral oil, 849
Scuba diver face mask, 751
Sculptors, occupational irritants and sensitisers, 880
Scurvy pea, phytophotodermatitis due to, 421
Secretaries, occupational irritants and sensitisers, 884
Selenium, 371
Sellotape, 786, 812
Semecarpus anacardium, 477
Sensitisation, active, by patch test, 15
Sequestrants in food, 178
Sesame oil, 265
Shampoos, 132
  containing formaldehyde, 790
  occupational dermatitis due to, 133
Shaving preparations, 140
Sheets (bed linen), 67
Shell splinters, cobalt dermatitis due to, 320
Shoe dermatitis, 72, 885
  alternative shoes, 74
  patch testing, 73
  sensitisation to, in children, 21
  sensitisers in 68
Shoemakers, occupational irritants and sensitisers, 884
Shrimps, 26, 172
Silica, 371
Silicone barrier creams, 873
Silk, 25, 26
Silver, 372

salts, 372
  -nickel surgical clips, 351
Sinningia speciosa, 515
Slaughterhouse workers, occupational irritants and sensitisers, 884
Smodingium argutum, 477, 478
Snakewood, 564
Soaps, 814
  containing turpentine, 804
Socks, 51–4
  elastic in, 751
Sodium benzoate, 173, 179
  bisulphite, 706
  ethylmercurithiosalicylate, 689
  hypochlorite, 889
  mercaptobenzothiazole, 845
  sulphide, 25
Soframycin, 207
Solanaceae, 534
Soldering fluxes, 787, 865
Soluble oils, occupational use, 841
  patch testing, 848
Solvent black, 852
  red, 145
  yellow, 33, 890
Solvents, chromate in, 305
  in dry cleaning, 76
Sorbates, 173
Sorbic acid, 173, 707
Sorbitan, 102
Spandex yarn, 745
Spearmint oil, 180
Spectacle frames, 577, 804
  cellulose, 644, 646
  epoxy resin, 608
  nickel, 348, 355
Spectra-Sorb UV 284, photosensitivity to, 454
Spectraban, photosensitivity to, 452
Spices, 25, 179
Spiramycin, 187
Sponge rubber, 753
Spruce wood, 565
Squaric-acid-diethylester, 890
Squash ball, rubber, 755
Stain repellants, 78
Stannous chloride, 890
Status eczematicus, effect on patch testing, 12
Stearyl alcohol, 25, 808
Steel, stainless, nickel release in, 349
Steering wheel, eczema due to monobenzoate in, 647
Sterculiaceae woods, 567
Sterilon, 696
Sterosan, 218
Stilbene whitening agent, 81, 84
Stilbenes, antigenic, in wood, 551
Stockings, 49–54
  elastic, 750
Storax, 267
Strawberry, 531
  flavouring, 179
Streptocarpus, 514
Streptomycin, 25, 27, 221

cross-reaction to neomycin, 214
Styrene, 629
Subtilisin, 820
Sudan III, 145
Sulisobenzone, 252, 454
Sulphanilamide, systemic, photosensitivity to, 450
Sulphapyridine, photo-allergy to, 439, 442, 443
Sulphate recovery process, cobalt dermatitis due to, 323
Sulphathiazole, 223
Sulphites, 174
Sulphonamides, 27, 222
    photo-allergy to, 439
1-Sulpho-β-naphthalene-azo-β-naphthol, 143
Sulphur, 890
    dioxide, 25, 174
Sunscreens, photosensitivity to, 450–54
Sunset yellow, 179
Surface active agents in foods, 178
Surfactants, 813
Surma, 114
Suspenders, 346, 747
Swietenia macrophylla, 563
Synadenium grantii, 513
Symmetrel, systemic, photosensitivity to, 447

Tabebuia, 554
Tagayasan wood, 558
Tagetes minuta, 510
Tannery workers, occupational irritants and sensitisers, 74, 884
Tanning, 793
Tartrazine, 179
Tasua wood, 563
Tattoos, 830
Toxaceae wood, 568
TBC, 845, 855
TBS, photosensitivity to, 434
TCC, photosensitivity to, 435
TCSA, photosensitivity to, 434
Teak, 26, 569
Tectonia grandis, 569
Television workers, occupational irritants and sensitisers, 884
Tellurium, 373
Terminalia superba, 554
Terpenes, 29, 797
    allergenic, in wood, 551
    irritancy, 800
α-Terpinene, 532
Terramycin, 224
    systemic, phototoxicity, 425, 427
Tetanus antitoxin, 25
Tetmosol, 398
Tetrabromofluorescein, 142
Tetracaine, 194
Tetrachloro-p-benzoquinone, 395
Tetrachlorodibenzodioxin, 890
Tetrachloroethylene, 76
Tetrachlorosalicylanilide, photosensitivity to, 432, 434, 437
    phototoxicity, 423, 442, 443

Tetracyclines, 224
    systemic, phototoxicity, 425, 427
Tetramethylene glycol diacrylate printing plates, 592
Tetraethylrhodamine, 145
Tetramethylthiuram disulphide, 398
    sensitiser in rubber, 69, 718, 726–9
    monosulphide, sensitiser in rubber, 718, 728, 729
Tetraphosphoric trisulphide, 890
Tetraphosphorus trisulphide, 825
Textiles, 36–92
    dermatitis, allergens, 886
        due to whiteners, 82
        phototoxic, 47
    dyes in, 36
    fibres, occupational dermatitis due to, 86
    industry, dermatitis in, 47, 48, 54
        occupational irritants and sensitisers, 884
    preservatives in, 85
    purpurea due to, 87
    resins in, 55, 63
    re-texing, 78
Thermofax copying, 855
Thiadazole, 268
Thiamine, 248
Thimerosal, 689
2,2'-Thiobis(4-chlorophenol), photosensitivity to, 433, 436
2,2'-Thiobis(4,6-dichlorophenol), photosensitivity to, 433, 436
Thiocarbamide, photo-allergy to, 441
Thioglycerol, 129
Thioglycollates, 129, 130, 134, 137
Thiomersal, 21, 689
Thioridazine, photosensitivity to, 444
Thiourea, photo-allergy to, 441
Thioxolone, 267
Thiram, 398
Thiurams, 28, 70, 75, 138
    in fungicides, 398
    patch testing, 766
    sensitisers in rubber, 718, 728, 726–9, 734, 735, 760
Thuja, 555
Thyme, 517
Thymelaeaceae wood, 568
Thymoquinone, 21
Tieghemella heckelii, 567
Tin-nickel alloy, 351
Tinactin, 231
Tinaderm, 231
Tineafax, 229
Tinopal, 83
Tinuvin P in face cream, 102
Tobramycin, cross-reaction to neomycin, 214
Tocopherols, 108, 177, 249
Toe-puffs, 72
Tolbutamide, systemic, photosensitivity to, 447
Tolmiea menziesii, 534
Tolnaftate, 231
Tolu balsam, 162
Toluene diisocyanate, 638, 640

p-Toluene sulphochloride, 890
Toluic acids, 890
α-Toluic aldehyde, 161
p-Toluoyl chloride phenylhydrazone, 890
Toluylene red, phototoxicity, 422
p-Toluylenediamine hair dye, 119, 120, 125, 137
Tomato, 535
Toney Red, 145
Toona sureni, 563
Toothpaste flavours, 180
Toporite, rubber, 556
Tourniquet, rubber, 752
Toxicodendron, 375, 467, 468, 475, 477
    cross-reactions, 478
    sensitisation in children, 20
Toys, rubber, 755
Trees, plant families and woods, 552
Trenimon, 239
Triacetyldiphenylisatin, systemic,
    photosensitivity to, 448
Triafur, 268
Triamcinolone, acetonide, 247
Triazine bacteriocide, 846
Triaziquone, 239
Tribromosalicylanilide, photosensitivity to, 433,
    434, 437
    phototoxicity, 423, 442, 443
Tribromsalan, photosensitivity to, 433, 434, 437
Tributyltin hydroxide, 401
    oxide, 85
Trichlormethyl propanol, 700
Trichlorocarbanilide, photosensitivity to, 432,
    433, 435, 442, 443
Trichloroethylene, 77, 890
Triclocarban, photosensitivity to, 433, 435, 442,
    443
Triclosan, 704
Tricresyl phosphate, 651, 852
Triethanolamine, 48, 100, 102
Triethylamine allergic contact dermatitis, 641
Triethylenetetramine, 603
Trifluorotrichloroethane, 77
Trilene, 77, 890
Trimeprazine, systemic, photosensitivity to, 445
Trimethyl hexamethylene diisocyanate, 641
Trimethylolpropane triacrylate, photosensitive
    ink, 593
Trimeton, 236
Triphenyl phosphate, 644
    tin acetate, 401
Triphenylmethane dyes, 240
Triplochiton scleroxylon, 568
Tris(2, 3-dibromopropyl)phosphate, 81
Trisoralen, photo-activity, 419
Triton, 268
Tromantidine hydrochloride, 225
Trouser pocket dermatitis, 39
Tulip, 519
    allergens, 520
    dermatitis, 521
        patch testing, 523
    irritants, 521
Tulipaline A, 520

Tuliposide A, 520
Turkey skin, 26
Turpentine, 22, 28, 797–805
    allergens, 800
    composition, 799
    contact sources, 802
    sensitising potential, 801
    sensitivity, incidence, 801
        patch testing, 804
    sources, 800
Turreanthus africanus, 563
Tylan, 187
Tylosin, 187
Typewriter correction papers, 619
Tyres, rubber, chemicals in, 755–66
    dermatitis due to, 757

Uajara wood, 567
Ulmaceae woods, 568
Ulmus procera, 538, 568
Ultraviolet light absorbers in cosmetic creams,
    102
    screens, 102, 450
Umbelliferae, 535
    phytophotodermatitis due to, 419
Unilax, systemic, photosensitivity to, 448
Uranium, 373
Urea, 55, 57, 63
    formaldehyde resin, 621, 789
Urtica dioica, 538
Urticaceae, 537
Urticaria, contact, 24
    immunologic, 26
    non-immunologic, 25
D-Usnic acid, 570
Utile wood, 562
Uval, photosensitivity to, 454
Uvinal MS-40, photosensitivity to, 454
Uvistat, photosensitivity, to, 453

Vallergan, systemic, photosensitivity to, 445
Vanicide BL, 393
Vanillism, 524
Varicose eczema and ulcers, lanolin sensitivity
    in, 779
Variotin, 230
Varnishes with phenol formaldehyde, 620
Vegetable oils, occupational use, 839
Veratrum album, 523
Verbenaceae woods, 569
Verifax copying, 855
Veterinarians, occupational irritants and
    sensitisers, 884
Vibramycin, systemic, phototoxicity, 425, 427
Vinblastine, phototoxicity, 425, 431
Vinyl carbazole, 654
    chloride disease, 652
        neoplasia due to, 652
    cyanide, 588
    polymers, 648–55
    pyridine, 654
Vioform, 218, 219
Violet 3567, 162

Virginiamycin, 188, 226
Vitallium, 351
Vitamin A acid 248
  B₁, 248
  B₁₂ cobalt, sensitivity to, 320
  E, 249
  K, 250
Vitex littoralis, 569
Vulval deodorants, 109

Wallflower, 511
Walnut, Brazilian, 557
  poison, wood, 557
  wood, 563
Warfarin, 411
Watch case and watch strap nickel dermatitis,
    348, 355
Water, 25
  nickel content, 352
Welding rods, chromate in, 307
Wheat, 25
Whitening agents, 81
  carcinogenicity and toxicity, 84
  patch testing, 83
  photosensitivity to, 82
Wigandia carcasana, 516
Wood, 25, 29, 548–74
  constituents, 549
  dermatitis, allergens, 551

causes, 549, 550
  incidence, 551
  management, 551
  irritant and sensitising chemicals, 551
  plant families with tree species, 552
Woodcutters' eczema, 556, 569
Woodworkers, occupational sensitisers, 885
Wool, 25, 40

Xerox photocopying, 855
Xerumenex, 268
X-ray developers, 863
  technicians, occupational irritants and
    sensitisers, 883
m-Xylene-azo-*β*-naphthol-3,6-disulphonic acid,
    144
Xylotox, 200

Yellow O B, 179
Yew wood, 568
Ylang-ylang oil, 161

Zephiran chloride, 693
Zinc, 374
  diethyldithiocarbamate, 720, 732, 786
Zineb, 396
Zingiberaceae, 538
Ziram, 396
Zirconium, 108, 374